Child and Adolescent Behavioral Health

A Resource for Advanced Practice Psychiatric
and Primary Care Practitioners in Nursing

Child and Adolescent Behavioral Health

A Resource for Advanced Practice Psychiatric and Primary Care Practitioners in Nursing

Editors

Edilma L. Yearwood, PhD, PMHCNS-BC, FAAN
Associate Professor
Georgetown University School of Nursing & Health Studies
Washington, DC

Geraldine S. Pearson, PhD, PMHCNS-BC, FAAN
Associate Professor
UCONN School of Medicine
Farmington, CT

Jamesetta A. Newland, PhD, FNP-BC, FAANP, DPNAP
Clinical Associate Professor
New York University College of Nursing
New York, NY

WILEY-BLACKWELL

A John Wiley & Sons, Ltd., Publication

This edition first published 2012 © 2012 by John Wiley & Sons, Inc

Wiley-Blackwell is an imprint of John Wiley & Sons, formed by the merger of Wiley's global Scientific, Technical and Medical business with Blackwell Publishing.

Registered Office
John Wiley & Sons, Ltd, The Atrium, Southern Gate, Chichester, West Sussex, PO19 8SQ, UK

Editorial Offices
2121 State Avenue, Ames, Iowa 50014-8300, USA
The Atrium, Southern Gate, Chichester, West Sussex, PO19 8SQ, UK
9600 Garsington Road, Oxford, OX4 2DQ, UK

For details of our global editorial offices, for customer services and for information about how to apply for permission to reuse the copyright material in this book please see our website at www.wiley.com/wiley-blackwell.

Library of Congress Cataloging-in-Publication Data

Child and adolescent behavioral health : a resource for advanced practice psychiatric and primary care practitioners in nursing / editors, Edilma L. Yearwood, Geraldine S. Pearson, Jamesetta A. Newland.
    p. ; cm.
  Includes bibliographical references and index.
  ISBN 978-0-8138-0786-7 (pbk. : alk. paper)
I. Yearwood, Edilma Lynch.   II. Pearson, Geraldine S.   III. Newland, Jamesetta A.
[DNLM: 1. Child.   2. Mental Disorders.   3. Adolescent.   4. Advanced Practice Nursing.
5. Nursing Assessment–methods.   6. Primary Care Nursing.   7. Psychiatric Nursing. WS 350]
  618.92–dc23

                          2011036443

A catalogue record for this book is available from the British Library.

Wiley also publishes its books in a variety of electronic formats. Some content that appears in print may not be available in electronic books.

Set in 10.5/12.5pt Minion by SPi Publisher Services, Pondicherry, India

1   2012

Dedication

To my children, Arayna and Matthew, and my parents, Edmund and Dorothy Lynch, for their love, support, understanding, and patience. Our special thanks to all the children, adolescents, and families who over the years served as the inspiration for this book.

Edilma

To Lloyd, Elizabeth, Neal, and David Pearson for their loving support throughout this project. And to my dear mother, Doris M. Sanner, R.N., for inspiring me to become a nurse.

Geri

To my husband and children, Lloyd, Kristina, Michael, Sonya, and Maya; my mother, Kather Lene Alexander; my sisters Sharon, Brenda, Sheila, and Michele; and my mother-in-law, Gloria Chang, for a lifetime of encouragement and support.

Jamie

Contents

About the Editors

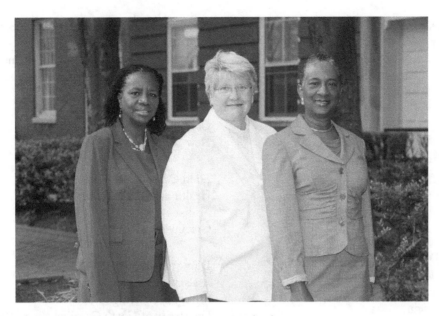

Left to right: Edilma Yearwood, Geraldine Pearson, and Jamesetta Newland

Edilma L. Yearwood, PhD, PMHCNS, BC, FAAN, is associate professor at the School of Nursing & Health Studies at Georgetown University, where she teaches psychiatric nursing. She is on the editorial board and is the column editor on cultural issues for the *Journal of Child and Adolescent Psychiatric Nursing*. She is a content expert reviewer for numerous nursing and psychology journals. Dr. Yearwood is ANCC certified as a clinical nurse specialist in child/adolescent psychiatric-mental health nursing and is a member of the International Society of Psychiatric Nurses.

Geraldine S. Pearson, PhD, PMHCNS, BC, FAAN, is past president of the International Society of Psychiatric Nurses and editor-in-chief of the journal *Perspectives in Psychiatric Care*. She is an associate professor in the Department of Psychiatry at the University of Connecticut School of Medicine and director of the Home Care Program, a community intervention for juvenile justice youth. Dr. Pearson is ANCC certified as a clinical nurse specialist in child/adolescent psychiatric-mental health nursing.

Jamesetta A. Newland, PhD, FNP-BC, FAANP, DPNAP, is clinical associate professor and director of the Doctor of Nursing Practice Program at New York University College of Nursing. She is the editor-in-chief of *The Nurse Practitioner: The American Journal of Primary Healthcare*. Dr. Newland, an ANCC certified family nurse practitioner, maintains practice at the NYU College of Nursing Faculty Practice, a primary care clinic serving a diverse inner city population.

Contributors

Angela Amar, PhD, RN, FAAN
Associate Professor
Robert Wood Johnson Nurse Faculty Scholar
Director, Forensic Nursing Program
William F. Connell School of Nursing
Boston College
Boston, MA

Robin Bartlett, PhD, RN
Associate Professor
School of Nursing
University of North Carolina at Greensboro
Greensboro, NC

Cecily L. Betz, PhD, RN, FAAN
Editor-in-Chief, *Journal of Pediatric Nursing*
Clinical Associate Professor
Keck School of Medicine
University of Southern California
Los Angeles, CA

Elizabeth Bonham, PhD, RN, PMHCNS, BC
College of Nursing and Health Professions
University of Southern Indiana
Evansville, IN

Susan Boorin, MSN, PMHNP-BC
Predoctoral Fellow
School of Nursing
Yale University
New Haven, CT

Eve Bosnick, MSN, APRN, PNP-BC
Director
Adolescent Health and Wellness Center
Advocare Mainline Pediatrics
Narberth, PA
Clinical Faculty
Primary Care Pediatric Nurse Practitioner Program
Division of Family and Community Health
School of Nursing
University of Pennsylvania
Philadelphia, PA

Penelope R. Buschman-Gemma, MS, RN, PMHCNS-BC, FAAN
Assistant Professor of Clinical Nursing
Director of the Psychiatric Nurse Practitioner
  Program
School of Nursing
Columbia University
New York, NY

Ellen Carroll, RN, CPNP, DNS(c)
Health Services Director
Abilis
Greenwich, CT

Diane M. Caruso, DNP, FNP-BC
Assistant Professor
School of Nursing
University of North Carolina Charlotte
Charlotte, North Carolina
Nurse Practitioner
Cleveland Pediatrics
Cleveland, NC

Judith Coucouvanis, MA, APRN, PMHCNS-BC
Clinical Nurse Consultant and Nurse Practitioner
Department of Psychiatry: Child and Adolescent
  Section
University of Michigan Health System
Ann Arbor, MI

Angela A. Crowley, PhD, APRN, PNP-BC, FAAN
Associate Professor
Yale University School of Nursing
Yale University
New Haven, CT

Tammi Damas, PhD, MBA, WHNP-BC, RN
Chair, Graduate Programs
Division of Nursing
College of Nursing & Allied Health Sciences
Howard University
Washington, DC

Janet A. Deatrick, PhD, FAAN, RN
Professor
School of Nursing
University of Pennsylvania
Philadelphia, PA

Kathleen R. Delaney, PhD, PMH-NP, FAAN
Professor and Specialty Coordinator – Psychiatric
    Mental Health—FNP Program
Department of Community Systems and Mental Health
    Nursing
College of Nursing
Rush University
Chicago, IL

Janiece DeSocio, PhD, RN, PMHNP-BC
Associate Dean for Graduate Education
Associate Professor of Nursing
Seattle University College of Nursing
Seattle, WA

Elizabeth Burgess Dowdell, PhD, CRNP, RN
Associate Professor
College of Nursing
Villanova University
Villanova, PA

Edith (Emma) Dundon, PhD, RN, CPNP
Clinical Assistant Professor
School of Nursing
University of Massachusetts Amherst
Amherst, MA

Kathryn K. Ellis, DNP, APRN, FNP-BC, ANP-BC
Assistant Professor and FNP Program Director
Department of Nursing
School of Nursing & Health Studies
Georgetown University
Washington, DC

Jean Nelson Farley, MSN, RN, PNP-BC,CRRN
Instructor
Department of Nursing
School of Nursing & Health Studies
Georgetown University
Washington, DC

Linda M. Finke, RN, PhD
Professor
College of Health and Human Services
Indiana University–Purdue University Fort Wayne
Fort Wayne, IN

Marie Foley, PhD, RN
Associate Professor
College of Nursing
Seton Hall University
South Orange, NJ

Pamela Galehouse, PhD, PMHCNS, BC
Associate Professor
Behavioral Science, Community and Health Systems
College of Nursing
Seton Hall University
South Orange, NJ

Judith Haber, PhD, APRN, BC, FAAN
Interim Dean, New York University College
    of Nursing
The Ursula Springer Leadership Professor in Nursing
College of Nursing
New York University
New York, NY

Donna Hallas, PhD, PNP-BC, CPNP
Clinical Associate Professor
Coordinator PNP Program
College of Nursing
New York University
New York, NY

Margaret Hardy, RN, MBA, JD
Attorney
Sands Anderson PC
Richmond, VA

Elizabeth Hawkins-Walsh, PhD, CPNP
Assistant Dean for Clinical Affairs and Community
    Partnerships
Clinical Associate Professor
Director of Pediatric Nurse Practitioner Programs
The Catholic University of America
Washington, DC

Laura C. Hein, PhD, RN, NP-C
Assistant Professor
College of Nursing
University of South Carolina
Columbia, SC

Charlotte A. Herrick, PhD, RN
Professor Emeritus
School of Nursing
University of North Carolina at Greensboro
Greensboro, NC

Judith Hirsh, NP-P, PMHCNS-BC, RPT-S
Psychiatric Nurse Practitioner
Registered Play Therapist and Supervisor
Private Practice
Rye, NY

M. Katherine Hutchinson, PhD, RN, FAAN
Associate Professor
College of Nursing
New York University
New York, NY

Barbara Schoen Johnson, PhD, RN, PMHNP
Psychiatric Mental Health Nurse Practitioner
Cook Children's Health Care System
Fort Worth, TX

Kathleen Kenney-Riley, APRN, PNP, EdD
Pediatric Nurse Practitioner & Clinical Coordinator of
    Pediatric Rheumatology Fellowship Program
Children's Hospital at Montefiore
Bronx, NY

Allison W. Kilcoyne, MS, RN, C-FNP
Family Nurse Practitioner and Site Manager
Teen Health Center at Lynn English High School
Lynn, MA

Maureen Reed Killeen, PhD, PMHCNS, BC, FAAN
Professor
Department of Biobehavioral Nursing
College of Nursing at Athens
Georgia Health Sciences University
Athens, GA

Eunjung Kim, PhD, RN, CPNP
Associate Professor
Department of Family and Child Nursing
School of Nursing
University of Washington
Seattle, WA

Carol Anne Marchetti, PhD, RN, PMHCNS-BC, SANE
Southeast Regional Coordinator
MA Sexual Assault Nurse Examiner Program
Massachusetts Office for Victim Assistance
Boston, MA

Natalie McClain, PhD, RN, CPNP
Assistant Professor
William F. Connell School of Nursing
Boston College
Boston, MA

Caroline R. McKinnon, PhD(c), PMHCNS, BC
PhD Candidate in Nursing
College of Graduate Studies
Georgia Health Sciences University
Augusta, GA

Mikki Meadows-Oliver, PhD, RN
Assistant Professor
School of Nursing
Yale University
New Haven, CT

Beth Muller, APRN
Nurse Clinician
University of Connecticut Health Center
Farmington, CT

Lois C. Powell, NP-P, PMHCNS
Nurse Practitioner in Psychiatry/Consultant
Private Practice
New York, NY

Cathy Quides, MSN
Pediatric Nurse Practitioner
Child Development Center
Division of Mental Health and Child Development
Children's Hospital & Research Center Oakland
Oakland, CA

Sally Raphel, MS, APRN/PMH, FAAN
University of Maryland
Johns Hopkins University
School of Nursing
Baltimore, MD

Amanda Reilly, MEd, MSN
Nurse Clinician
UCONN Health Center
Farmington, CT

Joan B. Riley, MS, MSN, FNP-BC, FAAN
Assistant Professor
Departments of Human Science and Nursing
School of Nursing & Health Studies
Nurse Practitioner
Student Health Center
Georgetown University
Washington, DC

Cynda H. Rushton, PhD, RN, FAAN
Associate Professor
School of Nursing
Johns Hopkins University
Baltimore, MD

Patricia Ryan-Krause, MS, RN, MSN, CPNP
Associate Professor
Pediatric Nurse Practitioner Specialty
Director of Clinical Education
Center for International Nursing Scholarship and
   Education
School of Nursing
Yale University
New Haven, CT

Lawrence D. Scahill, MSN, PhD, FAAN
Professor
Psychiatric-Mental Health Specialty
Professor
Yale Child Study Center
School of Nursing
Yale University
New Haven, CT

Kathleen Scharer, PhD, RN, PMHCNS-BC, FAAN
Associate Professor
College of Nursing
University of South Carolina
Columbia, SC

Karen G. Schepp, PhD, RN, PMHCNS, BC, FAAN
Associate Professor and Interim Chair
Department of Psychosocial & Community Health
School of Nursing
University of Washington
Seattle, WA

Carolyn Schmidt, BSN, RN
Community Health Nurse-Retired
Guilford County Department of Public Health
Greensboro, NC

Kathy Ann Sheehy, APRN, PCNS-BC
Advanced Practice Nurse
Division of Anesthesia and Pain Medicine
Children's National Medical Center
Washington, DC

Deborah Shelton, PhD, RN, NE-BC, CCHP, FAAN
E. Jane Martin Professor and Associate Dean
   for Research
West Virginia University
School of Nursing
Robert C. Byrd Health Sciences Center
Morgantown, WV

Sarah B. Vittone, RN, MSN, MA
Assistant Professor
School of Nursing & Health Studies
Ethics Consultant, Center for Clinical Bioethics
Georgetown University
Washington, DC

Sandra J. Weiss, PhD, DNSc, RN, FAAN
Professor and Eschbach Endowed Chair in Mental
   Health
Department of Community Health Systems
School of Nursing
University of California, San Francisco
San Francisco, CA

Stephanie Wright, PhD, FNP-BC, PNP-BC
Associate Professor
School of Nursing
The George Washington University
Washington, DC

Foreword by Janet A. Deatrick

We are often lectured as professionals about the importance of collaborating with individuals in other professions in order to optimize child and family outcomes. In addition, we are now being told to start those collaborative efforts during the educational process and to make interprofessional education a priority. While these efforts are most important, this book reminds us about the importance of collaboration within our own profession.

This book was written to enable the collaboration of nurses with each other. More specifically, the vision of the editors of this book is to provide a state-of-the-science guide regarding behavioral health that will be helpful not only for advanced practice psychiatric nurses but also for primary care nurse practitioners and to facilitate their communication with each other. Edilma Yearwood, Geraldine Pearson, and Jamesetta Newland are to be congratulated for this vision and for the grand success of this enormous undertaking.

My own journey within the profession of child psychiatric nursing has been rather circuitous. My education at the master's level in the early 1970s was avant-garde in the sense that I had the fortune of being educated by young, forward-looking clinicians who valued the importance of family and community in the lives of children. Throughout our classroom and clinical experiences, we were immersed in those phenomena. To this day, I use those understandings to frame my scholarship, as well as my own philosophy, values, and passion. During that time and throughout my career, I worked with many of the individuals who have contributed to this book. They have been a source of continued inspiration to me as I took a different road for my career outside of psychiatry into the world of pediatric nursing practice for my research regarding families and children with chronic conditions and cancer. During my travels,

I have had the opportunity to work with individuals from many professions and have been able to build upon my strong nursing identity and what I have learned about the purpose for our work from other child psychiatric nurses. Thus, I feel very strongly about the message of this book; that is, about the importance of collaboration within our profession.

We as nurses have a unique opportunity to become intimately involved in the lives of children, adolescents, and their families and therefore have a concomitant obligation to advocate for them. As outlined in this book, that advocacy may take many forms but all leads back to our desire for optimal functioning for everyone in the family system. I have always found that pediatric nursing gives me the best avenue for that advocacy. Thus, being given this opportunity to introduce this book also gives me the opportunity to go full circle, back to my roots, and allows me to lavish in the wisdom of my colleagues contained in these pages.

The book is organized according to issues of assessment, treatment, special populations, and special issues. Each section of text is written or reviewed collaboratively by a child and adolescent psychiatric advanced practice nurse and a pediatric or family nurse practitioner. Use it to build your wisdom, and may your travels be as rich as those whose work is reflected in this volume.

Janet A. Deatrick

Best,
Janet A. Deatrick, PhD, RN, FAAN

Foreword by Judith Haber

Nursing historically has been in the forefront in training health care professionals using a holistic framework that acknowledges a responsibility to address the needs of the whole person; individuals are not composed of parts that function independently of each other, to be separated for convenience or by virtue of the health care provider's educational preparation and training. Physical health and psychological well-being are intricately linked and, as such, the state of one influences the state of the other, and optimal health cannot be achieved if either one is overlooked or attended to without consideration for the other. In our nation's health care system, physical health and behavioral health have been traditionally rendered by different providers and in separate settings. Communication between the two groups often is either restricted or nonexistent. People are treated as two detachable and disconnected halves. This approach to patient care results in outcomes such as fragmented care; limited or no access to appropriate and timely care; the "falling through the cracks" phenomenon; disparate reimbursements between medical and mental health professionals; entrenched "silo" education, training, and practice; and patients with unmet needs, especially related to behavioral health. A paradox is reflected in the high demand for mental health services but a low supply of mental health professionals. There is an urgent need to prepare primary care nurses to be cognizant about and competent in assessing, treating, and managing mental health problems, and psychiatric mental health nurses to be knowledgeable about physical health problems of children and adolescents so they are prepared to address these through appropriate collaboration and referral.

The time is right, and the editors of this book—Edilma, Geri, and Jamie—had a vision to create a text that would be useful to primary care and psychiatric mental health advanced practice nurses in integrating primary care and behavioral health for children and adolescents. Children and adolescents represent one of the most vulnerable populations in our society, and to ensure a healthy future for the nation, we must address the needs of the young from a holistic as well as developmental perspective and initiate treatment in primary care settings. Many mental health problems and psychiatric disorders that begin in childhood are likely to persist and possibly worsen as the child reaches adulthood. The number of mental health professionals is not adequate to keep up with the demands of steadily increasing numbers of children with behavioral health needs. Thus, primary care professionals must take a more active and continuous role in identifying these children and facilitating access to appropriate interventions.

Putting together a text of this magnitude is a daunting task, but the editors, all highly accomplished experts who are recognized in their fields, selected authors from both primary and psychiatric mental health care to work together in writing the chapters. The intent was to make sure that both perspectives were represented and integrated in the discussions. This text will enhance the knowledge, assessment, and management skills of advanced practice nurses who care for children from infancy through adolescence. Because there is an emphasis on collaboration and integration of care throughout the book, readers will become acutely aware of the need to change systems of care to reduce barriers to the assessment and management of the behavioral health needs of this population. The advanced practice nursing role affords opportunities to continue moving nurses into positions of leadership on interprofessional teams and as innovators in developing new models to deliver primary care services to this special population of children and adolescents.

Warm regards,
Judith Haber, PhD, APRN, BC, FAAN

Preface

This book was conceptualized to help advanced practice nurses (APNs) working directly with children and adolescents in multiple care systems address the growing problem of unmet mental health needs of this population. The research on health disparities shows that early identification, access to care, and early treatment are lacking for vulnerable populations including children and adolescents. Children access primary medical care more frequently because of school requirements for regular immunizations, physical exams, and common childhood illnesses. There is no such requirement for mental health assessment. The result is a growing number of children and adolescents whose psychiatric symptoms largely go unrecognized and untreated. Research shows that many adult psychiatric disorders originate in childhood and adolescence and that these individuals have a poorer prognosis if not treated early. Physical health is a recognized public health issue; mental health, which is often not as visible or tangible, is often neglected. Another powerful barrier that cannot be overestimated is the powerful negative force of individual, group, and societal stigma toward mental illness and its effect on knowledge, understanding, treatment, inclusion/exclusion, and quality of life of those with a mental or behavioral disorder.

Early on in the process of developing this book, the commitment was to produce a body of work that was collaborative and reflected the work experience of child psychiatric, pediatric, and family APNs. Most chapters have been written through the joint efforts of both child psychiatric and primary care practitioners. All peer reviewers have reflected both psychiatric and primary care knowledge. Each chapter presents state-of-the-art, evidence-based knowledge about specific psychiatric and behavioral health issues presented by children and adolescents across health care settings.

It is our hope that any APN can use this book to understand behavioral disorders and their etiology, assessment guidelines, strategies for treatment in primary care settings, and indications for consultation, collaboration, and referral. The book is developmentally based and proposes strategies for working in partnership with children, adolescents, families, and other health care providers to improve mental health status of the vulnerable child population. The sections include assessment, treatment, special populations, and special issues. Chapters in each section focus on disorder and behavioral presentations. Chapters focused on disorders review clinical manifestation, etiology, nursing interventions, integration with primary care and implications for practice, research, and education. Chapters focused on issues describe the issue and the linkages with a behavioral/psychiatric profile of the child and associated risk and management issues.

The reality is that there are not enough child psychiatric providers to meet the burgeoning needs of the pediatric population for mental health services both in the United States and worldwide. Primary care is at the forefront of service provision and, as such, can play a significant role in mental health early case finding and supportive linkages to treatment. It is not the intent of this book to suggest that primary care providers treat complex mental health presentations. However, APNs in primary care can be instrumental in initial assessment and can and should continue to treat simple behavioral presentations, such as ADHD, affective disorders, and anxiety. As screening, collaboration, and referral are integral parts of the primary care practitioner's role, this book is intended to raise the awareness in primary care practitioners to consider behavioral health presentations in their assessment, then screen for severity, and work collaboratively with colleagues like APN child and adolescent psychiatric-mental health nurses, to ensure all children and adolescents receive treatment.

We endorse the view that nursing care is built on trust. Primary care nurses are in the unique position to have long-term relationships with children, adolescents, and their family. They can be the supportive bridge and catalyst to ensure that mental health treatment is both destigmatized and accessed.

Health care reform and development of innovative care delivery afford us an opportunity to forge new models of care including the integration of behavioral health into primary care treatment for children and adolescents. The ultimate goal is ensuring that children and adolescents presenting with mental health issues have access to timely care with the most appropriate health care provider. Healthy People 2020 goals advocate for all levels of prevention in pediatric care including early case finding, access to treatment, and increased awareness of mental health needs. It is our goal that this book facili- tates the work of all APNs who interact with children, adolescents, and families.

Edilma Yearwood
Geraldine Pearson
Jamesetta Newland

Peer Reviewers

Michelle Beauchesne, DNSc, RN, CPNP
Associate Professor Coordinator, Pediatric Nurse
 Practitioner Specialization
School of Nursing
Bouvé College of Health Sciences
Northeastern University
Boston, MA

Eve Bosnick, MSN, APRN PNP-BC
Director
Adolescent Health and Wellness Center
Advocare Mainline Pediatrics
Narberth, PA
Clinical Faculty
Primary Care Pediatric Nurse Practitioner Program
Division of Family and Community Health
School of Nursing
University of Pennsylvania
Philadelphia, PA

Angela A. Crowley, PhD, APRN, PNP-BC, FAAN
Associate Professor
Yale University School of Nursing
Yale University
New Haven, CT

Kathleen R. Delaney, PhD, PMH-NP, FAAN
Professor and Specialty Coordinator – Psychiatric
 Mental Health-FNP Program
Department of Community Systems and Mental Health
 Nursing
College of Nursing
Rush University
Chicago, IL

Edith (Emma) Dundon, PhD, RN, CPNP
Clinical Assistant Professor
School of Nursing
University of Massachusetts Amherst
Amherst, MA

Pamela Galehouse, PhD, PMHCNS, BC
Associate Professor
Behavioral Science, Community and Health Systems
College of Nursing
Seton Hall University
South Orange, NJ

Donna Hallas, PhD, PNP-BC, CPNP
Clinical Associate Professor
Coordinator PNP Program
College of Nursing
New York University
New York, NY

Vanya Hamrin, RN, MSN, APRN, BC
Associate Professor
Vanderbilt School of Nursing
Vanderbilt University
Nashville, TN

Laura C. Hein, PhD, RN, NP-C
Assistant Professor
College of Nursing
University of South Carolina
Columbia, SC

Judith Hirsh, NP-P, PMHCNS-BC, RPT-S
Psychiatric Nurse Practitioner
Registered Play Therapist and Supervisor
Private Practice
Rye, NY

Paula Deaun Jackson, MSN, CPNP, CCHC, LNC
Adjunct Nursing Instructor
Pediatric Urology Nurse Practitioner
Dysfunctional Elimination
Department of Surgery
Section of Urology
St Christopher's Hospital for Children
President Healthlinx, Ltd
Medical Legal Consultants
Philadelphia, PA

Barbara Schoen Johnson, PhD, RN, PMHNP
Psychiatric Mental Health Nurse Practitioner
Cook Children's Health Care System
Fort Worth, TX

Norman L. Keltner, EdD, RN, CRNP
Professor
School of Nursing
University of Alabama – Birmingham
Birmingham, AL

Kathleen Kenney-Riley, APRN, PNP, EdD
Pediatric Nurse Practitioner & Clinical Coordinator of
   Pediatric Rheumatology Fellowship Program
Children's Hospital at Montefiore
Bronx, NY

Allison W. Kilcoyne, MS, RN, c-FNP
Family Nurse Practitioner and Site Manager
Teen Health Center at Lynn English High School
Lynn, MA

Priscilla Killian, MSN, RN, MHPNP
Assistant Clinical Professor
Division of Undergraduate Nursing, R.N.-B.S.N.
   Completion Department
College of Nursing and Health Professions
Drexel University
Philadelphia, PA

Sandra L. Lobar, PhD, ARNP, PNP-BC
Associate Professor
Track Leader Advanced Child Health
College of Nursing and Health Sciences
Florida International University
Miami, FL

Teena M. McGuinness, PhD, CRNP, FAAN
Professor and Advanced Practice Psychiatric Nursing
   Specialty Coordinator
School of Nursing
University of Alabama at Birmingham
Birmingham, AL

Alison Moriarty-Daley, MSN, APRN, PNP-BC
Associate Professor
Pediatric Nurse Practitioner Specialty
Master's Program
Yale University School of Nursing
New Haven, CT

Beth Muller, APRN
Nurse Clinician
University of Connecticut Health Center
Farmington, CT

Jamesetta A. Newland, PhD, FNP-BC, FAANP, DPNAP
Clinical Associate Professor
College of Nursing
New York University
New York, NY

Geraldine S. Pearson, PhD, APRN
Associate Professor

Director, HomeCare Program
Department of Psychiatry
School of Medicine
University of Connecticut
Farmington, CT

Mary Jo Regan-Kubinski, PhD, RN (deceased)
Dean and Professor
College of Health Sciences
William and Kathryn Shields Endowed Chair
Indiana University – South Bend
South Bend, IN

Joan B. Riley, MS, MSN, FNP-BC, FAAN
Assistant Professor
Departments of Human Science and Nursing
School of Nursing & Health Studies
Nurse Practitioner
Student Health Center
Georgetown University
Washington, DC

Kathleen Scharer, PhD, RN, PMHCNS-BC, FAAN
Associate Professor
College of Nursing
University of South Carolina
Columbia, SC

Patti Varley, MN, ARNP, PMHCNS-BC
Seattle Children's Hospital
Seattle, WA

Roberta Waite, EdD, RN, PMHCNS-BC
Associate Professor and Assistant Dean of Academic
   Integration and Evaluation of Community Programs
Division of Graduate Nursing
Doctor of Nursing Practice Department
College of Nursing and Health Professions
Drexel University
Philadelphia, PA

Lois A. Wessel, RN, MS, CFNP
Family Nurse Practitioner
Department of Nursing
School of Nursing & Health Studies
Georgetown University
Washington, DC

Edilma Yearwood, PhD, PMHCNS, BC, FAAN
Associate Professor
Department of Nursing
School of Nursing & Health Studies
Georgetown University
Washington, DC

Beatrice Yorker, JD, RN, MS, FAAN
Dean
College of Health and Human Services
California State University, Los Angeles
Los Angeles, CA

Research Assistance from Jason Roffenbender, MS
O'Neill Institute for National and Global Health Law
Georgetown University
Washington, DC

SECTION 1
Assessment

1

Child, Adolescent, and Family Development

Stephanie Wright, Cecily L. Betz, and Edilma L. Yearwood

Objectives

After reading this chapter, APNs will be able to

1. Identify characteristics associated with each developmental stage that represent age-appropriate social and emotional behaviors of typically developing children and youth.
2. Determine at-risk behaviors in children and youth across the developmental span requiring referral for additional evaluation.
3. Describe behaviors manifested by children and youth with high secure self-esteem, high insecure self-esteem, and low self-esteem.
4. Compare and contrast models of cognitive development and their application to practice.
5. Understand child development within bio-psychosocial and environmental contexts.
6. Demonstrate an understanding of common characteristics of language (phonology, morphology, syntax, semantics, and pragmatics) and language development.
7. Identify normal patterns of family development.

Introduction

Knowledge of the behavioral characteristics of normal development in typically developing infants, children, and youth is a necessary precursor for recognizing behaviors that are considered atypical for the developmental stage. This knowledge is essential for advanced practice psychiatric and primary care practitioners in nursing who screen and monitor for the early signs of developmental delays, mental illness, or behavioral difficulties. These can be indicative of serious diagnostic conditions such as autism spectrum disorder (ASD) that can be ameliorated, although not cured, with intensive early intervention services. Understanding developmental norms aids in early recognition of mental health disorders such as depression in children and youth

(American Academy of Child and Adolescent Psychiatry, 2009). Depression is manifested by alterations in typical developmental behaviors such as social withdrawal and self-imposed isolation from peer relationships and group activities. To identify this, advanced practice nurses (APNs) must have the knowledge of developmental norms applicable to the children they treat.

Early assessment, case finding, and treatment of psychiatric disorders in a youngster may prevent acting out behaviors in the classroom and preserve the child's sense of self, competence, and relatedness to others. The areas of development chosen for review in this chapter reflect the topics discussed throughout this textbook. Descriptions of early brain development and typical social, emotional, and cognitive development spanning childhood to emerging adulthood are presented. In addition, because

Child and Adolescent Behavioral Health: A Resource for Advanced Practice Psychiatric and Primary Care Practitioners in Nursing,
First Edition. Edited by Edilma L. Yearwood, Geraldine S. Pearson, and Jamesetta A. Newland.
© 2012 John Wiley & Sons, Inc. Published 2012 by John Wiley & Sons, Inc.

child, adolescent, and family development are influenced by contextual and interactional factors, Bronfenbrenner's Bioecological Theory of Human Development is used to illustrate the dynamic nature of these interactions and how individuals and families are either propelled or impeded in their developmental trajectory by these factors. Finally, the family is on a developmental trajectory that can complement or conflict with the trajectory of the child or adolescent while influencing individual and or family outcomes. Therefore, family characteristics and dynamics are discussed as well.

Early Brain Development

The foundation for understanding child development begins with knowledge of early and progressive brain development and environmental, chemical, and biological factors that can interfere with normal brain growth. From birth to age two, brain development, while prolific, is uneven. Early brain development is characterized by several processes including birth of neurons, neuronal migration, neural pathway development, synaptogenesis, and pruning or shedding of unwanted parts (Berger, 2001; Marsh, Gerber, & Peterson, 2008). Neuronal and synaptic plasticity in the developing brain is believed to be either adaptive or maladaptive. Adaptive plasticity heralds an ability to learn new skills, store and retrieve information, respond to environmental stimuli, and maintain an intact memory. Maladaptive plasticity is implicated in neurological disorders, while excessive synaptic pruning is thought to contribute to psychiatric disorders such as schizophrenia (Belsky & Pluess, 2009; Johnston, 2009; Marsh et al. 2008).

At approximately two years of age, the size of the human brain is roughly 75 percent the weight of the adult brain (Berger, 2001). Myelination, or the process of nerve impulse transmission, occurs from a posterior to anterior direction, affecting sensory then motor pathways with enhanced myelination supporting greater intellectual functioning (Berger, 2001; Marsh, Gerber & Peterson, 2008). The largest part of the brain, the cerebral cortex, has two hemispheres, right and left, each responsible for different functions. The right hemisphere houses our ability to pay attention, intuition, spatial abilities, negative emotions, ability to process environmental challenges, ability to anticipate consequences, and whole to part processing (Berk, 2008; Schutz, 2005). The left hemisphere is responsible for positive emotions, oral and written language, analytic processing style, and part to whole processing abilities (Berk, 2008). The frontal lobe, where executive function originates, is involved with abstract thinking, motor activity, cognition, consciousness, planned behavior regulation, and impulse inhibition (Berk, 2008; Yaun & Keating, 2007). Seizure activity, attention deficit disorder, and learning difficulties have been attributed to damage in the frontal and parietal lobes (Yaun & Keating, 2007). The temporal lobe is the communication and emotional sensation center of the brain. Structural and physiological imaging techniques such as computed and positron emission tomography can identify anatomical and functional changes in the brain, assisting with a definitive psychiatric diagnosis in complex presentations. Utilization of imaging techniques, however, is neither routine nor recommended when diagnosing most children and adolescents.

Fetal exposure to *in utero* toxins, exposure to environmental toxins post birth, anoxia trauma, and genetic vulnerabilities are some of the factors affecting normal brain development and ultimate achievement of normal child and adolescent developmental milestones. While the brain is a unique and complex entity, structural or functional deviations in the brain can have profound emotional, social, intellectual, behavioral, or psychological impact on the developing individual both in the immediate and long term.

Social and Emotional Development

Infancy

The period of infancy is characterized by remarkable strides in social and emotional development. For example, beginning at birth through four months of age, the infant's behavior evolves from primarily reflexive behaviors. These include primitive infant reflexes (i.e., Moro and parachute reflexes) and the initial manifestations of voluntary or directed behaviors such as turning the head, brief tracking of an object with the eyes, the "freezing" response to an unfamiliar figure, and the emergence of smiling in response to the recognition of familiar care giving figures (Betz & Sowden, 2008; O'Reilly, 2007). As infancy concludes, the attachment to primary caregivers is evident by the infant's observable affectionate behaviors and the early use of language to acknowledge parents/primary caregivers (i.e., mama, dada) (National Institute on Deafness and Other Communication Disorders, 2000).

The insights pertaining to infant social and emotional development were first proposed by Sigmund Freud (1957) who suggested the infant's primary drive was motivated by need for oral satisfaction that could only be met by the mothering figure. This theoretical perspective was largely disregarded later in the work of Erik Erikson (1950, 1959) and subsequent developmental psychologists such as John Bowlby (1980, 1982) and Mary Ainsworth (1989) (Bretherton, 1992). Erikson's framework of psychosocial development conceptualized the period of infancy as the stage of *Trust vs. Mistrust*. Erikson (1950, 1959) theorized that the major developmental task to be achieved by the infant was the development of trust with the primary caregiver. This trusting awareness served as the foundation for the development of subsequent relationships. The infant's trust was the product of the primary caregiver's predictable and consistent cycle of response to the infant's needs for food, comfort, and security. In circumstances wherein the infant's needs were not met in this predictable and consistent fashion, then a sense of mistrust evolved instead.

Building on the earlier work of Erik Erikson, John Bowlby formulated additional insights about the process of attachment. Bowlby's work, relying heavily on ethological concepts, viewed attachment between the infant and mother (his focus was directed to the mothering figure) as predicated on instinctual mechanisms found in the imprinting behaviors of lower level species (Lorenz, 1937). According to Bowlby (1980, 1982), attachment, an innate survival behavior and as important as feeding and parturition, was described as a reciprocal process of interactions based upon the infant's need for safety, comfort, and protection, and the mother's care giving responses to address these infant needs. Furthermore, Bowlby (1980, 1982) suggested that disruptions in the attachment process would increase the risk of negatively affecting the child's psychosocial development.

Subsequent studies examining discordant attachment have supported Bowlby's original propositions (Madigan, Moran, Schuengel, Pederson, & Otten, 2007). Bowlby's work created the foundation for subsequent studies of this nascent mother-child relationship. These studies have attempted to describe the attributes, risk (i.e., maternal depression, extended mother-infant separation), and protective factors (i.e., mind-mindedness, maternal sensitivity) associated with adaptive and maladaptive attachment and the child's subsequent psychosocial development (Arnott, & Meins, 2007; Finger, Hans, Bernstein, & Cox, 2009; Larango, Bernier, & Meins, 2008; Niccols, 2008; Strathearn, Li, Fonagy, & Montague, 2009).

Mary Ainsworth, a contemporary of Bowlby, contributed to the study of attachment based upon the Strange Situation methodology that she developed and tested to identify three basic patterns of attachment: securely attached, avoidant, and resistant (Ainsworth, Blehar, Waters, & Wall, 1978). Later, another pattern of attachment was added to the original triad—disorganized/disoriented (Main & Solomon, 1990). According to Ainsworth, attachment refers to the affectional bond that develops between the mother and infant. Ainsworth (1989) characterized this bond as dependent on a persistent, consistent, and emotionally important caregiver who provided predictable care responses to meet the needs of the infant. Ainsworth's model has since been tested with divergent populations of children (i.e., premature infants, blind infants) and circumstances (i.e., foster care) to enlarge our understanding of the nature of infant and mother attachment (McMahon, Barnett, Kowalenko, & Tennant, 2006; Reyna & Pickler, 2009; Van Londen, Juffer, & van IJzendoorn, 2007). Other models of attachment have since been developed and refined in an effort to reconceptualize the attachment process as reciprocal rather than a unidimensional process between mother and baby (Goulet, Bell, St-Cyr Tribble, Paul, & Lang, 1998; Schenk, Kelley, & Schenk, 2005).

Toddlerhood

The sense of trust the infant develops sets the stage for the new psychosocial developmental challenge of toddlerhood: *Autonomy* versus *Shame and Doubt* (Erikson, 1950, 1959). It is during this stage that toddlers learn that the cautious excitement and curiosity of exploring, playing, and learning in new environments, such as at day care centers, are accompanied by unexpected limitations imposed on their behaviors by parents and other adults. The perceived barriers to pursuing these young desires and satisfying their basic needs create immediate feelings of frustration, bursts of temper, and other displays of unrestrained protest. A mantra ascribed to toddlers is that they "are long on will and short on skill" (Malley, 1991).

It is during this stage of development that physical abilities advance, enabling the obvious progression in gross and fine motor abilities. These advancements include newly acquired gross motor abilities of walking, running, and jumping together with recent fine motor achievements such as simple stacking of blocks and scribbling shapes. The emerging new motor abilities of the toddler, coupled with advances in cognitive development, enable the child to progress socially with noncustodial adults and other peers (California Department of Education [CDE], 2007).

Through their interactions with adults in their enlarging world, as defined in part by their child care arrangements, toddlers learn to interact with other adult figures by interpreting their social cues. Toddlers engage in the first efforts of social interactions with their peers. They engage in play activities that begin as parallel efforts and eventually loosely resemble cooperative play with the guided assistance of adults (CDE, 2007).

Knowledge of typical toddler development is a prerequisite for increasing understanding of this stage of childhood for research, clinical, and parenting purposes. It enables researchers to investigate the behavioral symptomatology and impact associated with chronic conditions and disabilities (Gray &

McCormick, 2005; Magiati, Charman, & Howlin, 2007; Peadon, Rhys-Jones, Bower, & Elliott, 2009). Knowledge of typical development facilitates APNs' abilities to screen and detect the early manifestations of delays for service referrals (Individuals with Disabilities Education Improvement Act of 2004). Additionally, understanding of typical social and emotional development enables APNs to suggest to parents age-appropriate activities to foster acquisition of domain-specific milestones.

Preschool Years

The preschool years extend from three to six years of age. Erikson (1950, 1959) referred to this period of childhood psychosocial development as *Initiative vs. Guilt*. One of the developmental challenges for the preschool child is to begin to learn how to integrate comparisons of his or her efforts that do not correspond to the same level of achievement by his peers. The preschooler's play increasingly evolves with the refinement and development of gross and fine motor skills, enabling more active participation in collective play with peers and evidence of preferred play interests. The preschool child learns to play more cooperatively with peers and is more aware of and sensitive to what are fair and unfair actions toward playmates (Betz & Sowden, 2008; Iannelli, 2006). Children's play takes on more dramatic overtones, with adaptation of adult roles of their parents or authority figures into their play and the incorporation of fantasy themes for acting out with their peers.

Knowledge and understanding of the typical psychosocial behaviors expected of preschool children are necessary to properly monitor, screen, and detect behaviors indicative of an actual or potential problem and for parental guidance regarding their child's development (Hagan, Shaw, & Duncan, 2008). It is during the preschool years that the child begins to move away from an egocentric orientation. The following stages of play table illustrates play activities that the child engages in based on developmental mastery, and which also serves to reinforce developmental skills (Table 1.1).

School-age Years

Erickson hypothesized that the psychosocial task of the school-age period (seven to eleven years), entitled *Industry vs. Inferiority*, was the learning and mastery of competencies associated with the child's expanding role expectations. During this stage, the child adopts the role of student, is delegated simple household responsibilities (i.e., making his bed and keeping his bedroom/sleeping area orderly), and engages in sports and recreational activities as a team member or competitor, whether formalized with Little League baseball, soccer teams, or loosely organized groups of peers (Betz & Sowden,

2008). The child's challenge is to achieve proficiency with new skills and knowledge to meet the expectations as a student, team member, and member of a peer group. Failure to do so leads to feelings of inferiority, low self-esteem, social isolation, and depression (Erikson, 1950, 1959). Investigating the impact of learning and behavior problems on typical psychosocial development in school-age children has been the focus of research interests. Researchers have also studied the impact of chronic illnesses and disabilities on this school-age developmental domain for the purpose of preventing and ameliorating this psychosocial co-morbidity (Grey & Sullivan-Bolyai, 1999; Koenning, Benjamin, Todaro, Warren, & Burns, 1995; Sullivan-Bolyai, Deatrick, Gruppuso, Tamborlane, & Grey, 2003; Woodgate & Degner, 2003).

Adolescence

By adolescence, the major psychosocial task of youth is to establish an identity. This identity represents the compilation and integration of intellectual, social, psychological, and physical domains of functioning that the youth has acquired and achieved during the preceding stages of development (Erikson, 1950, 1959). In turn, this development has been influenced and shaped by family membership, the social network of peers and adults, and the child- and youth-oriented community (i.e., school, youth groups, etc.).

The youth's developing identity is shaped in part by the company of peers she keeps. If the youth has developed an integrated identity without the painful and potentially destructive unresolved conflicts from the past, then peers will be chosen who reflect the current psychological and emotional status and future aspirations of the teen. If the conflicts and ensuing intrapersonal and psychosocial turmoil are not resolved appropriately, the adolescent is at risk for associating with other teens who engage in self-destructive, delinquent, and even criminal behavior (Erikson, 1950, 1959).

Although teens may espouse the beliefs and values of wanting independence, in truth, many seek first and foremost the acceptance of their peers as evidenced by their conformity in dress styles, physical appearance, colloquial expressions, and recreational and social interests (Bricker et al., 2009; Cin et al., 2009; Santor, Messervey, & Kusumakar, 2000). Peer-related activities are fortified in their importance by the collective formal and informal group activities that serve to create a group identity, as is found with sports teams, the celebrity-worship cults, and recreational interest groups.

For the first time, serious romantic relationships, some of which are based on physical attraction, develop (Nemours Foundation, 2008a, 2008b). Formerly, in past generations, these relationships were not seriously entertained until middle to late adolescence. In today's

Table 1.1 Stages of play

Infancy	Solitary or independent play: Infant's play is focused on activities that are dependent on reflexive and sensory actions. Play things that engage the infant by stimulating sensory motor behaviors are favored. These play things include: • Rattles • Mobiles • Toys that make sound • Colorful toys • Toys that can be mouthed • Bodily movements that create pleasurable sensations (i.e., sucking fingers, patting at mobile) • Responding to parental bonding and attachment behaviors
Toddler	Toddler play expands beyond the infant's body boundaries. The toddler's developing fine and gross motor abilities enable greater exploration of the environment and manipulation of play things. The toddler's developing language skills and cognitive skills enable parallel play activities, that is, play that is done in the presence of other children but does not involve other children. • Scribbling and coloring • Riding tricycles • Stacking and nesting toys • Playing with stuffed animals • Playing with dolls • Completing simple, large sized puzzles
Preschooler	The preschooler is developing social skills that enable the child to move beyond parallel play to play that involves the beginning of interacting with others. The child's developing cognitive abilities result in the emergence of fantasy play involving the adoption of imaginary roles such as storybook characters. Individual interests and preferences in play activities develop. • Playing with pretend toys such as costumes • Playing simple board games • Dancing • Playing with musical toys • Playing with high-tech toys (i.e., video games, movies) • Using wheel toys • Playing group games • Playing fantasy role-playing games • Gender-specific activities are not always evident.
School age	School-age children progress in the refinement of gross and fine motor skills associated with play. Their developing social network of classmates and friends provides the context for learning prosocial skills, learning to play by the rules, and making comparisons regarding their competencies in sports activities with their peers. Competitive sports activities emerge and flourish. Individual interests and preferences in play activities continue. • Team sports • Creative hobbies • Crafts • Video and computer games • Board games • Construction activities (making models, art objects, decorative items) • Outdoor sports (swimming, hiking, bicycling) • Special interest clubs • Technology recreational activities (use of the Internet)
Adolescent	While team sports are focused on gender-specific activities, development of opposite-sex activities can include dancing, music, clubs, and community advocacy/social justice activities. • Competitive team sports (i.e., football, baseball, volleyball, etc.) • Competitive individual sports (i.e., track and field, tennis) • Pleasure reading

(continued)

Table 1.1 (*cont'd*)

- Creative hobbies (i.e., drawing)
- Collection hobbies (i.e., baseball cards)
- Group outings
- Technology recreational activities (i.e., surfing the Internet)
- Computer games
- Outdoor sports (i.e., hiking, swimming)

Cincinnati Children's Hospital Medical Center. (2007–2009). Growth and development wellness: Stages of play. Retrieved from http://www.Cincinnatichildrens.org/health/info/growth/well/stages.Htm

Keith, K.L. (2009). Children's play. About.com. Retrieved from http://childparenting.about.com/od/activitiesandfun/u/kidsplay.htm?p=1

National Parent Teacher Association (2009). Play at different ages and developmental stages. Retrieved from http://school.familyeducation.com/games/growth-and-development/38382.html

Ramseyer, V. (2007). Stages of play. Retrieved from http://ezinearticles.com/?Stages-of-Play&id=900253&opt=print

society, younger adolescents engage in sexual relationships as evidenced by the lowering of the age of introduction to sexual intimacy (Abma, Martinez, Mosher, & Dawson, 2004; Guttmacher Institute, 2006). Yet, despite changing trends in adolescence pertaining to earlier initiation of active sexual behavior, the rate of adolescent pregnancy has dropped, due in part to the use of contraceptive options, including delaying sexual intercourse (Guttmacher Institute, 2006). Another interesting development is the trend of young adults to delay marriage, childbearing, and entry into the workforce until the late twenties. Formerly, the mean age for these developmental milestones of adulthood occurred earlier in the twenties (Arnett, 2000, 2001).

As societal and demographic trends change both nationally and globally, the characteristics associated with social and emotional development as well as all domains of development will be altered and revisited by developmental experts. Astute APNs in psychiatric and primary pediatric care settings will observe these shifting developmental paradigms in adolescents and respond in their typical clinical expert manner based on the evidence to determine what behaviors represent at-risk or actual concerns that need additional assessment and services.

This section has discussed the social and emotional development of children and youth across the lifespan. Characteristics associated with each developmental stage have been presented to illustrate the age-appropriate behaviors reflective of social emotional behaviors of typically developing children and youth. Knowledge of typical development is a foundation of knowledge needed to screen, detect, and refer for services those children and youth who require additional evaluation.

Self-Esteem

Self-esteem refers to an individual's perception of personal self-worth and it is a mutable view of self whose roots of development begin early in childhood (Rosenberg, 1965). A child's self-esteem, as measured by tools such as the Rosenberg Self Esteem Scale (1965) or the Coopersmith Self Esteem Inventory (Coopersmith, 1981), can be quantified on a continuum from high to low. High levels of self-esteem have been further conceptualized as high secure self-esteem and high insecure self-esteem.

Children who have high self-esteem are confident of their abilities to perform, whereas children with low self-esteem experience hesitancy and doubt about their competencies to function on a par with their peers or as expected by their parents and other responsible adults in their lives. Children with high secure self-esteem perform academically better in school and in athletics, engage in less risky behaviors, are healthier, have more effective coping skills, and are more socially competent (Biro, Striegel-Moore, Franko, Padgett, & Bean, 2006). There are some children with attention deficit hyperactivity disorder (ADHD) whose high self-esteem is typified as insecure and who are as at risk for problematic behaviors as children with low self-esteem (Menon et al., 2007). Those who have insecure self-esteem are described as inauthentic with feelings of entitlement narcissism. Children with high insecure self-esteem are particularly sensitive to criticism and react angrily to those who are perceived as criticizing them. They engage in high-risk behavior such as aggression and substance abuse but justify their behavior as appropriate (Menon et al.,

2007). In contrast, children with low self-esteem more frequently experience school failure, engage in antisocial, aggressive, and delinquent behaviors, and exhibit more health and mental health problems (Donnellan, Trzesniewski, Robins, Moffitt, & Caspi, 2005).

A child's self-esteem can be influenced negatively or positively by maturational, social, and environmental factors. The self-esteem of a child can be adversely affected amid periods of significant changes such as during pubertal growth, transition periods associated with enrollment in new schools (such as progressing from elementary to middle school), and the developmental challenges experienced during adolescence (Adler & Stewart, 2004; Biro et al., 2006). Increased levels of anxiety and poor or awkward social skills are additional factors that can contribute to low self-esteem. Researchers have been interested in studying self-esteem in children because it has been associated with adaptive and nonadaptive behaviors and alterable behavioral outcomes. Additionally, experts have recognized that self-esteem, a perceptual evaluation of our self-worth, is amenable to modification with the use of intervention strategies.

Understanding of self-esteem has evolved from estimates of global self-worth to its association with specific areas of functioning as it pertains to family, school, and peers. For example, researchers found that home and school areas of self-esteem were more strongly associated with teen drug use than was peer self-esteem (Donnelly, Young, Pearson, Penhollow, & Hernandez, 2008). Findings from this and other studies suggest that interventions targeting specific aspects of self-esteem may be more effective when the goal is global improvement of self-esteem (Donnelly, et al., 2008; Wilkinson, 2004; Young, Donnelly, & Denny, 2004).

A number of variables are associated with supporting higher levels of self-esteem. Family and parent variables associated with promoting higher self-esteem in children are secure family attachment, parental acceptance of the child, high parental self-esteem, and intact family structure (Adler & Stewart, 2004; Dalgas-Pelish, 2006; Donnelly et al., 2008; Edmondson, Grote, Haskell, Matthews, & White, n.d.). The profile of characteristics associated with high self-esteem in children includes productive school participation, protective peer activities, resiliency, and self-perceived physical attractiveness (Adler & Stewart, 2004; Donnelly et al., 2008; Edmondson et al., n.d; Manning, 2007; Veselska et al., 2009). Researchers have differed in their explanations of the factors that promote positive levels of self-esteem in children. For example, some argue that achievement outcomes are not the determining factors of self-esteem, but rather the consequence (Menon et al., 2007). That is, children who experience success with academics will, in turn, experience positive feelings about themselves.

The risk factors and consequences associated with low self-esteem have been examined as well. Associations have been reported between maternal and adolescent low self-esteem (Edmondson et al., n.d.). Peer activities may create the medium for at-risk behaviors (Veselska et al., 2009). That is, children and youth may feel encouraged to engage in at-risk activities such as substance abuse if that is an acceptable norm of the peer group (Donnelly et al., 2008). Gender differences have been reported in the behavioral manifestation of low self-esteem. Boys with low esteem exhibit more externalizing behaviors compared to girls with low self-esteem, who have the tendency to internalize problems (Veselska et al., 2009). Lower self-esteem in adolescents was associated with a number of at-risk behaviors including early sexual initiation, unprotected sex, teen substance abuse, and a history of risky partners (i.e., history of AIDS, HIV, and incarceration) in adolescent girls (Ethier et al., 2006). Although self-esteem can serve as a protective factor for at-risk health behaviors, a child who has low self-esteem is at risk for developing psychosocial and psychiatric problems such as social isolation, aggression, and delinquency (Veselska et al., 2009).

Self-esteem in children and youth warrants consideration by APNs in clinical practice. While it is unlikely that self-esteem would be formally assessed in clinical settings, it is appropriate to acknowledge its importance in determining the extent to which children and youth perceive their self-worth. Those who share feelings and/or demonstrate behaviors indicative of low self-esteem or high insecure self-esteem as described here should be referred for additional evaluations and services.

Cognitive Development

Understanding how cognitive development proceeds in children and being able to judge where a given child is on this timeline are important knowledge and skills for all pediatric health care providers. The understanding of aberrations or deviations from the "usual," "common," or "normal" pattern of development is, of course, firmly rooted in having developed an accurate understanding of normative patterns. Cognitive development is particularly challenging because so much of it is either unseen or inferred from a child's actions, language, or other indicators. Despite this, an understanding of how our current knowledge of human cognition developed and how children of various ages are both alike and different will assist readers in increasing knowledge about and skills with children.

Theoretical Considerations

Current developmental theory in the area of cognition is the product of a synthesis of thinking that began in the early part of the 20th century. Interest in child development in the United States evolved largely out of the child study movement, based in observational studies of child behavior. The development of theory began with the work of Arnold Gesell (1929), who based his descriptions of children's behavior on a theory of maturational unfolding. This unfolding resulted from innate abilities, a genetic template. For Gesell, the environment played a superficial or temporary role in influencing the unfolding of behaviors. While his theory would be regarded as overly simplistic today, what Gesell gave us was a template of development that formed the basis for future work in the field of human development.

Behaviorism developed in contrast to both Gesell's idea of maturationalism and Freud's theories of the mental mechanism, examining so carefully the function of the psyche. For behaviorists, the only important functions of the human organism were those that could be seen and recorded and these behaviors operated in clear response to certain fundamental rules. Behaviorist theory reduces cognitive development to learning behaviors, without regard for the internal processes that might enable one to learn.

Beginning his writing in the 1920s, Swiss psychologist Jean Piaget (1952) was the most dominant influence on a school of cognitive development commonly referred to as Constructivism. Piaget went largely undiscovered in the United States until the 1950s. His work was the basis for the study of cognitive development versus learning described by the behaviorists. Piaget's work revolves around the idea that individuals "construct" their own understanding of the world around them, organizing and reorganizing the structure of their knowledge. Piaget saw the cognitive structure as a product of the continuous interaction of the children's internal abilities and the world around them. Inherent in this thinking is the idea that we all attempt to create a meaning of the world around us and are constantly revising and remaking our interpretations or "schemas." This process takes place by way of the functions of assimilation or accommodation. We take in or assimilate things in our environment that match our internal schema or accommodate our internal schema if the reality does not match our schema.

Best known among Piaget's work are his major stages of development and their characteristics:

1. Sensorimotor period (birth to two years). Infants progress from being largely reflex beings to learning to associate their experiences with the outside world through the coordination of sensory input and motor functions. They begin to represent objects mentally and manipulate them.

2. Preoperational thought (ages two to seven). Children in this stage are still primarily dependent upon perception and have little developed logic. They begin to represent the world with words, ideas, and drawings. The period is characterized by egocentric speech and thought with children unable to appreciate another's point of view.

3. Concrete operations (ages seven to eleven). Logical thinking replaces intuition and children can perform basic logical operations on concrete objects and perform limited manipulation of mental objects. Piaget's classic tests for this period involved understanding reversibility and conservation.

4. Formal operations (ages eleven to fifteen). Individuals begin to think in more abstract ways. They understand hypothetical thinking, multiple causation, and other abstract concepts (Piaget, 1952).

Piaget's work with children, largely observational, had a profound impact on the development of modern cognitive psychology. His documentation of how cognition develops and the stages of development is what most who have a passing acquaintance with Piaget remember. Newer research suggests that his stages often underestimated the capabilities of children; however, what endures are his constructivist ideas about how individuals attempt to attach meaning to the external world and how the quality and form of thinking change over time.

Piaget largely ignored the influence of the context within which cognitive development occurred, but the Soviet psychologist Lev Vygotsky (1962) emphasized the importance of the social environment while maintaining a constructivist approach. He placed great emphasis on the importance of language and social interaction in cognitive development. Education for Vygotsky was a major tool in development, and the function of the adult as "teacher" was to assist the child in learning through the relational interactions. This then contributed to the overall development of the child. His idea of the Zone of Proximal Development proposed that adults as "teachers" provide supports or "scaffolding" for children, enabling them to grow from their basic capabilities to a higher level (Figure 1.1).

A newer approach to the study of cognition is the information processing approach. In some ways an information processing approach is a return to a more reductionistic view of cognitive development, in contrast to the constructivist views which are much more holistic and include the concept of metacognition (Kuhn, 1984). Information processing theory compares the functioning of the human mind to a computer model.

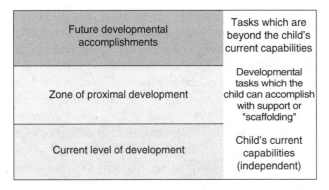

Figure 1.1 Vygotsky's Zone of Proximal Development.

Cognitive processes are thus reduced to a list of tasks processed using mechanisms of attention, encoding, representation, execution, decoding, and memory. Development is largely a growth in capacity, efficiency, or speed of processing in the individual. Information is taken in through the senses, encoded into electrochemical impulses, and stored in areas of short-term or working and/or long-term memory. Behavior is the result of processing of information by comparison to previous encoded experiences, arriving at a conclusion, and executing a decision via motor output (Figure 1.2).

Information processing theory has been helpful in clarifying some of the relationships between cognitive processes to physiologic mechanisms and states. It is also particularly useful in explaining and understanding some of the learning problems that develop in individuals and explaining where the usual methods of processing might have gone awry.

More recent developments in cognitive developmental theory include revisions of some of Piaget's classic ideas by the neo-Piagetians. Among these is Robbie Case, who relabeled and attempted to more accurately define some of Piaget's stages. Case (1996, p. 2) described the work of neo-Piagetian cognitive theorists in the following passage:

> Theorists began to assert that children's conceptual development was less dependent on the emergence of general logical structures than Piaget had suggested and more dependent on the acquisition of insights or skills that are domain, task and context specific.

In current thinking, the emergence of cognitive skills is more dependent on social interaction as described by Vygotsky (1962). Neo-Piagetian thinking also includes the idea that the general stages as described by Piaget are more of a "ceiling" or age-linked constraint. Within those constraints, children develop in unique ways more dependent upon their surroundings and interactions. Neo-Piagetian thinking has also included the idea that changes occurring in children's thinking are less general than originally described by Piaget. Instead, they are more specific or "modular" with children showing growth in cognition in a more piecemeal fashion, first in one area or domain and then in another (Goswami, 2008).

Infant Cognition

If there has been any area in which the capabilities of children have been underestimated over the years, it is in the area of infant development. This is a clearly understandable phenomenon, because infants have little in

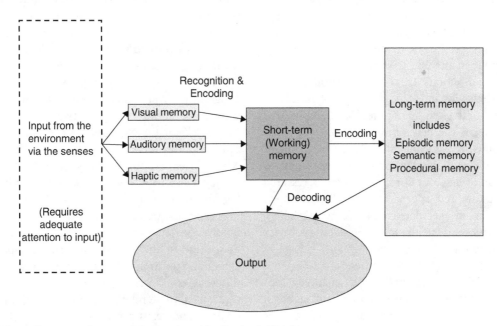

Figure 1.2 Information processing concepts. Developed by Stephanie Wright.

the way of language and motor skills to assist us in our assessment. The testing of infants is considerably more complex and requires some very clever experimental designs.

Infants are born predisposed to social interaction and constantly take in and process the world around them from the moment of birth. Infants are equipped with a set of primitive reflexes to assist them with their initial interactions with their environment, but these are rapidly replaced with reactions based on their developing awareness of the world around them. The sources of their information are their bodies and the senses. Infants, although physically immature, have intact sensory systems. Newborns can see, but have a short focal distance, likely the equivalent of someone quite nearsighted. They prefer high contrast and often scan to those areas of the human face. By two months of age, the eye has matured sufficiently so that the infant can focus about as well as an adult (McDonough, 1999). Depth perception, which requires the brain's coordination of two visual images, first appears around six to seven months of age and appears to be closely related to crawling (Trawick-Smith, 2010).

Touch is a crucial sense for newborns and they are well equipped to use this sense to interact with those caring for them. Newborns also have a well developed sense of pain. Newborns can distinguish basic tastes and will show this with facial responses. Smell is also well developed in newborns. Hearing is not terribly acute in newborns, likely related to delayed clearing of materials from the ear canal. However, their hearing capabilities are quite sensitive shortly after birth (Trawick-Smith, 2010).

Piaget's Sensorimotor Stage describes infants as inadvertently discovering new experiences through their sensual exploration and then trying to repeat those events or actions. This progresses to anticipation of events from cues, and then attempts to repeat interesting events through their own actions. This eventually leads to some goal-directed behavior and some simple problem solving toward the end of the first year of life. Piaget emphasized the importance of the development of object permanence in infants, recognizing that objects exist out of sight. Piaget claimed this appeared at about eight to twelve months of age, but current laboratory research indicates that this may appear much earlier, although it is not obvious in everyday events (Goswami, 2008). Imitation emerges early in infancy and is likely a primary source of learning for infants. Older infants engage in imitation of complex behaviors of others.

Piaget suggested that infants do not mentally represent their everyday experience until about eighteen months of age. Current research largely refutes this with infant research into memory showing that much

younger infants remember events, and later imitate or repeat actions and therefore must have mental representation of them (McDonough, 1999). Toward the end of the first year, infants show simple problem solving, such as flipping a light switch to turn on a light, and rapidly progress to problem solving that requires multiple steps.

By the second year, toddlers have well-developed object permanence, searching in multiple locations for objects. They develop excellent skills of deferred imitation of complex behaviors of others. They can actively sort objects.

While we now know that infants have the development of certain cognitive skills earlier than described by Piaget, there is still considerable discussion describing the actual capabilities of infants. Infant development is an area of ongoing rich research.

Early Childhood Cognitive Development

Piaget characterized the Preoperational Stage of development more by what children could not yet do than by what they could do. According to Piaget, the greatest change seen in this age group was the great capacity for mental representation (symbolic function), which permitted young children to separate the physical world from the world of thought. Their play then takes on the characteristics seen so commonly in children of this age: engagement in considerable make-believe and greater complexity in their play. Make-believe play serves a variety of functions for the child, including allowing them to express emotion, anticipate events, and become more socially competent. Children of this age also develop considerable fine motor coordination and use this to represent their ideas. Piaget pointed out several limitations of thought in children of this age. They engage in egocentric thinking, being unable to consider any other point of view or interpretation of the world than their own. Recent research questions this. Gelman and Schatz (1978) point out that young children adapt their language to their audience, at times showing clear appreciation for another's perspective. Several redesigns of Piaget's classic three mountains experiment have shown awareness of others' points of vantage during this preschool (preoperational) period (Borke, 1975).

Piaget also held that there were certain limitations of logic for preoperational children. The famous conservation experiments show difficulties of children appreciating the constancy of certain physical characteristics such as volume in the face of changes in appearance (the changing appearance of liquids of the same volume in different containers). Piaget felt this was related to centration, the tendency of preschool children to focus on one characteristic of a situation or object, while ignoring others. As with age-related limitations described by Piaget, preschoolers can overcome appearances and think more logically than he originally described, especially when the materials are familiar to them (Goswami, 2008).

Similarly, preschool children appear to be able to categorize with more sophistication than originally described by Piaget. In conclusion, preschool children gradually learn about relationships that involve interpreting appearances of objects, and this understanding is aided by their growing language abilities and their beginning to understand constancy of number. Like infants, preschoolers are considerably more capable than originally described by Piaget, but the steps they must pass through to achieve these milestones were accurately described by him.

Cognition in School-aged Children

Piaget (1952) described the school-age period as characterized by concrete operational thought, with thought becoming more logical and well organized. Children of this age understand concepts of conservation and reversibility and they grow to be able to perform classifications based in multiple characteristics of the items to be sorted. They can sort according to dimensions and can solve basic inferential problems. They understand spatial relationships and orient themselves in space. This allows them to learn basic directions from one place to another and to draw maps.

The limitation of concrete operations described by Piaget is that the logic of school-aged children is limited to what they perceive in the real world around them. They have difficulty considering abstract ideas and thinking about larger principles that might govern the real world.

School and culture heavily influence the growth of cognition in this age group; therefore, the achievement of the milestones of concrete operational thinking and the progression to formal operational thinking depend heavily upon the context within which the child grows. Some school-aged children show the beginnings of hypothetical thinking and deductive reasoning before Piaget's usual age for formal operational thinking (approximately eleven years), but this greatly depends upon their environment (Goswami, 2008).

Adolescent Cognitive Development

At about age ten or eleven, children begin to enter a period of formal operational thinking, according to Piaget. In this stage they develop the ability to think abstractly, going beyond the realm of their everyday experiences. Adolescents develop clear deductive reasoning, allowing them to solve problems based on logic and mental experimentation. The development of language is closely tied to this ability to perform abstract reasoning. Adolescents can consider problems that are counter to their everyday experience and engage in hypothetical thinking about possible outcomes.

Elkind (1967) described limitations on the newly developing cognitive skills of adolescents imposed by their dramatic changes in self-concept. This creates a kind of self-absorption, a new form of egocentrism, which tends to limit some areas of cognitive growth. While Elkind described four characteristics of adolescent egocentrism, his concepts should be examined for applicability within specific cultural contexts. His characteristics include:

Imaginary audience: Adolescents often believe that they are the center of others' attention, creating extreme self-consciousness and making them sensitive to criticism.

Personal fable: Adolescents, because they feel they are the center of others' attention, often feel that they are somehow unique and special, acting out extraordinary lives.

Invulnerability: Because they feel that they are somehow unique, adolescents may feel that are invulnerable to the usual consequences of everyday actions. Their ability to consider the long-term consequences of their actions may be severely limited by their egocentrism.

Idealism: Because they are able to go beyond the limits of reality and into the possible by their cognitive capabilities, adolescents may tend to be very idealistic and become quite critical of others who do not reach these ideals, parents in particular.

Recent research indicates that formal operational thinking is not always attained in all cultures and contexts, indicating that it is educationally and culturally transmitted. In addition, formal operational thinking does not emerge in all areas of thinking at once, but rather appears in relation to specific areas of learning (Keating, 2004).

Development and Information Processing Theory

As previously described, information processing theory ascribes the changes in cognition that occur as children grow in terms of growth in processing speed, ability to attend, short- and long-term memory, and organization of thinking. There are few age-related milestones to assist one in tying particular milestones to age. Older children have progressively faster processing speeds and are able to sustain selective attention for longer periods. Short-term memory, that is, retention of information for less than a minute without active memory retention strategies, is usually tested with digit span. Two- to three-year-olds can usually retain about two digits, seven-year-olds about five digits. This gradually increases to an adult level of about seven to eight digits. Changes in long-term memory may be more related to organization than to capacity, and children's abilities to retrieve information from long-term memory improve with age and with practice. Once children are in formal learning situations, they have many opportunities for improving memory and often learn organization and rehearsal strategies for improving memory (Santrock, 2007).

Development of Coping in Children

Responses to stress and imposed change have been extensively studied in adults. Physiologic and psychological response patterns to stress are well documented, but how those patterns develop is still unclear. Coping is defined to include all responses to stressful events. Most stress researchers would consider coping as falling into two categories: instinctive or reflexive reactions and those that are learned responses (Compas, 1987). In adult coping literature, there has been much research on coping as an adaptational response as evidenced by studies of coping function and style. As classically described by Lazarus and Folkman (1984), coping functions to both regulate the individual's emotional response and to engage in some problem solving around the crisis imposed by the stressor.

Individual variability in coping and the description of coping styles by various researchers (Krohne & Rogner, 1982; Miller & Green, 1984) lead to the question of how these patterns are developed in individuals and which individual differences and environmental issues play an important part in the development of these patterns. Included in these studies of individual differences is the question of why some children are more resilient and less vulnerable to stress than others (Garmezy, 1981).

While coping literature has built upon adult studies of stress psychology, it has important overlaps with traditional areas of child development research, including neurobiology, temperament, cognition, attention, emotion, and parental attachment. Because coping is such a complex phenomenon, no central theory has emerged, but several important principles have been reiterated related to the development of coping in children.

Early coping is embedded in neurobiology and the development of the brain and central nervous system. Early responses to stress seem to be particularly rooted in the temperamental characteristics related to arousal, reactions to novelty, attention, and affect (Rueda & Rothbart, 2009). As the child matures, experience contributes to the development or limiting of coping skills with different aspects of development playing more important roles at various ages. Early experiences with stress may in turn shape the development of the brain regions related to emotional regulation (Compas, 2009). Early experiences with uncontrollable stress have been associated with changes in the serotonin neurons and a pattern of learned helplessness (Maier & Watkins, 2005).

Parents are central figures in the child's development of coping skills, serving as important social support, role models for coping behaviors, and stress-absorbing figures. Parents can make demands on children that are early stressors that children must deal with. How parents support children in coping with their demands is an important variable. The availability and ability of parents to assist children in gaining a sense of control over the demands placed upon them help children develop a sense of mastery and control.

Age-graded shifts in coping have been described by Skinner and Zimmer-Gembeck (2007) and serve as a helpful developmental model for coping (Table 1.2). Within the first few months of life, infants progress from largely physiologic and temperamentally based reactions to learning self-soothing and use of distraction as early coping mechanisms. Children learn to regulate their own behavior with a shift occurring at about eighteen to twenty-four months of age, as mastery of motor skills and emotion come into play. A second major shift occurs at about five to seven years of age, when cognitive elements and social relations begin to play important parts in coping. A third shift is described at about age ten to twelve, marked by changes in patterns of thinking correlated with the growth of more sophisticated cognitive skills represented by formal operational thinking. At fourteen to sixteen years of age, autonomy and identity development begin to play salient roles in coping. New patterns again emerge between middle adolescence and the early twenties, when expanding social horizons provide challenging new experiences.

Acute and chronic stresses have been implicated in many physical and mental health problems in both children and adults. Documentation of patterns of coping in children has been a fairly recent field of research and one that will be extremely important as health care professionals attempt to understand and better treat the emotional and mental health problems of children as well as understand the behavior of all children.

Language Development

The exact reasons for humans' ability to communicate that is unrivaled by any other species are unclear. Piaget believed that language development was an extension of the intellectual development of humans; we speak

Table 1.2 Broad outlines of possible developmental shifts in means of coping

Developmental period	Approximate ages	Nature of coping	Role of social partners	Nature of regulation
Infancy	Birth to eighteen months	From reflexes to coordinated action schema	Carrying out coping actions based on infant's expressed intentions	Interpersonal co-regulation
Preschool age	Ages two to five	Coping using voluntary direct actions	Availability for direct help and participation	Intrapersonal self-regulation
Middle childhood	Ages six to eight	Coping using cognitive means	Cooperating with and supporting child's coping efforts	Coordinated self-regulation
Early adolescence	Ages ten to twelve	Coping using metacognitive means	Reminder coping	Proactive self-regulation
Middle adolescence	Ages fourteen to sixteen	Coping based on personal values	Backup coping	Identified self-regulation
Late adolescence	Ages eighteen to twenty-two	Coping based on long-term goals	Monitoring coping	Integrated self-regulation

Reprinted from Skinner and Zimmer-Gembeck (2007) with permission from Annual Review of Psychology.

because of superior intelligence. Noam Chomsky (1972), on the other hand, argued that humans are prewired for language and have a theoretical "language acquisition device." Regardless of which view is espoused, language development is a critical indicator of normal human development and delays or failure to develop language are an important sign that some pathology exists.

Language is a symbolic form of communication, spoken, written, or, in some cases, signed. Spoken communication can be further broken down into receptive language and expressive language, with expressive language being much easier to assess in children. Although there are many languages in the world, they all have common characteristics, described as phonology, morphology, syntax, semantics, and pragmatics.

Phonology describes the basic sounds of the language. Although there are many similar sounds in languages, there are sounds that are unique to some language structures. Research by Patricia Kuhl (1993) has shown that infants are capable of hearing all possible sounds for the first six months of life, but during the second half of the first year, infants improve their ability to recognize sounds in their own language and gradually lose the ability to hear sounds that do not occur in their native language.

We are more aware of infants developing an understanding of the morphology of language; that is, learning to recognize the meaning of sounds. During the second half of the first year, infants begin to recognize

the boundaries between words in spoken language (Brownlee, 1998; Jusczyk, 2000) and to attach meaning to words. By twelve or thirteen months, infants recognize about fifty words (Menyuk, Liebergott, & Schwartz, 1995), many more than they are capable of expressing. This pattern continues with receptive language exceeding expressive language for much of early childhood.

All children, regardless of the language spoken, generally follow a similar pattern of development of expressive language:

- All infants are capable of crying to signal distress and often have distinctive cries as signals for different states.
- Cooing predominantly refers to vowel sounds made by young infants, usually indicating a pleasurable state, but it is also seen in response to an interaction with another.
- Sometime around four to six months, infants begin adding consonant sounds and vocalize consonant-vowel combinations, called babbling.
- Later in infancy, these sounds are strung together and often have the intonation of human speech.

While this is occurring in infancy, infants are learning to communicate in other ways as well, often using gestures and head nods to communicate their wishes. Deaf children at this age often begin learning to sign

(Bloom, 1998). Signing has also been promoted for hearing children as a method for enhancing their ability to communicate while they are developing spoken language. Daniels (1994) has found that teaching hearing children sign language instruction had a number of benefits, including increased vocabulary among preschoolers.

Most children utter their first word sometime between ten and fifteen months of age, usually names of important people, animals, or common objects. While the acquisition of first words is gradual, most children experience a real spurt in growth of vocabulary sometime between thirteen and twenty-five months (Bloom, Lifter, & Broughton, 1985). During this period, young children often acquire multiple new words each day, a truly amazing feat of learning.

Most children begin to string words together in two-word phrases during the second year, and two-word phrases are expected in normal development by twenty-four months of age. These two-word phrases often have a characteristic commonly referred to as "telegraphic speech" in which children convey meaning with a very succinct use of words. Thus, a combination of two words expresses the desire to do or have something despite the absence of important nouns, articles, or verbs, such as "Bobby ice cream" to indicate that he wants ice cream or, alternately, that someone else is eating ice cream. Context is important in understanding telegraphic speech.

Children move rapidly from two-word sentences to more complex and longer structures between two and three years of age. During the entire preschool period, children develop further understanding of the morphology, syntax, semantics, and pragmatics of language. This includes understanding plural and possessive forms, correct word order in sentences, the meaning of sentences, and appropriate use of language in different contexts. Although children make many errors as they attempt to apply language rules, this is part of learning the complex rules of language. By the time children enter first grade, they have an extensive expressive vocabulary, estimated at more than 8,000 words (Rubin, 2006). During elementary school, children refine their grammar and continue a remarkable growth in vocabulary.

Environment influences language development in a number of important ways. Parental and caregiver response to the child in conversation has been shown to be critical in numerous studies. This begins with what is usually referred to as child-directed speech. Adults and older children around a young child alter their speech pattern for the young child, often reducing the number of syllables in words and the number of words in a sentence and changing the pitch of the speech. This has the important function of capturing the child's attention. Labeling familiar objects for the child serves to expand their vocabulary. In addition, parents and caregivers often use repeating of language as reinforcement, recasting something the child said, which may include correcting and expanding on what the child said. Infants whose mothers speak to them more often have been shown to have larger vocabularies (Huttenlocher, Haight, Bruk, Seltzer, & Lyons, 1991). Likewise, adults who read to children and later have their children read to them encourage language development.

While there is considerable variation in early language milestones, such as the first spoken word, the basic pattern of language learning applies to all children and to all spoken languages. Understanding this basic pattern assists practitioners in knowing when to seek help for children and their families. Emphasizing to parents their important role in language development, the APN can give them specific suggestions on ways to encourage their child's language development. These include reading to and talking with the child, singing songs to the child while emphasizing particular words or expressions, and providing age-appropriate explanations and descriptions of events.

Bronfenbrenner's Bioecological Theory of Human Development

As stated previously, child, adolescent, and family development is complex and occurs within environmental contexts in which multiple interactions transpire directly or indirectly, affecting the developing individual. In the 1970s, Bronfenbrenner developed and described the Ecology of Human Development Theory (1979). The original theory was composed of the microsystem, mesosystem, exosystem, and macrosystem. He later added the chronosystem. In 1994 he revised his theory and renamed it the Bioecological Theory of Human Development (Bronfenbrenner). Table 1.3 provides concepts from his original model, his evolved thinking, and additions to the model on human development.

The development of each individual is interdependent on multiple factors, genetics, experience, temperament, type and nature of reciprocal relationships, evolving complexity of interactions, context, time, attachments, quality of environments, and the emotional health of all individuals. A thorough nursing assessment of children, adolescents, and families must pay attention to all of these elements and understand how they affect the growth and development of each family member.

Table 1.3 Bronfenbrenner's evolving model of human development

Ecological Theory of Human Development: Original (individuals and settings)	Bioecological Theory of Human Development: Additional factors operating with original theoretical model
Microsystem: Individual, family, peers, school, and neighborhood; roles; where the individual lives; individual is an active actor in own development	Experience: Subjective feelings that are positive or negative; emotional and motivational in nature
Mesosystem: Connections and relationships between microsystem elements.	Proximal processes: Progressively complex and reciprocal interactions; the higher the levels of positive interactions between the parent/caretaker and the child, the lower the behavioral problems in the child
Exosystem: Connections and relationships between two or more systems, at least one of which does not contain the individual but can indirectly impact processes impacting the individual	Process-person-context-time : Characteristics of the developing person, the environment, changes over time, and developmental outcomes as a result of all interactions
Macrosystem: Customs, culture, ethnicity, beliefs, social fabric impacting the individual	Exposure: Multiple and complex activities must occur over time to promote emotional, social, moral, and intellectual development
Chronosystem: Change over time affecting the individual and the various environments the person experiences	Mutual emotional attachment: Such attachment with parent/caretaker that is internalized motivates child to engage with others
	"Third party": Children growing in environments where they are exposed to more than one caretaker have a greater variety of complex experiences that enriches development
	Future perspective: Psychological development (positive or negative) of caretakers influenced by behavior and development of the child

Bronfenbrenner, U. (1979). The ecology of human development. Cambridge, MA: Harvard University Press.
Bronfenbrenner, U. (1994). Ecological models of human development. *International Encyclopedia of Education, 3(2)*, 1643–1647.
Bronfenbrenner, U. & Ceci, S. (1994). Nature-nurture reconceptualized in developmental perspective: A biological model. *Psychological Review, 101*(4), 568–586.
Bronfenbrenner, U. (Ed.). (2005). Making human beings human. Thousand Oaks, CA: Sage.

Family Life Cycle Development

As individuals grow and develop, so to does the family in which they are nested. There is no one definition of a family; however, most would agree that a family is how the individuals involved define it and is composed of both biological and non-biological individuals as determined by the "family" unit. The Committee on the Science of Research on Families of the Institute of Medicine and the National Research Council further described families as, "members with very different perspectives, needs, obligations, and resources. The characteristics of individual family members change over time—within life spans, and across generations. Families exist in a broader economic, social, and cultural context that itself changes over time" (Olson, 2011, p. 7).

Contemporary family constellations are influenced by divorce, single parenting; remarriages; older parents; foster and adoptive status; lesbian, gay, bisexual, transgender, and questionable caretakers; economics; culture; mores; immigration status; co-parenting; and blended and geographic locations, among other factors (Olson, 2011; Wright & Leahey, 2009). Regardless of the family structure, family tasks include supporting the development of all its members; socialization; protection; providing food and shelter; communication; transmitting values, beliefs, and cultural norms; role development; and assisting with problem solving.

Two well known family development models are Duvall (1977) and McGoldrick and Carter (2003). Both models identify developmental stages that families go through over time. Adolescence, adulthood, launching (young adult leaving the nuclear family to live on his own or with a partner), marriage, addition of children (through birth, fostering, or adoption), midlife, and later life are specific times with specific characteristics that comprise the development of the family. While both models provide the APN with a foundation for understanding family development, families are increasingly viewed as dynamic with new configurations and processes that no longer fit into known traditional models. When conducting an assessment of the child or adolescent, it is important to understand factors that the family unit is dealing with because those factors and others beyond the immediate family unit impact the developing child or adolescent.

Assessment Tools

The American Academy of Pediatrics Policy Statement on *Identifying Infants and Young Children with Developmental Disorders in the Medical Home: An Algorithm for Developmental Surveillance and Screening* (2006), the American Academy of Child and Adolescent Psychiatry *Practice Parameter for the Assessment of the Family* (2007), and the adapted Calgary Family Assessment Model (CFAM) by Wright and Leahy (2009) are useful documents for both the primary care and child and adolescent APN to use when assessing child, adolescent, and family development.

Developmental surveillance is a longitudinal process whereby at each visit the provider assesses and documents the status of the child and family to determine developmental concerns, progress, individual or family risk or protective factors, educational needs, and effectiveness of prior health promotion or therapeutic regimen recommendations. Historical data; observation of the child, adolescent, and caretaker(s) alone or during interactions; family structure, functioning, adaptability, and stressors; cultural, gender, and ethnic information; and communication style are specific data that can be gathered using these tools.

CFAM looks at three aspects of the family: structural (internal, external, and context), developmental, and functional (instrumental and expressive). Structural characteristics include gender, ethnicity, class, family composition, and boundaries. Developmental characteristics include stages of family members, tasks performed by family members, and attachments. Functional characteristics include communication, roles, problem solving abilities, power, and beliefs (Wright & Leahy, 2009).

Case Exemplar

Both parents of thirteen-year-old twin boys Jason and Jeremy were killed in an automobile accident two months ago. Their unmarried aunt Tiffany who lived an hour away in another town assumed guardianship and moved the boys in to live with her. A divorced uncle with whom the boys have had minimal contact lives five hours away in another state. In the new school, the boys struggled with their loss of parents, school, friends, membership on sports teams and routine. Specific behaviors noted by teachers included sadness, isolation, lack of confidence and difficulty with school work. Both boys were referred to the school APN who met with them separately and then together. The APN was particularly struck by their sadness, tearfulness and anhedonia. He contacted the aunt to discuss his concerns about their clinical presentation and learned that she too was struggling with the loss of her sibling. With the consent of Tiffany and the assent of both Jason and Jeremy, a referral was made to a child and adolescent psychiatric APN. The twins and their aunt were assessed separately and a recommendation was made that they all attend weekly family meetings. The APN was able to help the newly configured family focus on their grieving, ways that the boys could reclaim some of their normal adolescent experiences and help the aunt assume a new role as parent. With the help of the APN, the new family began to talk openly with each other, were able to share their grieving and memories of the lost parents and sibling, the twins began to feel more secure and cared for and the aunt began to feel more confident in her new parenting role. The family developed the following plan:

1) The twins would continue in their new school and sign up for one after school activity with peers
2) The twins would maintain contact with long standing friends in their old community through weekend overnight visits, phone calls, emails and when possible, extended summer or holiday activities and visits.
3) The twins decided that they wanted to join the church their aunt attended and specifically wanted to participate in a youth bible study group.
4) The family decided to invite the uncle to visit during the Christmas holiday to develop that relationship and support system.
5) Tiffany and the boys realized that they all enjoyed swimming and decided to swim together once a week at the local indoor pool.
6) Tiffany discussed her behavioral and academic expectations with the twins and with support from the APN began to set limits around school performance.

As the family stabilized, the APN decreased the frequency of meetings and discharged the family with the stipulation that they could contact him in the future if needed. This case exemplar illustrates Bronfenbrenner's Bioecological Theory of Human Development and specifically the factors of experience, mutual emotional attachment, proximal processes, exposure, process-person-context-time and future perspective.

Summary

This chapter has provided a focused overview of social, emotional, and cognitive development in children and youth as a basis for understanding age-appropriate and typical behaviors. Bronfenbrenner's Bioecological Theory of Human Development and Family Development Theories remind us that children and adolescents grow in multiple contexts which impact their developmental trajectory. Emphasis was directed to presenting content on the developmental characteristics relevant to clinical understanding for the purposes of screening at-risk and problematic behavior requiring additional evaluation and services. To this end, subject matter on cognitive and social emotional development, self-esteem, coping, and language development was presented. Incorporated within the discussion of these developmental characteristics are the theoretical underpinnings and evidence that support these models of development.

References

Abma, J.C., Martinez, G.M., Mosher, W.D., & Dawson, B.S. (2004). Teenagers in the United States: Sexual activity, contraceptive use, and childbearing, 2002, *Vital and Health Statistics*, 2004, Series 23, No. 24.

Adler, N., & Stewart, J. (2004). Self esteem. John D. and Catherine T. MacArthur Research Network and Socioeconomic Status and Health.

Ainsworth, M.S. (1989). Attachment beyond infancy. *American Psychologist, 44*, 709–716.

Ainsworth, M.S., Blehar, M.C., Waters, E., & Wall, S. (1978). *The strange situation: Observing patterns of attachment*. Hillsdale, NJ: Erlbaum.

American Academy of Child and Adolescent Psychiatry. (2007). Practice parameters for the assessment of the family. *Journal of the American Academy of Child and Adolescent Psychiatry, 46*(7), 922–937.

American Academy of Child and Adolescent Psychiatry. (2009). *When to seek help for your child*. Retrieved from http://www.aacap.org/cs/root/facts_for_families/when_to_seek_help_for_your_child

American Academy of Pediatrics. (2006). Identifying infants and young children with developmental disorders in the Medical Home: An algorithm for developmental surveillance and screening. *Pediatrics, 118*(1), 405–420.

American Academy of Pediatrics. (2008). *Bright futures: Guidelines for health supervision of infants, children and adolescents*. (3rd edition). Retrieved from http://brightfutures.aap.org/pdfs/Guidelines_PDF/16-Early_Childhood.pdf

Arnett, J.J. (2000). Emerging adulthood: A theory of development from the late teens through the twenties, *American Psychologist, 55*, 469–480.

Arnett, J.J. (2001). Conceptions of the transition to adulthood: Perspectives from adolescence through midlife. *Journal of Adult Development, 8*, 133–143.

Arnott, B., & Meins, E. (2007). Links among antenatal attachment representations, postnatal mind-mindedness and infant attachment security: A preliminary study of mothers and fathers. *Bulletin of the Menninger Clinic, 71*, 132–149.

Belsky, J., & Pluess, M. (2009). The nature (and nurture?) of plasticity in early human development. *Perspectives on Psychological Science, 4*(4), 345–351.

Berger, K. (2001). *The developing person through the life span* (pp. 131–146). New York, NY: Worth Publishers.

Berk, L. (2008). Physical development in infancy and toddlerhood. In *exploring lifespan development* (pp. 90–114). Boston, MA: Pearson Education.

Betz, C.L., & Sowden, L. (2008). *Mosby's pediatric nursing reference* (6th edition). St. Louis: Mosby.

Biro, F.M., Striegel-Moore, R.H., Franko, D.L., Padgett, J., & Bean, J.A. (2006). Self-esteem in adolescent females. *Journal of Adolescent Health, 39*, 501–507.

Bloom, L. (1998). Language acquisition in its developmental context. In W. Damon (Ed.). *Handbook of child psychology* (5th edition). New York: Wiley.

Bloom, L., Lifter, K., & Broughton, J. (1985). The convergence of early cognition and language in the second year of life: Problems in conceptualization and measurement. In M. Barrett (Ed.). *Single word speech*. London: Wiley.

Borke, H. (1975). Piaget's mountains revisited: Changes in the egocentric landscape. *Developmental Psychology, 11*, 240–243.

Bowlby, J. (1980). *Attachment and loss: Vol. 5*. New York: Basic Books.

Bowlby, J. (1982). *Attachment and loss: Vol. 1*. Attachment. New York: Basic Books.

Bretherton, I. (1992). The origins of attachment theory: John Bowlby and Mary Ainsworth. *Developmental Psychology, 28*(5), 759–775.

Bricker, J.B., Rajan, K.B., Zalewski, M., Andersen, M.R., Ramey, M., & Peterson, A.V. (2009). Psychological and social risk factors in adolescent smoking transitions: A population-based longitudinal study. *Health Psychology, 28*(4), 439–447.

Brownlee, S. (1998). Baby talk. *US News & World Report* (June 15), 48–54.

Bronfenbrenner, U. (1979). *The ecology of human development*. Cambridge, MA: Harvard University Press.

Bronfenbrenner, U. (1994). Ecological models of human development. *International Encyclopedia of Education, 3*(2), 1643–1647.

Bronfenbrenner, U., & Ceci, S. (1994). Nature-nurture reconceptualized in developmental perspective: A bioecological model. *Psychological Review, 101*(4), 568–586.

Bronfenbrenner, U. (Ed.). (2005). *Making human beings human*. Thousand Oaks, CA: Sage.

California Department of Education. (2007). *California infant/toddler learning and developmental foundations*. Retrieved from http://www.cde.ca.gov/sp/cd/re/itf09intro.asp

Case, R. (1996). Introduction: The nature of children's conceptual structures and their development in middle childhood. In *The role of central conceptual structures in the development of children's thought* (pp. 1–26). Wiley-Blackwell.

Chomsky, N. (1972). *Language and mind*. New York: Harcourt Brace.

Cin, S.D., Worth, K.A., Gerrard, M., Gibbons, F.X., Stoolmiller, M., Wills, T.A. & Sargent, J. (2009). Watching and drinking: Expectancies, prototypes, and friends' alcohol use mediate the effect of exposure to alcohol use in movies on adolescent drinking. *Health Psychology, 28*(4), 473–483.

Cincinnati Children's Hospital Medical Center. (2007–2009). Growth and development wellness: Stages of play. Retrieved from http://www.Cincinnatichildrens.org/health/info/growth/well/stages.Htm

Compas, B.E. (1987). Coping with stress during childhood and adolescence. *Psychological Bulletin, 101*(3), 393–403.

Compas, B.E. (2009). Coping, regulation, and development during childhood and adolescence. In E.A. Skinner & M.J. Zimmer-Gemback (Eds.), *Coping and the development of regulation. New directions for child and adolescent development* (pp. 87–99, no. 124). San Francisco: Jossey-Bass.

Coopersmith, S. (1981). *Self-esteem inventories (SEI)*. Palo Alto, CA: Consulting Psychologists, Press, Inc.

Dalgas-Pelish, P. (2006). Effects of a self esteem intervention program on school-age children. *Pediatric Nursing, 32*, 341–348.

Daniels, M. (1994). The effect of sign language on hearing children's language development. *Communication Education, 43*, 291–298.

Donnellan, M.B., Trzesniewski, K.H., Robins, R.W., Moffott, T.E., & Caspi, A. (2005). Low self-esteem is related to aggression, antisocial behavior, and delinquency. *Psychological Science, 16*(4), 328–335.

Donnelly, J., Young, M., Pearson, R., Penhollow, T.M., & Hernandez, A. (2008). Area specific self-esteem, values, and adolescent substance use. *Journal of Drug Education, 28*, 289–403.

Duvall, E. (1977). *Marriage and family development (5th edition)*. Philadelphia, PA: Lippincott.

Edmondson, J., Grote, L., Haskell, L., Matthews, A., & White, M. (n.d.). Adolescent self-esteem: Is there a correlation with maternal self-esteem? *Citations, 3*, 1–8.

Elkind, D. (1967). Egocentrism in adolescence. *Child Development, 38*(4), 1025–1034.

Erikson, E. (1950). *Childhood and society*. New York: Norton.

Erikson, E. (1959). *Identity and the life cycle: Selected papers, psychological issues* (Monograph Vol. 1, No. 1). New York: International Press.

Ethier, K.A., Kershaw, T.S., Lewis, J.B., Milan, S., Niccolai, L.S., & Ickovics, J.R. (2006). Self-esteem, emotional distress and sexual behavior among adolescent females: Inter-relationships and temporal effects. *Journal of Adolescent Health, 38*, 268–274.

Finger, B., Hans, S.L., Bernstein, V.J., & Cox, S.M. (2009). Parent relationship quality and infant-mother attachment. *Attachment and Human Development, 11*, 285–206.

Freud, S. (1957). In J. Strachey (Ed.). *The standard edition of the complete psychological works of Sigmund Freud* (Vol. 18). London: Hogarth.

Garmezy, N. (1981). Children under stress: Perspectives on antecedents and correlates of vulnerability and resistance to psychopathology. In A.I. Rabin, J. Aronoff, A.M. Barclay & R.A. Zucker (Eds.). *Further explorations in personality* (pp. 196–269). New York: Wiley.

Gelman, R., & Schatz, M. (1978). Appropriate speech adjustments: the operation of conversational constraints on talk in two year olds. In M. Lewsi & L.A. Rosenblum (Eds.), *Interaction, conversation, and the development of language* (pp. 27–61). New York: Wiley.

Gesell, A. (1929). Maturation and infant behavior pattern. *Psychological Review, 36*, 307–319.

Goswami, U. (2008). *Cognitive development: The learning brain*. New York: Psychology Press.

Goulet, C., Bell, L., St-Cyr Tribble, D., Paul, D., & Lang, A. (1998). A concept analysis of parent-infant attachment. *Journal of Advanced Nursing, 28*, 1071–1081.

Gray, R., & McCormick, M.C. (2005). Early childhood intervention programs in the US: recent advances and future recommendations. *Journal of Primary Prevention, 26*(3), 259–275.

Grey, M., & Sullivan-Bolyai, S. (1999). Key issues in chronic illness research: lessons from the study of children with diabetes. *Journal of Pediatric Nursing: Nursing Care of Children and Families, 14*(6), 351–358

Guttmacher Institute. (2006). *In brief: Facts on American teen sexual and reproductive health*. Retrieved from http://www.guttmacher.org/pubs/fb_ATSRH.html

Hagan J.F., Shaw, J.S., & uncan, P.M. (Eds.). (2008). *Bright futures: Guidelines for health supervision of infants, children, and adolescents* (3rd edition). Elk Grove Village, IL: American Academy of Pediatrics.

Huttenlocher, J., Haight, W., Bruk, A., Seltzer, M., & Lyons, T. (1991). Early vocabulary growth: Relation to language input and gender. *Developmental Psychology, 27*, 236–248.

Iannelli, V. (2006). Preschoolers Child Development. About.com. *Pediatrics*. Retrieved from http://pediatrics.about.com/cs/growthdevelopment/a/child_dev_5.htm?=1

Individuals with Disabilities Education Improvement Act of 2004 (PL 108–446), U.S. Code, Vol. 20, secs.

Johnston, M. (2009). Plasticity in the developing brain: Implications for rehabilitation. *Developmental Disabilities Research Reviews, 15*, 94–101.

Jusczyk, P.W. (2000). *The discovery of spoken language*. Cambridge MA: MIT Press.

Keating, D.P. (2004). Cognitive and brain development. In R.M. Lerner & L. Steinberg (Eds.). *Handbook of adolescent psychology* (pp. 45–84). Hoboken, NJ: Wiley.

Keith, K.L. (2009). Children's play. About.com. Retrieved from http://childparenting.about.com/od/activitiesandfun/u/kidsplay.htm?p=1

Koenning, G.M., Benjamin, J.E., Todaro, A.W., Warren, R.W., & Burns, M.L. (1995). Bridging the "med-ed gap" for students with special health care needs: a model school liaison program. *Journal of School Health, 65*(6), 207–212.

Krohne, H.W., & Rogner, J. (1982). Repression-sensitization as a central construct in coping research. In H.W. Krohne & L. Laux (Eds.). *Achievement, stress, and anxiety* (pp. 167–193). Washington: Hemisphere.

Kuhl, P.K. (1993). Infant speech perception: A window on psycholinguistic development. *International Journal of Psycholinguistics, 9*, 33–56.

Kuhn, D. (1984). Cognitive development. In *Developmental psychology: An advanced textbook* (pp. 133–180). Hillsdale, NJ: Erlbaum.

Laranjo, J., Bernier, A., & Meins, E. (2008). Associations between maternal mind-mindedness and infant attachment security: Investigating the mediating role of maternal sensitivity. *Infant Behavior and Development, 31*, 688–695.

Lazarus, R., & Folkman, S. (1984). *Stress, appraisal and coping*. New York: Springer.

Lorenz, K.Z. (1937). The companion in the bird's work. *Auk, 54*, 245–273.

Madigan, S., Moran, G., Schuengel, C., Pederson, D.R., & Otten, R. (2007). Unresolved maternal attachment representations, disrupted maternal behavior and disorganized attachment in infancy: Links to toddler behavior problems. *Journal of Child Psychology and Psychiatry, 48*, 1042–1050.

Magiati, I., Charman, T., & Howlin, P. (2007). A two-year prospective follow-up study of community-based early intensive behavioural intervention and specialist nursery provision for children with autism spectrum disorders. *Journal of Child Psychology & Psychiatry & Allied Disciplines, 48*(8), 803–812.

Maier, S.F., & Watkins, L.R. (2005). Stressor controllability and learned helplessness: the roles of the dorsal raphae nucleus, serotonin, and corticotropin-releasing factor. *Neuroscience and Behavioral Reviews, 29*, 829–841.

Main, M., & Solomon, J. (1990). Procedures for identifying infants as disorganized/disoriented during Ainsworth Strange Situation.

In M.T. Greenberg, D. Cicchetti, & E.M. Cummings (Eds.). *Attachment in the preschool years* (pp. 120–160). Chicago: University of Chicago Press.

Malley, C. (1991). *Toddler development. National Network for Child Care*. Amherst, MA: University of Massachusetts. Retrieved from http://www.nncc.org/Child.Dev/todd.dev.html

Manning, M.A. (2007). *Self-concept and self esteem in adolescents. Student Services*, 11–15. Retrieved from http://www.nasponline.org/families/selfconcept.pdf

Marsh, R., Gerber, A., & Peterson, B. (2008). Neuroimaging studies of normal brain development and their relevance for understanding childhood neuropsychiatric disorders. *Journal of the American Academy of Child & Adolescent Psychiatry, 47*(11), 1233–1251.

McDonough, L. (1999). Early declarative memory for location. *British Journal of Developmental Psychology, 17*, 381–402.

McGoldrick, M., & Carter, B. (2003). The family life cycle. In F. Walsh, *Normal family processes growing diversity and complexity* (pp. 375–398). New York, NY: Guilford Press.

McMahon, C.A., Barnett, B., Kowalenko, N.M., & Tennant, C.C. (2006). Maternal attachment state of mind moderates the impact of postnatal depression on infant attachment. *Journal of Child Psychology and Psychiatry, 47*, 660–669.

Menon, M., Tobin, D.D., Corby, B.C., Menon, M., Hodgers, E., & Perry, D.G. (2007). The developmental costs of high self-esteem for antisocial children, *Child Development, 78*, 1627–1639.

Menyuk, P., Liebergott, J., & Schultz, M. (1995). *Early language development in full-term and premature infants*. Hilldale, NJ: Erlbaum.

Miller, S.M., & Green, M.L. (1984). Coping with stress and frustration: Origins, nature, and development. In M. Lewsi, & C. Saarni (Eds.). *The socialization of emotions*. New York, NY: Plenum Press.

National Institute on Deafness and Other Communication Disorders. (2000). *Speech and language developmental milestones*. Retrieved from http://www.nidcd.nih.gov/health/voice/speechandlanguage.asp#mychild

National Parent-Teacher Association (2009). Play at different ages and developmental stages. Retrieved from http://school.familyeducation.com/games/growth-and-development/38382.html

Nemours Foundation. (2008a). *Teen health: Sexual attraction and orientation*. Retrieved from http://kidshealth.org/parent/emotions/feelings/sexual_orientation.html

Nemours Foundation. (2008b). *Teen Health: Am I in a healthy relationship*. Retrieved from http://kidshealth.org/teen/your_mind/relationships/healthy_relationship.html#

Niccols, A. (2008). "Right from the start": Randomized trial comparing an attachment group intervention to supportive home visiting. *The Journal of Child Psychology and Psychiatry, 49*, 754–764.

Olson, S. (Edition). *Toward an integrated science of research on families: Workshop Report. Washington, DC: The National Academies*. Retrieved from http://www.nap.edu/catalog/13085.html

O'Reilly, D. (2007). *Infant reflexes*. Retrieved from http://www.nlm.nih.gov/medlineplus/ency/article/003292.htm

Peadon, E., Rhys-Jones, B., Bower, C., & Elliott, E.J. (2009). Systematic review of interventions for children with fetal alcohol spectrum disorders. *BMC Pediatrics, 9*(35).

Piaget, J. (1952). *The origins of intelligence in children*. New York: International Universities Press.

Ramseyer, V. (2007). Stages of play. Retrieved from http://ezinearticles.com/?Stages-of-Play&id=900253&opt=print

Reyna, B.A., & Pickler, R.H. (2009). Mother-infant synchrony. *Journal of Obstetric, Gynecologic, & Neonatal Nursing, 38*, 470–477.

Rosenberg, M. (1965). *Society and the adolescent self-image*. Princeton, NJ: Princeton University Press.

Rubin, D. (2006). *Gaining word power* (7th edition). Boston, MA: Allyn & Bacon.

Rueda, M.R., & Rothbart, M.K. (2009). The influence of temperament on the development of coping: The role of maturation and experience. In E.A. Skinner & M.J. Zimmer-Gemback (Eds.). *Coping and the development of regulation. New directions for child and adolescent development* (pp. 19–31, no. 124). San Francisco: Jossey-Bass.

Santor, D.A., Messervey, D., & Kusumakar, V. (2000). Measuring peer pressure, popularity, and conformity in adolescent boys and girls: Predicting school performance, sexual attitudes, and substance abuse. *Journal of Youth and Adolescence, 29*, 163–182.

Santrock, J.W. (2007). *A topical approach to lifespan development*. Boston: McGraw-Hill.

Schenk, L.K., Kelley, J.H., & Schenk, M.P. (2005). Models of maternal-infant attachment: A role for nurses. *Pediatric Nursing, 31*, 514–517.

Schutz, L. (2005). Broad-perspective perceptual disorder of the right hemisphere. *Neuropsychology Review, 15*(1), 11–27.

Skinner, E.A., & Zimmer-Gembeck, M.J. (2007). The development of coping. *Annual Review of Psychology, 58*, 119–144.

Strathearn, L., Li, J., Fonagy, P., & Montague, P.R. (2009). What's in a smile? Maternal brain responses to infant facial cues. *Pediatrics, 122*, 40–51.

Sullivan-Bolyai, S., Deatrick, J., Gruppuso, P., Tamborlane, W., & Grey, M. (2003). Constant vigilance: mothers' work parenting young children with type 1 diabetes. *Journal of Pediatric Nursing: Nursing Care of Children and Families, 18*(1), 21–29.

Trawick-Smith, J. (2010). *Early childhood development: A multicultural perspective*. Upper Saddle River, NJ: Pearson.

Van Londen, W.M., Juffer, F., & van IJzendoorn, M.H. (2007). Attachment, cognitive, and motor development in adopted children: Short-term outcomes after international adoption. *Journal of Pediatric Psychology, 32*, 1249–1258.

Veselska, Z., Geckova, A.M., Orosova, O., Gajdosova, B., van Dijk, J.P., & Reijneveld, S. (2009). Self-esteem and resilience: The connection with risky behavior among adolescents. *Addictive Behaviors, 34*, 287–291.

Vygotsky, L. (1962). *Thought and language*. Cambridge, MA: MIT Press.

Wilkinson, R.B. (2004). The role of parental and peer attachment in the psychological health and self-esteem of adolescents. *Journal of Youth Adolescents, 33*, 479–493.

Woodgate, R.L., & Degner, L.F. (2003). A substantive theory of keeping the spirit alive: The spirit within children with cancer and their families. *Journal of Pediatric Oncology Nursing, 20*(3), 103–119.

Wright, L.M., & Leahey, M. (2009). *Nurses and families: A guide to family assessment and intervention* (5th edition). Philadelphia, PA: F.A. Davis.

Yaun, A., & Keating, R. (2007). The brain and nervous system. In M. Batshaw, L. Pellegrino, & N. Roizen (Eds.). *Children with disabilities*. Baltimore, MD: Paul H. Brookes.

Young, M., Donnelly, J., & Denny, G. (2004). Area specific self-esteem, values and adolescent sexual behavior. *American Journal of Health Education, 35*, 282–289.

2

Temperament and Self-Regulation

Pamela Galehouse and Marie Foley

Objectives

After reading this chapter, APNs will be able to

1. Identify the key components of temperament and self-regulation
2. Assess temperament and self-regulation in children
3. Recognize the importance of "goodness of fit" between temperament and environment

4. Identify risk factors associated with temperament/self-regulatory abilities and mental health
5. Determine approaches for managing behaviors related to impaired self-regulatory skills

---

Introduction/Overview

This chapter focuses on two influential intrinsic constructs: temperament and self-regulation. Each influences how the child interacts with his or her environment and masters developmental tasks. Temperament can be simply described as innate, heritable, not easily changed patterns of behavioral responses to change or stress. Although present at birth, temperament is not believed to be consistent until about one year of age, when biological systems are more stabilized (Rothbart, 2007). Each individual has a unique temperament, and it is the interaction between temperament and the environment that affects the development of self-regulation and, ultimately, developmental task attainment.

Research indicates that children's unique temperament profiles influence the development of self-regulation, with some temperaments increasing the risk for inadequate or rigid self-regulation (Kochanska, Murray, & Harlan, 2000). Unlike temperament, the ability to self-regulate behavior and emotions develops in tandem with the child's brain until hardwiring is completed at about eight years (Posner & Rothbart, 2000). While temperament is usually viewed as a continuum of normal behavior which may challenge caretakers, the ability to self-regulate is critical to the individual's capacity to interact and function in society, and can be compromised by factors such as psychological and physiological stress. Persistent dysfunctional self-regulation is often associated with specific psychiatric disorders.

This chapter will describe both temperament and self-regulation, with attention to environmental influences and challenges, assessment, and intervention strategies to enhance self-regulation in young children and to manage dysfunctional self-regulatory skills. APNs can use this information as they assess children in pediatric and psychiatric settings.

Child and Adolescent Behavioral Health: A Resource for Advanced Practice Psychiatric and Primary Care Practitioners in Nursing,
First Edition. Edited by Edilma L. Yearwood, Geraldine S. Pearson, and Jamesetta A. Newland.
© 2012 John Wiley & Sons, Inc. Published 2012 by John Wiley & Sons, Inc.

Description of the Issue

Historical Context

Temperament

The concept of temperament is not a new one, but rather has ancient roots in both the study of animals and humans. In early Greco-Roman writings, temperament is linked to biology and bodily humors within individuals, which were seen as determinants of behavioral variations (Rothbart, Ellis, & Posner, 2004). Temperament also has evolutionary links to animal studies related to sensitivity and disposition, and continues to be a pertinent area of inquiry for those who study animals (Strelau, 2000). However, the premise of child temperament as significant to child-focused clinicians and researchers was introduced in the United States by Thomas and Chess (1977).

In their pioneering work known as the New York Longitudinal Study (NYLS), which began in 1953, these researchers examined individual personality traits of 133 subjects from infancy through adulthood. They defined temperament as constitutional characteristics that interact with the child's environment, are important in the child's development, and present regardless of context, ability, or motivation (Thomas & Chess, 1977).

Self-regulation

Self-regulation, as a psychological construct, has been traced back as far as William James, who in the eighteenth century included self-control in his principles of psychology (Mischel & Ayduk, 2004). Research and emerging theories in child development over the past thirty years include rigorously studying loss of self-control (Baumeister, Heatherton, & Tice, 1994). The seminal work by Barkley (1998) on attention deficit hyperactive disorder (ADHD) has inspired consideration in research and clinical work on specific aspects of attentional regulation or lack thereof. In addition, the work by Rothbart, Ellis, Rueda, and Posner (2003) has led to greater understanding of effortful control as a construct of temperament related to its role in attention and self-regulation.

Theoretical Approaches

Temperament

Different temperament theorists offer variations in their definitions of temperament. Emphasizing psychoneurobiological components, Rothbart and Bates (2006) have studied variability in reactivity, both physiological and psychological arousability, and its relationship to effortful control or the regulatory efforts to modulate reactivity. They believe this to be consistent across situations and stable over time. They go on to state that individuals' behavioral responses to change in their environment vary based on both reactivity and availability of strategies to regulate, either by strengthening or inhibiting, these reactions.

Plomin and Caspi (1999) conceptualized temperament, focusing on the heritable characteristics occurring early in life and being stable across time and circumstances. Kagan (1998) discussed temperament extremes in relation to shyness, which they termed "inhibited" and "uninhibited." They found that the child's environment could moderate these extremely shy behaviors. Through this evolution, most researchers agree that temperament can be defined as a child's behavioral style which he/she consistently exhibits in reaction to the environment. Temperament acts as a screen through which interpretation of the environment occurs.

Self-regulation

The roots of self-regulation are in temperament; for example, the ease with which a toddler takes assistance to dampen down strong emotions is one of the early influences on self-regulation. It is the counterbalancing "executive attentional system" proposed by Rothbart which begins to develop in late infancy and continues through the early school years (Posner & Rothbart, 2000). This allows the individual child to self-regulate by exerting effortful control over the reactive attentional system. Functionally, self-regulation can be described as childrens' capacities to control reactions to stress, maintain focused attention, and interpret their own mental states and those of others (i.e., empathy) (Fonagy & Target, 2002).

From a neurobiological perspective, self-regulation includes the ability to modulate behavior according to the emotional and social demands of a situation, governed by how the individual takes in, organizes, and uses information (Posner & Rothbart, 2000). Neurocognitive research identifies three separate brain network activities relating to attention, which evolve during these early years: orienting, the selection of information from sensory input; alerting, sensitivity to incoming stimulations and maintenance of a vigilant state; and executive control, monitoring and resolving thoughts, feelings, and physical responses (Fan & Posner, 2004). Viewed as the result of control of inhibitory and attentional processes, self-regulation consists of both conscious and unconscious processes that exercise control to meet certain goals (Calkins & Fox, 2002).

Because it involves self-monitoring of one's state in relation to one's goal and making the changes and adjustments required to attain that goal, the monitoring and control functions of attention play significant roles in self-regulation (Rothbart & Bates, 2006). The most successful self-regulators are children with inherent attention efficacy (Rueda, Posner, & Rothbart 2004). In other words, children born with certain temperaments tend to have better self-regulation.

Research indicates that the efficiency of executive attention shows improvement from ages two to seven (Chang & Burns, 2005; Rothbart et al., 2003). Studies of older children and adolescents found little change in skill from age eight to adulthood (Rueda et al., 2004; Simonds, Kieras, Rueda, & Rothbart, 2007). In summary, there appears to be a critical window of opportunity for laying the groundwork for executive attention.

Understanding how the mind directs attention and controls behavior so that children can respond appropriately to challenging situations has been advanced by modern neuroscience. It is beyond the task of this chapter to offer a comprehensive view of the current status of the science. See Chapter 3 for a more detailed account. However, a brief sequence of contemporary understanding of the neuroscience of the development of regulatory capacities will be outlined here, followed by a review of two specific areas of neurophysiology directly related to self-regulation development.

Affective neuroscience describes regulation as complex, hierarchical relations between the three core brain systems (brainstem, limbic, and cortical) that organize behavioral output (Tucker, Derryberry, & Luu, 2000). This is in agreement with earlier proposed neuropsychological models on brain maturation in its view of regulatory functions as evolutionary and vertically integrated (Panksepp, 1998). Feldman (2009) conducted a five-year study of premature infants that supports a hierarchical and integrative four-stage model of physiological, emotional, attentional, and self-regulatory development. These four stages include specific function/system relationships:

1. Physiological regulation associated with brainstem development (late fetal through early neonatal)
2. Emotional regulation, which is limbic mediated and serves to return to homeostasis (first year)
3. Attentional regulation (second year)
4. Self-regulation, which is determined by cortical control (preschool, three to five years). Self-regulation includes behavior adaptation, executive functions, and self-restraint.

Inherent in Feldman's model is evidence that while disruptions in lower level functions may lead to higher system dysfunction resulting in behavior problems at age five, the system is malleable. With sensitive, responsive care many infants made the transition over the first year of life from highly reactive preemies to toddlers with focused attention, typical of most two-year-olds.

This demonstrates both the dependence of the infant on regulatory context and the openness of regulatory functions to external influences (Bridgett et al., 2009). The process can be further explained by the concept of attunement, by which parents attach to their infants by reading and responding to signals for engagement or disengagement (Stern, 1985).

Supporting this notion is the work of Schore (1994), who found that facial expressions of the caregiver (demonstrating transactions) stimulates the production of opiates, which in turn activate dopamine neurons that trigger brain development, particularly in the orbital frontal cortex (OFC). The OFC serves to organize responses to threat by assessing signals of distress/danger, planning behavior, and modulating the timing of emotional responses. The right OFC is believed to be the primary regulator of the limbic system, managing how emotional experiences are handled (Scaer, 2005).

The brain's attentional system offers further explanations about how the complex systems of the brain interact and specifically how one system governs the reactions of another, allowing effortful control. The part of the brain actively participating in effortful control is the anterior cingulate cortex (ACC), a part of the frontal cortex whose dorsal portion is connected to the executive function center of the prefrontal cortex and whose ventral portion has pathways to the limbic section, where emotion is situated (Bush, 2004). This position links cognitive control functions with the emotional center. From a clinical standpoint, differentiation is made among the observed abilities to regulate attention, emotion, and behavior/inhibition (executive function). Although there are complex relationships among the three, each will be described separately.

Emotional Regulation

Emotional regulation is goal oriented and involves monitoring, evaluating, and modifying emotional reactions to accomplish goals (Thompson, Lewis & Calkins, 2008). Goals can be social (pleasing parents or others) or functional (gaining attention or having needs met). It is important to note that the efficiency of efforts to control emotions depends on the strength of the emotional processes against which effort is exerted (Eisenberg, Smith, Sadovsky, & Spinrad, 2004).

Early on, parents provide soothing, modeling a repertoire of soothing behaviors, and begin the process of helping the youngster attach names to his/her emotions. As the child matures, the parent or caregiver assists the young child in differentiating between similar feelings (happy: content, sad: nervous, angry: frustrated) and helps the child find ways to verbally express emotions and find suitable outlets for them. Emotional regulation is related to several dimensions of temperament. For example, high effortful control, high empathy, high guilt, and shame have been related to low aggressiveness (Rothbart, Ahadi, Hershey, & Fisher, 2001). Kochanska, Barry, Jimenez, and Hollatz (2009) explored effortful control and conscience development and found that fearful preschoolers internalize moral principles, especially when their mothers used gentle discipline.

Internalized control is higher in children who have effortful control (Kochanska, 1995; Kochanska, Murray, & Harlan, 2000; Kochanska, Murray, & Koy, 1997). Youngsters with good attentional control are more likely to deal with anger by using nonhostile verbal methods (Eisenberg, Fabes, Nyman, Bernzweig, & Pinuelas, 1994). When regulation is defective, or emotionally and cognitively based methods such as distraction or relaxation (self-soothing) are ineffective, the child may use certain behaviors to dampen down emotions. In these instances, negatively viewed behavioral regulation strategies such as tantrums, striking out, and venting are used by the youngster to reduce the amount of intense affect being experienced (Eisenberg, Fabes, & Guthrie, 1997).

Behavioral Regulation

The term behavioral regulation is often used interchangeably with inhibition and is also influenced by effortful control. It consists of five domains: attentional shifting, focusing, inhibitory control, low-intensity pleasure, and perceptual sensitivity (Rothbart, Ahadi, Hershey, & Fisher, 2001). Generally, regulating behavior requires the ability to suppress a dominant response in favor of a nondominant one.

Clearly, the ability to regulate behavior at an early age has positive consequences for children. For example, kindergarteners with higher levels of behavior regulation *have* stronger levels of achievement, especially in math, as well as higher teacher ratings of classroom self-regulation at the end of the year (Ponitz, McClelland, Matthews, & Morrison, 2009).

Attentional Regulation

Regulation of attention can be considered from two perspectives: modulating negative emotions or states and facilitating task completion and learning. Attention shifting and focusing are central to modulating internal psychological and physiological reactions and have been discussed previously under emotional regulation. Sustained attention, defined as the ability to filter out extraneous information and focus on the task at hand, has demonstrated importance for school readiness and achievement (Blair, 2002; NICHD, 2003; Sethi, Mischel, Aber, Shoda, & Rodriguez, 2000).

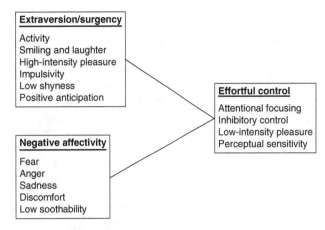

Figure 2.1 Factor analysis of the Children's Behavior Questionnaire; broad dimensions of temperament, six to seven years. [Reprinted from Rothbart, Ahadi, Hershey, and Fisher (2001) with permission from John Wiley & Sons, Inc.]

Closely aligned to the temperamental traits of task persistence (McClowry, 2003) and effortful control (Rothbart & Bates, 2006), attentional regulation skills can be facilitated by environmental inputs including parental sensitivity and maternal scaffolding (Belskey, Pasco Fearson, & Bell 2007; Deater-Deckard, Petrell, & Thompson, 2007; Harris, Robinson, Chang, & Burns, 2007). Maternal scaffolding, along with physical and verbal cues, assist a child in completing a task (Robinson, Burns, & Davis, 2009). Within this parent-child learning environment, demonstrated attention regulation in task completion is also influenced by intrinsic child factors: effortful control and motivation (Harris et al., 2007).

In summary, self-regulation is the child's ability to control reactions to stress, maintain focused attention, and interpret mental states in self and others by exercising emotional, behavioral, and attentional control. Whether one believes self-regulation to be rooted in temperament or to *be* temperament, there is agreement that its etiology is with two temperament components: reactivity and control (Rothbart & Bates, 2006). Development of self-regulation is determined by the strength of these two temperament domains and is enhanced or hindered by individual transactions with the environment (Figure 2.1).

Typologies and Variations
Temperament

In their seminal work on temperament, Chess and Thomas (1984) defined nine dimensions of temperament (Table 2.1). From these nine dimensions of temperament, they found that children tend to cluster in one of three temperamental constellations: easy, difficult, and slow to warm up. The easy child is characterized by having high rhythmicity and a positive mood, approaches new situations with moderate ease, and is easily adaptable.

Table 2.1 Theoretical approaches to temperament dimensions

Theorist	Dimensions of Temperament
Thomas & Chess (1977)	Activity (motor), rhythmicity (regularity), approach/withdrawal (initial response to new stimuli), adaptability (response to situations over time), threshold (intensity of stimulus to evoke response), intensity (energy level), mood (quality of pleasant behavior), distractibility (response to external stimuli), and persistence (continuation of activity through distraction)
Buss & Plomin (1984)	Emotionality (tendency to become psychologically aroused), activity (energy), and sociability (interactions with others)
Goldsmith & Campos (1982)	Activity (motor), anger, fearfulness (moving away), pleasure/joy (smiling/laughing), interest/persistence (attention)
Posner & Rothbart (2007), Rothbart & Bates (2006)	Surgency/extraversion (activity, positive affect, pleasure, impulsivity, smiling, outgoing), negative affectivity (inhibition, discomfort, fear, sadness, frustration, unable to be soothed), effortful control (attentional shifting, focusing, ability to suppress inappropriate responses, perceptual sensitivity) sociability/affiliation (social closeness, emotional empathy, empathetic guilt)
Kagan (1998)	Inhibited (shy) and uninhibited (outgoing)
Martin & Bridger (1999)	Negative emotionality (affect), activity (motor), persistence (attention), inhibition (shyness), and impulsivity (speed of response to stimuli)
McClowry (2002a)	Activity (motor), negative reactivity (intensity and frequency of negative affect), approach/withdrawal (initial response to new situations), and task persistence (attention span)

The difficult child is more irregular, has a negative mood, withdraws from new situations, and tends to require much time to adapt to the environment or situations. In contrast, the slow-to-warm-up child is more inhibited, withdraws from new situations, has occasional negative moods, and adapts slowly. These constellations represented 65% of their sample population: 10% were difficult, 40% easy, 15% slow to warm up, and the remaining 35% of the subjects did not fall into any of the three constellations (Thomas & Chess, 1977).

Building on the theoretical framework of Thomas and Chess (1977), McClowry and her colleagues (1995) examined the construct validity of the Middle Childhood Temperament Questionnaire and found that four factors emerged from the original nine dimensions (Hegvik, McDevitt, & Carey, 1982) (Table 2.1). Similar to the work of Thomas and Chess, McClowry (2002a) also identified temperament typologies or profiles based on combinations of dimensions: high maintenance and cautious/slow to warm up. The high maintenance child is high in negative reactivity, low in task persistence, and high in activity (8% of the sample). The cautious/slow to warm up child is high in negative reactivity and high in withdrawal (8% of the sample). McClowry then took the mirror images of these two profiles and named them

industrious and social/eager to try. The industrious child is high in task persistence, low in activity, and low in negative reactivity (6% of the original sample), and the social/eager to try child is high in approach and low in negative reactivity (9% of the sample). Four percent were both industrious and social/eager to try. Of the remaining 58%, all were found to be either high or low in at least one dimension, with the exception of 1.5% of the subjects.

From a psychobiological framework, Putnam and Rothbart (2006) studied child temperament and identified four factors: negative affectivity, surgency/extraversion, effortful control, and sociability/affiliation. The latter, sociability/affiliation, does not present itself until later adolescence and early adulthood.

As temperament theory has evolved, researchers seem to agree that four dimensions have emerged, understanding that as children grow and develop certain traits are no longer salient due to their ability to self-regulate themselves and their environments (Rothbart et al., 2001). For further clarification, see Table 2.1.

Self-regulation

Unfortunately, the only available incidence rates related to self-regulation are data collected when individuals lack adequate self-regulation. For example, the incidence of ADHD, depression, anxiety, conduct disorders, incarceration, and schizophrenia could be attributed to an individual's inability to self-regulate. According to the National Health Interview Survey, in 2007 slightly more than 5% of children ages four to seventeen were reported by a parent to have serious difficulties with emotions, concentration, behavior, or being able to get along with other people. More males were reported to have these conditions (Bloom & Cohen, 2009).

Assessment

The following section offers information about assessing infant, preschool, and school-age temperament and self-regulation with the intent of using this information for preventive interventions. In addition, guidelines for assessing the self-regulation abilities of children and adolescents who have diagnosed mental health problems in the context of a treatment or school facility will be presented. Routine temperament assessment of older children and adolescents will not be addressed: temperament in this age group is difficult to separate from personality. There are standardized instruments available for self-regulation measurement with this age group (e.g., Rothbart's); however, they are generally used in research rather than clinical practice.

In keeping with the definition and guidelines set by the American Academy of Pediatrics, assessment of infants must be part of a complete developmental and physical assessment (Gosling, Kwan, Hagan, Shaw, & Duncan, 2008). The importance of this is underscored by the similar behaviors presented by both the infant who is a challenge to care for because of health-related problems and the infant whose temperament presents a parenting challenge. Etiology aside, both groups require warm, responsive, soothing parenting, and support and education for the parents. Children with difficult temperaments will, however, require more attention throughout childhood.

Assessment of self-regulation in young children should be conducted to inform, assess risk, and consider interventions, as well as to diagnose (Mrakotsky & Heffelfinger, 2006). This developmental period is of critical importance to school and interpersonal success. A comprehensive assessment focusing on strengths/competencies as well as weaknesses/dysfunction is important and in agreement with the notion of health promotion held by nurses (Leddy, 2006; Pender, Murdaugh, & Parsons 2010). It is important to remember that there is a wide range of individual variability in regulatory skills of young children.

Both temperament and self-regulation are measured through parent report questionnaires, teacher report questionnaires, self-reports for older children, in-home and laboratory observations, and structured interviews.

All of these methods have both strengths and weaknesses for practice and research. The strengths of parent questionnaires include the parent's knowledge of the child and his/her typical behavior. The parent also knows how the child reacts on rare, but important occasions, and over time. Parent report questionnaires are inexpensive and easy to administer. The weaknesses are parental subjectivity, inaccurate memory of events, desire of acquiescence, and parental interpretation of behaviors (Rothbart & Bates, 2006). A historical timeline might be helpful in collecting information.

Teacher questionnaires can be more objective than parent reports, but not as broad reaching. Teachers can only measure a child's temperament and self-regulation within the school environment. Teacher questionnaires are inexpensive and easy to administer but can have the same biases as parent reports in relation to memory and interpretation.

The strengths of child observations are their objectivity. However, due to constraints of time and expense, they are often limited in number. There also may be a change in the child's behavior due to the presence of the observer. Moreover, the observer has restricted capacity to detect rare events.

Laboratory observations, while rarely used by clinicians, allow variable control, but are limited in the range of observations. Dependent upon available time and finances, a combination of techniques is most beneficial to the clinician or researcher in assessing child temperament and self-regulatory abilities. The use of multiple techniques provides an opportunity to obtain historical data as well as a report of child behavior on rare, but important, occasions.

There are many questions about the shortcomings of instruments measuring temperament and self-regulation in relation to validity and reliability (Rothbart & Bates, 2006). The researcher and clinician, after choosing a tool based on the theoretical framework that best conceptualizes their research or practice, must be cognizant of any limitations in measurement, in relation to both technique and instrumentation. For a description of tools commonly used to assess temperament and self-regulation, including the reported reliabilities, see Table 2.2.

As indicated in the preceding paragraphs, assessing a child's temperament and self-regulation can provide helpful information to the primary care practitioner who is advising parents and promoting healthy parenting practices. Information gathered will allow targeted parental education and support to be provided to those children most vulnerable to problems.

Potential risk for depressive and anxiety symptoms in childhood can be predicted for infants with difficult temperaments before six months as well as for future conduct

Table 2.2 Tools commonly used to assess temperament and self-regulation

Temperament scales	Age	Description	Reliability
Early Infancy Temperament Questionnaire (EITQ) (Medoff-Cooper, Carey, & McDevitt, 1993)	One to four months	76 items based on Thomas & Chess' nine dimensions of temperament	$\alpha = .42$ to .76
Infant Behavior Questionnaire Revised (IBQ-R) (Gartstein & Rothbart, 2003)	Three to twelve months	184 items based on Rothbart's neurobiological framework	$\alpha = .70$ to .90
Toddler Temperament Scale (TTS) (Fullard, McDevitt, & Carey, 1984)	One to three years	97 items based on Thomas & Chess' framework	$\alpha = .70$ to .81
EAS Temperament Survey for Children (EAS)* (Buss & Plomin, 1984)	One to three years	20 items based on Buss & Plomin's EAS dimensions	$\alpha = .80$ to .88
Toddler Behavior Assessment Questionnaire (TBAQ) (Goldsmith, 1996)	Fifteen to thirty-six months	108 items based on Emotion Systems approach by Goldsmith and Campos	$\alpha = .78$ to .89
Early Childhood Behavior Questionnaire (ECBQ) (Putnam, Gartstein, & Rothbart, 2006)	Eighteen to thirty-six months	267 items based on Rothbart's neurobiological framework	$\alpha = .56$ to .90
Colorado Childhood Temperament Inventory (CCTI) (Rowe & Plomin, 1977)	One to seven years	30 items based on Buss & Plomin's dimensions of EAS	$\alpha = .73$ to .88
Dimensions of Temperament Survey Revised (DOTS-R) (Windle & Lerner, 1986)	Preschool	54 items based on Thomas & Chess' framework	$\alpha = .70$ to .84
Temperament Assessment Battery (TAB)* (Martin & Bridger, 1999)	Two to seven years	35 items expanded upon Thomas & Chess' framework	$\alpha = .65$ to .86
Shortened Teacher Temperament Questionnaire (STTQ) (Keogh, Pullis, & Caldwell, 1983)	Three to six years	23 items based on Thomas & Chess' framework	$\alpha = .62$ to .92
EAS Temperament Survey for Children (EAS)* (Buss & Plomin, 1984)	Three to nine years	20 items based on Buss & Plomin's EAS dimensions	$\alpha = .65$ to .81
Children's Behavior Questionnaire (CBQ) (Rothbart, Ahadi, & Hershey, 2001)	Three to seven years	195 items based on Rothbart's neurobiological framework	$\alpha = .67$ to .94
Behavioral Style Questionnaire (BSQ) (McDevitt & Carey, 1978)	Three to seven years	100 items based on Thomas & Chess' framework	$\alpha = .48$ to .80
Middle Childhood Temperament Questionnaire (MCTQ) (Hegvik, McDevitt, & Carey, 1982)	Eight to twelve years	99 items based on Thomas & Chess' framework	$\alpha = .80$ to .93
Dimensions of Temperament Survey Revised (DOTS-R) (Windle & Lerner, 1986)	School age	54 items based on Thomas & Chess' framework	$\alpha = .54$ to .91
The Temperament in Middle Childhood Questionnaire, (TMCQ) (Simonds & Rothbart, 2004)	Seven to ten years	157 computer-generated items based on Rothbart's neurobiological framework	$\alpha = .50$ to .90
School-Age Temperament Inventory (SATI)* (McClowry, 1995)	Eight to twelve years	38 items based on Thomas & Chess' framework	$\alpha = .85$ to .90

Table 2.2 (cont'd)

Self-regulation scales	Age	Description	Reliability
Behavior Rating Inventory of Executive Function® Preschool Version (BRIEF®-P)* (Gioia, Espy, & Isquith, 2003)	Two to 5.11 years	63 items, Executive Functioning (5 aspects).	α = .80 to .95
Behavior Rating Inventory for Executive Function® (BRIEF®)* (Gioia, Isquith, Guy,& Kenworthy, 2000)	Five to eighteen years	86 items, 2 broad indexes: Behavioral Regulation (3 scales) and Metacognition (5 scales) plus a Global Executive Composite	α = .80 to .98

*Parent and teacher versions are available.

disorders with difficult infants (Côté et al., 2009; Lahey et al., 2005). Although not well studied, identifying problems such as maternal depression, accompanied by appropriate referrals for treatment, has potential to reduce the risk of the behavioral and mental health problems that develop in early childhood (Côté et al., 2009; Lahey et al., 2005).

While routine temperament assessment in clinical practice is most likely to take place during infancy, practitioners who assess behavior during routine health examinations and acute care episodes may consider temperament during preschool and school years, as well. As mentioned earlier, child temperament and delays in self-regulation are most apparent in situations that are stressful and during transitional periods, such as entering preschool or a new classroom, or when there are changes in the family structure. Assessing temperament at this time and referring back to earlier assessments and health histories will assist the practitioner in determining if this is a situation that requires referrals to either a parenting program or a mental health provider.

Observations in Context: Children with Serious Emotional or Behavioral Problems

Children and adolescents who require hospitalization or placement in special schools or residential facilities demonstrate behaviors that may be related to underlying deficits in emotional or behavioral self-regulation but are often misunderstood. Nurses, by virtue of their presence and understanding of self-regulation, are in an ideal position to recognize patterns of behavior and help other treatment team members understand possible underlying self-regulatory behaviors (Delaney, 2006a). Delaney (2006b, 2006c, 2006d) has taken a leading role in developing theoretically based guidelines for in-patient psychiatric observational assessments that consider specific child self-regulatory behaviors in context. In this section, we highlight Delaney's guidelines

for assessment that are directly related to self-regulation: emotional regulation, behavioral regulation/inhibitory control, and coping and stress responses.

Delaney's assessment of emotional regulation (2006b) is organized around two areas of inquiry: how well the patient regulates emotions, how well the patient understands his affect. Behavioral signs of emotional regulation (ER) are provided for each question, along with associated intervention strategies, which are not discussed here. One of six signs of well-regulated emotion is that the ability to "regulate the intensity of an affect, e.g., frustration, does not escalate to intense anger" (Delaney 2006b, p. 179). The behavioral signs of understanding affect include the ability to label affective states and to tie affect to the situation that generates it. Theoretical and empirical support for the individual domains and signs of emotional regulation are provided by Rothbart and Bates (2006), Eisenberg (Eisenberg, Champion, & Ma, 2004), Izard (Izard, Stark, Trentacosta, & Schultz, 2008), and Denham (2006).

Another part of self-regulation is behavioral control, or inhibitory control. This includes the ability to inhibit an action either at the idea stage or at the initiation of behavior, or to block incoming stimuli that might interfere with completion of the action (Barkley, 1998). The concept of inhibitory control is predicated on learning how to control direct attention and developing voluntary control over thoughts and actions (Posner & Rothbart, 2000). Delaney's assessment of behavioral control is organized around a single question, which asks how well the patient regulates impulses (Delaney, 2006c). Developmentally appropriate behavioral signs are given to differentiate expectations between younger children and latency age and adolescents. An example of the signs of good behavioral control, realistic for the young child, is the ability to contain oneself during quiet times; more advanced abilities, such as the ability to process troublesome situations, especially one's role in a conflict, is expected of older children.

Delaney's third observation assessment guideline related to self-regulation is the managing of stress and use of coping behaviors (Delaney, 2006d). Conceptually, coping skill requires multiple conscious efforts to regulate emotion, cognition, and behavior as well as physiological response when faced with stressful events (Compas, Connor-Smith, Saltzman, Thomsen, & Wadsworth, 2001). This area differs somewhat from the others because of event focus and diversity of coping strategies attempted (Eisenberg et al., 1997; Eisenberg, Spinard, & Smith, 2004). The observations are centered on a specific question asking "how well the patient cope[s] with stress and milieu expectations" (Delaney, 2006d, p. 200). This includes previously mentioned signs of emotional and behavioral self-regulation as well as items unique to this group. This area highlights the range of coping strategies, some of which are clearly signs of ineffective coping or inability to self-regulate. In addition, specific tendencies may not be evident unless provoked by a stressful situation which tips the balance of control. This phenomenon is explained by several temperament theories which suggest that as the individual develops strategies, temperament may only be visible in situations of stress (McClowry, 2003; Strelau, 2000).

Linkages with Behavioral/Psychiatric Profile

Temperament has been linked to physical, psychological, and social outcomes for children. In relation to physical outcomes, temperament has shown to be a predictor of general health of the child, frequency of sleep problems, and tendency for injury (Atkins & Matsuba, 2008; Darlington & Wright, 2006; Reid, Hong, & Wade, 2009). Psychopathology such as ADHD, anxiety, and depression have also been linked to temperament (Foley, McClowry, & Castellanos, 2008; Rothbart & Bates, 2006). The Diagnostic Statistical Manual, 5th Edition, (DSM-V) childhood and adolescent disorders work group is considering the inclusion of severe irritability as a subtype of both oppositional defiant disorder (ODD) and mood disorders (Pine, 2009). In addition, temperament has been linked to post-traumatic stress disorder (PTSD) in children following cardiac surgery (Connolly, 2002). Temperament also predicts individual differences in social outcomes in children (Blair, Denham, Kochanoff, & Whipple, 2004). Children's temperament influences parents' decisions to prepare children for medical procedures and compliance with therapeutic management of illnesses (Lee & White-Traut, 1996; Smitherman, 1996).

Temperament profiles of children with neurological and learning disabilities have also been examined. The profiles of children with autism suggest more problems with self-regulation than their typically developing peers (Gomez & Baird, 2005; Zwaigenbaum, et al., 2005). Parents of children with diagnoses of autism and fragile X syndrome rate their children as being lower in adaptability and persistence and higher in withdrawal (Bailey, Hatton, Mesibov, Ament, & Skinner, 2000). Schwartz et al. (2009) reported lower levels of surgency and higher levels of fear and negative affectivity in adolescents with high functioning autism. Others have reported similar results in relation to infants and children diagnosed with autism as having more difficult temperaments (Bryson, Zwaigenbaum, Roberts, Szatmari, Rombough, 2007; Zwaigenbaum et al., 2005). All of these confounding factors put children at additional risk for development of later mental health problems.

Dysregulation, encompassing underregulation and/or misregulation (exerting control but making an undesirable response), has been linked to a number of mental health problems including addiction (Fayette, 2004), alcohol abuse (Vaughn, Beaver, DeLisi, Perron, & Schelbe, 2009), eating disorders (Ohmann et al., 2008), sexual abuse (Yates & Kingston, 2006), compulsive spending, as well as involvement in criminal acts (Zeier, Maxwell, & Newman, 2009). In addition, relationships between self-regulation and personality disorders (Shiner, 2009), depression (Kovnacs, Joormann, & Gotlib, 2008), anxiety (Tincas, Benga, & Fox, 2006), and even schizophrenia (Koren, Seidman, Goldsmith, & Harvey, 2006) are suggested by some. Despite seemingly theoretical connections, the mechanisms are complex and in general are unstudied. In addition, it is often unclear if self-regulation deficits are causative or the result of the disorder itself. Although clarity is lacking, treatments based on self-regulation assessment and theory are presently being developed and studied by clinical researchers.

Contributing to the knowledge of developmental psychopathology and the linkage between temperament and self-regulation and childhood (including adolescence) behavioral and psychiatric problems are the prospective, longitudinal studies which found that children with extreme temperaments are at higher risk for behavior problems later in childhood (Chess & Thomas, 1984; Maziade et al., 1990; Prior, Sanson, Smart, & Oberklaid, 2000). These findings have been supported and expanded upon in contemporary studies which try to tease out the process and pathways of development and enhance understanding of not only how problems develop but, in some instances, to identify protective factors that allow so many of these at-risk children to accomplish successful development.

Research illustrates the influence of self-regulation skills on social competence and the ability to function in group settings. As early as preschool, even brief periods of observed inability to regulate emotions (crying,

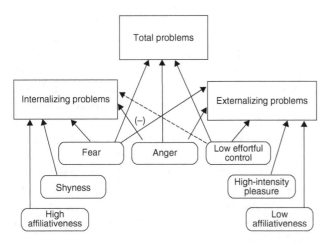

Figure 2.2 Rothbart's Model of Temperament and Problem Development. [Reprinted from Rothbart (2007) with permission from Wiley-Blackwell Publishing, London, UK.]

tantrums) and behavior (aggression, hyperactivity) predict later teacher reports of poor classroom adjustment and peer conflict (Miller, Gouley, Seifer, Dickstein, & Shields, 2004).

Rothbart (2007) has proposed an explanatory model that outlines the pathways between temperament (including self-regulation) and the development of both internalizing and externalizing problems in children. This model (Figure 2.2) is based upon Rothbart's temperament theory and research. As described earlier, her theory proposes the three dimensions of temperament: extraversion/surgency, negative affectivity, and effortful control. The later, effortful control (the child's ability to control reactive impulses), closely resembles self-regulation, although fear in the form of behavioral inhibition makes some regulatory contributions by controlling approach and aggression (Rothbart & Bates, 2006). The linkages are related to current temperament research findings. As can be noted, anger and fear relate directly to both internalizing problems and externalizing problems; however, anger is more strongly related to externalizing problems and fear to internalizing problems (it is low fear that relates to externalizing problems) (Rothbart, 2007). In contrast, the relationship between effortful control and internalizing problems is weak, while low effortful control is strongly related to externalizing problems.

It should be noted that Rothbart's developmental model illustrates direct and distinct relationships between several temperament dimensions and both categories of problems. High affiliativeness and shyness are related to internalizing problems; high-intensity pleasure and low affiliativeness relate to externalizing problems. Affiliativeness, the need for closeness and warmth, in preadolescence predicted problems during adolescence (Ormel et al., 2005). It must be noted that Rothbart's

theoretical model, like all such constructions, is general and marks the beginning of work to study the role temperament and self-regulation play in the development of problems. Clearly, it does not explore the context of the events or the various mediating and moderating factors, such as parenting stress, family psychopathology, stressful life events, and intelligence that influence development.

The inhibited (or shy) temperament has been linked to internalizing problems by many (Gladstone, Parker, Mitchell, Wilhelm, & Malhi, 2005; Hirshfeld-Becker et al., 2004). However, it is important to recognize that the identification of the proposed pathway between temperament and emotional dysregulation to serious anxiety and/or depression is ongoing. Much of the newest work investigating preschool children provides support and additional detail for Rothbart's model. Temperamental withdrawal (inhibition and low approach) at age five and parental internalizing problems predicted internalizing problems at age eleven (Mesman & Koot, 2000) and seventeen (Leve, Kim, & Peers, 2005).

Another study recognized the centrality of fear, finding that high fear emotionality and low fear regulation predicted internalizing problem behavior (Rydell, Berlin, & Bohlin, 2003); another found that functional impairment in young children may be attributed to the inability to refocus attention away from the source (executive attention) of sadness and distress (Cole, Luby, & Sullivan, 2008). The latter is in keeping with the thinking of Kovacs, Joormann, and Gotlib (2008), who proposed that emotional self-regulatory strategies used by children to attenuate sadness may develop atypically, serving to exacerbate rather than relieve distress.

A recent prospective study (Feng, Shaw, & Silk, 2008) has identified the divergent pathways that may influence why some children develop anxiety disorders while others with similar temperament profiles develop depressive disorders. This study uncovered four distinct trajectories in the development of anxiety: low, low increasing, high declining, and high increasing. In the presence of maternal negative control and maternal depression, boys who were shy were more likely to have high anxiety in middle childhood. Early shyness (anxiety) is associated with later depression only when it increases over childhood. These findings indicate that primary care nurses should take maternal histories, noting mothers who exhibit or have histories of depression and/or children who display high inhibition or withdrawal. Temperament-focused parent education and/or appropriate referrals to mental health providers may be warranted.

Externalizing behavior problems, ranging from serious misbehaviors to more extreme problems that characterize oppositional defiant disorders (ODD), conduct disorders (CD), and attention deficit hyperactive disorder (ADHD), have also been linked to specific temperaments and self-regulation. Young children whose temperaments are highly active respond negatively to events and who have low task persistence are at higher risk for developing disruptive behavior problems across childhood, and early conduct problems have been associated with delinquency and mental health problems in adolescence (Moffitt, Caspi, Harrington, & Milne, 2002). Again, as is true with internalizing problems, environmental, contextual, and child characteristics play an important part in determining whether temperamentally vulnerable children fail to develop the self-regulatory skills necessary to avoid disabling behavioral and mental health problems.

Studying developmental pathways to antisocial behaviors in low-income boys, Trentacosta and Shaw (2009) found that the inability to use active distraction as a means to regulate negative emotions in early childhood predicted peer rejection in middle childhood, which in turn predicted antisocial behavior in early adolescence. In another longitudinal, prospective study, Kochanska, Barry, Jimenez, Hollatz, and Woodard (2009), looking at the relationship between effortful control, guilt, and disruptive behaviors, found that children with no sense of guilt and poor effortful control were disruptive. However, children who displayed a strong sense of guilt avoided disruptive behaviors whether or not they demonstrated effortful control abilities. Well-child visits are an opportune time for primary care nurses to identify young children observed or reported to have difficulties complying with reasonable requests, ruling out sensory or perceptual problems. Preventive actions include referrals to temperament-based parenting programs that focus on providing warmth, structure, consistent rule enforcement, and noncoercive practices. For these youngsters, at each follow-up visit a thorough behavioral history update to track changes as well as ongoing parental guidance and support are necessary. Intractable and pervasive disruptive behaviors require a higher level of intervention.

Much work on temperament and self-regulation has been related to ADHD. Children who are low in self-regulation demonstrate difficulties organizing work, paying attention and staying on task at home and in school, making and retaining friends, moderating emotions, and controlling impulsive behaviors (Clark, Prior, & Kinsella, 2002; Miller, Gouley, Seifer, Dickstein, & Shields, 2004; Murphy, Shepard, Eisenberg, & Fabes, 2004). These behaviors are the same symptoms associated with a diagnosis of ADHD.

Nigg (2006) asserts that the temperamental traits of poor attentional focus, low inhibitory control, and high activity level are associated with and often serve as precursors of symptoms of ADHD. Researchers who examine the theoretical overlap between the constructs of ADHD and temperament conclude that children who are diagnosed with ADHD have temperaments that are high in negative reactivity, activity, and impulsivity, and low in task persistence, attentional focusing, and inhibitory control (Bussing, Gary, & Mason, 2003; Foley, McClowry, & Castellanos, 2008). Primary care nurses usually have little difficulty recognizing temperaments of children associated with or at risk for a diagnosis of ADHD. The challenge is to discern how much can be attenuated by encouraging environmental changes through parent education and parenting programs or ascertaining when other interventions may be necessary.

Temperament and self-regulation have also been associated with susceptibility for adverse reactions to trauma and stressful situations. For example, a study of children post 9/11, (Lengua, Long, Smith, & Meltzoff, 2005) found that temperament had a significant influence on the responses of children residing across country from the sites of the tragedy. They found that children who had poor inhibitory control (low self-regulation) prior to the attacks had higher levels of post-traumatic stress symptoms than their better regulated peers. This remained true after controlling for prior symptomatology, demonstrating the heightened vulnerability of children with poor self-regulatory abilities to traumatic events, even though not directly experienced. For primary care nurses seeing their patients longitudinally, this implies that they may be able to identify those patients in their caseload who are most vulnerable to traumatic events based on their temperament.

There is some evidence that youngsters may, because of their temperaments, particularly during early years, be more likely to be subjected to mistreatment and victimization (Famularo, Fenton, & Kinscherff, 1992). In addition, children with poor self-regulatory skills may be at higher risk for traumatic responses (including post-traumatic stress disorder [PTSD]) to abuse and maltreatment (Kruczek, Vitanza, & Salsman, 2008), with children subjected to maltreatment and abuse likely to have both altered capacities to regulate emotions and emotional dysregulation due to the abuse (Shipman et al., 2007). This emotional dysregulation is likely to influence cognition and impulse control (Cohen, Mannarino, & Deblinger, 2006). In the study by Shipman et al. (2007), physically maltreated children received less emotional socialization (emotional coaching, validation) by their mothers than non-maltreated children, making them less able to implement adaptive emotional regulation skills such as self-soothing and attentional control to manage emotional arousal constructively (Shipman et al., 2007). Non-adaptive self-regulation methods are dependent upon developmental level, and in extreme, may include self-mutilation, eating disorders, and substance abuse in older children and adolescents (van der Kolk, 1996). Long-range consequences of the affect dysregulation in relationship to interpersonal relatedness difficulties and PTSD have been noted in adults (Dietrich, 2007).

Goodness of Fit

A concept in temperament theory that is applicable to advanced practice nursing is goodness of fit (GOF). Chess and Thomas (1984) defined GOF as a match between the child's temperament and the expectations or demands of the environment. A good fit would be predictive of favorable outcomes; a poor fit, or incompatible relationship between the child's temperament and the environment, would result in risk of problem development (McClowry, Rodriquez, & Koslowitz, 2008; Zentner & Bates, 2008).

The usefulness of this concept is demonstrated in relation to family functioning and behavioral and psychiatric outcomes (Keiley, Lofthouse, Bates, Dodge, & Pettit, 2003; Lemery, Essex, & Smider, 2002) and, more specifically, to later adjustment (Lenuga & Kovacs, 2005; Morris et al., 2002). For example, children who were high negative reactors with mothers whose parenting was hostile demonstrated externalizing problems in middle childhood (Morris et al., 2002) while challenging children of parents who demonstrated supportive and consistent parenting were more likely to have fewer adjustment problems in later years (Pettit, Keiley, Laird, Bates, & Dodge, 2007).

Chess and Thomas (1984) also recognized that the child and the parent and/or the environment interact together and the effects on each are not unidirectional but rather transactional and nested in culture. For example, certain temperamental qualities are more valued in some cultures than others. Inhibition in China is seen positively and inhibited children are viewed favorably, whereas in Western cultures, children's inhibitions are viewed less favorably and efforts are made to teach the child to become more assertive. Likewise, parenting styles are nested within the cultural value system and affect child outcomes (Santisteban, Muir-Malcolm, Mitrani, & Szapocznik, 2002).

Furthermore, the influence of parental temperament and pathology affect the environments they create for their growing children (Churchill, 2003).

Depressed parents are often unable to be responsive and model self-regulatory activities for their children (Sethi et al., 2000).

Recent studies using longitudinal data from the National Institute of Child Health and Human Development (NICHD) illustrate the principle of GOF and the importance of environment for children with challenging temperaments. Pleuss and Belsky (2009) found that children described by their parent as difficult in infancy, when placed in excellent child care centers (with warm and encouraging teachers), did very well in preschool; in fact, in fifth and sixth grades were better behaved, got along better with their teachers, and had better reading skills. The reverse was true of children who had teachers who did not interact frequently, scolded, and had tense classrooms.

Evidence-based Implications for Practice

The increased developmental research in temperament and self-regulation has heightened interest in both assessing these areas in young children and integrating treatment strategies that target specific aspects of both temperament and self-regulation. Because parenting practices with children who have extreme temperaments (i.e., challenging, not so easy, high maintenance, slow to warm, feisty, spicy, spiritedness) are highly amenable to parental counseling, many pediatricians, nurses, and social workers have integrated temperament work into their clinical practices. Recognition of the effectiveness of early intervention has led to the creation of institutional programs to assess risk and educate parents. An example is a program, originally developed and tested at Kaiser Permanente (Preventive Ounce, 2007), which now independently provides online temperament assessments for parents of infants to six-year-olds along with "forecasts" of common behavior problems and management strategies. Typically, practitioners in health maintenance organizations alert new parent participants to this service. Once a profile is obtained, the information may be shared with providers and guidance and/or individualized counseling provided (H. Neville, personal communication, October 7, 2010).

Professionals who are committed to using temperament as the base of their interventions hold strong beliefs that most children with extreme temperaments will do well with sensitive parenting attuned to the child's individual needs and abilities. There is also recognition of the need to distinguish temperament issues from serious emotional and behavioral problems that interfere with functioning and attaining developmental goals and to refer those children to mental health professionals.

Models of Treatment

Temperament
INSIGHTS

While numerous interventions may be based on temperament theory and research, it is rare to find an intervention whose effectiveness has been empirically studied. One notable exception, the INSIGHTS program developed by McClowry (2003) for parents, teachers, and children, has demonstrated effectiveness in reducing disruptive behavior in young school-age children at home and demonstrated heightened efficacy with children who were at the diagnostic levels of three disruptive disorders: ADHD, oppositional defiant disorder, and conduct disorder (McClowry, Snow, & Tamis-LaMonda, 2005).

INSIGHTS was developed over the years as a preventive intervention for nonclinical populations (McClowry & Galehouse 2002; McClowry et al., 2005). It has an established protocol that, in the course of a series of group sessions, teaches parents and teachers to recognize the advantages and challenges of each temperament domain and use strategies to work with the child, as he or she is, to gain compliance and foster development. A quartet of puppets representing four common "profiles" of temperament is used to facilitate child understanding of temperament and encourage problem solving abilities (McClowry, 2002b). In addition to the puppets, McClowry has developed CDs to supplement materials and stimulate discussion for all three target groups. McClowry, Rodriguez, and Koslowitz (2008) propose that by helping parents and teachers tailor strategies to the child's unique temperament, GOF is achieved and abilities to self-regulate may be enhanced. Responding to the importance of intervention-culture concord, INSIGHTS is presently being adapted for other cultural groups (McClowry et al., 2008).

Self-regulation and Co-parenting

Empirically supported interventions that specifically target self-regulation abilities are also available but only a few have demonstrated efficacy and each targets different domains of self-regulation. Two of these programs, both designed for preschool children, are described here. One, Tools of the Mind program (Bodrova & Leong, 1996), focuses on enhancing the development of executive functions (also referred to as cognitive self-control) while the other, Emotions Course (Izard, 2001), seeks to foster emotional regulation abilities. A program focusing on co-parenting, Family Foundations, has also demonstrated effectiveness of increasing infants' self-regulation (Feinberg, Kan, & Goslin, 2009).

Tools of the Mind

Tools of the Mind is based on the work of Vygotsky (2004), whose theories underscore the importance of creative play with other children to develop self-regulation in three- to five-year-olds. Vygotsky believed that children develop habits of self-control by maintaining a role and pushing peers to follow the rules of make believe (Berk, Mann, & Ogan, 2006; Bodrova & Leong, 2005). While engaged in dramatic play, children have been found to be able to control impulses and to recall a greater number of new words than in traditional learning situations (Barnett et al., 2008).

Specific executive function targets for Tools are:

1. Inhibitory control by resisting habits, temptations, and distractions
2. Working memory demonstrated by the ability to mentally hold and use information
3. Cognitive flexibility in adjusting to change

Each of these is viewed as important for the effortful control of attention and behavior and as influencing and being influenced by the processes of emotional regulation (Clair & Diamond, 2008).

Preschool children from urban, low-income school districts receiving the Tools curriculum had significantly higher scores in each of the above three domains of executive function than did schoolmates receiving a different curriculum (Barnett et al., 2008; Diamond, Barnett, Thomas, & Munro, 2007).

The Emotions Course

Also designed for preschool children, the Emotions Course (EC) is based on Izard's conceptual model of emotion utilization (Izard, 2001). It endorses adaptive functioning such as substituting self-assertion for anger, identifying reasons, and seeking social support for sadness. The effectiveness of this program has been tested in two randomized cluster studies in Head Start settings (Izard et al., 2008), one rural and the other urban, and was found to increase emotion knowledge and emotional regulation in children receiving the EC. Other program outcomes included greater decreases in negative emotion expressions, aggression, anxious/depressed behavior, and negative peer and adult relationships than the control Head Start group.

Family Foundations

A new group program, Family Foundations, targets co-parenting, the way parents coordinate and support each other in the parenting role, during the important transitional time surrounding birth (Feinberg, 2002, 2003) and has demonstrated success in increasing infant self-regulation (self-soothing behaviors) as well as in diminishing parent depression and improving parenting quality (Feinberg, Kan, and Goslin, 2009).

Case Exemplar

While structured programs are excellent resources, the principal resource for families is the advanced practice nurse at point of contact. The following demonstrates what the individual practitioner can achieve.

Jana was a five-year-old girl displaying disruptive behaviors in her kindergarten classroom. Reported behaviors include inability to sit still, constantly moving about the classroom, yelling out answers, distractibility, failure to wait her turn in group activities, and being disrespectful to adults. Parental concerns were to maintain the child's fondness for school, achieve academic and social successes, and preserve self-concept and unique personality. They did not want the child labeled inappropriately and were adamantly against a medication evaluation, as suggested by the teacher. By history, Jana was a very active baby with precocious development, she was an irritable infant during the first six months, and had irregular wake/sleep patterns, but was responsive to parental attention and soothing behaviors. Since toddlerhood Jana had been friendly and played actively with others, but when disappointed could protest loudly. Parents found ignoring to be an effective management strategy. Mother reported that the child was more flexible than her older sibling and well behaved during religious services. At present she was able to read simple sentences and write the alphabet and her name.

An assessment revealed no changes in physical health status since prekindergarten assessment, six weeks prior. Parents reported no sleep problems; however, the child was difficult to wake and irritable on school mornings. Mom noted the child leaves personal items at school and frequently lost supplies. Mom often had to deliver items forgotten at home to school, making her late for work. Both parents noted a change in affect after school, and complaints that other children sometimes called her "the bad girl." Family assessment revealed an intact family, mom returned to work when the child started kindergarten, and dad worked long hours. Parents admitted to extending bedtime until 10 pm to allow for family time.

Classroom observation revealed the child's desk was located in the periphery of the classroom and many activities required students to work independently and make organized moves between learning centers. Observer noted that if the child spoke too loudly, the teacher yelled to her from across the classroom, ceasing the behavior yet puzzling the child. During reading time, the child was excited, enthusiastically commented on the story, and corrected others' interpretive errors.

Temperament assessment reveals the child was high in activity, low in task persistence, and responded negatively to change and frustration. On the Child Behavior Checklist (CBCL) assessment completed by the parent, she appeared to be approaching a diagnostic level of ADHD. In summary, her strengths appeared to be good intellectual capabilities, happiness, enjoyment in interacting with other children, and ability to identify feelings and express concerns. Parents were supportive, proactive, and cared about and were actively involved in her development and education. Despite parental responsiveness, neither the home nor school environment were a good fit with child's temperament at this time.

Temperament-based Intervention Plan

The broad goals are to alter the home and school environments and provide the best possible fit with Jana's temperament and ensure meeting developmental tasks.

The areas for change are:

- Ensure the parents' understanding of normal temperament and the importance of ignoring negativity, yet planning ahead to ensure compliance.
- Restructure the family's daily schedule to facilitate transitions for the child. For example, have the backpack at the door for easy pick-up in the morning and maintain an earlier bedtime.
- Develop parent strategies to encourage the child's ability to stay on task; for example, anticipatory planning using a timer to help the child understand how long she needs to be on task without distraction.
- Outline skills required of the child to successfully integrate into kindergarten, such as delaying gratification. Help the parents to set up a system of positive acknowledgement for goal achievement.
- Support parent advocacy in the school system, emphasizing the child's needs for teacher flexibility, consistent structure, and accommodation of energy expenditure during the day; for example, allowing the child to stand at her desk while working, but not walk around the classroom.

Jana's parents reported to the pediatric nurse practitioner (PNP) one month after their initial meeting, stating that they had successfully altered family routines to allow early bedtime and provide easy departures in the morning. In addition, they had instituted a simple reward system that acknowledged Jana's ability to complete tasks before playtime. The parents noted that talking with the teacher was less laden with complaints. The PNP spoke with the school nurse and described Jana's temperament, strengths, and challenges, and outlined effective temperament-based strategies to gain her compliance in the school setting. On follow-up three months later, the parents reported that they had been pleased with the teacher's responsiveness and report of Jana's improved classroom behavior. At the end of the school year, Jana's social status improved and she was promoted to first grade. They added that the school nurse had been an effective liaison in advocating for individualized management, and parental input was requested regarding next year's classroom assignment.

To summarize, the following steps were taken: assessment of age-appropriate self-regulatory abilities (i.e., behavior, attention, emotional regulation, sleep), assessment of parental perceptions of issues and understanding of temperament/self-regulation, assessment of goodness of fit issues between parent/child or parent/daycare provider-teacher/child, reframing issues of behavior in terms of regulation and temperament, providing anticipatory guidance to parents or more actively intervening when indicated around key regulatory areas, designing accommodation plans sensitive to gradually increasing demands for flexible responses, and recommending appropriate resources to parents.

Summary

Although child temperament is most easily recognized in infancy and in later situations of change or stress, temperament remains an important intrinsic factor throughout childhood. Children's unique temperaments contribute to self-regulation development and are viewed by many to be the foundation of personality. The ability to self-regulate emotion, behavior, and attention begins in infancy and is influenced by temperament (reactivity and effortful control) and by the warmth, support, modeling, and education provided by caregivers. Culture also plays a part, with some dimensions of temperament fostered by the cultures in which they are valued and those less valued heaped with criticism. Research suggests that there is a critical window of opportunity for regulation development and that capacities are in place by ages eight to ten, although it has been suggested that relationships between components of executive function may change as tasks become more complex.

Studies have demonstrated relationships between extreme temperaments and both externalizing and internalizing behaviors. High negative emotionality and high inhibition are two domains that are highly predictive of future problems in early childhood. However, it must be cautioned that the majority of children with these extreme temperaments do not develop behavior or mental disorders. There is some evidence that a lack of task persistence (poor self-regulation) is the strongest predictor of behavior problems in school-aged children.

It is important to remember that there is some evidence that children from impoverished homes are at most risk for having poor self-regulation skills.

Early assessment of temperament and continued assessment of age-appropriate self-regulatory abilities allow the APN to provide anticipatory guidance to parents and intervene when indicated. APNs must be cautioned, however, to present differences as unique human qualities, not as defects, and to provide realistic examples of how to secure goodness of fit for the youngster. Several promising new interventions based on temperament or self-regulation theory and research have been designed and are being empirically studied. While these new evidence-based programs focus exclusively on younger children, many professionals have experience working with older children and adolescents whose self-regulatory problems are prominent and dysfunctional. Assessing specific areas of regulatory dysfunction allows the APN to make environmental adjustments to reduce uncontrolled maladaptive behaviors within the setting. This nursing intervention, understanding the role of temperament in development and planning interventions, potentially improves the child's functioning and adjustment within the home and community.

Recommended Resources

Resources for Parents

Carey, W.B. (2005). *Understanding your child's temperament* (Rev. edition). New York: Macmillan/Simon & Schuster.

Kurcinka, M.S. (2006). *Raising your spirited child: A guide for parents whose child is more intense, sensitive, perceptive, persistent and energetic* (Rev. edition). New York: Harper Collins.

Kristal, J. (2004). *The temperament perspective: Working with children's behavioral styles.* Baltimore, MD: Brookes. Note: This is viewed by some as more for professionals than parents.

McClowry, S.G. (2003). *Your child's unique temperament: Insights and strategies for responsive parenting.* Champaign, IL: Research Press.

Probst, B. (2008). *When the labels don't fit: An approach to raising a challenging child.* New York: Three Rivers Press.

Resources for Professionals: Evidence-based and Empirically Tested Prevention Intervention Programs

Family Foundations
Mark Feinberg, PhD
Prevention Research Center
Penn State University
http://prevention.psu.edu/projects/Coparenting_Pubs.html

INSIGHTS
Sandee McClowry, PhD, RN
Steinhart School

New York University
http://www.insightsintervention.com/

Tools of the Mind
Deborah J. Leong, PhD
Metropolitan State College of Denver
http://www.mscd.edu/extendedcampus/toolsofthemind/

Emotions Course
Carroll Izard, PhD
University of Delaware

References

Atkins, R., & Matsuba, M. (2008). The association of personality and likelihood of serious unintentional injury during childhood. *Journal of Pediatric Nursing 23*(6), 451–459.

Bailey, D.B., Hatton, D.D., Mesibov, G., Ament, N., & Skinner, M. (2000). Early development, temperament, and functional impairment in autism and fragile X syndrome. *Journal of Autism and Developmental Disorders, 30*(1), 49–59.

Barkley, R.A. (1998). *Attention-deficit hyperactivity disorder: A handbook for diagnosis and treatment.* New York, NY: Guilford Press.

Barnett, W.S., Jung, K., Yarosz, D.J., Thomas, J., Hornbeck, A., Stechuk, R., & Burns, S. (2008). Educational effects of the Tools of the Mind curriculum: A randomized trial. *Early Child Research Quarterly, 23,* 299–313.

Baumeister, R.F., Heatherton, T.F., & Tice, D.M. (1994). *Losing control: How and why people fail at self-regulation.* San Diego, CA: Academic Press.

Belskey, J., Pasco Fearson, R.M., & Bell, B. (2007). Parenting, attention and externalizing problems: Testing mediation longitudinally, repeatedly and reciprocally. *Journal of Child Psychology and Psychiatry, 48*(12), 1233–1242.

Berk, L.E., Mann, T.D., & Ogan, A.T. (2006). Make-believe play: Wellspring for development of self-regulation. In D.G. Singer, R.M. Golinkoff, & K. Hirsh-Pasek (Eds.). *Play = learning: How play motivates and enhances children's cognitive and social-emotional growth* (pp.74–100). New York, NY: Oxford University Press.

Blair, C. (2002). Integrating cognition and emotion in a neurobiological conceptualization of children's functioning at school entry. *American Psychologist, 57,* 111–127.

Blair, K.A., Denham, S., Kochanoff, A., & Whipple, B. (2004). Playing it cool: Temperament, emotion regulation and social behavior in preschoolers. *Journal of School Psychology, 42*(6), 419–443.

Bloom, B. & Cohen, R.A. (2009). Summary health statistics for U.S. children: National Health Interview Survey, 2007. *Vital and Health Statistics, 10* (239). Hyattsville, MD: National Center for Health Statistics.

Bodrova, E., & Leong, D.J. (1996). *Tools of the Mind: The Zygotskian approach to early childhood education.* Upper Saddle River, NJ: Prentice-Hall.

Bodrova, E., & Leong, D.J., (2005). High quality preschool programs: What would Vygotsky say? *Early Education and Development, 16*(4), 435–444.

Bridgett, D.J., Gartstein, M.A., Putnam, S., McKay, T., Iddins, E., Robertson, C., Ramsay, K., & Rittmueller, A. (2009). Maternal and contextual influences and the effect of temperament development during infancy on parenting in toddlerhood. *Infant Behavior & Development, 32,* 103–116.

Bryson, S.E., Zwaigenbaum, L., Roberts, B., Szatmari, P., & Rombough, V. (2007). A prospective case series of high-risk infants who developed autism. *Journal of Autism and Developmental Disorders, 37,* 12–24.

Bush, G. (2004). Multimodal studies of cingulated cortex. In M.I. Posner (Ed.). *Cognitive neuroscience of attention* (pp. 207–218). New York, NY: Guilford Press.

Buss, A.H., & Plomin, R. (1984). *Temperament: Early developing personality traits.* Mahwah, NJ: Lawrence Erlbaum Associates.

Bussing, R., Gary, F.A., & Mason, D.M. (2003). Child temperament, ADHD, and caregiver strain: Exploring relationships in an epidemiological sample. *Journal of the American Academy of Child & Adolescent Psychiatry, 42*(2), 184–192.

Calkins, S.D., & Fox, N.A. (2002). Self-regulatory processes in early personality development: A multilevel approach to the study of childhood social withdrawal and aggression. *Development and Psychopathology, 14*(3), 477–498.

Chang, F., & Burns, B. (2005). Attention in preschoolers: Associations with effortful control and motivation. *Child Development, 76*(1), 247–263.

Chess, S., & Thomas, A. (1984). *Origins and evolution of behavior disorders: From infancy to early adult life.* Cambridge, MA: Harvard University Press.

Churchill, S.L. (2003). Goodness of fit in early childhood settings. *Early Childhood Education Journal, 31*(2), 113–118.

Clair, C., & Diamond, A. (2008). Biological processes in prevention and intervention: The promotion of self-regulation as a means of preventing school failure. *Development and Psychopathology, 20,* 899–911.

Clark, C., Prior, M., & Kinsella, G. (2002). The relationship between executive function abilities, adaptive behavior, and academic achievement in children with externalizing behavior problems. *Journal of Child Psychology and Psychiatry, 43,* 785–796.

Cole, P.M., Luby, J., & Sullivan, M.W. (2008). Emotions and the development of childhood depression: Bridging the gap. *Child Development Perspectives, 2*(3), 141–148.

Cohen, J.A., Mannarino, A.P., & Deblinger, E. (2006). *Treating trauma and traumatic grief in children and adolescents.* New York: Guilford Press.

Compas, B.E., Connor-Smith, J.K., Saltzman, H., Thomsen, A.H., & Wadsworth, M.E. (2001). Coping with stress during childhood and adolescence: Problems, progress, and potential in theory and research. *Psychological Bulletin, 127,* 87–127.

Connolly, D. (2002). Psychosocial responses of school-age children to cardiac surgery. Dissertation abstracts. New York University, New York, NY.

Côté, S., Boivin, M., Liu, X., Nagin, D.S., Zoccolillo, M., & Tremblay, R.E. (2009). Depression and anxiety symptoms: Onset, developmental course and risk factors during early childhood. *Journal of Child Psychology & Psychiatry, 50*(10), 1201–1208.

Darlington, A., & Wright, C. (2006). The influence of temperament on weight gain in early infancy. *Journal of Developmental Behavioral Pediatrics 27*(4), 329–335.

Deater-Deckard, K., Petrill, Stephen A., & Thompson, L.A. (2007). Anger/frustration, task persistence, and conduct problems in childhood: A behavioral genetic analysis. *Journal of Child Psychology and Psychiatry, 48*(1), 80–87.

Delaney, K.R. (2006a). Learning to observe in context. *Journal of Child and Adolescent Psychiatric Nursing, 19*(4), 170–174.

Delaney, K.R. (2006b). Following the affect: Learning to observe emotional regulation. *Journal of Child and Adolescent Psychiatric Nursing, 19*(4), 175–181.

Delaney, K.R. (2006c). Learning to observe cognition, mastery and control. *Journal of Child and Adolescent Psychiatric Nursing, 19*(4), 182–193.

Delaney, K.R. (2006d). Learning to observe relationships in context. *Journal of Child and Adolescent Psychiatric Nursing, 19*(4), 194–202.

Denham, S.A. (2006). Emotional competence: Implications for social functioning. In J.L. Luby (Ed.) *Handbook of preschool mental health: Development, disorders, and treatment* (pp. 23–44). New York, NY: Guilford Press.

Diamond, A., Barnett, W.S., Thomas, J., & Munro, S. (2007). Preschool program improves cognitive control. *Science, 318*(5855), 1387–1388.

Dietrich, A. (2007). Childhood maltreatment and revictimization: The role of affect dysregulation, interpersonal relatedness difficulties and posttraumatic stress disorder. *Journal of Trauma & Dissociation, 8*(4), 25–51.

Eisenberg, N., Champion C., & Ma, Y. (2004). Emotion-related regulation: An emerging construct. *Merrill-Palmer Quarterly, 50*, 236–259.

Eisenberg, N., Fabes, R.A., & Guthrie, J.K. (1997). Coping with stress: The role of regulation and development. In S.A. Wolchick, & I.N. Sandler (Eds.). *Handbook of children's coping: Linking the theory and intervention* (pp. 277–306). Mahwah, NJ: Lawrence Erlbaum.

Eisenberg, N., Fabes, R.A., Nyman, M., Bernzweig, J., & Pinuelas, A. (1994). The relations of emotionality and regulation to children's anger-related reactions. *Child Development, 65*, 109–128.

Eisenberg, N., Smith, C., Sadovsky, A., & Spinrad, T.L. (2004). Effortful control: Relations with emotional regulation, adjustment and socialization in childhood. In R.F. Baumeister, & K.D. Vohs (Eds.). *Handbook of self-regulation: Research, theory and applications* (pp. 259–282). New York, NY: Guilford Press.

Eisenberg, N., Spinard, T.L., & Smith, C. (2004). Emotional-related regulation: Its conceptualization, relations to social functioning and socialization. In P. Philippot, & R. S. Feldman (Eds.). *The regulation of emotion* (pp. 227–206). Mahwah, NJ: Lawrence Erlbaum.

Famularo, R., Fenton, T, & Kinscherff, R. (1992). Medical and developmental histories of maltreated children. *Clinical Pediatrics, 31*(9), 536–541.

Fan, J., & Posner, M. (2004). Human attentional networks. *Psychiatrische Praxis, Vol.31 (Suppl2)*, S210–S214.

Fayette, M.A. (2004). Self-regulatory failure and addiction. In R.F. Baumeister, & K.D. Vohs (Eds.). *Handbook of self-regulation: Research, theory, and applications* (pp. 447–465). New York, NY: Guilford Press.

Feinberg, M.E. (2002). Coparenting and the transition to parenthood: A framework for prevention. *Clinical Child and Family Psychology Review, 5*, 173–195.

Feinberg, M. (2003). The internal structure and ecological context of coparenting: A framework for research and intervention. *Parenting, Science and Practice, 3*, 95–132.

Feinberg, M.E., Kan, M.L., & Goslin, M.C. (2009). Enhancing coparenting, parenting, and child self-regulation: Effects of Family Foundations 1 year after birth. *Prevention Science, 10*, 276–285.

Feldman, R. (2009). The development of regulatory functions from birth to 5 years: Insights from premature infants. *Child Development, 80*(2), 544–561.

Feng, X., Shaw, D.S., & Silk, J.S. (2008). Developmental trajectories of anxiety symptoms among boys across early and middle childhood. *Journal of Abnormal Psychology, 117*(1), 32–47.

Foley, M., McClowry, S., & Castellanos, F. (2008). The relationship between attention deficit hyperactivity disorder and child temperament. *Journal of Applied Developmental Psychology, 29*, 157–169.

Fonagy, P., & Target, M. (2002). Early intervention and the development of self-regulation. *Psychoanalytic Quarterly, 22*, 307–335.

Fullard, W., McDevitt, S.C., & Carey, W.B. (1984). Assessing temperament in one- to three-year-old children. *Journal of Pediatric Psychology, 9*, 205–217.

Gartstein, M.A., & Rothbart, M.K. (2003). Studying infant temperament via the Revised Infant Behavior Questionnaire. *Infant Behavior and Development, 26*(1), 64–86.

Gioia, G.A., Espy, K.A., & Isquith, P.K. (2003). *The Behavior Rating Inventory for Executive Function—Preschool Version*. Lutz, FL: Psychological Assessment Resources.

Gioia, G.A., Isquith, P.K., Guy, S.C., & Kenworthy, L. (2000). Behavior Rating Inventory of Executive Function. *Child Neuropsychology, 6*(3), 235–238.

Gladstone, G.L., Parker, G.B., Mitchell, P.B., Wilhelm, K.A., & Malhi, G.S. (2005) Relationship between self-reported childhood behavioral inhibition and lifetime anxiety disorders in a clinical sample. *Depression and Anxiety, 22*(3), 103–113.

Goldsmith, H.H. (1996). Studying temperament via construction of the Toddler Behavior Assessment Questionnaire. *Child Development, 67*, 218–235.

Goldsmith, H.H., & Campos, J.J. (1982). Toward a theory of infant temperament. In R.N. Emde, & R.J. Harmon (Eds.). The development of attachment and affiliative systems (pp. 161–193). New York, NY: Plenum.

Gomez, C.R., & Baird, S. (2005). Identifying early indicators for autism in self-regulation difficulties. *Focus on Autism and Other Developmental Disabilities, 20*(2), 106–116.

Gosling, S.D., Kwan, V.S., Hagan, J.F., Shaw, J.S., & Duncan, P.M. (Eds.). (2008). *Bright futures: Guidelines for health supervision of infants, children, and adolescents* (3rd edition). Elk Grove Village, IL: American Academy of Pediatrics.

Harris, R.C., Robinson, J.B., Chang, F., & Burns, B.M. (2007). Characterizing preschool children's attention regulation in parent-child interactions: The role of effortful control and motivation. *Journal of Applied Developmental Psychology, 28*, 25–39.

Hegvik, R.L., McDevitt, S.C., & Carey, W.B. (1982). The Middle Childhood Temperament Questionnaire. *Journal of Developmental and Behavioral Pediatrics, 3*, 197–200.

Hirshfeld-Becker, D.R., Biederman, J., Fargone, S.V., Segool, N., Buchwald, J., & Rosenbaum, J.F. (2004). Lack of association between behavioral inhibition and psychosocial adversity factors in children at risk for anxiety disorders. *The American Journal of Psychiatry, 161*(3), 547–555.

Izard, C.E. (2001). The Emotions Course. Helping children understand and manage their feelings: An emotion-centered primary prevention program for Head Start. Newark, DE: University of Delaware.

Izard, C.E., King, K.A., Trentacosta, C.J., Laurenceau, J.P., Morgan, J.K., Krauthamer-Ewing, E.S., & Finlon, K.J. (2008). Accelerating the development of emotion competence in Head Start children. *Development & Psychopathology, 20*, 369–397.

Izard, C.E., Stark, K., Trentacosta, C., & Schultz, D. (2008). Beyond emotion regulation: Emotion utilization and adaptive functioning. *Child Development Perspectives, 2*(3), 156–163.

Kagan, J. (1998). Biology and the child. In W. Damon (Ed.), *Handbook of child psychology* (5th ed., pp. 177–235). New York, NY: Wiley.

Keiley, M.K., Lofthouse, N., Bates, J.E., Dodge, K.A., & Pettit, G.S. (2003). Differential risks of covarying and pure components in mother and teacher reports of externalizing and internalizing behavior across ages 5 to 14. *Journal of Abnormal Child Psychology, 31*, 267–283.

Keogh, B.K., Pullis, M.E., & Cadwell, J. (1982). A short form of the Teachers Temperament Questionnaire. *Journal of Educational Measurement, 19*, 323–329.

Kochanska, G. (1995). Children's temperament, mothers' discipline, and security of attachment: Multiple pathways in emerging internalization. *Child Development, 66*, 597–615.

Kochanska, G., Barry, R.A., Jimenez, N.B., Hollatz, A.L., & Woodard, J. (2009). Guilt and effortful control: Two mechanisms that prevent disruptive developmental trajectories. *Journal of Personality and Social Psychology, 97*(2), 322–333.

Kochanska, G., Murray, K.T., & Harlan, E.T. (2000). Effortful control in early childhood: Continuity and change, antecedents, and implications for social development. *Developmental Psychology, 36*, 220–232.

Kochanska, G., Murray, K., & Koy, K.C. (1997). Inhibitory control as a contributor to conscience in childhood: From toddler to early school age. *Child Development, 68*, 263–277.

Koren, D., Seidman, L.J., Goldsmith, M., & Harvey, P.D. (2006). Real-world cognitive—and metacognitive—dysfunction in *schizophrenia*: A new approach for measuring (and remediating) more 'right stuff.' *Schizophrenia Bulletin, 32*(2), 310–326.

Kovacs, M., Joormann, J., & Gotlib, I.H. (2008). Emotional (dys) regulation and links to depressive disorders. *Child Development Perspectives, 2*(3), 149–155.

Kruczek, T., Vitanza, S., & Salsman, J. (2008). Posttraumatic stress disorder in children. In T.P. Gullotta, & G.M. Blau (Eds.). *Handbook of childhood behavioral issues: Evidence-based approaches to prevention and treatment* (pp. 289–317). New York, NY: Routledge/Taylor & Francis.

Lahey, B.B., Van Hulle, C.A., Keenan, K., Rathouz, P.J., D'Onofrio, B.M., Rogers, J.L. & Waldman, I.D. (2005). Temperament and parenting during the first year of life predict future child conduct problems. *Journal of Abnormal Child Psychology, 36*(8), 1139–1158.

Leddy, S.K. (2006). Health promotion: Mobilizing strengths to enhance health, wellness, and well-being. Philadelphia, PA: F.A. Davis.

Lee, L.W., & White-Traut, R.C. (1996). The role of temperament in pediatric pain response. *Issues in Comprehensive Pediatric Nursing, 19*, 49–63.

Lemery, K.S., Essex, M.J., & Smider, N.A. (2002). Revealing the relation between temperament and behavior problem symptoms by eliminating measurement confounding: Expert rating and factor analyses. *Child Development, 73*, 867–882.

Lengua, L.L., & Kovacs, E.A. (2005). Bi-directional associations between temperament and parenting and the prediction of adjustment problems in middle childhood. *Applied Developmental Psychology, 26*, 21–38.

Lengua, L.J., Long, A.C., Smith, K.I., & Meltzoff, A.N. (2005). Pre-attack symptomatology and temperament as predictors of children's responses to the September 11 terrorist attacks. *Journal of Child Psychiatry and Psychology, 46* (6), 6331–645.

Leve, L., Kim, H.K., & Peers, K.C. (2005). Childhood temperament and family environment as predictors of internalizing and externalizing trajectories from ages 5 to 17. *Journal of Abnormal Child Psychology, 33*(5), 505–520.

Martin, R., & Bridger, R. (1999). *The Temperament Assessment Battery for Children-Revised.* Athens, GA: University of Georgia.

Maziade, M., Caron, C., Cote, R., Merette, C., Bernier, H., Laplante, B., Boutin, P., & Thivierge, J. (1990). Psychiatric status of adolescents who had extreme temperaments at age 7. *American Journal of Psychiatry, 147*(11), 1531–1536.

McClowry, S.G. (1995). The development of the School-Age Temperament Inventory. *Merrill Palmer Quarterly, 41*, 271–285.

McClowry, S.G. (2002a). The temperament profiles of school age children. *Journal of Pediatric Nursing, 17*, 3–10.

McClowry, S.G. (2002b). Transforming temperament profile statistics into puppets and other visual media. *Journal of Pediatric Nursing, 17*, 11–17.

McClowry, S.G. (2003). *Your child's unique temperament: Insights and strategies for responsive parenting.* Champagne, IL: Research Press.

McClowry, S.G., & Galehouse, P. (2002). A pilot study conducted to plan a temperament-based parenting program for inner city families. *Journal of Child and Adolescent Psychiatric Nursing, 15*, 97–108.

McClowry, S.G., Hegvik, R., & Teglasi, H. (1993). An examination of the construct validity of the Middle Childhood Temperament Questionnaire, *Merrill-Palmer Quarterly, 39*, 279–293.

McClowry, S.G., Rodriguez, E.T., & Koslowitz, R. (2008). Temperament-based intervention: Re-examining goodness of fit. *European Journal of Developmental Science, 2*, 120–135.

McClowry, S.G., Snow, D.L., & Tamis-LeMonda, C.S. (2005). An evaluation of the effects of INSIGHTS on the behavior of inner-city primary school children. *Journal of Primary Prevention, 26*, 567–584.

McDevitt, S. & Carey, W.B. (1978). The measurement of temperament in 3–7-year-old children. *Journal of Child Psychology and Psychiatry, 19*(3), 245–253.

Medoff-Cooper, B., Carey, W.B., & McDevitt, S.C. (1993). The Early Infancy Temperament Questionnaire. *Journal of Developmental and Behavioral Pediatrics, 14*(4), 230–235.

Mesman, J., & Koot, H.M. (2000). Common and specific correlates of preadolescent internalizing and externalizing psychopathology. *Journal of Abnormal Psychology, 109*, 367–374.

Miller, A.L., Gouley, K.K., Seifer, R., Dickstein, S., & Shields, A. (2004). Emotions and behaviors in the Head Start classroom: Associations among observed dysregulation, social competence and preschool adjustment. *Early Education and Development, 15*, 147–165.

Mischel, W., & Ayduk, O. (2004). Willpower in a cognitive-affective processing system: The dynamics of delay of gratification. In R.F. Baumeister, & K.D. Vohs (Eds.). *Handbook of self-regulation: Research, theory, and applications* (pp. 99–129). New York, NY: Guilford.

Moffitt, T.E., Caspi, A., Harrington, H., & Milne, B.J. (2002). Males on the life-course-persistent and adolescence-limited antisocial pathways: Follow-up at age 26 years. *Development and Psychopathology, 14*, 179–207.

Morris, A.S., Silk, J.S., Steinberg, L., Sessa, F.M., Avenevoli, S., & Essex, M.J. (2002). Temperamental vulnerability and negative parenting as interacting predictors of child adjustment. *Journal of Marriage and Family, 64*, 461–471.

Mrakotsky, C., & Heffelfinger, A.K. (2006). Neuropsychological assessment. In J.L. Luby (Ed.). *Handbook of preschool mental health: Development, disorders and treatment* (pp. 283–310). New York, NY: Guilford.

Murphy, B.C., Shepard, S.A., Eisenberg, N., & Fabes, R.A. (2004). Concurrent and across time prediction of young adolescent's social functioning: The role of emotionality and regulation. *Social Development, 13*, 56–86.

NICHD Early Child Care Research Network (2003). Do children's attention processes mediate the link between family predictors and school readiness? *Developmental Psychology, 39*(3), 581–593.

Nigg, J. (2006). Temperament and developmental psychopathology. *Journal of Child Psychology and Psychiatry, 47*(3–4), 395–422.

Ohmann, S., Schuch, B., König, M., Blaas, S., Fliri, C., & Popow, C. (2008). Self-injurious behavior in adolescent girls: Association with psychopathology and neuropsychological functions. *Psychopathology, 41*(4), 226–235.

Ormel, A.J., Oldenhinkel, A.J., Ferdinand, R.F., Harman, C.A., de Winter, A.F., & Veenstra, R. (2005). Internalizing and externalizing problems in adolescence: General and dimension-specific effects of familial loadings and preadolescent temperament traits. *Psychological Medicine, 35*(12), 1825–1835.

Panksepp, J. (1998). *Affective neuroscience: The foundations of human and animal emotions.* New York, NY: Oxford University Press.

Pender, N.J., Murdaugh, C.L., & Parsons, M.A. (2010). *Health promotion in nursing practice (6th edition)*. Upper Saddle River, NJ: Pearson Hall.

Pettit, G.S., Keiley, M.K., Laird, R.D., Bates, J.E., & Dodge, K.A. (2007). Predicting the developmental course of mother-reported monitoring across childhood and adolescence from early proactive parenting, child temperament, and parents' worries. *Journal of Family Psychology, 21(2)*, 206–217.

Pine, D. (April, 2009). Report of the DSM-V childhood and adolescent disorders work group. American Psychiatric Association. Retrieved from http://www.psych.org

Pleuss, M., & Belsky, J. (2009). Differential susceptibility to rearing experiences: the case of childcare. *Journal of Child Psychology and Psychiatry, 50(4)*, 396–404.

Plomin, R., & Caspi, A. (1999). Behavioral genetics and personality. In L.A. Pervin, & O.P. John (Eds.). *Handbook of personality: Theory and research (2nd edition)*. (pp. 251–276). New York: Guildford Press.

Ponitz, C.C., McClelland, M.M., Matthews, J.S., & Morrison, F.J. (2009). A structured observation of *behavioral self-regulation* and its contribution to kindergarten outcomes. *Developmental Psychology, 45(3)*, 605–619.

Posner, M.I., & Rothbart, M.K. (2000). Developing mechanisms of self-regulation. *Development and Psychopathology, 12*, 427–441.

Posner, M., & Rothbart, M. (2007). *Educating the human brain*. Washington, DC: American Psychological Association.

Preventive Ounce (2007). Retrieved from http://www.preventiveoz.org/aboutpoz.html

Prior, M., Sanson, A., Smart, D., & Oberklaid, F. (2000). *Pathways from infancy to adolescence: Australian temperament project 1983–2000*. Melbourne, Australia: Australian Institute of Family Studies.

Putnam, S.P., Garstein, M.A., & Rothbart, M.K. (2006). Measurement of fine-grained aspects of toddler temperament: The Early Childhood Behavior Questionnaire. *Infant Behavior and Development, 29*, 386–401.

Putnam, S.P., & Rothbart, M.K. (2006). Development of short and very short forms of the children's behavior questionnaire. *Journal of Personality Assessment, 87(1)*, 102–112.

Reid, G., Hong, R., & Wade, T. (2009). The relation between common sleep problems and emotional and behavioral problems among 2 and 3 year olds in the context of known risk factors for psychopathology. *Journal of Sleep Research,18(1)*, 49–55.

Robinson, J.B., Burns, B.M., & Davis, D.W. (2009). Maternal scaffolding and attention regulation in children living in poverty. *Journal of Applied Developmental Psychology, 30*, 82–91.

Rothbart, M.K. (2007). Temperament, development, and personality. *Current Directions in Psychological Science 16 (4)*, 207–212.

Rothbart, M.K., Ahadi, S.A., & Hershey, K.L. (1994). Temperament and social behavior in childhood. *Merrill-Palmer Quarterly, 40*, 21–39.

Rothbart, M.K., Ahadi, S.A., Hershey, K., & Fisher, P. (2001). Investigations of temperament at three to seven years: The Children's Behavior Questionnaire. *Child Development, 72(5)*, 1394–1408.

Rothbart, M.K., & Bates, J.E. (2006). Temperament. In W. Damon, R. Lerner, & N. Eisenberg (Eds.) *Handbook of child psychology: Vol 3. Social, emotional, and personality development* (6th ed., pp. 99–166). New York: Wiley.

Rothbart, M.K., Ellis, L.K., & Posner, M.I. (2004). Temperament and self-regulation. In R.F. Baumeister, & K.D. Vohs (Eds.), *Handbook of self-regulation: Research, theory, and applications* (pp. 357–370). New York: Guilford Press.

Rothbart, M.K., Ellis, L.K., Rueda, M.R., and Posner, M.I. (2003). Developing mechanisms of temperamental effortful control. *Journal of Personality, 71(6)*, 1113–1143.

Rowe, D.C., & Plomin, R. (1977). Temperament in early childhood. *Journal of Personality Assessment, 41*, 150–156.

Rueda, M.R., Posner, M.I., & Rothbart, M.K. (2004). Attentional control and self-regulation. In R.F. Baumeister, & K.D. Vohs (Eds.). *Handbook of self-regulation: Research, theory, and applications* (pp. 283–300). New York: Guilford Press.

Rydell, A.M., Berlin, L., & Bohlin, G. (2003). Emotionality, emotion regulation, and adaptation among 5- to 8-year-old children. *Emotion, 3(1)*, 30–47.

Santisteban, D.A., Muir-Malcolm, J.A., Mitrani, V.B., & Szapocznik, J. (2002). Integrating the study of ethnic culture and family psychology intervention science. In H. Liddle, D. Santisteban, R. Levant, & J. Bray (Eds.). *Family psychology: Science-based interventions* (pp. 331–352). Washington, DC: American Psychological Association Press.

Scaer, R. (2005). *The trauma spectrum: Hidden wounds and human resiliency*. New York: W.W. Norton.

Schore, A.N. (1994). *Affect regulation and the origin of the self: The neurobiology of emotional development*. Hillsdale, NJ: Erlbaum.

Schwartz, C.B., Henderson, H A., Inge, A.P., Zahka, N.E., Coman, D.C., Kojkowski, N.M., Hileman, C.M., & Mundy, P.C. (2009). Temperament as a predictor of symptomatology and adaptive functioning in adolescents with high-functioning autism. *Journal of Autism and Developmental Disorders, 39*, 842–855.

Sethi, A., Mischel, W., Aber, J.L., Shoda, Y., & Rodriguez, M.L. (2000). The role of strategic attention deployment in development of self-regulation: Predicting preschoolers' delay of gratification from mother-toddler interactions. *Developmental Psychology, 36*, 767–777.

Shiner, R.L. (2009). The development of personality disorders: Perspectives from normal personality development in childhood and adolescence. *Development and Psychopathology, 21*, 715–734.

Shipman, K., Schneider, R., Fitzgerald, M.M., Sims, C., Swisher, L., & Edwards, A. (2007). Maternal emotion socialization in maltreating and non-maltreating families: Implications for children's emotion regulation. *Social Development, 16(2)*, 268–285.

Simonds, J., Kieras, J., Rueda, R., & Rothbart, M.K. (2007). Effortful control, executive attention, and emotional regulation in 7- to 10-year-old children. *Cognitive Development, 22(4)*, 474–488.

Simonds, J. & Rothbart, M.K. (2004). The Temperament in Middle Childhood Questionnaire (TMCQ): A computerized self-report measure of temperament for ages 7–10. Poster session presented at the *Occasional Temperament Conference*, Athens, GA.

Smitherman, C.H. (1996). Child and caretaker attributes associated with lead poisoning in young children. *Pediatric Nursing, 22*, 320–326.

Stern, D. (1985). *The interpersonal world of the infant*. New York: Basic Books.

Strelau, J. (2000). *Temperament: A psychological perspective*. New York: Plenum.

Thomas, A., & Chess, S. (1977). *Temperament and development*. New York: Brunner & Mazel.

Thompson, R.A., Lewis, M.D., & Calkins, S.D. (2008). Reassessing emotional regulation. *Child Development Perspectives, 2(3)*, 124–131.

Tincas, I., Benga, O., & Fox, N.A. (2006). Temperamental predictors of anxiety disorders. *Cognitie Creier Comportament, 10(4)*, 489–515.

Trentacosta, C.J., & Shaw, D.S. (2009) Emotional self-regulation, peer rejection, and antisocial behavior: Developmental associations from early childhood to early adolescence. *Journal of Applied Developmental Psychology, 30(3)*, 356–365.

Tucker, D.M., Derryberry, D., & Luu, P. (2000). Anatomy and physiology of human emotion: Vertical integration of brain stem, limbic and cortical systems. In J.C. Borod (Ed.). *The neuropsychology of emotion: Series in affective science* (pp. 56–79). New York: Oxford University Press.

van der Kolk, B.A. (1996). The complexity of adaptation to trauma: Self-regulation, stimulus discrimination, and characterological development. In B.A. van der Kolk, A.C. McFarlane, & L. Weisaeth (Eds.). *Traumatic stress: The effects of overwhelming experience on mind, body, and society* (pp. 182–213). New York, NY: Guilford Press.

Vaughn, M.G., Beaver, K.M., DeLisi, M., Perron, B.E., & Schelbe, L. (2009). Gene-environment interplay and the importance of self-control in predicting polydrug use and substance-related problems. *Addictive Behaviors, 34*(1), 112–116.

Vygotsky, L.S. (2004). Imagination and creativity in childhood. *Journal of Russian & East European Psychology, 42*(1), 7–97.

Windle, M., & Lerner, R.M. (1986). Reassessing the dimensions of temperamental individuality across the life span: The Revised Dimensions of Temperament Survey (DOTS-R). *Journal of Adolescent Research, 1*, 213–230.

Yates, P.M., & Kingston, D.A. (2006). The self-regulation model of sexual offending: The relationship between offence pathways and static and dynamic sexual offence risk. *Sexual Abuse, 18*(3), 259–270.

Zeier, J.D., Maxwell, J.S., & Newman, J.P. (2009). Attention moderates the processing of inhibitory information in primary psychopathy. *Journal of Abnormal Psychology, 118* (3), 554–563.

Zentner, M., & Bates, J.E. (2008). Child temperament: An integrative review of concepts, research programs, and measures. *European Journal of Developmental Science, 2*, 7–37.

Zwaigenbaum, L., Bryson, S., Rogers, T., Roberts, W., Brian, J., & Szatmari, P. (2005). Behavioral manifestations of autism in the first year of life. *International Journal of Developmental Neuroscience, 23*, 143–152.

3

Neurobiology and Neurophysiology of Behavioral/Psychiatric Disorders

Lawrence D. Scahill and Susan Boorin

Objectives

After reading this chapter, APNs will be able to

1. Identify the significant neurobiological issues that influence the development of child/adolescent psychiatric disorders.
2. Identify the anatomy of the central nervous system and the brain that are involved in development of psychiatric disorders.

3. Note influences on the development of the brain.
4. Discuss implications of neurobiological issues on APN practice, education, and research.

Introduction

The mind, it may be said, is the product of physiological mechanisms within the nervous system that form the biological basis of behavior (Blumenfeld, 2002). The nervous system is composed of several cell types that are assembled into the central and peripheral systems during development. Abnormalities in the organization of the nervous system can occur due to genetic causes, environmental exposures (e.g., *in utero* or injury), or gene-environment interaction. Knowledge about the biological basis of behavior has accumulated through case studies that show a range of clinical abnormalities associated with specific brain injuries. More recently, animal studies and advances in neuroimaging have contributed to an explosion of information on neuronal circuitry. These advances have a bearing on several psychiatric disorders such as attention deficit hyperactivity disorder (ADHD), autism, anxiety disorders, depression, substance abuse, and schizophrenia, to name a few. The abnormalities associated with these disorders, although often subtle, may explain pathological activity in the absence of a specific lesion (Insel & Quirion, 2005). Understanding the etiology and treatment of major psychiatric disorders can be strengthened through examination of brain development, structures, and function.

This explosion of neurobiology is not only relevant to the etiology of child psychiatric disorders; it may guide the selection of treatment in the coming decade. This chapter begins with an examination of neuroanatomy and brain development that forms the foundation of understanding and discourse about the connection of neurobiology and behavior. It goes on to consider neurotransmission and specific neurotransmitters, which offers the possibility to discuss the role of neurobiology in selected psychiatric disorders and the rationale for treatment. The chapter concludes with implications for APN practice, education, and research.

Child and Adolescent Behavioral Health: A Resource for Advanced Practice Psychiatric and Primary Care Practitioners in Nursing,
First Edition. Edited by Edilma L. Yearwood, Geraldine S. Pearson, and Jamesetta A. Newland.
© 2012 John Wiley & Sons, Inc. Published 2012 by John Wiley & Sons, Inc.

Anatomy of the Central Nervous System

The central nervous system (CNS) comprises the brain and spinal cord; the peripheral nervous system includes the twelve pairs of cranial nerves and all the remaining nerves of the body. The CNS evolves from the neural tube, which emerges from the neural plate early in fetal development through an organized process of cellular folding called neurulation. Neurulation appears to be similar in all vertebrates. The adult brain is organized according to its embryonic scheme with the anterior portion of the neural tube developing into the brain and the posterior portion developing into the spinal cord. The fluid-filled cavities within the neural tube develop into ventricles, which contain cerebral spinal fluid. Because the brain grows more rapidly than the membranous skull that contains it, the cerebral hemispheres are forced to grow posteriorly and laterally. This causes the growing brain to crease and fold, producing convolutions that increase the surface area. The cerebral hemispheres of the newborn resemble a mushroom enveloping a stem of the diencephalon and midbrain (Marieb, 2004). Brain development continues rapidly in the postnatal period. By the age of six years the total size of the brain is approximately 90% of its adult size. As the child matures into an adolescent, there are age-related changes in white and gray matter volume which continues into young adulthood (Tamnes et al., 2010).

Cranial Vault and Meninges

The brain is protected by hard bones that form the skull and three meningeal layers: pia, arachnoid, and dura. These can be remembered by the mnemonic "PAD" from the interior layer to the outer layer. The word dura means "hard," and like its name the dura is composed of two fibrous layers. The arachnoid is a wispy meningeal layer. The pia adheres closely to the surface of the brain, and follows the folds of the brain. The major arteries of the brain run between the arachnoid and pia layers, and this area is called the subarachnoid space (Blumenfeld, 2002). Recent advances in diagnostic imaging have enhanced the understanding of neurovascular anatomy. The arterial and venous vascular network is extensive with notable individual differences (Borden, 2007).

Blood-Brain Barrier, Blood-CSF Barrier

The blood-brain barrier (BBB) is formed by endothelial cells that line an extensive capillary system in the brain (Abott, Ronnback, & Hanson, 2006). The BBB has a large surface area, and regulates what enters and exits the CNS. The distinguishing feature of the BBB endothelial cells—compared to endothelial cells in the periphery—is the presence of tight junctions between the cells. Because

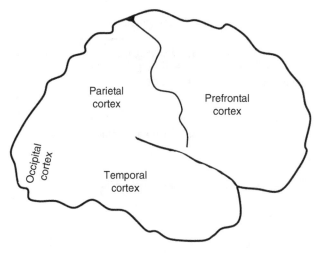

Figure 3.1 Lobes of the cerebral cortex. [Adapted from Arnsten & Castellanos (2011), with permission from Oxford University Press.]

the BBB has continuous tight junctions, molecules are forced to cross the BBB. Certain drugs and small gases can cross an intact BBB; however, specific transport systems regulate much of the traffic (Deeken & Loscher, 2007).

The choroids plexus (CP) is located in all four cerebral ventricles and produces cerebral spinal fluid (CSF). Together with the arachnoid membrane it constitutes the blood-CSF barrier. Increasing evidence indicates that the integrity of the brain tissue-blood barriers plays an important role in brain immune response and neuro-inflammation (Hickey, 2001; Szmydynger-Chodobska, Stazielle, Zink, Ghersi-Egea, & Chodobski, 2009). For example, oxidative stress, which is a common feature in the pathogenesis of many neuroinflammatory conditions, may contribute to the disruption of the BBB. Blood-brain barrier breakdown plays an important role in the pathogenesis of HIV–1 associated dementia (Chaudhuri, Duan, Morsey, Persidsky, & Kanmogne, 2008).

Cerebral Cortex

The cerebral cortex (Figure 3.1) is the outer layer of the cerebral hemispheres, and it is responsible for sensory perception, movement, language, thinking, memory, consciousness, and certain aspects of emotion (Hendelman, 2006). Comprised of billions of neurons and vast interconnections, it is divided into four major lobes (Table 3.1). The majority of the cerebral cortex is composed of neocortex, which has six cell layers labeled I through VI, counting from the surface inward. Neurons in each layer differ in their functional contribution to cerebral processing. The cerebral cortex was mapped out based on fifty-two cytoarchitectonic regions by the neuroanatomist Brodmann in 1909. For example, specifically numbered Brodmann areas located in the somatosensory

Table 3.1 Major divisions of the cerebral cortex

Lobes	Selected structure	Primary function	Symptoms related to damage
Frontal lobes	Prefrontal cortex	Attention, working memory, impulse control	Deficits in working memory, lack of ability to plan for the future, lack of executive functioning (insight, reasoning, judgment, concept formation)
	Primary motor cortex	Voluntary movement	
	Supplementary motor cortex	Planning movement	
	Broca's area	Speech production	
Parietal lobes	Primary somatosensory cortex	Processing of sensory input, orienting attention	Complex sensory deficits; decreased spatial cognition, sustained attention, and visual selective attention; difficulty understanding actions of others
Occipital lobes	Primary visual cortex	Processing visual input	Decreased visual integration of information, color vision
Temporal lobes	Auditory cortex	Processing auditory input	Deficits in auditory processing, word finding difficulties, impaired language production, prosopagnosia facial (blindness)
	Wernicke's area	Language production	
	Fusiform gyrus	Facial and object recognition	

cortex play a role in touch (Blumenfeld, 2002). It is generally agreed that the human neocortex has increased a 1,000-fold in surface size and cytoarchitectonic areas since early mammalian ancestors. However, because cortical neurons are not generated within the cortex itself, questions remain regarding how each neuron reaches its appropriate position (Rakic, Ayoub, Breunig, & Dominguez, 2009). A visual animation of Rakic's model of neuronal migration in the development of the cerebral cortex can be found at his Yale University website: rakiclab.med.yale.edu/

Cortical-Subcortical Connections

Over the past twenty-five years, a substantial amount of research has focused on brain pathways that connect cortical and subcortical structures. Table 3.2 lists the major subcortical structures, primary functions, and connections. Brain circuitry is a vast topic that is beyond the scope of this chapter. However, the principles and structural components can be illustrated through a brief review of dopamine circuits. In a landmark paper, Alexander, DeLong, and Strick (1986) described five parallel, minimally overlapping dopamine circuits. These circuits have a common architectural loop from the cortex to the striatum, globus pallidus, thalamus, and back to cortex. The communication between the striatum and thalamus is through the globus pallidus, which regulates the connection between the striatum and thalamus. The names of these cortico-striatal-thalamic-cortical loops

are derived from their cortical origin. For example, the motor circuit arises from the primary motor strip (Figure 3.2). The dorsolateral prefrontal circuit has its origin in the dorsolateral prefrontal region and plays an important role in attention, impulse control, and planning. The circuit emanating from the anterior cingulate plays a role in emotion regulation (Alexander et al., 1986).

Another way to describe dopamine circuits is to trace the pathway from the subcortical origin to the cortex. For example, the nigro-striatal circuit arises from the substantial nigra to the striatum, with connections proceeding to the globus pallidus, thalamus, and motor cortex. Similarly, the mesolimbic circuit has its origin in the ventral tegmental area and courses to the nucleus accumbens (often called the reward circuit). The mesocortical circuit also has its origin in the ventral tegmental area, but it projects directly to the prefrontal cortex. The tuberoinfundibular pathway is yet another dopamine circuit that warrants mention due to its relevance to antipsychotic medications. Signals from the hypothalamus influence secretion of prolactin. Potent D2 blocking agents such as haloperidol or risperidone result in an increase in prolactin due to blockade of D2 receptors in the tuberoinfundibular system (Findling, McNamara, & Gracious, 2003).

Synaptic Organization of the Brain

Brain circuits integrate vast amounts of information to guide biological, behavioral, and cognitive functions.

Table 3.2 Major subcortical structures, primary functions, and connections

Structure	Location	Primary function	Primary connections
Thalamus	Telencephalon	Sensory-motor integration	Cortex, basal ganglia, amygdala
Hypothalamus	Diencephalon	Appetite, temperature regulation, sleep, mood regulation	Pituitary, hippocampus, amygdala
*Basal ganglia	Telencephalon	Motor	Cortex, thalamus
Hippocampus	Temporal region	Learning and memory	Cortex, cingulate, amygdala, thalamus
Amygdala	Temporal region, anterior to hippocampus	Emotion regulation, coordination of fear response	Thalamus, cortex, locus coeruleus
Ventral tegmental area	Midbrain (inferior to the diencephalon)	Behavioral reinforcement, motivation	Nucleus accumbens, cortex
Substantia nigra	Midbrain (just inferior to the diencephalon)	Motor	Putamen, caudate

*The basal ganglia are gray matter structures that are highly connected to the cortex and other subcortical structures such as the thalamus and hypothalamus.

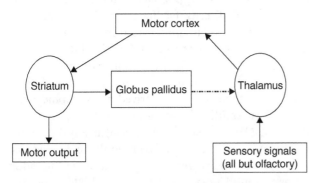

Figure 3.2 The motor circuit, which is one of five dopamine circuits traversing specific regions of the cortex through the striatum, globus pallidus, thalamus, and back to the cortex.

These neural circuits change and develop as a child matures, influenced not only by genetic predispositions but also by unique environmental exposures and experiences. Neurons, dendrites, axons, and supporting glial cells are important components of these neural circuits (Tau & Peterson, 2010).

The Neuron

There are 10^{11} (one hundred billion) neurons in the central nervous system that process information (Heckers, Konradi, & Anderson, 2011). Although neurons include the same organelles found in all cells,

their structure is specialized to enable intercellular communication. The neuron, which is composed of a cell body, dendrites, and axons, has the ability to receive and integrate information from multiple inputs. In addition, neurons can send information to other neurons, muscles, and organs. Communication between neurons takes place at the synapse via chemical neurotransmitter molecules.

Dendrites and Dendritic Spines

Dendrites, which are the primary target for synaptic input from other neurons, appear as a vast branching structure also known as the dendritic arbor. The smallest structural unit of the dendritic arbor is the dendritic spine. These small (1 to 2 μm) thorn-like projections play a key role in post-synaptic signaling. The morphology of a mature spine consists of an expanded head connected to a thinner stalk. The maturity of the dendritic spine influences the strength and number of neuronal connections (Kasai, Matsuzaki, Noguchi, Yasumatsu, & Nakahara, 2003). The central role of dendritic spines in learning and memory is illustrated by fragile X, which a genetically inherited mental retardation syndrome characterized by intellectual deficits. In fragile X, dendritic spines are few in number and fail to mature (Dolen & Bear, 2008).

Axons and Cerebral White Matter

Axons are myelinated fiber pathways that constitute cerebral white matter. White matter tracts can be grouped into five bundles: association fibers, striatal fibers, commissural fibers, thalamic fibers, and pontine fibers. These tracts reflect the anatomical location of the cortical connection. Association fibers are cortical-cortical connections within the hemisphere; commissural fibers are also cortical-cortical connections, but across hemispheres. The names of the other tracts directly refer to location (Schmahmann, Smith, Eighler, & Filley, 2008). During development, axons migrate through the CNS guided by cues from the surrounding cellular environment, and follow behind the leading edge of their structure known as growth cones (Gitai, Zu, Lundquists, Tessier-Lavigne, & Bargmann, 2003). In addition to linking brain structures that are relatively far apart, axons also form relatively short circuits (interneurons) (Purves et al., 2008).

Glia astrocytes and oligodendrocytes are the two main types of glial cells in the CNS. Historically, the function of glial cells has been relegated to the provision of support for neurons. Research conducted over the last decade shows that these cells have an important role in synaptic transmission and the modulation of neuronal activity (Halassa, Fellin, & Hayden, 2006). For example, oligodendrocytes provide insulation and support for axons, which improves the efficiency of nerve signals along the axon. Astrocytes play a role in glutamate transmission, which in turn plays an essential role in learning and memory (Halassa et al., 2006). Emerging evidence also suggests that astrocytes play a key role in the integration of neuronal and vascular activity (Barres, 2008). Thus, increases in local neuronal activity promote changes in cerebral blood flow to sustain the neuronal activity (Haydon & Carmignoto, 2006). This local physiological action is exploited in functional magnetic resonance imaging (fMRI). Changes in astrocyte activation may contribute to the pathophysiology of Lyme disease, Alzheimer's disease, and amyotrophic lateral sclerosis (Dotevall, Hagberg, Karlsson, & Rosengren, 1999; Rossi & Volterra, 2009).

Learning and Memory: Synaptic Plasticity

Learning and memory are concepts used to explain how experience influences behavior (Rudy, 2008). The brain is able to capture and store the range of content from our experiences. There are two broad types of memory: declarative memory and procedural memory. Declarative memory is specific recall of events, facts, and figures. Procedural memory involves skill acquisition such as riding a bicycle, playing the violin, or pitching a curve ball. Learning and memory involve an impressive array of brain structures and connections including the cortex, medial temporal lobe, striatum, amygdala, cerebellum, and hippocampus (Milner, Squire, & Kandel, 1998). At the center of learning and memory is the synapse. In 1973, Bliss and Lomo showed that synaptic connections can be modified by experience. For example, an isolated weak stimulus evokes commensurate synaptic activity in a specialized region of the hippocampus called the dentate gyrus. When a stronger stimulus is delivered, it evokes a larger synaptic response. If this stronger stimulus is followed by repeated stimuli (even a weaker stimulus) down the same pathway, the evoked response will also be large. This is because repeated neuron-to-neuron connection strengthens the communication (called Hebb's rule). Ultimately, as the connection strengthens, the signal required to "send the message" is reduced (long-term potentiation).

Development of the Central Nervous System

Development is a series of progressive changes that results in elaboration of specialized cell types from a single cell. All types of somatic cells retain all of the genes that are present in the fertilized egg (nuclear equivalence). However, genetically identical cells differentiate over time under the influence of specific genes during development. Genes control development through transcription factors and growth factors (signals from neighboring cells). Transcription factors reside in the neuron cell body and directly facilitate protein transcription. The rare mental retardation syndrome called Rubstein-Taybi syndrome is due to a mutation that interferes with transcription factor activity resulting in dysmorphic features, skeletal abnormalities, and intellectual disability.

The growth factor brain-derived neurotrophic factor (BDNF) is essential for the growth of axons and dendrites. BDNF also plays a role in learning and memory. For many years, there was a commonly held belief that neurons were incapable of regeneration in the adult human brain. Under the influence of BDNF, however, it is clear that neurogenesis does occur in the mature brain, at least in the specialized cells of the dentate gyrus. Recent studies have shown that successful treatment of depression with antidepressant medications promotes neurogenesis in this region (Duman, 2009).

Early Gestational Events in the Development of the Nervous System

There is rapid cell proliferation but little gene differentiation following fertilization. Within weeks, however, cells coalesce into the blastocyte to form three primary layers: the endoderm, mesoderm, and ectoderm. This critical stage of development is called gastrulation. Gastrulation involves migration of cells, which permits opportunities for one cell to influence the development of a neighboring cell. Soon after gastrulation, the growing ball of cells begins to fold and extend to form the neural tube. This eventually orients the brain anteriorly and the spinal cord posteriorly. The closure of the tube is subject to environmental impact. For example, folate deficiency in pregnancy increases the risk of spina bifida. By week four of gestation, the neural tube is separated into regions called the proencephalon (forebrain), mesencephalon (midbrain), and rhombencephaplon (hindbrain) (Gilbert, 2006).

This anterior to posterior scheme for the developing brain is under genetic control (Vaccarino & Leckman, 2011). Neuronal migration peaks at gestational weeks twelve and twenty and is largely completed by gestational weeks twenty-six to twenty-nine (Tau & Peterson, 2010). As axons continue to grow and synapses are formed, more complex neuronal circuits emerge. Apoptosis, defined as programmed cell death, helps to regulate brain development and specialization.

Brain Development and Synaptogenesis

Total brain volume increases throughout the first years of life and then stabilizes. By the age of six, the total size of the brain is about 90% of its adult size. Growth in gray matter volume is rapid in early childhood followed by a decline in adolescence (Ostby et al., 2009). This expansion of gray matter in the first few years of life is coincident with intensive axonal growth and dendritic arborization. By contrast, white matter volume increase follows a more linear path (Tamnes et al, 2010). Using MRI in both cross-sectional and longitudinal studies of typically developing children between four and twenty years of age, investigators have shown an increase in white matter of 12% to 25% during this time interval (Ment, Hirtz, & Huppi, 2009). The volume and density of white matter usually increase with age until the fifth decade (Kumar & Chugani, 2009).

Synaptogenesis, or formation of synaptic connections in the human cortex, begins *in utero* and continues during the first two postnatal years. Peak synaptic density is reached at different times throughout the cortex. For example, the prefrontal cortex achieves maximum density at about fifteen months of age; primary sensory areas achieve maximum density at an even younger age (Huttenlocher & Dabholkar, 1997). After peaking in the first few postnatal years, synaptic density stabilizes and then starts to decline around seven years of age. Synaptic density reaches adult levels in the auditory cortex by twelve years and the prefrontal cortex by mid-adolescence (Tau & Peterson, 2010). Early synaptogenesis appears to be intrinsically regulated (controlled by the cell itself). By contrast, is the formation of new synapses that occurs later in life are related to learning and memory (Huttenlocher & Dabholkar, 1997).

Development of Neural Circuits: Age-Related Maturation

Executive function (EF) is a commonly used term that reflects the role of the prefrontal cortex in the regulation of attention and impulse control, as well as planning and working memory (the short-term memory we use in everyday life to guide behavior). Studies using fMRI have shown that an improving capacity for cognitive control with advancing age is associated with increasing activation of frontal-subcortical circuits involving the striatum and thalamus (Tau & Peterson, 2010). As children progress through developmental stages, the capacity of the frontal lobe to regulate and monitor behavior increases. The period of greatest expansion in executive function is probably between six and eight years of age, with continued expanded capacity in adolescence (Ellison & Semrud-Clikeman, 2007).

Measurement of EF has most often been represented by pencil and paper tests during a structured testing session. Two issues relevant to test results should be considered. First, a child can score within the normal range for one aspect of EF and yet sustain deficits in another. This may be due to developmental differences or an actual lag in specific aspects of EF. Second, pencil and paper testing of working memory or attention performed in a structured environment may not reflect the child's strengths or weaknesses in real world settings (Goulden & Silver, 2009). For clinicians, this highlights the importance of gathering information from multiple settings to make judgments about EF in home and school settings.

Neurotransmission

In the previous sections we examined the gross anatomy of the brain, the architecture of the neuron, and the capacity of the neuron to receive and transmit information. At the center of neurotransmission is the synapse (Shepherd, 2004). It is fitting to describe brain connections as circuits that are dedicated to particular brain activities. Although the image of circuitry conjures up a notion of electrical connections, the circuitry of the brain is both electrical and neurochemical. Unlike wiring in a house or in electronic devices, the pathways in the brain do not have "wire-to-wire connection." Indeed, the final transmission of the signal is through a neurochemical. There are several neurochemicals in the brain. In this section, we review the neurotransmitters that are most common to illustrate general principles of neurotransmission and to provide brain-behavior connection. The selected neurotransmitters for this review include dopamine, norepinephrine, serotonin, acetylcholine, GABA, and glutamate (Cooper, Bloom, & Roth, 2003).

Signal Transduction

Before considering these specific neurotransmitter systems, we examine how neurotransmitters carry out their functions. In a simplified model, neurotransmission begins with the firing of the neuron (e.g., the dopamine firing neurons of the substantia nigra). This causes the stimulus to travel down the axon, and release of the neurotransmitter at the terminal nerve ending into the synapse. Once released, the neurotransmitter binds to postsynaptic receptors. Binding of the neurotransmitter to the postsynaptic receptor is often the first of many events. For example, binding may promote the passage of ions across the membrane of the postsynaptic receptor, resulting in depolarization and an action potential. Thus, the first, simplest classification of receptors is presynaptic and postsynaptic (Heckers, Konradi, & Anderson, 2011; Rudy, 2008) (Figure 3.3).

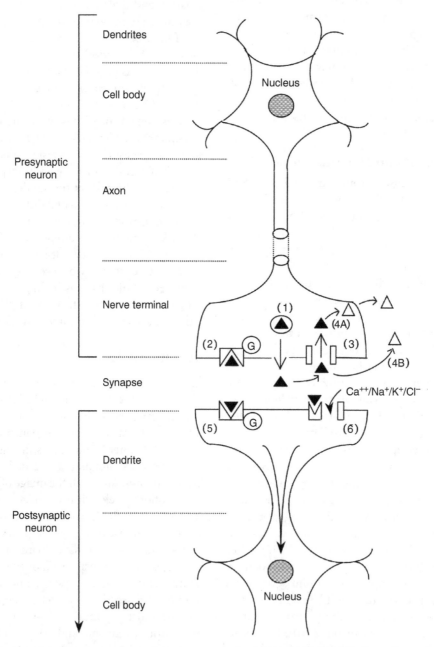

Figure 3.3 Basic structure of the neuron. The figure shows the presynaptic and postsynaptic junction (synapse). The solid triangles illustrate neurotransmitter release from the presynaptic neuron (1), binding at the postsynaptic neuron (5,6), autoreceptor (2), and reuptake transporter (3); open triangles depict enzymatic degradation (4). The figure also shows the movement of ions into the postsynaptic nerve ending (6) and metabotropic or G-coupled receptor binding (5) (see text for details). [Adapted from Heckers, Konradi, & Anderson (2011), with permission from Oxford University Press.]

However, there are several other systems that need to be considered in this simplified model. For example, once a neurotransmitter is released into the synaptic space, there must be various systems to return that synapse back to its resting state. This is accomplished by several actions. Perhaps the most active method is through reuptake of the released transmitter by the transporter. The transporter resides on the presynaptic nerve ending and, through active transport, recovers the released neurotransmitter and pulls it back into the presynaptic nerve ending.

Other important regulatory receptors include autoreceptors and enzymatic breakdown. Autoreceptors take readings on the amount of transmitter in the synapse and regulate synthesis and release of the neurotransmitter through signaling back to the presynaptic nerve ending. A familiar example of enzymatic breakdown is monoamine oxidase (MAO), which inactivates dopamine, norepinephrine, and serotonin. MAO resides in the synaptic cleft and in greater amounts inside the presynaptic nerve ending.

Many neurotransmitters in the presynaptic nerve ending reside in vesicles, which protect the neurotransmitter from degrading enzymes such as monoamine oxidase. In addition, they are an effective way to control the amount of released neurotransmitter. When the signal moves down the axon to the terminal end, it causes the vesicle to migrate to the surface of the presynaptic nerve ending and releases its contents into the synapse. Therefore, we expand our simple receptor type 2 postsynaptic and presynaptic to include the transporter and the autoreceptor (Cooper et al., 2003).

Another way to classify receptor subtypes includes ionotropic and metabotropic receptors. Ionotropic, also called ligand gated, receptors are marked by their capacity to mediate rapid effects when activated by a neurotransmitter. The ionotropic receptors are directly linked to an ion channel. Ion channels are actual pores that allow specific ions to move across the membrane of the postsynaptic receptor. In the resting state, the intracellular environment is enriched with potassium and the extracellular environment is enriched with sodium. When there is a movement of sodium ions from outside the cell to inside the cell, there is a change in electrical potential. In this example, the change in electric potential is called depolarization (the voltage difference across the cell membrane is less negative compared to the resting state). The general structure is composed of four or five subunits, or leaves. When there is binding to the receptor, there is a conformational change in the receptor, which allows the movement of ions across the membrane. These ions' channels are specific. The biological effects depend on whether the ion is positive or negative. The movement of sodium ions into the intercellular fluid causes depolarization. Hyperpolarization occurs when there is a movement of negative ions into the cell (e.g., chloride ions), which makes the voltage difference between the external environment and the internal environment more negative. Hyperpolarization inhibits signal transduction (Cooper et al., 2003).

The other, and much larger, brain receptor family is the metabotropic type. In contrast to ionotropic receptors, the metabotropic receptors exert biological activity on a slower time course. The metabotropic receptors are also called G-coupled protein receptors, reflecting their general structure. The metabotropic receptors have several features in common as well as differences. As with the ionotropic receptors, metabotropic receptors have an extracellular and intracellular terminal. The structure of the internal terminal is complex and composed of so-called alpha, beta, and gamma subunits at rest. These subunits are bound inside the cell membrane and to each other. When there is binding at the receptor, the alpha unit separates away from its companion beta and gamma subunits and begins one or more specific intracellular events. For example, it may initiate the opening of an ion channel as described above with ionotropic receptors. By contrast, the alpha subunit may bind to specific proteins inside the cell and begin a cascade of intracellular activities resulting in turning on a gene for protein synthesis (Cooper et al., 2003).

Neurotransmitters

Dopamine

The primary neurons that produce dopamine firings are the substantia nigra and ventral tegmental area. The projections on the substantia nigra are central to the motor system, sending projections to the striatum (caudate and putamen). The projections of the ventral tegmental area go to the ventral striatum (nucleus accumbens) and cortical regions. When these dopamine neurons fire, they cause the signal to move along specific axonal pathways organized to carry out specific functions. When the signal makes it way to the terminal end, dopamine is released. As shown in Table 3.3, all dopamine receptors are metabotropic.

Table 3.3 Major families of receptors in the central nervous system

Transmitter	Ionotropic	Metabotropic
Dopamine		DA1-5
Norepinephrine		Alpha-1, -2, beta -1, -2, -3
Serotonin	5-HT3	5-HT1, 2, 4, 5, 6, 7
Acetylcholine	Nicotinic	Muscarinic
Glutamate	AMPA, NMDA	mGluR1-5
Gamma-aminobutyric acid	GABAA	GABAB

Dopamine is central to many functions in the brain. Perhaps most familiar is its role in movement. The loss of dopamine-firing neurons in the substantia nigra over time is directly related to the onset and course of Parkinson disease. The nigrostrial (s. nigra to striatum) pathway plays a central role in the coordination of movement. Other dopaminergic pathways have their origin in the neighboring nuclei of the ventral tegmental area (Green & Ostrander, 2009).

There are two main families of dopamine receptors, called D1 type and D2 type. Over time it has been discovered that the D1 type includes D1 and D5 receptor types; D2 receptors, D2, D3, and D4. It is not surprising, given the multiple actions of dopamine in the brain, that these dopamine receptor subtypes are located in specific areas of the brain. For example, D1 and D2 receptors are distributed liberally in the striatum, but few are found in the cortex. By contrast, D4 receptors are more commonly found in the cortex.

Alterations in dopamine transmission have been implicated in several major psychiatric disorders including schizophrenia, substance abuse, and attention deficit hyperactivity disorder, and neuropsychiatric conditions such as Tourette syndrome, Parkinson disease, and Huntington chorea. The role of dopamine in these disorders varies by disorder. For example, symptoms of Parkinson disease begin when there is a 70% reduction in dopamine-firing neurons in the substantia nigra (Jankovic & Tolosa, 2007). Similarly, the well-known Parkinsonian adverse effects in patients treated with potent D2 blockers such as haloperidol are due to blockade of D2 receptors in the striatum. In the case of antipsychotic medications, the substantia nigra may be firing, but dopamine is not allowed to bind with these receptors, resulting in a picture that mimics Parkinson disease (Findling et al., 2003).

The evidence of the role of dopamine in schizophrenia emerged primarily from the observation that potent D2 blockers reduce positive symptoms of schizophrenia such as hallucinations and delusions. In addition, repeated use of dopamine enhancing agents such as amphetamine can mimic the positive symptoms of schizophrenia. As will be discussed later, however, the dopamine hypothesis of schizophrenia does not sufficiently account for the negative symptoms (poverty of thought, low motivation, etc.) of schizophrenia. At the risk of oversimplification, the negative symptoms of schizophrenia appear to be due to abnormality in the mesocortical circuit and the positive symptoms due to abnormality in the mesolimbic circuit (Cooper et al., 2003).

The support for the role of dopamine in drug addiction is emerging as a complex interaction between dopamine and other neurotransmitter systems, especially glutamate.

Dopamine is known to play a central role in the reward circuit (the mesolimbic circuit mentioned earlier). Not surprisingly, many drugs of abuse cause a release of dopamine and stimulate the reward circuit. Over the past decade, mounting evidence from animal and human studies indicates that glutamatergic input from the cortex to the striatum appears to play a role in craving and the actual drug-seeking behavior (Kalivas, 2009).

The evidence of the supporting role of dopamine in attention deficit hyperactivity disorder (ADHD) is substantial. The positive effects of stimulant drugs, which enhance dopamine function in the brain, provide indirect evidence that dopamine plays a role in ADHD. Of particular interest is the dorsolateral prefrontal circuit, which is known to play an important role in the executive functions of attention and planning (Arnsten, 2009). Data from more than one MRI study have shown a slight but significant decrease in cortical volume for children with ADHD (Castellanos & Proal, 2009). Functional MRI studies also show reduced activity in the prefrontal region during the performance of neuropsychological tasks of attention and impulse control in children with ADHD compared to controls (Pliszka et al., 2006).

Given the effectiveness of methylphenidate in treating ADHD (MTA Cooperative Group, 1999) and the strong evidence supporting the role of dopamine in attention and impulse control, there has been tremendous interest in various dopamine genes as candidate genes that could underlie ADHD (Banaschewski, Becker, Scherag, Franke, & Coghill, 2010). For example, much interest has been focused on the dopamine transporter gene (*DAT1* gene). The action of this gene may influence the efficiency of the dopamine transporter in clearing out dopamine to the synapse. This possibility is supported by the pharmacological action of methylphenidate, which promotes release and blocks reuptake of dopamine at the transporter.

Another gene of great interest is the dopamine D4 receptor (*DRD4*) gene. This receptor resides in the cortex and quite likely plays a role in attention and impulse control. Several genetic association studies have shown that individuals with ADHD are more likely to have a particular variant of the gene (Li, Sham, Owen, & He, 2006). This variant of the *DRD4* has also been associated with the personality trait of novelty seeking, though this finding has not always been replicated (Gelernter et al., 1997). Another potentially important gene is the *SNAP-25* gene (Li et al., 2006). This gene affects the release of dopamine from presynaptic vesicles (where the neurotransmitter is contained prior to release). These genes reflect areas of active research that may inform treatment in the future.

In many ways, the term "inattention" is somewhat ambiguous. Presumably it refers to the inability to pay attention. However, discussion with many parents of children with ADHD often results in comments such as, "He can spend hours on playing video games, but can't pay attention in school." This common observation suggests that there is something fundamentally different about the attention required for highly stimulating video games versus the attention required to listen in the classroom or read a book. This difference has been described as bottom-up versus top-down attention. In bottom-up attention, the bright lights and catchy sound effects of video games engage parietal and temporal cortices, which do not require great mental effort. By contrast, a teacher's lecture requires top-down attention and engagement of the prefrontal cortex (Arnsten, 2009). In this model, children with ADHD have difficulty engaging the prefrontal cortex to select and maintain focus on tasks requiring mental effort (e.g., a teacher's lecture).

The right inferior prefrontal cortex is specialized for behavioral inhibition. Impaired functioning in this region presumably contributes to impulsiveness and hyperactivity. The ventral medial prefrontal cortex is specialized for emotional regulation. At the risk of oversimplification, it might be said that impaired prefrontal cortical function contributes to aggression, obsessional behavior, and perhaps even conduct disorder. The regulation of attention involves the inhibition of external stimuli other than the chosen stimuli, and inhibition of internal stimuli as well.

Norepinephrine

The above discussion on ADHD focused on the relevance of dopamine in ADHD. It should be noted, however, that norepinephrine also likely plays an important role in attention-deficit hyperactivity disorder (Arnsten, 2009). The effectiveness of norepinephrine affecting medications such as guanfacine and atomoxetine further supports the notion that norepinephrine also influences ADHD symptoms (Arnsten, 2009).

Norepinephrine-firing neurons are located in the locus coeruleus situated at the top of the brainstem. These neurons send signals to virtually all areas of the brain and are involved in basic physiological functions such as heart rate, blood pressure, breathing, and higher cortical functions (Arnsten, 2009). Norepinephrine is known to play a central role in the so-called fight-or-flight reaction. The projections from the locus coeruleus go to the prefrontal cortex, cingulate, amygdala, hypothalamus, and cerebellum. There are two major types of norepinephrine receptors: alpha-receptors and beta-receptors. Alpha-receptors are further subdivided into alpha-1 and alpha-2 subtypes, each of which also has subtypes. For example, the alpha-2A receptor plays a role in attention and impulse control and is implicated in the action of the medication guanfacine (Arnsten, 2009). All

norepeinephrine receptors belong to the metabotropic family of receptors.

For both dopamine and norepinephrine, there appears to be a "just right" spot for neurotransmitter levels and prefrontal cortex (PFC) function. Low levels of norepinephrine are associated with inattention and impaired impulse control. Likewise, high levels of norepinephrine are also associated with decreased attention and decreased working memory. In the fight-or-flight reaction, there is a dramatic rise in the amount of norepinephrine released, which takes the PFC offline (Arnsten, 2009).

Practically speaking, threatening situations are not moments for weighing options. Rather, these are times for action. Thus, it makes sense for the PFC to go offline. Given this model, it is clear that norepinephrine function is relevant to ADHD and anxiety disorders. In ADHD, it is possible that a failure to regulate norepinephrine levels in the PFC contributes to difficulties with attention, impulse control, and planning.

Recent evidence suggests that the alpha-2A agonist, guanfacine, stimulates these receptors in the prefrontal brain, which may improve prefrontal function (Arnsten, 2009). An extended release form of the drug is now approved for the treatment of attention deficit hyperactivity in children (Scherer & SPD503 Study Group, 2008).

The potential role of norepinephrine in anxiety disorders such as generalized anxiety, panic, and post-traumatic stress disorder (PTSD) is well accepted (Geracioti et al., 2001; Goddard et. al, 2010). For example, perhaps due to genetic vulnerability, environmental exposure, or the interaction of genes and environment, the patient with anxiety disorder is too easily tripped into the fight-or-flight state, mediated by release of norepinephrine. Further support for the role of norepinephrine in anxiety disorders is the direct connection between the locus coeruleus and the amygdala. The amygdala plays an important role in fear and fear conditioning (Davis, 1992). Norepinephrine is certainly not the only player in the complex network of circuitry involved in fear and anxiety. However, a reciprocal connection between the amygdala and the locus coeruleus fits with the fight-or-flight reaction.

The neuroscientist Joseph LeDoux has articulated two amygdala pathways that play a role in mammalian fear response (LeDoux, 2000). LeDoux's model describes a low road (rapid response) and a high road (slower response). In this model, the sensory input goes to the anterior thalamus, which has a direct connection to the amygdala. The output of the amygdala goes to the hypothalamus and locus coeruleus. This causes direct and rapid physiological effects such as increased heart rate, blood pressure, and increased respiration. The slower mode (or the so-called high road) involves a connection from the thalamus to the cortex. In this mode, the sensory input to the anterior thalamus not only signals the amygdala as discussed previously, but it also sends a signal to the cortex. This signal allows consideration of the current threat compared with past events to make an appraisal of threat. The cortex has input to the amygdala, which can then modulate the alarm signals from the amygdala. This is clearly relevant to cognitive behavior therapy, which promotes cortical appraisal of threat to modulate the automatic or rapid mode response.

This idea of perceived threat versus actual threat in generalized anxiety disorder also may be relevant to obsessive-compulsive disorder (OCD) and even to some extent PTSD. For many patients with generalized anxiety disorder (GAD), OCD, or PTSD, life is unpredictable and feels fundamentally unsafe (Woody and Rachman, 1994). The perception of threat is high and perception of safety is low. This overestimation of risk gives rise to increased vigilance and avoidance. In the case of GAD, the focus is on worries of upcoming events and situations. In OCD, particular themes often are the focus of potential harm. For example, worries about contamination prompts washing rituals, or concerns about harm coming to the self or others gives rise to checking compulsions and avoidance. In PTSD, a past experience of trauma heightens the perception of threat and decreases the sense of safety.

The circuitry for fear conditioning has been informed greatly through preclinical studies on acoustic startle. Many mammalian species show a startle reaction to loud noises. The startle reaction has been shown to involve a simple three-synapse sequence that is at least partially mediated by norepinephrine (Davis, 1986). The auditory nerve fibers signal the cochlea, which sends signals to a specialized area in the temporal lobe. From the temporal lobe, the signal travels directly to facial motor neurons (producing the startled expression) and spinal cord (e.g., arching of the back in the frightened cat) (Davis, 1986). Startle can be highly influenced by context. For example, a car backfiring in midday on a busy street would likely induce a startle response for those nearby. The same loud noise at night on a deserted street would produce a larger response. This is called fear-potentiated startle.

Another relevant animal model demonstrates the role of learning in fear responses. In rodents, foot shock produces a characteristic freezing behavior. If a rodent is placed in an environment in which a flash of light (or horn blast) is paired with a foot shock, over time, the light flash alone will induce freezing. If the experiment is continued such that the light flash is repeatedly delivered without the foot shock, the freezing behavior in response to the light flash alone will extinguish. Finally, if the light

flash is once again paired with the foot shock, the freezing response to the light flash alone will occur after fewer repetitions than the original behavioral response (Rogan, Leon, Perez, & Kandel, 2005).

Serotonin

Serotonin (also called 5-hydroxytryptamine or 5-HT) is also a monoamine (like dopamine and norepinephrine). Unlike dopamine and norepinephrine, however, it is not a catecholamine. Serotonin-firing neurons are located in the raphe nucleus, which sits at the top of the brainstem. Examination of the serotonin circuitry shows that it has projection to every area of the brain. Not surprisingly then, it plays a role in several human functions including regulation of mood, emotions, anxiety, memory, aggression, body temperature, sleep, and appetite.

As with the dopamine and norepinephrine receptors, there are multiple types of serotonin receptors. Once again, the location of these receptors is deliberate so that specific serotonin receptor subtypes are dedicated to specific functions. Currently, there are seven major types of serotonin receptors and many of these 5-HT receptors have subtypes. All but one type (5-HT3 receptor) are metabotropic receptors.

A detailed description of these various subtypes and their location is beyond the scope of this discussion. For illustration, however, we note that the serotonin receptor, 5-HT2, resides in the cortex and hippocampus. This receptor subtype is relevant to the action of the atypical antipsychotic medications, which have an antagonist effect at these receptors. The 5-HT7 receptor is located in the thalamus, hippocampus, and amygdala. This receptor is presumed to play a role in fear conditioning and anxiety, as discussed above. Serotonin is believed to play an important role in OCD, depression, and other anxiety disorders. Evidence supporting a role of serotonin in these disorders emanates from the demonstrated effectiveness of the selective serotonin reuptake inhibitor medications in these disorders.

The introduction of the selective serotonin reuptake inhibitors (SSRIs) revolutionized the treatment of depression, OCD, and other anxiety disorders. As suggested by the name, the SSRIs block reuptake at the serotonin transporter, thereby allowing serotonin to remain in the synapse longer. This pharmacological effect of the SSRIs is evident with the very first dose. However, the benefit of the SSRIs in depression, OCD, or other anxiety disorders in children is generally not evident for several weeks (Geller et al., 2003; Hammerness, Vivas, & Geller, 2006; TADS, 2007; Walkup et al., 2008). The explanation of this lag is not clear. The SSRIs have been proposed to be helpful in autism spectrum disorders. When tested in a large-scale, randomized trial, the SSRI citalopram was no better than a placebo in reducing repetitive behavior in children with autism spectrum disorders (King et al., 2009).

Acetylcholine

Acetylcholine is derived from choline and is not an amine. In addition to its role in the CNS, acetylcholine plays a central role in the peripheral nervous system. There are two major classes of acetylcholine receptors, referred to as muscarinic (metabotropic) and nicotinic (ionotropic). This nomenclature is based on their preferential binding to muscarine (poison in mushrooms) or nicotine. There are five identified subtypes of muscarinic receptors and two major subtypes of nicotinic receptors (Cooper et al., 2003; Purves et al., 2008). The organization of the acetylcholine circuitry in the brain is somewhat different from those previously discussed. The primary source of acetylcholine firing is the basal nucleus, which is in the forebrain. It has connections to the prefrontal cortex and parietal cortex. There are also acetylcholine-firing neurons in the brainstem that project to the thalamus and hypothalamus. Finally, there are specialized interneurons in the striatum that appear to play an important role in regulating movement. Acetylcholine pathways have become of great interest due to their potential role in Alzheimer's disease (Hardy, 2009; Hernandez, Kayed, Zheng, Sweatt, & Dineley, 2010).

GABA and Glutamate

The two most common neurotransmitters in the central nervous system are glutamate and gamma-aminobutyric acid (GABA). Glutamate is the major excitatory neurotransmitter and GABA is a major inhibitory transmitter in the central nervous system. Glutamate is synthesized from glucose and GABA is synthesized from glutamate. Glutamate is presumed to play an important role in several disorders including drug addiction, Tourette syndrome, schizophrenia, and the mental retardation syndrome fragile X (Abi-Dargham, 2009; Dolen & Bear, 2008; Kalivas, 2009; Lombroso, Bloch, & Leckman, 2009). In drug addiction, glutamatergic excitatory signals from the cortex to striatum appear to play a role in craving and drug-taking behavior (Kalivas, 2009). Similarly, in Tourette syndrome, signals from the cortex to a different region of striatum may play a role in the dysregulation of the motor circuit and give rise to tic behaviors.

Ionotropic glutamate receptors include NMDA and AMPA receptor types. The NMDA (N-methyl-D-aspartate) receptor is widely distributed in the brain, especially in the cortex and hippocampus, and plays an important role in learning and memory (Berger-Sweeney, Schaevitz, & Frick, 2009). Its molecular structure is complicated with multiple binding sites for glutamate as well as drugs such as phencyclidine (PCP) and ketamine. When stimulated, positive sodium and calcium ions move across the cell membrane, resulting in an excitatory effect. When an impulse travels down the axon and causes a release of glutamate, a series of steps follows that involves first the movement of sodium ions and then calcium ions into the cell. The passage of calcium into the postsynaptic cell produces a large action potential which tends to strengthen the connection between the presynaptic and postsynaptic neuron (Cooper et al., 2003). This enhanced connection is now more ready to respond to subsequent stimulation, even signals of lower magnitude.

The potential role of glutamate in psychiatric disorders can be reviewed by examining the role of glutamate in schizophrenia and fragile X. The role of glutamate in schizophrenia is an exciting and still emerging story. First, the compound PCP is an antagonist of the glutamate NMDA receptor. This drug induces both the positive and negative symptoms of schizophrenia. In contrast, as noted above, dopaminergic compounds, such as high doses of amphetamine, mimic the positive but not the negative symptoms of schizophrenia. PCP has now been recognized to promote dopamine release in the mesolimbic circuit (positive symptoms) and decrease dopaminergic tone in the prefrontal cortex (negative symptoms). These observations suggest an interaction between dopamine and glutamate (Seeman, 2009).

Evidence from cerebrospinal fluid studies indicates a decreased amount of glutamate in schizophrenia compared to control subjects. Postmortem studies have also shown decreased glutamate concentration in the prefrontal cortex and hippocampus in schizophrenia versus controls. Preclinical studies show that NMDA-deficient mice exhibit hyperactivity, stereotypic behavior, and social isolation. These transgenic mice show improvement in hyperactivity and stereotypic behaviors with haloperidol, and show improvement in social isolations when treated with clozapine. These observations have also raised questions about the potential relevance of glutamate in the neurobiology of autism.

The potential role of glutamate in schizophrenia has prompted interest in the development of a glutamate agonist to treat schizophrenia. In a study of 193 adults with schizophrenia, Patil et al. (2007) reported that a novel glutamate agonist was superior to a placebo in reducing both positive and negative symptoms. The positive results of this compound were similar in magnitude to the group that was randomly assigned to olanzapine. These results, although preliminary, show promise that manipulation of the glutamate system could be a useful treatment for schizophrenia. Noting the dynamic interaction of glutamate and dopamine, however, Seeman (2009) proposes dopamine blocking effects (the mechanism of currently available antipsychotics) may also play a role in these observed benefits.

The metabotropic glutamate receptors (mGluRs) include five subtypes (Cooper et al., 2003). Little was known about these metabotropic glutamate receptors until the early 1990s. It is now clear that some of these mGluRs play key roles in learning and memory. This is illustrated by recent findings in fragile X syndrome, an inherited syndrome characterized by intellectual deficits caused by a mutation in the X chromosome in which a specific series of DNA nucleotides is expanded in number. This expansion results in a failure to produce the FMR1 protein. FMR1 appears to play a regulatory role in the maturation of dendritic spines (Dolen & Bear, 2008). As noted above, the maturation of dendritic spines is essential for learning and memory. Recent work by Dolen and Bear has shown that antagonists to mGluRs remediate deficits in fragile X knockout mice from several of the markers of the fragile X syndrome in these animals. These mGluR antagonists are now just beginning to be studied in humans and are an area of great interest. Because there is a relatively high percentage of children with fragile X that also meet diagnostic criteria for autism, there is also interest in whether mGluR antagonists may also be useful in autism.

Conclusions and Implications for Primary Care and Mental Health Nursing Practices

The burgeoning of information on neurobiology over the past twenty-five years is extraordinary and will have an increasing impact on nursing practice in the next decade. In the discourse of primary care practice, we can expect to hear discussion about brain circuitry and the mechanisms of action for psychotropic medications. Primary care providers and mental health clinicians who prescribe medication have an ethical imperative to expand their knowledge about brain function and behavior to practice effectively in this rapidly changing landscape. For example, although we are not quite to the point that genotypes will guide medication selection, this possibility may not be far off. For example, cytochrome P450 enzyme genotypes may be used in the future to identify slow metabolizers of commonly used medications. More specific to the pharmacological action of medication, genotyping of serotonin receptors may enter into the selection of antipsychotics that are related to weight gain or adverse effects of SSRIs (Anderson, Veenstra-Vadner, Weele, Cook, & McCracken, 2011).

In the next decade, it is likely that medications used in the treatment of mental illness in children and adolescents will be guided by a clearer understanding of the underlying neurobiology. For example, as noted above, recent discoveries regarding the pathophysiology of fragile X have led to the development of compounds that may counteract this pathophysiology.

Above and beyond psychopharmacology, clinicians will also be charged with integrating the neurobiology of anxiety with the rationale for cognitive behavioral therapy. To meet the challenges of the coming decade, primary care providers and mental health clinicians in child and adolescent psychiatry have a responsibility to become conversant with clinical neurobiology. This chapter offers an introduction and an invitation for interested readers to learn more.

References

Abi-Dargham, A. (2009). The neurochemistry of schizophrenia: a focus on dopamine and glutamate. In D. Charney, & E. Nestler (Eds.). *Neurobiology of mental illness* (3rd edition; pp. 321–329). New York: Oxford University Press.

Abott, N., Ronnback, L., & Hansson, E. (2006). Astrocyte–endothelial interactions at the blood-brain barrier. *Nature Reviews Neuroscience, 7*, 41–53.

Alexander, G., DeLong, M., & Strick, P. (1986). Parallel organization of functionally segregated circuits linking basal ganglia and cortex. *The Annual Review of Neuroscience, 9*, 357–81.

Anderson, G.M., Veenstra-Vander Weele, J., Cook, E.H., & McCracken, J.T. (2011). Pharmacogenetics. In A. Martin, L. Scahill, & D. Kratchovil (Eds.). *Pediatric psychopharmacology: Principles and Practice* (2nd edition; pp. 81–91). New York: Oxford University Press.

Arnsten, A. (2009). Toward a new understanding of attention-deficit hyperactivity disorder pathophysiology: an important role for prefrontal cortex dysfunction. *CNS Drugs, 23*(1), 33–41.

Arnsten, A.F.T., & Castellanos, F.X. (2011). Neurobiology of attention regulation and its disorders. In A. Martin, L. Scahill, & C.J. Kratochvil (Eds.), *Pediatric psychopharmacology: Principles and practice* (2nd edition; pp. 95–111). New York: Oxford University Press.

Banaschewski, T., Becker, K., Scherag, S., Franke, B., & Coghill, D. (2010). Molecular genetics of attention-deficit/hyperactivity disorder: An overview. *European Child & Adolescent Psychiatry, 19*(3), 237–57.

Barres, B. (2008, November 6). The mystery and magic of glia: A perspective on their roles in health and disease. *Neuron, 60*, 430–440.

Berger-Sweeney, J., Schaevitz, L., & Frick, K. (2009). Neurochemical systems involved in learning and memory. In D. Charney, & E. Nestler (Eds.). *Neurobiology of mental illness* (3rd edition; pp. 927–935). New York: Oxford University Press.

Bliss, T.V.P., & Lomo, T. (1973). Long-lasting potentiation of synaptic transmission in the dentate area of the anaesthetized rabbit following stimulation of the perforant path. *Journal of Physiology, 232*, 331–356.

Blumenfeld, H. (2002). *Neuroanatomy through clinical cases*. Sunderland, MA: Sinauer Associates.

Borden, N. (2007). *3D angiographic atlas of neurovascular anatomy and pathology*. New York: Cambridge University Press.

Castellanos, F.X., & Proal, E. (2009). Location, location, and thickness: volumetric neuroimaging of attention-deficit/hyperactivity disorder comes of age. *Journal of the American Academy of Child and Adolescent Psychiatry, 48*(10), 979–981.

Chaudhuri, A., Duan, F., Morsey, B., Persidsky, Y., & Kanmogne, G.D. (2008). HIV-1 activates proinflammatory and interferon-inducible genes in human brain microvascular endothelial cells: putative mechanisms of blood-brain barrier dysfunction. *Journal of Cerebral Blood Flow & Metabolism, 28*, 697–711.

Cooper, J., Bloom, F. & Roth, R. (2003). *The biochemical basis of neuropharmacology* (8th edition). New York: Oxford University Press.

Davis, M. (1986). Pharmacological and anatomical analysis of fear conditioning using the fear-potentiated startle paradigm. *Behavioral Neuroscience, 100*(6), 814–824.

Davis, M. (1992). The role of the amydala in fear and anxiety. *Annual Review in Neuroscience, 15*, 353–375.

Deeken, J., & Loscher, W. (2007). The blood-brain barrier and cancer: transporters, treatment, and Trojan horses. *Clinical Cancer Research, 13*(6), 1663–1674.

Dolen, G., & Bear, M. (2008). Role for metabotropic glutamate receptor 5 (mGluR5) in the pathogenesis of fragile X syndrome. *Journal of Physiology, 586*, 1503–1508.

Dotevall, L., Hagberg, L., Karlsson, J., & Rosengren, L. (1999). Astroglial and neuronal in cerebrospinal fluid as markers of CNS involvement in Lyme neuroborreliosis. *European Journal of Neurology, 6*(2), 169–178.

Duman, R. (2009). Neurochemical theories of depression: preclinical studies. In D. Charney, & E. Nestler (Eds.). *Neurobiology of mental illness* (3rd edition). New York: Oxford University Press.

Ellison, P., & Semrud-Clikeman, M. (2007). *Child neuropsychology. Assessment and interventions for neurodevelopmental disorders.* New York: Springer Science & Business Media.

Findling, R., McNamara, N., & Gracious, B. (2003). Antipsychotic agents: traditional and atypical. In A. Martin, L. Scahill, D. Charney, & J. Leckman (Eds.). *Pediatric psychopharmacology* (pp. 328–341). New York: Oxford University Press.

Gelernter, J., Kranzler, H., Coccaro, E., Siever, L., New, A., & Mulgrew, C.L. (1997). D4 dopamine-receptor (DRD4) alleles and novelty seeking in substance-dependent, personality-disorder, and control subjects. *American Journal of Human Genetics, 61*, 1144–1152.

Geller, D., Biederman, J., Stewart, S., Mullin, B., Martin, A., Spencer, T., & Faraone, S. (2003). Which SSRI? A meta-analysis of pharmacotherapy trials in pediatric obsessive-compulsive disorder. *American Journal of Psychiatry, 160*, 1919–1928.

Geracioti, T., Baker, D., Ekhator, N., West, S., Hill, K., Bruce, A., Schmidt, D., Rounds-Kugler, B., Yehuda, R., Keck, P., & Kasckow, J. (2001). CSF norepinephrine concentrations in posttraumatic stress disorder. *American Journal of Psychiatry, 158*, 1227–1230.

Gilbert, S. (2006). *Developmental biology* (8th edition). Sunderland, MA: Sinauer Associates.

Gitai, Z., Yu, T., Lundquist, E., Tessier-Lavigne, M., & Bargmann, C. (2003). The netrin receptor UNC-40/DCC stimulates axon attraction and outgrowth through enabled and, in parallel, Rac and UNC-115/AbLIM. *Neuron, 37*, 53–65.

Goddard, A., Ball, S., Martinez, J., Robinson, M., Yang, C., Russell, J., & Shekhar, A. (2010). Current perspectives of the roles of the central norepinephrine system in anxiety and depression. *Depression and Anxiety, 27*, 339–350.

Goulden, L., & Silver, C. (2009). Concordance of the children's executive functions scale with established tests and parent rating scales. *Journal of Psychoeducational Assessment, 27*(6), 439–451.

Green, R., & Ostrander, R. (2009). *Neuroanatomy for students of behavioral disorders.* New York: W.W. Norton & Company.

Halassa, M., Fellin, T., & Haydon, P. (2006). The tripartite synapse: roles for gliotransmission in health and disease. *Trends in Molecular Medicine, 13*(2), 54–63.

Hammerness, P., Vivas, F., & Geller, D. (2006). Selective serotonin reuptake inhibitors in pediatric psychopharmacology: A review of the evidence. *The Journal of Pediatrics, 148*(2), 158–165.

Hardy, J.A. (2009). The genetics and pathogenesis of Alzheimer's disease and related dementia. In D. Charney & E. Nestler (Eds.). *Neurobiology of mental illness* (3rd edition; pp. 883–895). New York: Oxford University Press.

Haydon, P., & Carmignoto, G. (2006). Astrocyte control of synaptic transmission and neurovascular coupling. *Physiological Reviews, 86*, 1009–1031.

Heckers, S., & Konradi, C. (2003). Synaptic function and biochemical neuroanatomy. In A. Martin, L. Scahill, D. Charney, & J. Leckman (Eds.). *Pediatric psychopharmacology* (pp. 20–32). New York: Oxford University Press.

Heckers, S., Konradi, C., & Anderson, G.M. (2011). Synaptic function and biochemical neuroanatomy. In A. Martin, L. Scahill, & C.J. Kratochvil (Eds.) *Pediatric psychopharmacology: Principles and practice* (2nd edition; pp. 23–37). New York: Oxford University Press.

Hendelman, W. (2006). *Atlas of functional neuroanatomy.* New York: Taylor and Francis.

Hernandez, C., Kayed, R., Zheng, H., Sweatt, J., & Dineley, K. (2010). Loss of α7 nicotinic receptors enhances β-amyloid oligomer accumulation, exacerbating early-stage cognitive decline and septohippocampal pathology in a mouse model of Alzheimer's disease. *The Journal of Neuroscience, 30*(7), 2442–2453.

Hickey, W. (2001). Basic principles of immunological surveillance of the normal central nervous system. *Glia, 36*, 118–124.

Huttenlocher, P., & Dabholkar, A. (1997). Regional differences in synaptogenesis in human cerebral cortex. *The Journal of Comparative Neurology, 387*, 167–178.

Insel, T., & Quirion, R. (2005). Psychiatry as a clinical neuroscience discipline. *Journal of the American Medical Association, 294*, 2221–2224.

Jankovic, J., & Tolosa, E. (2007). *Parkinson's disease & movement disorders* (5th edition). Philadelphia: Lippincott Williams & Wilkins.

Kalivas, P. (2009). The glutamate homeostasis hypothesis of addiction. *Nature Reviews Neuroscience, 10*, 561–572.

Kasai, H., Matsuzaki, M., Noguchi, J., Yasumatsu, N., & Nakahara, H. (2003). Structure-stability-function relationships of dendritic spines. *Trends in Neuroscience, 26*(7), 360–367.

King, B., Hollander, E., Sikich, L., McCracken, J., Scahill, L., Bregman, J., Donnelly, C., Anagnostou, E., Dukes, K., Sullivan, L., Hirtz, D., Wagner, A., Ritz, L. for the STAART Psychopharmacology Network (2009). Lack of efficacy of citalopram in children with autism spectrum disorders and high level of repetitive behaviors. *Archives of General Psychiatry, 66*(6), 583–590.

Kumar, A., & Chugani, H. (2009). PET in the assessment of pediatric brain development and developmental disorders. *PET Clinics, 3*, 487–515.

LeDoux, J. (2000). Emotion circuits in the brain. *Annual Review in Neuroscience, 23*, 155–184.

Li, D., Sham, P.C., Owen, M.J., & He, L. (2006). Meta-analysis shows significant association between dopamine system genes and attention deficit hyperactivity disorder (ADHD). *Human Molecular Genetics, 15*, 2276–2284.

Lombroso, P., Bloch, M., & Leckman, J. (2009). Tourette's syndrome and tic-related disorders in children. In D. Charney, & E. Nestler (Eds.). *Neurobiology of mental illness* (3rd edition; pp. 1218–1229). New York: Oxford University Press.

Marieb, E. (2004). *Human anatomy & physiology* (6th edition). New York: Pearson Education.

Ment, L., Hirtz, D., & Huppi, P. (2009). Imaging biomarkers of outcome in the developing preterm brain. *Lancet Neurology, 8*, 1042–55.

Milner, B., Squire, L., & Kandel, E. (1998). Cognitive neuroscience and the study of memory. *Neuron, 20*, 445–468.

MTA Cooperative Group. (1999). A 14-month randomized trial of treatment strategies for attention-deficit/hyperactivity disorder. *Archives of General Psychiatry, 56*, 1073–1086.

Ostby, Y., Tamnes, C., Fjell, A., Westlye, L., Due-Tonnessen, P., & Walhovd, K. (2009). Heterogeneity in subcortical brain development: A structural magnetic resonance imaging study of brain maturation from 8 to 30 years. *The Journal of Neuroscience, 29*(38), 11772–11782.

Patil, S.T., Zhang, L., Martenyi, F., Lowe, S.L., Jackson, K.A., Andreev, B.V., Avedisova, A.S., Bardenstein, L.M., Gurovich, I.Y., Morozova, M.A., Mosolov, S.N., Neznanov, N.G., Reznik, A.M., Smulevich, A.B., Tochilov, V.A., Johnson, B.G., Monn, J.A., & Schoepp, D.D. (2007). Activation of mGlu2/3 receptors as a new approach to treat schizophrenia: A randomized Phase 2 clinical trial. *Nature Medicine, 13*, 1102–1107.

Pliszka, S., Glahn, D., Semrud-Clikeman, M., Franklin, C., Perez, R., Xiong, J., & Liotti, M. (2006). Neuroimaging of inhibitory control areas in children with attention deficit hyperactivity disorder who were treatment naïve or in long-term treatment. *American Journal of Psychiatry, 163*, 1052–1060.

Purves, D., Augustine, G., Fitzpatrick, D., Hall, W., LaMantia, A., McNamara, J., & White, L. (2008). *Neuroscience* (4th edition). Sunderland, MA: Sinauer Associates.

Rakic Lab (2007). *Rakic Laboratory, Yale University.* Retrieved from rakiclab.med.yale.edu/pages/radial/Migration.php

Rakic, P., Ayoub, A., Breunig, J., & Dominguez, M. (2009). Decision by division: Making cortical maps. *Trends in Neuroscience, 32*(5), 291–301.

Rogan, M., Leon, K.S., Perez, D., & Kandel, E. (2005). Distinct neural signatures for safety and danger in the amygdale and striatum of the mouse. *Neuron, 46*, 309–320.

Rossi, D., & Volterra, A. (2009). Astrocyte dysfunction: Insights on the role in neurodegeneration. *Brain Research Bulletin, 80*, 224–232.

Rudy, J. (2008). *The neurobiology of learning and memory.* Sunderland, MA: Sinauer Associates.

Scherer, N., & SPD503 Study Group (2008). A randomized, double-blind, placebo-controlled study of guanfacine extended release in children and adolescents with attention-deficit/hyperactivity disorder. *Pediatrics, 121*(1), e73–e84. Retrieved from http: www.pediatrics.aappublications.org/cgi/?content/full/121/1/e73

Schmahmann, J., Smith, E., Eichler, F., & Filley, C. (2008). Cerebral white matter. *Annals of the New York Academy of Sciences, 1142*, 266–309.

Seeman, P. (2009). Glutamate and dopamine components in schizophrenia. *Journal of Psychiatry & Neuroscience, 34*(2), 143–149.

Shepherd, G. (2004). *The synaptic organization of the brain* (5th edition). New York: Oxford University Press.

Szmydynger-Chodobska, J., Stazielle, N., Zink, B., Ghersi-Egea, J., & Chodobski, A. (2009). The role of the choroid plexus in neutrophil invasion after traumatic brain injury. *Journal of Cerebral Blood Flow & Metabolism, 29*, 1503–1516.

TADS Team. (2007). The treatment for adolescents with depression study (TADS) long-term effectiveness and safety outcomes. *Archives of General Psychiatry, 64*(10), 1132–1144.

Tamnes, C., Ostby, Y., Fjell, A., Westlye, T., Due-Tonnessen, P., & Walhovd, K. (2010). Brain maturation in adolescence and young adulthood: regional age-related changes in cortical thickness and white matter volume and microstructure. *Cerebral Cortex, 20*(3), 534–548.

Tau, G., & Peterson, B. (2010). Normal development of brain circuits. *Neuropsychopharmacology, 35*, 147–168.

Vaccarino, F., & Leckman, J. (2011). In A. Martin, L. Scahill, and D. Kratchovil (Eds.). *Pediatric psychopharmacology: Principles and practice* (2nd edition; pp. 3–19). New York: Oxford University Press.

Walkup, J., Albano, A., Piacentini, J., Birmaher, B., Compton, S., Sherrill, J., Ginsburg, G., Ryan, M., McCracken, J., Waslick, B., Iyengar, S., March, J., & Kendall, P. (2008). Cognitive behavioral therapy, sertaline, or a combination in childhood anxiety. *The New England Journal of Medicine, 359*(26), 2753–2765.

Woody, S., & Rachman, S. (1994). Generalized anxiety disorder (GAD) as an unsuccessful search for safety. *Clinical Psychology Review, 14*(8), 743–753.

4

Integration of Physical and Psychiatric Assessment

Barbara Schoen Johnson and Jamesetta A. Newland

Objectives

After reading this chapter, APNs will be able to

1. Discuss the elements of a psychiatric assessment of children and adolescents by the advanced practice nurse.
2. Describe the essential elements of a comprehensive medical history and physical exam of children and adolescents seen in primary care to determine presence or absence of medical conditions.
3. Identify common screening tools used to assess mental health and behavioral disorders in children and adolescents.
4. Recognize indications for consultation, referral, and collaboration between primary care and mental health professionals for children and adolescents with mental health care needs.

Overview of Chapter

Mental health impacts children's physical health, social relationships, and learning. Early and thorough assessment of children and adolescents with psychiatric-mental health disorders is the most effective way to begin timely treatment, diminish the severity of mental disorders, and decrease the likelihood of chronic mental disorders in adulthood. A report by the National Research Council and Institute of Medicine (2009) reinforced the need for behavioral health screening to take place in primary care settings and schools to detect risk factors in children and adolescents and the appearance of early symptoms of disorder. Early identification and treatment can ameliorate the effects of mental illness in children and adolescents as well as adults.

This chapter will describe the elements that make up a comprehensive psychiatric-mental health assessment of

children and adolescents. This assessment can be used in primary care settings to help identify children and adolescents in need of mental health services. Key areas include history taking, physical exam process, risk and protective factors, teaching needs of the child or adolescent and family, and ways to communicate the assessment findings to the patient and family so that they are able to pursue appropriate treatment as needed.

Approximately 20% of youth in the United States are estimated to have a mental or behavioral disorder, which translates to a cost of $247 billion plus the emotional, social, and economic costs for the child and family (National Research Council and Institute of Medicine, 2009). While that statistic demonstrates the high rate of mental health disorders in this age group, the actual percentage of children with psychiatric disorders who are being diagnosed and/or receiving treatment is low. This is despite the fact that early detection and treatment

Child and Adolescent Behavioral Health: A Resource for Advanced Practice Psychiatric and Primary Care Practitioners in Nursing,
First Edition. Edited by Edilma L. Yearwood, Geraldine S. Pearson, and Jamesetta A. Newland.
© 2012 John Wiley & Sons, Inc. Published 2012 by John Wiley & Sons, Inc.

of child and adolescent mental disorders result in the best outcomes. Furthermore, according to the 1999 U.S. Surgeon General's report on child mental health, approximately 70% of American children and adolescents who need treatment for mental and behavioral health disorders do not receive any type of treatment (American Academy of Child and Adolescent Psychiatry [AACAP], 2009; AACAP & American Academy of Pediatrics [AAP], 2009; Melnyk & Moldenhauer, 2006). These statistics help highlight the need for primary care practitioners (PCPs), including advanced practice nurses (APNs), to be able to evaluate children and adolescents for mental health problems and appropriately refer them for services.

A major contributing factor to these startling numbers has been the lack of or inadequate screening for mental health problems by primary care providers (Cawthorpe, 2005; Olson, et al., 2001; Ozer et al., 2009; Williams, Klinepeter, Palmes, Pulley, & Meschan Foy, 2004). Cawthorpe (2005) found that 87% of a group of Canadian physicians felt unprepared to address the psychosocial needs of children younger than six years of age, stating that they had neither the knowledge nor support to identify and manage mental health problems in young children. Another group of pediatricians identified time (56% to 68%) and training or knowledge (38% to 56%) as major barriers to diagnosing and managing depression in children and adolescents (Olson et al., 2001).

Not only do PCPs state that they are unprepared to evaluate children for mental health problems, a U.S. study of adolescents aged thirteen to seventeen years found that only one-third of the adolescents interviewed stated their PCPs had ever had a discussion with them about their emotions and mood during a routine visit (Ozer et al., 2009). PCPs must be trained in methods to evaluate children and adolescents for psychiatric problems, as well as recognize that moods and emotions are a mainstay of one's well-being and should be incorporated into every primary care visit.

Compounding the problem of so few children and adolescents in need not receiving mental health screening and identification in primary care settings is the severe shortage physicians, APNs, and others who are skilled and willing to treat children and adolescents with mental disorders (National Technical Assistance Center for Children's Mental Health, 2005; Huang, Macbeth, Dodge, & Jacobstein, 2004; Koppelman, 2004). According to data from 2000, there was a projected need for 30,000 child and adolescent psychiatrists, yet only 6,300 were realized with no promise of any significant increase. Currently, the federal Bureau of Health Professions projects that the nation will need another 12,624 by 2020 to maintain current utilization rates for psychiatric services. The anticipated number who will be available, however, is just over 8,000 (Koppelman, 2004). These numbers do not address the number of psychiatric caregivers that would be needed if all children and adolescents with mental health issues were identified in primary care settings.

Another discouraging fact in this growing need for mental health care providers is the declining enrollment of nurses in graduate psychiatry training programs (Huang, Macbeth, Dodge, & Jacobstein, 2004). According to the American Academy of Nurse Practitioners (2010), only 2.9% of the more than 135,000 practicing nurse practitioners (NPs) choose psychiatric mental health as their specialty. The U.S. Department of Health and Human Services (USDHHS) (2010) data analysis for the 2008 National Sample Survey of Registered Nurses found that only 6.3% of practicing NPs were working in psychiatric mental health settings, whereas 36.1% were employed in primary care; furthermore, the only group of APNs that declined in numbers was the psychiatric clinical nurse specialist, who is part of the mental health workforce.

These realities have generated a growing interest in including and integrating mental health screening into primary care settings. Incorporating mental health assessment into each primary care visit increases the likelihood of identifying children in need earlier and allowing for early intervention in order to decrease long-term complications from mental health disorders. Assessment during critical periods of a child's or adolescent's development is most likely to result in effective treatment. The need to provide PCPs with the appropriate knowledge and skills so they are able to screen for mental and behavioral health problems in children and adolescents who present in their practices for routine health care has been acknowledged (AACAP, 2009; Evans, 2009; Koppelman, 2004; National Research Council and Institute of Medicine, 2009). PCPs must be able to use history taking and the physical exam to differentiate physical problems/conditions from mental health issues in order to offer these children appropriate interventions and support.

The World Health Organization (WHO) and the World Organization of Family Doctors (Wonca, 2008) stated, "Certain skills and competencies are required to effectively assess, diagnose, treat, support and refer people with mental disorders: it is essential that primary care workers are adequately prepared and supported in their mental health work" (p. 1). The National Technical Assistance Center for Children's Mental Health (2005) stated, "We must train professionals to have attitudes, behaviors, and skills that are congruent with the changing children's mental health field" (p. 3).

WHO and Wonca also emphasized how a child's cognitive and emotional developmental levels impact his ability to understand and communicate his mental health issues. Therefore, PCPs/APNs must be cognizant of their expected developmental ability to differentiate normal developmental issues from mental health problems. Additionally, children's and adolescents' responses and reactions are influenced by issues such as fatigue, hunger, and lack of comfort with the people examining them. It is important for PCPs to consider the possibility of drug and alcohol problems mimicking mental health conditions and should screen children and adolescents when appropriate.

Finally, the child or adolescent may not be aware of or understand that her feelings or symptoms are related to her mental health; thus she will not tell the PCP that she is depressed, anxious, etc. PCPs should interview the parents as well as the child or adolescent and obtain information from school personnel whenever possible. Often it is the parents or school personnel who recognize the child or adolescent is having psychiatric symptoms. APNs must be sure to evaluate the child's or adolescent's social environment such as his family dynamics, living situation, friends, and school issues to help evaluate the child fully. These are important sources of information that can help in making a diagnosis.

When caring for children and adolescents in primary care, in addition to the psychiatric-mental health assessment, a thorough medical history and physical examination to determine the presence or absence of underlying medical conditions that might be treatable is warranted. Although the assessment guidelines in this chapter will purposefully be general rather than specific, readers are referred to other chapters in the text that cover each grouping of mental disorders for more in-depth information. The chapter will provide APNs and other PCPs in primary care and mental health settings a way to systematically approach the assessment of behavioral and mental health of their patients.

Integrating Psychiatric and Physical Assessment Approaches

Primary care providers are often the first individuals who face parents' concerns about their child's mental health. The National Center for Health Statistics reported that between 2005 and 2006, 15% of U.S. children aged four to seventeen years had parents who sought guidance from a health care provider or school staff about their child's emotional or behavioral difficulties (Simpson, Cohen, Pastor, & Reuben, 2008).

Often families do not know where to turn when they become aware of their child behavioral or mental problems; they may realize that "something's not right" with their child, but little else.

Almost four of ten children received treatment at school, while approximately 25% received services from a pediatric or general medicine practice (Simpson, Cohen, Pastor, & Reuben, 2008). In an urban practice, Hacker, Myagmarjav, Harris, Franco Suglia, Weidner and Link (2006) found that parental/personal concern was 40% sensitive for a positive score on the Pediatric Symptom Checklist, while parental/personal concern regardless of score identified 4.5%. These patients were between four years eleven months and nineteen years of age. In the Netherlands, researchers found similar results in children aged five to fifteen years; identification of psychosocial problems and subsequent referral were six times more likely in children with serious parent-reported problem behavior, based on total scores on the parent-completed Child Behavior Checklist (Brugman, Reijneveld, Verhulst, & Verloove-Vanhorick, 2001). These three reports support a strong association between a parent's concern and the presence of mental or behavioral health issues in a child. The PCP's role in detecting behavioral or psychiatric disorders, initiating treatment, and referring for further treatment is paramount in assuring timely and appropriate help for the child.

Alternatively, PCPs are often in the position of having to inform parents who are not aware, ignore, or deny the signs and symptoms of behavioral problems that "something's not right." The long-term relationship developed between child, parent, and PCP can be beneficial in approaching sensitive areas for discussion. PCPs can support parents who do not believe in or trust mental health providers. If the parents have a strong connection with their PCP they are more likely to follow her suggestions, even if they fear or distrust psychiatric health care providers. One of this chapter's goals is to assist PCPs with the knowledge and confidence to proceed with their evaluation of the child's history, behavior, complaints, school performance, social skills, family functioning, and available resources for care.

One barrier to asking questions about mental health issues is what to do with the information received. It is, therefore, essential for PCPs to develop strong relationships with mental health care providers to whom a child or adolescent and family can be referred (Lemmon & Stafford, 2007). Pediatric PCPs also promote protective resilience by building on the child's or adolescent's strengths through reinforcement of competence, confidence, connection to family and community, sense of control over one's actions, and positive coping (Lemmon & Stafford).

Who Initially Assesses the Child?

Children and adolescents with mental disorders or problems often first appear in the office of their primary care APN, who might be an NP or other APN. Many of the "new morbidities" such as ADHD and learning problems, drug and alcohol abuse, anxiety and mood problems, suicide and homicide, HIV and AIDS, and violence and sexual activity have been added to the responsibilities of pediatrics (Lemmon & Stafford, 2007). Because PCPs are now being asked to care for children with these chronic conditions it is even more important for mental health evaluations to be a part of routine care. Evans (2009) recommended screening children at risk for mental health problems, particularly children expelled from day care and preschool settings, children of depressed parents, children with disabling or chronic illnesses, children in military families, and children in foster care or juvenile justice systems. The AACAP (2009) supports the initiation of services in primary care by PCPs for emerging developmental and behavioral problems and common mental health disorders such as ADHD, depression, and anxiety disorders in children and adolescents. The pediatricians, pediatric NPs, and family NPs must possess the necessary skills to complete a thorough and sensitive assessment of the "problem." Primary care practices are the optimal settings for screening for mental health disorders in children and determining the next step in treatment. But just as important, providers must know when mental health specialty care or referral is indicated.

Elements of an Assessment

Several considerations should precede the APN's gathering of information about the "problem" that prompted the family to seek care for their child or adolescent. The APN must realize that a thorough assessment does not consist of a checklist to be completed in a robotic way but that the child and family are facing a difficult situation that needs to be approached in a calm, sensitive, and caring manner. The unknown is generally perceived as frightening and the perceptions of children, adolescents, and families regarding the unknown assessment process are no different. The assessment of these children and adolescents must include a comprehensive medical, environmental, and social history from multiple sources to gain insight into all aspects of the child's problem. Once a comprehensive history has been completed the APN must complete a full physical assessment. The PCP must take the history, physical exam, and any lab tests that are done and consider whether this child or adolescent has a mental health issue that is causing their symptoms. If the APN/PCP thinks the diagnosis is a mental/behavioral health problem, then she must help the family understand what is going on and connect them with appropriate providers to allow optimal treatment for the child.

Observation of the Child, Adolescent, and Family

The APN must be skillful in observing and interpreting the child's or adolescent's and family members' verbal behavior and in listening to their spontaneous verbalizations and their answers to questions. Observation includes attention to the family members' interactions, relationships, responses to the child, concerns about the problem at hand, and openness to learn new ways to help their child. It also includes focusing on the child's activity level, interruptions, interaction with parents and siblings, responses to the parents' words and actions, and willingness to separate from the parents to talk privately with the APN.

Impact of the Problem or Disorder

The child's or adolescent's mental health problem makes an impact, sometimes a significant one, on all family members. Siblings worry about their troubled brother or sister and may wonder why he or she has this problem and whether they will develop it too. Parents often admit, "We are all affected" or "We are all suffering," when describing the impact of the child's problem on the family. The emotional problem or mental disorder has an impact on the child and her friends, classmates, teachers, grandparents, extended family, and often neighbors. Sometimes the impact seems to be more "internal," such as the suffering of the child or adolescent with anxiety or depression. Other times, the impact is "external" as in children with ADHD, oppositional defiant disorder, conduct disorder, and other disruptive behavior disorders. In any case, the behavior of children and adolescents affects others in their environment, particularly when they have chronic conditions, whether psychiatric or physical (Knafl & Santacroce, 2010). The primary care APN must encourage open communication with family members and others in the child's life to assess the need for family interventions in order to maximize the child's health and child's and family's quality of life.

Eliciting Information

The most thorough psychiatric-mental health assessments are based on information from all relevant parties, including the child or adolescent, parents/grandparents/guardians, extended family members, school personnel, and past and present treating providers. Often it is not possible to gather information from all these sources and the APN must proceed with whatever data are available. These data may include emails from teachers, phone calls from other treating professionals (with consent), and testing results from psychologists. It is important for the APN to attempt to get as much information from as many sources as possible to help in identifying sources of stress or anxiety or the impact the mental health issue is having on the child/adolescent. Each child/adolescent should be interviewed alone to allow him to feel free to speak about any issues or concerns. Parents should also be interviewed without the child present to ensure that they can speak freely and not withhold information because the child is present. During the history taking it is important for the PCP to observe all reactions by the child/adolescent and parents when being questioned, as well as interactions between them throughout the exam process.

Ways Children and Adolescents Communicate

Children and adolescents communicate in their own ways according to their ages, stages of development, and life circumstances. They use not just verbalizations, but also interactions with others, drawings, play, music, engagement versus withdrawal, appearance, facial expression, eye contact, and other forms of verbal communication. For example, a child may play out feelings of helplessness and fear about being abused; an adolescent may draw pictures of the "devils" he remembers from nightmares or a picture of the torment he wants to inflict on a peer. APNs should use many forms of communication from the child/adolescent to elicit as much information as possible to aid in making a diagnosis.

Age- and Development-Specific Considerations

When evaluating children of various ages for mental health issues, the APN must recognize the different developmental stages and how these influence the evaluation process. Mental health assessment must use questioning and other methods appropriate to the child's age and developmental level.

Typically children and adolescents undergo rapid developmental change. Each age and developmental stage, from a very young age through adolescence, presents its own challenges to the evaluator. When working with toddlers and preschoolers, much of the verbal information is received from parental reports, but the APN should use multiple sources and resources to gather all the needed information. For example, assessment of a preschooler has usually relied on parent reports, but the APN can gain more information by watching the par-

ent-child interaction, getting feedback from a preschool teacher, and by watching the child's interactions with others. Additionally, there has been recent evidence of the usefulness of the Preschool Age Psychiatric Assessment, a standardized structured diagnostic tool (Egger et al., 2006). School-aged children may not be able to verbalize what they are feeling; rather, they may have physical symptoms that are caused by a mental health issue. Here again, gathering information from the child, parents, teachers, and other resources can help in the evaluation. Adolescents may be able to discuss their feelings, but some adolescents might balk and refuse to talk; trust building may take some time. The use of standardized evaluative tools can assist in the assessment of children of all ages with a range of disorders. APNs conducting mental health assessments of children and adolescents must consider developmental levels and adapt accordingly.

Personal Factors Influencing the Assessment

No matter what field of practice, APNs must all recognize the influence of their own biases, anxieties and fears, life experiences, and needs when working with other people. Whatever their own cultural background, APNs must be culturally sensitive to the experiences of others. They must accept and celebrate the things that make each child, adolescent, and family unique and capable (Dunn, 2010a). In addition, APNs' views of children as vulnerable makes it especially poignant and difficult when they suffer from either internal challenges such as heightened anxiety or external stressors such as family disruption. These are troublesome concerns for all APNs to deal with in helping people. One of the most positive messages the APN can communicate to a child or adolescent and the family is a sense of hopefulness for the child's or adolescent's future.

Areas of Psychiatric Assessment of Children and Adolescents

A thorough assessment of a child presenting with a mental disorder or behavioral problem must include certain points, such as chief complaint, review of systems, developmental history, school history, mental status examination, physical exam, and formulation of diagnoses and treatment plan. In addition, other elements may need to be assessed in depth in relation to the child's presenting behavior or complaint, such as suicidal behavior and plan, risk for violence, mood lability, or hallucinations. Keep in mind, however, that the child might present to the primary care APN or other provider with no complaint of psychiatric etiology. Rather, children may present with physical or somatic complaints that mimic a physical problem. The APN must remember that physical symptoms may represent mental health problems; therefore, they should always consider a mental or behavior health diagnosis among the differentials. Many of the following elements of the psychiatric assessment also apply to the medical assessment and will guide additional actions performed in the physical examination (Burns & Kodadek, 2010).

Chief Complaint or Presenting Symptoms and Behaviors

The APN must first ask, "Why are you here today?" Any complaints or concerns of the child or adolescent and parents should be assessed. A young child may respond, "I don't know," "Because my stomach hurts," or "The teacher yells at me," and thus open the door for reassurance such as, "It sounds like sometimes you get in trouble for your behavior" or another simple explanation. Adolescents may be angry that they were "dragged" to the appointment or they may feel guilty about their problems or too anxious or depressed to be able to express their concerns.

Parents may present a list of complaints or problems which have surfaced recently or which have been present for many years; they may bring with them a brief or lengthy list of their child's signs and symptoms. Some parents may not recognize that their child is having mental health problems and may not connect their symptoms with their mental well-being. The APN should evaluate all children presenting in the primary care office for any signs of mental or psychiatric distress.

Medically unexplained symptoms can be an important sign that underlying mental problems exist because emotional distress can cause pain and other physical symptoms (Lemmon & Stafford, 2007). The primary care ANP also must remember that children or adolescents with chronic illness experience an increased risk of behavioral and emotional problems (Hysing et al., 2007). If the presenting complaint is a medical concern, additional information about onset, location, duration, character, aggravating factors, relieving factors, and current self-treatment measures should be elicited. The APN should evaluate the child/adolescent for sources of distress to help differentiate medical causes of physical symptoms from emotional sources.

A comprehensive subjective review of systems is helpful in working through physical complaints about the child. Asking questions about general well-being, including energy level, excessive fatigue, rashes, eye pain, throat pain, difficulty swallowing, chest pain or palpitations, shortness of breath, abdominal pain, nausea or vomiting, diarrhea or constipation, body aches, or headaches are helpful in working through the differential diagnoses. Addressing possible sources of stress in the child's or adolescent's life is also important when eliciting a history. This includes asking about school, friends, social activities, and home life.

Prior Treatment

The APN questions whether and where the child or adolescent has been previously treated for a mental health disorder. The child may have received inpatient care (the most intensive level of treatment), partial hospitalization or day treatment (which is less intensive), and/or outpatient care such as medication management (the least intensive level of care). The child may have been in therapy, sometimes over a period of years and with various therapists. All of the information about prior treatment gives the assessing APN a picture of the extent to which the family has already sought help for their child and the perceived success or failure of the treatment.

Developmental History

A child's or adolescent's developmental history begins with the mother's age and health during pregnancy and moves on to include any parental health or emotional problems, difficult life circumstances, and drug or alcohol use during pregnancy. This part of the assessment includes information gathering about the labor and birth, any neonatal complications, difficulties in the early weeks and months of life, and whether or not the child met developmental milestones. The APN must acknowledge that normal development falls somewhere within an identified span of time, with some children meeting developmental milestones earlier or later than others. For younger children, height and weight should be recorded on the CDC growth chart to track how his growth compares to previous measurements and standardized norms. With adolescents, it is important to assess the development of secondary sex characteristics. Because of the wide variability in physical appearance and the psychosocial developmental stage of the adolescent, repeated reassurance that she is developing within the normal spectrum might be necessary.

It is imperative that APNs know normal growth and developmental milestones because often mental health problems may be related to common developmental stages that are not achieved or are not completed. When parents of a child having temper tantrums present to the primary care office it is important for the APN to recognize that this is a common issue among toddlers as they learn to control their environment or are overwhelmed in a situation. Alternatively, if a child is seven years old and having temper tantrums, this may represent a mental health issue because by this age, the child should be able to communicate her frustrations to others and/or control her emotions better. Parental expectations of the child are also an important part of the developmental assessment. If parents have expectations of the child that are above what the child can cognitively achieve, they may reprimand the child or punish him inappropriately, causing anxiety or fear.

The importance of understanding growth and development by the primary care provider cannot be emphasized enough. Lack of achievement of specific milestones or lack of progression along the developmental trajectory may be early signs of mental health problems for the PCP. A comprehensive developmental assessment is a key part of the mental health evaluation.

Family History

Assessment of mental health problems in children and adolescents always includes a thorough family history of mental illness. Because the initial reaction of most people is to deny the presence of mental illness in their families, the primary care NP or the psychiatric-mental health APN (PMH-APN) must carefully assess whether family members have certain disorders. For example, instead of just asking, "Is there anyone in the family with depression?" it is helpful to ask, "On either side of the biological parents' families, is there anyone who has depression, takes an antidepressant, used to take an antidepressant, should take an antidepressant, committed suicide, or tried to commit suicide?" Instead of asking, "Is there anyone in the family with anxiety," it is helpful to ask, "On either side of the biological parents' families, is there anyone who has anxiety, takes a medication for anxiety, has anxiety attacks, has panic attacks, worries all the time, or can't leave home?"

Construction of a genogram and pedigree and an ecomap is useful to visually display the structure and pattern of family relationships, medical (and psychiatric) conditions that have affected family members across several generations, and interactions among family members inside and outside the family system (McGuiness, Noonan, & Dyer, 2005). As McGuiness et al. state, "Viewing clients from an ecological perspective yields a much richer understanding of the pathways linking psychosocial and biophysiological mechanisms" (p. 122). These diagrams can help the APN and family view the multiple influences on the child's mental and physical health status as well as the child's and family's responses to these influencing factors. The visual revelation may assist in guiding decisions about the appropriate referrals and interventions.

Medical History

Initial questions the primary care APN will ask the family when taking the medical history include whether the child's immunizations are up to date; if there is any history of a loss of consciousness or head injury; whether there have been any surgeries or hospitalizations, accidents, chronic illnesses, and recent acute illnesses, and if there are any allergies to medicine, food, or environmental allergens. Chronic illnesses are often associated with mental health issues such as anxiety or depression. If there is a diagnosis, the APN should ask parents when it was made, what the child/adolescent knows about the diagnosis, and how he is coping with it. Past head trauma is also known to be associated with mental health problems later in life. Children with multiple head injuries should have cognitive testing evaluate for subtle declines in their mental abilities. Chronic allergies can present as crankiness or moodiness in children. APNs should evaluate children/adolescents who have mood changes during certain seasons or when exposed to certain environments. Children with histories of trauma and/or abuse are also at increased risk for mental health problems; therefore, these questions should be asked when reviewing a child/adolescent's past medical history.

Activities of Daily Living

Primary care visits are a time when the PCP should evaluate children's activities of daily living, including nutrition and sleep patterns. Parents might not be aware that their child is overeating or eating too little or consuming unhealthy food and drink. In addition, the family's cultural patterns related to diet and eating must be considered. Eating disorders may include anorexia nervosa and bulimia, overweight or obesity, and severe allergies to foods; drug-induced conditions such as malnutrition can lead to slowed growth or altered metabolism of many vital nutrients (Dunn, 2010b). Children who are hypoglycemic may present with a depressed mood or affect. Conversely, those with diets high in sugar or caffeine may present with symptoms of hyperactivity or anxiety. Obesity in children/adolescents has been associated with depression. APNs must be cognizant of how the child/adolescent feels about her appearance, which influences her emotional well-being.

Parents often do not know how much sleep a child needs each day or realize the importance of a regular bedtime, even for older adolescents. Sleep requirements per twenty-four hours vary according to age, ranging from sixteen to twenty hours for a newborn to eleven hours for a six-year-old to eight hours for a fifteen-year-old. Very young children manifest the effects of insufficient sleep with hyperactivity, emotional lability, irritability, and aggressiveness. School-age children may experience inattention, restlessness, emotional lability, or daydreaming at school; symptoms overlap with those of ADHD. Adolescents with inadequate sleep may exhibit excessive sleepiness, difficulties with mood regulation, impaired academic performance, and increased risk for accidents (Burns, 2010). Disordered sleep can lead to physical and mental health issues. Sleep problems may also be related to something that is happening in the family. Children and adolescents with depression or anxiety may be unable to sleep due to worry or obsessive thoughts that keep them awake, which in turn adds to their feelings of fatigue or moodiness.

Medication History

It is important to know past and present medications taken by the child, when they were taken, their effects, side or adverse effects, and why they were discontinued and by whom. Many over-the-counter medications cause symptoms that may be misdiagnosed as anxiety or depression. Pseudophedrine may cause difficulty in concentrating, palpitations, anxiety, or tremors in children. Asthma medications, including albuterol, may make a child jittery, hyperactive, or aggressive. Benadryl may cause a child/adolescent to appear sad, disinterested, sleepy, or moody. When evaluating children/adolescents for possible psychiatric conditions, the APN should have parents stop all medications prior to the evaluation so that the medications have been excreted from the system.

For those children/adolescents for whom psychotropic medications are warranted, parents and children/adolescents must know that all medications have potential side effects and that parents should be responsible for both administering the medication and observing the children for any negative effects. There are certain risk factors to assess when considering specific psychotropic medications, such as the risks associated with the use of stimulant medications in the presence of cardiac structural defect in a child or adolescent or a family member who died of sudden cardiac death at a young age. APNs must emphasize the importance of taking psychotropic medications as ordered to avoid overdosing and/or decreasing complications from side effects.

Social History

The child's or adolescent's social history should state with whom the child lives and the relationship to the child; the city in which the child lives; whether there has been a recent move; where a separated or divorced parent lives; sources of support from extended family and their proximity to the child; and family dynamics, strengths, and needs. Relationships with parents/grandparents or guardians and with siblings are part of a thorough assessment. In addition, any legal problems or involvement in the juvenile justice system should be included. The occupations of parents, guardians,

or primary caretakers; family financial resources; and access to health care services are factors that can affect the mental and physical health of a child and family.

Peer relationships, in terms of whether the child has any friends and how she interacts with peers, are important. Sometimes a child or adolescent will report that he has plenty of friends but the parent will report that he is not invited to peers' birthday parties or not asked to join peer activities. Determining how the child views himself in comparison to his peers can help in understanding his view of himself. Children who state "I am not popular" or "I am just a loser" should alert the PCP for possible mental health issues. The APN should ask the child/adolescent what she likes to do for fun. Asking children/adolescents what they want to do when they grow up can provide a view of how the child/adolescent views her future. Children who say they have no fun, or don't have any activities, or don't think about a future for themselves should be evaluated for depression or mental health problems. Social relationships and activities are key components of the lives of children/adolescents that often are directly related to their mental well-being.

School History

Information to gather about the child's or adolescent's school history includes the school grade; name of the school; and whether the child receives regular education or special education services for a specific learning problem such as ADHD, learning differences, or another behavioral issue that interferes with the educational process. Parents can often identify the years which were "good" for the child related to a particularly excellent teacher versus the year or years which were not as productive. The school-related data are essential to examine carefully because school is often associated with stressful events for the child and family.

Substance Use/Abuse History

The APN should ask children and adolescents about drug and alcohol use or abuse. Adolescents, in particular, will often not volunteer information about their use of drugs and alcohol. Some don't consider marijuana a drug. Surprisingly, though, adolescents will often answer direct questions from the APN assessor honestly and openly. The APN must not forget that children, even young children, may be using drugs and alcohol, especially when they are part of the parents' lifestyle; therefore, they too must be evaluated. Access to medications in the home should also be part of the evaluation process. Parents who take antidepressants or narcotics should be asked where they keep their medications, if they are locked up, and/or if any of their medications have gone missing. Over-the-counter medications may also be used by children/adolescents who are dealing with mental health issues, so access to these medications should also be included when taking a history.

Risk Behaviors

Every child and adolescent should be assessed for high-risk behaviors involving sex, drugs, alcohol, association with unsavory individuals, and dangerous, thrill-seeking behaviors. Parents may not be aware of their child's behavior and this can be shocking and very upsetting to them. It is important to keep in mind the level of sensitivity and absence of judgment or condemnation needed to discuss risk behaviors.

Abuse and Trauma History

Assessing the child's or adolescent's experience of abuse, whether physical, emotional, or sexual, requires a great deal of sensitivity and care so as not to further traumatize the young patient. It often helps to remark that the abuser's behavior was wrong and that the victim is not to blame. Natural or manmade disasters, family violence, neglect, betrayal, and/or abandonment can also be traumatic. These experiences may contribute to a variety of symptoms including re-experiencing the trauma, sleep disruptions, and fears, which are collectively known as post-traumatic stress disorder or acute stress disorder.

Mental Status Examination (MSE)

The mental status examination (MSE) provides a snapshot of the child's or adolescent's cognitive functions. The MSE explores psychiatric symptoms and their severity and effect on the patient's and family's lives. The presenting symptoms, such as excessive worries or consuming sadness, and the family history indicate areas to be examined in depth. The MSE and mini-MSE can be easily incorporated into primary care visits without adding significant time requirements. This tool can provide the PCP with an initial evaluation of the mental well-being of the child or adolescent.

Initially, the child's or adolescent's appearance is examined; this may include the head size, stature, facial expressions, eye contact, nutritional state, bruising, open sores that have been "picked" by the child, dress, motor mannerisms or tics, signs of anxiety such as chewing on fingernails, or evidences of self-harm such as scratches or knife marks. When a mark is observed, such as a burn on the hand or a scratch on the arm or leg, the child or adolescent should be asked about it ("How did this happen?") to determine if the child was burned by a cigarette, caused himself an "eraser burn," has been cutting herself, etc. Also initially, during the child's or adolescent's separation from the parent to talk with the APN privately, the child should be observed to determine if she has excessive difficulty in separating or an inability to do so in relation to her developmental stage. On the other hand, it should be noted if there is too much ease in separating, which is not expected in young children.

The MSE also assesses the child's or adolescent's orientation to time, place, person, and circumstances, although these may be limited in young children. That said, even young children can usually identify a big holiday that is coming up or the season of the year. Impaired orientation may be related to low intelligence, organic brain problems, or thought disorders such as schizophrenic illnesses.

Central nervous system (CNS) functioning is assessed through observing gross (throwing a ball) and fine (copying a circle, cross, triangle) motor coordination, abnormal movements, right-left discrimination, cerebellar functioning (finger-to-nose test), gait (heel-to-toe walking), and symmetry (squeezing hands of examiner). Sensory difficulties may lead to problems in school performance and should be assessed by hearing screening, audiometric testing, and vision screening or other means to determine problems in visual acuity.

Attention span is assessed through the child's ability to focus and follow through, distractibility, and disorganization. Poor attention span can be caused by other factors, such as fatigue, anxiety, language difficulties, disorders on the autism spectrum, and sedation or other effects of medication.

Activity level is a tricky issue to assess because at times a parent or grandparent may comment that a child is "hyperactive," when in fact, she has a developmentally normal activity level. Reports of the child's activity level are most helpful when they come from multiple sources, such as different classes in school and from different parenting figures. Excess activity can be due to anxiety, hypomania or mania, psychosis, or even oppositionalism.

Academic performance should be assessed by observing the child read and write; evaluating language fluency; and noting the patient's own words about his ability to read, write, and do mathematical computations. Letter and word reversals are common in first graders and other young children learning to read and do not necessarily indicate the presence of a learning difference.

Speech and language difficulties may be noted because of a developmentally small vocabulary, overuse of concrete verbs and nouns, underuse of abstract words, or nodding the head instead of clarifying through speech. Receptive language problems can also be due to a sensory impairment, mental retardation, or a pervasive developmental disorder. Expressive language problems, such as echolalia, misuse of pronouns, or difficulty using language as a means of social interaction, can be due to a language delay or impairment in speech production.

Intelligence is evaluated through the child's or adolescent's use of vocabulary, responsiveness, level of comprehension, curiosity, identification of body parts, and ability to subtract serial sevens or threes for younger children.

Memory difficulties can be due to several causes including attention problems, anxiety, or organic brain problems. Memory is assessed by having the child repeat three items five minutes after the words are presented. Younger children can be asked what they had for supper yesterday and the names of teachers.

The quality of thinking and perception is related to both thought content and thought process or form. The child's or adolescent's disordered thought content could include hallucinations, delusions, excessive concreteness, or the use of neologisms. His disordered thought process could be seen by slowness of thinking, pressured speech, flight of ideas, muteness, or loose associations. His fantasies and feelings are assessed through his three wishes and spontaneous play or speech, including information offered about dreams and his drawings.

Affect and mood are often misinterpreted terms. When assessing affect, the APN is looking for the objective manifestation of the child's or adolescent's emotional state, range of affect, predominant affects, and her appropriateness to the situation or content being discussed. Mood, on the other hand, is a subjective internal state and is elicited by asking the child or adolescent directly about feelings and emotions.

The risk of harm to self and others is a serious issue to explore in both children and adolescents. Even very young children can have fantasies about their death and not grasp its finality. APNs must assess any suicidal ideation and behavior, the intent to self harm, any attempts to self harm, and self-injurious behavior such as cutting oneself. The APN can help the patient to differentiate by asking, "Are you cutting to bleed or to die?" In addition, the APN should assess whether the suicidal attempt was planned versus impulsive, performed out of desperation or depression, and whether it was a lethal act in the child's mind.

The child's or adolescent's typical defenses and ways to cope with conflicts may become evident. For example, is the adolescent's usual response avoidant, angry, phobic, inhibited, depressed, or frustrated? Interests are potential strengths for the child and adolescent. These could be hobbies, sports, favorite subjects in school, and career goals. Nurses must identify positive attributes which may include coping skills, cooperativeness, cognitive flexibility, friendliness and social skills, academic success and interests, intelligence, positive self-esteem, and supportive family members. Information is gathered about children's or adolescents' perception of their relationships with family, peers, and teachers and other authority figures.

Subjective Review of Systems

A complete review of systems should be conducted to elicit any report of signs or symptoms consistent with medical conditions: general, skin, head; eyes, ears, nose, and throat; and respiratory, cardiovascular, genitourinary, gastrointestinal, musculoskeletal, neurologic, endocrine. Many physical complaints may be symptoms of a mental health problem. In asking about a child's/adolescent's general health, the APN should ask what the child's general well-being is and how his health compares to children of the same age. Children with various psychiatric conditions may complain of frequent blinking or difficulty swallowing, or they may hear voices. When children complain of shortness of breath the APN should clarify when these symptoms occur. If the child/adolescent states that she feels short of breath when sitting alone or before a test rather than with activity, the APN should consider a psychiatric cause rather than a medical one. Children who complain of chest pains and/or palpitations often have issues with anxiety. The longer the symptoms of chest pain or palpitations have been going on, the more likely they are related to mental health problems. Chronic abdominal pain, nausea, vomiting and/or diarrhea, and constipation are frequently related to mental health conditions. The child who has these symptoms with no physical cause should be referred for a psychiatric evaluation. Headaches are another common complaint that may represent mental health problems in children or adolescents.

When conducting a review of systems from children/adolescents, the APN should ask when these symptoms present. Physical symptoms that are associated with specific environments such as only during the school week or during testing times should alert the APN to possible emotional causes. Symptoms that occur more often when people are present than when the child is alone are also concerning for psychosomatic causes. When children with multiple physical complaints are found to have a normal exam and normal laboratory tests, the APN should consider the possibility of a psychological cause. Any physical complaints from the child/adolescent should be fully evaluated during the physical exam to determine whether the child's feelings are associated with physical findings in the patient.

Physical Examination

The primary care APN performs a comprehensive age-appropriate physical examination, recording height, weight, body mass index, and vital signs. Screening tests for hearing and vision and laboratory data are included.

Elements of the examination depend on the child's age and information gathered during the review of systems and problems under consideration. A full head-to-toe physical evaluation should be performed by the APN. It should include a neurologic evaluation with a developmental assessment. The provider should test reflexes, fine and gross motor skills, and mood. Any complaints the child had during the review of systems such as palpitations should be evaluated during the physical exam, with additional evaluation tools available.

For example, children who complain of chest pain or palpitations should have their heart sound ausculated as well as an ECG, and if needed a 24-hour halter monitor to be sure there is no cardiac cause for these symptoms. Throughout the physical exam the APN should demonstrate to the parents and child the normal findings in order to help them begin to recognize that these symptoms are not related to a physical condition. When appropriate the APN should order laboratory tests to augment the physical evaluation; such tests might include hematocrit or other blood tests, lead level, and urinalysis.

Data from other disciplines, such as nutrition and social work, should be incorporated with other objective data. The primary care APN uses her knowledge, experience, and clinical decision-making skills to develop diagnoses that reflect any identified disease states, daily living and developmental needs, and family issues. Evidence-based practice guidelines direct the APN in the management of the child's physical health within the context of family and culture. Once the APN has completed the history and physical exam and has collected all the necessary information, he must introduce the possibility of a psychological cause of the child's/adolescent's symptoms. Mental health is managed in collaboration with the PMH-APN after psychiatric assessments are completed.

Use of Assessment Tools

The purposes of assessment tools are to further the understanding of the child or adolescent experiencing the mental disorder, to accurately diagnose, and to plan treatment recommendations (Cohen et al., 2008; Warnick, Weersing, Scahill, & Woolston, 2009). Assessment tools can augment the history and physical exam for the APN to aid her in making the diagnosis. In busy pediatric and primary care practices, the use of brief and straightforward assessment tools can help the provider gather a wide variety of data in a relatively short amount of time. Making use of time before and after the visit increases efficiency and effectiveness (Melnyk & Moldenhauer, 2006; Schor, 2004). Parents and/or children can complete screening tools before the visit, which might help them organize their concerns and questions to maximize time-limited visits. The completed questionnaires can be mailed or sent electronically to the office before the visit, allowing the provider (primary care or psychiatric-mental health) the opportunity to review it in preparation for discussing the results with the parent and child or adolescent. One advantage of using parent-completed questionnaires is that the process might improve parent-provider communication (Squires, Nickel, & Eisert, 1996). Providers benefit when both the children/adolescents and parents complete the forms because they gain information from both sides to optimize their evaluation process.

Optimal mental health screening tools should be brief and focused on the child's psychosocial functioning and the degree of interference of the child's behaviors and problems in her and the family's life. An example of an assessment tool that meets these criteria is the Brief Mental Health Screening Questionnaire for children and adolescents, which can be used in primary care settings. This tool requires parents to answer "yes" or "no" to only six questions about their child's behavior and functioning in the family, at school, with friends, and his personal well-being (de la Osa, Ezpeleta, Granero, & Domenech, 2009). These few questions cover the child's success in school and how he gets along with friends. Warnick et al. (2009) compared several other tools—the Child Behavior Checklist (CBCL); the Strengths and Difficulties Questionnaire (SDQ); and the Ohio Youth Problem, Functioning, and the Satisfaction Scales (OHIO)—using caregivers of 211 children referred to the Yale Child Study Center Outpatient Psychiatric Clinic. OHIO proved the optimal measure to assess needed services, whereas the CBCL and SDQ demonstrated better assessment for specific disorders (Warnick et al., 2009).

Some computer-based screening tools for children/adolescents can be used in primary care settings. In a study evaluating the usefulness of computer-based screening, many adolescents stated that they felt comfortable answering questions on a computer screen and appreciated the privacy that computerized screening afforded. The computer-assisted screening tool demonstrated improvement in the quality and quantity of health history collected and current symptoms expressed; identification of adolescents (eleven to twenty years old) with risk behaviors; and increased identification and referral for behavioral health services for depression, substance use, or suicidal thoughts (Chisolm, Gardner, Julian, & Kelleher, 2008). Perceived ease of use and usefulness of the technological approach to gather sensitive information were significantly associated with satisfaction in both low-risk and high-risk patients and in all topical areas asked (Chisolm et al., 2008). Primary care settings may choose to have adolescents use these tools while they are waiting to be seen.

Ethnic Differences Using Behavioral Rating Scales

Behavioral rating scales are helpful to the practitioner if the scale is brief; easy to use and interpret; and valid across different ages, genders, and ethnic and racial groups. The normative population, cultural sensitivity, comprehensiveness, utility in medical settings, and attractiveness to children should be considered when selecting assessment tools for use with a specific population, and not just the established psychometric properties of the tools (Squires, Nickel, & Eisert, 1996). Behavioral rating scales are only useful if they validly reflect the phenomena being examined, i.e., the child's or adolescent's behavior and difficulties.

Review of Specific Evaluation Tools for Use in Primary Care

The following section reviews common tools that can be used in the pediatric and adolescent population in primary care settings as screening tools. They should be used in conjunction with the history and physical findings to aid the PCP to identify children and adolescents who should be referred for psychiatric evaluation and treatment.

Pediatric Symptom Checklist (PSC)

The PSC (Jellinek & Murphy, 1988) is a one-page thirty-five-item questionnaire designed to help the practitioner identify cognitive, emotional, and behavioral problems as perceived by a parent or other caretaker. It is appropriate for children and adolescents aged four to eighteen years. Items are rated as "never", "sometimes," or "often" present and scored as 0, 1, and 2, respectively. The PSC is easy to complete and easy to score. The PSC-Youth Report (Y-PSC), a youth self-reported version of the scale, is available for older adolescents. The cutoff score of 28 or higher is indicative of psychological impairment in children and adolescents ages six through sixteen. For children ages four and five, the PSC cutoff score is 24 or higher. For the Y-PSC, the cutoff score is 30 or higher. Items that are left blank are simply ignored; however, the questionnaire is invalid if four or more items are left blank (Jellinek & Murphy, 1988; Jellinek, Murphy, Robinson et al., 1988).

A positive score suggests the need for further evaluation by a qualified health or mental health professional.

Because false positives and false negatives occur, there should be no substitute for interpretation by an experienced clinician; parents and other lay people who administer the form should consult with a licensed professional if their child receives a positive score. These scales are in the public domain and can be downloaded for use at http://www2.massgeneral.org/allpsych/psc/psc_home.htm. Users are encouraged to read information about the scales and scoring before first use. Copies of both the PSC and Y-PSC are included at the end of this chapter (Appendix 4.A).

Child Behavior Checklist (CBCL)

Parents or other individuals such as teachers, social workers, or other significant adults in the child's or adolescent's life can use the CBCL (Achenbach, 1991) to rate a child's problem behaviors and competencies. This tool can be self-administered or through an interview with the parent. It can be used for further evaluation if a positive score is found on the PSC. There are two versions, both of which were revised from the original: one for children eighteen months to five years of age (CBCL/1-1/2–5) (Achenbach, 2010a) and another for ages six to eighteen years (CBCL/6–18) (Achenbach, 2010b). The CBCL-Youth Self Report (YSR) can be completed by the adolescent eleven to eighteen years of age. Included with the CBCL for preschoolers is a Language Development Survey (LDS), and teacher report forms (TRF) for each age group (version of the CBCL) are also available. The CBCL consists of two sections with items on competence and behavior or emotional problems; the individual completing the scale rates how true each item is now and within the past six months (Achenbach & Ruffle, 2000). The CBCL has been found to be a valid and reliable tool with African American, Caucasian, and Hispanic/Latino children across all socioeconomic levels. Manual or computer scoring is available and permission is required to use the instrument, which can be ordered at www.ASEBA.org. See Appendices 4.B, 4.C, and 4.D.

Diagnostic Interview for Children and Adolescents (DICA)

The DICA (Reich, 2000) was originally developed in the 1970s as a highly structured interview, but later versions have been created for use in a semistructured format. Training is required for anyone who administers the instrument. The latest version is based on the Diagnostic and Statistical Manual of Mental Disorders (DSM-IV™) and designed for administration to six- to seventeen-year-olds, either through interview or by self-report or parent-completed reports. Items cover six categories: conduct disorder, street drugs, marijuana, post-traumatic stress disorder, alcohol, and major depressive disorder.

Each category takes about five to twenty minutes to complete, and up to two hours for the entire tool (Reich, 2000). Because of length and time involved, it might be too burdensome for use with younger children. This tool might also be difficult to use in primary care settings due to the length of time it takes to complete and time constraints during primary care visits. The DICA-IV has established validity and reliability and relates highly to other psychopathology scales, such as the CBCL (Sala, Granero, & Ezpeleta, 2005). Information about the scale and how to obtain it and the training is available from the publisher Multi-Health Systems, Inc. at www.mhs.com.

Child and Adolescent Psychiatric Assessment (CAPA)

The CAPA is an "interview-based structured psychiatric interview that collects data on the onset dates, duration, frequency, and intensity of symptoms of a wide range of psychiatric diagnoses according to DSM-IV™, DSM-III-R™, or ICD-10™ (International Classification of Diseases) criteria" (Angold & Costello, 2000, p. 39). CAPA is glossary-based, with detailed definitions of symptoms provided. Core sections include psychiatric symptoms, functional impairment, demographics, family structure, and functioning. The tool is intended for use with nine- to seventeen-year-old children and adolescents, either by child self-report or parent report. It can be completed in about one and a half hours. The interviewer decides whether a symptom is present after intensive questioning of the patient through three levels of probing—screening questions, mandatory probes, and discretionary probes—and finally noting which of sixty-seven glossary-defined terms of observable behaviors were observed with the child or adolescent (Angold et al., 1995). Interviewers must first undergo one to two weeks of classroom/practice training before administering the tool; scoring is also learned. Reliable data can be obtained from well-trained and supervised lay interviewers. Other special versions are available for use with younger children and young adults. This tool is difficult to use in the primary care setting due to the length of time it takes to complete as well as the need for specialized training for the provider. Information about CAPA training and tools can be found at http://devepi.duhs. duke.edu/capa.

Global Assessment

Several tools have been developed to allow for an evaluation of the child's overall assessment, or global assessment. Because there is no international consensus regarding the best scale for global assessment, Haugen Schorre and Vandvik (2004) conducted an overview of the empirical evidence published in 103 articles about the three most common unidimensional scales used in child and adolescent psychiatry with children ages zero to eighteen years old: the Global Assessment of Psychosocial Disability (GAPD), Children's Global Assessment Scale (CGAS), and the Global Assessment of Functioning Scale (GAF).

Differences in instructions given to the assessor, coding, meaning of scores, and age ranges for use were found for each tool. The authors made several conclusions:

1. Global assessment scales help reduce biases inherent in the subjective responses of self-report scales
2. The patient's total situation is evaluated, versus a "target symptom"
3. All three scales were easy to use and score after training and could be used on psychiatric as well as normal populations
4. Global assessment of psychosocial functioning should be done with an appropriate scale and in combination with clinical judgment
5. International consensus on the use of one scale for global assessment would improve reliability of scales in clinical practice

Identifying Risk and Protective Factors

When evaluating children and adolescents for mental health problems, the APN should assess the child and family for risk factors as well as protective factors. Risk factors are conditions in the child's life, family, environment, or personality that increase the likelihood of negative outcomes, such as the development of mental disorders. Factors that put children and adolescents at higher risk include family history of psychiatric illness and substance abuse, poor physical health, limited intelligence, weak family support, limited family resources, poverty, parental conflict and marital disruption, history of being abused or neglected, community violence (Evans, 2009), and damaged bonding with primary caregivers. Although the significance of genetic factors in determining the occurrence of mental illness is recognized, it is important to remember that genetic influences are modulated by environmental factors (Evans, 2009).

An assessment that focuses solely on the weaknesses, problems, and limitations of children and adolescents is not a useful one, for it is their and the families' strengths and abilities which will help them develop the adequate skills needed to build resilience, reduce symptoms, and, if possible, recover from mental disorders. Identifying these protective factors is, therefore, essential. Examples of protective factors, that is, factors that decrease the likelihood of mental illness and help protect the child or adolescent from its negative effects, include healthy parenting, strong family connections, physical health, normal or higher intelligence, strong relationships with parents, and family support and resources.

Teaching Needs

Throughout the assessment process, the APN should look for and take advantage of opportunities for mental health teaching of the child, adolescent, and family members. This includes clear, concise explanations of the assessment process and findings, reinforcing the positive actions already taken by the child or adolescent and family, and strengthening the competencies of all the family.

Communicating Findings to Children, Adolescents, and Families

Discussing issues regarding the mental health care of children and adolescents can be overwhelming to the primary care provider. Williams et al. (2004) conducted a study with forty-seven pediatricians who worked in urban primary care settings, 87% of whom used checklists or other screening tools to diagnose mental health problems, the most frequent of which was ADHD. Reasons given for not making other behavioral health diagnoses were the perceived [negative] impact of a diagnosis on the child and family, possible negative effects of labeling a child, and lack of parental readiness to accept the diagnosis. Lack of personal comfort in making behavioral health diagnoses and lack of experience and training were influential pediatrician characteristics (Williams et al., 2004). Melnyk (2006) recommended using caution in placing psychiatric diagnoses on children and adolescents, especially if the diagnosis is not accurate, because of the added burden that stigma and labeling might place on the family.

There is nothing magical or mystical about psychiatric assessments, nor should the assessment findings be conveyed to parents as though there is something to be feared or that their child or adolescent is "mental." It is helpful to remember the words of Jensen et al. (1999, p. 118):

> …it is all too easy to reify the diagnostic labels and to forget that the labels are temporary abstractions that do not capture the complex presentation of a human being who is suffering from some mental, behavioral, or emotional difficulty within a developmental context.

Parents, grandparents, or guardians should receive clear and accurate explanations of assessment findings in a way that does not alarm them, but rather, offers hopeful ideas about treatment options. Parents must have sufficient information to make informed decisions about which treatment option or options to select.

Establishing Trust with the Child or Adolescent and Family

Bringing a child or adolescent to a PCP or psychiatric health care provider for a mental health issue is typically an unfamiliar event, wrought with anxiety and fear. The parent, as well as the child or adolescent, may feel defeated, hopeless, and frightened. Parents may believe that their child's problem behavior indicates that they have not been good parents and wonder whether they will be judged as inadequate or weak parents. The child or adolescent may be confused or disheartened by the looming encounter and wonder if they are "bad," "stupid," "in trouble", or whether their parents are angry at them.

On the other hand, the primary care setting is a familiar experience, one that is less likely to be threatening. The primary care APN is usually already familiar with the family, has a trusting relationship with them, and is knowledgeable of multidisciplinary community resources that can provide further treatment for the child or adolescent and family. The importance of establishing trust cannot be overemphasized. Trust is reinforced when the APN is calm, supportive, and knowledgeable about the types of disorders children commonly experience and their treatment, including the fact that treatment is available, because many people do not realize that mental health disorders and behavioral problems are treatable.

Referral to Mental Health Professionals

Many children and adolescents with mental health disorders are successfully treated by primary care APNs, physicians, and others with training in treating certain disorders. The AACAP (2010) has prepared a statement, *When to Seek Referral or Consultation with a Child Adolescent Psychiatrist*, that identifies circumstances under which referral to a trained child and adolescent mental health practitioner is appropriate and preferred. Referrals can be formal—according to procedure—or informal, occurring via telephone, email, or mail consultation.

The decision to refer can be determined by a number of factors such as "the clinical presentation of the patient, training, skill and experience of the practitioner, family and environmental situation, availability of support services and personnel, and availability of a child and adolescent psychiatrist with relevant experience" (AACAP, 2010, paragraph 1).

Report of the following behaviors in children and adolescents are examples of circumstances in primary care that mandate referral (AACAP, 2009, p. 6):

1. A significant change in his emotional or behavioral functioning for which there is no obvious or recognized precipitant, e.g., sudden onset of school avoidance.

2. A problem that constitutes a threat to the safety of the child/adolescent or the safety of those around her, e.g., severe aggressive behavior.
3. Significant disruption in day-to-day functioning or reality contact, e.g., repeated severe tantrums with no apparent reason.
4. Difficulty with school performance and no significant improvement after attempts by the PCP and school personnel to remediate the problems.

Emergency situations, such as suicidal behavior or suicide attempt, would not be initially managed in the primary care setting.

In a secondary analysis of Child Behavior Study data, Rushton, Bruckman, and Kelleher (2002) examined PCP referral patterns for patients with psychosocial problems. Clinicians from primary care offices in the United States, Canada, and Puerto Rico screened patients aged four to fifteen years, identifying 19% with a psychosocial problem at the index visit. Watchful waiting/no treatment was decided for 38.4%, and 16.2% were referred at the index visit (27.4% for newly diagnosed) to a mental health professional, most commonly for psychotic episodes, substance abuse, emotional problems, and adjustment reaction. The most common reason for referral was the ability of the clinician to manage the patient in her practice for conditions such as ADHD, developmental delays, and mental retardation. At the six-month follow-up, less than half of newly diagnosed patients had seen a mental health care provider. Adherence to management recommendations should be considered serious by PCPs and addressed at every primary care visit through counseling on the importance of follow-through with referrals. Rushton, Bruckman, and Kelleher (2002) recommended that PCPs establish and maintain strong communications and relationships with their mental health colleagues to increase referral completions. The ultimate goal is to make sure the children receive the appropriate care from the most qualified professionals to improve long-term outcomes.

After screening in primary care, children and adolescents who have been identified with mental health disorders and behavioral problems should be referred to PMH-APNs or other qualified mental health professionals for further evaluation and appropriate intervention, as indicated. Interventions might include care that can be directed by the PCP with consultation from the psychiatric experts. Improving patient outcomes requires the integration of collaboration between mental health experts and the primary care providers working together to promote the well-being of the child/adolescent and family (AACAP, 2010). Developing efficient and effective referral systems and maintaining open communication with the various specialists, primary care providers, and family are integral in assisting families as they attempt to optimize the mental health of their children.

Implications for Nursing Practice, Research, and Education

Assessment of children and adolescents for mental health disorders and behavior problems is within the scope of practice of primary care and PMH-APNs, and every opportunity to screen should used, especially during pediatric visits for routine primary care. APNs must be sure to listen to parental concerns and follow through with the appropriate screening. Easy-to-use scales are available and should be accessible in all pediatric practices. The primary care APN should refer more complex assessments to the PMH-APN or other psychiatric provider.

Training for APNs should include more purposeful content for physical and psychiatric assessments in undergraduate and graduate curricula. A mental health history has significant overlap and commonalities with a child's primary care health history. Teaching more critical observation skills of child behavior to students and practicing APNs is also key to increasing the numbers of children actually being screened. Studies about child and adolescent mental health by authors from other disciplines far outnumber those conducted by nurses; more nurses must become principal or co-investigators on teams to document how effective nurses are at assessing and identifying children with mental health needs. Testing models in primary care, where nursing takes the lead, might improve access and increase opportunities for screening and early identification of children and adolescents with mental health needs.

Case Exemplar

Mary, a ten-year-old girl, entered the fifth grade in September. In mid-December her mother made an appointment with the pediatric NP at the primary care clinic to discuss her concern about Mary's intermittent complaints of abdominal pain over the past two months. The pain would occur in the morning shortly after eating breakfast and was severe enough that Mary would cry and hold her stomach. She often had to return to bed for two to three hours while the pain resolved. At the time her mother came in for an evaluation, she was missing several days of school each week. Her mother also noted that these pains occurred during the week and never on weekends or school holidays.

Although the teacher described Mary as a model student, her mother had noticed that she had become moodier and did not want to spend time with her friends as before. Prior to this year Mary had always loved going to school, rarely missed a day due to illness, and frequently had play dates after school. During the history, the PNP learned that Mary had had no weight loss, no fever, no nausea or vomiting, no diarrhea or constipation, and no blood in her stool. There was no history of headaches, chest pain, or shortness of breath. She did state that when her abdomen hurt her sometimes she could also feel her heart "racing in my chest." She denied any dizziness or syncope with these symptoms.

Her mother stated she had been trying new foods in her diet but when these symptoms started she returned to her regular diet with no improvement. She denied any history of recent trauma or loss in the family. Her mother reported no changes in the family or home situation. Mary was taking no medications, had no known allergies, and had not started menstruating.

Mary sat quietly in the exam room but was in constant motion in the chair and biting her fingernails. She was able to answer the PNP's questions when asked. She stated her stomach pains felt like someone was "punching me in the stomach." She could not identify anything that would make the pains worse but did state if her mother massaged her abdomen the pains would subside. When asked how she liked school, she did not offer much information; rather, she simply stated, "I guess it is OK." When asked if anything or anyone was bothering her, she said, "No."

The PNP proceeded with the physical examination to check for any obvious signs of disease. Her height, weight, blood pressure, pulse, and temperature were all in normal range. Her height and weight were in the 45% for her age. Her physical exam was normal, with a regular heart rate and rhythm and a normal abdominal exam. The PNP arranged for Mary to have laboratory work including a CBC, chemistry, urinalysis, and a stool guiac, which were all normal. Mary's mother completed the Pediatric Symptom Checklist (PSC) in another room while the PNP interviewed Mary without her mother. The PNP again asked Mary if anyone or anything was bothering her and if she felt safe at home. Mary did not disclose any new information during the time alone with the PNP.

The results of the PSC were positive for possible anxiety disorder. Because Mary's score on the PSC was positive, the PNP referred her to a psychiatric-mental health NP colleague who conducted a comprehensive psychiatric assessment a few days later, including administration of the Child Behavior Checklist (CBCL/6–18) along with other targeted scales for anxiety and depression. She closely observed Mary in her interactions with her mother and all the staff at the clinic for any behavioral

signs of functional impairment. Mary was diagnosed with anxiety disorder and a treatment plan was developed.

By April, her abdominal pains were significantly improved and she was no longer missing school due to the pain. She also reported her palpitations had resolved. Her mother informed the school so they could offer support to Mary when she appeared anxious. With the counseling and support from her parents and the school, her anxiety was better controlled and she was slowly beginning to engage again in activities with her friends.

Resources for Primary Care Providers and Families

This list includes a number of resources available for APNs in primary care to aid in evaluating children and families. It provides access to the tools discussed in this chapter, and offers some educational and support services for families:

American Academy of Child and Adolescent Psychiatry (AACAP), http://www.aacap.org

American Academy of Pediatrics (AAP), http://www.aap.org

American Psychiatric Nurses Association (APNA), http://www.apna.org

Achenbach System of Empirically Based Assessment (ASEBA), http://www.aseba.org

Ages and Stages Questionnaire, http://www.agesandstages.com

Bright Futures, http://www.brightfutures.org

International Society of Psychiatric-Mental Health Nurses, http://www.ispn-psych.org

MGH Pediatric Symptom Checklist, http://www2.massgeneral.org/allpsych/psc/psc_home.htm

National Association of Pediatric Nurse Practitioners (NAPNAP), http://www.napnap.com

References

Achenbach, T. (1991). *Integrative guide to the 1991 CBCL/4–18, YSR, and TRF profiles.* Burlington, VT: University of Vermont, Department of Psychology.

Achenbach, T. (2010a). *Preschool (Ages 1 1/2–5) assessments.* Retrieved November 6, 2010, from http://www.aseba.org/preschool.html

Achenbach, T. (2010b). *School-age (Ages 6–11) assessments.* Retrieved November 6, 2010, from http://www.aseba.org/schoolage.html

Achenbach, T. (2010c). *YSR (Ages 11–18) assessment.* Retrieved November 6, 2010, from http://www.aseba.org/schoolage.html

Achenbach, T.M., & Ruffle, T.M. (2000). The child behavior checklist and related forms for assessing behavioral/emotional problems and competencies. *Pediatrics in Review, 21*, 265–271.

American Academy of Child and Adolescent Psychiatry. (2010). *When to seek referral or consultation with a child adolescent psychiatrist.* Retrieved on November 2, 2010, from http://www.aacap.org/cs/

root/member_information/practice_information/when_to_seek_referral_or_consultation_with_a_child_adolescent_psychiatrist

American Academy of Child and Adolescent Psychiatry. (2009). Improving mental health services in primary care: Reducing administrative and financial barriers to access and collaboration. *Pediatrics, 123,* 1248–1251.

American Academy of Child and Adolescent Psychiatry and American Academy of Pediatrics. (2009). *Improving mental health services in primary care: Reducing administrative and financial barriers to access and collaboration—Background.* Retrieved from http://www.aacap.org/galleries/LegislativeAction/Final%20Background%20paper%203-09.pdf

American Academy of Nurse Practitioners. (2010). *Nurse practitioner facts.* Retrieved November 2, 2010, from http://aanp.org/NR/rdonlyres/54B71B02-D4DB-4A53-9FA6-23DDA0EDD6FC/0/NPFacts2010.pdf

Angold, A., & Costello, J. (2000). The child and adolescent psychiatric assessment (CAPA). *Journal of American Academy of Child & Adolescent Psychiatry, 39,* 39–48.

Angold, A., Prendergast, M., Cox, A., Harrington, R., Simonoff, E., & Rutter, M. (1995). The child and adolescent psychiatric assessment (CAPA). *Psychological Medicine, 25,* 739–753.

Brugman, E., Reijneveld, S.A., Verhulst, F.C., & Verloove-Vanhorick, P. (2001). Identification and management of psychosocial problems by preventive child health care. *Archives of Pediatric & Adolescent Medicine, 155,* 462–469.

Burns, C.E. (2010). Sleep and rest. In C.E. Burns, A.M. Dunn, M.A. Brady, N.B. Starr, & C.G. Blosser (Eds.). *Pediatric primary care* (4th edition; pp. 304–319). St. Louis, MO: Saunders.

Burns, C.E., & Kodadek, S.M. (2009). Child and family health assessment. In C.E. Burns, A.M. Dunn, M.A. Brady, N.B. Starr, & C.G. Blosser (Eds.). *Pediatric primary care* (4th edition; pp. 12–40). St. Louis, MO: Saunders.

Cawthorpe, D. (2005). Primary care physician ability to identify pediatric mental health issues. *The Canadian Child and Adolescent Psychiatry Review, 14*(4), 99–102.

Chisolm, D.J., Gardner, W., Julian, T., & Kelleher, K.J. (2008). Adolescent satisfaction with computer-assisted behavioural risk screening in primary care. *Child and Adolescent Mental Health, 13*(4), 163–168. doi:10.1111/j.1475-3588.2007.00474.x

Cohen, L.L., LaGreca, A.M., Blount, R.L., Kazak, A.E., Holmbeck, G.N., & Lemanek, K.L. (2008). Introduction to special issue: Evidence-based assessment in pediatric psychology. *Journal of Pediatric Psychology, 33,* 911–915.

de la Osa, N., Ezpeleta, L., Granero, R., & Domenech, J.M. (2009). Brief mental health screening questionnaire for children and adolescents in primary care settings. *International Journal of Adolescent Medicine and Health, 21*(1), 91–100.

Dunn, A.M. (2010a). Cultural perspectives for pediatric primary care. In C.E. Burns, A.M. Dunn, M.A. Brady, N.B. Starr, & C.G. Blosser (Eds.). *Pediatric primary care* (4th edition; pp. 41–50). St. Louis, MO: Saunders.

Dunn, A.M. (2010b). Nutrition. In C.E. Burns, A.M. Dunn, M.A. Brady, N.B. Starr, & C.G. Blosser (Eds). *Pediatric primary care* (4th edition; pp. 191–234). St. Louis, MO: Saunders.

Egger, H.I., Erkanli, A., Keeler, G., Potts, E., Walter, B.K., & Angold, A. (2006). Test-retest reliability of the Preschool Age Psychiatric Assessment (PAPA). *Journal of American Academy of Child & Adolescent Psychiatry, 45,* 538–549.

Evans, M.E. (2009). Prevention of mental, emotional, and behavioral disorders in youth: The Institute of Medicine report and implications for nursing. *Journal of Child and Adolescent Psychiatric Nursing, 22,* 154–159.

Hacker, K.A., Myagmarjav, E., Harris, V., Franco Suglia, S., Weidner, D., & Link, D. (2006). Mental health screening in pediatric practice: Factors related to positive screens and the contribution of parental/personal concern. *Pediatrics, 118,* 1896–1906. doidoi:10.1542/pedsw.2006-0026

Haugen Schorre, B.E., & Vandvik, I.H. (2004). Global assessment of psychosocial functioning in child and adolescent psychiatry. *European Child & Adolescent Psychiatry, 13,* 273–286. doi:10.1007/s00787-004-0390-2

Huang, L., Macbeth, G., Dodge, J., & Jacobstein, D. (2004). Transforming the workforce in children's mental health. *Administration and Policy in Mental Health, 32,* 167–187.

Hysing, M., Elgen, I., Gillberg, C., Lie, S.A., & Lundervold, A.J. (2007). Chronic physical illness and mental health in children: Results from a large-scale population study. *Journal of Child Psychiatry and Psychology, 48,* 785–792.

Jellinek, M.S., & Murphy, J.M. (1988). Screening for psychosocial disorders in pediatric practice. *American Journal of the Diseases of Children, 142,* 1153–1157.

Jellinek, M.S., Murphy, J.M., Robinson, J., Feins, A., Lamb, S., & Fenton, T. (1988). Pediatric symptom checklist: Screening school-age children for psychosocial dysfunction. *Journal of Pediatrics, 112,* 201–209.

Jensen, P.S., Brooks-Gunn, J., & Graber, J.A. (1999). Introduction—Dimensional scales and diagnostic categories: Constructing crosswalks for child psychopathology assessments. *Journal of American Academy of Child and Adolescent Psychiatry, 38,* 118–120.

Knafl, K.A., & Santacroce, S.J. (2010). Chronic conditions and the family. In P.J. Allen, J.A. Vessey, & N.A. Schapiro (Eds). *Primary care of the child with a chronic condition* (5th edition; pp. 74–89). St. Louis, MO: Mosby Elsevier.

Koppelman, J. (2004, October 26). *The provider system for children's mental health: Workforce capacity and effective treatment* (NHPF Issue Brief No. 801). Washington, DC: The George Washington University. Retrieved from http://76.12.169.157/library/issue-briefs/IB801_ChildMHProvider_10-26-04.pdf

Lemmon, K.M., & Stafford, E.M. (2007). Recognizing and responding to child and adolescent stress: The critical role of the pediatrician. *Pediatric Annals, 36,* 225–234.

McGuiness, T.M., Noonan, P., & Dyer, J.G. (2005). Family history as a tool for psychiatric nurses. *Archives of Psychiatric Nursing, 19,* 116–124. doi:10.1016/j.apnu.2005.04.003

Melnyk, B. (2006). Section 2: Diagnosing, managing, and preventing mental health disorders. In B.M. Melnyk, & Z. Moldenhauer, *The KySS^SM (Keep your children/yourself Safe and Secure): Guide to child and adolescent mental health screening, early intervention and health promotion* (pp. 49–56). Cherry Hill, NJ: National Association of Pediatric Nurse Practitioners.

Melnyk, B.M. (Ed.), & Moldenhauer, Z. (Asst. Ed.). (2006). *The KySS^SM(Keep your children/yourself Safe and Secure): Guide to child and adolescent mental health screening, early intervention and health promotion.* Cherry Hill, NJ: National Association of Pediatric Nurse Practitioners.

National Research Council and Institute of Medicine. (2009). *Preventing mental, emotional, and behavioral disorders among young people: Progress and possibilities.* Washington, DC: The National Academies Press.

National Technical Assistance Center for Children's Mental Health. (2005, February). *Transforming the workforce in children's mental health* (Issue Brief No. 1). Washington, DC: Georgetown University Center for Child and Human Development.

Olson, A.L., Kelleher, K.J., Kemper, K.J., Zuckerman, B.S., Hammond, C.S., & Dietrich, A.J. (2001). Primary care pediatricians' roles and perceived responsibilities in the identification and management of depression in children and adolescents. *Academic Pediatrics, 1*(2), 91–98.

Ozer, E.M., Zahnd, E.G., Adams, S.H., Husting, S.R., Wibbelsman, C.J., Norman, K.P., et al. (2009). Are adolescents being screened for emotional distress in primary care? *Journal of Adolescent Health, 44,* 520–527.

Reich, W. (2000). Diagnostic interview for children and adolescents (DICA). *Journal of American Academy of Child & Adolescent Psychiatry, 39,* 59–66.

Rushton, J., Bruckman, D., & Kelleher, K. (2002). Primary care referral of children with psychosocial problems. *Archives of Pediatric Adolescent Medicine, 156,* 592–598.

Schor, E.L. (2004). Rethinking well-child care. *Pediatrics, 114,* 210–216. doidoi:10.1542/peds.114.1.210

Sala, R., Granero, R., & Ezpeleta, L. (2005). Dimensional analysis of a categorical diagnostic interview: the DICA-IV. *Psicothema, 18,* 123–129. Retrieved from http://redalyc.uaemex.mx/pdf/727/72718119.pdf

Simpson, G.A., Cohen, R.A., Pastor, P.N., & Reuben, C.A. (2008, September). *Use of mental health services in the past 12 months by children aged 4–17 years: United States, 2005–2006* (NCHS Data Brief No. 8). Hyattsville, MD: National Center for Health Statistics.

Squires, J., Nickel, R.E., & Eisert, D. (1996). Early detection of developmental problems: Strategies for monitoring young children in the practice setting. *Developmental and Behavioral Pediatrics, 17,* 420–427.

U.S. Department of Health and Human Services, Health Resources and Services Administration. (2010). *The registered nurse population: Findings from the 2008 national sample survey of registered nurses.* Retrieved from http://bhpr.hrsa.gov/healthworkforce/rnsurvey/initialfindings2008.pdfhttp://bhpr.hrsa.gov/healthworkforce/rnsurvey/initialfindings2008.pdf

Warnick, E.M., Weersing, V.R., Scahill, L., & Woolston, J.L. (2009). Selecting measures for use in child mental health services: A scorecard approach. *Administration and Policy in Mental Health and Mental Health Services Research, 36,* 112–122.

Williams, J., Klienpeter, K., Palmes, G., Pulley, A., & Foy, J. M. (2004). Diagnosis and treatment of behavioral health disorders in pediatric practice. *Pediatrics, 114,* 601–606. doidoi:10.1542/peds.2004-0090

World Health Organization (WHO) and World Organization of Family Doctors (WONCA). (2008). *Integrating mental health into primary care: A global perspective.* Geneva, Switzerland: WHO Press.

Appendix 4.A

Pediatric Symptom Checklist (PSC)

Emotional and physical health go together in children. Because parents are often the first to notice a problem with their child's behavior, emotions or learning, you may help your child get the best care possible by answering these questions. Please indicate which statement best describes your child.

Please mark under the heading that best describes your child:

	NEVER (0)	SOMETIMES (1)	OFTEN (2)
1. Complains of aches and pains			
2. Spends more time alone			
3. Tires easily, has little energy			
4. Fidgety, unable to sit still			
5. Has trouble with teacher			
6. Less interested in school			
7. Acts as if driven by a motor			
8. Day dreams too much			
9. Distracted easily			
10. Is afraid of new situations			
11. Feels sad, unhappy			
12. Is irritable, angry			
13. Feels hopeless			
14. Has trouble concentrating			
15. Less interested in friends			
16. Fights with other children			
17. Absent from school			
18. School grades dropping			
19. Is down on him or herself			
20. Visits the doctor with doctor finding nothing wrong			
21. Has trouble sleeping			
22. Worries a lot			
23. Wants to be with you more than before			
24. Feels he or she is bad			
25. Takes unnecessary risks			
26. Gets hurt frequently			
27. Seems to be having less fun			
28. Acts younger than children his or her age			
29. Does not listen to rules			
30. Does not show feelings			
31. Does not understand other people's feelings			
32. Teases others			
33. Blames others for his or her troubles			
34. Takes things that do not belong to him or her			
35. Refuses to share			

Total score

Does your child have any emotional or behavioral problems for which she/he needs help?--------- __No __Yes
Are there any services that you would like your child to receive for these problems?----------------- __No __Yes

If yes, what type of services? _____

Pediatric Symptom Checklist - Youth Report (Y-PSC)

Please mark under the heading that best fits you:

	Never	Sometimes	Often
1. Complain of aches and pains	___	___	___
2. Spend more time alone.............................	___	___	___
3. Tire easily, little energy..........................	___	___	___
4. Fridgety, unable to sit still	___	___	___
5. Have trouble with teacher	___	___	___
6. Less interested in school	___	___	___
7. Act as if driven by motor	___	___	___
8. Daydream too much.................................	___	___	___
9. Distract easily	___	___	___
10. Are afraid of new situations	___	___	___
11. Feel sad, unhappy.................................	___	___	___
12. Are irritable, angry	___	___	___
13. Feel hopeless	___	___	___
14. Have trouble concentrating.........................	___	___	___
15. Less interested in friends.........................	___	___	___
16. Fight with other children	___	___	___
17. Absent from school.................................	___	___	___
18. School grades dropping	___	___	___
19. Down on yourself..................................	___	___	___
20. Visit doctor with doctor finding nothing wrong........	___	___	___
21. Have trouble sleeping.............................	___	___	___
22. Worry a lot	___	___	___
23. Want to be with parent more than before.............	___	___	___
24. Feel that you are bad.............................	___	___	___
25. Take unnecessary risks...........................	___	___	___
26. Get hurt frequently................................	___	___	___
27. Seem to be having less fun.........................	___	___	___
28. Act younger than children your age................	___	___	___
29. Do not listen to rules..............................	___	___	___
30. Do not show feelings	___	___	___
31. Do not understand other people's feelings............	___	___	___
32. Tease others......................................	___	___	___
33. Blame others for your troubles...............	___	___	___
34. Take things that do not belong to you...............	___	___	___
35. Refuse to share...................................	___	___	___

Appendix 4.B

Please print. Be sure to answer all items.	CHILD BEHAVIOR CHECKLIST FOR AGES 1½-5	For office use only ID #

| CHILD'S FULL NAME | First | Middle | Last | **PARENTS' USUAL TYPE OF WORK, even if not working now.** *Please be specific — for example, auto mechanic, high school teacher, homemaker, laborer, lathe operator, shoe salesman, army sergeant.* |

CHILD'S GENDER ☐ Boy ☐ Girl	CHILD'S AGE	CHILD'S ETHNIC GROUP OR RACE

FATHER'S TYPE OF WORK _____

MOTHER'S TYPE OF WORK _____

TODAY'S DATE Mo. ____ Day ____ Year _____	CHILD'S BIRTHDATE Mo. ____ Day ____ Year ____

THIS FORM FILLED OUT BY: (print your full name)

_____

Please fill out this form to reflect *your* view of the child's behavior even if other people might not agree. Feel free to write additional comments beside each item and in the space provided on page 2. **Be sure to answer all items.**

Your relationship to child:

☐ Mother   ☐ Father   ☐ Other (specify):

Below is a list of items that describe children. For each item that describes the child **now or within the past 2 months**, please circle the **2** if the item is **very true or often true** of the child. Circle the **1** if the item is **somewhat or sometimes true** of the child. If the item is **not true** of the child, circle the **0**. Please answer all items as well as you can, even if some do not seem to apply to the child.

0 = Not True (as far as you know)   1 = Somewhat or Sometimes True   2 = Very True or Often True

0 1 2 1. Aches or pains (without medical cause; *do not* include stomach or headaches)	0 1 2 30. Easily jealous
0 1 2 2. Acts too young for age	0 1 2 31. Eats or drinks things that are not food—*don't* include sweets (describe): _____
0 1 2 3. Afraid to try new things	_____
0 1 2 4. Avoids looking others in the eye	0 1 2 32. Fears certain animals, situations, or places (describe): _____
0 1 2 5. Can't concentrate, can't pay attention for long	_____
0 1 2 6. Can't sit still, restless, or hyperactive	
0 1 2 7. Can't stand having things out of place	0 1 2 33. Feelings are easily hurt
0 1 2 8. Can't stand waiting; wants everything now	0 1 2 34. Gets hurt a lot, accident-prone
0 1 2 9. Chews on things that aren't edible	0 1 2 35. Gets in many fights
0 1 2 10. Clings to adults or too dependent	0 1 2 36. Gets into everything
0 1 2 11. Constantly seeks help	0 1 2 37. Gets too upset when separated from parents
0 1 2 12. Constipated, doesn't move bowels (when not sick)	0 1 2 38. Has trouble getting to sleep
	0 1 2 39. Headaches (without medical cause)
0 1 2 13. Cries a lot	0 1 2 40. Hits others
0 1 2 14. Cruel to animals	0 1 2 41. Holds his/her breath
0 1 2 15. Defiant	0 1 2 42. Hurts animals or people without meaning to
0 1 2 16. Demands must be met immediately	0 1 2 43. Looks unhappy without good reason
0 1 2 17. Destroys his/her own things	0 1 2 44. Angry moods
0 1 2 18. Destroys things belonging to his/her family or other children	0 1 2 45. Nausea, feels sick (without medical cause)
	0 1 2 46. Nervous movements or twitching (describe): _____
0 1 2 19. Diarrhea or loose bowels (when not sick)	
0 1 2 20. Disobedient	
0 1 2 21. Disturbed by any change in routine	0 1 2 47. Nervous, highstrung, or tense
0 1 2 22. Doesn't want to sleep alone	0 1 2 48. Nightmares
0 1 2 23. Doesn't answer when people talk to him/her	0 1 2 49. Overeating
0 1 2 24. Doesn't eat well (describe): _____	0 1 2 50. Overtired
	0 1 2 51. Shows panic for no good reason
0 1 2 25. Doesn't get along with other children	0 1 2 52. Painful bowel movements (without medical cause)
0 1 2 26. Doesn't know how to have fun; acts like a little adult	
	0 1 2 53. Physically attacks people
0 1 2 27. Doesn't seem to feel guilty after misbehaving	0 1 2 54. Picks nose, skin, or other parts of body (describe): _____
0 1 2 28. Doesn't want to go out of home	
0 1 2 29. Easily frustrated	*Be sure you answered all items. Then see other side.*

Reprinted from Achenbach, 2010, with permission from the author.

Please print your answers. Be sure to answer all items.

0 = Not True (as far as you know)	1 = Somewhat or Sometimes True	2 = Very True or Often True

0	1	2	55. Plays with own sex parts too much	0 1 2	79.	Rapid shifts between sadness and excitement
0	1	2	56. Poorly coordinated or clumsy	0 1 2	80.	Strange behavior (describe): _____
0	1	2	57. Problems with eyes (without medical cause) (describe): _____ _____			_____
				0 1 2	81.	Stubborn, sullen, or irritable
0	1	2	58. Punishment doesn't change his/her behavior	0 1 2	82.	Sudden changes in mood or feelings
0	1	2	59. Quickly shifts from one activity to another	0 1 2	83.	Sulks a lot
0	1	2	60. Rashes or other skin problems (without medical cause)	0 1 2	84.	Talks or cries out in sleep
				0 1 2	85.	Temper tantrums or hot temper
0	1	2	61. Refuses to eat	0 1 2	86.	Too concerned with neatness or cleanliness
0	1	2	62. Refuses to play active games	0 1 2	87.	Too fearful or anxious
0	1	2	63. Repeatedly rocks head or body	0 1 2	88.	Uncooperative
0	1	2	64. Resists going to bed at night	0 1 2	89.	Underactive, slow moving, or lacks energy
0	1	2	65. Resists toilet training (describe): _____ _____	0 1 2	90.	Unhappy, sad, or depressed
				0 1 2	91.	Unusually loud
0	1	2	66. Screams a lot	0 1 2	92.	Upset by new people or situations (describe): _____ _____
0	1	2	67. Seems unresponsive to affection			
0	1	2	68. Self-conscious or easily embarrassed			
0	1	2	69. Selfish or won't share	0 1 2	93.	Vomiting, throwing up (without medical cause)
0	1	2	70. Shows little affection toward people	0 1 2	94.	Wakes up often at night
0	1	2	71. Shows little interest in things around him/her	0 1 2	95.	Wanders away
0	1	2	72. Shows too little fear of getting hurt	0 1 2	96.	Wants a lot of attention
0	1	2	73. Too shy or timid	0 1 2	97.	Whining
0	1	2	74. Sleeps less than most kids during day and/or night (describe): _____ _____	0 1 2	98.	Withdrawn, doesn't get involved with others
				0 1 2	99.	Worries
0	1	2	75. Smears or plays with bowel movements	0 1 2	100.	Please write in any problems the child has that were not listed above.
0	1	2	76. Speech problem (describe): _____ _____	0 1 2		_____
				0 1 2		_____
0	1	2	77. Stares into space or seems preoccupied	0 1 2		_____
0	1	2	78. Stomachaches or cramps (without medical cause)			

Please be sure you have answered all items.
Underline any you are concerned about.

Does the child have any illness or disability (either physical or mental)? ☐No ☐Yes—Please describe:

What concerns you most about the child?

Please describe the best things about the child:

LANGUAGE DEVELOPMENT SURVEY FOR AGES 18-35 MONTHS

The Language Development Survey assesses children's word combinations and vocabulary. By carefully completing the Language Development Survey, you can help us obtain an accurate picture of your child's developing language. ***Please print your answers. Be sure to answer all items.***

I. Was your child born earlier than the usual 9 months after conception?

☐ No   ☐ Yes—how many weeks early? _____ weeks early.

II. How much did your child weigh at birth? _____ pounds _____ ounces; or _____ grams.

III. How many ear infections did your child have before age 24 months?

☐ 0-2   ☐ 3-5   ☐ 6-8   ☐ 9 or more

IV. Is any language beside English spoken in your home?

☐ No   ☐ Yes—please list the languages: _____ _____

_____ _____

V. Has anyone in your family been slow in learning to talk?

☐ No   ☐ Yes—please list their relationships to your child; for example, brother, father:

_____

VI. Are you worried about your child's language development?

☐ No   ☐ Yes—why? _____

_____

VII. Does your child spontaneously say words in any language? (not just imitates or understands words)?

☐ No   ☐ Yes—if yes, please complete item VIII and page 4.

VIII. Does your child combine 2 or more words into phrases? For example: "more cookie," "car bye-bye."

☐ No   ☐ Yes—please print 5 of your child's longest and best phrases or sentences.

For each phrase that is not in English, print the name of the language.

1. _____

2. _____

3. _____

4. _____

5. _____

Be sure you have answered all items. Then see other side.

Please circle each word that your child says SPONTANEOUSLY (not just imitates or understands). If your child says non-English versions of words on the list, circle the English word and write the first letter of the language (e.g., S for Spanish). Please include words even if they are not pronounced clearly or are in "baby talk" (for example: "baba" for bottle).

FOODS
1. apple
2. banana
3. bread
4. butter
5. cake
6. candy
7. cereal
8. cheese
9. coffee
10. cookie
11. crackers
12. drink
13. egg
14. food
15. grapes
16. gum
17. hamburger
18. hotdog
19. ice cream
20. juice
21. meat
22. milk
23. orange
24. pizza
25. pretzel
26. raisins
27. soda
28. soup
29. spaghetti
30. tea
31. toast
32. water

TOYS
33. ball
34. balloon
35. blocks
36. book
37. crayons
38. doll
39. picture
40. present
41. slide
42. swing
43. teddy bear

OUTDOORS
44. flower
45. house
46. moon
47. rain
48. sidewalk
49. sky
50. snow
51. star
52. street
53. sun
54. tree

ANIMALS
55. bear
56. bee
57. bird
58. bug
59. bunny
60. cat
61. chicken
62. cow
63. dog
64. duck
65. elephant
66. fish
67. frog
68. horse
69. monkey
70. pig
71. puppy
72. snake
73. tiger
74. turkey
75. turtle

BODY PARTS
76. arm
77. belly button
78. bottom
79. chin
80. ear
81. elbow
82. eye
83. face
84. finger
85. foot
86. hair
87. hand
88. knee
89. leg
90. mouth
91. neck
92. nose
93. teeth
94. thumb
95. toe
96. tummy

VEHICLES
97. bike
98. boat
99. bus
100. car
101. motorcycle
102. plane
103. stroller
104. train
105. trolley
106. truck

ACTIONS
107. bath
108. breakfast
109. bring
110. catch
111. clap
112. close
113. come
114. cough
115. cut
116. dance
117. dinner
118. doodoo
119. down
120. eat
121. feed
122. finish
123. fix
124. get
125. give
126. go
127. have
128. help
129. hit
130. hug
131. jump
132. kick
133. kiss
134. knock
135. look
136. love
137. lunch
138. make
139. nap
140. open
141. outside
142. pattycake
143. peekaboo
144. peepee
145. push
146. read
147. ride
148. run
149. see
150. show
151. shut
152. sing
153. sit
154. sleep
155. stop
156. take
157. throw
158. tickle
159. up
160. walk
161. want
162. wash

HOUSEHOLD
163. bathtub
164. bed
165. blanket
166. bottle
167. bowl
168. chair
169. clock
170. crib
171. cup
172. door
173. floor
174. fork
175. glass
176. knife
177. light
178. mirror
179. pillow
180. plate
181. potty
182. radio
183. room
184. sink
185. soap
186. spoon
187. stairs
188. table
189. telephone
190. towel
191. trash
192. T.V.
193. window

PERSONAL
194. brush
195. comb
196. glasses
197. key
198. money
199. paper
200. pen
201. pencil
202. penny
203. pocketbook
204. tissue
205. tooth brush
206. umbrella
207. watch

PLACES
208. church
209. home
210. hospital
211. library
212. park
213. school
214. store
215. zoo

MODIFIERS
216. all gone
217. all right
218. bad
219. big
220. black
221. blue
222. broken
223. clean
224. cold
225. dark
226. dirty
227. dry
228. good
229. happy
230. heavy
231. hot
232. hungry
233. little
234. mine
235. more
236. nice
237. pretty
238. red
239. stinky
240. that
241. this
242. tired
243. wet
244. white
245. yellow
246. yucky

CLOTHES
247. belt
248. boots
249. coat
250. diaper
251. dress
252. gloves
253. hat
254. jacket
255. mittens
256. pajamas
257. pants
258. shirt
259. shoes
260. slippers
261. sneakers
262. socks
263. sweater

OTHER
264. any letter
265. away
266. booboo
267. byebye
268. excuse me
269. here
270. hi, hello
271. in
272. me
273. meow
274. my
275. myself
276. nightnight
277. no
278. off
279. on
280. out
281. please
282. Sesame St.
283. shut up
284. thank you
285. there
286. under
287. welcome
288. what
289. where
290. why
291. woofwoof
292. yes
293. you
294. yumyum
295. any number

PEOPLE
296. aunt
297. baby
298. boy
299. daddy
300. doctor
301. girl
302. grandma
303. grandpa
304. lady
305. man
306. mommy
307. own name
308. pet name
309. uncle
310. name of TV
     or story
     character

Other words your child says, including non-English words:

_____

_____

_____

_____

PAGE 4

Appendix 4.C

☑ **Please print**   CHILD BEHAVIOR CHECKLIST FOR AGES **6-18**

For office use only
ID #

CHILD'S FULL NAME	First	Middle	Last

PARENTS' USUAL TYPE OF WORK, even if not working now.
(Please be specific — for example, auto mechanic, high school teacher, homemaker, laborer, lathe operator, shoe salesman, army sergeant.)

FATHER'S
TYPE OF WORK _____

CHILD'S GENDER	CHILD'S AGE	CHILD'S ETHNIC GROUP OR RACE
☐ Boy ☐ Girl		

MOTHER'S
TYPE OF WORK _____

THIS FORM FILLED OUT BY: (print your full name)

_____

TODAY'S DATE

Mo. ____ Day ____ Year _____

CHILD'S BIRTHDATE

Mo. ____ Day ____ Year ____

Your gender: ☐ Male   ☐ Female

Your relation to the child:

GRADE IN SCHOOL _____

NOT ATTENDING SCHOOL   ☐

Please fill out this form to reflect *your* view of the child's behavior even if other people might not agree. Feel free to print additional comments beside each item and in the space provided on page 2. **Be sure to answer all items.**

☐ Biological Parent   ☐ Step Parent   ☐ Grandparent

☐ Adoptive Parent   ☐ Foster Parent   ☐ Other (specify)

I. Please list the sports your child most likes to take part in. For example: swimming, baseball, skating, skate boarding, bike riding, fishing, etc.

None ☐

Compared to others of the same age, about how much time does he/she spend in each?

Compared to others of the same age, how well does he/she do each one?

	Less Than Average	Average	More Than Average	Don't Know	Below Average	Average	Above Average	Don't Know
a. _____	☐	☐	☐	☐	☐	☐	☐	☐
b. _____	☐	☐	☐	☐	☐	☐	☐	☐
c. _____	☐	☐	☐	☐	☐	☐	☐	☐

II. Please list your child's favorite hobbies, activities, and games, other than sports. For example: stamps, dolls, books, piano, crafts, cars, computers, singing, etc. (Do **not** include listening to radio or TV.)

None ☐

Compared to others of the same age, about how much time does he/she spend in each?

Compared to others of the same age, how well does he/she do each one?

	Less Than Average	Average	More Than Average	Don't Know	Below Average	Average	Above Average	Don't Know
a. _____	☐	☐	☐	☐	☐	☐	☐	☐
b. _____	☐	☐	☐	☐	☐	☐	☐	☐
c. _____	☐	☐	☐	☐	☐	☐	☐	☐

III. Please list any organizations, clubs, teams, or groups your child belongs to.

None ☐

Compared to others of the same age, how active is he/she in each?

	Less Active	Average	More Active	Don't Know
a. _____	☐	☐	☐	☐
b. _____	☐	☐	☐	☐
c. _____	☐	☐	☐	☐

IV. Please list any jobs or chores your child has. For example: paper route, babysitting, making bed, working in store, etc. (Include both paid and unpaid jobs and chores.)

None ☐

Compared to others of the same age, how well does he/she carry them out?

	Below Average	Average	Above Average	Don't Know
a. _____	☐	☐	☐	☐
b. _____	☐	☐	☐	☐
c. _____	☐	☐	☐	☐

Be sure you answered all items. Then see other side.

Reprinted from Achenbach, 2010, with permission from the author.

Please print. Be sure to answer all items.

V. 1. About how many close friends does your child have? (Do *not* include brothers & sisters)

☐ None   ☐ 1   ☐ 2 or 3   ☐ 4 or more

2. About how many times a week does your child do things with any friends outside of regular school hours?

(Do *not* include brothers & sisters)   ☐ Less than 1   ☐ 1 or 2   ☐ 3 or more

VI. Compared to others of his/her age, how well does your child:

	Worse	Average	Better	
a. Get along with his/her brothers & sisters?	☐	☐	☐	☐ Has no brothers or sisters
b. Get along with other kids?	☐	☐	☐	
c. Behave with his/her parents?	☐	☐	☐	
d. Play and work alone?	☐	☐	☐	

VII. 1. Performance in academic subjects.   Does not attend school because _____

Other academic subjects–for example: computer courses, foreign language, business. Do *not* include gym, shop, driver's ed., or other nonacademic subjects.

Check a box for each subject that child takes	Failing	Below Average	Average	Above Average
a. Reading, English, or Language Arts	☐	☐	☐	☐
b. History or Social Studies	☐	☐	☐	☐
c. Arithmetic or Math	☐	☐	☐	☐
d. Science	☐	☐	☐	☐
e. _____	☐	☐	☐	☐
f. _____	☐	☐	☐	☐
g. _____	☐	☐	☐	☐

2. Does your child receive special education or remedial services or attend a special class or special school?

☐ No   ☐ Yes—kind of services, class, or school:

3. Has your child repeated any grades?   ☐ No   ☐ Yes—grades and reasons:

4. Has your child had any academic or other problems in school?   ☐ No   ☐ Yes—please describe:

When did these problems start? _____

Have these problems ended?   ☐ No   ☐ Yes–when?

Does your child have any illness or disability (either physical or mental)?   ☐ No   ☐ Yes—please describe:

What concerns you most about your child?

Please describe the best things about your child.

Be sure you answered all items.

Please print. Be sure to answer all items.

Below is a list of items that describe children and youths. For each item that describes your child *now or within the past 6 months*, please circle the *2* if the item is *very true or often true* of your child. Circle the *1* if the item is *somewhat or sometimes true* of your child. If the item is *not true* of your child, circle the *0*. Please answer all items as well as you can, even if some do not seem to apply to your child.

0 = Not True (as far as you know)   1 = Somewhat or Sometimes True   2 = Very True or Often True

0 1 2 1. Acts too young for his/her age	0 1 2 32. Feels he/she has to be perfect
0 1 2 2. Drinks alcohol without parents' approval (describe): _____	0 1 2 33. Feels or complains that no one loves him/her
	0 1 2 34. Feels others are out to get him/her
0 1 2 3. Argues a lot	0 1 2 35. Feels worthless or inferior
0 1 2 4. Fails to finish things he/she starts	
0 1 2 5. There is very little he/she enjoys	0 1 2 36. Gets hurt a lot, accident-prone
0 1 2 6. Bowel movements outside toilet	0 1 2 37. Gets in many fights
	0 1 2 38. Gets teased a lot
0 1 2 7. Bragging, boasting	0 1 2 39. Hangs around with others who get in trouble
0 1 2 8. Can't concentrate, can't pay attention for long	
0 1 2 9. Can't get his/her mind off certain thoughts; obsessions (describe): _____	0 1 2 40. Hears sound or voices that aren't there (describe): _____
	0 1 2 41. Impulsive or acts without thinking
0 1 2 10. Can't sit still, restless, or hyperactive	0 1 2 42. Would rather be alone than with others
0 1 2 11. Clings to adults or too dependent	0 1 2 43. Lying or cheating
0 1 2 12. Complains of loneliness	0 1 2 44. Bites fingernails
0 1 2 13. Confused or seems to be in a fog	0 1 2 45. Nervous, highstrung, or tense
0 1 2 14. Cries a lot	0 1 2 46. Nervous movements or twitching (describe): _____
0 1 2 15. Cruel to animals	
0 1 2 16. Cruelty, bullying, or meanness to others	
0 1 2 17. Daydreams or gets lost in his/her thoughts	0 1 2 47. Nightmares
0 1 2 18. Deliberately harms self or attempts suicide	0 1 2 48. Not liked by other kids
0 1 2 19. Demands a lot of attention	0 1 2 49. Constipated, doesn't move bowels
0 1 2 20. Destroys his/her own things	
0 1 2 21. Destroys things belonging to his/her family or others	0 1 2 50. Too fearful or anxious
	0 1 2 51. Feels dizzy or lightheaded
0 1 2 22. Disobedient at home	0 1 2 52. Feels too guilty
	0 1 2 53. Overeating
0 1 2 23. Disobedient at school	
0 1 2 24. Doesn't eat well	0 1 2 54. Overtired without good reason
	0 1 2 55. Overweight
0 1 2 25. Doesn't get along with other kids	
0 1 2 26. Doesn't seem to feel guilty after misbehaving	56. Physical problems *without known medical cause:*
	0 1 2 a. Aches or pains (*not* stomach or headaches)
0 1 2 27. Easily jealous	0 1 2 b. Headaches
0 1 2 28. Breaks rules at home, school, or elsewhere	0 1 2 c. Nausea, feels sick
	0 1 2 d. Problems with eyes (*not* if corrected by glasses) (describe): _____
0 1 2 29. Fears certain animals, situations, or places, other than school (describe): _____	
	0 1 2 e. Rashes or other skin problems
0 1 2 30. Fears going to school	0 1 2 f. Stomachaches
0 1 2 31. Fears he/she might think or do something bad	0 1 2 g. Vomiting, throwing up
	0 1 2 h. Other (describe): _____

PAGE 3   *Be sure you answered all items. Then see other side.*

Please print. Be sure to answer all items.

0 = Not True (as far as you know)   1 = Somewhat or Sometimes True   2 = Very True or Often True

0 1 2 57. Physically attacks people

0 1 2 58. Picks nose, skin, or other parts of body (describe): _____

0 1 2 59. Plays with own sex parts in public
0 1 2 60. Plays with own sex parts too much

0 1 2 61. Poor school work
0 1 2 62. Poorly coordinated or clumsy

0 1 2 63. Prefers being with older kids
0 1 2 64. Prefers being with younger kids

0 1 2 65. Refuses to talk
0 1 2 66. Repeats certain acts over and over; compulsions (describe): _____

0 1 2 67. Runs away from home
0 1 2 68. Screams a lot

0 1 2 69. Secretive, keeps things to self
0 1 2 70. Sees things that aren't there (describe):

0 1 2 71. Self-conscious or easily embarrassed
0 1 2 72. Sets fires

0 1 2 73. Sexual problems (describe): _____

0 1 2 74. Showing off or clowning

0 1 2 75. Too shy or timid
0 1 2 76. Sleeps less than most kids

0 1 2 77. Sleeps more than most kids during day and/or night (describe): _____

0 1 2 78. Inattentive or easily distracted

0 1 2 79. Speech problem (describe): _____

0 1 2 80. Stares blankly

0 1 2 81. Steals at home
0 1 2 82. Steals outside the home

0 1 2 83. Stores up too many things he/she doesn't need (describe): _____

0 1 2 84. Strange behavior (describe): _____

0 1 2 85. Strange ideas (describe): _____

0 1 2 86. Stubborn, sullen, or irritable
0 1 2 87. Sudden changes in mood or feelings

0 1 2 88. Sulks a lot
0 1 2 89. Suspicious

0 1 2 90. Swearing or obscene language
0 1 2 91. Talks about killing self

0 1 2 92. Talks or walks in sleep (describe): _____

0 1 2 93. Talks too much

0 1 2 94. Teases a lot
0 1 2 95. Temper tantrums or hot temper

0 1 2 96. Thinks about sex too much
0 1 2 97. Threatens people

0 1 2 98. Thumb-sucking
0 1 2 99. Smokes, chews, or sniffs tobacco

0 1 2 100. Trouble sleeping (describe): _____

0 1 2 101. Truancy, skips school

0 1 2 102. Underactive, slow moving, or lacks energy
0 1 2 103. Unhappy, sad, or depressed

0 1 2 104. Unusually loud
0 1 2 105. Uses drugs for nonmedical purposes (**don't** include alcohol or tobacco) (describe):

0 1 2 106. Vandalism
0 1 2 107. Wets self during the day

0 1 2 108. Wets the bed
0 1 2 109. Whining

0 1 2 110. Wishes to be of opposite sex
0 1 2 111. Withdrawn, doesn't get involved with others

0 1 2 112. Worries

113. Please write in any problems your child has that were not listed above:

0 1 2 _____
0 1 2 _____
0 1 2 _____

Please be sure you answered all items.

Appendix 4.D

				For office use only
Please print	**YOUTH SELF- REPORT FOR AGES 11-18**			ID #

YOUR FULL NAME	First	Middle	Last	**PARENTS' USUAL TYPE OF WORK, even if not working now.** *(please be specific — for example, auto mechanic, high school teacher, homemaker, laborer, lathe operator, shoe salesman, army sergeant.)*

YOUR GENDER ☐ Boy ☐ Girl	YOUR AGE	YOUR ETHNIC GROUP OR RACE	FATHER'S TYPE OF WORK _____ MOTHER'S TYPE OF WORK _____

TODAY'S DATE Mo._____ Date _____ Yr. _____	YOUR BIRTHDATE Mo._____ Date _____ Yr. _____	

GRADE IN SCHOOL _____ NOT ATTENDING SCHOOL ☐	IF YOU ARE WORKING, PLEASE STATE YOUR TYPE OF WORK: _____ _____	Please fill out this form to reflect *your* views, even if other people might not agree. Feel free to print additional comments besdie each item and in the spaces provided on pages 2 and 4. **Be sure to answer all items.**

I. Please list the sports you most like to take part in. For example: Swimming, baseball, skating, skate boarding, bike riding, fishing, etc.

☐ None

	Compared to others of your age, about how much time do you spend in each?				Compared to others of your age, how well do you do each one?		
	Less Than Average	Average	More Than Average		Below Average	Average	Above Average
a._____	☐	☐	☐		☐	☐	☐
b._____	☐	☐	☐		☐	☐	☐
c._____	☐	☐	☐		☐	☐	☐

II. Please list your favorite hobbies, activities, and games, other than sports. For example: cards, books, piano, cars, computers, crafts, etc. (Do *not* include listening to radio or watching TV.)

☐ None

	Compared to others of your age, about how much time do you spend in each?				Compared to others of your age, how well do you do each one?		
	Less Than Average	Average	More Than Average		Below Average	Average	Above Average
a._____	☐	☐	☐		☐	☐	☐
b._____	☐	☐	☐		☐	☐	☐
c._____	☐	☐	☐		☐	☐	☐

III. Please list any organizations, clubs, teams, or groups you belong to.

☐ None

	Compared to others of your age, how active are you in each?		
	Less Active	Average	More Active
a._____	☐	☐	☐
b._____	☐	☐	☐
c._____	☐	☐	☐

IV. Please list any jobs or chores you have. For example: paper route, babysitting, making bed, working in store, etc. (Include **both** paid and unpaid jobs and chores.)

☐ None

	Compared to others of your age, how well do you carry them out?		
	Below Average	Average	Above Average
a._____	☐	☐	☐
b._____	☐	☐	☐
c._____	☐	☐	☐

Be sure you answered all items. Then see other side.

Please print. Be sure to answer all items.

V. 1. **About how many close friends do you have?** (Do not include brothers & sisters)

☐ None   ☐ 1   ☐ 2 or 3   ☐ 4 or more

2. **About how many times a week do you do things with any friends outside of regular school hours?**
(Do not Include brothers & sisters)   ☐ Less than 1   ☐ 1 or 2   ☐ 3 or more

---

VI. Compared to others of your age, how well do you:

	Worse	Average	Better	
a. Get along with your brothers & sisters?	☐	☐	☐	☐ I have no brothers or sisters
b. Get along with other kids?	☐	☐	☐	
c. Get along with your parents?	☐	☐	☐	
d. Do things by yourself?	☐	☐	☐	

VII. 1. Performance in academic subjects.   ☐ I do not attend school because _____

Other academic subjects–for example: computer courses, foreign language, business, Do **not** include gym, shop, driver's ed., or other nonacademic subjects.

Check a box for each subject that you take	Failing	Below Average	Average	Above Average
a. English or Language Arts	☐	☐	☐	☐
b. History or Social Studies	☐	☐	☐	☐
c. Arithmetic or Math	☐	☐	☐	☐
d. Science	☐	☐	☐	☐
e. _____	☐	☐	☐	☐
f. _____	☐	☐	☐	☐
g. _____	☐	☐	☐	☐

Do you have any illness, disability, or handicap?   ☐ No   ☐ Yes—please describe:

Please describe any concerns or problems you have about school:

Please describe any other concerns you have:

Please describe the best things about yourself:

Be sure you answered all items.

Please print. Be sure to answer all items.

Below is a list of items that describe kids. For each item that describe you *now or within the past 6 months*, please circle the *2* if the item is *very true or often true* of you. Circle the *1* if the item is *somewhat or sometimes true* of you. If the item is *not true* of you, circle the *0*

0 = Not True   1 = Somewhat or sometimes True   2 = Very True or Often True

0 1 2	1. I act too young for my age	0 1 2	33. I feel that no one loves me
0 1 2	2. I drink alcohol without my parents' approval (describe): _____	0 1 2	34. I feel that others are out to get me
		0 1 2	35. I feel worthless or inferior
	_____	0 1 2	36. I accidentally get hurt a lot
0 1 2	3. I argue a lot	0 1 2	37. I get in many fights
0 1 2	4. I fail to finish things that I start	0 1 2	38. I get teased a lot
0 1 2	5. There is very little that I enjoy	0 1 2	39. I hang around with kids who get in trouble
0 1 2	6. I like animals	0 1 2	40. I hear sounds or voices that other people think aren't there (describe): _____
0 1 2	7. I brag		
0 1 2	8. I have trouble concentrating or paying attention		_____
0 1 2	9. I can't get my mind off certain thoughts; (describe): _____		_____
		0 1 2	41. I act without stopping to think
	_____	0 1 2	42. I would rather be alone than with others
0 1 2	10. I have trouble sitting still	0 1 2	43. I lie or cheat
0 1 2	11. I'm too dependent on adults	0 1 2	44. I bite my fingernails
0 1 2	12. I feel lonely	0 1 2	45. I am nervous or tense
0 1 2	13. I feel confused or in a fog	0 1 2	46. Parts of my body twitch or make nervous movements (describe): _____
0 1 2	14. I cry a lot		
0 1 2	15. I am pretty honest		_____
0 1 2	16. I am mean to others		_____
0 1 2	17. I daydream a lot	0 1 2	47. I have nightmares
0 1 2	18. I deliberately try to hurt or kill myself	0 1 2	48. I am not liked by other kids
0 1 2	19. I try to get a lot of attention	0 1 2	49. I can do certain things better than most kids
0 1 2	20. I destroy my own things	0 1 2	50. I am too fearful or anxious
0 1 2	21. I destroy things belonging to others	0 1 2	51. I feel dizzy or lightheaded
0 1 2	22. I disobey my parents	0 1 2	52. I feel too guilty
0 1 2	23. I disobey at school	0 1 2	53. I eat too much
0 1 2	24. I don't eat as well as I should	0 1 2	54. I feel overtired without good reason
0 1 2	25. I don't get along with other kids	0 1 2	55. I am overweight
0 1 2	26. I don't feel guilty after doing something I shouldn't		56. Physical problems *Without known medical cause*:
0 1 2	27. I am jealous of others	0 1 2	a. Aches or pains (*not* stomach or headaches)
0 1 2	28. I break rules at home, school, or elsewhere	0 1 2	b. Headaches
0 1 2	29. I am afraid of certain animals, situations, or places, other than school (describe): _____	0 1 2	c. Nausea, feels sick
		0 1 2	d. Problems with eyes (*not* if corrected by glasses) (describe): _____
	_____	0 1 2	e. Rashes or other skin problems
0 1 2	30. I am afraid of going to school	0 1 2	f. Stomachaches
0 1 2	31. I am afraid I might think or do something bad	0 1 2	g. Vomiting, throwing up
0 1 2	32. I feel that I have to be perfect	0 1 2	h. Other (describe): _____
			_____

PAGE 3   *Be sure you answered all items. Then see other side.*

Please print. Be sure to answer all items.

0 = Not True	1 = Somewhat or Sometimes True	2= Very True or Often True

0 1 2   57. I Physically attack people

0 1 2   58. I pick my skin or other parts of my body (describe):_____

0 1 2   59. I can be pretty friendly

0 1 2   60. I like to try new things

0 1 2   61. My school work is poor

0 1 2   62. I am poorly coordinated or clumsy

0 1 2   63. I would rather be with older kids than kids my own age

0 1 2   64. I would rather be with younger kids than kids my own age

0 1 2   65. I refuse to talk

0 1 2   66. I repeat certain acts over and over (describe):_____

0 1 2   67. I run away from home

0 1 2   68. I scream a lot

0 1 2   69. I am secretive or keep things to myself

0 1 2   70. I see things that other people think aren't there (describe):_____

0 1 2   71. I am self-conscious or easily embarrassed

0 1 2   72. I set fires

0 1 2   73. I can work well with my hands

0 1 2   74. I show off or clown

0 1 2   75. I am too shy or timid

0 1 2   76. I sleep less than most kids

0 1 2   77. I sleep more than most kids during day and/or night (describe):_____

0 1 2   78. I am inattentive or easily distracted

0 1 2   79. I have a speech problem (describe):_____

0 1 2   80. I stand up for my rights

0 1 2   81. I steal at home

0 1 2   82. I steal from places other than home

0 1 2   83. I store up too many things I don't need (describe):_____

0 1 2   84. I do things other people think are strange (describe):_____

0 1 2   85. I have thoughts that other people would think are strange (describe):_____

0 1 2   86. I am stubborn

0 1 2   87. My moods or feelings change suddenly

0 1 2   88. I enjoy being with people

0 1 2   89. I am suspicious

0 1 2   90. I swear or use dirty language

0 1 2   91. I think about killing myself

0 1 2   92. I like to make others laugh

0 1 2   93. I talk too much

0 1 2   94. I tease others a lot

0 1 2   95. I have a hot temper

0 1 2   96. I think about sex too much

0 1 2   97. I threaten to hurt people

0 1 2   98. I like to help others

0 1 2   99. I smoke, chew, or sniff tobacco

0 1 2   100. I have trouble sleeping (describe):_____

0 1 2   101. I cut classes or skip school

0 1 2   102. I don't have much energy

0 1 2   103. I am unhappy, sad, or depressed

0 1 2   104. I am louder than other kids

0 1 2   105. I use drugs for nonmedical purposes (**don't** include alcohol or tobacco) (describe):_____

0 1 2   106. I like to be fair to others

0 1 2   107. I enjoy a good joke

0 1 2   108. I like to take life easy

0 1 2   109. I try to help other people when I can

0 1 2   110. I wish I were of the opposite sex

0 1 2   111. I keep from getting involved with others

0 1 2   112. I worry a lot

Please write down anything else that describes your feelings, behaviour, or interests. *Please be sure you answered all items.*

5

Child and Adolescent Sexual Development and Sexual Identity Issues

Tammi Damas, Laura C. Hein, Lois C. Powell, and Edith (Emma) Dundon

Objectives

After reading this chapter, APNs will be able to

1. Identify normal adolescent secondary sex characteristics and sexual behavior.
2. Assess external influences (social and environmental) that may affect child and adolescent sexual development.
3. Identify and assess issues related to sexual and gender identity.
4. Describe the unique challenges that sexual minority youth face.
5. Develop strategies for providing care for all youth during times of sexual and gender identity development.

Introduction

This chapter will discuss normal and abnormal sexual development during childhood and adolescence and issues experienced by sexual minority youth as they navigate their sexual and gender identity. The advanced practice nurse (APN) will be provided with biological data that will serve as a guide during physical assessment and screening and will be helpful when conducting child, adolescent, or family psychoeducation. The chapter will also include a brief discussion of pregnancy and sexually transmitted infections (STIs) in heterosexual and nonheterosexual youth and clinical strategies for the APN during all levels of preventive efforts. Nurses are frequently at the forefront to intervene with youth during times of crisis involving sexual development, gender identity, and any mental health issues related to these developmental challenges. The authors want to stress the importance of assessment and screening in primary care, of APN management of minor psychosocial issues associated with sexual development, and of having sensitivity and knowledge of factual information when working with sexual minority youth. As will be stated throughout this text, early case findings of more complex mental health challenges must be referred immediately to a trained mental health professional, including APNs, when screening reveals serious emotional, behavioral, or psychological consequences of abnormal sexual development or sexual minority youth in turmoil.

Sexuality in Childhood

Healthy parent-child interaction during infancy, toddlerhood, and beyond involves physical contact (hugging, stroking, and kissing) and responsiveness, activities needed for the establishment of trust (Gerlt, Blosser, & Dunn,

Child and Adolescent Behavioral Health: A Resource for Advanced Practice Psychiatric and Primary Care Practitioners in Nursing,
First Edition. Edited by Edilma L. Yearwood, Geraldine S. Pearson, and Jamesetta A. Newland.
© 2012 John Wiley & Sons, Inc. Published 2012 by John Wiley & Sons, Inc.

2009). Preschool and school-aged children are curious about their bodies and will engage in self-stimulation and self-exploration without erotic meaning. The fact that their self-stimulation results in a pleasurable feeling prompts repeating the behavior. Parents should be taught that this is normal behavior and that they should not belittle or over-react when this occurs. Instead, they should talk to their youngsters about appropriate names for body parts, one's body being private, good touch/bad touch, and the importance of respectfully conducting self-stimulating activities in private. Children may engage in more provocative behaviors by using language or behaviors centered around sexual exploration to test parental reaction. Parents should be encouraged to minimize reactivity and punishing or condemning these behaviors as that may give the child the impression that there is something wrong with his or her sexual expressions. Parents and primary care APNs should be open to discussing sexuality and answering any questions children may have without exhaustive and complicated responses. The use of simple language and visual aids to help explain normal sexual development, at age-appropriate times, is helpful in educating children, responding to questions they might have, and minimizing anxiety around their development.

School-aged and preadolescent children vacillate between inhibition and disinhibition of their sexual fantasies. Adults may notice more silliness around discussing body parts or gender differences, embarrassment over body changes or new attraction to peers, attentiveness to media information about sexual development, and a desire for more privacy when changing clothes. Hornor (2004) provided a comprehensive review of the literature on normal and abnormal sexual behavior in children along with nursing intervention strategies. During primary care visits, both the child and the parent should be asked questions about normal sexual curiosity and if the child is engaging in behaviors of concern to the child, parent, or school. If sexual behaviors are worrisome or causing concerns with other peers or the school, further assessment and evaluation may be warranted to rule out an inappropriate sexual event. Often children will be able to use dolls, drawings, or other play therapy techniques to divulge an inappropriate sexual act that they had experienced (see Chapter 15 in this text for more information about play therapy purpose and techniques).

Sexual Development

Adolescence is a time of great confusion for today's youth as they make the transition from childhood to adulthood. Erickson's fifth stage of psychosocial development (Identity versus Role Confusion) takes place during adolescence (Erickson, 1950). It is during this time that the individual's life has reached a crossroads at which radical changes are taking place. The emotional stress of trying to find oneself and establish a place in society is coupled with the physical stress of the new changes the body is going through. Due to a number of factors, the adolescent of today is developing at a much faster pace compared to decades ago, when the physical characteristics of adolescence were reached at a later age. APNs must be knowledgeable of the physical changes and emotional stressors that teens experience. Failure to achieve a sense of identity and to stay true to self may lead to a weak sense of self and role confusion. This failure ultimately places teens at risk for substance abuse and violent behaviors. The physical changes that herald the onset of adolescence typically occur earlier in girls than in boys.

Hormonal Development

One of the milestones of adolescent development is achieving puberty. **Puberty,** with origins from the Latin *pubertas,* meaning "adulthood," is defined as the process in which a child's body goes through physical, sexual, and psychosocial maturation in order to reach adulthood and become capable of reproduction (Blondell, Foster, & Kamlesh, 1999). The initial physical manifestations of puberty are adrenarche (involving the adrenal glands) and gonadarche (involving the ovaries and testes), which are initiated by hormonal signals from the hypothalamus. Adrenarche marks changes in the adrenal gland that lead to the development of secondary sex characteristics such as increased body odor, axillary and pubic hair growth, increased testicular size, and growth in height (Lalwani, Reindollar, & Davis, 2003; Pinyerd & Zipf, 2005).

Gonadarche occurs when the hypothalamus produces gonadotropin-releasing hormone (GnRH), which triggers the development of the ovaries in girls and testes in boys. In turn, GnRH signals the pituitary gland to secrete the gonadotropins follicle-stimulating hormone (FSH) and luteinizing hormone (LH). In girls, both FSH and LH are necessary for ovulation. FSH and LH stimulate the production of estrogen, progesterone, and testosterone, which are necessary for the initiation of menstruation. In boys, FSH promotes sperm production, while LH causes testosterone production.

Physical Development in Females

Until puberty the bodies of boys and girls are similar except for the genitalia. The timing of puberty differs between the sexes, with girls starting puberty around the age of ten and boys following two years later. Tanner stages describe the sequence of pubertal development including breast development for girls, genital

Table 5.1 Tanner stages of female puberty

Stage	Breasts	Pubic Hair
1 (Preadolescent)	Elevation of papilla only	No pubic hair/vellus hair only and hair is similar to development over abdominal wall
2	Elevation of breast and papilla as a small mound; diameter of areola is enlarged	Sparse growth of long, slightly pigmented, downy hair, or slightly curled, appearing along labia
3	Further enlargement of breast and areola with no separation of contours	Darker, coarser, more curled and spreads over the pubic junction
4	Areola and papilla are enlarged to form a secondary mound above the level of the breast	Adult-type hair; area covered is less than in most adults; there is no spread to the medial surface of thighs
5 (Mature)	Adult breast; projection of papilla due to recession of areola to the mound of breast tissue	Adult-type hair in quantity and type; distribution as an inverse triangle; spread to medial surface of thighs

Reprinted from Marshall and Tanner, 1969, with permission from BMJ Publishing Group Ltd.

development for boys, and the growth of pubic hair for both sexes (Marshall & Tanner, 1969).The Tanner stages of female puberty are found in Table 5.1.

The sequence of pubertal development in girls generally begins with the emergence of breast buds (thelarche) followed by the appearance of pubic hair (puberache). In a small population of girls puberache will occur before thelarche. Menarche, the initiation of the first menstrual cycle, usually occurs two years after the onset of puberty. Historically, this has occurred during mid-adolescence between the ages of thirteen and fourteen. However, the age of menarche has declined over time with twelve and one-half years being the average age of menarche in the United States (Anderson, Dallal, & Must, 2003). It is not uncommon for a female to have irregular cycles during the initial stages of menarche. The first year after menarche is marked with a majority of anovulatory cycles. By the third year post menarche, half of the teen's cycles will be anovulatory. The majority of the cycles will be ovulatory by the sixth year post menarche.

Amenorrhea is the absence of menstruation, either transiently or permanently, due to either pregnancy or a variety of endocrine or anatomical anomalies, and can be classified as either primary or secondary. Primary amenorrhea is failure of the menses to occur by either the age of sixteen or two years after the onset of puberty or absence of menses by age thirteen in the absence of secondary sex characteristics. Presence of secondary sexual characteristics indicates normal hormonal function suggesting that the amenorrhea is ovulatory and due to an obstruction. If secondary sex characteristics

are absent, amenorrhea is anovulatory and is likely due to a genetic or hormonal disorder.

Secondary amenorrhea is diagnosed when there is an absence of menses for six months after previously normal periods and is usually secondary to another disorder. A careful history is necessary to help determine the cause. For example, galactorrhea in the absence of periods may be due to hyperprolactinemia, symptoms of estrogen deficiency (i.e., hot flashes, vaginal dryness, night sweats) may signal premature ovarian failure, and virilization may indicate an androgen excess. The most common causes of amenorrhea are pregnancy (for those of reproductive age), constitutional delay of puberty, functional hypothalamic anovulation, use or abuse of certain medications, breastfeeding, or polycystic ovarian syndrome. Pregnancy should not be ruled out based on history only; testing is required for secondary amenorrhea. Pregnancy can occur prior to the first menstrual period.

Anovulatory amenorrhea is due to a disruption of the hypothalamic-pituitary-ovarian axis. Causes can be due to a hypothalamic or pituitary disorder, ovarian failure, or androgen excess. **Ovulatory amenorrhea** is due to chromosomal abnormalities or other congenital anatomical abnormalities that could cause an obstruction in the menstrual flow. Treatments are based on the underlying cause. A patient with secondary amenorrhea and normal hormonal levels may be given a trial of progesterone to stimulate withdrawal bleeding. If bleeding occurs, amenorrhea suggests a hypothalamic-pituitary dysfunction, ovarian failure, or estrogen excess. If bleeding does not occur, amenorrhea could be due to an obstruction or endometrial lesion.

On the opposite end of the spectrum, an adolescent female may present with complaints of **menorrhagia** (heavy menstrual bleeding), which may be caused by organic, endocrine, or anatomical factors. Bleeding disorders, such as von Willebrand disease, should be considered in teens who present with complaints of heavy bleeding since menarche. A detailed history is important to assess for number of pads used per day on heaviest day, total pads used during cycle, length of cycle, quality of life, and number of school days missed. Evaluation should include a von Willebrand profile and complete blood count. If a diagnosis is made, treatment would include intranasal desmopressin (Werner et al., 1993).

The onset of puberty in females varies by individual and between populations. A number of factors, such as race, genetics, and nutritional status, influence the development of secondary sex characteristics. The most prominent genetic factor that affects the onset of puberty is race. African American females tend to start puberty at an earlier age than their Latino and White counterparts (Chumlea et al., 2003; Wu, Mendola, & Buck, 2002). African American females tend to achieve menarche 2.1 months earlier than white females. Breast development also occurs months earlier in African American and Mexican females compared to white females (Sun et al., 2002). While the most influential environmental factor to affect puberty is nutrition, a model proposed by Ellis and Garber (2000) suggested that stresses within the family, such as maternal depression or stepfather presence, contributed to earlier pubertal maturation. Research has found increased body fat/elevated body mass index (BMI) leads to an earlier onset of menses and breast development (Kaplowitz, Slora, Wasserman, Pedlow, & Herman-Giddens, 2001; Qing & Karlberg, 2001). In a typical ten-year-old girl, the body fat concentration is 6% higher than that of her male counterpart. Overweight children tend to experience puberty early (Wu et al., 2002). On the opposite end of the spectrum, female athletes with a low BMI and increased levels of physical activity have slower rates of puberty. Poor nutrition can lead to a delayed onset of menses, and vegetarian diets consisting of low protein and high dietary fiber are also associated with a delayed onset of menses and puberty.

Physical Development in Males

For boys, the first physical sign of puberty is the enlargement of the testes (gonadarche), accompanied by the appearance of pubic hair. Until this time there has been very little growth in the size of the penis since infancy. After the onset of puberty, the testes continue to grow until reaching mature adult size, which usually occurs within six years. Within a year after the testes have reached maturity, the length and width of the shaft of the penis grow to adult size, followed by growth of the glans penis. Sperm and hormone production occur about a year after the first signs of puberty. Upon the production of sperm, fertility is reached, occasionally occurring at the age of thirteen years. Full fertility is reached by the age of sixteen years. Tanner stages for males are based on the growth of the genitals and pubic hair. The Tanner stages of male puberty are found in Table 5.2.

Shortly after the growth of a male's pubic hair, body and facial hair also begin to grow. This development varies between individuals and populations with no distinct timeline regarding the growth patterns. The typical order would be axillary, perianal, upper lip, periauricular (sideburns), periareolar, and the beard. Hair growth on the upper and lower extremities along with the abdomen and back tends to grow thicker than the hair on the rest of the body. Facial hair grows thicker over a number of years.

Physical changes occurring during puberty may lead the adolescent male to feel self-conscious and uncomfortable. Gynecomastia (enlargement of breast tissue) occurs in some boys during puberty, lasting eighteen to twenty-four months and then slowly regressing. There is no treatment required unless the condition persists beyond two years. This condition may be distressing for the adolescent; reassurance that the symptoms will most likely go away and provision of emotional support are called for. The APN can also recommend loose-fitting clothing and encourage maintenance of a healthy weight.

Another physical characteristic of puberty in males is the voice change, which is caused by the hormonal effects on the larynx. Although this effect occurs in both sexes, the effect on the male is more prominent. The longer and thicker vocal cords cause the male's voice to become deeper and drop one octave. The voice change usually occurs during Tanner Stage 3 and reaches full adult level around the age of fifteen years. As the male reaches the end of puberty, his skeletal features have grown heavier and he has on average double the muscle mass of a female. The muscular growth will continue even into adulthood.

Adolescents going through the physical changes of puberty need reassurance that they are normal. Teens may be ashamed of their development, whether they are overdeveloped or underdeveloped, compared to their peers. APNs can help teens by providing anticipatory guidance regarding the physical and emotional changes that are a normal part of puberty.

This brief overview provides a context of the typical pubertal changes in adolescence. Awareness of these changes serves as a guide when conducting history and physical examinations (H&P) with this population. It is

Table 5.2 Tanner stages of male puberty

Stages	Genitals	Pubic Hair
1 (Preadolescent)	Testes, scrotum, and penis are about the same size and proportion as in early childhood	No pubic hair; vellus over the pubes is no further developed than that over the abdominal wall
2	Scrotum and testes have enlarged, there is a change in the texture of scrotal skin and some reddening of scrotal skin	Sparse growth of long, slightly pigmented, downy hair, straight or slightly curled, appearing at the base of penis
3	Growth of the penis has occurred, at first mainly in length but with some increase in breadth. There has been further growth of the testes and the scrotum	Hair is considerably darker, coarser, and more curled and spreads sparsely over junction of pubes
4	Penis is further enlarged in length and breadth, with development of glans penis. The testes and the scrotum are further enlarged. There is also further darkening of scrotal skin	Hair is adult type, but the area covered is smaller than that in most adults; no spread to the medial surface of the thighs
5 (Adult)	Genitalia are adult in size and shape. No further enlargement takes place after Stage 5 is reached	Hair is adult quantity and type, distributed as an inverse triangle. Spread to medial surface of the thighs but not up linea alba or elsewhere above the base of the inverse triangle

Reprinted from Marshall and Tanner, 1970, with permission from BMJ Publishing Group Ltd.

not uncommon for an individual to experience pubertal changes outside of the timeline discussed.

Abnormal Puberty

There are two types of abnormal puberty: early puberty and delayed puberty. It is critical for APNs to assess the age of onset of pubertal development due to the risk of adjustment problems that may occur in individuals who reach puberty earlier or later than their peer group. Early puberty is when puberty begins before age eight for girls and before age nine for boys. Delayed puberty occurs when sexual maturation is not evident by thirteen years of age in girls and fourteen years of age in boys. Puberty is also delayed if there is an absence of menarche by the age of sixteen or five years from pubertal onset (Rosen & Foster, 2001).

Early Onset

Early puberty is not usually due to an underlying pathological cause if other physical characteristics are within the normal pubertal growth and development. For diagnostic purposes, a radiograph to determine the child's skeletal age is indicated. If the skeletal age is within two years of the chronological age, the findings are benign. However, if other physical characteristics are outside of the normal Tanner stage—for example, a nine-year-old boy with penile enlargement or scrotal thinning—a formal evaluation is necessary.

Precocious puberty occurs when there is overstimulation of the GnRH hormone. Precocious puberty presents as breast development or menarche in girls younger than eight years (Kaplowitz, Oberfield, & the Drug and Therapeutics and Executive Committees of the Lawson Wilkins Pediatric Endocrine Society, 1999). In boys, signs of precocious puberty include enlarged testicles and penis, facial hair (usually on the upper lip), or a deepening voice. Symptoms that can occur in both genders are pubic or underarm hair, rapid growth in height, acne, or an adult body odor. The potential reason for the cause of these symptoms will determine how the diagnosis is classified. Due to racial disparities in sexual maturation among girls, a provider may revise criteria for referral before diagnosing a child with precocious puberty (Herman-Giddens et al., 1997).

The two types of precocious puberty are central and peripheral. **Central precocious puberty (CPP)** occurs when the entire hypothalamic-pituitary-gonadal (HPG) axis starts too soon. The pattern of growth and development is the same and follows the normal sequence; however, it occurs earlier than normal. Usually the cause of CPP is idiopathic. In a few rare cases, these symptoms are due to a central nervous system (CNS) lesion caused by neurofibromatosis, hydrocephalus, a CNS infection, or an intracranial neoplasm. Other causes of CPP are McCune-Albright syndrome, congenital adrenal hyperplasia, and hypothyroidism. CNS lesions affect both boys and girls equally. However, among children who present with precocious puberty who do not have an underlying pathology, girls are diagnosed 10 to 1 compared to their male counterparts (Carel & Leger, 2008).

Peripheral precocious puberty (PPP) is due to the release of estrogen or testosterone into the body as a result of problems with the ovaries, testicles, or adrenal or pituitary glands. GnRH is not involved in the development of PPP. Upon assessment a patient may present with a tumor of the adrenal or pituitary gland that is secreting either estrogen or testosterone (McCune-Albright syndrome) or exposure to a topical estrogen or testosterone cream. Female patients may be diagnosed with either an ovarian cyst or tumor. Male patients may have a tumor in the germ cells (cells that make sperm) or Leydig cells (cells that make testosterone). A rare gene mutation may also be the result of a disorder called familial gonadotropin-independent sexual precocity, which results in the production of testosterone between the ages of one and four (Muir, 2006).

The prevalence of precocious puberty varies depending on the age limits used by researchers but is approximately 4% to 5%. Risk factors for developing precocious puberty are being female, African American, and/or obese; having exposure to sex hormones; or having a disorder such as McCune-Albright syndrome or congenital adrenal hyperplasia (Muir, 2006). Complications of precocious puberty are development of polycystic ovarian syndrome or short stature. Polycystic ovarian syndrome may be recognized at the time of diagnosis of early menarche. Short stature is the result of rapid bone mineralization, which causes decreased linear growth.

Diagnosing the type of precocious puberty may be accomplished with a history, physical examination, and hormonal blood tests. A radiograph to measure bone age may also be indicated. Hormonal blood tests are done following a GnRH injection. Increase in FSH and LH levels indicates CPP, whereas in PPP the FSH and LH levels will remain constant. If a diagnosis of CPP is made, magnetic resonance imaging (MRI) may be performed to identify potential CNS lesions. A thyroid test is done to rule out hypothyroidism if a child presents with signs such as sensitivity to cold, dry skin, fatigue, or constipation. Treatment for CPP is focused on medications aimed at preventing further pubertal development. The treatment of choice is a GnRH analog (typically leuprolide). The medication is given monthly to delay the pubertal process until the child reaches the appropriate age. Once the medication is discontinued, the process of puberty resumes.

Delayed Onset

Delayed puberty is more common in boys than in girls and is defined as a lack of testicular enlargement by the age of fourteen, lack of pubic hair by the age of fifteen, or a five-year time lapse from beginning to end of genital enlargement in boys. In girls, delayed puberty is diagnosed when there is an absence of breast development by the age of thirteen or a five-year time lapse from the beginning of breast development to menarche, or menarche occurring after the age of sixteen. Boys may experience increased pressure and embarrassment from their peers due to the delay. A girl who is smaller or less physically mature may not have the same level of embarrassment.

Less than 3% of adolescents will be diagnosed with delayed puberty and it is usually deemed to be a constitutional delay. In most cases when puberty does occur, it progresses normally. Referral to a pediatric endocrinologist will rule out any genetic or systemic causes due to a hypothalamic, pituitary, or gonadal condition. Other causes of delayed puberty are radiation or chemotherapy treatment secondary to a cancer diagnosis and excessive dieting or exercise. Less common causes of delayed puberty are **Turner syndrome** in girls or **Klinefelter syndrome** in boys. Both Turner and Klinefelter syndromes are due to congenital bilateral gonadal failure and present with elevated serum gonadotropin levels (Rosen & Foster, 2001). Girls who present with Turner syndrome usually have a short stature and a variation in sexual development or incomplete development. Often the diagnosis is not made until there is an inconsistency in pubertal development. Turner syndrome also presents with primary ovarian failure. Some girls may experience menarche, but most girls with a diagnosis of Turner syndrome will require long-term estrogen replacement therapy.

Klinefelter syndrome is a common disorder in males carrying the 46,XXY genotype. Due to the variation in pubertal development in males, the diagnosis often is not made until puberty or in adulthood. Unlike girls with Turner syndrome, who present with a smaller stature, boys affected by Klinefelter syndrome tend to be taller than their peers. Their height may mask their physical immaturity. Upon examination, testosterone levels will be extremely low, FSH levels will be elevated, and there will be decreased or absent sperm production.

Any tumor that damages the pituitary or hypothalamus can potentially decrease or stop production of the gonadotropins. In diagnosing delayed puberty, a complete history and physical examination, including laboratory tests and hormonal levels, should be obtained. Family history may reveal that the child's parents or siblings experienced a similar developmental delay. The exam is usually unremarkable except for a decreased bone age inconsistent with biological age. A chromosomal analysis may be performed. Computed tomography (CT) or MRI may be used to rule out a brain tumor. Treatment is based on the underlying cause of the delay. If it is a natural (constitutional) delay, no treatment is warranted, and the APN can elect to reassess every six months to ensure puberty is developing normally. If the patient is emotionally stressed by the delay, supplemental hormones can be prescribed to initiate the process sooner. If a boy does not show any signs of pubertal developmental or bone growth by early adolescence, testosterone may be considered as a treatment option (Rogol, 2005). The supplemental testosterone will trigger puberty to begin without negatively affecting the boy's height. If the cause is due to an underlying disorder, puberty will not begin until the disorder has been treated. Prescribing hormones may help with the development of sex characteristics if a genetic disorder is the cause. If a tumor is present, surgery may be warranted.

Clinical Implications

Adolescence marks an important time for the individual to feel accepted. If puberty is not progressing at a similar rate to the peer group, anxiety may develop. Adolescents with early or delayed puberty may present with symptoms of withdrawal, depression, and/or anxiety. Young teens who develop earlier or later than their peers are at risk for social isolation and teasing or bullying. Counseling and education on normal growth and development can help alleviate some of the anxiety. Knowledge of developmental milestones for both normal and delayed puberty will help the APN provide the appropriate counseling and intervention for the patient. Continuous monitoring of pubertal development, in addition to assessing for high-risk behaviors that could have negative consequences, is crucial for APNs when caring for adolescents.

In addition to physical development, adolescents may begin to experience sexual feelings. Early physical development in females can also bring untoward attention from members of the opposite sex. APNs can provide counseling on safe sex practices and stress that risk of pregnancy and/or STIs exists.

Sexual Behaviors

Changes in hormonal levels during puberty lead adolescents to begin to feel a physical attraction to others. During adolescence, it is normal for teens to begin to have questions about sexual development and develop a curiosity about relationships and sexual behaviors. These conversations usually begin first with their peers. It is abnormal for a teen to perform adultlike sexual acts or display signs of sexuality in public places. However, sexual experimentation between adolescents of the same age and gender is common. Another uncommon behavior is having sexual interest in someone much younger. Not all teens are knowledgeable about normal sexual behaviors. A parent may present with complaints or questions regarding a child's sexual behavior as a result of observation or complaints from school. Assessing a child's sexual behavior must be done in the context in which the behavior occurs. Children's sexual behavior is not intrinsic; it is learned from interactions with adults and other children (Essa & Murray, 1999). A child's home environment plays a significant role in the development of his or her sexual behavior. Certain sexual behaviors are considered normal in young children, such as self-stimulation, invasion of personal boundaries (i.e., standing too close, rubbing against another, or touching the mother's breasts or the father's genitals), and exposing body parts (Friedrich, Fisher, Broughton, Houston, & Shafran, 1998).

Normal child sexuality is differentiated from adult sexuality by the focus on curiosity and play, whereas adult sexuality presents with a mature understanding of the sexual behavior and its consequences. A child's sexual behavior is open, spontaneous, and sensual; while adult behavior is private, passionate, or erotic. Curiosity, playfulness, spontaneity, and sensuality are all a part of normal sexual development in the child. When caring for children, the APN must consider normal sexual behavior and view the behavior in context. Johnson (1991) developed a continuum of sexual behaviors, ranging from normal to pathological, which may help APNs determine their level of concern.

Group I. The majority of children fall into this category and exhibit natural and healthy sexual play. They may play "house" or "doctor" and develop scenarios to include sexual exploration. The play is voluntary, fun, and spontaneous. Neither of the parties feels fear, shame, or anxiety. There is mutual touch and exploration as a way of learning. The child's level of interest in sexuality is not any different than other aspects of their lives. The child should show an equal balance in their interest of sexual matters and other areas and people in their environment.

Group II. Children in this group engage in more sexual behaviors than their counterparts in Group I. They will sometimes admit to feeling guilty and ashamed about their sexuality. These children have usually been either sexually abused or exposed to sexually explicit materials. A parent may complain about their excessive masturbation, conversations about sexual acts, or their overtly sexual behaviors around adults. These may be signs of the child trying to work through their confusion regarding their sexual experiences.

Group III. Children in this group engage in all aspects of adult sexual behaviors with a consenting child partner. These children are usually physically and/or sexually abused. They consent to participating in sexual acts but are private about their sexual behaviors. Due to their betrayal, usually by adults, adults are not a part of their sexual world. Psychologically, these children do not exhibit emotions like the light-heartedness of Group I or the anxiety of Group II. They often present with a blank affect.

Group IV. Unlike the consenting partners in Group III, children in Group IV coerce others into sexual acts. This behavior can be classified as molestation. These children are usually acting out the aggressor role from their own personal experience of being a victim of child molestation in the past. These children have very little impulse control and suffer from a number of social-behavioral problems.

In addition to the four categories that Johnson (1991) classified, she also developed a "RED FLAG" checklist to identify inappropriate sexual behaviors in children. These include:

1. Interest in sex that is out of proportion with their interest in other aspects of the world.
2. Interest in sex that is compulsive, to the exclusion of interest in other developmentally appropriate activities.
3. A level of sexual knowledge that is greater than other same-age children from similar socioeconomic backgrounds and neighborhoods.
4. Approaching unfamiliar children instead of peers to engage in sexual acts.
5. Attempting to bribe or force other children to engage in sexual acts.
6. Other children complain about the sexual behavior of the child.
7. When sexual conversations are raised the child becomes anxious, fearful, or angry.

As APNs, if any of these symptoms are identified, the family should be counseled to seek professional help. There is also an ethical duty to report any episodes of suspected sexual abuse to the authorities.

Consequences of Abnormal Sexual Development

Early sexual experimentation can lead to an early sexual debut that places the adolescent at risk for multiple consequences, some of which can have lifelong implications.

Adolescents with complex mental health diagnoses such as depression, anxiety, or substance abuse are at risk for engaging in unprotected sexual activity. It is common for an adolescent not to practice safe sex when engaging in sexual acts, risking pregnancy, or acquiring an STI. Adolescents are very egocentric and do not believe that they can become infected or pregnant despite the media messages to the contrary. An adolescent's decision-making may be irrational at times, leading to poor decision-making rather than faulty decision-making. This behavior is due to immature cognitive processing skills. Immature cognitive development, along with the influence of various intense emotions, can lead to unplanned sexual encounters that would have otherwise required preplanning for the use of contraception (Herman, 2007).

Pregnancy

Teenage pregnancy continues to be an area of concern for educators, lawmakers, and health care professionals due to the adverse consequences associated with a pregnancy during adolescence. Teenagers who give birth are more likely to deliver a preterm (Martin, Osterman, & Sutton, 2010a) or low birth weight infant compared to older women, and their babies are more at risk of dying during infancy (Mathews & MacDorman, 2010). In addition, teen mothers are more at risk for interrupting or stopping their education. The initiation of prenatal care during the first trimester usually increases with age. The annual U.S. birth rate has steadily increased from 1998 through 2007 to 4.3 million. Despite the 2% decrease in 2008 to 4.2 million, the United States still has one of the highest teen birth rates in the world. Although the birth rate in 2008 declined to 41.5 births per 1000 women aged fifteen to nineteen years (Martin et al., 2010b), Hispanic (41.0 per 1000) and non-Hispanic black (32.1 per 1000) teen pregnancy rates remain higher than those of their non-Hispanic white (11 per 1000) counterparts (Ventura & Hamilton, 2011).

Adolescent pregnancy is a societal concern due to the potential increase in the socioeconomic burden of teen pregnancy and childbearing. The APN in primary care should assess for a potential pregnancy in teens who are sexually active, have lack of access to or poor use of contraception, live in poverty, have parents with low levels of education, are growing up in a single parent household, and are performing poorly in school (Singh & Darroch, 2000; Ventura, Abma, Mosher, & Henshaw, 2008).

Understanding the complex cognitive processes of adolescence will help the APN overcome the multiple challenges faced when providing care for this population. With the knowledge that adolescents do not see their sexual behavior as being risky, it is best practice to assess all adolescents' sexual behavior regardless of the reason for their visit. The APN must keep in mind that all female adolescent patients are potentially at risk for an adverse consequence of sexual behavior. A young female may be unaware of the possibility of being pregnant, may be in denial about being pregnant, or may be reluctant to initiate a conversation about fears of being pregnant. Therefore, it is best for the APN to initiate the conversation around sexuality and sexual behaviors at all primary care visits.

Diagnosing a pregnancy in an adolescent may come with many challenges such as vague symptoms, unreliable menstrual history, and the teen's reluctance to disclose her sexual activity (Polaneczky & O'Connor, 1999). Health care providers will need the necessary skills for accurate diagnosis, assessment, and counseling options (Aruda, Waddicor, Frese, Cole, & Burke, 2010). An adolescent will not disclose her concern or accurate information if she does not feel comfortable with or trust the provider. With that in mind, it is imperative that rapport be established and confidentiality be explained (McKee, Karasz & Weber, 2004). Conducting the history in private without a parent or guardian present helps in the development of trust.

Establishing the date of the last menstrual period (LMP) is crucial to diagnosing a pregnancy. Adolescents tend to have difficulty remembering their LMP and whether it was a normal period. Any female who has achieved menarche and presents with amenorrhea should have a pregnancy test performed, despite denying sexual activity or endorsing the persistent use of condoms (Nicolletti, 2005). The most likely cause of amenorrhea in adolescents is pregnancy (Aruda, 2010). Implantation bleeding may be mistaken for a light period. Additional symptoms that should be assessed for are breast soreness or enlargement, nausea, vomiting, abdominal cramping, urinary frequency, fatigue, appetite changes, or aversion to certain smells. Research shows that only a third of adolescents have performed a home pregnancy test prior to presenting to the clinic for confirmation (Shew, Hellerstedt, Sieving, Smith, & Fee, 2000). Potential barriers to the use of home pregnancy kits are cost and fear of privacy concerns. In a clinical setting, urine pregnancy tests can detect the pregnancy hormone, human chorionic gonadotropin (HCG), 10 to 14 days post conception. Serum HCG levels are more sensitive and can be detected by day 7, but this testing is more costly and takes longer to get results.

While waiting for the test results the APN should assess the adolescent's desire for pregnancy by asking what her feelings would be if a result were positive or negative. If a positive result occurs, counseling should be performed (Simmonds & Likis, 2005) and options discussed. If a negative result occurs, contraceptive counseling should

be given or reinforced. Studies show females under the age of 17 with a negative pregnancy test result are more likely to carry a pregnancy to term 18 months after the negative result compared to a new teen mom or a female who recently had an abortion (Zabin, Sedivy, & Emerson, 1994). Counseling should also include assessment of whether a condom is used. In addition to a lack of condom use, adolescents are at risk for improper condom use. If unprotected sex occurred or there is faulty condom use, she should also be assessed for symptoms of an STI, such as vaginal discharge, odor, or dysuria (Daley, Sadler, Leventhal, Cromwell, & Reynolds, 2005; Ickovics, Niccolai, Lewis, Kershaw, & Ethier, 2003). The patient should also have a follow-up appointment for a repeated urine pregnancy test within a month.

SEXUALITY

As teens try to navigate adolescence and define who they are, this is also a time in which they will experiment with defining who they are sexually. It is not uncommon for teens to engage in sexual experiments with both members of the opposite sex and same-sex population. This should be assessed in primary care during routine physical examinations. This experimentation does not predict their sexual orientation. Assessments should also be made regarding their practice of safe sex behaviors, and routine STI screenings should be conducted. The identification of risk factors should be assessed including the number of lifetime sexual partners, participation in various sexual acts, alcohol or drug use, and mental health status. While a teen may not have engaged in sexual intercourse at the time of examination, there are multiple behaviors such as heavy petting and being alone with their partner that can eventually lead to the initiation of sexual activity. During the assessment, the teen's attitude toward sex should be assessed regarding their beliefs about premarital sex and engaging in oral and anal intercourse. Due to the growing rate of HIV infection and other STIs, early education, detection, and intervention are prudent.

Sexual and Gender Identity

This section of the chapter will discuss issues sexual minority youth experience. It will serve as a guide for all APNs who provide care for lesbian, gay, bisexual, and transgender (LGBT) youth. The term "youth" is used here because recognition of differentness, which is later attributed to nonheterosexuality or gender-incongruence, often begins in early childhood (Zucker, 2010). Issues related to sexual and gender identity will be viewed through the lens of growth and development framed within the broader context of society.

Definitions

Before proceeding, several important terms need to be defined. **Sexual minority** is a synonym for "nonheterosexual." While there are numerous self-identifications and sexual practices, within the context of this chapter its meaning is limited to lesbian, gay, bisexual, and transgender (LGBT) behaviors and identities. The terms **gay** (♂♂♀♀) and **lesbian** (♀♀) refer to an exclusive physical and emotional attraction to members of one's own sex. In the past, **homosexual** was used to refer to gay and lesbian persons. However, due to the association of this term with the earlier editions of the Diagnostic and Statistical Manual of Mental Disorders (DSM), it has acquired pathological connotations and is considered offensive to many LGBT people. **Bisexual** people are physically and emotionally attracted to members of both sexes. **Transgender** (gender identity ⚥) refers to a person who feels his or her body is not the sex it should be, regardless of transformational hormones or surgical status. Table 5.3 presents other important definitions.

Prevalence

The exact prevalence of same-sex behavior, attraction, or gender incongruence is unknown. Divergent results have been reported in the literature depending on whether self-identification or sexual behavior is measured. Prevalence of LGBT self-identification is lower than the prevalence of sexual behavior. One in five, or 21%, of all males in the United States reported either homosexual behavior or homosexual *attraction* since age 15 (Sell, Wells, & Wypij, 1995). In another study, 5% of youth self-identified as gay, lesbian, or bisexual and/or reported same-sex sexual contact (Massachusetts Youth Risk Behavior Survey, 2001). Self-identification rates varied from 3% (Massachusetts Youth Risk Behavior Survey, 2001) to 6% of adolescent males self-identifying as gay or bisexual (Remafedi, Resnick, Blum, & Harris, 1992).

Many sexual minority youth are very comfortable with their sexuality and move into adulthood uneventfully; others struggle with their sexual orientation/gender identity and experience myriad obstacles. Over the last decade lesbian and gay youth have become more visible. Being comfortable with their sexual orientation and gender identity can not only be liberating, but it can also cause difficulties when concealment is necessary (Rieger, Linsenmeier, Gygax, Garcia, & Bailey, 2010; Sylva, Rieger, Linsenmeier, & Bailey, 2009).

These youth are members of all racial, ethnic, socioeconomic, and religious groups and may be indistinguishable from their heterosexual peers. Savin-Williams (2000) described a new generation of youth who rejected all gender categories and were attracted to and intimate with both same and opposite sexes without shame or guilt. He pointed out that the entertainment industry's normalizing same-sex desire has had a dramatic impact on the ability of adolescents to understand their own emerging sexual desires.

Increasing societal acceptance, the availability of older LGBT role models, access to resources for nonheterosexual youth, the Internet, television shows that portray positive same-sex relationships, and school and community–based gay/straight alliances have played a role in the possibility of youth "coming out" or disclosing that they are LGBT at an earlier age (Walls, Kane, & Wisneski, 2010). Despite the probability of successfully navigating childhood while LGBT, individual and collective biases have created a minefield of barriers to their success. Heterosexist beliefs and institutions effectively create a myriad of barriers that LGBT youth must traverse.

Oppression: Heterosexism and Homophobia

Although many youth are comfortable with identifying themselves as LGBT and discussing it openly, some youth are confused and frightened by their same-sex feelings and attractions at times due to feelings of conflict with their family's beliefs and religious values. These youth are often acutely aware of the stigma associated with being LGBT. Historically, the term "homophobia" was used to describe the loathing of nonheterosexuals. However, inclusion of "phobia" in the term created a misnomer related to the loci of hating homosexuals. Phobia or fear did not play a role in these feelings (Herek, 2002). Heterosexism, however, was the belief and the actions related to feeling that being heterosexual was the only acceptable way of existing (Herek, 1990). Although some segments of society were more tolerant of sexual minorities, a large portion of society continued to stigmatize and perpetuate hatred (Fish, 2010). Tolerance is not acceptance. Sexual minorities have been adversely affected by this hatred and intolerance, at home, in school, in the workplace, and in their places of worship (Hatzenbuehler, McLaughlin, Keyes, & Hasin, 2010). The negative effects can in many instances be profound. Fear and stigma may lead them to resort to nonhealthy methods of coping such as drinking, using drugs, eating disorders, engaging in unprotected sex, self-harm behavior, and running away from home.

Not all primary care and psychiatric-mental health APNs are comfortable working with lesbian, gay, bisexual, transgender, and youth who are questioning their sexual identity. They may be conflicted about their own feelings, thoughts, and religious beliefs related to homosexuality. The APN must address his or her own beliefs and values, anxieties, lack of knowledge about LGBT-related issues, and any discomfort about providing care for these youth in order to work effectively

Table 5.3 Definitions

Term	Definition
Bisexual	Physical and emotional attraction to members of one's own sex, as well as to members of the opposite sex (Kinsey, Pomeroy, & Martin, 1948; Nycum, 2000).
Gay	Having an exclusive physical and emotional attraction to members of one's own sex (Kinsey et al., 1948; Nycum, 2000). This term may be used for both men and women.
Gender identity	The psychological counterpart of biological sex, a social construction.
Heterosexism	An ideological system that denies, denigrates, and stigmatizes any nonheterosexual form of behavior, identity, relationship, or community (Herek & Berrill, 1990, p. 315).
Homophobia	A fear of homosexuals.
Homosexual	A pathology-derived term for a person with same-sex attractions and/or behaviors.
Intersex	A person born with biological characteristics of both sexes (Barrow, 2008). A contemporary synonym for hermaphrodite.
Lesbian	A woman with an exclusive physical and emotional attraction to other women (Nycum, 2000).
LGBT	Lesbian, gay, bisexual, and transgender.
Queer	Any category of gender and sexuality other than strictly heterosexual, including gay, lesbian, bisexual and transsexual, and transgender. Queer was historically a derogatory term used by homophobes against nonheterosexual people that has been appropriated and is used affectionately among nonheterosexual people (Nycum, 2000, p. 148; Ridge, Minichiello, & Plummer, 1997).
Reparative therapy	Reparative or conversion therapy refers to a collection of treatments intended to change the sexual orientation of nonheterosexuals to heterosexual (Hein & Matthews, 2010).
Sex work	The performance of sexual acts, in exchange for food, shelter, money, protection, or drugs (Greene, Ennett, & Ringwalt, 1999; McNamara, 1994; Rotheram-Borus, Mahler, & Rosario, 1995). Synonyms: Survival sex, prostitution, rent.
Straight	Contemporary, nonclinical term for heterosexual.
Transgender	A term inclusive of people who cross-dress for sexual (transvestite) or theatrical (drag queen) reasons and people who feel his or her body is not the sex it should be (regardless of transformational surgical status) (transsexual) (Barrow, 2008; Califia, 1997; Nycum, 2000).
Transsexual	A person who feels his or her body is not the sex it should be (regardless of transformational surgical status) (Nycum, 2000).
Transman	A person with female sex and male gender: a female-to-male (FtM) transsexual (regardless of transformational surgical status). Use the pronoun "he" when referring to this person.
Transwoman	A person with male sex and female gender: A male-to-female (MtF) transsexual (regardless of transformational surgical status). Use the pronoun "she" when referring to this person.

Modified from Hein, 2006, with permission from Vanderbilt University, Nashville, Tennessee.

with them and their families. In a 2006 study, nurse researchers assessed nurses from several national nurse associations and found that approximately 70% of the respondents indicated low levels of knowledge on LGBT issues, while only 27% expressed high interest in further training (Saewyc, Bearinger, McMahon, & Evans, 2006). The role of the therapist is to understand LGBT adolescents' sense of their own sexuality within the context of their own self-labels. This understanding will hopefully enable a healthy integration of the adolescent's sexuality into his or her own identity. If the health care provider is unable to address his or her own issues about adolescent sexuality and sexual identity and is uncomfortable working with sexual minority adolescents, it is best for the provider to refer these youth to another provider who is skilled and comfortable working with nonheterosexual youth (Hoffman, Freeman, & Swann, 2009).

Double Minorities: LGBT Minority Youth

Challenges are magnified in LGBT youth from minority backgrounds involving race and ethnicity, possibly resulting in them being doubly marginalized youth (Mays, Yancey, Cochran, Weber, & Felding, 2002). Many of these youth and/or their parents have religious affiliations that rely on interpretations of the Bible that traditionally condemn same-sex behavior (Wheeler, 2003). There are specific gender roles, family values, and expectations that contribute to the identity development process within different cultural groups. And same-sex relationships are rejected in many minority cultures (Parks, Hughes, & Matthews, 2004). In the African American and Latino communities, many members believe that the nonreproductive nature of homosexuality can be a threat to the survival of the group (Diaz, Ayala, & Bein, 2004; Garcia, Gray-Stanley, & Ramirez-Valles, 2008). Asian Americans traditionally reject same-sex relations because of Confucianism and traditions, and the perception that homosexuality threatens family and gender roles, viewing the continuation of the family through marriage and child rearing as a primary obligation (Chan, 1989). Openly disclosing homosexuality is seen as a threat to these cultural values (Berry, 2001).

Racial and ethnic minority youth face challenges that are similar to those of their white peers; however, there are also significantly different challenges that they must confront, possibly making them doubly marginalized. These youth have the burden of not only racism but also homophobia and religious and/or cultural condemnation. At times, they also encounter racism in the lesbian and gay community. Pressured by the cultural expectations of family and community related to marriage and childbearing, these young people experience high levels of stress. These youth do not have the benefit of their families reframing racial or ethnic stereotypes in order to support healthy development. Instead, many ethnic minority families and communities reinforce negative cultural perceptions of homosexuality (Ryan & Futterman, 1998). Ethnic minority youth are often unable to cope with the stress of trying to handle the stigma of racial, ethnic, and sexual identity and as a result, they become invisible. In hiding, they lose the ability to fully integrate key aspects of their identity. This puts them at risk for a host of mental health problems and for victimization.

Victimization

LGBT youth recognize their vulnerability to victimization and the absence of resources to assist them (Grossman & D'Augelli, 2006). Sexual minorities are twice as likely to have been a victim of child abuse and traumatic events and to experience post-traumatic stress disorder (PTSD) than are heterosexual adults (Roberts, Austin, Corliss, Vandermorris, & Koenen, 2010). Additionally, recent hate crime data indicate LGBT people are proportionally more than twice as likely to be victims of hate crimes as any other group (Potok, 2010). Hate crimes target someone just because of who they are. Being a victim of a hate crime carries longer-lasting psychological feelings of vulnerability than other victimization (Herek, 2009; Willis, 2008).

For many LGBT youth, attending school feels like torture due to near-constant overt and covert harassment from peers and adults (Craig, Tucker, & Wagner, 2008; Grossman & D'Augelli, 2006; Wyss, 2004). Sexual minorities are often the victims of bullying at school (Berlan, Corliss, Field, Goodman, & Bryn Austin, 2010). Additionally, when LGBT youth break rules at school or laws, they tend to receive harsher punishments than heterosexual youth (Himmelstein & Bruckner, 2010). However, schools with gay-straight alliances (GSAs) have a more positive school climate for all children, even those not involved in the GSA (Walls et al., 2010).

Mental Health

Many gay and lesbian youths live a life of isolation, alienation, depression, and fear because of negative stereotypes, religious taboos regarding homosexuality, family and cultural beliefs about homosexuality, and their own fears about being lesbian or gay. These youth are at risk for depression, suicidal ideation, low self-esteem, sexual risk taking, and substance abuse.

When LGBT youth access primary care services, APNs are in a unique position to provide counseling, support, and health care to them and their families. The National Association of Pediatric Nurse Practitioners (NAPNAP) developed a position statement titled

"Health Risks and Needs of Gay, Lesbian, Bisexual, Transgender, and Questioning Adolescents" (2006), which advocates for reducing risks to LGBT youth by promoting physical health and social and emotional well-being. Although behavioral, psychosocial, and lifestyle problems are major causes of morbidity and mortality within this population, adolescents rarely choose to seek help from mental health care providers, including APNs. They do not see a connection between psychosocial issues such as depression, drug use/abuse, sexual behaviors, family/school problems, victimization and abuse, and mental health. Adolescents are often referred for mental health evaluations by school personnel, law enforcement personnel, or other concerned individuals.

APNs in primary care should also refer these youngsters to psychiatric-mental health APNs who are trained to manage more complex mental health and behavioral concerns. Parents may first bring their concerns to the attention of the primary care APN, who should initiate an assessment with appropriate screening tools. Parents can be the greatest advocate for their child (Ryan, Huebner, Diaz, & Sanchez, 2010) or a source of danger (Balsam, Rothblum, & Beauchaine, 2005). The psychiatric-mental health APN provides expert care that is based on current, factual nonjudgmental information in a confidential manner. The most effective tools all nurses can use when interacting with LGBT youth or their parents are compassion and genuineness.

Self-realization and Coming Out

Realization that one is different from heterosexual peers is a common experience for LGBT youth. This perception of difference is often more acute for transgender youth. Transgender youth tend to become consciously aware of their sex-gender incongruence when they enter school (Grossman & D'Augelli, 2006); for some youth, other-gender play and interests begin as early as the age of two (American Psychiatric Association, 2000a, p. 536). Male-to-female transgender youth tend to come out as preteens or adolescents (Grossman & D'Augelli, 2006). Savin-Williams and Diamond (2000) identified slightly different developmental trajectories for lesbian, gay, and bisexual males and females. Girls tended to develop an emotional attachment to another girl leading to self-identification (around eighteen years old). Boys often pursued sexual relations (at around sixteen years old) several years before self-identifying as gay (Savin-Williams & Diamond, 2000).

All youth are similar in that they must develop a sense of self, individuate, make decisions about their future and about social and ethical issues, establish independence from their parents, and have a clear sense of their own identity and sexuality. The coming out process is defined as a developmental process in which gay people recognize their sexual orientation within a social context and choose to integrate this knowledge into their personal and social lives (Kaufman & Johnson, 2004; Savin-Williams & Diamond, 2000). Several theorists describe coming out as a life-long process with stage-like sequencing. Several models (Cass, 1984; Coleman, 1982; Troiden, 1988) have described the coming out process which involves five interrelated areas of development: (1) a growing awareness of homosexual feelings; (2) developing intimate same-sex romantic relationships; (3) developing social ties with gay and lesbian peers or community; (4) developing a positive evaluation of homosexuality; and (5) self-disclosure and disclosure to others. These theorists described the coming out process as occurring in stages. However, during this coming out process, the person could go back to a previous stage if issues had not been resolved.

Coming out is stressful under the best of circumstances (Barrow, 2008). LGBT youth have to cope with not only the complexities of mastering developmental tasks but also with the daily stresses of realizing that they are different. A major source of stress is the fear that a parent, friend, or teacher might unexpectedly find out about his or her sexual orientation/gender identity. There are times when the lesbian or gay youth might experience feelings of conflict or confusion over his or her sexuality. Some youth might experience pressure to disclose their identity as a result of having inaccurate information about sexual orientation. APNs should assess the level of information the youth has regarding homosexuality and coming out and provide information about the coming out process and the potential ramifications of disclosure.

Some youth have been put out of their homes; leaving them at risk for depression, suicide, drug abuse, violence, and sexual victimization (Hein, 2010). Many youth become targets of bullying and harassment at school and in their communities. They are left to cope with isolation, depression, fear, and rejection. If their parents and community are religious, they may be subjected to reparative therapies, which are also known as conversion therapies (Hein & Matthews, 2010). Some youth who disclose their sexual/gender identity to parents or friends are rejected by them and subsequently by their faith communities. Faced with being told they no longer have value to their families or to their God, it is no wonder these youth struggle with depression and self-injurious behaviors including suicide. Ryan, Huebner, Diaz, and Sanchez (2009) found that youth who experienced high levels of family rejection during adolescence were six times more likely to be depressed and eight times more likely to have attempted suicide.

The coming out process for LGBT adolescents is related to developmental issues faced by all adolescents. Adolescents need supportive and affirming adults in their lives as they move toward independence. It is important for these youth to establish social ties with peers and learn to safely interact within their communities. Due to the barriers these youth face at home, in school, and in the community, many of them will experience deficits in development. These youth have the same needs and developmental expectations as heterosexual youth. Unfortunately, secondary to environmental constraints, LGBT youth may need assistance in revisiting and reintegrating skipped developmental tasks into their current stage. They will need the support and affirmation of adults who are accepting of their sexual orientation. Developing social ties with healthy LGBT adults and peers through school and other social activities is important. However, identifying what resources are safe and helpful can sometimes be difficult. One unsafe "treatment" or "therapy" available to LGBT people is reparative therapy.

Reparative or Conversion Therapy

Reparative or conversion therapy refers to a collection of treatments intended to change the sexual orientation of nonheterosexuals to heterosexual (Hein & Matthews, 2010). At times the parent(s) of LGBT youth or even the youth themselves might ask the APN to assist in changing the youth's sexual orientation or gender identity. In some cases parents are pressured by their religious leaders so seek reparative/conversion therapies to "cure" their child's same-sex attractions. In other cases, the adolescent becomes frightened by his or her same-sex attractions and seeks help from a provider to "fix the problem" or make him or her "normal" (Fox, 2009, p. 61). Encouraging adolescents to change their sexual orientation conveys a message that there is something intrinsically wrong with them (Hein & Matthews, 2010). Reparative therapy to change one's sexual orientation has been deemed harmful and/or unethical by most professional organizations (American Psychiatric Association, 2000b; Blackwell, 2008; Hein & Matthews, 2010). The inherent belief is that homosexuality is a mental illness that can be cured; however, to date, there is no clinical evidence that reparative therapies cure individuals of homosexuality.

However, partially due to the continued DSM diagnosis of "gender identity disorder" (GID) (American Psychiatric Association, 2000a), therapies to change a person's gender identity continue (Coates, 2008). Proposed changes to the DSM (DSM V) would change the name of the diagnosis to "gender incongruence" (American Psychiatric Association, 2009; Zucker, 2010). Many of the therapies used to "cure" children of their transsexual feelings are those now discredited for "curing" LGBT persons. There is debate about whether a diagnosis of GID carries some benefit related to insurance and assistance with transitioning. Insurance companies have been quick to explicitly exclude treatments for GID from pharmaceutical, mental health, and other coverage (Aetna, 2010). Additionally, there is some evidence that gender atypical behavior in childhood is more predictive of being lesbian, gay, or bisexual than transgender (Bailey & Zucker, 1995; Bartlett & Vasey, 2006). Consequently, the utility and benefit of a GID diagnosis or GID treatment of children are uncertain.

Substance Abuse

Many youth use alcohol and drugs to cope with stress and depression. Gay and lesbian youth may use substances to manage feelings of depression, isolation, shame, and low self-esteem. A thorough assessment that includes sexuality issues can assist the youth and the APN in opening the door to discussion about sexual identity. This may be the first opportunity for the youth to talk about concerns and confusion and/or ask questions. However, it is important for the APN who regularly works with LGBT youth to acquaint himself or herself with same-sex sexual behaviors and any related risks. Additionally, developing a strong referral network within the community will improve the ability to provide quality comprehensive care. Similar to questions about sexual behaviors, APNs who inquire about substances of abuse should familiarize themselves with drugs used in the LGBT community and LGBT clubs/venues, or risk alienating their patients.

Sexual Behavior

It is important to ask the patient about sexual activity. The APN who on assessment discovers that a youth is engaging in sexual behavior should assess the type of behaviors to help the youth understand how premature sexual behavior (before the youth has concluded the nature of his or her sexual attractions) complicates his or her ability to move through the developmental tasks of adolescence and the development of a healthy sense of self. Nonthreatening questions about any symptoms the youth might be experiencing should be asked and, based on those findings, appropriate lab work should be ordered (e.g., screening for STIs, human papillomavirus [HPV], and HIV). However, the APN should prepared to comfortably answer questions about any/all sexual activities. For both the sexually active and nonsexually active LGBT youth, counseling about protection for sexual activities that put them at risk for STIs, HIV infection, and possible pregnancy should be provided. Some LGBT youth engage in heterosexual sex as a way of coping with pressure they perceive from peers or family members about dating. They may use heterosexual sex as a way of warding off suspicion about their sexuality or to prove to themselves that they are not lesbian or gay if they are in conflict about their sexual identity. Another risk of this behavior is unwanted pregnancy. Pregnancy can occur as a result of rape, failure to practice safe sex, drug use/abuse, or survival sex. It is also important to be particularly sensitive to the needs of transgender youth. If you are unwilling to assist them with halting the onset of puberty (Asscheman, 2009; Cohen-Kettenis, Delemarre-van de Waal, & Gooren, 2008) into the wrong sex, they will find another way to transition through street hormones, silicone parties, and occasionally self-mutilation. Although sexual activity and unconventional transitioning activities can convey HIV, it is important to be clear you do not see the youth as merely a vector of disease.

It is essential that LGBT youth are provided with information about adolescent sexuality, sexual and gender identity, and resources that are able to meet their needs. Unfortunately, some states (Alabama, South Carolina, and Texas) criminalize teaching about sexual orientation outside of the context of sexually transmitted diseases (STDs) ("Comprehensive Health Education Act," 1988), and eighteen states mandate teaching that sexual activity should *only* occur within the context of marriage (Guttmacher Institute, 2011). It is important for APNs to be aware that only five states and the District of Columbia issue marriage licenses to same-sex couples at this time (Human Rights Campaign, 2011). So not only does the sexual education provided in some states ignore the existence of sexual minorities through their emphasis on marriage (something these same states are simultaneously denying to sexual minorities), other states overtly vilify nonheterosexual sex. It is important for APNs to be aware of the content and context of the sex education their patients may have received.

Depression, Anxiety, and Suicide

It is important to assess LGBT youth for depression, anxiety, and suicidal ideation. Inquiring about suicide ideation and attempts should be part of your assessment. Suicide is the third leading cause of death in adolescents in the United States (Hamilton et al., 2007). Data on suicide and suicidal ideation in LGBT youth are inconclusive; however, evidence from one study indicated a slightly elevated level of suicidal ideation among LGBT youth (Clements-Nolle, Marx, & Katz, 2006; Savin-Williams, 2001). A relationship has also been reported between victimization, gender nonconformity, and suicide attempts (Clements-Nolle et al., 2006; D'Augelli et al., 2005).

LGBT youth who are conflicted about their sexual orientation; who have been subjected to harassment, violence, and/or rejection; and who have used addictive substances have a greater chance of becoming depressed and of experiencing suicidal ideation. The stress of being lesbian or gay can also exacerbate existing problems such as sexual acting out, a significant decrease in school grades, social isolation, and arguments with parents and peers. When these issues are addressed with youth, it helps them to feel safe. Depressed LGBT youth tend to be invisible, and they do not usually seek help for fear of being discovered and rejected. When they do come to the attention of APNs, they do not announce that they are lesbian, gay, or bisexual. They may present with symptoms of depression. Discussion can help them to address the stressors that affect their well-being such as confusion about their sexuality, fear of rejection by family and peers, and the stress of leading a double life and having to hide their sexual identity. Some adolescents who have disclosed their sexual orientation/gender identity or have had it discovered by peers or family become depressed when they sense little support. Conversely, others find disclosure cathartic and freeing.

Safe Health Care

LGBT youth may perceive health care services and providers as intolerant and consequently unsafe (Grossman & D'Augelli, 2006). Transgender youth may be unable to access needed health care services due to unavailability—for example, lack of providers willing to prescribe hormone treatment to delay puberty or to assist with transitioning or simply gynecological services that are not harassing to masculine lesbians. Compounding the general absence of safe services outside of very large urban areas, youth have no legal standing to provide independent consent to treatment. There are ways the affirming APN can demonstrate safety in their practice. Figure 5.1 summarizes key points.

- Acknowledge LGBT youth exist (Grossman & D'Augelli, 2006). Post a sticker with a rainbow flag or other symbol of the LGBT community on the door to the office.
- Stay informed about LGBT and youth (Hoffman et al., 2009).
- Include LGBT-affirming reading material in the waiting room.
- Modify the intake form to include "partnered" beside checkboxes for "married, single, divorced."
- When discussing relationship status with your client, ask everyone (whether male or female) if they have a "boyfriend or girlfriend."

- Ask what pronoun (he/she) they would like you to use.
- In the event the youth needs referral: Be careful where you refer so that you do not make things worse. Confirm the provider is LGBT affirming before referring.
- Carefully consider whether parental involvement in your patients' care will be helpful or harmful. Many youth prefer to receive care without parental involvement (Hoffman et al., 2009). Are their parents aware of their sexual orientation/gender identity? Will you endanger the youth if you disclose their sexual orientation/gender identity (physical safety, housing, etc.)?
- Assist the youth to create a safety plan (Barrow, 2008). Where can they go and who can assist them if their physical safety (abuse) or housing is compromised?

Once the adolescent has decided that he or she is ready to disclose, the APN has an important role in the process. The decision to disclose involves several steps:

1. Weigh the risks and benefits, which include parental response. Coming out to parents can be upsetting for parents, siblings, and the disclosing adolescent. The nurse should be prepared to support both the adolescent and the family during their adjustment to the disclosure. Anticipatory guidance for adolescents and parents involves providing information on adolescent sexuality and practices, resources such as gay and lesbian youth centers, school support networks, and support networks for parents such as Parents, Families and Friends of Lesbian and Gays (PFLAG). The Gay and Lesbian Medical Association (GLMA), an interdisciplinary professional organization of health care providers, offers an online directory of gay-affirming health care providers.
2. Examine the youth's motivation for disclosure. While some youth may not be able to clearly identify their motives, they need to be explored to determine whether disclosure originated from anger, self-preservation, or self-destruction.
3. Assist the youth to explore what being LGBT means to them and the resources and social support that are available.
4. Explore the youth's relationship with parents and the family cultural/ethnic, moral, and religious views. For reasons of safety, it is important to help the youth recognize his or her social milieu—to gain insight into the situation and environment. Explore with the youth what resources are available outside the home in the event that there is parental, family, and peer disapproval and/or rejection.
5. Offer anticipatory guidance, which will be helpful. For instance, what do parents, family, and friends think about homosexuality? How will he or she respond to negative comments about LGBT people and when the comments are directed at her or him? What are some ways to respond if these comments are made by someone in authority? Assisting the youth to think through and answer these questions will not only assist with the coming out process but will help the youth to be safer once out.

The APN must help the youth consider their parents' reaction in the event they came out. The APN can be a source of strength and support for the youth if they wish to come out. The APN must be careful not to push the youth toward resolution and disclosure, particularly if they express conflict or confusion about their sexuality. Additionally, youth must be cautioned to seriously consider their parents' potential reaction; they are still minors and consequently very vulnerable. The youth may need to be encouraged to consider delaying their disclosures until they are self-supporting and living independently.

Conclusion

All children and adolescents progress through stages of sexual development, with most achieving comfort with their sexuality and their choice of sexual behaviors and partner(s). However, for some this journey is painful and worrisome and results in emotional and mental health distress. APNs working with the pediatric population are in a position to educate children, adolescents, and families about sexual development and appropriate childhood expression of sexuality. This includes helping sexual minority youth and LGBT youth achieve safety and comfort with their sexual choices.

The provision of quality sexual health care to children and adolescents has been difficult to achieve because it tends to engender discomfort in the people who must provide it. Although in recent years there has been an emphasis on sexual health, many APNs are uncomfortable broaching the subject with youth. Controversy exists about who should discuss and educate youth about sexuality and sexual health. The fact is that today's youth engage in early sexual behavior, question their own

---

- It's not a lifestyle – it's who they are
- It's not a "sexual preference" – use "sexual orientation" or "sexual identity"
- Families of Choice – Respect who they consider their family
- Don't Out Someone – You many endanger their safety, shelter and continued employment

Figure 5.1 Take-home points.

sexuality, and are frequent victims of sexual abuse, rape, and sexual victimization.

Health needs of LGBT youth are seldom met because they rarely seek help and their issues are generally dismissed when they do seek help. LGBT youth may present for therapy for issues other than their sexual orientation. It is important for the APN to address the presenting problem even if it is known that the youth is LGBT. Engaging youth in a nonjudgmental, nonthreatening manner is essential to developing a therapeutic relationship with them. Sexual minority youth need to be able to explore what being nonheterosexual means and how their lives are affected by it. They need to be able to talk about how they are feeling and coping in a safe and open environment. Nurse therapists who work with LGBT youth have a responsibility to become knowledgeable about adolescent sexuality and sexual orientation development.

APNs will encounter adolescents who are moving through the different stages of their physical, psychosocial, and sexual development. Some of these youth will be heterosexual, others will be homosexual, and some of them will be questioning their sexual identity. The APN will encounter these youth in a variety of environments; therefore, it is important for the clinician to be educated and knowledgeable about various sexualities and gender identities as well as the issues that arise as youth move through developmental stages. APNs must be comprehensive in their assessment of child and adolescent health and illness issues, which includes assessment of physical, psychosocial, and sexual development. APNs can be pivotal in helping all youth fully integrate developmental tasks while supporting youth comfort with their sexuality through appropriate education and linkages to needed services.

Resources on Adolescent Sexual Development

Resources for Patients and Families

Harris, R.H. and Emberley, M. 2005. It's Perfectly Normal: Changing Bodies, Growing Up, Sex, and Sexual Health. Massachusetts: Candlewick.

Gravelle, K. and Gravelle, J. 1996. The Period Book: Everything You Don't Want to Ask but Need to Know.

Mayle, P. 1981. What's Happening to Me? An Illustrated Guide to Puberty.

American Academy of Pediatrics
141 Northwest Point Boulevard
Elk Grove Village, IL 60007-1098
Tel 847 434-400
www.healthychildren.org

Office of Public Health and Science, www.4parents.gov
Sexuality Information and Education Council of the United States, www.siecus.org

Resources for Precocious Puberty

Resources for Patients and Families

Magic Foundation
1327 N. Harlem Avenue
Oak Park, IL 60302
Tel 708 383 0808
www.magicfoundation.org

National Adrenal Diseases Foundation
505 Northern Boulevard
Great Neck, NY 11021
Tel 516 487 4992
www.nadf.us

Healthscout: Precocious Puberty
www.healthscout.com

KidsHealth.org (The Nemours Foundation)
KidsHealth:Precocious Puberty
www.kidshealth.org

Resources for Clinicians

American Academy of Pediatrics
141 Northwest Point Boulevard
Elk Grove Village, IL 60007-1098
Tel 847 434-4000
www.aap.org

NIH/National Institute of Child Health and Human Development
31 Center Drive
Building 31, Room 2A32
MSC2425
Bethesda, MD 20892
Tel 301 496 5133
www.nichd.nih.gov

Society for Adolescent Medicine
1916 Copper Oaks Circle
Blue Springs, MO 64015
Tel 816 224-8010
www.adolescenthealth.org

Resources on Homosexuality and Adolescents

Resources for Clinicians

Washington, DC
National Gay and Lesbian Task Force
1325 Massachusetts Avenue NW, Suite 600
Washington D.C. 20005-4171
Tel 202 393 2241

New York, NY
121 West 27th Street, Suite 501
New York, NY 1001
Tel 212 604 9831

Los Angeles, CA
5455 Wilshire Boulevard, Suite 1505
Los Angeles, CA 90036
Tel 323 954 9597

Cambridge, MA
1121 Massachusetts Avenue,
Cambridge, MA 02138
Tel 617 492 6393
ngltf@ngltf.org
www.ngltf.org

Gay and Lesbian Medical Association
www.glma.org

Gay and Lesbian and Straight Education Network
www.glsen.org

International Society of Psychiatric–Mental Health Nurses
www.ispin-psych.org

Society for Adolescent Medicine
www.adolescenthealth.org

Sexuality Information and Education Counsel of the United States (SIECUS)
90 John Street, Suite 402
New York, NY 10038
212 819 9770
www.siecus.org

Resources for Lesbian and Gay Adolescents and Families

Books

"Prayers for Bobby" by Leroy Arrons -A mother's coming to terms with religious intolerance. Also adapted for a TV movie on the Lifetime Network.
"The God Box" by Alex Sanchez. Addresses religion and conflict related to being gay.
"The Misfits" by James Howe. Addresses bullying of gay youth.
"The Bermudez Triangle" by Maureen Johnson. Addresses conflict and struggle with sexuality and sexual orientation in girls.
"Absolutely Positively Not" by David Larochell. Addresses coming out issues.
"Annie on My Mind" by Nancy Garden. Addresses the relationship of a young lesbian.

Other Resources

Parents, Families and Friends of Lesbians and Gays (PFLAG.) Offers support for families and individuals, provides training and education about LBGT issues.
National Office
1828 L Street Suite 660
Washington DC 20036
202 467-8180
www.community.pflag.org

Advocates for Youth. Advocates for youth and helps them to make informed and responsible decisions about their sexual and reproductive health.
www.advocatesforyouth.org

Sexuality Information and Education Council of the United States
90 John Street Suite 402
New York, NY 10038
212 819-9770
www.siecus.org

References

Aetna. (2010, February 5). Gender reassignment surgery. *Clinical Policy Bulletin.* Retrieved from http://www.aetna.com/cpb/medical/data/600_699/0615.html

American Academy of Pediatrics (AAP), Committee on Adolescence. (1993). Policy statement (rev.): Homosexuality and adolescence. *Pediatrics, 113,* 1827–1832.

American Psychiatric Association. (2000a). *Diagnostic and statistical manual of mental disorders, fourth revised edition.* Washington, DC: American Psychiatric Association.

American Psychiatric Association. (2000b). *Therapies focused on attempts to change sexual orientation (reparative or conversion therapies): Position statement.* Retrieved from http://www.psych.org/Departments/EDU/Library/APAOfficialDocumentsandRelated/PositionStatements/200001.aspx

American Psychiatric Association. (2009). 302.6 Gender identity disorder in children. In *DSM-5 development.* Arlington, VA: American Psychiatric Association.

Anderson, S.E., Dallal, G.E., & Must, A. (2003). Relative weight and race influence average age at menarche: Results from two nationally representative surveys of US girls studied 25 years apart. *Pediatrics, 111,* 844–850.

Aruda, M.M., McCabe, M., Litty, C., & Burke, P. (2008). Adolescent pregnancy diagnosis and outcomes: A six year clinical sample. *Journal of Pediatric and Adolescent Gynecology, 21,* 17–19.

Aruda, M.M., Waddicor, K., Frese, L., Cole, J.C.M., & Burke, P. (2010). Early pregnancy in adolescents: Diagnosis, assessment, options counseling, and referral. *Journal of Pediatric Health Care, 24,* 4–13.

Asscheman, H. (2009). Gender identity disorder in adolescents. *Sexologies, 18,* 105–109.

Bailey, J.M., & Zucker, K.J. (1995). Childhood sex-typed behavior and sexual orientation: A conceptual analysis and quantitative review. *Developmental Psychology, 31,* 43–55.

Balsam, K.F., Rothblum, E.D., & Beauchaine, T.P. (2005). Victimization over the life span: A comparison of lesbian, gay, bisexual, and heterosexual siblings. *Journal of Consulting and Clinical Psychology, 73,* 477–487.

Barrow, K.L. (2008). *Achieving optimal gender identity integration for transgender female-to-male adult patients: An unconventional psychoanalytic guide for treatment* (Doctoral dissertation). Available through ProQuest Dissertations Abstracts. (AAT 3326610)

Bartlett, N., & Vasey, P. (2006). A retrospective study of childhood gender-atypical behavior in Samoan fa'afafine. *Archives of Sexual Behavior, 35,* 659–666. doi:10.1007/s10508-006-9055-1

Berlan, E.D., Corliss, H.L., Field, A.E., Goodman, E., & Bryn Austin, S. (2010). Sexual orientation and bullying among adolescents in the growing up today study. *Journal of Adolescent Health, 46,* 366–371. doi:10.1016/j.jadohealth.2009.10.015

Berry, C. (2001). Asian values, family values: Film, video, and lesbian and gay identities. *Journal of Homosexuality, 40*(3–4), 211. doi:10.1300/J082v40n03_04

Blackwell, C.W. (2008). Nursing implications in the application of conversion therapies on gay, lesbian, bisexual and transgender clients. *Issues in Mental Health Nursing, 29,* 651–665.

Blondell, R.D., Foster, M.B., & Kamlesh, C.D. (1999). Disorders of puberty. *American Family Physician, 60*(1), 209–224.

Califia, P. (1997). *Sex changes: The politics of transgenderism.* San Francisco, CA: Cleis Press.

Carel, J.C., & Leger, J. (2008). Precocious puberty. *New England Journal of Medicine, 358,* 2366–2377.

Cass, V. (1984). Homosexual identity formation: Testing a theoretical model. *Journal of Homosexuality, 20,* 143–167.

Centers for Disease Control and Prevention. (2009). Sexual and reproductive health of persons aged 10–24 years: United States, 2002–2007. *MMWR, 58* (SS-6), 1–58.

Chan, C. (1989). Issues of identity development among Asian-American lesbians and gay men. *Journal of Counseling and Development, 68*, 16–20.

Chumlea, W.C., Schubert, C.M., Roche, A.F., Kulin, H.E., Lee, P.A., Himes, J.H., & Sun, S.S. (2003). Age at menarche and racial comparisons in US girls. *Pediatrics, 111*, 110–113.

Clements-Nolle, K., Marx, R., & Katz, M. (2006). Attempted suicide among transgender persons. The influence of gender-based discrimination and victimization. *Journal of Homosexuality, 51*, 53–69.

Coates, S.W. (2008). Intervention with preschool boys with gender identity issues. *Neuropsychiatrie de l'enfance et de l'adolescence, 56*, 392–397.

Cohen-Kettenis, P.T., Delemarre-van de Waal, H.A., & Gooren, L. J.G. (2008). The treatment of adolescent transsexuals: Changing insights. *Journal of Sexual Medicine, 5*, 1892–1897.

Coleman, E. (1982). Developmental stages of the coming out process. *Journal of Homosexuality, 7*, 157–176.

Comprehensive Health Education Act, SC ST SEC 59-32-30, South Carolina Code of Laws (1988).

Craig, S.L., Tucker, E.W., & Wagner, E.F. (2008). Empowering lesbian, gay, bisexual, and transgender youth: Lessons learned from a safe schools summit. *Journal of Gay & Lesbian Social Services, 20*, 237–252.

Daley, A.M., Sadler, L.S., Leventhal, J.M., Cromwell, P.F., & Reynolds, H.D. (2005). Negative pregnancy tests in urban adolescents: An important and often missed opportunity for clinicians. *Pediatric Nursing, 31*, 87–89.

D'Augelli, A.R., Grossman, A.H., Salter, N.P., Vasey, J.J., Starks, M.T., & Sinclair, K.O. (2005). Predicting the suicide attempts of lesbian, gay, and bisexual youth. *Suicide and Life-Threatening Behavior, 35*, 646–660.

DeMonteflores C., & Schultz, S. J. (1978). Coming out: Similarities and differences for lesbians and gay men. *Journal of Social Issues, 34*, 59–72.

Diaz, R. M., Ayala, G., & Bein, E. (2004). Sexual risk as an outcome of social oppression: Data from a probability sample of Latino gay men in three U.S. cities. *Cultural Diversity & Ethnic Minority Psychology, 10*, 255–267.

Ellis, B.J., & Garber, J. (2000). Psychosocial antecedents of variation in girls' pubertal timing: Maternal depression, stepfather presence, and marital and family stress. *Child Development, 71*, 485–501.

Erickson, E.H. (1950). *Childhood and society*. New York, NY: Norton.

Essa, E., & Murray, C.I. (1999). Sexual play: When should you be concerned? *Childhood Education, 75*, 231–234.

Fish, J. (2010). Conceptualising social exclusion and lesbian, gay, bisexual, and transgender people: The implications for promoting equity in nursing policy and practice. *Journal of Research in Nursing, 15*, 303–312. doi:10.1177/1744987110364691

Fontaine, J.H. (1998). Evidencing a need: School counselors' experiences with gay and lesbian students. *Professional School Counseling, 1*, 18–24.

Fox 61 (Producer). (2009, July 14). *Connecticut church posts controversial gay exorcism video on YouTube*. Retrieved from http://www.youtube.com/watch?v=L9v2uk99o2E

Frankowski, B.L., & Committee on Adolescence. (2004). Sexual orientation and adolescents: Cinical report. *Pediatrics, 113*,1827–1832.

Friedrich, W.N., Fisher, J., Broughton, D., Houston, M., & Shafran, C.R. (1998). Normative sexual behavior in children: A contemporary sample. *Pediatrics, 101*, 1–13.

Friedrich, W.N., Grambush, P., Broughton, D., Kuiper, J., & Beilke, R.L. (1991). Normative sexual behavior in children. *Pediatrics, 88*, 456–464.

Garcia, D. I., Gray-Stanley, J., & Ramirez-Valles, J. (2008). "The priest obviously doesn't know that I'm gay": The religious and spiritual journeys of Latino gay men. *J Homosex, 55*, 411–436.

Gerlt, T., Blosser, C., & Dunn, A. (2009). Sexuality. In C. Burns, A. Dunn, M. Brady, N. Starr, & C. Blosser. *Pediatric primary care* (fourth edition, pp. 395–410). St. Louis, MO: Saunders Elsevier.

Green, B. (1994). Lesbian women of color: Triple jeopardy. In Comas-Diaz, L, Green, B. (Eds.), *Women of color: Integrating ethnic and gender identities in psychotherapy*. New York, NY: Guilford Press.

Greene, J. M., Ennett, S. T., & Ringwalt, C. L. (1999). Prevalence and correlates of survival sex among runaway and homeless youth. *American Journal of Public Health, 89*, 1406–1409.

Goldenring, J.M., & Rosen, D. S. (2004). Getting into adolescent heads: An essential update. *Contemporary Pediatrics, 21*, 64–90.

Grossman, A.H., & D'Augelli, A.R. (2006). Transgender youth: Invisible and vulnerable. *Journal of Homosexuality, 51*, 111–128.

Guttmacher Institute. (2011). *Sex and HIV Education* [State Policies in Brief]. New York, NY: Guttmacher Institute.

Hamilton, B.E., Minino, A.M., Martin, J.A., Kochanek, K.D., Strobino, D.M., & Guyer, B. (2007). Annual summary of vital statistics: 2005. *Pediatrics, 119*, 345–360.

Hatzenbuehler, M.L., McLaughlin, K.A., Keyes, K.M., & Hasin, D. S. (2010). The impact of institutional discrimination on psychiatric disorders in lesbian, gay, and bisexual populations: A prospective study. *American Journal of Public Health, 100*, 452–459. doi:10.2105/ajph.2009.168815

Hein, L.C. (2006). *Survival among male homeless adolescents* (Doctoral dissertation). Available from ProQuest Dissertation Abstracts database. (AAT 3230568)

Hein, L.C. (2010). Where did you sleep last night? Homeless male adolescents: Gay, bisexual, transgender and heterosexual compared. *Southern Online Journal of Nursing Research, 10*(1). Retrieved from http://snrs.org/publications/SOJNR_articles2/Vol10Num01Art09.pdf

Hein, L.C., & Matthews, A.K. (2010). Reparative therapy: The adolescent, the psych nurse and the issues. *Journal of Child and Adolescent Psychiatric Nursing, 23*, 29–35.

Herek, G.M. (1990). The context of anti-gay violence: Notes on cultural and psychological heterosexism. *Journal of Interpersonal Violence, 5*, 316–333.

Herek, G.M. (2002). Heterosexuals' attitudes toward bisexual men and women in the United States. *The Journal of Sex Research, 39*, 264–274.

Herek, G.M. (2009). Hate crimes and stigma-related experiences among sexual minority adults in the United States. *Journal of Interpersonal Violence, 24*(1), 54–74.

Herek, G.M., & Berrill, K.T. (1990). Documenting the victimization of lesbians and gay men: Methodological issues. *J Interpers Violence, 5*, 301–315. doi:10.1177/088626090005003005

Herman, J.W. (2007). Repeat pregnancy in adolescence intentions and decision making. *MCN: The American Journal of Maternal Child Nursing, 32*, 89–90.

Herman-Giddens, M.E., Slora, E.J., Wasserman, R.C., Bourdony, C.J., Bhapkar, M.V., Koch, G.G., & Hasemeier, C.M. (1997). Secondary sexual characteristics and menses in young girls seen in office practice: A study from the pediatric research in office settings network. *Pediatrics, 99*, 505–512.

Himmelstein, K.E.W., & Bruckner, H. (2010). Criminal-justice and school sanctions against nonheterosexual youth: A national longitudinal study. *Pediatrics, 127*, 49–57. doi:10.1542/peds.2009–2306

Hoffman, N.D., Freeman, K., & Swann, S. (2009). Healthcare preferences of lesbian, gay, bisexual, transgender and questioning youth. *The Journal of Adolescent Health: Official Publication of the Society for Adolescent Medicine, 45,* 222–229. doi:10.1016/j.jadohealth.2009.01.009

Hornor, G. (2004). Sexual behavior in children: Normal or not? *Journal of Pediatric Health Care, 18*(2), 57–64.

Human Rights Campaign. (2011). *Marriage and relationship recognition.* Retrieved from http://www.hrc.org/issues/marriage/marriage_introduction.asp

Ickovics, J.R., Niccolai, L.M., Lewis, J.B., Kershaw, T.S., & Ethier, T.A. (2003). High postpartum rates of sexually transmitted infections among teens: pregnancy as a window of opportunity for prevention. *Sexually Transmitted Infections, 79,* 469–473.

International Society of Psychiatric Nurses (ISPN). (2009). *Position statement on reparative therapy.* Retrieved from http://www.ispn-psych.org/docs/PS-ReparativeTherapy.pdf

Johnson, T.C. (1991, August/September). Understanding the sexual behaviors of young children. *SIECUS Report,* 8–15.

Kaplowitz, P.B., Oberfield, S.E., & the Drug and Therapeutics and Executive Committees of the Lawson Wilkins Pediatric Endocrine Society (1999). Reexamination of the age limit for defining when puberty is precocious in girls in the United States: Implications for evaluation and treatment. *Pediatrics, 104,* 936–941.

Kaplowitz, P.B., Slora, E.J., Wasserman, R.C., Pedlow, S.E., & Herman-Giddens, P.A. (2001). Earlier onset of puberty in girls: Relation to increased body mass index and race. *Pediatrics, 108,* 347–353.

Kaufman, J.M., & Johnson, C. (2004). Stigmatized individuals and the process of identity. *Sociological Quarterly, 45,* 807–833. doi:10.1111/j.1533-8525.2004.tb02315.x

Kinsey, A.C., Pomeroy, W.B., & Martin, C.E. (1948). *Sexual behavior in the human male.* Philadelphia, PA: W.B. Saunders.

Lalwani, S., Reindollar, R.H., & Davis, A.J. (2003). Normal onset of puberty have definitions of onset changed? *Obstetrics and Gynecology Clinics of North America, 30,* 279–286.

Marshall, W.A., & Tanner, J.M. (1969). Variations in pattern of pubertal changes in girls. *Archives of Disease in Childhood, 44,* 291–303.

Marshall, W.A., & Tanner, J.M. (1970). Variations in pattern of pubertal changes in boys. *Archives of Disease in Childhood, 45,* 13–23.

Martin, J.A., Osterman, M.K., & Sutton, P.D. (2010a). Are preterm births on the decline in the United States? Recent data from the National Vital Statistics System. NCHS Data Brief. Hyattsville, MD: National Center for Health Statistics.

Martin, J.A., Hamilton, B.E., Sutton, P.D., Ventura, M.A., Mathews, M.S., & Osterman, M.S. (2010b). Births: Final data for 2008. *National Vital Statistics Reports, 59*(1). Hyattsville, MD: National Center for Health Statistics.

Massachusetts Youth Risk Behavior Survey. (2001). *Massachusetts high school students and sexual orientation.* Retrieved from http://www.doe.mass.edu/cnp/hprograms/yrbs/01/results.pdf

Mathews, T.J., & MacDorman, M.F. (2010). Infant mortality statistics from 2006 period linked birth/infant death data set. *National Vital Statistics Reports, 58*(17). Hyattsville, MD: National Center for Health Statistics.

Mays, V.M., Yancey, A.K., Cochran, S.D., Weber, M., & Felding, J.E. (2002). Heterogeneity of health disparities among African American, Hispanic, and Asian American women: Unrecognized influences of sexual orientation [Research]. *American Journal of Public Health, 92,* 632–639.

McKee, M.D., Karasz, A., & Weber, C.M. (2004). Health care seeking among urban minority adolescent girls: The crises at sexual debut. *Annals of Family Medicine, 2,* 549–554.

McNamara, R. (1994). *The Times Square hustler: Male prostitutes in New York City.* Westport, CT: Praeger.

Muir, A. (2006). Precocious puberty. *Pediatrics in Review, 27,* 373–381.

National Association of Pediatric Nurse Practitioners (NAPNAP). (2006). Position statement on health risks and needs of gay, lesbian, bisexual, transgender, and questioning adolescents. *Journal of Pediatric Health Care, 20*(1), 29A–30A.

Nycum, B. (2000). *XY Survival guide. Everything you need to know about being young and gay.* San Francisco, CA: XY Publishing.

Parks, C., Hughes, T., & Matthews, A. (2004). Race/Ethnicity and sexual orientation: Intersecting identities. *Cultural Diversity and Ethnic Minority Psychology, 10,* 241–254.

Pinyerd, B., & Zipf, W.B. (2005). Puberty—Timing is everything. *Journal of Pediatric Nursing, 20,* 75–82.

Polaneczky, M., & O'Connor, K. (1999). Pregnancy in the adolescent patient: Screening, diagnosis, and initial management. *Pediatric Clinics of North America, 46,* 649–70.

Potok, M. (2010). Anti-gay hate crimes: Doing the math. In Southern Poverty Law Center Center (Ed.), *Intelligence Report,* 140. Montgomery, AL: Southern Poverty Law Center.

Qing, H., & Karlberg, J. (2001). BMI in childhood and its association with height gain, timing of puberty, and final height. *Pediatric Research, 49,* 244–251.

Remafedi, G., Resnick, M., Blum, R., & Harris, L. (1992). Demography of sexual orientation in adolescents. *Pediatrics, 89,* 714–721.

Ridge, D., Minichiello, V., & Plummer, D. (1997). Queer connections: Community, "the scene," and an epidemic. *Journal of Contemporary Ethnography, 26,* 146–181.

Rieger, G., Linsenmeier, J., Gygax, L., Garcia, S., & Bailey, J. (2010). Dissecting "gaydar": Accuracy and the role of masculinity-feminity. *Archives of Sexual Behavior, 39, 124–140.*

Roberts, A.L., Austin, S.B., Corliss, H.L., Vandermorris, A.K., & Koenen, K.C. (2010). Pervasive trauma exposure among US sexual orientation minority adults and risk of posttraumatic stress disorder. *American Journal of Public Health,* preprint, doi:10.2105/ajph.2009.168971

Rogol, A.D. (2005). New facets of androgen replacement therapy during childhood and adolescence. *Expert Options in Pharmacotherapy, 6,* 1319–1336.

Rosen, D.S., & Foster, C. (2001). Delayed puberty. *Pediatrics, 22,* 309–315.

Rotheram-Borus, M.J., Mahler, K.A., & Rosario, M. (1995). AIDS prevention with adolescents. *AIDS Education and Prevention, 7,* 320–336.

Ryan, C., & Futterman, D. (1998). *Lesbian and gay youth: Care and counseling,* New York, NY: Columbia University Press

Ryan, C., Huebner, D., Diaz, R.M., & Sanchez, J. (2009). Family rejection as a predictor of negative health outcomes in white and Latino lesbian, gay, and bisexual young adults. *Pediatrics, 123,* 346–352.

Ryan, C., Huebner, D., Diaz, R.M., & Sanchez, J. (2010). Family acceptance in adolescence and the health of LGBT young adults. *Journal of Child and Adolescent Psychiatric Nursing, 23,* 205–213.

Saewyc, E., Bearinger, L., McMahon, G., & Evans, T. (2006). A national needs assessment of nurses providing health care to adolescents. *Journal of Professional Nursing, 22,* 304–313.

Saewyc, E.M., Poon, C.S., Homma, Y., & Skay, C.L. (2008). Stigma management? The links between enacted stigma and teen pregnancy trends among gay, lesbian, and bisexual students in British Columbia. *Canadian Journal of Human Sexuality, 17*(3), 123–139.

Savin-Williams, R.C. (2009). Gay and lesbian adolescents. In F.W. Bozett & M.B. Sussman (Eds.), *Homosexuality and family relations.* Binghamton, NY: Harrington Park Press.

Savin-Williams, R.C. (2005). *The new gay teenager.* Cambridge, MA: Harvard University Press.

Savin-Williams, R.C. (2001). Suicide attempts among sexual-minority youths: Population and measurement issues [Review article]. *Journal of Consulting and Clinical Psychology, 69*, 983–991.

Savin-Williams, R.C., & Diamond, L.M. (2000). Sexual identity trajectories among sexual-minority youths: Gender comparisons. *Archives of Sexual Behavior, 29*, 607–627.

Sell, R.L., Wells, J.A., & Wypij, D. (1995). The prevalence of homosexual behavior and attraction in the United States, the United Kingdom and France: Results of national population-based samples. *Archives of Sexual Behavior, 24*, 235–248.

Shew, M.L., Hellerstedt, W.L., Sieving, R.E., Smith, A.E., & Fee, R.M. (2000). Prevalence of home pregnancy testing among adolescents. *American Journal of Public Health, 90*, 974–976.

Simmonds, K., & Likis, F. (2005). Providing options counseling for women with unintended pregnancy. *Journal of Obstetric, Gynecologic, and Neonatal Nursing, 34*, 373–379.

Singh, S., & Darroch, J. (2000). Adolescent pregnancy and childbearing: Levels and trends in developed countries. *Family Planning Perspectives, 32*(1), 14–23.

Sun, S.S., Schubert, C.M., Chumlea, W.C., Roche, A.F., Kulin, H.E., Lee, P.A., Himes, J.H., & Ryan, A.S. (2002). National estimates of the timing of sexual maturation and racial differences among US children. *Pediatrics, 110*, 911–919.

Sylva, D., Rieger, G., Linsenmeier, J., & Bailey, J. (2010). Concealment of sexual orientation. *Archives of Sexual Behavior, 39*, 141–152.

Troiden, R. (1988). Homosexual identity development. *Journal of Adolescent Health Care, 9*, 15–113.

Ventura, S.J., & Hamilton, B.E. (2011). U.S. teenage birth rate resumes decline. *NCHS Data Brief*, No. 58. Hyattsville, MD: National Center for Health Statistics.

Ventura, S.J., Abma, J.C., Mosher, W.D., & Henshaw, S.K. (2008). Estimated pregnancy rates by outcomes for the United States, 1990–2004. *National Vital Statistics Reports, 56*(15). Hyattsville, MD: National Center for Health Statistics.

Walls, N.E., Kane, S.B., & Wisneski, H. (2010). Gay straight alliances and school experiences of sexual minority youth. *Youth and Society, 41*, 307–322. doi:10.1177/0044118X09334957

Werner, E.J., Broxson, E.H., Tucker, E.L., Giroux, D.S., Shults, J., & Abshire, T.C. (1993). Prevalence of von Willebrand disease in children: A multiethnic study. *Journal of Pediatrics, 123*, 893–898.

Wheeler, D.P. (2003). Methodological issues in conducting community-based health and social services research among urban black and African American LGBT populations. *Journal of Gay & Lesbian Social Services, 15*(1), 65–78.

Willis, D.G. (2008). Meanings in adult male victims' experiences of hate crime and its aftermath. *Issues in Mental Health Nursing, 29*, 567–584.

Wu, T., Mendola, P., & Buck, G. (2002). Ethnic differences in the presence of secondary sex characteristics and menarche among US girls: The third national health and nutrition examination survey, 1988–1994. *Pediatrics, 110*, 752–757.

Wyss, S.E. (2004). 'This was my hell': The violence experience by gender non-conforming youth in US high schools. *International Journal of Qualitative Studies in Education, 17*, 709–730.

Zabin, L.S., Sedivy, V., & Emerson, M.R. (1994). Subsequent risk of child-bearing among adolescents with a negative pregnancy test. *Family Planning Perspectives, 26*, 212–217.

Zucker, K. (2010). The DSM diagnostic criteria for gender identity disorder in children. *Archives of Sexual Behavior, 39*, 477–498.

SECTION 2
Treatment

6

Issues in Prescribing Psychiatric Medication to Children and Adolescents

Geraldine S. Pearson, Beth Muller, and Amanda Reilly

Objectives

After reading this chapter, APNs will be able to

1. Identify principles of psychotropic medication management applicable to a pediatric primary care population.
2. Perform mental health assessments in the primary care setting and develop treatment plans that include medication referrals for diagnostic clarity and further treatment.
3. Identify commonly used psychotropic medications, indications for use, dosing, contraindications, and side effect profiles.
4. Discuss collaboration between advanced practice nurses in pediatric primary care and child/adolescent psychiatry regarding medication evaluation, medication stabilization, and mediation maintenance strategies.

Introduction

In the United States, approximately one in four children have a mental health problem affecting their functioning at home and/or school (U.S. Office of the Surgeon General, 1999). This raises the likelihood that the vast majority of children requiring mental health assessment and treatment may initially present with these issues to their pediatric primary care provider (PCP). Of all children affected by mental health issues, it is estimated that 70% do not receive treatment of any kind (Melnyk et al., 2002). This creates the potential for a significant negative impact on all aspects of development, including physical, social, cognitive, and emotional health. The costs of untreated mental health issues in the United States have been estimated to be as much as $150 billion annually (http://www.kingcounty.gov/healthservices/MentalHealth/Information.aspx). These estimates do not incorporate the additional costs for long-term consequences to the child and family from untreated mental health issues. Delays in providing mental health treatment lead to exponentially more expensive interventions due to chronic complications from untreated conditions that occur over time.

A major contributing factor to these unidentified children is the lack of mental health providers having direct contact and/or access to these children. Bernal (2003) noted that only 2% of children with mental health difficulties were seen by mental health specialists while as many as 75% of children seen by PCPs required some type of mental health care. Opportunities for PCPs to identify, assess, and intervene in childhood mental health problems are significantly higher because they are usually the main point of contact for families to the health care system. The early identification and treatment of mental health issues lessen the

---

Child and Adolescent Behavioral Health: A Resource for Advanced Practice Psychiatric and Primary Care Practitioners in Nursing,
First Edition. Edited by Edilma L. Yearwood, Geraldine S. Pearson, and Jamesetta A. Newland.

degree of disruption across all domains of development. Therefore, it is imperative that PCPs help children with mental health issues gain access to mental health providers and become more adept at understanding many of the treatments modalities, including medications used to care for children with mental health conditions. Many PCPs not only feel uncomfortable diagnosing children with mental health conditions but also feel they do not have the knowledge or skills to prescribe treatments and medications for these children. These factors, combined with the current national shortage of child psychiatric specialists, has placed the PCP on the frontline of not only identifying these children but also caring for young patients with serious mental health problems (Theoktisto, 2009). While many mental health issues can be addressed with targeted interventions at the individual, family, academic, or community level, the judicious use of psychopharmacological interventions in some child psychiatric disorders is still indicated. This chapter will explore these issues as they apply to prescribing medication for mental health disorders in children and adolescents.

Challenges in Prescribing Psychotropic Medications

Even though pediatric pharmacology presents challenges to the APN caring for a pediatric population, "the use of psychotropic medication is a therapeutic option worthy of consideration for the treatment of a substantial number of children and adolescents" (Miller & Findling, 2010, p. 667). Risks of untreated psychiatric illness are thought to be much greater than the known and potentially known risks and side effects of medication (Vitiello, 2008). Prescribing any psychotropic medication should be done carefully and judiciously and with the full consent and understanding from parents/ caregivers and assent/consent from the pediatric patient. Psychopharmacology intervention is the treatment of first choice for some of the most prevalent disorders, so familiarity with these agents/diagnoses is essential for the PCP. Connor and Meltzer (2006) noted that pediatric psychopharmacology came of age in the 1970s and marked the beginning of the use of psychiatric medications to treat neuropsychiatric disorders in children and adolescents. Since that time, acceptance of psychotropic medication management for a variety of pediatric disorders has slowly grown among clinicians, physicians, teachers, parents, and children. The debate continues, however, and a wide range of individual preferences influence the use of biochemical treatments.

Psychiatric nurse practitioners, family nurse practitioners, pediatric nurse practitioners, and clinical nurse specialists are among the widening array of people who are able to prescribe psychotropic medication. Their level of independent practice, from supervisory with a physician to independent practice, is determined by each state's practice laws. Similarly, the ability to write prescriptions for different levels of controlled substances, such as stimulants, is also determined by individual state statutes. Finally, the educational programs of these primary care clinicians often do not include specific information on prescribing psychiatric medications to children and adolescents. Prescribing medications for the treatment of mental health conditions for children requires that the clinician possess the knowledge and skills to assess these children appropriately, identify the condition, and then develop a treatment plan.

Assessment

Assessment of a psychiatric disorder in a child or adolescent might occur differently in a pediatric primary care environment versus in a more traditional psychiatric service. Primary care nurses tend to provide well-child care and ambulatory acute care to their population. Behavioral health issues are likely to come up during these visits. Psychiatric evaluation, in its most traditional form, requires knowledge of psychiatric assessment to conduct the evaluation, scheduled time to facilitate this, followed by case formulation, and then treatment planning involving medication choice, dose, and adjunct treatment recommendations. Most pediatric appointments are brief and focused on the physical health issues presented by the patient. Few pediatric practices routinely schedule the time needed to conduct a complete psychiatric evaluation. It is not an expectation of the role. Yet, primary care pediatric providers, including advanced practice nurses (APNs), routinely make treatment decisions regarding using stimulants and antidepressants for children in their practice. This practice is influenced by many factors including limited specialized psychiatric resources for children and adolescents and family comfort levels and trust with PCPs (Williams, Klinepeter, Palmes, Pulley, & Foy, 2004; Melnyk, Brown, Jones, Kreipe, & Novak, 2003). The professional comfort line between treating common conditions related to mental health and managing more complex psychiatric disorders seems to vary by provider. Prescribing practices of PCPs might also vary according to type of setting, type of community, and degree of access to child psychiatric consultation.

A comprehensive psychiatric assessment integrates information from many sources including direct interview with the parents/caregivers and child or adolescent and collateral information from day care providers, schools, medical providers, and other members of the treatment team. Given time restraints and skills needed by primary providers, it is not possible to conduct a traditional psychiatric assessment in this setting. DiMarco and Melnyk (2009) advocate that pediatric APNs be given the skills to conduct prevention, screening, early intervention, and follow-up for their patients with mental health needs. They strongly urge that child psychiatric and pediatric APNs collaborate to better meet the mental health needs of pediatric patients in primary care.

Specifically, the use of evaluation tools can augment the evaluation process in the primary care setting. Tools that have been approved for use and are relatively easy to administer in this setting include structured rating scales such as the Child Behavior Checklist (CBCL), the Vanderbilt Scale, or Conners Rating Scales, used specifically for assessing symptoms of attention deficit hyperactivity disorder (ADHD). Connor and Meltzer (2006) noted, "Rating scales can supplement categorical diagnoses by providing information on symptom severity, compared to non-referred children and adolescents" (p. 25). It is important for the clinician to recognize that rating scales cannot replace a direct interview with a child and parent/guardian but can be used in conjunction with it to help make a diagnosis.

Performing the Psychiatric Interview

Psychiatric interviews with children and adolescents traditionally involve a comprehensive history and evaluation of the child and parent(s). Reviewing the presenting problem and chief complaint introduces the practitioner to what may be going on. Important to understand also is what the child and/or parent hope to achieve by a psychiatric evaluation or beginning medication to treat a behavior problem. The evaluation should identify the spheres including home, school, and/or community in which the child is having difficulties. Gaining information regarding when and how these problems first presented and what the parents noticed, as well as what the child perceives happened, is helpful in formulating a diagnosis. Understanding how long the child has been experiencing difficulties helps determine whether this is an acute or long-term issue. Finally, gaining an understanding of any preceding or concurrent stressors, trauma, or historical events that may have occurred within the child's environment will help in understanding what may be going on.

The evaluation by the provider should include a full psychiatric history, which should include any related prior treatment. The provider should ask if there is a history of psychiatric hospitalizations or other specialized psychiatric care such as IOP (intensive outpatient) or PHP (partial hospitalization) and any prior history of medications used to treat behavior problems. Additionally, the psychiatric history should include a review of any family history of psychiatric diagnoses. This information will help the provider not only in making the diagnosis but also in understanding the family's past interactions and possible trust/mistrust of mental health treatments.

The child's history must also contain an in-depth medical history including any chronic conditions, surgeries, cardiac history, head injuries, loss of consciousness, and/or hospitalization. The history should also include a review of any medications the child is or has taken and any allergies to medications.

The developmental history for the child might offer many clues in the diagnostic picture. This history should be comprehensive and include the mother's pregnancy history, birth history, developmental progress up to the current age and developmental delays, history of school performance including special education status, and any behavioral/developmental areas of concern the parent(s) have had for the child or adolescent.

A social history offers insight into the child's relationships and ability to interact with others and might help identify additional sources of stress or trauma. A comprehensive social history should include discussions about the child's relationships with adults, peers, teachers, and friends; history of arrests or involvement in the juvenile justice system; and involvement in community activities and/or team sports.

Physical Exam

Once the history has been completed, the provider must perform a full physical and mental status exam. The mental status exam includes the child's appearance, behavior, affect, thinking, suicidal/homicidal ideation, ability to relate to others, language, estimation of cognitive issues, and evidence of any substance abuse/use. A full neurological exam including testing reflexes and gross and fine motor skills should also be performed to assure the ability to rule out a physical cause of the child/adolescent's behavior. See Table 6.1 for a listing of physical assessment parameters that should be considered before beginning psychotropic medication.

Formulation of a Diagnosis and Plan

Once the provider has accumulated all of the abovementioned information, he or she must integrate this into a clinical understanding of the child and his or her developmental stage, and then summarize the assessment to guide the treatment planning.

Table 6.1 Physical parameters and lab guidelines for medication monitoring in child and adolescent pharmacologic management

Prior to medication initiation: Baseline physical examination (within 6–12 months) and medical history. (Please obtain a copy from the pediatrician and place in the UCHC medical record.)
  Informed consent and child/adolescent assent
  Review contraindications of medication to be started and check for interactions with any current medications.
  Vital signs (VS)
  Height (Ht), Weight (Wt), and body mass index (BMI; www.cdc.gov/growthcharts)
  Consider beta-HCG (in females of child-bearing age who are sexually active)

If not available in prior records:
  For age 7 and under: Lead level within 1 year
  For children with a concern about sexual abuse: consider testing for STDs (Genprobe for Chlamydia and gonorrhea, RPR, and HIV if risk factors present)
  PPD and TB evaluation

Uncomplicated care without medications (provided by the pediatrician):
  Every 6 months: VS, Ht, Wt, BMI
  Every year: Physical exam, dental exam, eye exam, hearing exam

The following are protocols for monitoring individual medications:

Psychostimulants
Methylphenidate (Ritalin, Concerta, Metadate, Methylin), dextroamphetamine (Dexedrine), mixed amphetamine salts (Adderall), dexmethylphenidate (Focalin), and lisdexamfetamine (Vyvanse):
  Baseline: Ht, Wt, and BMI
  Every 3 months: Ht, Wt, and BMI

Antidepressants
SSRIs:
  Baseline: Ht, Wt, and BMI
  Every 6 months: Ht, Wt, and BMI

Venlafaxine (Effexor):
  Baseline: VS, Ht, Wt, and BMI
  Every visit: VS (monitor for HTN)
  Every 3 months: Ht, Wt, and BMI

Bupropion (Wellbutrin):
  Baseline: VS, Ht, Wt, and BMI
  Every 3 months: VS, Ht, Wt, and BMI
  Contraindications: seizure disorder, bulimia, anorexia

Trazadone (Desyrel):
  Baseline: Ht, Wt, and BMI
  Every year: Ht, Wt, and BMI

Mirtazapine (Remeron):
  Baseline: Ht, Wt, and BMI
  Every year: Ht, Wt, and BMI

Antipsychotics
Typical antipsychotic agents:
  Baseline: VS, Ht, Wt, BMI, CBC, LFTs, AIMS. Baseline ECG for chlorpromazine, thioridazine, haloperidol, pimozide
  ECG parameters:
    Sinus rhythm: every QRS complex is preceded by a P wave and a PR interval
    Rate: 60–110 beats per minute

Table 6.1 (*cont'd*)

PR interval <200 msec
QRS interval <120 msec and no more than 30% over baseline (before drug initiation)
QTc interval <460 msec
Stabilizing dose: VS, ECG (chlorpromazine, thioridazine, haloperidol, pimozide)
Every 3 months: VS, Ht, Wt, and BMI
Every 6 months: AIMS and ECG (chlorpromazine, thioridazine, haloperidol, pimozide)
Every year: CBC and LFTs

Atypical antipsychotic agents (all but clozapine):
Baseline: VS, Ht, Wt, BMI, CBC, LFTs, fasting lipid panel and glucose, AIMS
Every visit: Ht, Wt, BMI (www.cdc.gov/growthcharts), activity levels and diet. If 7% or greater weight gain on drug relative to baseline, then clinician must address wt loss interventions.
Every 3–6 months: fasting lipid panel and glucose, LFTs, and AIMS
Every year: consider HgbA1c

Clozapine (Clozaril):
Baseline: VS, Ht, Wt, BMI, CBC (ANC), LFTs, fasting lipid panel and glucose, ECG, and AIMS. Enroll in Clozaril monitoring system through the pharmacy.
First 6 months: CBC (ANC – www.curehodgekins.com) every week per monitoring system (see below).
Second 6 months: CBC (ANC) every 2 weeks
Thereafter: CBC (ANC) every month
Every visit: VS, Ht, Wt, and BMI
Every 6 months: LFTs, fasting lipid panel and glucose, ECG, AIMS

Clozapine hematology monitoring for the first 6 months of therapy:

WBC (mm^3)	ANC (mm^3)	Action
Baseline: > or = 3500	Baseline: > or = 1500	Weekly monitoring.
>3000	>1500	Continue weekly monitoring.
Drop in count > or = 3000 and total count between 3000–3500	>1500	Start twice weekly monitoring.
2000–3000	>1500	D/C clozapine; start daily blood monitoring; observe for signs/symptoms of flulike illness.
< or = 2000	< or = 1000	Hematology consult; consider BM aspiration.
—	< or = 500	Agranulocytosis – Med ER.

Mood Stabilizers

Lithium (Eskalith, Lithobid):
Clarify if NSAID is used (will increase lithium level)
Baseline: VS, Ht, Wt, BMI, CBC, LFTs, electrolytes, BUN, creatinine, TSH, freeT4, urinalysis, and ECG
Stabilizing dose: Lithium level
Every 6 months: VS, Ht, Wt, BMI, lithium level, CBC, LFTs, electrolytes, BUN, creatinine, TSH, free T4, and urinalysis
Every year: ECG

Valproate (Depakote, Depakene):
Baseline: VS, Ht, Wt, BMI, CBC, LFTs, electrolytes, and amylase
Stabilizing dose: Valproate level, CBC, and LFTs
Every 3 months: VS, Ht, Wt, BMI, valproate level, CBC, and LFTs
Every year: carnitine (free, total, and acyl) and amylase

(continued)

Table 6.1 (*cont'd*)

Carbamezapine (Tegretol):
  Baseline: VS, Ht, Wt, BMI, CBC, LFTs, and electrolytes
  Stabilizing dose: Carbamezapine level, CBC, and LFTs
  Every 3 months: VS, Ht, Wt, BMI, carbamzapine level, CBC, and LFTs
  Contraindication: Concomitant clozapine use (bone marrow suppression)

Oxycarbazepine (Trileptal):
  Baseline: VS, Ht, Wt, BMI, CBC, LFTs, electrolytes, BUN, and creatinine
  Stabilizing dose (every 1–2 months): VS
  Every 3 months: VS, Ht, Wt, BMI, CBC, and electrolytes

Gabapentin (Neurontin):
  Baseline: VS, Ht, Wt, BMI, CBC, LFTs, BUN, creatinine, and urinalysis
  Stabilizing dose: VS
  Every 3 months: VS, Ht, Wt, and BMI
  Every year: CBC and LFTs

Lamotrigine (Lamictal):
  Baseline: VS, Ht, Wt, BMI, CBC, and LFTs. Clarify if any history of rash reactions to medications.
  Stabilizing dose: VS
  Every 3 months: VS, Ht, Wt, and BMI
  Every year: CBC and LFTs
    Note: slow titration decreases risk for rash

Topirimate (Topamax):
  Baseline: VS, Ht, Wt, BMI, CBC, LFTs, bicarbonate and urinalysis. Clarify if any history of preexisting eye disease/glaucoma
    or kidney stones.
  Stabilizing dose: VS
  Every 3 months: VS, Ht Wt, BMI, and bicarbonate
  Every year: CBC and LFTs

Alpha 2 Agonists
Clonidine (Catapres) and guanfacine (Tenex):
  Baseline: VS, Ht, Wt, and BMI
  Stabilizing dose: VS
  Every 3 months: VS, Ht, Wt, and BMI
  Contraindication: history of syncope, cardiovascular disease, Raynaud's syndrome

Anxiolytics
Benzodiazapines and buspirone (Buspar):
  Baseline: VS, Ht, Wt, and BMI
  Stabilizing dose: VS
  Every 6 months: VS, Ht, Wt, and BMI

Benedryl, Atarax, Vistaril:
  Baseline: VS, Ht, Wt, and BMI
  Stabilizing dose: VS
  Every 6 months: VS, Ht, Wt, and BMI

Other Agents
Non-BZD Hypnotics – eszopiclone (Lunestra), zolpidem (Ambien), zaleplon (Sonata):
  Baseline: Ht, Wt, and BMI
  Every 6 months: Ht, Wt, and BMI

Table 6.1 (cont'd)

Beta blockers:
    Baseline: VS, Ht, Wt, BMI, CBC, LFTs, and ECG
    Stabilizing dose: VS, ECG
    Every 3 months: VS, Ht, Wt, and BMI
    Every 6 months: CBC, LFTs, and ECG

Strattera (Atomoxitine):
    Baseline: VS, Ht, Wt, and BMI
    Stabilizing dose: VS
    Every 6 months: VS, Ht, Wt, and BMI

Source: Connor DF, Meltzer BM. (2006). *Pediatric Psychopharmacology Fast Facts.* New York: WW Norton Professional Books.

This process will lead to a final diagnosis, which will then allow the practitioner to develop a management plan.

Diagnoses

Psychiatric diagnoses are organized on Diagnostic and Statistical Manual of Mental Disorders (DSM) or International Classification of Diseases (ICD) taxonomy created through the World Health Organization. For DSM-IV-TR (Fourth Edition, Text Revision) (American Psychiatric Association [APA], 2000) there are five diagnostic axes. The diagnoses listed should guide the decisions regarding medication management.

Treatment Plan

The treatment plan should flow from the diagnostic axes. Target symptoms, a problem list, and planning for adjunct clinical services should be included, along with recommendations about type of psychiatric medication. The type or class of medication chosen to treat a disorder needs to follow the evaluation information and the working diagnoses. For example, it is not good practice to give a depressive disorder diagnosis and prescribe stimulant medication. The treatment extends from the formulation of the problem. The choice of medication evolves from this information.

Cultural Considerations

Cultural considerations regarding pharmacological management of pediatric psychiatric problems have to be considered on at least two levels. The growing field of cultural psychopharmacology acknowledges that there is variability among ethnic groups regarding the pharmacokinetics of drug absorption, distribution, metabolism, and excretion (Dell, 2010). For example, Hispanic individuals may require lower doses of antidepressants and antipsychotics. Similarly, African Americans may respond to lower doses of selective serotonin reuptake inhibitors (SSRIs). Asians may also respond to lower doses of antipsychotic medication (Munoz, Primm, & Ananth, 2007). Equally important as the biochemical considerations regarding using medication is the cultural meaning of psychotropic medication held by parents. Meaning is often linked to bias and stigma regarding mental health issues and to belief systems regarding the efficacy of psychotropic medication (Munoz et al.). Careful assessment of cultural views is essential to effective medication management with a pediatric population.

Decision Making

The decision to begin a medication trial to treat a behavioral health issue is a complex one for pediatric and psychiatric providers. For pediatric providers, the realization that a symptom constellation might benefit from medication requires an assessment of the disorder and type of medication that is most useful for the disorder. For the primary care APN, the decision regarding which medication would provide the best outcome for the child/adolescent's specific issue should be based upon certain aspects of the medication's profile. Issues to be considered include use of a medication that is expected to be time limited, has a low safety risk defined by evidence-based assessment, and involves a simple treatment plan with clear interventions and follow-up.

Some conditions treated with psychotropic medication in primary care might include:

- ADHD (no comorbid issues identified such as trauma, anxiety, obsessive-compulsive disorder [OCD], or mood disorder)

- Uncomplicated anxiety
- Depression (without other psychiatric comorbidities)

Conditions that might necessitate referral to a psychiatric APN or child psychiatrist include:

- Any untoward response to current or past psychotropic medication trial
- Comorbid symptoms or the presence of two or more psychiatric disorders
- Trauma history
- Previous treatment with no improvement in symptoms
- Any high-risk symptom or behavior such as hallucinations (auditory, visual, tactile, or olfactory) or suicidal or homicidal ideation
- Substance abuse or addiction

Need for Consultation

The recognition by the PCP that mental health consultation is needed will likely depend on several factors. The ability to differentiate between situationally driven, lower-level mental health issues versus major mental health disorders or complex symptom clusters will influence referral. The complexity of mental health issues presented by children and adolescents, the interplay between providers, and the need for coordination of multiple systems involved with the child necessitate a team approach to psychotropic prescribing. The psychiatric APN may be consulting with a variety of other health professionals including PCPs, psychiatric providers, school systems, and neurology specialists. The process of prescribing is not simple or easy. The skill set necessary for the PCP to appropriately treat mental health issues is complex and requires additional time and knowledge within the primary care setting. A complex skill set encompasses the ability to quickly perform a brief assessment, make an informed diagnosis of the problem, develop a sequential plan of care, facilitate referrals and consultations to appropriate care agencies, and apply knowledge of the various agents that can be used to treat a disorder. When an issue is identified as appropriate to primary care settings, this may include lifestyle interventions, parenting ideas, or psychopharmacological interventions. If presenting symptoms are complex and not appropriate to the primary care setting, the pediatric APN can assist and support the patient and family in connecting with an available mental health provider to facilitate a positive treatment relationship. Mental health services can run the gamut of traditional psychodynamic individual and family therapy, in-home services, parent management training, or behavioral models such as cognitive-behavioral therapy (CBT). The prescriber, whether a PCP or a mental health specialist, needs to have an understanding of how psychotropic medication fits into the other treatment needs presented by a child or adolescent. Rarely does a pill fix the mental health problems of a child presenting to the APN in a primary or psychiatric care setting. The PCP needs to recognize that along with medications, the child/adolescent and possibly the family require comprehensive treatment—therapy, stress management, and close follow-up care. It is imperative to emphasize that medications alone are not the answer to the mental health issues.

Patient Family Education

An essential aspect of medication management is the careful patient/family education process that occurs with both primary care and psychiatric APNs. A clear, focused description of the presenting problem and its possible etiology, trajectory, and possible treatment should be shared with parents and guardians. If the treatment involves medication, there must be written consents from parent/guardian and assent from the pediatric patient. Consent might be noted in the nursing progress note or, depending on the agency, involve a formal document. Whenever possible, medication information should be given to the parent with sensitivity to cultural and language issues. Parents/guardians need to be given an informed choice regarding psychotropic medication management for their child and, if appropriate, the child/adolescent should be included in conversations about medications to be used.

Parents/guardians need to have a time frame for the intervention, a follow-up plan, and a clear explanation of the risks, benefits, and side effects of the proposed medication. Parents need to participate in the decision making regarding seeking a psychiatric opinion when behavior problems are beyond the scope of the pediatric primary care APN. DiMarco and Melnyk (2009) noted that mental health needs of children and adolescents could not be met by any one discipline or specialty. They proposed that synergism between primary care and psychiatric APNs will result in better care and more coordinated services. For those pediatric patients who have been treated with psychiatric medication, the next step is returning to their PCP for continued medication management. The psychiatric APN remains a consultative and treating back-up if needed.

Review of Common Psychiatric Medications

Stimulants and Nonstimulants for ADHD
Pharmacology

Stimulants are sympathomimetic agents structurally similar to endogenous catecholamines that influence the central nervous system by activating the level of activity, arousal, and alertness (Spencer, Biederman, & Wilens, 2010). These medications can be obtained in short-, intermediate-, and long-acting preparations of methylphenidate and mixed amphetamine salts. Efficacy and safety have been widely studied (Pliszka, 2010). They are Schedule II drugs, which are closely regulated and controlled by the U.S. Drug Enforcement Agency (DEA). Stimulants are highly effective when used to treat symptoms of ADHD. Nonstimulant medications include atomoxetine, a norepinephrine reuptake inhibitor, and alpha-adrenergic agents including clonidine and guanfacine.

Indications for Use

Stimulant medication is used for core ADHD symptoms of inattention and motoric hyperactivity. Nonstimulant medication may be indicated as adjuncts to stimulant treatment or part of monotherapy to reduce hyperactivity, distractibility, and impulsiveness (Scahill, Poncin, & Westphal, 2010).

Contraindications

There are concerns that stimulant treatment might trigger mood instability in patients at risk for mood disorder. The general view is that ADHD can be safely treated with a stimulant provided the mood disorder has been stabilized first (Merkel, 2010). Careful psychiatric assessment is imperative given the high prevalence of other comorbid psychiatric disorders in individuals with ADHD. Blood pressure, pulse, and weight/BMI (body mass index) must be monitored regularly.

Side Effects

The only black box warning for stimulant medication involves their abuse potential (Spencer, Biederman, & Wilens, 2010). The most commonly reported side effects involve appetite suppression and sleep disturbances. Difficulties falling asleep and lack of noontime appetite can be specifically targeted as potential side effects of stimulants. While there have been concerns about the effects of stimulants on growth, research has shown that treatment with stimulant medication into adolescence may lead to only modest delays in growth. The greater deficit tends to involve weight rather than height (Faraone, 2000). Some children may develop mild and transient behavior tics. The literature suggests that tics are not a serious side effect and in most instances will disappear (Merkel, 2010). Decisions about continuing or stopping medication should be based on status of tics, how much they concern the parents or the child/adolescent, and a careful evaluation of the benefits versus adverse effects of the medications should be considered.

Drug-drug Interactions

Drug-drug interactions between stimulants and other agents are rare (Wolraich & Doffing, 2004). There are two instances when care must be taken when administering a stimulant. The first involved the use of concomitant monoamine oxidase inhibitors (MAOIs), used to treat adults, and the second is stimulant use with furazolidone (antibiotic). Both of these can result in a life-threatening hypertensive crisis (Spencer, Biederman, & Wilens, 2010).

Before prescribing a stimulant or any medication to treat ADHD, it is imperative that a list of all medications including vitamins, herbals, energy drinks, and over-the-counter preparations be obtained from parents. Monitoring of drug-drug interactions is best done with a complete list of all substances being taken by the child or adolescent.

Monitoring

Stimulant medications have been linked to causing arrhythmias in certain patient populations. Prior to beginning a stimulant, the APN needs to conduct a thorough screen for any history of sudden death in a first-degree relative or for a history of cardiac arrhythmias or abnormalities in the patient. If the patient has a preexisting cardiac condition, the APN should consult with a cardiologist before initiating treatment. While an electrocardiogram (ECG) is an effective screen for cardiac symptoms in all patients beginning stimulant treatment, the American Academy of Pediatrics has stated that it is not routinely indicated in otherwise healthy youth (Perrin, Friedman, & Knilans, 2008). Similarly, routine lab work is not required prior to beginning stimulant medication. Atomoxetine has a black box warning for increased suicidal ideation in young children.

Dosing

Stimulants are the first line of treatment for children with ADHD and the usual dose range is 0.3 to 2 mg/kg/day for methylphenidate and half of this for Dexedrine derivatives; these agents are approximately twice as potent as methylphenidate (Spencer et al., 2010). These agents have a short half-life and must be given twice a day approximately four hours apart. Longer-term agents can be given once a day in the morning. Some children will require a cover dose of a short-acting stimulant after school in addition to the longer-term preparation in the morning. The risk of this afternoon dose is decreased appetite at dinnertime and difficulties falling sleep. Abrupt discontinuation of a stimulant can precipitate transient behavior problems. It is not recommended that "drug holidays" be taken from medication.

Long-term Use

There is growing evidence that the adverse effects of untreated ADHD on behavior and functioning suggest that long-term stimulant treatment is warranted. While many adolescents stop taking their medication, ADHD symptomatology continues to persist and influence functioning. Risks regarding automobile accidents, academic difficulties, and interpersonal problems related to untreated ADHD in adulthood are well documented (Pliszka, 2010). No studies to date suggest that long-term stimulant use has adverse effects on health (Pliszka, 2010). See Table 6.2 for stimulant and nonstimulant medications.

Antidepressants
Pharmacology

Traditionally, tricyclic antidepressants (TCAs) were the first antidepressants used with children and adolescents and were characterized by a lack of efficacy, cardiotoxic side effects, and lethal overdose risk (Connor & Meltzer, 2006). They have been mostly replaced by the use of SSRIs, a class of medication with a safer side effect profile. The primary mode of action for SSRIs is "thought to be presynaptic inhibition of serotonin reuptake. Chronic treatment also down regulates serotonin receptors in most cases and modulates serotonergic transmission" (Emslie, Croarkin, & Mayes, 2010, p. 703). Atypical antidepressants are widely used in adults but limited data regarding use in children and adolescents exist. They will not be discussed in this chapter. However, desyrel (Trazodone), while an atypical antidepressant, is often used at low doses (<50 mg at bedtime) for managing sleep disturbances in pediatric populations. There are no studies citing efficacy for sleep.

Indications for Use

SSRIs have become the first-line pharmacological treatment for major depressive disorders, OCDs, and other anxiety disorders in pediatric populations (Connor & Meltzer, 2006). They are used in both primary care and child psychiatric settings with positive effectiveness. While there has been controversy in the past regarding the risks of suicidal ideation/suicidal attempts with pediatric use of antidepressants, benefits outweigh risks (Emslie et al., 2010). Sharing of black box warning information with patients and parents is indicated when medication is being considered for treatment (Bridge et al., 2007). Use of rating scales (such as Beck Depression Inventory) is encouraged prior to initiating SSRI use and during treatment to measure progress in symptom amelioration.

Contraindications

SSRIs should not be taken with MAOI medication or pimozide. Taking tryptophan along with an SSRI can result in headache, nausea, sweating, and dizziness. While a rare side effect, there is documentation of seizures when SSRIs are given with the analgesic tramadol hydrochloride.

Side Effects

The most prominent side effects from SSRI use include gastrointestinal (GI) complaints of nausea or diarrhea, motor restlessness, and behavioral activation (Emslie, Croarkin, & Mayes, 2010). Prescribers should watch for symptoms of hypomania and mania and discontinue the SSRI trial if these occur. Sexual side effects, notable in sexually active adolescents, include erectile dysfunction, delayed ejaculation, and anorgasmia (Scahill, Oesterheld, & Martin, 2007). Adolescents should be informed of these risks.

Monitoring

Before beginning an antidepressant trial, a routine pediatric physical exam is indicated. Baseline assessment of suicide risk and level and severity of depression or anxiety should occur. It takes between 2 and 12 weeks for a positive response to antidepressant treatment and the lowest dose should be given first with gradual increases every five to seven days. No specific lab work is required during an antidepressant trial (Connor & Meltzer, 2006). Weight and vital signs should be regularly evaluated, and the child or adolescent should be seen frequently while the dose of medication is being titrated upwards.

Dosing

SSRIs are generally started at the lowest possible dose and slowly titrated upwards with medication increases every one to two weeks to optimal dose. Duration of treatment of depression with an SSRI is usually set at one year after resolution of symptoms. OCD and anxiety symptoms may require a longer period of treatment (Scahill et al., 2007). When discontinuing the medication, patients and parents need to be cautioned to slowly decrease the dose to avoid SSRI discontinuation syndrome. Abrupt stoppage of an SSRI can result in flu-like symptoms such as dizziness, nausea, vomiting, myalgia, fatigue, and moodiness. See Table 6.3 for a listing of antidepressants.

Mood Stabilizers
Pharmacology

Mood stabilizers include lithium and anticonvulsants such as divalproex/valproic acid (Depakote), carbamazepine (Tegretol), oxcarbazepine (Trileptal), lamotrigine

Table 6.2 Stimulant and nonstimulant medications to treat ADHD

Medications indicated for the treatment of ADHD

Generic Name	Trade Name	Approved Age (yr)	Dosing	Common Adverse Events
Amphetamine	Adderall	3+	Once/twice daily	Headache, abdominal pain, insomnia, decreased appetite, nervousness, dizziness
Amphetamine	Adderall XR	6+	Once daily	Headache, loss of appetite, insomnia, abdominal pain, weight loss, xerostomia, tachycardia, nervousness, emotional lability, dizziness
Methylphenidate HCL Extended release tablets	Concerta	6+	Once daily	Headache, abdominal pain, insomnia, decreased appetite, nervousness, dizziness
Methylphenidate HCL Transdermal system	Daytrona	6+	Removed 9 hr after application; frequency based on need and response	Decreased appetite, insomnia, nausea, vomiting, emotional lability, weight loss, tics
Methamphetamine HCL tablets	Desoxyn	6+	Once/twice daily	Tachycardia, tremors, insomnia, abdominal pain, xerostomia, decreased appetite, headache, dizziness, weight loss
Destroamphetamine sulfate spansule Sustained-release capsules and tablets	Dexedrine	3–16	Once/twice/3X daily	Tachycardia, tremors, insomnia, abdominal pain, xerostomia, decreased appetite, headache, dizziness, weight loss
DEX methylphenidate HCL tablets	Focalin	6–17	Twice daily	Abdominal pain, nausea, decreased appetite, fever
DEX methylphenidate HCL extended-release capsules	Focalin XR	6+	Once daily	Decreased appetite, headache, abdominal pain, anxiety, insomnia, xerostomia, dizziness, nervousness
Methylphenidate HCL Extended-release capsules	Metadate CD	6–15	Once daily	Headache, abdominal pain, decreased appetite, insomnia, nervousness, dizziness
Methylphenidate HCL Oral solution	Methylin Oral Solution	6+	Twice daily	Nervousness, insomnia, headache, abdominal pain, tachycardia, nausea, decreased appetite, dizziness, weight loss
Methylphenidate HCL Chewable tablets	Methylin chewable tablets	6+	Twice daily	Nervousness, insomnia, headache, abdominal pain, tachycardia, nausea, decreased appetite, dizziness, weight loss
Methylphenidate HCL tablets	Ritalin	6+	Twice daily	Headache, abdominal pain, insomnia, nausea, decreased appetite, nervousness
Methylphenidate HCL Sustained-release tablets	Ritalin-SR	6+	Twice daily	Headache, abdominal pain, insomnia, nausea, decreased appetite, nervousness
Methylphenidate HCL Extended-release capsules	Ritalin LA	6+	Once daily	Headache, abdominal pain, decreased appetite, insomnia

(continued)

Table 6.2 (cont'd)

Generic Name	Trade Name	Approved Age (yr)	Dosing	Common Adverse Events
Atomoxetine HCL	Strattera	6+	Once/twice daily	Headache, abdominal pain, appetite decreased, vomiting, cough
Lisdexamfetamine dimesylate	Vyvanse	6–12	Once daily	Decreased appetite, insomnia, abdominal pain, headache

Reprinted from Vierhile, Robb, Ryan-Krause, 2009, with permission from Elsevier Publishing.

Nonstimulant drugs for treatment of ADHD

Drug (Generic/Trade Name)	Relevant Pharmacokinetic Parameters	Recommended Dosage Regimen	Comments
Atomoxetine (Strattera)	Half-life: 5 hrs (extensive metabolizers) 20 hrs (poor metabolizers)	Children: 0.5 mg/kg/day; increase dosage weekly until achieve response (optimum 1.2 mg/kg/day, maximum 1.8 mg/kg/day); b.i.d. or 20 mg q.d.; increase dosage weekly until achieve response (maximum 100 mg/day)	No abuse potential, less insomnia and growth effects than stimulants Delayed onset (2–4 weeks), lower efficacy rates than stimulants
Bupropion (Wellbutrin) Also available as extended release daily dose	Half-life: 12 hrs (adolescents) 21 hrs (adults)	3 mg/kg/day or 150 mg/day, whichever is less; dosed b.i.d. or t.i.d. (maximum 6 mg/kg/day or 300 mg/day with no single dose > 150 mg)	Rash, lowers seizure threshold, insomnia if given too late in the day
Clonidine (Catapres)	Half-life: 6–16 hrs	≤ 45 kg: 0.05 mg h.s., then titrate in 0.05 mg increments b.i.d., t.i.d., or q.i.d. > 45 kg: 0.1 mg h.s., then titrate in 0.1 mg increments b.i.d., t.i.d., or q.i.d.	Used alone or as an adjunct to stimulants to manage insomnia, tics, or aggressive behavior
Guanfacine (Tenex) Guanfacine Extended Release (Intuniv)	Half-life: 10–30 hrs	≤ 45 kg: 0.5 mg h.s., then titrate in 0.5 mg increments b.i.d., t.i.d., or q.i.d. > 45 kg: 1 mg h.s., then titrate in 1 mg increments b.i.d., t.i.d., or q.i.d. Extended release: begin with 1 mg q am and taper up in 1 mg increments weekly	Delayed onset (2–4 weeks) Review personal and family cardiovascular history Taper to prevent rebound hypertension Extended release formulation also available (1–4 mg)

Pliszka, Bernet, Bukstein et al., 2007; Pliszka, Crismon, Hughes, 2006; Prince, 2006; Wolraich et al., 2007; Caballerro & Nahata, 2003
Reprinted from Dopheide & Pliszka, 2009, with permission from Pharmocotherapy Publications.

(Lamictal), and topiramate (Topomax). Lithium has the most extensively documented mechanism of action, affecting multiple neurotransmitter systems including serotonin, dopamine, and gamma aminobutyric acid (GABA) and modulating signal transduction via second messenger systems (Berns & Nemeroff, 2003). Exact mechanisms of action for the anticonvulsant agents used in pediatric psychiatry have not been fully established. However, anticonvulsants used for mood stabilization ultimately affect many of the same signaling pathways believed to mediate lithium's therapeutic effects (Manji & Chen, 2000).

Indications for Use

Use of mood stabilizers includes symptom management for acute mania, bipolar depression, and aggressive behavior associated with conduct and other behavioral disorders (Amaladoss, Roberts, & Amaladoss, 2010; Correll, Sheridan, & DelBello, 2010). Data for the efficacy for these medications in the pediatric population are mixed. An early open-label trial of the most commonly used mood stabilizers—lithium, divalproex, and carbamazepine—evinced large effect sizes (Cohen's $d > 1.0$) for the treatment of acute pediatric mania (Kowatch, Suppes, & Carmody, 2000). More recent monotherapy trials of

Table 6.3 Antidepressants

Formulations and Dosing for Selective Serotonin Reuptake Inhibitors (SSRIs)

Medication	Formulations	Initial dose, mg	Target Dose, mg		Maximum Dose, mg
			Children	Adolescents	
Citalopram (Celexa)	Tablet: 10 mg, 20 mg, 40 mg Solution: 10 mg/5 mL	10	20–40	20–40	60
Escitalopram (Lexapro)	Tablet: 5 mg, 10 mg, 20 mg Solution: 5 mg/5 mL	5–10	10–20	10–20	30
Fluoxetine (Prozac)	Capsule: 10 mg, 20 mg, 40 mg Tablet: 10 mg Solution: 20 mg/5 mL	10	20	20–40	60
Fluvoxamine (Luvox)	Tablet: 25 mg, 50 mg, 100 mg	25	50–200	50–200	200 300
Paroxetine (Paxil)	Tablet: 10 mg, 20 mg, 30 mg, 40 mg Tablet CR: 12.5 mg, 25 mg, 37.5 mg Suspension: 10 mg/5 mL	10	10–30	20–40	50
Sertraline (Zoloft)	Tablet: 25 mg, 50 mg, 100 mg Solution: 20 mg/mL	12.5–25	50–200	50–200	200

Note: CR = controlled release.
Reprinted with permission from Emslie, Croarkin, & Mayes, 2010, Dulcan's Textbook of Child & Adolescent Psychiatry published by American Psychiatric Publishing, Inc.
Adverse effects for all of the above medications include irritability, akathisia, insomnia, change in appetite, GI symptoms, flu-like symptoms with abrupt discontinuation, black box warning around exacerbation of existing or new suicidal ideation (Scahill, Oesterheld, & Martin, 2007).

U.S. Food and Drug Administration (FDA) (2011) Indications for SSRIs

Medication	FDA-Approved Indication	Indication Age Range
Citalopram (Celexa)	Depression	Adults
Escitalopram (Lexapro)	Depression	Adults
Fluoxetine (Prozac)	Depression OCD Bulimia	8 years to adult 7 years to adult Adults
Fluvoxamine (Luvox)	OCD	8 years to adult
Paroxetine (Paxil)	Depression OCD PD SOC GAD PTSD	Adults Adults Adults Adults Adults Adults

(continued)

Table 6.3 (cont'd)

Medication	FDA-Approved Indication	Indication Age Range
Sertraline (Zoloft)	Depression	Adults
	OCD	6 years to adult
	PMDD	Adults
	PD	Adults

Note: GAD = generalized anxiety disorder; OCD = obsessive-compulsive disorder; PD = panic disorder; PMDD = premenstrual dysphoric disorder; PTSD = posttraumatic stress disorder; SOC = social anxiety disorder.

lithium, divalproex, and carbamazapine have shown more moderate symptom reduction (Correll et al.). Combination therapy, using two mood stabilizers or a mood stabilizer plus an antipsychotic, has generally demonstrated more significant symptom reduction than the monotherapeutic use of these mood-stabilizing agents (Nandagopal, DelBello, & Kowatch, 2009). Lamotrigine may be more effective for bipolar depression than for pediatric aggression or acute mania (Chang, Saxena, & Howe, 2006; Pavuluri et al., 2009). Topiramate, oxcarbazapine, and divalproex ER have not shown efficacy in randomized controlled trials of children with psychiatric disorders (DelBello et al., 2005; Wagner et al., 2006, 2009).

Contraindications

In general, mood stabilizers should be used with caution in patients with renal, cardiovascular, or hepatic impairment. Lithium uniquely requires cautious use in patients with thyroid dysfunction but may be a good choice for patients with liver disease (Kowatch, Strawn, & Danielyan, 2010). Each mood stabilizer has different properties and may be more or less appropriate depending on a patient's medical history and co-occurring medical conditions.

Providers should counsel females of childbearing age regarding the risks and benefits of these medications. Although divalproex has the only U.S. FDA black box warning regarding teratogenic effects (FDA, 2011), carbamazepine has also demonstrated teratogenic effects (Jones, Lacro, Johnson, & Adams, 1989), and lithium has been associated with fetal cardiac defects (Cohen, Friedman, Jefferson, Johnson, & Weiner, 1994). Although no specific birth defects have been consistently associated with lamotrigine use during pregnancy, caution is warranted (Tennis, Eldridge, & International Lamotrigine Pregnancy Registry Scientific Advisory Committee, 2002). Divalproex additionally presents an increased risk of polycystic ovarian syndrome (PCOS) in female patients (Isojarvi & Tapanainen, 2000).

Side Effects

Many mood stabilizers have black box warnings (FDA, 2011). Carbamazapine has black box warnings for dangerous skin conditions, increased suicidality, and blood dyscrasias. Lamotrigine has black box warnings for dangerous skin conditions and aseptic meningitis. Divalproex has black box warnings for hepatotoxicity, life-threatening pancreatitis, and teratogenic effects. Lithium requires close monitoring due to the risk of lithium toxicity, its only black box warning. Signs of lithium toxicity include nausea, vomiting, slurred speech, altered mental status, and poor motor coordination (Okusa & Crystal, 1994).

Common side effects of all mood stabilizers include nausea, vomiting, diarrhea, dizziness, increased appetite, weight gain, sedation, tremor, and headache. Lithium may additionally contribute to acne, hypothyroidism, neurotoxicity, and kidney dysfunction, whereas divalproex use may lead to thrombocytopenia or hyperammonemia (Nandagopal et al., 2009). Although carbamazapine has the only black box warning for increased suicidality, worsening mood and increased thoughts of suicide may be side effects of any of these agents. Hepatotoxicity is also a potential side effect of mood stabilizers, with the exception of lithium (Kowatch et al., 2010).

Drug-Drug Interactions

Both divalproex and carbamazapine are metabolized by the cytochrome P450 system, and therefore interact with many other medications. Unrecognized drug-drug interactions may lead to toxicity or treatment failure. The following represents a partial list of drug-drug interactions most relevant to pediatric patients (Danielyan & Kowatch, 2005). Carbamazepine has an extensive list of interactions with other medications including other antiepileptics, lithium, oral contraceptives, guanfacine, all classes of antidepressants, and some antipsychotics (aripiprazole, haloperidol, and risperidone). Divalproex interacts with other antiepileptic medications—guanfacine, risperidone, tricyclic antidepressants, and salicylates.

Lamotrigine interacts with other antiepileptics—desmopressin, olanzapine, and oral contraceptives. Lithium may increase the neurotoxic effects of both tricyclic antidepressants and antipsychotics. Lithium also interacts with carbamazepine, MOAI antidepressants, and nonsteroidal anti-inflammatory drugs (NSAIDs).

Monitoring

Ongoing and careful monitoring is required with all mood stabilizers. Periodically checking serum drug levels may be useful to evaluate patient compliance and possible toxicity for all mood stabilizers, with the exception of lamotrigine. Weight gain and signs/symptoms of suicidality or worsening depression should also be monitored with all mood-stabilizing agents. Prior to beginning mood stabilizers, baseline labs including complete blood cell count (CBC), liver function tests (LFTs), electrolytes, blood urea nitrogen (BUN), and creatinine should be drawn. They should be repeated after three months on the medication and, if within normal limits, yearly (Connor & Meltzer, 2006).

Dosing

See Table 6.4 for a list of mood stabilizers and dosing strategies.

Anxiolytics

Introduction

All primary care practitioners will need to address anxiety in their pediatric population at some point in time. Anxiety is the most common mental health issue in childhood and a normative state under many situations. The degree of anxiety and persistence of symptoms under specific conditions are correlated with the individual's hard-wired, anxiety traits (temperament), experiences, developmental stage, and parental response sets and expectations. Reactions can result from normative, fear-inducing situations (i.e., medical or dental procedures) to high-intensity responses to typically low-stress phenomenon. There are also the more functionally challenging anxiety response patterns that appear more within the boundary of a mental health condition than a normative response (but of higher intensity) to general life events. As anxiety is a universal, basic emotion experienced by almost everyone at some point in time, the primary care practitioner will be required to evaluate the presenting picture and be confident in addressing the symptoms at the appropriate level. Chapter 8, on anxiety disorders, discusses anxiety seen as a particular, mental health disorder and does not address the more transient states that accompany daily caseloads in the primary care setting.

Anxiety that is more trait-dependent, crosses domains and significantly disturbs normal developmental function, and is sustained over time is more appropriately addressed by mental health specialists who would be able to develop comprehensive treatment plans utilizing CBT treatment, desensitization, SSRIs (covered under "Antidepressants"), or a combination of these strategies. Anxiolytics, on the other hand, are the typical choice in primary care to provide short-term intervention for a specific, circumscribed anxiety provoking situation that is time-limited. Screening is essential to assess whether the symptoms represent a more embedded pattern of emotional responsiveness or a normative, situation-dependent response that provokes an untoward level of anxiety before prescribing an anxiolytic. Anxiolytics are useful in medical or dental procedures that are fear-inducing or for life events that pose a brief but significant challenge to the coping skills of the child (a death of a family member) or to disrupt a phobic response (i.e., travel by plane). Anxiolytics are also useful for short-term bridging for rapid symptom relief after starting an SSRI, particularly in situations that can rapidly become a mental health crisis such as phobic school refusal. A traumatic event can overwhelm anyone depending on the power of the experience to overturn a child's world. Anxiolytics should only be used in the immediate aftermath of an event and typically should not be used for durations greater than two weeks or dependency (e.g., benzodiazepines [BZDs]) or decreased efficacy (e.g., antihistamines) might become problematic.

Assessment

It is necessary to assess the presenting symptoms (internal experience and behavioral manifestations) and whether they are present now, or anticipatory. Determining the trigger as specific or diffuse, expected or out of proportion, the duration, variability across time/environments, intensity (created scale of 1 to 10) and baseline temperament is the key to deciding to address this within a primary care setting or to refer for more specialized mental health services. Identifying how long the symptoms have been present, what helps (self-soothing strategies), what does not help, and what the child and/or parent believes the behavior/symptom is about (cultural variables and values) is very useful in gathering enough information to justify the use of an anxiolytic. The risk of what could happen if the anxiety is not addressed (i.e., not obtaining necessary blood test with a needle phobia) should also be heavily factored into the treatment plan. There are many situations that can be addressed, after a good assessment, by providing information and reassurance about the fear-inducing issue. Please note that the most typical presentation of anxiety in the primary

Table 6.4 Mood stabilizers

Medication Generic Name and (Trade)	FDA Approved Age (yr)	Dosing (Range)	Side Effects	Duration of Medication	Pros	Precautions
Lithium carbonate (Lithobid, Eskalith, Cibalith-S)	>12 yr	Start 25 mg/kg/day, BID–TID Target: 30 mg/kg/day or 900–1200 mg/day div. doses, serum level 0.6–1.2, after meals	Common: nausea, vomiting, diarrhea, increased appetite, weight gain, sedation, tremor, acne. Uncommon: hypothyroidism, neurotoxicity, kidney dysfunction, lithium toxicity, nausea, vomiting, slurred speech, altered mental status, ataxia, lack of coordination, polyuria, polydipsia	half-life 24 hr	Good for bipolar mania in adolescence, better choice if liver problems	Initial: BMI %, HCG/UCG, thyroid, chem. screen, CBS, renal function, ECG, weight and height check, sun sensitivity, avoid during pregnancy. Therapeutic index, blood level absolutely necessary, neurotoxicity
Divalproex sodium and valproic acid (Depokote, Depokote DR, Depokote ER)	>2 yr	Start 15 mg/kg/day, BID–TID, serum level 50–120 mg/L, range 15–60 mg/kg/day- divided doses	Common: nausea, vomiting, diarrhea, constipation, weight gain, sedation, tremor, blurred vision. Uncommon: PCOS, hepatotoxicity, pancreatitis, thrombocytopenia, hyperammonemia	half-life 6–16 hr	Good for bipolar in childhood both mania and depression. Anticonvulsant, may be useful for aggression.	Initial: BMI %, HCG/UCG, thyroid, chem. screen, CBC with differential, ECG, weight and height check, BP, P, LFTs, serum ammonia, POCS, hepatotoxic, risk of pancreatitis, teratogenic Depokote ER: no efficacy shown, CYP450 system: lots of interactions
Carbamazepine (Tegretol) Carbamazepine XR (Tegretol XR)	>6 yr	Start 10–20 mg/kg/day, BID–TID, Target: response, serum level 8.9–11 mg/L, range 100–1200 mg/day div. doses	Common: vomiting, diarrhea, weight gain, sedation, tremor, dry mouth, dizziness, trouble urinating. Uncommon: increased SI, blood dyscrasias, Steven-Johnson syndrome, renal failure, SAIDH, auto induces own metabolism and many other medications	half-life 25–65 hr	Moderate for BPD in childhood. May be useful for rapid cycling, anticonvulsant.	BMI %, HCG/UCG, thyroid, chem. screen, CBC with differential, ECG, weight and height check, BP, P, LFTs, monitor CYP450 system interactions, teratogenic, black box, caution with Asian children increased risk of hypersensitivity, increased suicidality, blood dyscrasias, bone marrow suppression; warnings around dangerous skin conditions; assess for rash

128

Drug	Approval/Age	Dosing	Side effects	Half-life	Comments	Monitoring
Lamotrigine (Lamictal)	>16 yr	Start 12.5 mg/wk up to once a day, range 25–300 mg/day div. doses. Titrate carefully and slowly	Common: headache, nausea, vomiting, ataxia, sedation, blurred vision, sedation, dizziness. Uncommon: Steven-Johnson syndrome, aseptic meningitis, amnesia, hepatic failure, anemia	half-life 33 hr	Anticonvulsant, may be useful in pediatric BPD and depression, not associated with weight gain, no frequent labs needed, adult BPD	HCG/UCG, thyroid, chem. screen, CBC with differential, ECG, weight and height check, BP, P, LFTs, monitor for aseptic meningitis (anytime), Steven-Johnson syndrome (rash), many drug-drug interactions
Oxcarbazepine (Trilepal)	No approval for adults and children with BPD	Start 2–20 mg/kg/day BID, range 150–1800 mg/day, serum level, NA	Common: nausea, vomiting, ataxia, sedation, blurred vision, sedation, dizziness., GI upset, tremor. Uncommon: rash, hyponatremia, nystagmus, Increased risk for URI		No evidence of efficacy for mood in children, no need for frequent blood draws	HCG/UCG, thyroid, chem. screen, CBC with differential, ECG, weight and height check, BP, P, LFTs, monitor for hyponatremia
Topiramate (Topamax)	No approval for adults and children with BPD	Start 25–50 mg, BID, range 50–400 mg div. doses	Common: nausea, vomiting, sedation, decreased appetite, fatigue, tingling, change in taste, nervousness Uncommon: sudden decreased vision, diaphoresis, fever, suicidal thoughts, agitation, restlessness, insomnia, irritability, anger, aggression, alopecia		No evidence of efficacy for mood in children, anticonvulsant, may facilitate weight loss or be weight neutral	HCG/UCG, chem. screen, CBC with differential, vision changes, metabolic acidosis, hyperammonemia, cognitive dulling, neurology problems, inattention, word retrieval difficulty, caution with oral contraceptives

Developed by B. Muller from Connor & Meltzer, 2006; Danielyan & Kowatch, 2005; Kowatch, Strawn, & Danielyan, 2010.

care environment is often a somatic picture and frequently does not include affective symptoms in the first round of assessment. For many cultures, anxiety is only expressed through somatic constellations of symptoms, partly because there is no recognition of the connection between the two domains and partly due to stigmatization. Before considering a medication for the symptoms, assess for substance abuse (for child or parent), pregnancy, medical problems that may mimic anxiety, especially endocrine, cardiac, or autoimmune disorders. Recently, the use of caffeine/energy drinks and supplements also can cause anxiety-like symptoms that resolve almost immediately after stopping the offending item.

Anxiety is known to be comorbid with many serious mental health disorders or part of the prodromal trajectory for others. This is a caution about treating anxiety that appears with any other prominent emotional/behavioral symptoms that are not subsumed under the anxiety itself. This is also important when assessing any untoward effects of using an anxiolytic as it may portend complications of another mental health problem that is present or evolving developmentally.

Pharmacology

There are three commonly used groups of anxiolytics used cautiously for short-term anxiety management with children and adolescents: BZDs, antihistamines, and one azaspirone (buspirone). BZDs have been in widespread use since the 1960s as they were less toxic, better tolerated, and safer medications for use in anxiety than the earlier antianxiety agents. They are a Controlled Substance Schedule IV group, which indicates moderate potential for abuse when used with other central nervous system (CNS) depressant agents, or used alone in doses that are higher or taken more frequently than prescribed. Tolerance develops rapidly (sometimes in as little as 1 to 2 weeks), so short-term use is essential and rapid withdrawal is not recommended. The BZDs work at the GABA-A receptor sites in the spinal cord (muscle relaxation), brainstem (anticonvulsant effects), brainstem reticular formation (sedation), cerebellum (ataxia), and cortical and limbic CNS (anxiolytic effect) to enhance CNS inhibitory effects. BZDs bind to the GABA-A receptors, facilitating the opening of chloride channels, which reduce cellular excitability leading to greater general neuronal inhibition throughout the CNS.

Antihistamines have many uses (as do the BZDs) and were developed to suppress anaphylactic shock; for allergies, pruritis, insomnia, nausea, and vomiting; and for preoperative sedation. They are used primarily in primary care for their medical efficacy in a wide variety of problems. The two mostly commonly used antihistamines for anxiety in children are diphenhydramine (Benadryl) and hydroxyzine hydrochloride or hydroxyzine pamoate (Atarax or Vistaril). The antihistamines act as competitive inhibitors of histamine at H1 receptors both within the CNS and outside the CNS. The anxiolytic effects stem from the effects within the CNS. Side effects are experienced (though generally mild) from within the CNS and peripherally. They are not a controlled substance so the use is much easier as there is no concern about dependency. Tolerability does happen after approximately 2 weeks of consistent use (Scahill, Poncin, & Westphal, 2010).

Azaspirones (Buspirone [Buspar] is the only one available in the United States.) are a more recently derived group of medications developed for mental health conditions. Unlike the previous two groups, the response to buspirone takes one to four weeks, so it is not a good choice for immediate problems with anxiety. Buspirone has action as an agonist at presynaptic 5-HT1A autoreceptors, some antagonistic effects on postsynaptic 5-HT1A receptors, and down-regulation of 5-HT2 receptors. This is similar to SSRIs approved for anxiety and depression in children. It also has dopaminergic effects at the D2 receptors (although it has not been effective as an antipsychotic agent) and enhances noradrenergic release in the locus coeruleus (it may be helpful for ADHD). It does not have any site of action in the GABA system (though it may have some minor antagonistic effect, leading to possibility of activation).

Indications for Use

BZDs are indicated for adult anxiety, for detoxification from drugs and alcohol, and for short-term use for anxiety in children. Due to the risk for dependency, little research has been done on the use of BZDs for children so few are used. Uses of various agents depend on purpose intended, whether a shorter-acting agent for insomnia or longer-acting agent for temporary anxiety relief is selected. Uses for mental health other than for brief anxiety relief include augmentation for mania and schizophrenia, acute agitation or aggression, somnambulism, sleep terrors (pavor nocturnus), tic disorders, brief sleep induction (less than two weeks), or preoperatively for medical or dental procedures. BZDs are approved for seizure disorders and as muscle relaxants as well, which may play a role in some mental health treatment. Significant caution should be used for BZDs in adolescence due to abuse potential, including use with other CNS depressants, which increases risks of overdose and risk of unplanned pregnancy (Connor & Meltzer, 2006).

Antihistamines can be used as sedatives, anxiolytics, and to manage extrapyramidal symptoms (EPS). They are not effective in treating chronic anxiety, and tolerance builds quickly to sedative effects so daily use is not helpful. They can also be used for angry/aggressive outbursts in an acute situation. Their unpleasant side effects at higher doses make them unlikely agents for abuse. Azaspirones (buspirone/Buspar) currently has no indication for children younger than eighteen years. Other agents that have been developed with good efficacy in adults have failed to provide clear evidence of significant effects on anxiety or depression in children and even adolescents. Few studies have been completed at this time as other agents with stronger profiles of efficacy are still in the early stages of being analyzed. Buspirone may be a good candidate for the future, due to high-safety/low-risk profile, for the treatment of longer-term anxiety. Its timeline of action, however, makes it of minimal use at this time for immediate or acute episodes of anxiety (Scahill, Poncin, & Westphal, 2010).

Contraindications

BZDs are contraindicated for any child or family with a substance abuse history. While the use of BZDs alone is relatively safe, many overdose situations involve the combination of BZDs with other CNS depressants. Children who have a history of suicidal ideation, worsening depression, or significant signs of other major mental health disorders should not be treated with BZDs in a primary practice due to risk of worsening of mood and behavioral disinhibition leading to dangerous behavior. Teratogenic effects during pregnancy are known, also infants exposed to BZDs in utero, especially in the third trimester, may experience withdrawal. Birth control must be assessed and a serum pregnancy test (human chorionic gonodatropin [hCG]) should be obtained for females of child-bearing age. Sedative properties can affect driving ability, so special caution is needed with adolescent drivers or with adolescents involved in activities that require high levels of attention. Be aware of need to taper gradually to avert withdrawal syndrome for use of more than one to two weeks.

Antihistamines are relatively safe, but any hypersensitivity to the class of drugs, especially akathesia or history of a paradoxical reaction, should be noted and an agent from a different class of medications would be indicated. Antihistamines are contraindicated for several medical conditions less likely to affect youth but are still unsafe and include narrow-angle glaucoma, urinary outlet obstruction, GI obstruction, acute asthma, and use of other CNS depressants. Use during pregnancy and breastfeeding is not recommended. Contraindications for azaspirones are primarily those associated with other serotonergic agents and include concurrent or recent use of MAOIs, known hypersensitivity to the drug, history of behavioral activation on other serotonergic agents, elevated prolactin levels, and hepatic or renal disease.

Side Effects

Benzodiazepines

Common side effects include sedation, dizziness, ataxia, blurry vision, cognitive dulling, decreased REM sleep, suppression of sleep stage 4, and lack of coordination. Uncommon side effects include paradoxical disinhibition with agitation, activation, insomnia, anxiety, and increased risk behaviors. *Caution:* In combination with other CNS depressants, BZDs can cause fatal respiratory depression.

Antihistamines

Common side effects include sedation, "hangover," dizziness, hypotension, diarrhea, constipation, dry mouth, blurred vision, and urinary retention. Uncommon side effects may include lowered seizure threshold, blood dyscrasias, tachycardia, involuntary movement disorders, and cholinergic rebound/withdrawal symptoms (high doses of antihistamine). The same risk of akathesia and paradoxical response exists with this medication group.

Azaspirones

Common side effects include dizziness, headache, and fatigue/sedation (less than the others). Uncommon side effects include nervousness and increased activation (increased irritability, restlessness, insomnia).

Drug-Drug Interactions

Benzodiazepines

All BZDs are metabolized in the liver by the CYP450 cytochrome enzymatic pathway. They are also highly lipid soluble, quickly cross the blood-brain barrier, and collect readily in lipid tissue. They interact with a variety of agents, especially increased CNS depression in combination with any other CNS depressing agent leading to increased sedation, decreased cognitive functioning, lack of coordination, and risk of overdose. Commonly prescribed medications that can have drug-drug interactions that decrease metabolism of BZDs are isoniazid (diazepam), erythromycin (diazepam), and oral contraceptives (diazepam). Antacids reduce/delay absorption of BZDs from the GI tract. Bronchodilators can antagonize the effects of diazepam and lorazepam.

Antihistamines

All antihistamines interact with other CNS depressants to increase the symptoms of CNS depression: sedation, lack of coordination, and decreased psychomotor speed. Combined with any other anticholinergic, these agents are also additive in exacerbating anticholinergic side effects.

Azaspirones

Buspirone (Buspar) has a few significant drug-drug interactions. Cimetidine may increase buspirone plasma levels. Buspirone may increase levels of plasma haldol when taken together. Caution is advised when using it with trazodone as this may lead to an increase in risk for hepatic toxicity. This is a partial list of possible drug-drug interactions.

Monitoring

Benzodiazepines

For brief treatment (less than two weeks) with BZDs, screen for substance use for the child and family, sexual activity, and pregnancy. Otherwise human chorionic gonadotropin (serum or urine hCG), blood pressure, pulse, LFTs, and CBC are standard before beginning a longer-term treatment with BZDs.

Dosing

Dosing should start low, approximately 20% to 25% of the usual daily adult dose (Connor & Meltzer, 2006). Titration should progress very slowly and with clear outcome measures for the anxiety to prevent overshooting the necessary dose for the achievement of the treatment goal. Physiological dependence can occur quite quickly (within one to two weeks of steady use). Any requests for additional doses prior to the next anticipated prescription, lost prescriptions, and requests for increased dose without validated need could be an indication that the medication may be misused or that dependency is occurring. Withdrawal should be carefully controlled. If used for any length of time, taper dose at approximately 25% every five to seven days.

Withdrawal symptoms include dysphoria, anxiety, insomnia, tremor, pain, restlessness, diaphoresis, and hallucinations and disturbances of perception. Signs of overdose (usually in conjunction with other CNS depressants) are drowsiness, ataxia, confusion, slurred speech, tremor, depressed reflexes, diploplia, and, finally, respiratory depression/death. Typically, the protocol involves careful planning to provide a prescription for coverage of a specific number of days with a specific purpose. At the end of the time expected to elicit a particular outcome, the child should be seen again before renewing a prescription for a BZD.

Antihistamines

Initial assessment for any extended use should include blood pressure, pulse, and any history of untoward reactions. If the child has never used an antihistamine and it is being prescribed to manage pre-procedure anxiety, a parent can give a "test" dose prior to the procedure to ensure that the child does not have a paradoxical reaction or akathesia. Caution adolescents using these agents while driving or during the school day when sedative effects can impair cognitive functioning and attention. For longer-standing use (not recommended), a gradual taper is helpful to avoid cholinergic rebound.

Dosing. For children, diphenhydramine (Benadryl) can be given at a dose of 5 mg/kg/day divided into four individual doses every six hours.

Azaspirones

There are no indications for short-term use in adults or children. Obtain a baseline for anxiety before considering a trial of buspirone (Buspar). Typically, other medications that have indications for use in children should be trialed before considering buspirone. The benefit of not being sedating, addicting, or a controlled substance make it appealing, but the lack of firm evidence puts this medication further down the algorithm in treating more global types of anxiety disorders such as separation anxiety, generalized anxiety disorder, or social phobia.

Monitoring. Before initiating this medication, useful laboratory tests would include liver enzymes (SGOT, SGPT) and a CBC to monitor for a decrease in platelet count or white blood cell count. Like all psychiatric medications, utilizing the start low, go slow strategy is always best. Table 6.5 lists all anxiolytics, dosing, and side effects.

Antipsychotics

Pharmacology

Antipsychotic medication was first introduced to adult populations in the 1950s and since then has evolved to use with pediatric populations. They are classified according to typical (first generation antipsychotics) versus atypical type (second generation antipsychotics) and also according to their potency of dopamine blockade and management of symptoms (Scahill et al., 2007). Typical antipsychotics used with pediatric populations are chlorpromazine and haloperidol. Atypical antipsychotics used with children and adolescents are clozapine, olanzapine, risperidone, ziprasidone, quetiapine, and aripiprazole (Correll, 2010). Typical antipsychotics, while as effective in symptom management as atypical, have a higher side effect profile resulting in more movement disorders and tardive dyskinesia.

Atypical antipsychotics are used most often with pediatric populations. They act on the dopamine and serotonin systems. Antipsychotics have an ability to block the dopamine D2 receptor site. This is associated with antimanic, antipsychotic, and antiaggressive effects of this medication (Correll et al., 2010).

Table 6.5 Anxiolytics

Medication Generic Name and (Trade)	FDA Approved Age (yr)	Form	Dosing (Range)	Side Effects	Duration of Medication	Pros	Precautions
Benzodiazepine							
Diazepam (Valium)	>6 mo	PO, IV, IM	Start 0.1–0.3 mg/kg Start age 5–12 y = 1 mg, age 12 + = 2 mg, range 1–10 mg	Drowsiness, dizziness, sedation, cognitive blunting, ataxia	Onset 15–30 min Long acting 20–100 hr half-life, duration 2–3 hr	Safe, effective, works rapidly, produces night terrors, less euphoria, somnambulism	Short-term use if possible, behavior disinhibition, consider potential for developing addiction, discontinuation requires gradual taper to avoid seizures or withdrawal high risk for teens
Clonazepam (Klonopin)	2 yr	tabs, melts, wafers	Start 0.25–0.5 mg, dose 0.2–0.8 mg/kg, BID–TID, range 0.25–2 mg, PO, <10 yr 0.01–0.03 mg/kg/day in div. doses, max 0.05 mg/kg/day		Long-acting—15–50 hr half-life, peak 1–2 hr, duration 6–12 hr	Safe, effective, works rapidly, better for panic disorder and anticonvulsant	drug-drug interactions—oral contraceptives, antacids, erythromycin, isoniazid
Lorazepam (Ativan)	12 yr	PO, IV, IM	Start 0.5–1.0 mg BID–QID q4–8hr, 0.03–0.08 mg/kg, range 0.5–4 mg		Immediate—30 min onset, peak 60–90 min, duration 12–24 hr	Safe, effective, works rapidly	Not recommended during pregnancy or breastfeeding
Alprazolam (Xanax)	18 yr	PO	Start 0.25–0.5 mg, once only 0.25, 0.07–0.08 mg/kg BID–TID		Immediate—30 min onset, peak 1–2 hr, duration 4–6 hr, 12–15 hr half-life	Safe, effective, works rapidly	Highest risk for abuse

(continued)

133

Table 6.5 (cont'd)

Medication Generic Name and (Trade)	FDA Approved Age (yr)	Form	Dosing (Range)	Side Effects	Duration of Medication	Pros	Precautions
Antihistamines							
Diphenhydramine (Benadryl)	Avoid <2–6 yr	capsules, elixir, IM,IV	<6 yr, 12.5 mg @hs 6–12 yr, 5 mg/kg/day >12 yr, 25–100 mg BID–QID (up to 300 mg), range, 5–300 mg PO	Common: sedation, dizziness, dry mouth, constipation, blurry vision Uncommon: lower seizure threshold, EPS, tachycardia, hypotension, blood dyscrasias, hypotension	Onset 30 min, peak 1–3 hr, duration 4–7 hr	Not a controlled substance	Taper to avoid cholinergic rebound, not for neonates, tolerance can develop to sedation; urinary obstruction, careful driving and avoid breastfeeding
Hydoxyzine Pamoate (Vistaril)	6 yr	capsules, elixir, IM	Start 10–25 mg <6 yr, 50mg/day div. doses >6, 50–100 mg div. doses	Common: sedation, dizziness, dry mouth, constipation, blurry vision Uncommon: lower seizure threshold, EPS, tachycardia, hypotension, blood dysgrasias, hypotension	onset 15–60 min, duration 4–6 hr		Taper to avoid cholinergic rebound, not for neonates, tolerance can develop to sedation; urinary obstruction, careful driving and avoid breastfeeding
Azaspirone							
Buspirone (Buspar)	18 yr		Start 2.5–5 mg BID. Max dose <12 yr, 40 mg >12 yr, 60 mg 0.2–0.6/mg/kg/day, range: 10–60 mg	Dizziness, fatigue, headache, nausea, vomiting, depression, ataxia, nervousness, activation	onset 1 hr, Peak 40–90 min, 2–3 hr half-life	May help with generalized anxiety disorder, separation anxiety, social phobia, not sedating, not addicting, not a controlled substance, no muscle relaxation	*Avoid grapefruit juice*, not effective for panic, takes 1–2 wk for clinical effect, avoid during pregnancy and breastfeeding

Developed by B. Muller & A. Riley, from Connor & Meltzer , 2006; Emslie, Croarkin, & Mayes, 2010.

Table 6.6 Typical and atypical antipsychotics

Typical (Traditional) Antipsychotics

Drug	Mechanism of Action	Main Indications and Clinical Uses	Dosage (mg/day)	Schedule	Adverse Effects	Comments	Select Brand Names and Preparations Available
Phenothiazines: Low Potency							
Chlorpromazine	D2 receptor blockade. All agents in the family have similar efficacy, but different potency based on the dosage required to achieve a similar effect. 100 mg of chlorpromazine are equivalent to: Thioridazine:95 mg, Perphenazine: 8 mg, Fluphenazine: 2 mg, Thiothixene: 5 mg, Molomdone: 10 mg, Pimozide: 1 mg	Psychosis, mania, aggressive behavior, agitation, self-injurious behavior, autism	25–400	QD/BID/TID	Anticholinergic (dry mouth, constipation, blurred vision, hypotension—more common with low potency agents), weight gain, extrapyramidal reactions (dystonia, rigidity, tremor, akathisia, greater risk with high potency), drowsiness, risk for tardive dyskinesia with long-term administration, withdrawal dyskinesia, hypotension, especially when administered IM	A warning label from the FDA was introduced for thioridazine in 2000, advising against its use as a first-line drug, given concerns over QTc interval prolongation. Traditional agents are not as effective in treating the negative or affective symptoms of psychosis. Low potency agents have high anticholinergic profiles (e.g. sedation, hypotension), whereas high potency agents are likely to cause extrapyramidal side effects (EPS)	Chlorpromazine: 10,25, 50, 100, 200 mg t; elixir; suppositories; injectable
Thioridazine							Thioridazine: 10, 15, 25, 50, 100, 150, 200 mg t; elixir
Phenothiazines: Medium and High Potency							
Perphenazine			4.0–32.0 (Perphenazine) 0.5–10 (Fluphenazine)				Perphenazine: 2, 4, 8, 16 mg t; elixir, injectable
Fluphenazine							Fluphenazine: 1, 2, 5, 10 mg; elixir,injectable, long acting
Other Traditional Antipsycotics–Potency							
Haloperidol—high (butyrophenone)			0.5–10		Lowest weight gain liability among traditional agents		Haloperidol: 0.5, 1, 2.5, 10, 20 mg t; elixir, injectable, long acting
Thiothixene—medium (thiothixene)		Same as the other antipsychotics,	1–20		Cardiac arrhythmias (ECG prolonged QTc), seizures, extrapyramindal reactions, drowsiness, tardive dyskinesia.		Thiothixene: 1, 2, 5, 10, 20 mg t, elixir, injectable
Molindone—medium (indole derivative)		Tourette disorder	5–150				Molindone: 5, 10, 25, 50, 100 mg t, elixir
Pimozide—high			1–4				Orap: 1, 2 mg t

Note: Doses are provided as general guidelines only, and are not meant to be definitive. All doses must be individualized and monitored through the appropriate clinical and/or laboratory means. Abbreviations: c (capsule); t (tablet); FDA (Food and Drug Administration).

Reprinted from Scahill, L., Oesterheld, J. R., Martin, A. 2007, with permission from Lippincott Williams & Wilkins.

(continued)

Table 6.6 (cont'd)

Atypical Antipsychotics

Drug	Mechanism of Action	Main Indications and Clinical Uses	Dosage (mg/day)	Schedule	Adverse Effects	Comments	Select Brand Names and Preparations Available
Risperidone	Dopamine and 5HT receptor blockade. Atypical antipsychotics in general have high 5HT2a/D2 affinity ratios: Risperidone 8:1, Olanzapine 5:1, Quetiapine 1:1, Aripiprazole 10:1, Clozapine 30:1	Psychosis: positive and negative symptoms, TS. Augmentation in OCD. Bipolar disorder, autism, and PDDs aggression and agitation.	0.25–4	QD/BID	Sedation, appetite increase, weight gain, metabolic syndrome (glucose intolerance, dyslipidemia). Low incidence of extrapyramidal adverse effects, Insomnia. Mild activation more likely with Aripiprazole		Risperdal: 0.25, 0.5, 1, 2, 3, 4 mg t, injectable
Olanzapine			2.5–10				Zyprexa: 2.5, 5, 7.5, 10, 15, 20 mg t, oral disintegrating tablet: 5, 10, 15, 20 mg t, injectable
Quetiapine			100–600				Seroquel: 25, 50, 100, 200, 300, 400 mg t
Aripiprazole			5–40				Abilify: 2, 5, 10, 15, 20, 30 mg t
Ziprasidone			40–160			Monitoring of QTc interval recommended	Geodon: 20, 40, 60, 80 mg c
Clozapine		Treatment: refractory psychosis	50–400	BID/TID	Low incidence of extrapyramidal adverse effects; does not induce dysonia. Low risk for tardive dyskinesia. Granulocytopenia/agranuloctosis (treatment requires constant monitoring of blood count). Higher risk of seizures (dose related)	Weekly blood counts mandatory (monitoring for WBC >3000, ANC >2000). Possibility of going to qoWk monitoring by 6 months, qM by 12 months. Seizure prophylaxis (with valproate or gabapentin) recommended at high doses (>300mg/d)	Clozaril: 25, 100 mg t

Reprinted from Scahill, L., Oesterheld, J. R., Martin, A. 2007, with permission from Lippincott Williams & Wilkins.

Indications for Use

Atypical antipsychotic medication is typically used in children and adolescents to treat psychosis, severe behavioral issues associated with autism and other developmental disorders, along with aggression, bipolar disorder, and tics. They can be used as monotherapy or in conjunction with mood stabilizers. Recently, the FDA approved use of aripiprozale (Abilify) for pediatric bipolar disorders. Antipsychotic medication is used in early onset schizophrenia, bipolar disorders, aggressive behaviors, and Tourette syndrome.

Contraindications

Antipsychotics can affect the QTc prolongation of the heart. In patients with a family history of early sudden death, irregular heartbeat, shortness of breath, or dizziness, a cardiac screen is warranted (Correll et al., 2010). Antipsychotics should be used carefully in patients at risk for metabolic syndrome because of either family history or current obesity. These medications can precipitate metabolic syndrome in pediatric patients.

Monitoring

Prior to initiating any antipsychotic medication, the prescriber must obtain baseline physical examination information and do a careful history of metabolic disorders and/or diabetes in the family. Fasting blood glucose, cholesterol, and lipid panel are required prior to initiating therapy. A baseline weight, BMI, and Abnormal Involuntary Movement Disorder (AIMS) scale score should be obtained. Weight must be followed monthly with a follow-up AIMS conducted every six months. Psychoeducation regarding weight management and exercise must be part of the treatment process. Other risks involve hyperprolactinemia and neutropenia. Weight and metabolic difficulties can be the outcome of long-term use of psychotropic medication. All should be encouraged to manage weight with diet, exercise, and frequent monitoring. Vital signs, height, weight, and BMI should be measured every three months. Fasting metabolic profiles and LFTs should be done every six months after obtaining the baseline.

Side Effects

One of the risks of antipsychotic medication is a rare but serious disorder, neuroleptic malignant syndrome (NMS). It can occur after a single dose of medication but most often occurs within two weeks of initiation of antipsychotic medication or a dose increase. This is to be considered a medical emergency with symptoms of severe muscular rigidity, altered mental status, consciousness, stupor, labile pulse and blood pressure, and fever. All antipsychotic medication must be discontinued immediately, and the individual might require

hospitalization for supportive measures. Males and young children are considered most at risk (Correll, 2010; Connor & Meltzer, 2006).

Dosing

The goal is symptom management on the lowest possible dose of medication. Table 6.6 lists traditional and nontraditional anti-psychotic medications, dosing, and side effects.

Summary

This chapter has given an overview of issues of evaluating and treating children and adolescents for psychiatric conditions in primary care and of psychiatric medication use with children and adolescents. It has delineated the differing prescribing roles between APNs in primary care and APNs in psychiatric practice. Major classes of medication are summarized, and prescribing considerations, side effects, drug interactions, and monitoring have been discussed. APNs in both primary care and psychiatric settings are taking an increasingly important role in prescribing psychiatric medications to children and adolescents. The goal is always evidence-based practice considering safety and welfare of the pediatric patient based within a professional nursing practice model that provides high-quality care.

References

Amaladoss, A., Roberts, N., & Amaladoss, F. (2010). Evidence for use of mood stabilizers and anticonvulsants in the treatment of nonaffective disorders in children and adolescents. *Clinical Neuropharmacology, 33*, 303–311.

American Psychiatric Association (APA). (2000). *Diagnostic and statistical manual of mental disorders,* fourth edition, text revision. Washington, DC: Author.

Bernal, P. (2003). Hidden morbidity in pediatric primary care. *Pediatric Annals, 32*, 413–418.

Berns, G.S., & Nemeroff, C.B. (2003). The neurobiology of bipolar disorder. *American Journal of Medical Genetics. Part C: Seminars in Medical Genetics, 123C*, 76–84.

Bridge, J.A., Iyengar, S., Salary, C.B., Barbe, R.P., Birmaher, B., Pincus, H.A., & Brent, D.A. (2007). Clinical response and risk for reported suicidal ideation and suicide attempts in pediatric antidepressant treatment: A meta-analysis of randomized controlled trials. *Journal of the American Medication Association, 297*, 1683–1696.

Chang, K., Saxena, K., & Howe, M. (2006). An open-label study of lamotrigine adjunct or monotherapy for the treatment of adolescents with bipolar depression. *Journal of the American Academy of Child & Adolescent Psychiatry, 45*, 298–304.

Cohen, L.S., Friedman, J.M., Jefferson, J.W., Johnson, E.M., & Weiner, M.L. (1994). A reevaluation of risk of in utero exposure to lithium. *JAMA, 271*, 146–150.

Connor, D.F., & Meltzer, B.M. (2006). *Pediatric psychopharmacology fast facts.* New York, NY: W. W. Norton.

Correll, C.U. (2010). Antipsychotic medications. In M.K. Dulcan (Ed.), *Dulcan's textbook of child and adolescent psychiatry* (pp. 743–774). Washington, DC: American Psychiatric Publishing, Inc.

Correll, C.U., Sheridan, E.M., & DelBello, M.P. (2010). Antipsychotic and mood stabilizer efficacy and tolerability in pediatric and adult patients with bipolar I mania: A comparative analysis of acute, randomized, placebo-controlled trials. *Bipolar Disorders, 12*, 116–141.

Danielyan, A., & Kowatch, R.A. (2005). Management options for bipolar disorder in children and adolescents. *Paediatric Drugs, 7*, 277–294.

Delbello, M.P., Findling, R.L., Kushner, S., Wang, D., Olson, W. H., Capece, J.A., & Rosenthal, N.R. (2005). A pilot controlled trial of topiramate for mania in children and adolescents with bipolar disorder. *Journal of the American Academy of Child & Adolescent Psychiatry, 44*, 539–547.

Dell, M.L. (2010). Ethnic, cultural, and religious issues. In M.K. Dulcan (Ed.), *Dulcan's textbook of child and adolescent psychiatry* (pp. 517–529). Washington, DC: American Psychiatric Publishing.

DiMarco, M.A., & Melnyk, B. (2009). The mental health needs of children and adolescents. *Archives of Psychiatric Nursing, 23*, 334–336.

Dopheide, J.A., & Pliszka, S.R. (2009). Attention-deficit-hyperactivity disorder: an update. *Pharmacotherapy, 29*, 656–679.

Emslie, G.J., Croarkin, P., & Mayes, T.L. (2010). Antidepressants. In M.K. Dulcan (Ed.), *Dulcan's textbook of child and adolescent psychiatry* (pp. 701–723). Washington, DC: American Psychiatric Publishing.

Faraone, S.V. (2000). Genetics of childhood disorders, XX, ADHD, Part 4: Is ADHD genetically heterogeneous? *Journal of the American Academy of Child and Adolescent Psychiatry, 39*, 1455–1457.

Isojarvi, J.I., & Tapanainen, J.S. (2000). Valproate, hyperandrogenism, and polycystic ovaries: A report of 3 cases. *Archives of Neurology, 57*, 1064–1068.

Jones, K.L., Lacro, R.V., Johnson, K.A., & Adams, J. (1989). Pattern of malformations in the children of women treated with carbamazepine during pregnancy. *New England Journal of Medicine, 320*, 1661–1666.

Kowatch, R.A., Strawn, J.R., & Danielyan, A. (2010). Mood stabilizers: Lithium, anticonvulsants, and others. In A. Martin, L. Scahill, & C. Kratochivil (Eds.), *Pediatric psychopharmacology* (pp. 297–311). New York, NY: Oxford University Press.

Kowatch, R.A., Suppes, T., Carmody, T.J., Bucci, J.P., Hume, J.H., Kromelis, M., & Rush, A.J. (2000). Effect size of lithium, divalproex sodium, and carbamazepine in children and adolescents with bipolar disorder. *Journal of the American Academy of Child & Adolescent Psychiatry, 39*, 713–720.

Manji, H.K., & Chen, G. (2000). Post-receptor signaling pathways in the pathophysiology and treatment of mood disorders. *Current Psychiatry Reports, 2*, 479–489.

Melnyk, B.M., Brown, H.E., Jones, D.C., Kreipe, R., & Novak, J. (2003). Improving the mental/psychosocial health of U.S. children and adolescents: Outcomes and implementation strategies from the National KySS Summit. *Journal of Pediatric Health Care, 17*, S1–S24.

Melnyk, B.M., Feinstein, N.F., Tuttle, J., Moldenhauer, Z., Herendeen, P., Veenema, T.G., et al. (2002). Mental health worries, communication, and needs of children, teens, and parents during the year of the nation's terrorist attack: Findings from the national KySS survey. *Journal of Pediatric Health Care, 16*, 222–234.

Merkel, R.L. (2010). Safety of stimulant treatment in attention deficit hyperactivity disorder: Part II. *Expert Opinion Drug Safety, 9*, 917–935.

Miller, N.L., & Findling, R.L. (2010). Principles of psychopharmacology. In M.K. Dulcan (Ed.), *Dulcan's textbook of child and adolescent psychiatry* (pp. 667–679). Washington, DC: American Psychiatric Publishing, Inc.

Munoz, R., Primm, A., & Ananth, J. (2007). *Life in color: Culture in American psychiatry.* Chicago, IL: Hilton.

Nandagopal, J.J., DelBello, M.P., & Kowatch, R. (2009). Pharmacologic treatment of pediatric bipolar disorder. *Child & Adolescent Psychiatric Clinics of North America, 18*, 455–469.

Okusa, M.D., & Crystal, L.J. (1994). Clinical manifestations and management of acute lithium intoxication. *American Journal of Medicine, 97*, 383–389.

Pavuluri, M.N., Henry, D.B., Moss, M., Mohammed, T., Carbray, J.A., & Sweeney, J.A. (2009). Effectiveness of lamotrigine in maintaining symptom control in pediatric bipolar disorder. *Journal of Child & Adolescent Psychopharmacology, 19*, 75–82.

Perrin, J.M., Friedman, R.A., & Knilans, T.K. (2008). Cardiovascular monitoring and stimulant drugs for attention-deficit/hyperactivity disorder. *Pediatrics, 122*, 451–453.

Pliszka, S.R. (2010). Attention-deficit/hyperactivity disorder. In M.K. Dulcan (Ed.), *Dulcan's textbook of child and adolescent psychiatry* (pp. 205–221). Washington, DC: American Psychiatric Publishing.

Scahill, L., Oesterheld, J.R., & Martin, A. (2007). General principles, specific drug treatments, and clinical practice. In A. Martin and F.R. Volkmar (Eds.), *Lewis's child and adolescent psychiatry: A comprehensive textbook* (4th ed.) (pp. 754–789). Philadelphia, PA: Lippincott Williams & Wilkins.

Scahill, L., Poncin, Y., & Westphal, A. (2010). Alpha-adrenergics, beta-blockers, benzodiazepines, buspirone, and desmopressin. In M.K. Dulcan (Ed.), *Dulcan's textbook of child and adolescent psychiatry* (pp. 775–785). Washington, DC: American Psychiatric Publishing, Inc.

Spencer, T.J., Biederman, J., & Wilens, T.E. (2010). Medications used for attention-deficit/hyperactivity disorder. In M.K. Dulcan (Ed.), *Dulcan's textbook of child and adolescent psychiatry* (pp. 681–700). Washington, DC: American Psychiatric Publishing.

Tennis, P., Eldridge, R.R., & International Lamotrigine Pregnancy Registry Scientific Advisory Committee. (2002). Preliminary results on pregnancy outcomes in women using lamotrigine. *Epilepsia, 43*, 1161–1167.

Theoktisto, K.M. (2009). Pharmacokinetic considerations in the treatment of behavioral issues. *Pediatric Nursing, 35*, 369–377.

U.S. Food and Drug Administration (FDA). (2011). *Drug safety labeling changes.* Retrieved from http://www.fda.gov/Safety/MedWatch/SafetyInformation/Safety-RelatedDrugLabelingChanges/default.htm

U.S. Office of the Surgeon General, Department of Health and Human Services. (1999). *Mental health: A report of the Surgeon General (chapter 3).* Retrieved from http://www.surgeongeneral.gov/library/mentalhealth/home.html

Vierhile A., Robb, A., & Ryan-Krause, P. (2009). Attention-deficit/hyperactivity disorder in children and adolescents: closing diagnostic, communication, and treatment gaps. *Journal of Pediatric Health Care, 23*, S5–S21.

Vitiello, B. (2008). Developmental aspects of pediatric psychopharmacology. In R.L. Findling (Ed.), *Clinical manual of child and adolescent psychopharmacology* (pp. 1–31). Washington, DC: American Psychiatric Publishing.

Wagner, K.D., Kowatch, R.A., Emslie, G.J., Findling, R.L., Wilens, T.E., McCague, K., & Linden, D. (2006). A double-blind, randomized, placebo-controlled trial of oxcarbazepine in the treatment of bipolar disorder in children and adolescents. *American Journal of Psychiatry, 163*, 1179–1186.

Wagner, K.D., Redden, L., Kowatch, R.A., Wilens, T.E., Segal, S., Chang, K., & Saltarelli, M. (2009). A double-blind, randomized, placebo-controlled trial of divalproex extended-release in the treatment of bipolar disorder in children and adolescents. *Journal of the American Academy of Child & Adolescent Psychiatry, 48*, 519–532.

Williams, J., Klinepeter, K., Pamles, G., Pulley, A., & Foy, J. M. (2004). Diagnosis and treatment of behavioral health disorders in pediatric practice. *Pediatrics, 114*, 601–606.

Wolraich, M.L., & Doffing, M.A. (2004). Pharmokinetic considerations in the treatment of attention-deficit hyperactivity disorder with methylphenidate. *CNS Drugs, 18*, 243–250.

7

Attention Deficit Hyperactivity Disorder (ADHD)

Geraldine S. Pearson and Angela A. Crowley

Objectives

After reading this chapter, APNs will be able to

1. Define the epidemiology and prevalence statistics of ADHD,
2. Discuss theories of etiology associated with ADHD including family dynamics and neurobiological, genetic, and psychosocial factors.
3. Define and describe the presenting signs and symptoms of ADHD and common comorbid disorders in children and adolescents.
4. Describe evidence-based interventions for children and adolescents diagnosed with ADHD.
5. Describe care management of ADHD and differentiate roles of primary care practitioners and advanced practice psychiatric nurses in the diagnosis and treatment of children and adolescents with ADHD.
6. Discuss implications for nursing practice, research, and education.

Introduction

Attention deficit hyperactivity disorder (ADHD) is a commonly occurring disorder that is probably treated equally by child psychiatric advanced practice nurses (APNs), pediatric nurse practitioners, and family nurse practitioners. ADHD is a neurodevelopmental disorder that progresses and changes at different life stages. Treatment options can be dependent on the age of the child and severity of symptoms as well as many other factors, including family stability and support of treatment (Young & Amarasinghe, 2010). APNs see children and adolescents at all stages of development and are uniquely positioned to plan care based on developmental needs and symptom presentation.

The diagnosis of ADHD is made after obtaining history and behavior rating scales, carefully listening to caregivers' descriptions of behaviors, and directly observing the child. After careful assessment, the first line of treatment should be psychosocial interventions aimed at promoting parent management of behavior. Medication treatment, if used, should ideally be combined with educational and behavioral interventions (Vierhile, Robb, & Ryan-Krause, 2009). With significant effect sizes related to efficacy, stimulant treatment can make a significant difference in symptom presentation. Treatment and diagnostic complexity emerges when other disorders are comorbid with ADHD and when behavioral issues presented by the child or adolescent become too psychiatrically based or acute for primary care management.

This chapter will discuss historical perspectives of ADHD and will review presenting signs and symptoms, common comorbid conditions, and evidence-based

Child and Adolescent Behavioral Health: A Resource for Advanced Practice Psychiatric and Primary Care Practitioners in Nursing,
First Edition. Edited by Edilma L. Yearwood, Geraldine S. Pearson, and Jamesetta A. Newland.
© 2012 John Wiley & Sons, Inc. Published 2012 by John Wiley & Sons, Inc.

Table 7.1 Diagnostic criteria for attention deficit hyperactivity disorder (APA, 2000)

Criterion	Clinical Presentation
Inattention	Often fails to give close attention to details or makes careless mistakes in schoolwork or other activities
	Often has difficulty sustaining attention in tasks or play activities
	Often does not seem to listen when spoken to directly
	Often does not follow through on instructions and fails to finish schoolwork, chores, or duties in the workplace
	Often has difficulty organizing tasks and activities
	Often avoids, dislikes, or does not want to do things that take a lot of mental effort for a long period of time (e.g., schoolwork, homework)
	Often loses things necessary for tasks or activities
	Is often easily distracted by extraneous stimuli
	Is often forgetful in daily activities
Hyperactivity	Often fidgets with hands or feet or squirms in seat
	Often leaves seat in classroom or in other situations in which remaining seated is expected
	Often runs about or climbs excessively in situations in which it is inappropriate
	Often has difficulty playing or engaging in leisure activities quietly
	Is often "on the go" or often acts as if "driven by a motor"
	Often talks excessively
Impulsivity	Often blurts out answers before questions have been completed
	Often has difficulty awaiting turn
	Often interrupts or intrudes on others

The presence of six symptoms causing functional impairment in at least two different settings (i.e., home, school) over 6 months is necessary to confirm the diagnosis. Symptoms must be present before age 7 years.
Reprinted from Pliszka et al., 2006, with permission from Elsevier.

interventions. The chapter will differentiate the roles of primary care pediatric and family nurse practitioners and advanced practice psychiatric nurses and present indications for referral to a psychiatric provider. The chapter will conclude with a case study describing management issues, with implications for nursing practice, research, and education.

Historical Perspective

As noted by Pliszka (2010), the first clinical description of ADHD occurred in 1902 by George Still in which he related problematic behavior to a lack of moral control in children. Early observers of the disorder suggested that behavior disorders, such as hyperkinesis, explosive behavior, fatigability, and attention deficit behaviors, were related to some biologic etiology such as encephalitis and cerebral trauma in children (Ebaugh & Franklin, 1923; Strecker & Ebaugh, 1924).

In the 1930s, the term "minimal brain dysfunction" was coined to describe hyperkinesis, impulsivity, learning disability, and short attention span (Spencer, Biederman, & Mick, 2007). By the 1950s, the terms

"hyperactive child syndrome" and "hyperkinetic reaction of childhood" were present in the Diagnostic Statistical Manual of Mental Disorders (DSM-II) that was published in 1968 (APA, 1968).

The focus shifted in DSM-III to inattention as a major component of the disorder (Spencer et al., 2007). There was recognition that the disorder could look different at various developmental stages. DSM-III also identified a residual form of ADHD that could continue to cause impairment into adulthood. DSM-IV-TR defines three subtypes of ADHD: predominantly inattentive, predominantly hyperactive-impulsive, and combined. Table 7.1 outlines the predominant DSM-IV criteria for ADHD.

The proposed DSM-V revisions, while not finalized, suggest that only one diagnostic code could be assigned to ADHD with an additional code of attention-deficit disorder (ADD) having its own code and criteria. Age of onset would be broadened up to age twelve with the indicator of onset changed from impairment to symptom. Autism spectrum or pervasive developmental disorders would no longer be exclusionary of an ADHD diagnosis (APA, 2010).

Epidemiology and Prevalence of ADHD

ADHD has a prevalence estimated at 6% to 9% in children aged five to twelve years with 60% to 80% showing symptoms into adolescence and 50% with symptoms persisting into adulthood (Pliszka and AACAP Child and Adolescent Work Group on Quality Issues, 2007). In the National Comorbidity Survey, the adult prevalence of ADHD was 4.4% (Kessler et al., 2006). The lifetime prevalence of ADHD implies influence of ADHD at all stages of the life cycle and includes family functioning, academic and occupational success, and the heritable aspects of the disorder.

International prevalence rates of ADHD are estimated at 5.3% with the highest rates in Africa (8.5%) and South America (11.8%); Asia, Europe, and North America have lower rates. Study method variability and diagnostic accuracy may account for the differences (Polanczyk, Lima, Horta, Biederman, & Rohde, 2007). Despite these regional differences, ADHD is an international disorder.

Matza, Paramore, and Prasad (2005) found during a longitudinal study of children diagnosed with ADHD who were re-interviewed 15 years later that the involved group was more likely to fail to finish high school and more likely to father children early, have more automobile accidents, and have more unemployment. Similar longitudinal research showed an increased likelihood of meeting criteria for antisocial disorders (conduct, oppositional defiant), major psychiatric disorders (mood disorders and psychosis), and substance dependence disorders when compared to matched controls at a 10-year follow-up point (Biederman et al., 2006). Having a childhood diagnosis of ADHD puts an individual at risk for developing other comorbid psychiatric diagnoses. This risk of adverse psychiatric outcomes makes it essential that APNs who encounter ADHD in their young pediatric patients proactively provide effective treatment aimed at reducing the risk of other disorders developing as the child grows and matures.

Etiology

Genetics

The etiology of ADHD is complex and not defined by any single issue. Genetic studies have explored etiology with family/adoption studies, twin studies, and molecular genetics research (Pliszka, 2010). While candidate genes have been identified for ADHD, studies have been unable to identify the specific genes responsible for ADHD. It is known that if a child has ADHD, 10% to 35% of first-degree relatives are likely to also have the disorder (Biederman et al., 1992). Similarly, if a child has a parent with ADHD, the risk of developing the disorder can run as high as 57% (Biederman et al., 1995). ADHD is considered a polygenetic disorder (Pliszka, 2010).

Neurobiology

Research suggests that individuals with ADHD may have alterations in specific areas of the brain, including the ventral medial prefrontal cortex, posterior cingulated cortex, and precuneus (Weissman, Roberts, Visscher, & Woldorff, 2006). Other research suggests that adults with ADHD have less functional connectivity between some areas of the brain resulting in anterior regions failing to suppress the default mode network. This, in turn, results in impaired ability to focus and pay attention (Castellanos et al., 2008).

Research also suggests that atypical consolidation of the brain's default network could be a causative factor of ADHD beginning in childhood (Fair et al., 2010). This shift marks a change in research focused on determining the neurobiological cause of ADHD from a view that regional brain abnormalities caused the disorder to a dysfunction in distributed network organization. This specifically involves research identifying the dopamine receptors and transporters associated with ADHD (Sterigiakouli & Thapar, 2010). Additional research is necessary to further define the brain processes that precipitate development of ADHD in children (Konrad & Eickhoff, 2010).

Brain imaging such as PET or MRI is not recommended for the assessment of ADHD (http://archive.psych.org/edu/other_res/lib_archives/archives/200501.pdf). While children with ADHD have an increased number of subtle nonfocal neurological symptoms, these should not determine treatment (Pliszka, 2010; Pine, Shaffer, & Schonfeld, 1993). More research is needed in the area of brain imaging used to diagnose ADHD.

Environmental

A variety of environmental factors are also likely to influence the development of ADHD. These can include severe traumatic brain injury, maternal smoking during pregnancy, prenatal stress and low birth weight, twin births, early social deprivation, and exposure to lead (Braun, Kahn, Froehlich, Auinger, & Lanphear, 2006; Kreppner, O'Connor, & Rutter, 2001; Linnet et al., 2003; Mick, Biederman, Faraone, & Sayer, 2002). Greater environmental adversity including exposure to family conflict, parental psychopathology, and poverty may influence the development of ADHD but are not thought to contribute to the etiology of ADHD (Pliszka, 2010). ADHD is a brain-based disorder that can be mediated by environmental factors but is not directly caused by such factors.

Table 7.2 Attention deficit hyperactivity disorder symptoms across the life span

Developmental Stage	Symptoms
Preschool	Excessive motor activity or mobility, low frustration tolerance, impulsivity, inability to sustain attention, distractibility, poorly organized behavior, aggressiveness, noncompliance, inappropriate or demanding behaviors, negative social behavior, less adaptive behaviors
School-age	Symptoms similar to those in preschool-aged children, with the emergence of academic difficulties, rejection by peers, oppositional behavior, lying, stealing, poor self-esteem, poor sleep patterns
Adolescence	Inattention, impulsiveness, inner restlessness, continued academic difficulties, problems with authority, increased risky behavior (e.g., smoking, substance abuse, early sexual activity, driving accidents/traffic violations), excessively aggressive and antisocial behavior, overall feelings of worthlessness
Adulthood	Exacerbation of underlying psychiatric conditions, frequent job changes and job losses, marital discord, multiple marriages, problems with the law, substance abuse

Armstrong & Nettleton, 2004; Harpin, 2005; Woodard, 2006.
Adapted from: Vierhile, Robb, Ryan-Krause, 2009, with permission from Elsevier Publishing.

Implications for Adulthood

It is likely that children and adolescents with ADHD continue to show symptoms of the disorder into adulthood and may require pharmacological and psychosocial treatment interventions throughout their lives. The key to adult psychopathology seems to be in identifying comorbid disorders that accompany the ADHD symptomatology along with the degree of impairment that may extend into adulthood.

Adults with a history of ADHD as children tend to have a higher rate of antisocial behavior, injuries and accidents, and employment and marital difficulties (Barkley, 2004; Biederman et al., 2006). ADHD symptoms that carry into adulthood have implications for parenting effectiveness and family stability. Assessment of parental history of diagnosed and undiagnosed ADHD should routinely occur when assessing a child for the disorder. ADHD is a disorder whose etiology and presentation are influenced by a complex interplay between genetic and environmental factors. It has a clear influence on adult vocational and social functioning.

Presenting Signs and Symptoms of ADHD

A diagnosis of ADHD is made after careful assessment of the child and family and determination that inattention, or impulsivity and hyperactivity, or both, is impairing functioning on multiple domains of the child's life for at least six months. When diagnosing a child with ADHD it is essential to consider other disorders, including learning disabilities, disruptive behavior disorders, substance abuse disorder, and Tourette's disorder (Pliszka et al.,

2007). The child's level of maturity, developmental history, family situation, and physical health must all be considered. Diagnosing ADHD requires careful attention to assessment details, processing with parents what symptoms they are concerned about, and, most important, understanding the parental attitudes, culture, and potential bias that will influence how they view any type of disorder in their child. Table 7.2 details ADHD symptoms across the life span.

The symptoms of ADHD rarely occur without some other mediating disorder or factor influencing functioning. In the young child, this can include learning disorders, mood disorders, autistic spectrum disorders, and oppositional defiant disorders. In adolescents, the diagnosis of ADHD can be complicated by substance use, learning disorders, and other psychiatric disorders. Table 7.2 describes the diagnostic criteria for ADHD based on DSM IV-TR criteria (APA, 2000).

Assessment tools are useful to use with parents and teachers in identifying the symptoms of ADHD through a normative, well-defined, reliable, and valid scale. It is best to use screening tools that assess across disorders especially since comorbidity exists between disorders. The cautions of using scales with parents can involve over-reporting or underreporting of symptoms based on attitudes about ADHD and stigma around having the disorder. Teacher ratings must be considered based on familiarity with the child (Vierhile & Robb, 2009). Rating scales performed before and after treatment intervention can offer APNs a concrete measurement of change in symptoms and can inform interventions. Table 7.3 gives four common rating scales used in primary care that are also useful in psychiatric settings.

Table 7.3 Comparison of common ADHD rating scales used in primary care

Scale	Age Range	Description	Advantages	Disadvantages
Connors Rating Scale Revised (CRS-R)	3–17 yr	• Based on DSM-IV criteria • Assesses wide variety of common behavior problems (e.g., sleep, eating, peer group problems) • Revised scale updates, age, and sex-normative data and factor structure • Available in both short and long, parent, teacher, and self-report versions	• Large normative base • Multiple observer forms • Abbreviated forms aid in treatment monitoring • French version	• Few items regarding comorbidities • Somewhat redundant • Complete version is lengthy
Brown Attention Deficit Disorder Scale for Children and Adolescents (BADDS)	3–12 yr, parent and teacher report; 8–12 yr self-report; 12–18 yr self-report	• Unlike other scales based on DSM-IV criteria, BADDS measures executive functioning associated with ADHD • Also measures developmental impairments • Separate rating scales for 3–7 yr, 8–12 yr, 12–18 yr	• Measures inattentive ADHD • Only scale that accounts for inattentive behavior as a function of age • Strong psychometrics	• Minimal data about use in clinical settings
Vanderbilt ADHD Rating Scale	6–12 yr, parent and teacher forms	• Newer scale based on DSM-IV criteria • Both parent and teacher forms • Similar to CRS-R and SNAP-IV • Assesses for comorbidities and school functioning	• Screens for comorbidities (oppositional-defiant disorder, anxiety, depression) • Spanish and German versions • Available online • Psychometrically strong scales	• Newer scales that lack sufficient data to establish their validity • Normative data from only one US region • No self-report scales
Swanson, Nolan, and Pelham IV (SNAP)	5–11 yr, parent and teacher rating scale	• One of the first scales based on DSM-IV criteria • Frequently used in ADHD research	• Scoring available online • Same scale used for both parent and teacher • Measures comorbidity	• Lack of published psychometrics and normative data • Brief assessment of comorbidities

Adapted from Vierhile, Robb, and Ryan-Krause, 2009, with permission from Elsevier Publishing.

Common Comorbid Conditions and Treatment

Comorbid psychiatric conditions are common in patients with ADHD. Successful management of ADHD involves identification and treatment of comorbid conditions (Connor & Meltzer, 2006). Comorbid conditions in childhood can include oppositional defiant disorder, conduct disorder, depression, cigarette smoking, anxiety disorder, learning disorders, and tic disorders. In adolescents, the most common comorbidities are substance use disorders, cigarette smoking, conduct disorder, depression, anx-

iety disorder, and bipolar disorder. In adults with ADHD, the comorbid disorders can include substance use disorders, antisocial personality disorder, depression, anxiety disorders, and bipolar disorder (Connor & Meltzer, 2006).

Oppositional Defiant Disorder and Conduct Disorder

It is estimated that between 30% to 50% of children diagnosed with ADHD also have oppositional defiant disorder (ODD) or some other form of a conduct disorder

(CD) (Armenteros, Lewis, & Davalos, 2007). Behavior difficulties in conduct problems include aggression, impulsivity, and oppositional problems beyond the diagnosis of ADHD. However, several studies have shown that treating the ADHD with a stimulant medication will help improve the oppositional behaviors (Pliszka et al., 2007). A review of 28 studies looking at the antiaggressive effects of stimulants found that aggressive symptoms diminished with the use of stimulants (Connor, Glatt, Lopez, Jackson, & Melloni, 2002). Dopheide and Pliszka (2009) found no evidence that stimulants increased aggression or antisocial behavior.

If aggression persists even if the ADHD symptoms are improved, bipolar disorder has to be ruled out (Pliszka, Crismon, & Hughes, 2006). Pliszka et al. recommend consideration of an atypical or second generation antipsychotic medication to manage behavior. Considerations with these medications involve carefully monitoring of metabolic effects and side effects such as extrapyramidal symptoms.

Bipolar Disorder

Bipolar disorder in children with ADHD is difficult to diagnose. Core symptoms of inattention, hyperactivity, impulsivity, and aggression can occur in both disorders (Kowatch & DelBello, 2006), yet children with an ADHD diagnosis do not tend to exhibit manic symptoms such as elated mood, grandiosity, decreased need for sleep, or racing thoughts. When children present with symptoms of both ADHD and a mood disorder, it is recommended that initial treatment with medication focus on mood stabilization followed by treatment of the ADHD (Kowatch & Debello, 2006).

Major Depression

The first step in treating a child who meets diagnostic criteria for both major depression and ADHD is determining which disorder is causing the most functional impairment and symptom distress (Pliszka et al., 2006). Depressive symptoms respond best to a combination of cognitive-behavioral therapy (CBT) with medication management with a selective serotonin reuptake inhibitor (SSRI) (Dopheide, 2006). The APN must carefully and continuously assess the risk of suicide in any child who suffers from a depressive disorder. Treatment of ADHD symptoms could be considered after some resolution of the depressive symptoms.

Anxiety Disorders

Children with ADHD and comorbid anxiety disorders suffer more impairment when both disorders are present. Research suggests that 25% to 35% of the children with ADHD also have an anxiety disorder (Bowen, Chavira, Baily, Stein, & Stein, 2008). APNs treating ADHD in an anxious child should be aware that the benefits of stimulant treatment might be mixed, causing increased anxiety even if ADHD symptoms have improved (Goez, Back-Bennet, & Zelnik, 2007). Anxiety disorders are best treated first with CBT, followed by pharmacologic interventions if CBT is not helpful.

Tic Disorders or Tourette's Disorder

Tic disorders and ADHD are frequently comorbid with up to 75% of children with Tourette's disorder also suffering from ADHD (Jankovic, 2001). Research has shown that combination therapy of a stimulant and alpha-agonist resulted in improving ADHD in children with comorbid tic disorders (The Tourette's Syndrome Study Group, 2002). Studies show that use of methylphenidate and atomoxetine can effectively manage ADHD symptoms without worsening the tic disorder (Pliszka, Crismon, & Hughes, 2006).

Effects of ADHD on Peer Relationships

Recent research has looked at developmental process as it involves peer problems in children diagnosed with ADHD. Compared to a nondiagnosed group, researchers found that, over a six-year study period, children with ADHD exhibited difficulties with aggression, social skills, inaccurate self-perceptions, and peer rejection (Murray-Close et al., 2010). They found that the peer problems in the children with ADHD reflected their failure to successfully negotiate developmental tasks. The authors described "multiple vicious cycles and cascading effects among areas of functioning across development. These findings suggest that there are a number of indirect effects among overly positive self-perceptions, social skills, aggression, and peer rejection. As a result, failure in one area may have both direct and indirect effects on functioning in other areas across development" (p. 799).

These findings have implications for intervention strategies aimed at better peer relationships for the child with ADHD. The researchers recommend intervening at multiple levels, with a social behavioral curriculum that emphasizes skill building from elementary through high school. The notion that impairments from ADHD have a cascading effect on development is beginning to emerge in the literature and requires more research, especially around effective mediating interventions.

Evidence-Based Interventions

Nonpharmacological

Nonpharmacological interventions have been shown to have positive influence on ADHD symptoms and include behavioral therapy models, including CBT and parent management training. Young and Amarasinghe (2010), in their review of nonpharmacological treatment for ADHD, organized by developmental stage, note that in very young children the predominant intervention is parent training. Assessment of risk is recommended since many young children with ADHD are difficult to manage and may engage in an early, damaging, negative relationship with parents.

For young school-aged children, they recommend continued indirect models of treatment involving parent training and classroom interventions. Parent management training specifically helps parents and caregivers learn to manage difficult, impulsive behaviors in a structured, reward-oriented system. Children with learning disabilities require specialized educational programs that consider the role ADHD symptoms play in academic difficulties. Some form of special education services might be needed to maximize use of the classroom. School-focused interventions include academics, peer relationships, a structured classroom environment, and accommodations such as untimed tests or small class size (Connor & Meltzer, 2006).

By middle and high school, nonpharmacological treatment becomes more complex, involving parents, classroom, and, for the adolescent, social skills training or CBT. Tutoring support, use of assistive electronic devices, and planning for special accommodations beyond high school in technical school or college are important for the middle and high school patient with ADHD. Until adulthood the recommendation is for a multimodal approach. By adulthood, the recommended psychosocial intervention is CBT (Young & Amarasinghe, 2010). By adulthood, most individuals with ADHD will have had at least a trial of stimulant medication. Ideally, this is part of a comprehensive treatment regimen involving psychosocial interventions with parents, teachers, and the patient.

Pharmacological Interventions

Use of stimulant medication has generally been the first-line pharmacological intervention for individuals with diagnosed ADHD. Methylphenidate and amphetamine preparations have been shown to enhance dopaminergic and noradrenergic neurotransmission peripherally and in the central nervous system (Volkow et al., 2001). Clinical trials have consistently shown these medications to be effective and safe in symptom management with children, adolescents, and adults who have ADHD (Pliszka, 2010).

Other medications have also been used in treating ADHD and include nonstimulant agents (atomoxetine), antidepressants (buproprion), and alpha-agonist preparations (clonidine, guanfacine). These medications tend to be second-line agents and are used if stimulants are poorly tolerated, there is a partial response to stimulant medication, or there are comorbid disorders contraindicating the use of stimulants (Connor & Meltzer, 2006). Table 7.4 lists stimulant medications indicated for the treatment of ADHD. Table 7.5 lists nonstimulant medications.

Approach to Management

Symptoms of ADHD usually emerge as behavioral concerns revealed by parents during well-child primary care visits, or a parent may schedule an appointment to discuss concerns about the child's behavioral issues. With the proliferation of media related to ADHD, parents often present with a question or potential diagnosis of ADHD to explain their child's symptomatology. Teachers frequently encourage parents to seek health care assessments and may suggest a diagnosis of ADHD when impulsive and inattentive behavior is observed in the classroom. One of the most important roles of primary care APNs is to accurately diagnose ADHD by gathering an extensive history and assessments, conducting a thorough physical examination, gathering data from multiple sources (school, home, observations), and ruling out other diagnoses.

Once the diagnosis of ADHD is established, the clinician should determine if the patient has a comorbid condition, such as ODD. Patients with comorbid conditions are more likely to require referral to a child guidance clinic for individual and family therapy. However, the therapist may not be a prescriber and comanagement with the primary care provider can be arranged.

Table 7.4 Medications indicated for the treatment of attention-deficit/hyperactivity disorder

Generic Name	Trade Name	Approved Age (yr)	Dosing	Common Adverse Events
Amphetamine	Adderall	3+	Once/twice daily	Headache, abdominal pain, insomnia, decreased appetite, nervousness, dizziness
Amphetamine	Adderall XR	6+	Once daily	Headache, loss of appetite, insomnia, abdominal pain, weight loss, xerostomia, tachycardia, nervousness, emotional lability, dizziness

(continued)

Table 7.4 (*cont'd*)

Generic Name	Trade Name	Approved Age (yr)	Dosing	Common Adverse Events
Methylphenidate HCl extended-release tablets	Concerta	6+	Once daily	Headache, abdominal pain, insomnia, decreased appetite, nervousness, dizziness
Methylphenidate HCl transdermal system	Daytrona	6+	Removed 9 hr after application; frequency based on need and response	Decreased appetite, insomnia, nausea, vomiting, emotional lability, weight loss, tics
Methamphetamine HCl tablets	Desoxyn	6+	Once/twice daily	Tachycardia, tremors, insomnia, abdominal pain, xerostomia, decreased appetite, headache, dizziness, weight loss
Destroamphetamine sulfate spansule sustained-release capsules and tablets	Dexedrine	3–16	Once/twice/3X daily	Tachycardia, tremors, insomnia, abdominal pain, xerostomia, decreased appetite, headache, dizziness, weight loss
DEX methylphenidate HCl tablets DEX methylphenidate	Focalin	6–17	Twice daily	Abdominal pain, nausea, decreased appetite fever
HCl extended-release capsules	Focalin XR	6+	Once daily	Decreased appetite, headache, abdominal pain, anxiety, insomnia, xerostomia, dizziness, nervousness
Methylphenidate HCl extended-release capsules	Metadate CD	6–15	Once daily	Headache, abdominal pain, decreased appetite, insomnia, nervousness, dizziness
Methylphenidate HCl oral solution	Methylin oral solution	6+	Twice daily	Nervousness, insomnia, headache, abdominal pain, tachycardia, nausea, decreased appetite, dizziness, weight loss
Methylphenidate HCl chewable tablets	Methylin chewable tablets	6=	Twice daily	Nervousness, insomnia, headache, abdominal pain, tachycardia, nausea, decreased appetite, dizziness, weight loss
Methylphenidate HCl tablets	Ritalin	6+	Twice daily	Headache, abdominal pain, insomnia, nausea, decreased appetite, nervousness
Methylphenidate HCl sustained-release tablets	Ritalin-SR	6+	Twice daily	Headache, abdominal pain, insomnia, nausea, decreased appetite, nervousness
Methylphenidate HCl extended-release capsules	Ritalin LA	6+	Once daily	Headache, abdominal pain, decreased appetite, insomnia
Atomoxetine HCl	Strattera	6+	Once/twice daily	Headache, abdominal pain, appetite decreased, vomiting, cough
Lisdexamfetamine dimesylate	Vyvanse	6–12	Once daily	Decreased appetite, insomnia, abdominal pain, headache

Adapted from Vierhile, Robb, Ryan-Krause, 2009, with permission from Elsevier Publishing.

Table 7.5 Comparison of nonstimulant drugs for treatment of attention deficit hyperactivity disorder

Drug (Generic/ Trade Name)	Relevant Pharmacokinetic Parameters	Recommended Dosage Regimen	Comments
Atomoxetine/ Strattera	Half-life: 5 hr (extensive metabolizers) 20 hr (poor metabolizers)	Children: 0.5 mg/kg/day; increase dosage weekly until achieve response (optimum 1.2 mg/kg/day, maximum 1.8 mg/kg/day); BID or 20 mg q.d.; increase dosage weekly until achieve response (maximum 100 mg/day)	No abuse potential, less insomnia and growth effects than stimulants Delayed onset (2–4 weeks), lower efficacy rates than stimulants
Bupropion/ Wellbutrin	Half-life: 12 hr (adolescents) 21 hr (adults)	3 mg/kg/day or 150 mg/day, whichever is less; dosed BID or TID (maximum 6 mg/kg/day or 300 mg/day with no single dose > 150 mg)	Rash, lowers seizure threshold, insomnia if given too late in the day
Clonidine/ Catapres	Half-life: 6–16 hr	≤ 45 kg: 0.05 mg h.s., then titrate in 0.05 mg increments BID, TID, or QID >45 kg: 0.1 mg h.s., then titrate in 0.1 mg increments BID, TID, or QID	Used alone or as an adjunct to stimulants to manage insomnia, tics, or aggressive behavior
Guanfacine/ Tenex	Half-life: 10–30 hr	≤ 45 kg: 0.5 mg h.s., then titrate in 0.5 mg increments BID, TID, or QID >45 kg: 1 mg h.s., then titrate in 1 mg increments BID, TID, or QID	Delayed onset (2–4 weeks) Review personal and famly cardiovascular history Taper to prevent rebound hypertension Extended release formulation also available (1–4 mg)

Pliszka, Bernet, Bukstein et al., 2007; Pliszka, Crismon, Hughes, 2006; Prince, 2006; Wolraich et al., 2007; Caballerro & Nahata, 2003. Adapted from Dopheide & Pliszka, 2009, with permission from Pharmocotherapy Publications.

Best practice advocates that parents and adolescents give written permission so that both clinicians can share confidential information. However, there may be variations across states about the legality of formal consent prior to communication between health care providers.

Parents, children, and adolescents require at least one full visit to discuss the diagnosis of ADHD and recommended evidence-based management. The clinician should determine the parents' and child's understanding of the diagnosis and the cultural meaning of the disorder (Dell, 2010). Previous to diagnosis, parents may view the child's behavior as intentionally "lazy" or difficult. Children in turn are often baffled, sometimes hopeless, and resigned to criticism from parents, teachers, and peers. For some parents the diagnosis is a relief, but others may be fearful that controlled substances will lead to drug dependence. Health care providers should not speak only to parents but should also fully engage children and adolescents at their developmental level in the discussion. Adolescents require time alone with the provider to address their specific concerns and in recognition of their growing independence and responsibility

to begin managing their health care. Despite an in-depth initial discussion, some parents are not prepared to include medication as a component of therapy. The clinician should remain open to the parents' need to explore other options and resources. In many instances, when other therapies have failed, parents will return and accept pharmacotherapy as part of the therapeutic plan. If psychosocial therapies are successful in managing symptoms, medication may not be necessary.

Health care providers should explain that effective management of ADHD requires a multifaceted approach including behavior management at home, at school, and when engaged in other activities; communication with school personnel, and pharmacological therapy. *ADHD: A Complete and Authoritative Guide,* published by the American Academy of Pediatrics (2004), is a useful comprehensive resource for parents, older children, and adolescents.

Selecting the stimulant dose is not based on weight, which is the standard for most pediatric medications. The provider should start with the lowest dose, and explain that the dose will be increased every one to two weeks as needed depending on the child's response. Beginning with the lowest dose provides some assurance to parents, who may be reluctant to consider pharmacotherapy. Parents and children should be advised of common side effects, such as anorexia and insomnia, which occur with some but not all patients, and plan accordingly. Parents may prefer to give the first dose on a weekend so they can monitor both positive responses as well as potential side effects. Routine and ongoing visits are critical to monitor progress, reinforce patient and family education about ADHD, pharmacotherapy, and other components of the treatment. Parent and teacher progress forms, such as the Vanderbilt Rating Scale follow-up form, are useful in monitoring changes in behavior (Wolraich et al., 2003). Weight, height, blood pressure, and pulse should be monitored at each visit. After one to two weeks, if no change in behavior is noted and no significant side effects emerge, increase the stimulant dose slowly and incrementally, such as Concerta 18 mg to Concerta 27 mg. Once the child has demonstrated positive behavioral changes, the dose can be maintained and periodically reevaluated. Stimulants are Schedule II controlled substances and refills are not allowed. However, the DEA rules (http://www.deadiversion.usdoj.gov/fed_regs/rules/2006/fr0906.htm) permit prescribers to give multiple prescriptions up to a 90-day supply. This option is appropriate once a child is stabilized on a stimulant dose and the management plan is effective. Importance of monitoring over time as the child grows and develops is countered by the realization that ADHD is a chronic condition. New challenges emerge for the APN as children mature to adolescence and adulthood and must make choices about use of medication, dosing, and continuing treatment.

A useful guide for managing ADHD resulted from the Texas Children's Medication Algorithm Project (Pliszka et al., 2006). Revised several times, the project began in 1998 to develop an algorithm for choosing ADHD treatments. Guidelines for treating conditions comorbid with ADHD were also developed. The algorithm general guidelines for managing ADHD treatment are included in Figure 7.1.

Case Exemplars

Case 1

At a five-year-old well-child visit, Joseph's mom reported that he was very active and had a short attention span. He was a healthy, well-developed, and happy child. Mother decided to monitor his behavior at school and home. The same symptoms were reported at the six- and seven-year well-child visits. By age seven years, Mom had successfully advocated for additional school services although

no indication of a learning disorder was revealed. Mom stated that she did not want to consider any additional screening or treatment. At the eight-year visit, Mom reported that Joseph was having difficulty concentrating, he had a diagnosed learning disorder, and his behavior, primarily "talking back" and "not listening," was an issue at school and home. His parents were ready to discuss his symptoms in depth. Based on his symptoms, comprehensive assessment, and screening, he was diagnosed as positive for ADHD.

Joseph was an only child. His mother was treated for stomach cancer at age forty years and expected that she would never conceive. She gave birth to Joseph a year later. He was born at twenty-eight weeks' gestation and was discharged from the neonatal intensive care unit three months later. Joseph received birth-to-three services primarily for a language and communication disorder. His parents were married and in a stable relationship. They were competent loving parents. Family history was negative for mental health disorders.

Both parents initially met with the primary APN alone. The mother was prepared for the diagnosis and beginning a comprehensive management plan including medication. The father was fearful that stimulants would lead to drug dependence. The pediatric APN explained the action of the drugs, safety profile, and evidence. In addition, she described the potential consequence of not treating ADHD—that is, the increased likelihood of school failure and drug or alcohol dependence due to low self-esteem and frustration with personal and work relationships.

Once both parents were in agreement, Joseph joined his parents for a discussion of the diagnosis and plan for pharmacotherapy, behavior management, and communication with school personnel. Concerta 18 mg once a day was started on a Saturday morning. A follow-up visit was scheduled each week for four weeks. The parents and teachers reported some improvements in attention and behavior during the first two weeks. The dose was increased to Concerta 27 mg by week three. Follow-up assessments (Vanderbilt) by the parents, teacher, and child were consistent in reporting reduction of impulsivity and prolonged attention. No significant side effects were reported. Parents and child were pleased with progress and they noted that there was less tension in their relationship. Once stabilized, quarterly visits with the primary care pediatric APN were scheduled with continued monitoring of progress.

Case 2

At a three-year well-child visit, Juan's mother reported that he was very active and continued to have temper tantrums. His father was incarcerated two years previously for selling drugs and a new sibling was born.

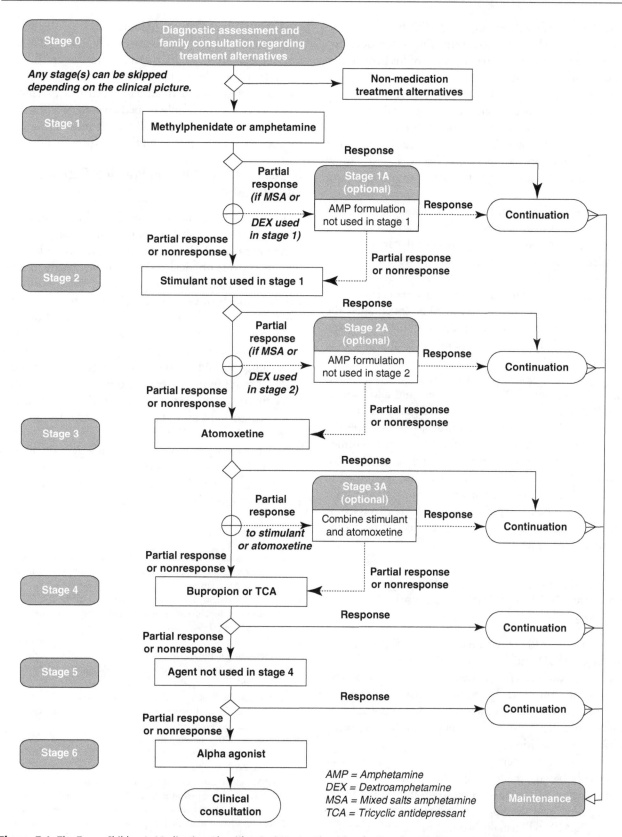

Figure 7.1 The Texas Children's Medication Algorithm Project: An Algorithm for Treating ADHD. Reprinted from Pliszka et al., 2006, with permission from Elsevier.

A stepfather was actively involved with both children. The pediatric APN provided counseling about developmental expectations and management of his behavior in view of family transitions.

Juan was the first child of an eighteen-year-old single mother. Though young, she was mature and appropriately attached to Juan. She was not aware of any family history of mental health problems but did report that his father did not complete high school. Her family provided consistent loving support to the mother and children.

By five years of age, Juan's inattention, impulsivity, and temper tantrums increased in frequency and teachers urged his mother to contact his health care provider. Vanderbilt scores by both the mother and teacher were positive for ADHD and ODD. A plan of care included Concerta 18 mg daily and behavior management at home and school. The pediatric APN encouraged the mother to contact a child guidance clinic to manage this child's intense outbursts. Juan and his mother were followed weekly for six weeks. At two-week intervals, dosing was increased with little effect. Medication was changed to Adderall XR 10 mg. The child and mother enrolled in weekly therapy at the child guidance clinic.

During the next two years, due to the complexity of this child's symptoms, a child psychiatrist assumed management with the therapist. The pediatric APN discontinued managing the medications but continued to monitor his progress with his mother at well visits. He continued to be managed on Adderall XR 10 mg in the morning and at noon with positive effects reported by mom and teacher.

Role Differentiation Between Primary Care and Child Psychiatric Advanced Practice Nurses

Primary care APNs are educationally well prepared to manage ADHD and it is a practice expectation for the nurse practitioner. The presence of comorbid psychiatric conditions usually requires consultation with a psychiatric APN. The complexity of the comorbid conditions may determine solo management by the psychiatric nurse practitioner.

The ultimate determination of who manages care is usually based on the complexity of the ADHD and the response of the child/adolescent and family to the therapeutic plan developed to manage symptoms. The pediatric APN will usually begin stimulant treatment. If ADHD symptoms do not resolve or if disorders other than ADHD are diagnostically present, it is advised that the pediatric APN seek referral, with resulting psychiatric evaluation, followed by a management plan. Psychiatric medications, including stimulants, may become the sole responsibility of the psychiatric APN. They may also transfer back to the pediatric APN when the child is stable. Either way, the pediatric APN should continue to monitor progress and treatment. Even if a psychiatric referral occurs, the family or pediatric APN will still be providing well-child care and would resume management of the ADHD if the child's condition stabilizes.

Implications for Nursing Practice, Research, and Education

ADHD occurs commonly in pediatric populations and is generally responsive to both pharmacological and nonpharmacological interventions. APNs, who frequently provide physical and mental health care to these children, are in an excellent position to practice comprehensive models of care utilizing both primary care and child psychiatry specialties. The seamless transition back and forth between these two nursing specialties as determined by the patient's presenting problems and degree of stability should be the ultimate goal of treatment and will result in improved care outcomes. All pediatric APNs need to have extensive knowledge of this disorder, its comorbidities, and evidence-based interventions. Nurses are in an excellent position to research the most effective treatment models, especially ADHD that is comorbid with other conditions requiring combination treatment. The goal is always provision of excellent care resulting in improved functioning.

References

American Psychiatric Association. (1968). *Diagnostic and statistical manual of mental disorders (2nd ed.)*. Washington, D.C.: American Psychiatric Association.

American Psychiatric Association. (2010, September 21). DSM V: The future of psychiatric diagnosis. Retrieved from http://www.dsm5.org/Pages/Default.aspx

Armenteros, J.L., Lewis, J.E., & Davalos, M. (2007). Risperidone augmentation for attention-deficit/hyperactivity disorder. *Journal of the American Academy of Child Adolescent Psychiatry, 46*, 558–565.

Armstrong, M.B., & Nettleton, S.K. (2004). Attention deficit hyperactivity disorder and preschool children. *Seminars in Speech and Language, 25*, 225–232.

Barkley, R.A. (2004). Driving impairments in teens and adults with attention-deficit/hyperactivity disorder. *Psychiatric Clinics of North America, 27*, 233–260.

Biederman, J., Faraone, S.V., Keenan, K., Benjamin, J., Krifcher, B., Moor, C., Sprich-Buckminster, S., Ugaglia, K., Jellinek, M.S., & Steingard, R. (1992). Further evidence for family-genetic risk factors in attention deficit hyperactivity disorder: patterns of comorbidity in probands and relatives psychiatrically and pediatrically referred samples. *Archives of General Psychiatry, 49*, 728–738.

Biederman, J., Faraone, S.V., Mick, E., Spencer, T., Wilens, T., Kiely, K., Guite, J., Ablon, J. S., Reed, E., & Warburton, R. (1995). High risk for attention deficit hyperactivity disorder among children of parents with childhood onset of the disorder: a pilot study. *American Journal of Psychiatry, 152*, 431–435.

Biederman, J., Monuteaux, M.C., Mick, E., Spencer, T., Wilens, T.E., Silva, J.M., Snyder, L.E., & Faraone, S.V. (2006). Young adult outcome of attention deficit hyperactivity disorder: a controlled 10 year follow-up study. *Psychological Medicine, 36*, 167–179.

Bowen, R., Chavira, D.A., Baily, K., Stein, M.T., & Stein, M.B. (2008). Nature of anxiety comorbid with attention deficit hyperactivity disorder in children from a pediatric primary care setting. *Psychiatry Research, 157*, 201–208.

Braun, J.M., Kahn, R.S., Froehlich, T., Auinger, P., & Lanphear, B.P. (2006). Exposures to environmental tosxicants and attention-deficit-hyperactivity disorder in U.S. children. *Environmental Health Perspectives, 114*, 1904–1909.

Castellanos, F.X., Margulies, D.S., Kelly, C., Uddin, L.Q., Ghaffari, M., Kirsch, A., Shaw, D., Shehzad, Z., DiMartino, A., Biswal, B., Sonuga-Barke, E.J.S., Rotrosen, J., Addler, L.D., & Milham, M.P. (2008). Cingulate-precuneus interactions: A new locus of dysfunction in adult attention-deficit/hyperactivity disorder. *Biological Psychiatry, 63*, 332–337.

Connor, D., Glatt, S.J., Lopez, I.D., Jackson, D., & Melloni, R. (2002). Psychopharmacology and aggression: I, a meta-analysis of stimulant effects on overt/covert aggression-related behaviors in ADHD. *Journal of the American Academy of Child and Adolescent Psychiatry, 41*, 253–261.

Connor, D.F., & Meltzer, B.M. (2006). *Pediatric psychopharmacology fast facts.* New York: W. W. Norton & Co.

Dell, M.L. (2010) Ethnic, cultural, and religious issues. In M.K. Dulcan (Ed.), *Dulcan's Textbook of child and adolescent psychiatry* (pp. 517–529). Washington, D.C.: American Psychiatric Publishing, Inc.

Dopheide, J.A. (2006). Recognizing and treating depression in children and adolescents. *American Journal of Health-System Pharmacy, 63*, 233–243.

Ebaugh, F., & Franklin, G. (1923). Neuropsychiatric sequelae of acute epidemic encephalitis in children. *American Journal of Diseases of the Child, 25*, 89–97.

Fair, D.A., Posner, J., Nagel, B.J., Bathula, D., Dias, T.G., Mills, K.L., Blythe, M.S., Giwa, A., Schmitt, C.F., & Nigg, J.T. Atypical default network connectivity in youth with attention-deficit/hyperactivity disorder. *Biological Psychiatry.* doi:10.1016/j.biopsych.2010.07.003

Goez, H., Back-Bennet, O., & Zelnik, N. (2007). Differential stimulant response on attention in children with comorbid anxiety and oppositional defiant disorder. *Journal of Child Neurology, 22*, 538–542.

Harpin, V.A. (2005). The effect of ADHD on the life of an individual, their family, and community from preschool to adult life. *Archives of Disease in Childhood, 90(suppl. 1)*, 12–17.

Jankovic, J. (2001). Medical progress: Tourette's syndrome. *New England Journal of Medicine, 345*, 1184–1192.

Kessler, R.C., Adler, L., Barkley, R., Biederman, J., Conners, C.K., Demler, O., Faraone, S.V., Greenhill, L.L., Howes, M.J., Secnik, K., Spencer, T., Ustun, T.B., Walters, E.E., & Zaslavsky, A.M. (2006). The prevalence and correlates of adult ADHD in the United States: Results from the National Comorbidity Survey Replication. *American Journal of Psychiatry, 163*, 716–723.

Konrad, K., & Eickhoff, S.B. (2010). Is the ADHD brain wired differently? A review on structural and functional connectivity in attention deficit hyperactivity disorder. *Human Brain Mapping, 31(6)*, 904–916.

Kowatch, R.A., & DelBello, M.P. (2006). Pediatric bipolar disorder: Emerging diagnostic and treatment approaches. *Child and Adolescent Psychiatric Clinics of North America, 15*, 73–108.

Kreppner, J.M., O'Connor, T.G., & Rutter, M. (2001). Can inattention/overactivity be an institutional deprivation syndrome? *Journal of Abnormal Child Psychology, 29*, 513–528.

Linnet, K.M., Dalsgaard, S., Obel, C., Wisborg, K., Henriksen, T.B., Rodriguez, A., Kotimaa, A., Moilanen, I., Thomsen, P.H., Olsen, J., & Jarvelin, M.R. (2003). Maternal lifestyle factors in pregnancy risk of attention deficit hyperactivity disorder and associated behaviors: review of the current evidence. *American Journal of Psychiatry, 160*, 1028–1040.

Mataz, L.S., Paramore, C., & Prasad, M. (2005). A review of the economic burden of ADHD. *Cost Effectiveness and Resource Allocation, 3*, 5. doi 10.1186/1478-7547-3-5

Mick, E., Biederman, J., Faraone, S.V., Sayer, J., & Kleinman, S. (2002). Case-control study of attention-deficit hyperactivity disorder and maternal smoking, alcohol use, and drug use during pregnancy. *Journal of the American Academy of Child and Adolescent Psychiatry, 41*, 378–385.

Murray-Close, D., Hoza, B., Hinshaw, S.P., Arnold, L.E., Swanson, J., Jensen, P.S., Hechtman, L., & Wells, K. (2010). Developmental processes in peer problems of children with attention-deficit/hyperactivity disorder in The Multimodal Treatment Study of Children With ADHD: Developmental cascades and vicious cycles. *Development and Psychopathology, 22*, 785–802.

Pine, D., Shaffer, D., & Schonfeld, I. (1993). Persistent emotional disorder in children with neurological soft signs. *Journal of the American Academy of Child and Adolescent Psychiatry, 32*, 1229–1236.

Pliszka, S.R. (2010). Attention-deficit/hyperactivity disorder. In M.K. Dulcan (Ed.), *Dulcan's Textbook of child and adolescent psychiatry* (pp. 205–221). Washington, D.C.: American Psychiatric Publishing.

Pliszka, S.R., & AACAP Child and Adolescent Work Group on Quality Issues. (2007). Practice parameter for the assessment and treatment of children and adolescents with attention-deficit-hyperactivity disorder. *Journal of the American Academy of Child and Adolescent Psychiatry, 46*, 894–921.

Pliszka, S.R., Crismon, M.L., Hughes, C., Corners, C.K., Emslie, G.J., Jensen, P.S., McCracken, J. T., Swanson, J.M., & Lopez, M. (2006). The Texas children's medication algorithm project: revision of the algorithm for pharmacotherapy of attention-deficit/hyperactivity disorder. *Journal of the American Academy of Child and Adolescent Psychiatry, 46*, 642–657.

Polanczyk, G., de Lima, M.S., Horta, B.L., Biederman, J., & Rohde, L.A. (2007). The worldwide prevalence of ADHD: A systematic review and metaregression analysis. *American Journal of Psychiatry, 164*, 942–948.

Reiff, M.I. & Tippins, S. (2004). *ADHD: A complete and authoritative guide.* Elk Grove Village, IL: American Academy of Pediatrics.

Spencer, T.J., Biederman, J., & Mick, E. (2007). Attention-deficit/hyperactivity disorder: Diagnosis, lifespan, comorbidities, and neurobiology. *Ambulatory Pediatrics, 7(1)*, 73–81.

Stergiakouli, E., & Thapar, A. (2010). Fitting the pieces together: Current research on the genetic basis of attention-deficit/hyperactivity disorder (ADHD). *Neuropsychiatric Disease and Treatment, 6*, 551–560.

Strecker, E., & Ebaugh, F. (1924). Neuropsychiatric sequelae of cerebral trauma in children. *Archives of Neurology and Psychiatry, 12*, 443–453.

The Tourette's Syndrome Study Group. Treatment of ADHD in children with tics: A randomized controlled trial. *Neurology, 58*, 527–535.

Vierhile, A., Robb, A., & Ryan-Krause, P. (2009). Attention deficit/hyperactivity disorder in children and adolescents: Closing diagnostic, communication, and treatment gaps. *Journal of Pediatric Health Care, 23*, S5–S21. doi:10.1016/j.pedhc.2008.10.009

Volkow, N.D., Wang, G., Fowler, J.S., Logan, J., Gerasimov, M., Maynard, L., Ding, Y., Gatley, S.J., Gifford, A., & Franceschi, D. (2001). Therapeutic doses of oral methylphenidate significantly increase extracellular dopamine in the human brain. *Journal of Neuroscience, 21*, RC121.

Weissman, D.H., Roberts, K.C., Visscher, K.M., & Woldorff, M. G. (2006). The neural bases of momentary lapses in attention. *Nature Neuroscience, 9*, 971–978.

Wolraich, M.L., Lambert, W., Doffing, M.A., Bickman, L., Simmons, T., & Worley, K. (2003). Psychometric properties of the Vanderbilt ADHD diagnostic parent rating scale in a referred population. *Journal of Pediatric Psychology, 28*, 559–568.

Woodard, R. (2006). The diagnosis and medical treatment of ADHD in children and adolescents in primary care: A practical guide. *Pediatric Nursing, 32*, 363–370.

Young, S., & Amarasinghe, J.M. (2010). Practitioner review: Non-pharmacological treatments for ADHD: A lifespan approach. *The Journal of Child Psychology and Psychiatry, 51*, 116–133. doi:10.1111/j.1469-7610.2009.02191.x

8

Anxiety Disorders

Geraldine S. Pearson and Kathleen Kenney-Riley

Objectives

After reading this chapter, APNs will be able to

1. Describe normal developmental stages from infancy through adolescence that are associated with anxiety.
2. Define the epidemiology, prevalence statistics, and theories of etiology related to anxiety disorders.
3. Describe types, common presenting signs, and symptoms of anxiety disorders in children and adolescents.
4. Discuss comorbid conditions associated with anxiety.
5. Define pharmacological and nonpharmacological evidence-based interventions.
6. Differentiate roles of primary care practitioners and advanced practice psychiatric nurses in the diagnosis and treatment of children and adolescents with anxiety.

Introduction

"Anxiety" is a broad term referring to the brain's response to perceived or actual danger. It can be characterized by fear, concern, or dread related to a specific event, or it can be pervasive (Gregory & Eley, 2007). The capacity for the basic emotion of anxiety is present in infancy and persists throughout childhood. Anxiety is a normal part of life and is experienced to some degree by all people. Anxious reactions can range from mild to severe (Beesdo, Knappe, & Pine, 2009). Anxiety disorders occur when anxiety becomes so severe that it interrupts and/or disrupts the child's ability to function. When anxiety disorders present in early childhood, the result may be disruption of the normal growth and developmental trajectory. This sets a course of problems that can extend into adulthood for these children. It is challenging for advanced practice nurses (APNs) to differentiate anxiety that is a normal part of development from that which has the potential to disrupt functioning. Anxiety disorders in adulthood have nearly always had their symptomatic roots in childhood or adolescence, lending credence to the need for early identification and intervention.

Anxiety can be characterized by two distinctly different entities of worry and fear. Worry "involves anxious apprehension and thoughts focused on the possibility of negative future events, while fear is related to the response to threat or danger that is perceived as actual or impending" (Connolly & Suarez, 2010, p. 299). Nurses are likely to see children and adolescents presenting for basic well-child care or psychiatric care who have symptoms of anxiety. Again, the challenge is distinguishing between developmentally normal worries about life and worries that debilitate and inhibit accomplishment of normal developmental milestones.

Child and Adolescent Behavioral Health: A Resource for Advanced Practice Psychiatric and Primary Care Practitioners in Nursing,
First Edition. Edited by Edilma L. Yearwood, Geraldine S. Pearson, and Jamesetta A. Newland.
© 2012 John Wiley & Sons, Inc. Published 2012 by John Wiley & Sons, Inc.

Anxiety disorders are a common presenting problem in pediatric primary care and within child/adolescent psychiatric practices. Many children and adolescents with anxiety disorders are psychosocially complex with associated family difficulties, exposure to trauma, and/or negative life events. While symptoms can range from transient and mild to extreme and debilitating, they are rarely simple disorders to treat and often are associated with comorbid psychiatric disorders. Conditions such as attention deficit hyperactivity disorder (ADHD), depression, oppositional defiant disorder, and motor tics can be accompanied by varying degrees of anxiety.

Anxiety disorders diagnosed in the Diagnostic and Statistical Manual of Mental Disorders (DSM-IV-TR) (American Psychiatric Association, 2000) include separation anxiety disorder, generalized anxiety disorder, obsessive-compulsive disorder, and social phobia in children and adolescents. Additional categories include specific phobias, agoraphobia, selective mutism, and panic attacks. Post-traumatic stress disorders are also part of the anxiety spectrum of symptoms. There is considerable heterogeneity in diagnostic subsets of anxiety disorders. This can be challenging to the primary care provider (PCP) who is trying to assess the child or adolescent who presents with symptoms of anxiety and to identify its cause and specific manifestation.

This chapter describes anxiety as it is manifested across the pediatric life span. Evidence-based assessments and psychosocial interventions and associated psychopharmacological treatments are presented. The chapter concludes with a case exemplar that illustrates chapter concepts and nursing interventions. Implications for nursing practice, education, and research are discussed.

Normative Anxiety as Part of Development

APNs who see children with anxiety have to carefully distinguish normative, transient worries and fears that are developmentally appropriate from anxiety disorders that are a constellation of symptoms interfering with functioning. Connelly and Suarez (2010) noted that common fears among infants include loud noises, being dropped, stranger anxiety, and, later, separation from the caregiver. Stranger anxiety begins around seven months of age, when infants are able to recognize persons who are different than their normal caregiver. Separation anxiety represents an infant's inability to recognize that even if his or her parent is not visible, they still exist. Issues such as separation anxiety can be concerning for parents; thus, the APN must be adept at understanding when separation anxiety is part of the normal development of late infancy versus when it becomes pathological. Separation anxiety should be resolved in children around the time of the preschool years before they prepare for school.

As babies move onto toddlerhood, common fears include fears of monsters or darkness. Toddlers who previously seemed fascinated by animals may now become anxious around animals such as dogs, demonstrating significant fear. Preschoolers may worry about physical well-being, pleasing their parents and teachers, as well as natural events such as bad weather. Most anxiety reactions are transient and considered a normative part of preschool development (Connolly & Suarez, 2010).

The school-aged years bring about a time when children must separate from their parents, spending more and more time away from their main source of support. While some anxiety regarding starting school is normal, school anxiety can become severe in a small subset of children. Anxiety-related school avoidance occurs in school-aged children when they are excessively worried about grades, being disliked by others, and/or have persistent separation anxiety. Children who are at risk for significant school anxiety include children with a shy or sensitive temperament, those with overprotective parents, or children who are being teased by other children (Phillips, 1968). Additionally, school-aged children are now able to understand what others think of them, which may be different from how they think of or see themselves. This cognitive ability results in fear of what their friends or teachers think of them. They also begin to worry about their appearance and abilities compared to their peers. Older school-aged children may also have fears about the dark, peers, school, and sports performance. These children develop anxiety regarding scary things they see on television or hear about from others, such as natural disasters or accidents.

In adolescence, the most common sources of anxiety involve social competence, evaluation, and psychological well-being (Albano & Hayward, 2004). Additional fears include issues regarding sexual development, uncertainty regarding sexual identity, and fear of not being accepted by those they find attractive. Late adolescence is a time when children are told they must begin to think about who they will become later in life. This pressure to choose a career, decide on a college, or get a job can result in adolescent worry and anxiety.

While fear and anxieties are common among different age groups, PCPs must recognize that in certain children and adolescents these fears/anxieties become so great that they interrupt the child's normal activities and development. PCPs should ask children during health care visits what they worry about and assess children for signs of distress and anxieties that are overwhelming to them. During the visit, it is important for the provider to ask the child how he or she deals with their anxiety and to whom they turn for help and support. When these anxieties interrupt their daily functioning, it is imperative to provide these children with appropriate evaluation and treatment.

Epidemiology and Prevalence of Anxiety Disorders

An international review of epidemiological studies regarding diagnosed rates of anxiety among male and female preadolescent children of different races and ethnicities noted that the prevalence had a wide range from 2.6% to 41.2% (Cartwright-Hatton, McNicol, & Doubleday, 2006). The prevalence of generalized anxiety disorders across all ages and genders is 3% with a lifetime prevalence of 4% to 6%. Estimates for development of any type of anxiety disorder in one's lifetime are 15% to 20%. While strongly influenced by assessment and diagnostic variance (Beesdo et al., 2009), lifetime rates across gender and ethnicity for developing any type of anxiety disorder are estimated to also be between 15% and 20%. The mean age of onset for anxiety disorders in children is 8.8 years old; twice as many females are diagnosed as males (Costello, Egger, & Angold, 2004). As the most common psychiatric disorders in children and adolescents, they are also the disorders that can precede manifestation of other developmental and psychiatric difficulties, including disruptive behavior disorders and depression (Connolly & Suarez, 2010). All of these prevalence rates are impacted by the ability of the provider to identify and diagnosis patients with anxiety disorders. As a precursor to other psychiatric disorders, it is imperative to address pediatric anxiety when it is identified.

Genetics and Environmental Risk Factors

Anxiety disorders can be present in families; there is documented heritable risk along with psychosocial factors that determine the transmission of anxiety disorders in families (Gregory & Eley, 2007; Moore, Whaley, & Sigman, 2004). Whaley, Pinto, and Sigman (1999) found that clinically anxious mothers had higher levels of criticism and a tendency to catastrophize or predict dire outcomes, modeling a fearful cognitive style for their children. Moore et al. found that mothers of anxious children were less warm toward their children, regardless of their own anxiety. They also found a tendency for mothers of anxious children to be overprotective. They raised the question of whether a child's temperament shaped parental behavior or parental behavior resulted in anxiety among children, suggesting that familial anxiety is a complex multifaceted bidirectional process.

Genetics are not the sole cause of anxiety disorders in children. Environmental factors are significant variables that can result in increased rates of anxiety disorders. Parental rearing style can support the development of anxiety disorders in children. Research has found that parents with more negative affect and criticism toward children resulted in higher rates of anxiety in the child. Leis and Mendelson (2010) found that maternal major depression resulted in greater risk for offspring developing a lifetime mood or anxiety disorder. They suggested that major and minor parental depressive symptoms put offspring at psychiatric risk. Additionally, researchers found parents who worried more about their child exerted more control over her or him, such as not allowing the child time to experience certain anxiety-producing situations. This deprived these children of the ability to develop effective coping skills, resulting in an increased risk of developing anxiety (Lindhurst et al., 2009). Children who have a diminished sense of personal control can become anxious when faced with unpredictable situations (Suarez, Bennett, Goldstein, & Barlow, 2009).

Research has also demonstrated that children who grew up in families with a parent or sibling who was chronically ill had higher rates of anxiety both during childhood and as an adult (Batte, Watson, & Amess, 2006). Other risk factors can include temperamental and personality traits and psychosocial adversities such as loss, abuse, or parental divorce (Beesdo et al., 2009), as well as life events such as health problems and poverty (Hirshfeld-Becker, Micco, Simoes, & Henin, 2008). Being rejected by peers was found to make the individual more prone to social anxiety. In contrast, being teased or bullied did not predispose children as highly to anxiety disorders (Storch, Masia-Warner, Crisp, & Klein, 2005).

Anxiety disorders in children and adolescents are likely the result of a complicated meshing of biologic, personality, and psychosocial risk factors. Egger and Angold (2006) found that a childhood diagnosis of anxiety was associated with greater risk of developing a range of psychiatric disorders across the life span. Thus, APNs need to realize that environmental factors also play a significant role in the type of anxiety disorder that may develop, the degree of psychopathology, and the resulting degree of developmental impairment. It is important to recognize that these disorders can continue throughout the child's life if not addressed early.

Role of Trauma in the Development of Anxiety

Children experiencing childhood adversities, including trauma such as abuse and neglect, have been found to be at risk for developing psychopathology, including anxiety disorders (Benjet, Borges, & Medina-Mora, 2010). Children who experience traumas such as early loss of a parent, living with a mentally ill parent, and/or loss of a brother or sister suddenly have been found to be at increased risk of anxiety disorders both in childhood and as an adult (Heim & Nemerof, 2001). As PCPs evaluate children who have experienced a trauma of any kind, they must recognize the significant impact trauma can have on the development of anxiety disorders, assess for symptoms of anxiety in these children, and provide access to support for these children as early as possible. Children showing symptoms of anxiety after trauma should be referred for psychological care as soon as possible in order to intervene before the anxiety disrupts the child's life and becomes pathological.

Types and Symptoms of Anxiety Disorders

Anxiety disorders occur within a context that produces anxiety symptoms (Sakolsky & Birmaher, 2008). While assessing symptoms, the APN must consider whether presenting anxiety symptoms are situation specific or generalized. The most widely identified childhood anxiety disorders are generalized anxiety disorder (GAD), obsessive-compulsive disorder (OCD), social phobia, selective mutism (SM), panic disorder, specific phobia, separation anxiety disorder (SAD), and school refusal behavior (APA, 2000). Each will be specifically discussed.

Generalized anxiety disorder: GAD is characterized by "chronic, excessive worry in a number of areas such as schoolwork, social interactions, family, health/safety, world events, and natural disasters with at least one associated somatic symptom" (American Academy of Child and Adolescent Psychiatry [AACAP], 2007, p. 268). *Exemplar:* Kate, age twelve years, vomits her breakfast on the days she is going to have a written test or oral classroom presentation. She is fearful that she will forget the studied information and fail the test.

Obsessive-compulsive disorder: OCD involves the presence of either obsessions/worries or compulsions/rituals. It usually begins before puberty, affects more boys than girls, and can involve secretive washing or checking rituals (Geller, 2010). *Exemplar:* Juan, age six years, washes his hands three times—when he touches the doorknob and both before and after using the toilet. He states that he is afraid he will get sick if he doesn't wash his hands; his grandmother was recently hospitalized for an infection.

Social phobia: Social phobia involves feeling scared or uncomfortable in one or more social settings or situations where the individual is required to perform. Exemplar: Tony, age seven years, refuses to go outside and play with peers. His teacher reports that he is reticent to speak up in class and avoids unstructured, social situations.

Selective mutism: SM, part of social phobia, is a failure to speak aloud in a social situation. These individuals may whisper or gesture with peers or adults. *Exemplar:* Serena, age seven years, has refused to speak at school or at home for the past two years. With no clear precipitant or trauma, she communicates in monosyllabic whispers to her parents only.

Panic disorder: Panic disorder involves unexpected but recurrent and intense episodes of fear (AACAP, 2007). Panic disorder may occur with or without agoraphobia, an anxiety of social situations or places where escape might be difficult. This agoraphobia may inhibit activities of daily life and restrict the child's or adolescent's environment, causing impairment in functioning (Connor & Meltzer, 2006). *Exemplar:* Anne, age thirteen years, is frightened of large groups of people. She refuses to go to the grocery or mall but manages to go to school, although she is unable to attend large school assemblies. She reports sweating, rapid pulse, and feeling like she will physically die in a group setting.

Specific phobia: Specific phobias involve "excessive, specific, persistent fear of a stimulus that is then avoided or endured with significant distress" (Connor & Meltzer, 2006, p. 411). These include reactions that are disproportionate to the situation and are not logical. Insects, blood, clowns, or thunderstorms are all examples of phobia-inducing objects or situations. *Exemplar:* Joe, age ten years, is frightened of elevators and refuses to ride in them. He expresses an extreme fear of being enclosed in a moving "box."

Separation anxiety disorder: SADs involve a high level of fear, worry, and anxiety around separation from home or the primary attachment. The fear of separation must be considered in light of the child's developmental stage (Connor & Meltzer, 2006). For example, separation anxiety is normative in a very young child (younger than six years) but inappropriate for a teenager (Connolly & Suarez, 2010). *Exemplar:* Tom, age fifteen years, has not attended school for the past two years despite juvenile justice interventions around truancy. His mother has chronic emphysema, and he refuses to leave her.

School refusal: School refusal is also part of social phobia and involves fear of going to school. *Exemplar:* Ed, age five years, cries and clings to his father's leg when taken to kindergarten. Dad has been unsuccessful in getting him to attend a full session of kindergarten.

Assessment of Anxiety

APNs must recognize that anxiety disorders may present in primary care offices as common physical or behavioral complaints seen in children and adolescents that represent many actual physical conditions. Therefore, APNs must become adept at understanding common symptoms that may represent anxiety disorders to ensure that these children are identified and offered treatment as early as possible. Children with anxiety disorders often present with physical symptoms such as headache, abdominal pain, and sleep difficulties. The goal of assessment by any provider is helping the child and parent understand the meaning of the symptoms and to rule out a physical cause unrelated to the anxiety (AACAP, 2007).

Common Presenting Signs and Symptoms of Anxiety

Anxiety in childhood can present with many common signs and symptoms seen in primary care offices. The APN must be able to recognize when symptoms represent somaticizing rather than a specific physical condition. Somatic complaints that interfere with daily functioning are the hallmark features of anxiety disorders in children (Ginsburg, Riddle, & Davies, 2006). Common symptoms of anxiety include frequent recurrent abdominal pain, muscle aches and pains, chest pain, palpitations, sweating, dizziness, shortness of breath, and headaches (Dufton, Dunn, & Compas, 2009; Ginsburg et al., 2006; Last, 2002). Anxious symptoms can also be manifested as nonspecific complaints such as irritability, somatic complaints, acting out behaviors, and frequent crying (Connor & Meltzer, 2006). Additionally, often these patients have other psychosocial pressures or demands that make the diagnostic picture cloudy. While many of these symptoms may be signs of an actual physical condition, when the health care provider finds no evidence of physical findings consistent with a specific diagnosis, anxiety must be considered as a possible cause.

When children present with any of these complaints along with frequent absences from school and/or an inability to perform routine daily activities, it is of utmost importance that the APN consider anxiety as a possible cause of these symptoms. Making the diagnosis of anxiety disorders in children and adolescents is not always clear cut. APNs have to keep in mind that children and young adolescents may not recognize their symptoms of anxiety and may struggle with reporting how they feel. Additionally, many of the physical symptoms, including vomiting, abdominal pain, and/or frequent headaches, are concerning to many providers because of possible physical causes, making the possibility that anxiety is the cause even more difficult to identify.

The goals of assessment by any APN are to help the child and parent understand the meaning of the symptoms and to rule out a physical cause unrelated to the

anxiety (AACAP, 2007). When an APN is presented with these symptoms in the face of a normal physical exam and normal test results, anxiety must be considered. APNs should be sure to include in all of their assessments a comprehensive history that addresses possible sources of stress and anxiety in the child and/or family.

The following questions can help guide the assessment:

1. What are the symptoms?
2. Are the symptoms stimulus specific, spontaneous, or anticipatory?
3. Are the symptoms out of the realm of normal functioning?
4. When did the presenting symptoms begin to cause problems for the youngster?
5. How is this influencing daily functioning? Assess the specific spheres of home, school, occupation, interpersonal, and social.
6. Who is expressing concerns about this child or adolescent? Assess teachers, day care providers, other family members, or probation officers (if the juvenile justice system is involved).

When evaluating these children, the answers to these questions can help guide the APN in determining the cause of somatic complaints. Symptoms that happen more often on school days than on weekends or those that seem to be stimulus specific should alert the provider to a possible anxiety disorder. Symptoms that appear to be severe in view of a normal physical exam and lab tests are concerning for anxiety. Additionally, when symptoms influence the child's or adolescent's daily functioning, an anxiety disorder should be included as a possible diagnosis. In trying to discriminate normal, adaptive, and protective fear from pathological anxiety, the APN will find that pathological anxiety is more diffuse, lacks specificity, and occurs in the absence of a stimulus (Krain et al., 2007). While many of these symptoms are common complaints among children and adolescents, when the cause is an anxiety disorder, the exam and lab results will be normal. APNs must be aware of the common somatic complaints seen in anxiety disorders in order to accurately identify and diagnose this condition and provide appropriate treatment for these children and adolescents.

Younger children may not be able to verbalize their symptoms of anxiety; therefore, the APN should observe for behavioral symptoms such as crying, irritability, avoidance, clingy behaviors, or somatic complaints (AACAP, 2007). Medical causes of anxiety should be ruled out first. Medical conditions that mimic anxiety include hyperthyroidism, asthma, seizure, caffeinism, migraines, hypoglycemia, and lead intoxication.

Prescription drugs such as antiasthmatics, steroids, sympathomimetics, and selective serotonin reuptake inhibitors can also induce anxiety (Krain et al., 2007).

Diagnostic Screening Instruments

Once the APN considers that a child or an adolescent patient may be suffering from anxiety, he or she may use one of the available screening tools to aid in making the final diagnosis. Assessment is best accomplished with a careful assessment of all symptoms combined with standardized symptom measures. While a variety of standardized instruments exists for evaluating anxiety in children and adolescents, none are comprehensive enough to fully evaluate this disorder (Beesdo et al., 2009). Beginning with open-ended questions is the best way to begin assessing anxiety in a child or adolescent, followed by use of standardized instruments that confirm or deny a suspected anxiety disorder.

The most commonly used standardized assessments include the MASC (Multidimensional Anxiety Scale for Children), a self-report tool for youngsters aged eight to nineteen years old that is available for purchase for use with children and parents (March, Parker, Sullivan, Stallings, & Conners, 1997). The clinician-rated PARS (Pediatric Anxiety Rating Scale) is for children aged six to seventeen years. Both of these tools measure anxiety severity and are sensitive to symptom changes (Myers & Winters, 2002). The PARS is available for free online. The Screen for Child Anxiety Related Emotional Disorders (SCARED) scale is a forty-one-item self-report questionnaire that is administered to both the child and parent (Birmaher et al., 1999). Child and parent versions can be purchased online. Also useful in identifying pediatric anxiety and symptom changes is the CBCL (Child Behavior Checklist), available in a parent form, a youth self-report form, and a teacher form (Achenbach, 2001). In addition, the Anxiety Disorders Interview Schedule for DSM-IV–Child Version is another anxiety-specific interview tool for assessing children (Silverman & Albano, 1996). Standardized rating scales should never be used alone to diagnose anxiety disorders but are a useful adjunct to open-ended interviewing available to primary providers.

Making the Diagnosis

While APNs may not feel comfortable making the final diagnosis of anxiety disorder, one should be able to identify those children whose symptoms are related to anxiety and refer them appropriately to a psychiatric provider. In evaluating all children, APNs must be cognizant of common complaints that may represent anxiety as well as understand normal developmental anxieties of children. When presented with a child with physical complaints with no identifiable physical diagnosis, anxiety must be part of the differential. Use of approved tools for identifying anxiety can help the provider in assessing these children. Discussion of possible stressors in the child or family can aid in making the diagnosis as well. APNs should interview the child alone when considering anxiety as a possible diagnosis because children may not feel free to discuss their worries when parents are in the room. Additionally, if abuse is causing the anxiety, the child may be unable to discuss the abuse with the parent present. The primary provider should also interview the parent(s) without the child present to assess for any stressors within or outside the family that may be impacting the child. If no cause is found for any of the child's complaints, APNs must consider anxiety as a possible diagnosis even if the child and parent deny any source of anxiety.

APNs providing primary health care should refer any child or adolescent with sustained or complex symptoms of anxiety for a full evaluation by a psychiatric clinician. Helping parents understand the importance of seeing a psychiatric clinician is an important part of the diagnostic process as often parents are reluctant to seek psychological help. The relationship between the parent and APN is an important aspect of the workup as many parents are unable to accept a psychiatric diagnosis as a cause of their child's problem and refuse to follow up when referred. Using the approved diagnostic tools in the primary care setting may help APNs demonstrate to parents that anxiety is a diagnosis that requires treatment the same way that a throat infection does. The stigma of psychological diagnosis is often a barrier to parents and families seeking and/or following through with treatment. Part of the primary care APN's role is in connecting the families with the appropriate source for care and helping them recognize the importance of getting psychological help for their child in order to promote the child's optimal health and well-being.

Comorbidities of Anxiety Disorder with Other Psychiatric Disorders

The most diagnostically challenging patients are those who present with unclear symptoms of anxiety that are interfering with functioning or anxiety that, while defined, are comorbid with other psychiatric disorders. There is a high rate of comorbidity between anxiety and other psychiatric disorders (Kendall, Brady, & Verduin, 2001). Depression (Angold & Costello, 1993), ADHD (MTA Cooperative Group, 2001), oppositional defiant disorder, and learning disorders (Manassis & Monga, 2001) are commonly comorbid with anxiety disorders. Additional comorbid conditions include panic disorders, selective mutism, and separation anxiety disorder (Last & Strauss, 1989; Warren, Umylny, Aron, & Simmens, 2006). The risk of developing alcohol abuse in adolescence is increased after experiencing a childhood anxiety disorder (Schuckit & Hesselbrock, 1994).

The issue of comorbidity is important from a symptom severity standpoint and from the diagnostic complexities presented by a child who suffers from more than two psychiatric disorders. Overlapping symptoms can make accurate diagnosis difficult (AACAP, 2007). Comorbidity, once defined by the APN in primary care settings, might necessitate a referral for more comprehensive psychiatric evaluation.

Models of Treatment

Psychological Management of Anxiety Disorders

Anxiety disorders in childhood are predictors of psychiatric disorders in adolescence and later in life (Bittner et al., 2007). A multimodal treatment approach for pediatric anxiety disorders involves parent and child education about the disorder; consultation with all involved school, health care, and community professionals; and a treatment plan that considers behavioral interventions (AACAP, 2007). The severity and degree of impairment from anxiety symptoms will determine the use of medication management as an adjunct to behavioral/psychological treatment. Anxiety can be a lifelong impairment and may require long-term treatment.

From an evidence-based perspective, the treatment of choice for anxiety in children and adolescents is cognitive-behavioral therapy (CBT) (Compton et al., 2004). Originally, behavior therapy resulted from theoretical frameworks involving classical and operant conditioning. Over time it was increasingly recognized that person-environment interactions were influenced by thinking. The premise of behavior therapy was that changing behaviors would result in altering distressing thoughts and feelings (Compton et al.). Cognitive models work to connect negative self-talk and negative cognitive schemas, while correcting cognitive distortions. Psychiatric APNs teach children a new set of adaptive coping skills for specific symptoms of anxiety. These new coping skills include relaxation training, feeling identification, confronting rather than avoiding fears, and decreasing emotional arousal of anxiety cues (Kendall, 2006). This can include social skills training, assertiveness training, and positive reinforcement. Systematic desensitization, problem-solving skills, and extinction are all part of the skill set that can be taught to an anxious child.

CBT is actually a term that encompasses several models of treatment. Nevertheless, there are five shared premises among most CBT treatment models (Compton et al., 2004). They include:

1. Adherence to the scientist-clinician model, whereby treatments are chosen based on demonstrated evidence or are applied within a case evaluation format to determine efficacy
2. A thorough idiographic assessment (e.g., functional analysis) of target behaviors and the situational, cognitive, and behavioral factors that have established or are managing the symptoms of interest
3. An emphasis on psychoeducation that identifies the specific triggers to the anxiety and the meaning of the anxious symptoms to physical and emotional health
4. Problem-specific treatment interventions designed to ameliorate the symptoms of concern
5. Relapse prevention and generalization training at the end of treatment (p. 930)

Models of CBT treatment are a good choice for managing pediatric anxiety. Understanding the symptoms in the context of the child's life becomes the challenge when planning treatment. The goal is normal development that is not hindered by anxiety symptoms. There are specific interventions for trauma-based anxiety in children and adolescents. Cohen, Mannaino, and Debling (2006) have developed a manualized treatment that includes psychoeducation, parenting skills, relaxation skills, affect expression, and development of coping skills through writing a trauma narrative. Research has found that this model is highly effective in youth with post-traumatic stress disorders. The Coping Cat Workbook (1992) was developed by Philip Kendall and is an excellent manualized treatment lasting sixteen to twenty weeks that APNs can use. It has demonstrated excellent results for treating anxiety in children and adolescents.

Psychotropic Medication Management of Anxiety Disorders

It is strongly recommended that a course of psychosocial treatment be considered for patients with mild to severe symptoms of anxiety prior to initiating medication management. Behavior therapy is seen as the most effective mediator of symptoms and has the highest rate of success (Compton et al., 2004). If the patient has had six to eight weeks of behavior therapy with no resolution of symptoms, has comorbid psychiatric disorders, or has daily impairment of functioning, medication should be considered. Spheres of child assessment include home, school, occupational, interpersonal, and social. Impairment of functioning in three or more of these spheres might necessitate consideration of a medication trial. Consideration of psychotropic medication for anxiety disorders generally occurs after the child and family have participated in CBT or if the symptoms of anxiety are severe and unrelenting and unresponsive to less invasive treatment. Medication is ideally used as an adjunct to CBT and should not be used in isolation.

While APNs and other health care providers may be pressured by family members to prescribe medications for pediatric anxiety disorder symptoms, the decision to medicate anxiety requires careful consideration of several factors. Connor and Meltzer (2006) note the importance of distinguishing anxious symptoms from anxiety syndromes or disorders. Disorders are "clusters of symptoms that exist together over time, have a discrete onset and longitudinal course, cause subjective stress and impairment in functioning, and may have a familial heritability" (p. 411 to 412). Children with some symptoms of anxiety alone should not be medicated; rather, only children who meet the criteria for an anxiety disorder and those who have also tried CBT or are receiving CBT should be prescribed medications (Connor & Meltzer).

When making the decision of whether to medicate, a number of questions should be asked. Are there associated medical conditions that could precipitate the anxiety? Is the anxiety related to a medical condition or is the medical condition part of a generalized anxiety disorder? What medication, herbal supplements, and over-the-counter preparations are the child taking? Herbal supplements and over-the-counter medications may cause symptoms that mimic anxiety, such as heart palpitations or restlessness. Always carefully assess ALL over-the-counter, herbal, and prescribed medication being taken by the child. Additionally, health care providers must inform parents of the potential interactions between antianxiety medications and herbs or over-the-counter medications for those children requiring medications to treat their anxiety. Is there any current or past substance use by the child or family members living in the immediate household? Medications used to treat anxiety disorders can have a high abuse/misuse potential (Hernandez & Nelson, 2010); other family members may access the child's prescribed medication for illicit use.

Note any history of cardiac problems or seizure disorder in the child. These conditions could be influencing the presence of anxiety symptoms and could influence the choice of medications selected to treat the disorder (Connor & Meltzer, 2006). Certain medications can affect the electrical circuit of the heart, increasing the possibility of arrhythmias. Any child with a history of congenital heart defects or rhythm disturbances should be evaluated by a cardiologist prior to starting medications for medical clearance. Some medications may alter the seizure threshold; thus, these children should also be evaluated by neurology for clearance.

What are the family attitudes about use of psychotropic medication? Certain cultural and family beliefs do not condone the use of psychotropic medications. While research has been conducted regarding cultural beliefs and psychiatric medications, little research has been completed regarding cultural effects on the treatment of children with medications for psychiatric diagnoses. The National Stigma Study (Pescosolido, Perry, Martin, McLeod, & Jensen, 2007) was one of the first to evaluate society's feelings regarding medication and mental health issues in children. Preliminary findings demonstrated that while feelings of the importance of identifying and treating mental health issues with children with therapy were evenly split, more than two-thirds of the respondents had negative feelings regarding the use of medications to treat children. Sixty-eight percent of the respondents believed that the medications negatively affected child development, delayed solving behavior-related problems, and prevented families from working out problems. More significantly, 86% of the respondents stated that physicians tended to overmedicate children for what they believed were "common behavioral problems." The biggest issues were related to the safety of these medications in children and the level of distrust in the physicians prescribing the medications. Finally, this study found that persons in cultures that were less likely to trust physicians or have negative beliefs toward psychiatric diagnoses had more negative attitudes toward medicating children (Pescosolido et al.).

A study by Schnittke (2003) found that African Americans were less likely to use psychiatric medications themselves or to give them to their children regardless of socioeconomic status, knowledge, religious beliefs, or trust in the medical field. As a result, these patients were being diagnosed later and treated later, complicated by their distrust in the use of medications to treat mental health problems. Similarly, Asian patients with psychological distress were more likely to present with somatic complaints as it was more acceptable to have physical conditions than to admit to psychological or emotional distress. The stigma associated with mental health problems within the Asian culture negatively impacted their compliance with medications recommended by psychiatric personnel. They often sought alternative treatments and used healing traditions and herbal remedies before seeking psychiatric care and medications for mental health problems (Lin & Cheung, 1999).

Cultural beliefs are essential issues for APNs when considering pediatric anxiety. The family's beliefs and level of trust in the mental health field have a strong impact on a child's treatment. Addressing the family's concerns and repeatedly answering questions are important in helping to ensure adherence with the prescribed treatment plan. The effect that cultural beliefs have on the diagnosis and treatment of children with anxiety disorders cannot be ignored. APNs, who have likely fostered a level of trust with parents, are able to work closely with the psychiatric provider to support choice of treatment options. This collaboration may increase the likelihood of the family following through with the plan of care.

If the family does decide to allow the child to be treated with medication, other considerations include the following: Does the family have sufficient organization to safely manage giving and storing a psychiatric medication? If the anxiety disorder is comorbid with depression, is suicide a risk? This makes development of a safety plan with the family and safe storing of medication even more essential.

Medications

The most studied and widely used medications for anxiety are selective serotonin reuptake inhibitors (SSRIs). These include Prozac (fluoxetine), Zoloft (Sertraline), Celexa (citalopram), and Paxil (paroxetine). The general side effects of these medications include nausea, vomiting, diarrhea, headaches, dizziness, sleep disorders, weight changes (gain and loss), and skin rashes. Side effects can vary by individual (Emslie, Croarkin, & Mayes, 2010). SSRIs may also carry a risk of increased suicidal thinking and behavior. Psychoeducation must focus on the side effects and potential risk of these medications. See Chapter 6 for a description of medications used to treat anxiety disorders.

Benzodiazepines are a class of medication usually used to treat adult anxiety disorders; they are rarely used to manage long-term pediatric anxiety given the lack of evidence-based efficacy and the abuse potential for both the patient and family members. Benzodiazepines may be administered for short-term use as well as with event-specific sources of anxiety such as medical procedures to help alleviate anxiety or for severe panic disorder. Similarly, tricyclic antidepressants, while effective with pediatric anxiety, are rarely used because of their side effect profile and adverse cardiac effects. Currently, SSRIs are the first pharmacological choice for treating pediatric anxiety disorders (Connor & Meltzer, 2006).

Combined CBT and SSRI treatment is an effective, evidence-based strategy for treating children and adolescents with anxiety disorder. Walkup et al. (2008) evaluated 488 children and adolescents with separation anxiety disorder, generalized anxiety disorder, or social phobia who received either fourteen sessions of CBT, sertraline, combined CBT and sertraline, or a placebo for twelve weeks. Results showed those who received the combined therapy of CBT and sertraline had an 80% improvement on the Clinical Global Improvement Scale compared to 59% for the CBT-alone group and 54% for the sertraline-alone group. The placebo group had a 23% ratio of improvement in symptoms of anxiety.

Case Exemplar

Sonja is a seven-year-old Hispanic girl who has received her primary health care at the well-child clinic in her community. Her mother made an appointment outside the parameters of normal check-ups to discuss Sonja's difficulty in going to school. A second grader in a local public elementary school, she began the school year with no problems. In December, she began refusing to go to school at least two days of the week. It is now mid-January and she was refusing to attend school every day. Her mother had responded by walking her to the classroom, putting her to bed earlier, and having food treats available at home upon her return on the days she went to school. Sonja came into the office in a quiet, withdrawn manner, with her thumb in her mouth. This was quieter and somewhat more regressed than previously noted at well-child checkups. She clung to her mother and twirled her hair while you and mom spoke.

When you asked what had changed for Sonja since you last saw her in August of the previous year, the mom initially stated that nothing was different. Mom complained about the problems getting Sonja to school and how distressing this had been to her. You again asked about who was living in the family unit and mom admitted that Sonja's father had been incarcerated in the fall and was likely to remain in prison for several years. This had caused a financial crisis in the family as mom had not been employed. Mom also shared that she was overwhelmed with raising Sonja, her older brother, and two younger preschool siblings. She emphasized that everyone else was "fine" and that Sonja was the one "giving me trouble."

Sonja was physically healthy but had gained 10 pounds since you last saw her. Mom stated that her appetite had increased and she was eating more junk food. Mom described increasing nightmares and difficulties going to sleep, especially since her dad went to jail. While the children had not visited him there, they knew he has gone away for a long time after doing something bad.

As the primary care practitioner you placed a call to the school and found out they were very worried about her. The school stated that Sonja had become more withdrawn in school, isolated herself on the playground, and cried for one hour each morning after her mother dropped her off.

Her teacher stated that prior to December Sonja would run into the classroom, had many friends, and seemed well adjusted to school. Mom initially disagreed with psychiatric evaluation, stating she thinks "this is just a phase." She further stated she did not believe in therapy for children because "they always say it is the mother's fault when children have problems." After discussion with the primary provider, who assured Sonja's mother that her school anxiety was outside the realm of developmental anxiety regarding school and that the stress of her father's incarceration and subsequent family changes were having an impact on Sonya, her mother agreed to an evaluation and possible behavior treatment.

Mom agreed to a psychiatric evaluation and possible behavioral treatment to ascertain the nature of the school refusal. After an evaluation and recommendation for sixteen weeks of CBT, Sonja began treatment. Medication was not prescribed for her anxiety and within five weeks she showed a 50% improvement in symptoms at school. By the end of the sixteen weeks of treatment, her symptom improvement was 75% as rated by the Clinical Global Improvement Scale. She was attending school four or five days a week. The clinician continued to see her monthly for three months and then discharged her from care at the mother's request. At that time she was regularly attending school five days a week. Psychoeducation was performed with her mother and Sonja about the risk of future problems with anxiety and depression when she is confronted with school and environment stress or change.

Integration with Primary Care and Referral

The role of the APN in primary care is to identify those children or adolescents with symptoms of an anxiety disorder. While the APN may not be able to make the actual diagnosis, he or she must be able to identify those patients who present with symptoms of anxiety that are outside of the normal developmental anxieties of childhood and are causing ongoing stress that interferes with normal developmental tasks. Once a patient has been identified with symptoms of a possible anxiety disorder, he or she should be referred for further evaluation and testing by an appropriate child psychiatric APN or other psychiatric provider. The APN can play an integral role in helping parents understand the importance of seeking out psychiatric care for their child because of the relationship they have developed over time with the families. APNs can help with facilitating the connection with a child psychiatric specialist and with continued evaluation and care of the child throughout their treatment.

Management of Anxiety Disorders and Implications for Practice, Research, and Education

Anxiety in children and adolescents is a common presentation to pediatric primary care practices. Psychiatric resources are essential for referring patients to psychiatric care when their anxiety becomes debilitating and interferes with functioning and development. Primary care APNs are likely to see these children first during well-child visits. They have an opportunity to evaluate and intervene in a potentially debilitating disorder. The high rate of anxiety disorders among children makes it imperative that APNs understand the disorder, how to evaluate symptoms, and how to plan care. The challenge comes in ensuring that primary care APNs have the basic assessment skills and the clinical time to assess anxiety while also having access to child psychiatric services that will support their assessment and provide needed psychiatric treatment. The partnership between primary care APNs and child psychiatric APNs will result in more comprehensive care for children and adolescents presenting with anxiety that disrupts their development.

Summary

This chapter has given an overview of anxiety in children and adolescents, focusing on normal development, epidemiology, theories of etiology, and the types of anxiety disorders that children and adolescents present when seen in pediatric primary care. Comorbid conditions and evidence-based assessments and interventions have been presented, along with the role differentiation between APNs focused on psychiatric treatment versus those focused on primary care management. Whenever possible, behavior interventions such as CBT should be used to treat symptoms of anxiety. Implications for research and practice were also discussed.

Resources for Practitioners and Families

Anxiety Disorders Association of American (www.adaa.org)
Mental Health American (Children's Mental Health Resource List) (www.nmha.org/children)
National Institute of Mental Health (Anxiety Disorders) (www.nimh.nih.gov/publicat/anxiety.cfm)
International OCD Foundation (www.ocfoundation.org)

References

Achenbach, T.M. (2001). *Manual for the child behavior checklist/4-18 and 1991 profile.* Burlington, VT: University of Vermont Department of Psychiatry.

Albano, A.M., & Hayward, C. (2004). Social anxiety disorder. In T.H. Ollendick (Ed.), *Phobic and anxiety disorders in children and adolescents* (pp. 198–235). New York, NY: Oxford University Press.

American Academy of Child and Adolescent Psychiatry (AACAP). (2007). Practice parameter for the assessment and treatment of children and adolescents with anxiety disorders. *Journal of the American Academy of Child and Adolescent Psychiatry, 46*, 267–283.

American Psychiatric Association (APA). (2000). *Diagnostic and statistical manual of mental disorders,* fourth edition, text revision. Washington, DC: American Psychiatric Association.

Angold, A., & Costello, E.J. (1993). Depressive comorbidity in children and adolescents: Empirical, theoretical, and methodological issues. *American Journal of Psychiatry, 150,* 1779–1791.

Batte, S., Watson, A.R., & Amess, K. (2006). The effects of chronic renal failure on siblings. *Pediatric Nephrology, 21,* 246–250.

Beesdo, K., Knappe, S., & Pine, D.S. (2009). Anxiety and anxiety disorders in children and adolescents: Developmental issues and implications for DSM-V. *Psychiatric Clinics of North America, 32,* 483–524.

Benjet, C., Borges, G., & Medina-Mora, M.E. (2010). Chronic childhood adversity and onset of psychopathology during three life stages: Childhood, adolescence and adulthood. *Journal of Psychiatric Research, 44,* 732–740.

Birmaher, B., Brent, D.A., Chiappetta, L., Bridge, J., Monga, S., & Baugher, M. (1999). Psychometric properties of the Screen for Child Anxiety Related Emotional Disorders (SCARED): A replication study. *Journal of the American Academy of Child and Adolescent Psychiatry, 38,* 1230–1236.

Bittner, A., Egger, H.L., Erkanil, A., Jane Costello, E., Foley, D.L., & Angold, A. (2007). What do childhood anxiety disorders predict? *Journal of Child Psychology and Psychiatry, 48,* 1157–9.

Cartwright-Hatton, S., McNicol, K., & Doubleday, E. (2006). Anxiety in a neglected population: Prevalence of anxiety disorders in preadolescent children. *Clinical Psychology Review, 26,* 817–833.

Cohen, J.A., Mannarino, A.P., & Deblinger, E. (2006). *Treating trauma and traumatic grief in children and adolescents.* New York, NY: Guilford Press.

Compton, S.N., March, J.S., Brent, D., Albano, A.M., Weersing, V.R., & Curry, J. (2004). Cognitive-behavioral psychotherapy for anxiety and depressive disorders in children and adolescents: an evidence based medicine review. *Journal of the American Academy of Child and Adolescent Psychiatry, 8,* 930–959.

Connolly, S.D., & Suarez, L.M. (2010). Generalized anxiety disorder, specific phobia, panic disorder, social phobia, and selective mutism. In M. Dulcan (Ed.), *Dulcan's textbook of child and adolescent psychiatry* (pp. 299–323). Arlington, VA: American Psychiatric Association.

Connor, D.F., & Meltzer, B.M. (2006). *Pediatric psychopharmacology fast facts.* New York, NY: W.W. Norton & Company.

Costello, E.J., Egger, H.L., & Angold, A. (2004). Developmental epidemiology of anxiety disorders. In T. H. Ollendick & J. S. March (Eds.), *Phobic and anxiety disorders in children and adolescents* (pp. 334–380). New York, NY: Oxford University Press.

Dufton, L.M., Dunn, M.J., & Compas, B.E. (2009). Anxiety and somatic complaints in children with recurrent abdominal pain and anxiety disorders. *Journal of Pediatric Psychology, 34,* 176–186.

Egger, H.L., & Angold, A. (2006). Common emotional and behavioral disorders in preschool children: presentation, nosology, and epidemiology. *Journal of Child Psychology and Psychiatry, 47,* 1451–1459.

Emslie, G.J., Croarkin, P., & Mayes, T.L. (2010). Antidepressants. In M. Dulcan (Ed.), *Dulcan's textbook of child and adolescent psychiatry* (pp. 701–723). Arlington, VA: American Psychiatric Association.

Geller, D.A. (2010). Obsessive compulsive disorder. In M. Dulcan (Ed.), *Dulcan's textbook of child and adolescent psychiatry* (pp. 349–363). Arlington, VA: American Psychiatric Association.

Ginsburg, G.S., Riddle, M.A., & Davies, M. (2006). Somatic complaints in children and adolescents with anxiety disorders. *Journal of the American Academy of Child and Adolescent Psychiatry, 45,* 1179–1187.

Gregory, A.M., & Eley, T.C. (2007). Genetic influences on anxiety in children: What we've learned and where we're heading. *Clinical Child and Family Psychology, 10,* 199–212.

Heim, C., & Nemerof, C. (2001). The role of childhood trauma in the neurobiology of mood and anxiety disorders: Preclinical and clinical studies. *Society of Biological Psychiatry, 49,* 1023–1039.

Hernandez, S.H., & Nelson, L.S. (2010). Prescription drug abuse: Insight into the epidemic. *Clinical Pharmacology and Therapeutics, 88,* 307–317.

Hirshfeld-Becker, D.R., Micco, J.A., Simoes, N.A., & Henin, A. (2008). High risk studies and developmental antecedents of anxiety disorders. *American Journal of Medical Genetics, 148C,* 99–117.

Kendall, P.C. (2006). Guiding theory for therapy with children and adolescents. In P. C. Kendall (Ed.), *Child and adolescent therapy, cognitive-behavioral procedures* (3rd edition; pp. 3–32). New York, NY: Guilford Press.

Kendall, P.C. (1992). *Coping cat workbook.* Ardmore, PA: Workbook Publishing.

Kendall, P.C., Brady, E.U., & Verduin, T.L. (2001). Comorbidity in childhood anxiety disorders and treatment outcome. *Journal of the American Academy of Child and Adolescent Psychiatry, 40,* 787–794.

Krain, A., Ghaffari, M., Freeman, J., Garcia, A., Leonard, H., & Pine, D.S. (2007). Anxiety disorders. In A. Martin & F. R. Volkman (Eds.), *Lewis' child and adolescent psychiatry: A comprehensive textbook* (4th edition; pp. 538–547). Philadelphia, PA: Lippincott Williams & Wilkin.

Last, C.G. (2002) Somatic complaints in anxiety disordered children. *Journal of Anxiety Disorders, 5,* 125–138.

Last, C.G., & Strauss, C.C. (1989). Panic disorder in children and adolescents. *Journal of Anxiety Disorders, 3,* 87–95.

Leis, J.A., & Mendelson, T. (2010). Intergenerational transmission of psychopathology: Minor versus major parental depression. *Journal of Nervous and Mental Disorder, 198,* 356–61.

Lin, K.M., & Cheung, F. (1999). Mental health issues for Asian Americans. *Psychiatric Services, 50,* 774–780.

Lindhurst, I.E., Marcus, M.T., Borst, S.R., Hoogendijk, T.H., Dingemans, P.M., & Boer, F. (2009). Childrearing style in families of anxiety disturbed children: Between family and within family differences. *Child Psychiatry and Human Development, 40,* 197–202.

Manassis, K., & Monga, S. (2001). A therapeutic approach to children and adolescents with anxiety disorders and associated comorbid conditions. *Journal of the American Academy of Child and Adolescent Psychiatry, 40,* 115–117.

March, J.S., Parker, J.D., Sullivan, K., Stallings, P., & Conners, C.K. (1997). The Multidimensional Anxiety Scale for Children (MASC): Factor structure, reliability, and validity. *Journal of the American Academy of Child and Adolescent Psychiatry, 36,* 1645–1646.

Moore, P.S., Whaley, S.E., & Sigman, M. (2004). Interactions between mothers and children: Impacts of maternal and child anxiety. *Journal of Abnormal Psychology, 113,* 471–476.

MTA Cooperative Group (2001). ADHD comorbidity findings from the MTA study: Comparing comorbid subgroups. *Journal of the American Academy of Child and Adolescent Psychiatry, 40,* 147–158.

Myers, K., & Winters, N.C. (2002). Ten-year review of rating scales. II: Scales for internalizing disorders. *Journal of the American Academy of Child and Adolescent Psychiatry, 41,* 634–659.

Pesocosolido, B., Perry, B.L., Martin, J.K., McLeod, J.D., & Jensen, P.S. (2007). Stigmatizing attitudes and beliefs about treatment and psychiatric medications for children with mental illness. *Psychiatric Services, 58,* 613–618.

Phillips, B.N. (1968). The nature of school anxiety and its relationship to children's school behavior. *Psychology in the Schools, 5,* 195–204.

Sakolsky, D., & Birmaher, B. (2008). Pediatric anxiety disorders: Management in primary care. *Current Opinion in Pediatrics, 20,* 538–543.

Schuckit, M.A., & Hesselbrock, V. (1994). Alcohol dependence and anxiety disorders: What is the relationship? *American Journal of Psychiatry, 151,* 1723–1734.

Schnittker, J. (2003). Misgivings of medicine?: African Americans' skepticism of psychiatric medication. *Journal of Health and Social Behavior, 44,* 506–524.

Silverman, W.K., & Albano, A.M. (1996). *Anxiety Disoreders Interview Schedule for DSM-IV: child Version, Child and Parent Interview Schedules.* San Antonio, TX: Psychological Corporation.

Storch, E.A., Masia-Warner, C., Crisp, H., & Klein, R.G. (2005). Peer victimization and social anxiety in adolescence: A prospective study. *Aggresssive Behavior, 31,* 437–452.

Suarez, L.M., Bennett, S.M., Goldstein, C.R., & Barlow, D.H. (2009). Understanding anxiety disorders from a "triple vulnerability" framework. In M.M. Anthony, & M.B. Stein (Eds.), *Oxford handbook of anxiety and related disorders* (pp. 153–172). New York, NY: Oxford University Press.

Walkup, J.T., Albano, A.M., Piacentini, J., Birmaher, B., Compton, S.N., Sherrill, J.T., & Kendall, P.C. (2008). Cognitive behavioral therapy, sertraline, or a combination in childhood anxiety. *New England Journal of Medicine, 359,* 2753–2766.

Warren, S.L., Umylny, P., Aron, E., & Simmens, S.J. (2006). Toddler anxiety disorders: A pilot study. *Journal of American Academy of Child and Adolescent Psychiatry, 45,* 859–866.

Whaley, S.E., Pinto, A., & Sigman, M. (1999). Characterizing interactions between anxious mothers and their children. *Journal of Consulting and Clinical Psychology, 67,* 826–836.

9

Mood Dysregulation Disorders

Edilma L. Yearwood and Mikki Meadows-Oliver

Objectives

After reading this chapter, APNs will be able to

1. Describe clinical presentations of children and adolescents experiencing a variety of mood disorders.
2. Examine neurobiological, environmental, relational, and other etiological risk factors of mood dysregulation.
3. Analyze the evidence related to assessment and management of mood dysregulation in children and adolescents.
4. Identify potential consequences of untreated mood dysregulation.
5. Differentiate between the roles and responsibilities of primary care and child and adolescent psychiatric-mental health APNs in managing mood dysregulation in children, adolescents, and their families.

Introduction

Nearly 20% of children and adolescents have an emotional, mental, or behavioral disorder at some time during their formative years with symptoms preceding the diagnosis of a disorder by up to four years (Institute of Medicine [IOM], 2009). The annual cost of treatment or lost productivity due to a psychiatric or behavioral disorder is estimated at $247 billion (IOM). In its timely publication, *Preventing Mental, Emotional and Behavioral Disorders among Young People,* the IOM recommended a focus on evidence-based treatment research and prevention and wellness promotion in early childhood and adolescence. To be effective, these efforts must be comprehensive to include the individual, the family, schools, and communities rallying around a central goal of mental health promotion.

This chapter will focus on mood dysregulation, one of the most common psychological symptoms seen in children and adolescents that, if left untreated, can progress to a diagnosable disorder, self-medication with substances, self-injurious and risk-taking behaviors, suicide, and impairment in social, relational, and cognitive development (Jeffery, Sava, & Winters, 2005). Mood dysregulation refers to behavioral, psychological, and physiological impairment in the normal regulatory mechanisms associated with mood or affective states. In the individual it can manifest as a state of disequilibrium or emotional extremes resulting in a clinical picture of depression, dysthymia, hypomania, or mania. Mood dysregulation is dynamic, influenced by internal and external stimuli and reactive to real-life settings and contextual events, whether real or perceived (Ebner-Priemer & Trull, 2009; Siever & Davis, 1985).

Child and Adolescent Behavioral Health: A Resource for Advanced Practice Psychiatric and Primary Care Practitioners in Nursing,
First Edition. Edited by Edilma L. Yearwood, Geraldine S. Pearson, and Jamesetta A. Newland.
© 2012 John Wiley & Sons, Inc. Published 2012 by John Wiley & Sons, Inc.

When mood disorders first occur in childhood or adolescence, they have a long-term impact on quality of life, relationships, self-esteem, and emotional and psychological integrity. Unfortunately, early onset can be a predictor of long-term episodic and chronic turmoil with the disease of depression (unipolar or bipolar) continuing into and throughout adulthood (Kessler, Avenevoli, & Merikangas, 2001). The World Health Organization (WHO) estimates that unipolar depressive disorders will rise from having been the third cause of global burden of disease (GBD) among the noncommunicable diseases in 2004 to become the leading cause of GBD by 2030 (2008).

The prevalence rate of mood disorders in children is less well known than in adults, with estimates of 1% to 3% in children under the age of twelve years and between 4.6% and 14% in thirteen- to eighteen-year-olds (Costello, Erkanli, & Angold, 2006; Merikangas et al., 2010). However, epidemiological data from Kessler et al. (2001) indicated that depression was experienced by as many as 25% of adolescents at some point during adolescence. It is believed that most episodes of depression in childhood are untreated and that untreated depressive events can last up to nine months. What is equally concerning is that approximately 50% of children and adolescents who experience a depressive episode relapse and 70% have a recurrence of symptoms within five years, a harbinger of a cycle of chronicity with the disorder (Jeffery et al., 2005). Depression rates between boys and girls under the age of twelve are comparable. However, at puberty there is a dramatic shift with girls experiencing mood disorders at a 2:1 ratio when compared to boys (Costello et al., 2006). Data are less robust on the accuracy of prevalence rates of bipolar mania in children and adolescents. In addition, it is difficult to accurately assess how many children and adolescents under the age of eighteen experience nondiagnosable mood symptoms that significantly impact their normal developmental trajectory and quality of life.

All humans experience periods of sadness or elation in the normal course of growth and development. It is when these emotions are prolonged, interfere with day-to-day functioning, threaten relationships with others, impact the progress of normal development, and affect self-esteem and quality of life that they become problematic. Mood disorders include major depression (MDD), bipolar I (MDD and mania), bipolar II (MDD and hypomania), dysthymia, mood disorder not otherwise specified (NOS), substance induced mood disorder, and mood disorder due to a general medical condition. *The Diagnostic and Statistical Manual of Mental Disorders,* Fourth Edition, Text Revision (DSM-IV-TR) (American Psychiatric Association [APA], 2000)

diagnostic criteria for the various mood disorders are applied to children, adolescents, and adults. It is anticipated that DSM-V (expected to be released in 2013) will have some child and adolescent – specific modifications in descriptors and diagnostic criteria for pediatric mood disorders. Preliminary indications are that the presence and quality of the characteristic *irritability* will be a key element of the differential diagnosis within the pediatric population (APA, 2009).

This chapter will include DSM-IV symptoms of mood dysregulation in children and adolescents, risk factors for mood disorders, etiology of mood disorders, screening and assessment tools for use in primary care, evidence-based management strategies, the advanced practice nurse (APN)'s role in caring for children and adolescents presenting with mood symptoms, potentially lethal consequences of untreated mood disorders, and implications for nursing research with this population. What is abundantly clear from the data on mood disorders is that prevention, early detection, and evidence-based treatment can positively influence the quality of life of those at risk for or affected by these disorders.

Symptom Recognition in Children and Adolescents

Accurately diagnosing mood disorders in childhood and adolescence can be difficult due to frequent prevalence of comorbid disorders in this population and the rapid growth and maturational shifts characteristic of individuals under the age of eighteen years. Mood disorders should be viewed as a spectrum of disorders that range from unipolar depression on one end to bipolar mania at the other end. While controversy around diagnosing bipolar disorder in children continues, APNs are encouraged to stay informed about the latest evidence from the National Institute of Mental Health (NIMH) and the DSM-V Child and Adolescent Disorders Work Group.

Clinical and research experts on bipolar disorder in children and adolescents recommend that practitioners apply the existing DSM-IV-TR criteria when making a diagnosis and pay particular attention to the issues of "distinct episodes of mania or hypomania" (Baroni, Lunsford, Luckenbaugh, Towbin, & Leibenluft, 2008; Brotman et al., 2006; Kowatch et al., 2005). The APN should be alert for prodromal symptoms, which are the early signs of a disorder seen before an acute episode and which precede the appearance of the full range of symptoms associated with the disorder by weeks to months (Fava & Tossani, 2007). It is also important for the APN to keep in mind the difference between a cluster of mood symptoms and the presence of enough

Table 9.1 Common symptoms associated with depressed mood

Young Children	Adolescents	Both
Somatization (headaches, GI disturbances, stomachaches, malaise)	Anhedonia	Suicidal ideation or attempt
Sad affect	Apathy	Irritability/Anger
Social withdrawal	Hopelessness	Insomnia/Hypersomnia
Soft spoken/Quiet	Delusions	Poor concentration
Poor self-esteem	Psychomotor retardation	Appetite disturbance
Helplessness	Neglect of hygiene	Fatigue/Lethargy
Auditory hallucinations	Suicidal ideation and/or attempt(s)	Impaired academic functioning
	Behavioral problems	Impaired social functioning
		Rumination
		Negative self-talk/negative self-attributes
		Verbal outbursts/tantrums
		Social isolation

Adapted from APA (2000); Sadock and Sadock (2009); U.S. Preventive Services Task Force (2009a).

symptoms to meet the diagnostic threshold. In addition, the APN must rule out the possibility that the symptoms are due to a medical condition such as hypothyroidism (depression), substance abuse of a central nervous system depressant such as alcohol (depression), use of a stimulant such as cocaine or amphetamines (mania/hypomania), head trauma (depression or hypomania/mania), hyperthyroidism (hypomania/mania), or side effects from a *prescribed* medication such as an anticonvulsant, oral contraceptive, or alpha adrenergic agonists like clonidine (depression) (Hamrin & Magorno, 2010; Rockhill, Hlastala, & Myers, 2005).

Depression

Unipolar depression is an affective disorder characterized by periods when the individual feels "down" internally and exhibits external symptoms of that mood state (Stahl, 2008). Unipolar depression in children is chronic and recurrent with many adults tracing the start of their mood symptoms to their childhood. For a diagnosis of major depression to be made, there has to be a change from previous functioning and a two-week duration of symptoms accompanied by five of the nine behavioral criteria for the disorder (APA, 2000).

Common comorbid psychiatric diagnoses include anxiety (25% to 50%), substance abuse, conduct disorder, eating disorder, and attention deficit hyperactivity disorder (ADHD) (Anderson & Hope, 2008; Kessler et al., 2001). Medical comorbidities can include obesity, heart disease, cancer, or HIV/AIDS (Jeffery et al., 2005).

Psychosocial comorbidities can include trauma, loss, parent-child difficulties, and poor academic achievement (Coyle et al., 2003; Jeffery et al., 2005). Table 9.1 provides the APN with symptoms of depressed mood seen in young children or adolescents and symptoms that may be found in both age groups.

Depression in children and adolescents is usually classified as mild, moderate, or severe. In mild depression, there are fewer symptoms experienced or seen, scores on standardized screening tools are lower, and duration of symptoms is brief with minimal impact on the individual's functioning. If the depression is assessed as moderate, there are more symptoms accompanied by functional impairment. In severe depression, the individual has significant impairment in functioning and is considered to be in an acute state with symptoms exceeding those needed to make the diagnosis (APA, 2000). The individual may present as actively suicidal, significantly regressed, or psychotic (Hamrin & Magorno, 2010; Jeffery et al., 2005). Table 9.2 contains a comparison of diagnostic and clinical criteria for major depression and dysthymia established by the DSM-IV-TR. Table 9.2 also includes lists of other applicable disorders associated with depression with which children and adolescents might be diagnosed.

Bipolar Disorder

Bipolar disorder is also an affective mood spectrum disorder in which the individual experiences *both* "up" and "down" mood states in varying levels of intensity (Stahl,

Table 9.2 Criteria for major depression and dysthymia

Major Depression	Dysthymia
Five or more symptoms present during the same 2-week period demonstrating a change from prior functioning where there is depressed mood or anhedonia.	Depressed mood most of the day for more days than not for *at least 2 years*. In children and adolescents, it can be irritable mood of at least 1 year duration. Two or more of the following must be present:
– depressed mood most of the day by report or observation. *In children and adolescents can appear as irritability* – lack of interest in activities nearly all day most days – weight loss (without dieting) or weight gain. *In children can manifest as failure to achieve expected weight gain* – insomnia or hypersomnia nearly each day – psychomotor agitation or retardation self-report or observed – fatigue or anergia – feelings of worthlessness or guilt – difficulty with concentration; indecisive – suicidal ideation without a plan or suicide attempt	– poor appetite or overeating – insomnia or hypersomnia – low energy/fatigue – low self-esteem – poor concentration; difficulty with decision making – feelings of hopelessness Person is never without symptoms for more than 2 months Does not meet the criteria for major depression, has not experienced a manic episode Not due to medical illness, substance abuse Causes significant distress and impairment in functioning
Symptoms result in distress and impairment in functioning, cannot be explained by bereavement, medical condition or substance use	

Reproduced with permission from: APA (2000). Diagnostic and Statistical Manual of Mental Disorders, Fourth Edition, Text Revision). Washington, DC: Author.

2008). At times children exhibit what has been termed "affective storms," which are severe violent outbursts of irritability, anger, and attacking behaviors (Stahl). The mood states in pediatric bipolar disorder (PBD) can manifest as either distinct entities or overlapping symptom experiences. The diagnosis of PBD using the DSM-IV-TR criteria used for adults has been controversial. Reasons include difficulty identifying duration of episodes (as this is often difficult to accurately pinpoint from the child and/or caretakers) to meet the diagnostic criteria in youth and the similarity of several symptoms that are also seen in ADHD. In an effort to capture the variability of behaviors seen in children and adolescents who appear to have bipolar disorder but do not meet the DSM-IV TR criteria for diagnosis and to distinguish pediatric symptoms from true adult bipolar disorder, Leibenlauf, Charney, Towbin, Bhangoo, and Pine (2003) described criteria for a syndrome that they termed *severe mood dysregulation* (SMD).

SMD is characterized by chronic irritability, hyperarousal, impairment, anger, sadness that is present most of the time and noticeable to others, and outbursts at least three times per week. Symptoms must start before age twelve, persist for at least one year, and result in impairment in two of the three domains with which the child interfaces (school, home, or peers). In addition, the child must screen positive for three or more of the following—insomnia, racing thoughts, distractibility, pressured speech, restlessness, flight of ideas, and intrusiveness (Baroni et al., 2008). Youth who meet the criteria for SMD do not meet the DSM-IV TR criteria for PBD. Of note, hypersexuality, a criterion for adult bipolar disorder, is seen in approximately 40% of PBD, and psychosis is characteristic of less than 45% of youth with a diagnosis of bipolar disorder (Kowatch, Youngstrom, Danielyan, & Findling, 2005). Other symptoms that the APN should be aware of include increased talkativeness and "affective storms," which are severe and dramatic mood eruptions (Hamrin & Pachler, 2007).

Prevalence rates of bipolar disorder in children and adolescents are difficult to accurately identify because of the lack of good epidemiological studies and the controversy over using the diagnosis in the pediatric population. However, estimates in children under the age of twelve are believed to be approximately 0.1%, with rates during adolescence increasing to between 1% and 3% (Merikangas et al., 2010; NIMH, n.d.).

Pediatric bipolar disorder can present as a comorbid disorder with other disruptive disorders such as ADHD, conduct disorder (CD), or oppositional defiant disorder (ODD); making effective treatment more complex (Rockhill et al., 2005). In addition to the DSM-IV criteria for making a diagnosis, the Child Psychiatric Workgroup on Bipolar Disorder recommends using the acronym FIND to assess for manic symptoms (Kowatch, Fristad, et al., 2005, p. 215).

Table 9.3 Criteria for pediatric bipolar disorder (Must meet criteria for mania or hypomania)

Severe mood dysregulation	Hypomania	Mania
Onset before age 12 with range of 7–17 Abnormal mood (anger or sadness) Hyperarousal (need 3) – insomnia – agitation – racing thoughts/flight of ideas – distractibility – intrusiveness – pressured speech – restlessness Verbal or behavioral reactivity, frustration, tantrums or aggression at least 3 times/week Presence of symptoms for at least 12 months with absence of symptoms no longer than 2 months Severe symptoms in at least 2 domains (home, school or with peers) ***Cannot meet criteria for bipolar as described in columns 2 and 3***	Distinct period of elevated, expansive or irritable mood *lasting at least 4 days* and different than usual mood Must have 3 or more of the following: – grandiosity/inflated self-esteem – decreased need for sleep – talkative more than usual – flight of ideas – distractibility – increase in goal-directed activity – excessive involvement in pleasurable activities Changes in mood and functioning observable by others Absence of psychotic features Behavioral change does not necessitate hospitalization Not due to use of substances, a medical condition, or a medication	Abnormal and persistent elevated, expansive or irritable mood *lasting at least 1 week* Must have 3 or more of the following: – inflated self-esteem or grandiosity – decreased need for sleep Talkative more than usual – flight of ideas – distractibility – increase in goal-directed activity – excessive involvement in pleasurable activities Symptoms are severe and cause marked impairment in all areas and may lead to hospitalization to prevent harm to self or others May have psychotic features Not due to substance use, medical condition, or the effects of nedication

Reprinted with permission from: APA (2000); Baroni et al. (2009); Brotman et al. (2006); Diagnostic and Statistical Manual of Mental Disorders, Fourth Edition, Text Revision. Washington, DC: Author.

Frequency (symptoms occur most days in a week)
Intensity (severe symptoms that significantly impact one domain or moderately affect two or more domains)
Number (symptoms occur three or more times each day)
Duration (symptoms occur 4 or more hours per day)

Table 9.3 provides a comparison between the DSM-IV-TR criteria for hypomania and mania and the Leibenluft et al. (2003), Baroni et al. (2008), and Brotman et al. (2006) criteria for severe mood dysregulation.

Etiology

The science behind the etiology of mood disorders points to multiple factors interacting at critical times on vulnerable individuals to cause affective dysregulation. While the causation in children and adolescents appears to be similar to the causation in adults, onset before age eighteen poses a risk for both presence of comorbidities and recurrence in adulthood. Garber (2006), Nemeroff and Vale (2005), Lewinsohn, Rohde, and Seeley (1998), and Sadock and Sadock (2009) provide excellent reviews of the biological, genetic, cognitive, personality, and environmental (internal, external, and relational) factors that have been implicated in the development and maintenance of mood dysregulation. The type of factor, combination of factors, intensity, chronicity, and onset during critical developmental periods determine the disease pathway (U.S. Preventive Services Task Force [USPSTF], 2009a).

Biological Evidence

The monoamine hypothesis of depression identifies three neurotransmitters as playing a key role in depression. Inefficient or dysregulated serotonin, norepinephrine, and dopamine activity in the amygdala, prefrontal cortex, nucleus accumbens, and hypothalamus explain the symptoms of depressed mood, difficulty with information processing, psychomotor retardation or agitation, emotion regulation, and sleep disturbances (Neuroscience Educational Institute [NEI], 2009; Stahl, 2008). Antidepressants target specific neurotransmitters to alleviate specific problematic presenting symptoms. In a study conducted by Caspi et al. (2003), the researchers found that individuals with one or two copies of the short variant of the serotonin transporter gene (*5-HTTLPR*) instead of the long form demonstrated higher levels of depression when exposed to life stressors.

Dysregulation of the hypothalamic-pituitary-adrenal (HPA) axis has long been identified as a factor in depression. In response to physical or psychological stress, the adrenal gland releases the hormone cortisol and the hypothalamus releases corticotrophin-releasing hormone, which triggers a further increase in production of cortisol. Hypercortisolism is believed to cause the cognitive impairment seen in depressed individuals (Howland, 2010). Watamura, Donzella, Alwin, and Gunnar (2003) conducted a study on fifty-five low-risk children (twenty infants and thirty-five toddlers), looking at salivary cortisol levels of the sample in two contexts: during full-day center-based child care and home. They found that cortisol levels increased over the course of the day in toddlers to 71% and 35% in infants during center-based stays. Teacher-reported social fearfulness temperament style predicted increases in afternoon cortisol levels. At home, 71% of the same infants and 64% of the same toddlers showed a decrease in cortisol levels across the day. This finding led the researchers to question the relationship between cognitive and social challenges in context-specific environments and the development of psychopathology. They recommend conducting similar studies with infants and toddlers in high-risk environments and among a larger sample size. These results beg the question of whether remittance of high cortisol levels during critical developmental periods in childhood postpones the onset of psychopathology. And do the numbers of remittances that occur affect intensity and characteristics of symptoms once they develop?

Hypothyroidism

Hypothyroidism occurs when the thyroid gland fails to respond to the thyroid-stimulating hormone (TSH) and increases levels of circulating T_3 (triiodothyronine) and T_4 (thyroxine). Primary hypothyroidism can mimic some of the classic symptoms seen in depression such as hypersomnia, fatigue, psychomotor and cognitive slowing, anxiety, mood instability, weight gain, constipation, and depression. The individual with severe hypothyroidism presents with aggression, agitation, and paranoia. Blood serum T_3 and T_4 levels are usually low but TSH is elevated above 3.5 mlU/mL. In subclinical hypothyroidism, T_3 and T_4 are within normal range but TSH is elevated (Geracioti, 2006; Harvard Mental Health Letter, 2007). In a retrospective study conducted in Germany by Holtmann, Duketis, Goth, Poustka, and Boelte (2009), thyroid function data were analyzed from 114 children

ages four to seventeen years who were referred to both outpatient and inpatient psychiatric care. Children ($n = 53$) who met the criteria on the Child Behavior Checklist for Dysregulation Profile (CBCL-DP) had scores in the definite clinical range in three of the eight subscales of attention problems, aggression, and anxious/depressed. The TSH levels of the CBCL-DP group was elevated compared to the psychiatric control group ($n = 61$) who did not meet the criteria for dysregulation. In addition, when looking at the entire sample ($N = 114$) for those who met the criteria for subclinical hypothyroidism only, there were twice as many youth who met the criteria for CBCL-DP (45.3%) with elevated TSH than in the control group (23%).

Genetic Evidence

Children and adolescents who have one first-degree biological relative with unipolar or bipolar disorder have up to a 24% chance of also having a mood disorder (APA, 2000), and the chances increase if both parents have mood disorders. Luby, Belden, and Spitznagel (2006) conducted a six-month (Time 1 and Time 2) study on 119 preschool-aged children (three years to five years and seven months old) looking at risk factors for preschool depression. Data obtained included family history of psychiatric disorders, caregiver interviews to obtain a structured diagnostic assessment of the child's depression severity score, child assessment, and caregiver response to a stressful life events tool aimed at capturing stressful events for the child within the past year. The researchers found that both family history and stressful life events predicted depression scores at Time 2. Duffy, Alda, Hajek, and Grof (2009) conducted a longitudinal study of 207 offspring, aged eight to twenty-five years, of parents with bipolar disorder. During the fifteen years of the study, 32% of the sample met the DSM-IV criteria for at least one major mood event with the average onset of symptoms occurring at age seventeen. The researchers also noted that during the course of the study, over 60% of the sample had a recurrence of mood episodes within five years.

Cognitive Evidence

Maladaptive negative cognitive factors have been implicated in mood dysregulation and appear to be a learned pattern of distorted thinking triggered by stressful events that then activate a cascade of negative thought processes. Beck (1967) first identified cognitive vulnerabilities, which he associated with depression, as including negative interpretation of events, perceived incompetence, poor self-schema, helplessness, hopelessness, and a pessimistic view of the world. In more recent research, Beck (2008) and Clark and Beck (2010) stated that "dysfunctional schemas about the self are due to early adverse childhood events such as parental loss, rejection or neglect that sensitizes the individual to later losses" (p. 419). Individuals in whom this negative schema is continuously activated develop entrenched and more elaborate negative self-schemas that become more easily triggered by milder stressors. APNs are urged to evaluate cognitive distortions within the context of pervasiveness, intensity, and developmental sense of self (Horowitz & Marchetti, 2009). Garber (2006) and Jacobs, Reinecke, Gollan, and Kane (2008) provide a good review of the evidence related to cognitive susceptibilities in the pediatric population.

Evidence from the Tripartite Model

Clark and Watson (1991) proposed the tripartite model to illustrate the relationship between anxiety and depression. The three dimensions of the model include negative affect (NA) [anger, guilt, distress, irritability, and insomnia], positive affect (PA) [*absence* of fatigue or anhedonia], and physiological hyperarousal (PH) [muscle tension, tachycardia, shortness of breath, and dry mouth]. Presence of NA and elevated PH are characteristic of anxiety disorders, and NA and lack of PA are characteristic of depression. The model serves to remind practitioners of the overlap between the two disorders, their high comorbid risk, and the importance of assessing for the presence of both disorders (Anderson & Hope, 2008; De Bolle & De Fruyt, 2010).

Environmental Evidence

Environmental factors have also been implicated in the development of mood dysregulation in children and adolescents. These include family and peer relationships, maltreatment, school performance, and real or perceived neighborhood threats or risk exposure. Bronfenbrenner's ecological systems theory is a useful framework for understanding systems with which human beings interact and that contribute to proximal processes involved with development including development of psychopathology (1979, 1994). For example, the microsystem is made up of the individual, family, peers, school, and neighborhood. The relationships (attachment and support) and interactions (teasing or bullying) that a child has with individuals within that system during development will affect not only mood but also self-esteem and ability to successfully navigate developmental tasks.

Oland and Shaw (2005) conducted an extensive review of the literature looking at factors that contribute to internalizing and externalizing behaviors in children and adolescents. They found that across research findings, depression correlated with failure to form social relationships, failure to attain developmental milestones of independence and autonomy from parents, maternal depression, overinvolved and controlling parents, parental psychopathology, psychosocial difficulties, negative self-evaluation, low self-esteem, and behavioral inhibition. Within microsystem dynamics, children who display externalizing behaviors tend to have difficulty with social skills, in understanding social cues, and with self-reflection; have had low or inconsistent parental supervision; may have parents who are antisocial; and had exposure to community violence.

The risk for mood psychopathology in the developing child or adolescent may also be affected by linkages and processes occurring between two or more settings (mesosystem), one of which includes the developing child. An example would include conflicts between the school and the parents over the child's behavior at school or the impact of community violence on the developing child. Mrug and Windle (2010) conducted a longitudinal study with a community sample of 603 boys and girls recruited at the fifth grade and followed for sixteen months. At baseline the Birmingham Youth Violence Study Violence Exposure self-report tool was administered. The tool measures witnessing violence, being the victim of violence, or having been threatened by violence, including when a weapon was involved. The context of the violence was also assessed at baseline. At Time 2 of the study, the participants completed a self-report measure of aggression assessing for pure, reactive, and instrumental overt aggression on a Likert 4-point scale. The researchers found that violence exposure in more than one setting, such as at home and at school, was a predictor of adjustment problems; witnessing violence at school and victimization at home were related to depression; witnessing violence and victimization at home was associated with aggression (externalizing symptom); and witnessing violence in the community predicted delinquency. A more detailed discussion of Bronfenbrenner's theory is found in Chapter 1 of this text.

Internalizing and Externalizing Symptoms in the Context of Mood Dysregulation

The Child Behavior Checklist (CBCL) developed by Achenbach and proved reliable across cultures assesses for two distinct youth behavioral profiles: internalizing and externalizing. Externalizing youth have been described as undercontrolled with inadequate regulation in that they are aggressive, hostile, and irritable; have low frustration tolerance; and tend to break rules. Internalizing youth have been referred to as overcontrolled in that they exhibit symptoms of anxiety, depression, social withdrawal, more psychosomatic distress, and rumination (Achenbach, 1991; Eisenberg et al., 2001; Tackett, 2010; Verhulst et al., 2003). Eisenberg and colleagues conducted a study on 214 children aged four and a half to eight years of age looking at the relationship between internalizing and externalizing child behaviors and negative emotion, regulation, and control. Data collection measures included parent and teacher version of the CBCL and child observations. While they found that these two distinct behavioral profiles had separate characteristics, they can co-occur, and sadness was a common shared characteristic.

Risk Factors for Mood Dysregulation

As stated previously, risk factors for mood disorders are extensive and include history of parental depression, family history of bipolar disorder, female gender, anxiety, being a victim of abuse, stressful life experiences, health problems, one or more traumatic events, negative cognitions, loss, subsyndromal depression, negative affect temperament style; exposure to family or environmental violence, substance abuse, and interpersonal conflicts (Garber, 2006; Moldenhauer, 2006; Prager, 2009). Factors contributing to mood dysregulation are complex and multifactorial, often posing a challenge to the APN who works with children and adolescents. The child's presentation, history, significant current and past experiences, relationships at home and at school, blood serum levels, and physiological status are important components of the comprehensive assessment that must be conducted.

In a study conducted in Canada on a sample of 2014 children aged twelve and thirteen years, researchers wanted to identify the most salient risk factors for depression in youth from among the common predictors (MacPhee & Andrews, 2006). Researchers looked at self-report data from nine measures available from the National Longitudinal Survey of Children and Youth (NLSCY) study, which collects data on health and well-being every two years on a randomly selected group of children, following them into adulthood. The most salient risk factors for depression were low self-esteem, perceived parental rearing behaviors of rejection or nurturance, peer relationships, conduct problems, inattention, and hyperactivity. Conduct problems manifested as externalizing behaviors were more predictive in girls than in boys. The researchers recommended centering prevention efforts around developing and maintaining healthy self-esteem/self-concept in children and supporting effective parenting behaviors to strengthen the parent-child bond, which is a protective factor in healthy child self-concept (MacPhee & Andrews).

A thorough review of family risk factors contributing to and maintaining youth depressive symptoms was conducted by Restifo and Bogels (2009), who likewise included a road map on validated family-based depression interventions.

Protective Factors

Research has shown that there are several protective factors against the development of mood disorders. One of the most studied protective factors has been participation in sports. As sports participation increased, the odds of suffering from depression decreased by 25% among adolescents, and the odds of suicidal ideation decreased by 12%. Adolescents who participated in sports were at decreased risk for substance abuse, which has been associated with both depression and suicidal ideation. Participation in sports also increases physical activity, which has been shown to be protective against depression, suicidal ideation, and obesity. The protective effects were mediated by increases in self-esteem and social support (Babiss & Gangwisch, 2009).

Assessing Mood Dysregulation in Primary Care

The importance of assessing and treating mood dysregulation early in the pediatric population cannot be stressed enough (Sala, Axelson, & Birmaher, 2009). Recognition of pediatric mood disorders often presents a challenge for pediatric APNs who often lack sufficient time, training, and/or referral sources for management of more complex presentations by these youngsters. As a result, mood disorders are often underdiagnosed and undertreated in pediatrics (Emslie, Mayes, Kennard, & Hughes, 2006). The typical duration of pediatric office visits can be a barrier to completing a comprehensive psychiatric screen. The amount of time required to perform a psychiatric interview with both a child and a parent would be difficult to find in a busy pediatric primary care practice (Schlesinger, 2008).

These disorders significantly affect a child's emotional, cognitive, relational, and social development and, unfortunately, can have a long-lasting negative impact on quality of life. Evidence shows that screening for mood disorders improves the identification of depressed patients and that effective follow-up and treatment decrease clinical morbidity and associated psychosocial complications such as substance use, self-injuring behaviors, suicide, school difficulties, and eating disorders (Chang, Singh, Wang, & Howe, 2010; Yackel, McKennan, & Fox-Deise, 2010). APNs are in an ideal position to conduct routine screening, recognize the warning signs of mild to severe mood dysregulation, and provide initial management (Singh, Pfeifer, Barzman, Kowatch, & DelBello, 2007).

Families may be more likely to present to the primary care setting with a complaint about a mental health problem because they may have a long-term relationship with their health care provider and the primary care office is a place where they are comfortable (Brunk, 2010). Depressive illnesses, bipolar disorder, and other mood disorders that are seen in patients in primary care settings may be less severe than those directly admitted to mental health settings. Thus, the short-term prognosis, the chance of recovery, and the response to treatment may be greater in those children and adolescents who are initially identified in primary care settings early during the course of their symptoms.

Nonetheless, pediatric health care providers frequently encounter youths who exhibit symptoms of or are at risk for mood dysregulation. For example, families may present to the pediatric APN with concerns about childhood sleep problems or adolescent complaints of fatigue, both of which may be symptoms of depression. Unfortunately, without proper tools and support, it may be more feasible (and convenient) to recommend a sleep aid or to order blood tests than to diagnose an underlying and often treatable mental health disorder. This approach, while expedient, does not address the real underlying problem and further delays appropriate interventions.

History

A detailed and thorough history is essential to create an accurate timeline for onset of symptoms that may be related to a mood disorder and to help guide treatment decisions. For the pediatric patient, multiple informants—such as the child, parents, teachers, and other caregivers—are needed to gather adequate information to determine symptoms, severity, and course of illness (Emslie et al., 2006). When the APN is assessing a child for a mood disorder, the history can be structured similarly to a well-child history. After determining the chief complaint, a complete history should include a history of the present illness, a past medical and surgical history (including a list of medications and allergies), a family medical history, a psychosocial history, and a review of systems (including diet, sleep, and elimination).

In addition, a comprehensive physical examination including laboratory blood work is needed to determine the child/adolescent's general health status and to rule out medical conditions that may mimic mood disorders. When working with children and adolescents who present with symptoms of a mood disorder, the APN should remember that many of these children may often have comorbid psychiatric conditions such as ADHD, ODD,

substance abuse disorders, and/or anxiety disorders. Successful treatment of mood disorders requires effective treatment for the co-occurring conditions (Singh et al., 2007). An additional comorbidity that may present with PBD is overweight and obesity. Overweight/obesity among youth with bipolar disorder may be associated with increased psychiatric burden (Goldstein et al., 2008).

History of the Present Illness

When conducting a history of the present symptoms, it is important to note the duration and severity of symptoms. It is also important to determine what, if anything, triggers or improves the symptoms. APNs should be aware that in children and adolescents, the presenting symptoms for mood disorders may differ from those seen in adults (Garzon, Nelson, & Figgemeier, 2009). The age and developmental level of the pediatric patient must be considered when assessing for these disorders. Again, while the core symptoms of major depressive disorder (MDD) in adolescents are similar to those in adults, younger children are less likely to identify sadness and more commonly present with irritability or auditory hallucinations compared with adults (Tables 9.1 and 9.2). PBD also differs from the adult form of the disorder. In children, bipolar disease may be marked by longer episodes, rapid cycling, prominent irritability, and high rates of comorbid ADHD and anxiety disorders (Carbray & McGuiness, 2009).

It is clear that children with mood disorders may present differently than adults. However, even within the pediatric population, there are differences in presentation based on the child's age and developmental status. An adolescent will likely have a different presentation of a mood disorder than a younger child. For example, adolescents may engage in risky behaviors such as alcohol and drug use, dangerous driving, and/or promiscuous sex. Adolescents may also present with antisocial behavior exemplified by stealing, vandalism, and/or running away from home. Such behaviors may be the presenting symptoms of mood dysregulation in this age group (Garzon et al., 2009). Adolescents may also commonly present with severe mood swings, hypersexuality, irritability, distractibility, decreased need for sleep, impulsivity, and racing thoughts (Singh et al., 2007). Younger children may present with somatic complaints such as a headache or upset stomach, causing the APN to treat these symptoms without fully realizing that they may be initial signs of a mood disorder such as depression (Garzon et al.). Regarding the presentation of PBD, the manic and depressive symptoms that occur in young children often occur simultaneously, as in a mixed state, or they cycle several times within a day (Newman, 2006).

A child or adolescent who presents to the primary care setting with recurrent depressive symptoms, persistently irritable or agitated behaviors, hyperactivity, labile mood, reckless or aggressive behaviors, or psychotic symptoms may be experiencing the initial symptoms of bipolar disorder. Dysthymic disorder is not likely to be present in infancy or early childhood. In middle childhood and adolescence, it may present with decreased interest in or participation in activities, feelings of inadequacy, and/or low-esteem. Children with dysthymic disorder may also present with symptoms of social withdrawal, guilt or brooding, irritability, and increases or decreases in sleep or appetite (Jellinek, Patel, & Froehle, 2002).

In infancy and early childhood, depression may present to the primary care setting with a variety of symptoms including failure to thrive, speech and motor delays, decreased ability to interact, and poor attachment. The child may also display repetitive self-soothing behaviors, withdrawal from social contact, and a loss of previously learned skills (e.g., self-soothing skills). An increase in temper tantrums or irritability, separation anxiety, and phobias may also be noted (Jellinek et al., 2002). Older children and adolescents may present with poor self-esteem, reckless and destructive behavior (e.g., unsafe sexual activity, substance abuse), somatic complaints, poor social and academic functioning, hopelessness, boredom, emptiness, and loss of interest in activities (Jellinek et al.).

Although PBD is not diagnosed until later in childhood, research has found that children with PBD were reported to experience increased difficult temperament during infancy (West, Schenkel, & Pavuluri, 2008). It is known that manic symptoms characterized as elevated, expansive, or irritable are key features of bipolar disorder (APA, 2000) However, manic symptoms present differently during childhood. In children, a persistently irritable mood may be noted more than a euphoric mood. Children may also have aggressive uncontrollable outbursts and agitated behaviors with hyperactivity and impulsivity. Extreme fluctuations in mood may be noted. These mood fluctuations can occur on the same day over the course of days or weeks. Children with PBD may also present with reckless behaviors, dangerous play, and inappropriate sexual behaviors. Adolescents with bipolar disorder may present to the primary care office with sleep disturbances, labile mood, agitated behaviors, and pressured speech. They may also have racing thoughts and reckless behaviors such as dangerous driving, substance abuse, and sexual indiscretions. Adolescents may also report illicit activities such as impulsive stealing or fighting, spending sprees, and psychotic symptoms (e.g., hallucinations, delusions, irrational thoughts).

Past Medical History

When gathering information regarding the past medical history, pertinent birth history information should be obtained. The APN should be sure to inquire about any history of psychiatric conditions, hospitalizations, surgeries, and/or medical disorders/chronic illnesses. The ages at which conditions occurred should be noted. It should also be noted whether the child is up to date on immunizations. Included in the history should be an assessment of medications that the child or adolescent is taking, since some medications may cause depression-like symptoms such as sedation (Garzon et al., 2009). The medication history should also note not only prescription medications but over-the-counter and herbal medications as well. The APN should assess allergies to medications, foods, or the environment.

Family Medical History

Children are at higher risk of developing a mood disorder at an earlier age if there is a history of a mood disorder in the family (Mick & Faraone, 2009; Singh et al., 2007). The APN should inquire about the family's mental health history (e.g., anxiety/mood disorders). Ideally, the family medical history should be obtained for three generations of family members (the child [and his or her siblings], the parents [and their siblings], and the grandparents). A family history of parental mental health diagnoses should be determined. A history of maternal depression has been shown to be more predictive of depression for female children (Mazza et al., 2009). If a parent has been diagnosed with a mental health condition and confirms taking prescribed medications, the APN should record parental responses to those psychiatric medications. Data about the ethnic background of each parent would also be important to obtain since ethnopharmacological research has revealed that ethnicity significantly affects psychotropic drug response. A family history of medical conditions such as headaches, chronic illness (obesity, diabetes, dyslipidemia, and cardiovascular disease), or recurrent pain should also be noted (Moldenhauer, 2006).

Psychosocial History

When a child presents to the primary care office with symptoms of a mood disorder, a thorough psychosocial history should be obtained. This section should describe members of the current household, their relationships to the child, and the familial sources of stress and support. If the visit involves an adolescent, consider gathering this information separately from both the adolescent and the parent. The adolescent should be assured that what is shared in the health care encounter is confidential and that only certain information will be shared.

Information that cannot be held confidential includes if the adolescent reveals that he or she is considering harming him- or herself, that someone is harming him or her, or if he or she is or is planning to harm someone else. The questioning during this portion of the history should proceed from least to most sensitive questions, giving the APN a chance to first establish rapport with the patient.

Family risk factors such as marital and family conflict and parent stress should be noted. Such factors have been shown to impact the nature of the parent-child relationship. Family conflict has been shown to be a strong predictor of adolescent depression (Mazza et al., 2009). Parent-child relationships may also have a significant effect on children with pediatric mood disorders and these relationships may, in turn, be affected by the child's illness. A parent with an active mood disorder may have a negative effect on family interactions. The mood disorder may interfere with the parent's ability to nurture, show affection, and support the child. Compared to controls, parent-child relationships in the mood disorders group were characterized by significantly less warmth, affection, and intimacy and more quarreling and forceful punishment. Living in a single-parent home was also associated with greater parent-child relationship difficulties (Schenkel, West, Harral, Patel, & Pavuluri, 2008). Further, stressful life events such as parental loss through death, incarceration, or substance abuse may put children at greater risk for developing psychological or behavioral disorders (Horwitz & Marchetti, 2009).

Peer relationships should be explored, as well as information about the child's social environment. Children with mood disorders may have trouble relating to peers. Problematic peer relationships should be noted with particular attention paid to negative interactive patterns such as ongoing bullying or hurtful teasing, social exclusion, physical violence or threats, sexual and racial harassment, and public humiliation. Anhedonia in the child may limit engagement in social activities, which may interfere with mastery of social and peer relatedness skills. Irritability may make children difficult to be around and tends to push others away. Disruptive behavior can cause safety problems and interfere with group activities. A history of victimization including poly-victimization and cyber-bullying should also be obtained as these types of bullying activities are more pervasive and may lack a clearly defined source, resulting in increased anxiety and depression (Finkelhor, Ormrod, & Turner, 2007; Moldenhauer, 2006).

Information regarding school and day care should be gathered since children and adolescents spend more time in day care and school than in any other setting outside of the home. This actuality makes appropriate school adjustment crucial to every child (Fields &

Fristad, 2009). When conducting a history about school, be sure to inquire about academic, athletic, social, relational, and behavioral functioning. The APN should also note the child's pattern of attendance and school nurse visits. Children and adolescents with mood disorders may experience difficulty in school, since successful school performance requires concentration, alertness, proper behavior, and teamwork. Poor concentration, irritability, disorganization, and a lack of self-confidence may interfere with academic work. Low academic achievement and poor social competency have been shown to be related to depression during adolescence (Jaycox et al., 2009; Lazaratou, Dikeo, Anagnostopoulos, & Soldatos, 2010). A drop in grades, difficulty managing school-related activities, and behavior problems in the classroom may be indicators that students might be experiencing a mood disorder. These symptoms may also be associated with other health-related problems and often will not trigger evaluation for a mood disorder. It is important for the APN to try to determine the cause of these issues since school-related problems often escalate and may lead to academic failure and dropping out of school (Mazza et al., 2009).

In addition to affecting the ability to relate to peers, symptoms of mood dysregulation may interfere with the adolescent's capacity to develop intimate relationships and to manage responsibilities—important tasks for the transition to adulthood. Obtaining occupational preparation and holding a consistent job may be challenges for these youth. APNs can and should play an important role in helping families plan for educational and occupational preparation of these youth (Horowitz & Marchetti, 2009).

Mood disorders may affect sexuality in adolescents by reducing their interest and by altering their performance ability. Adolescence is a time when the development and maintenance of peer relationships are of the utmost importance. Adolescents with mood dysregulation often have difficulty in establishing close relationships, which may, in turn, interfere with the development of healthy sexuality. In adolescents with bipolar disorder, manic episodes may be associated with poor judgment and may lead to impulsive sexual behavior. Adolescents with impulsive sexual behaviors may not use condoms or other contraception and be at increased risk for unwanted pregnancy and sexually transmitted infections (STIs). During the visit, the APN should be sure to discuss dating and sexual behavior while also providing early contraception education. Testing for pregnancy and STIs should be available as needed. Some medications used to manage mood disorders may reduce the effectiveness of hormonal contraceptives (e.g., topiramate). Conversely, some oral contraceptives may reduce the effectiveness of medications used to treat mood disorders (e.g., lamotrigine) (Townsend, 2009). For the adolescent using hormonal contraception while being treated for a mood disorder, alternative or dual contraceptive methods should be encouraged.

Review of Systems

The review of systems can provide a comprehensive and methodical overview of the child's health. This structured approach provides an additional opportunity to identify signs and symptoms that may be associated with mood disorders. This approach can cover topics such as diet, sleep, and elimination. This process will also assist the APN in covering important areas related to safety and anticipatory guidance. When discussing the child's or adolescent's diet, it is important to note that changes in eating patterns may occur with mood dysregulation. Both an increase and a decrease in appetite can be an early symptom associated with mood disorders. Excessive eating may signal an attempt to self-soothe. During mania, children may be "too busy" to stop for a meal. This may result in an inadequate intake of calories and nutrients. The APN should inquire about a history of hoarding or binge eating. Poor nutrition may result from binge eating because the child may be filling up on junk foods and sweets. Increases or decreases in appetite may be important clues and require additional evaluation.

Asking questions about sleep or elimination is important when conducting the history. The APN should elicit an account of the child's or adolescent's recent sleep patterns, including any changes from their usual pattern. Sleep disturbances are noteworthy and may include hypersomnia, insomnia, disrupted sleep, or poor quality of sleep. These sleep disturbances may contribute to irritability, agitation, and poor school performance. It is also important for the APN to ask about changes in elimination patterns. Problems with bedwetting and soiling have been seen in children with mood disorders (Papolos & Papalos, 2006).

Safety and Anticipatory Guidance

Discussions of safety and anticipatory guidance play an important role when dealing with a child or adolescent with symptoms of a mood disorder. The APN must assess the child's potential for self-injury secondary to poor judgment and risky behavior. Driving violations, such as speeding, place the adolescent at risk for self-injury and harming others. The use of seat belts in children of all ages should be encouraged at all times. For children already taking psychotropic medications, there may be additional safety considerations. The risk of overdose and potential for adverse medication reactions require that the APN provide education regarding

medications at every health care encounter. For children with medical conditions taking psychotropic medications, the APN must monitor for medication interactions. For example, inhaled steroids used to treat asthma may have potentially harmful interactions with some antidepressants.

During primary care encounters, an assessment of substance use is especially important in those youth at risk for a mood disorder. The APN should ask about drug and alcohol use since youth with symptoms of mood disorders may attempt to self-medicate. When inquiring about drugs, the APN must ask about prescription medications as well as illicit drugs. It is important to remember that substance use can mask symptoms of mood disorders while simultaneously placing youth at risk for overdose, accidents, impulsive sexual activity, sexual assault, and aggression toward others (Horowitz & Marchetti, 2009).

Anticipatory guidance regarding mood disorders consists of education and information that will assist families in preparing for expected changes during their child's or adolescent's assessment and treatment. It will be important to provide information regarding discipline since children with symptoms of a mood disorder may have interaction problems. A child with depressive symptoms may be quiet and withdrawn. However, these behaviors may be viewed as uncooperative. Children with PBD may demonstrate aggressive behaviors and outbursts. These behaviors may serve to alienate them from other children and adults. Irritability displayed by a child with mood disorder symptoms may be seen as a lack of cooperation and lack of respect. In these cases, discipline will not be effective if the underlying disorder is not addressed. Also, inappropriate discipline may intensify undesired behaviors. Consistent limit setting and clear explanation of behavioral contingencies are appropriate discipline strategies for youth with symptoms of mood disorders. Enforcing rules regarding safety is critical (Horowitz & Marchetti, 2009).

Physical Examination

Mood disorders are not associated with specific alterations in normal physical growth and development. Therefore, regular age-appropriate growth screening is recommended for these youth. Vital signs, including height, weight, and blood pressure should be monitored at each visit. A body mass index (BMI) should also be calculated. Height, weight, and BMI should be plotted on the appropriate growth chart. Screenings should be done for hearing and vision to ensure that impaired attention, irritability, distractibility, and low self-esteem are not caused by impaired sight or hearing. When conducting the physical examination, it is important to assess for objective signs of depression such as weight gain or loss and hypoactivity or hyperactivity. A complete physical examination should be conducted, including a thorough neurological examination.

Importance of Differentials

Several problems that have overlapping presentations with mood disorders present to APNs in primary care settings. If a mood disorder is suspected from information gathered in the history, there are several medical diagnoses that should be ruled out. Examples include weight loss, somatic complaints, fatigue, recurrent injuries, and school failure. Weight loss and reduced appetite might present similarly to anorexia nervosa. Binge eating or poor food intake may occur with mania. While somatic complaints may be expressions of emotional distress, they may also be signs of a physical illness or a medical problem. For example, a child presenting to the primary care clinic with a stomachache may have an emotional issue or a gastrointestinal disorder. Fatigue is associated with depression but it is also associated with many physical illnesses. Before attributing a physical symptom to mood disorder, the APN should be sure to investigate possible physical causes of the complaints (Horwitz & Marchetti, 2009).

Youth presenting with recurrent injuries require not only a thorough evaluation but also safety education. Such a presentation might indicate impulsiveness, a propensity for self-injurious behaviors, or a physical problem such as neurological disorders. Poor school performance may be the result of a learning or developmental disorder or may be caused by an exacerbation of a mood disorder (Horowitz & Marchetti, 2009). Sleep problems may also be indicative of either a physical or emotional disorder. Younger children (those younger than nine years of age) who are depressed may present with restlessness or irritability that can be misdiagnosed as ADHD (Moldenhauer, 2006).

Laboratory tests may help the APN rule out other medical conditions that cause symptoms similar to those of a mood disorder. If a patient presents with fatigue, consider ordering thyroid function tests and a complete blood count (with differential) to rule out hypothyroidism and anemia. Mononucleosis can be ruled out by ordering a monospot or heterophile test or Epstein-Barr virus (EBV) antibody titers, in correlation with clinical symptoms. Although there is no definitive laboratory test for chronic fatigue syndrome, this condition should be included in the differential. Diabetes can also cause fatigue. If the patient is thought to have diabetes, obtain a fasting blood glucose level. If substance use or withdrawal is suspected, the APN may order a toxicology screen. Sudden behavioral changes may indicate head trauma or a central nervous system (CNS) lesion. Lead intoxication may also be associated with behavior changes. A blood lead level should be obtained if lead intoxication is suspected. If the youth is taking any medications, the APN should review medication side effects to ensure that the youth is not suffering from adverse effects (Moldenhauer, 2006).

Surveillance and Screening

Any youth who presents to primary care and child and adolescent psychiatric-mental health APNs with an emotional problem as the primary complaint should be screened for a mood disorder. After the initial history and review of symptoms, a formal screening can be conducted. When screening for a mood disorder, it is important to remember that depressed mood falls along a continuum. Short periods of sadness or irritability in response to disappointment or loss are a normal developmental reaction in youth. In a supportive environment, these feelings typically resolve promptly. However, some children and adolescents experience intense or long-lasting sadness or irritability that may interfere with self-esteem, friendships, family life, or school performance. Youths who experience long-lasting or intense feelings of sadness may be depressed and should be monitored and further evaluated.

Evidence has shown that patients with depression or depressive symptoms who present to primary care offices often have a greater chance of receiving treatment, responding to that treatment, and achieving recovery if primary care providers screen for depression using a short self-administered questionnaire during the office visit (Yackel et al., 2010). Surveillance and screening can begin with open-ended questions such as, "How are things at home? How are things at school?" After asking these questions, consider using a validated depression screening instrument to screen for depressive symptoms. There are several validated screening instruments that can be used to screen children and adolescents for depressive symptoms. Primary care APNs should note that positive screens should be followed up with referral to a mental health provider for further assessment using standardized provider-administered tools such as the Kiddie Schedule for Affective Disorders and Schizophrenia (K-SADS) or the NIMH Diagnostic Interview Schedule for Children (DISC-IV).

The Children's Depression Inventory (CDI) (Kovacs, 1992) was developed for use with children aged seven to seventeen years. It is written at the first-grade level, the lowest of any measure of depression for children. There are twenty-seven multiple choice self-report items that take ten to fifteen minutes to complete. A short form with ten items can be used when a quick screening is necessary. While both forms are reported to give comparable results, the longer form generally gives a more robust description of the child's symptoms. Internal consistency reliability has been found to be good, with alpha coefficients ranging from .71 to .89 with various samples. The CDI was developed from the Beck Depression Inventory (BDI).

The BDI II (Beck, Steer, & Brown, 1996) is a twenty-one-item self-report questionnaire, written at a six-grade reading level, that measures depressive symptoms. The BDI II includes the three subdomains of somatic, cognitive, and affective symptoms and has been found to accurately discriminate between depressed and nondepressed youth based on diagnostic criteria. Disadvantages of the tool are that it does not measure school functioning and that there are no accompanying teacher or parent forms.

The Center for Epidemiologic Studies – Depression Scale (CES-D) (Radloff, 1977) is a reliable and valid instrument that may be used to screen adolescents for depression (Wilcox, Field, Prodromidis, & Scafidi, 1998). The CES-D is a twenty-item self-report questionnaire designed for the general population, with an administration time of five to ten minutes. With responses ranging from "0" ("rarely") to "3" ("most of the time"), participants rate the frequency with which each of the twenty items occurs. Total scores range from 0 to 60, with scores of 16 or higher indicating possible depression.

Center for Epidemiological Studies – Depression Scale for Children (CES-DC) (Weissman, Orvaschel, & Padian, 1980) was adapted from the adult version to be more easily understood by children and adolescents (Faulstich, Carey, Ruggiero, Enyart, & Gresham, 1986). Also a twenty-item self-report questionnaire, the responses range from "0" ("not at all") to "3" ("a lot") and yield total scores ranging from 0 to 60. A score of 15 or higher may indicate possible depression. Alpha coefficients for this scale used in adolescent samples range from .84 to .90 (Faulstich et al.).

The Reynolds Child/Adolescent Depression Scales (RCDS/RADS) are ten-minute self-report scales for children aged seven to twelve years old (RCDS) and adolescents aged eleven to twenty years (RADS). The screening tool assesses cognitive, somatic, psychomotor, and interpersonal symptoms. While the tool is brief and psychometrically sound, it is not as robust as the BDI-II (Elmquist, Melton, Croarkin, & McClintock, 2010).

The Mood and Feelings Questionnaire (MFQ) (thirty to thirty-five items) and Mood and Feelings Short Form (SMFQ) (thirteen items) are self-report tools that assess

for symptoms of depression, loneliness, feeling unloved and ugly, and cognitive/affective symptoms. The tool is psychometrically sound with a brief administration time of between five and fifteen minutes (Elmquist et al., 2010).

The Patient Health Questionnaire-Adolescent Version (PHQ-9) is a nine-item self-administered screening tool for depression among thirteen- to seventeen-year-olds. The tool uses DSM-IV-TR criteria for depression and is highly sensitive and specific. Items receive a score of from "0" ("not at all") to "3" ("nearly every day"). A score of 11 or higher correlates with the DSM criteria for major depression (Richardson et al., 2010).

While the formal screening tools are available for screening for depression, it has been found that screening with two questions about mood and anhedonia may be as effective as using a longer screening instrument (USPSTF, 2009b; Whooley, Avins, Miranda, & Browner, 1997): (1) Over the past two weeks, have you been down, depressed, or hopeless? (2) Have you felt little interest or pleasure in doing things?

When screening for PBD, there are several screening instruments that significantly discriminate bipolar disorder from nonbipolar conditions in youths aged five to eighteen years. Parents may be asked to complete the Parent Mood Disorder Questionnaire (P-MDQ), the ten-item short form of the Parent General Behavior Inventory (PGBI-SF10), and the Parent Young Mania Rating Scale (P-YMRS). Adolescent self-report measures, such as the Adolescent Self-Report MDQ, have been shown to be significantly less efficient, sometimes performing no better than chance at detecting bipolar cases (Youngstrom et al., 2005). The Child Behavior Checklist – Pediatric Bipolar Disorder (CBCL-PBD) profile has been shown to help identify children at high risk for developing bipolar disorder (Biederman et al., 2009).

Role of APNs

In the primary care office, APNs need to promote mental health, engage the family early and effectively in order to address emerging problems, and collaborate with mental health specialists when needed (Brunk, 2010). APNs should be able to recognize the signs and symptoms of mood disorders and establish a basic plan that provides for safety, a therapeutic relationship, and ongoing social support for the child, adolescent, and family (Garzon et al., 2009). The APN must find out from the family how they perceive the problem. This may help to address potential and actual barriers (e.g., stigma) that the family may experience when deciding to seek mental health services. It is important to remember that any treatment plan for youth with mood disorders must involve active participation of the whole family. APNs may instruct youth and/or their caregivers to keep a daily record of the level of depressive and/or manic symptoms ("mood charting") to help monitor symptom presence and patterns (Singh et al., 2007). Families of youth with depressive symptoms must also be educated about the signs and risk of suicide and other self-injurious behaviors. Families with youth at risk for suicide should be told about the need to remove weapons and other means of carrying out lethal intentions (e.g., ropes, medications, poisons, alcohol) from the home.

Children with mood disorders may require special accommodations in the school setting, as required by federal law. The APN may assist the child's school with the development of an individualized education plan (IEP). IEPs are discussed further in Chapter 29 of this text. In addition, the APN may be asked to participate in school planning meetings to develop behavioral care plans. Primary care APNs should become familiar with the child and adolescent APNs in their area in order to facilitate referrals when needed. A transitional meeting between the APNs, the child or adolescent in need of more intensive treatment, and the family may facilitate a smoother transfer and help to define the unique differences in the two practice roles.

When the youth with symptoms of a mood disorder has problems falling asleep or staying asleep, the APN can encourage the youth or family members to keep a sleep diary. The implementation of good sleep habits, such as a regular bedtime, avoidance of caffeine in the evening, and instituting a relaxing routine before sleep, may assist in normalizing sleep patterns. Nutritional counseling may be needed to ensure that the child or adolescent maintains an adequate dietary intake (Horowitz & Marchetti, 2009).

APNs should connect youth and their families with needed services and also coordinate their care. APNs should be aware of resources and referral sources that are available in the community. They should also be aware of insurance sources and know how to code and bill for mental health services (Brunk, 2010). Referral to psychiatric practitioners to initiate medication use and to provide periodic evaluation is essential for youth with symptoms of mood disorders.

Evidence-Based Treatment

Effective treatment of children and adolescents diagnosed with a mood spectrum disorder usually involves use of more than one treatment modality. Individual, family, or group therapy is frequently combined with use of medications and switching modality based on child readiness is not unheard of. Readers are urged to read Chapters 6, 15, 16, and 17 in this text for a more in-depth discussion of effective, evidence-based mental health treatment approaches with the pediatric population. Of paramount concern for all APNs is assessing for suicide risk when presented with youth who are depressed or manic as both are at risk for self-injury. For the youngster who presents with acute symptoms, the goals of treatment center on safety and stabilization. For youngsters with ongoing nonacute symptoms, treatment goals include ensuring medication along with treatment adherence and relapse prevention.

The Treatment for Adolescents with Depression Study (TADS) randomized clinical trial was conducted between 2000 and 2003 at twelve sites with a total sample size of 439 male and female adolescents. Inclusion criteria were age of twelve to seventeen years, a diagnosis of mild to severe depression, impairment in at least two settings, not on an antidepressant, and an IQ greater than 80. Participants were randomly assigned to one of four groups—fluoxetine only, cognitive-behavioral therapy (CBT) only, a combination of antidepressant and CBT, or placebo for twelve weeks. Responders to treatment were continued on the treatment protocol for an additional six months. The Children's Depression Rating Scale – Revised, the Clinical Global Impressions Improvement Scale, the self-report Reynolds Adolescent Depression Scale, and the self-report Suicidal Ideation Questionnaire were the outcome measures used. The most effective initial treatment for adolescent depression was found to be a combination of an SSRI (selective serotonin reuptake inhibitor) such as fluoxetine and CBT. However, over time both fluoxetine alone and CBT alone were comparable to the combination of medication and CBT (March, Silva, & Vitiello, 2006; Vitiello, 2009).

Cognitive-Behavioral Therapy

As previously discussed in Chapter 17, one goal of CBT is to change negative thinking and cognitive distortions. Specific to mood dysregulation, CBT uses psychoeducation to teach the child or adolescent about his or her depression or bipolar disorder, challenges his or her negative thinking, promotes emotion regulation, teaches problem-solving techniques, and teaches/models the importance of engaging in positive relationships and social skills building.

Pharmacological Intervention

As discussed in Chapter 6, SSRIs are the drugs of choice for treating depression with fluoxetine (Prozac) approved for the treatment of depression in children and adolescents. While SSRIs have a safer side effect profile, there is a black box warning with this category of medications and clinicians are urged to assess for suicidality (see Chapter 10) at each pediatric visit in those patients prescribed an antidepressant. It would also be prudent to enlist the support of the parent or caretaker in monitoring for suicidal ideation at home, requiring more frequent "touch-in" visits by these youngsters to the clinic, telephone contacts if in-person contacts are delayed, limiting the amount of antidepressant refills that can be obtained without an office visit, and flagging the chart to remind all providers about the importance of conducting suicide and mood changes assessments (Cheung, Dewa, Levitt, & Zuckerbrot, 2008).

For those youngsters diagnosed with bipolar disorder, the two most frequently prescribed categories of medication are mood stabilizers and atypical antipsychotics. Both the anticonvulsants like divalproex and carbamazepine and lithium are used for their mood-stabilizing properties. More recently, several atypical antipsychotics such as olanzapine, risperidone, and quetiapine have been approved for monotherapy use in children and adolescents diagnosed with bipolar disorder with good results (Hamrin & Pachler, 2007; Kowatch et al., 2005). Medication augmentation can occur when treating PBD. For example, if the adolescent was started on divalproex but effective management of all symptoms could not be achieved, the provider would consider adding a low dose of an atypical agent. Medication algorithms for treating PBD can be found in *Treatment Guidelines for Children and Adolescents with Bipolar Disorder: Child Psychiatric Workgroup on Bipolar Disorder* by Kowatch et al. (2005). Again, APNs are urged to monitor the use and effectiveness of these medications, assess for mood changes along with suicidality, and educate both the youth and parents or caretakers about potential side effects and the importance of contacting the provider should behavioral or physiological concerns arise.

Child and Family Therapy

All youth who are assessed with mood dysregulation in primary care should be evaluated further for referral to individual, group, and/or family therapy. As previously stated, the etiology of mood dysregulation is multifactorial and assaults on self-esteem from one or more sources perpetuate the disorder. Family therapy can enhance parent-child communication, promote attachment/bonding, and develop family skills around behavioral management. Group therapy can place the child or adolescent with peers experiencing similar challenges (universality). Groups can also teach personal symptom management skills, promote healthy peer interactions, and serve as a mechanism for supporting appropriate social development. Interpersonal Therapy for Adolescents (IPT-A) is a short-term (approximately twelve sessions) focused therapy used to educate the adolescent about depression and explore sources of his or her stress/conflict with others. The five areas that become the focus of therapy include authority problems, issues of separation from parents, developing dyadic relationships, loss of relatives and friends, and being in a single parent family. Once the mood state and problem areas are identified, the adolescent is taught skills around problem solving, effective communication, and maintaining relationships (Gallagher, 2005).

Implications for Practice and Nursing Research

The increased morbidity and mortality associated with mood disorders call for APNs to be involved as a central part of the health care team. APNs are instrumental in screening for mood disorders in the primary care setting and for treating minor mood dysregulation in children and adolescents across a variety of settings. Primary care APNs will also be instrumental in working with mental health APNs and making appropriate referrals for behavioral and psychiatric disorders that are beyond the management strategies of their scope of practice. Establishing collaborative treatment partnerships with mental health providers can ensure timely and appropriate treatment of youth and reduce the treatment wait times and difficulty with access that currently exists. Adhering to recommended routine screening for mental, emotional, and behavioral disorders during primary care visits will result in early case-finding and appropriate referrals for care. Building on a previously established relationship with children and their parents, knowledge of the patient's background, and being among the first line of care that children routinely access, APNs can bring about positive outcomes for youth with mental health challenges including mood disorders (Garzon et al., 2009). APNs working with youth should work to foster and fortify relationships with mental health advocates, school officials, human services agencies, mental health and substance abuse providers, and developmental specialists. The best results for youth and their families are obtained when screening for mood disorders is linked to collaborative models of care (Sanci, Lewis, & Patton, 2010).

Most of the randomized controlled trials and large-sample research on mood dysregulation in youth have been conducted by providers in other disciplines. Therefore, more nursing research is needed in the area of pediatric mood dysregulation, especially with preschool, school-aged, and preadolescent populations. Table 9.4 provides examples of nursing research that has been conducted with adolescents.

With mental health screening strongly recommended in primary care, APNs are in a unique position

Table 9.4 Examples of nursing research on mood disorders

Researcher (s)	Title and Source	Year Published	Type of Study	Findings
Dundon, E.	Adolescent depression: A Metasynthesis. *Journal of Pediatric Health Care, 20*(6), 384–392.	2006	Qualitative	A metasynthesis of six qualitative studies was conducted by the researcher who identified 6 themes in the process of adolescent depression. 1) Beyond the blues, 2) spiraling down and within, 3) breaking points, 4) seeing and being seen, 5) seeking solutions and 6) taking control.
Mahon, N., & Yarcheski, A.	Outcomes of depression in early adolescents. *Western Journal of Nursing Research, 23*(4), 360–375.	2001	Quantitative	Study conducted on 144 adolescents to examine the relationship between depressed mood and depressive symptomatology and their influence on four other variables. Depressed mood and depressive symptoms contributed negatively to well-being and perceived health status. In addition, depressed mood and symptoms disrupt relationships and social supports.
Puskar, K., Bernardo, L., Fertman, C., Ren, D., & Stark, K.	The relationship between weight perception, gender, and depressive symptoms among rural adolescents. *Online Journal of Rural Nursing and Health Care, 8*(1).	2008	Quantitative	Data from 75 male and female adolescents with depressive symptoms were analyzed in this study. Researchers concluded that female adolescents who perceived a problem with their weight had higher depressive scores compared to females who did not perceive a problem with their weight. No differences were noted in the male adolescents in the study.
Puskar, K., Sereika, S., & Tusaie-Mumford, K.	Effect of the teaching kids to cope (TKC) program on outcomes of depression and coping among rural adolescents. *Journal of Child and Adolescent Psychiatric Nursing, 16*(2), 71–80.	2003	Quantitative	This randomized controlled study tested the effectiveness of a group administered cognitive-behavioral intervention on 89 rural adolescents. Subjects in the TKC group showed improvement in depressive symptoms and higher use of problem-solving coping skills.
Yarcheski, A., & Mahon, N.	A causal model of depression in early adolescents. *Western Journal of Nursing Research, 22*(8), 879–894.	2000	Quantitative	This theory testing causal model examined depression, gender, state anxiety, self-esteem, and perceived stress in 225 early adolescents. Results indicated that perceived stress had the strongest direct, indirect, and total effect on depression.

to conduct research related to assessment and treatment of minor symptoms by primary care APNs, to test effectiveness of collaborative efforts, and to collect longitudinal data on the well-being of children with mood dysregulation who are able to be maintained in "real world" environments. It is also an opportunity to design collaborative empirical and naturalistic research between primary care APNs and child and adolescent mental health APNs to advance the science within the discipline of nursing.

Case Exemplar

Ann was a thirteen-year-old Caucasian girl who was brought into the pediatric office by her mother for her well-child check. Both Ann and her mother were historians for this interview. When asked if there are any concerns, Ann's mother revealed that Ann has had a decrease in her school performance and grades over the past two months. The family moved into a new home three months ago and Ann has had to change schools. Since changing schools, she has not made many friends and her grades have begun to decline. Other aspects of the history revealed that Ann has begun to eat more than usual since the move and had gained weight. Ann's nutrition history revealed that she had a balanced diet with sufficient sources of dairy, protein, fruits, and vegetables. However, she had begun to eat more junk food and to drink more sugary drinks such as soda. Ann was on the field hockey team at her previous school but had not been participating in sports at her new school.

Ann had also been sleeping more. She did not have any problems falling asleep. She slept approximately twelve hours each night but did not have a set bedtime or a regular bedtime routine. She slept in her own bed and shared a room with her younger brother. Within the past month, Ann had begun to take a daily nap. There had been no changes in her elimination pattern. She was voiding well with no complaints of dysuria or enuresis. She had one bowel movement daily and denied constipation or diarrhea.

The social history revealed that Ann lived at home with her mother and her younger brother (three years old). Her parents had recently gone through a divorce and her father no longer lived in the home. Ann's mother worked as a restaurant waitress. Ann attended an after-school program until her mother got home from work. The family had no pets. There were no smokers in the home. There were no weapons in the home, per mother's report.

Ann's past medical history revealed no use of substances and no recent trauma. She had never been hospitalized and did not have any chronic illnesses. Ann was currently taking no over-the-counter, prescription, or herbal medications. She has no known allergies to medication, food, or the environment and she was up to date for required immunizations.

The family medical history revealed that Ann's mother (thirty-seven years old) and father (thirty-six years old) were both healthy. Ann's mother was diagnosed with depression after the divorce. She was in therapy and was taking medication to treat her depression. Ann's three-year-old sibling also had no history of chronic medical conditions. Her maternal grandmother (age sixty-four years) had a history of asthma. Her maternal grandfather (sixty-five years old) had a history of high cholesterol. Ann's paternal grandmother (sixty-two years old) had a history of hypertension. Her paternal grandfather (sixty-two years old) had a history of hypertension and had a stroke at age fifty-seven years.

A comprehensive physical examination was conducted. When observing Ann's general appearance, the APN noticed that her shoulders were slumped and that Ann did not make eye contact. Ann's neurological examination revealed no abnormalities. The remainder of the physical examination was unremarkable.

Upon further discussion, Ann revealed that she feels that her parents' divorce was her fault and that she felt sad because of that. Taking into account Ann's general appearance, her feeling of sadness, decreasing grades, changes in her weight and sleep, and the family history of depression, the APN decided that Ann should be screened for depressive symptoms at this visit. Ann was screened for depressive symptoms with the CES-DC. Her score revealed that Ann was experiencing depressive symptoms, with a score of 18.

The primary care APN ordered a complete blood cell count with differential in the initial laboratory evaluation to rule out infection and anemia as causes for Ann's symptoms. Thyroid function tests (T_3, T_4, and TSH) were ordered to rule out a thyroid dysfunction. Imaging studies are usually not conducted as part of the initial work-up for an adolescent with depressive symptoms. However, if the neurological examination reveals findings that may indicate a brain abnormality, a magnetic resonance imaging (MRI) test can be performed to examine the brain. MRI is the preferred imaging test in youths because it does not involve ionizing radiation or radioactive isotopes.

The primary care APN should establish a basic plan with Ann and her mother that provides for safety and ongoing social support for the family. The APN must determine if Ann is experiencing suicidal ideation. If she is, Ann must be referred immediately for emergency psychiatric evaluation.

To assist with sleep problems, Ann can be encouraged to keep a sleep diary. The implementation of good sleep habits should be discussed. Nutritional and fitness counseling may be needed to ensure that the Ann maintains an adequate dietary intake and has an appropriate amount of daily physical activity.

Ann and her family should be referred to a pediatric psychiatric mental health APN for a full evaluation and confirmatory diagnosis of depression. The psych-mental health APN will determine the treatment program. The primary care APN will work together with that clinician and family to provide support and to ensure that the family adheres to the treatment guidelines.

The following are some sources of guidelines for identifying and treating adolescents with depression in primary care.

Cheung, A.H., Zuckerbrot, R.A., Jensen, P.S., Ghalib, K., Laraque, D., Stein, R.E., & GLAD-PC Steering Group. (2007). Guidelines for adolescent depression in primary care (GLAD-PC): II. Treatment and ongoing management. *Pediatrics, 120*(5), e1313–e1326.

Zuckerbrot, R.A., Cheung, A.H., Jensen, P.S., Stein, R.E., Laraque, D.., & GLAD-PC Steering Group. (2007). Guidelines for adolescent depression in primary care (GLAD-PC): I. Identification, assessment, and initial management. *Pediatrics, 120*(5), e1299–s1312.

Outcome

Ann was referred for an evaluation with a child/adolescent psychiatric APN in a local clinic. After assessment, she began a trial of CBT and her mother and brother began working in family therapy with a social worker around issues surrounding the parental divorce. After six weeks of outpatient treatment, with continuing high scores on the depression inventory, a trial of Prozac 20 mg was instituted with good response. When therapy finished, Ann was referred back to her pediatric APN with a continuation of the Prozac, now at a 40-mg dose. A follow-up appointment with the psychiatric APN occurred three months later and Prozac was discontinued at Ann's and her mother's request. Ann had experienced one year free of depressive symptoms. Both she and her mother were given information about risk for recurring depression and the pediatric APN will monitor this.

Conclusion

This chapter has described the symptoms, etiology, and management of mood dysregulation in children and adolescents with a focus on depression, severe mood dysregulation, and PBDs. The chapter also acknowledges the unique opportunity for pediatric primary care APNs to become even more pivotal in the screening, early case finding, and referral process for children in need of mental health treatment. All too often there has been a time frame of two to four years between onset of symptoms, diagnosis, and initiation of treatment. During that gap, mood symptoms can interfere with normal development, relationships, academic performance, self-esteem, and the safety of the child who is at risk for engaging in self-injurious behaviors. APNs who have a sound knowledge base regarding recognizing pediatric mood dysregulation and when to refer to mental health providers will improve the mental health care that children and adolescents receive when they access the primary care system.

Resources

American Academy of Child and Adolescent Psychiatry available at www.aacap.org

Behavioral assessment tools available for purchase at http://www.pearsonassesments.com

Bright Futures in Practice. (2002). Mental Health, Volume I: Practice Guide. Washington, DC: National Center for Education in Maternal and Child Health at Georgetown University.

Bright Futures in Practice. (2002). Mental Health, Volume II: Tool Kit. Washington, DC: National Center for Education in Maternal and Child Health at Georgetown University. Available at http://www.brightfutures.org/mentalhealth/pdf/professionals/ped_symptom_chklst.pdf

Guidelines for Adolescent Depression in Primary Care (GLAD-PC) Tool Kit available to download at http://www.gladpc.org. Contains screening tools and psychoeducation materials (depression facts, medications, counseling, self-management, etc.) for healthcare providers to use with children, adolescents and parents.

Melnyk, B., & Moldenhauer, Z. (2006). KYSS Guide to Child and Adolescent Mental Health Screening, Early Intervention and Health Promotion. Cherry Hill, NJ: NAPNAP.

Neuroscience Educational Institute (NEI). Annual membership fee to access materials. Available at http://www.neiglobal.com

TeenScreen National Center for Mental Health Checkups at Columbia University. Available at http://www.teenscreen.org

U.S. Preventive Services Task Force (2009a). Screening for child and adolescent depression in primary care settings: A systematic evidence review. Available at http://www.uspreventiveservicestaskforce.org/uspst09/depression/chdeprat.htm

References

Achenbach, T. (1991). *Manual for the youth self-report and 1991 profiles.* Burlington, VT: University of Vermont Department of Psychiatry.

American Psychiatric Association (APA). (2000). *Diagnostic and statistical manual of mental disorders: DSM-IV-TR* (4th ed., text revision). Washington, DC: Author.

American Psychiatric Association. (2009). *Report of the DSM-V childhood and adolescent disorders workgroup.* Retrieved from http://www.psych.org/MainMenu/Research/DSMIV/DSMV/DSMRevisionActivities/DS M.

Anderson, E., & Hope, D. (2008). A review of the tripartite model for understanding the link between anxiety and depression in youth. *Clinical Psychology Review, 28,* 275–287.

Babiss, L., & Gangwisch, J. (2009). Sports participation as a protective factor against depression and suicidal ideation in adolescents as mediated by self-esteem and social support. *Journal of Developmental & Behavioral Pediatrics, 30,* 376–384.

Baroni, A., Lunsford, J., Luckenbaugh, D., Towbin, K., & Leibenluft, E. (2008). Practitioner review: The assessment of bipolar disorder in children and adolescents. *Journal of Child Psychology and Psychiatry, 50*(3), 203–215.

Beck, A. (1967). *Depression: Clinical, experiential, and theoretical aspects.* New York, NY: Harper& Row.

Beck, A. (2008). The evolution of the cognitive model of depression and its neurobiological correlates. *American Journal of Psychiatry, 165*(8), 969–977.

Beck, A., Steer, R., & Brown, G. (1996). *BDI-II manual*. San Antonio, TX: Psychological Corporation.

Biederman, J., Petty, C., Monuteaux, M., Evans, M., Parcell, T., Faraone, S., & Wozniak, J. (2009). The child behavior checklist-pediatric bipolar disorder profile predicts a subsequent diagnosis of bipolar disorder and associated impairments in ADHD youth growing up: A longitudinal analysis. *Journal of Clinical Psychiatry, 70*, 732–740.

Bronfenbrenner, U. (1979). *The ecology of human development: Experiments by nature and design.* Cambridge, MA: Harvard University Press.

Bronfenbrenner, U. (1994). Nature-nurture reconceptualized in developmental perspective: A bioecological model. *Psychological Review, 101*(4), 568–586.

Brotman, M., Schmajuk, M., Rich, B., Dickstein, D., Guyer, A., Costello, E., & Leibenluft, E. (2006). Prevalence, clinical correlates, and longitudinal course of severe mood dysregulation in children. *Biological Psychiatry, 60*, 991–997.

Brunk, D. (2010). AAP task force report offers guide to enhance delivery of mental health services. *Pediatric News, 44*,1,5.

Carbray, J., & McGuinness, T. (2009). Pediatric bipolar disorder. *Journal of Psychosocial Nursing and Mental Health Services, 47*(12), 22–26.

Caspi, A., Sugden, K., Moffitt, T., Taylor, A., Craig, I., & Harrington, H. (2003). Influence of life stress on depression: Moderation by a polymorphism in the 5-HTT gene. *Science, 301*, 386–389.

Chang, K., Singh, M., Wang, P., & Howe, M. (2010). Management of bipolar disorders in children and adolescents. In T. Ketter (Ed). *Handbook of diagnosis and treatment of bipolar disorders.* Arlington, VA: American Psychiatric Publishing, Inc.; US. pp. 389–424.

Cheung, A., Dewa, C., Levitt, A., & Zuckerbrot, R. (2008). Pediatric depressive disorders: Management priorities in primary care. *Current Opinion in Pediatrics, 20*, 551–559.

Cheung, A.H., Zuckerbrot, R.A., Jensen, P.S., Ghalib, K., Laraque, D., Stein, R.E., & GLAD-PC Steering Group. (2007). Guidelines for adolescent depression in primary care (GLAD-PC): II. Treatment and ongoing management. *Pediatrics, 120*(5), e1313–e1326.

Clark, D., & Beck, A. (2010). Cognitive theory and therapy of anxiety and depression: Convergence with neurobiological findings. *Trends in Cognitive Sciences, 14*, 418–424.

Clark, L., & Watson, D. (1991). Tripartite model of anxiety and depression: Psychosomatic evidence and taxonomic implications. *Journal of Abnormal Psychology, 100*, 316–336.

Costello, E. J., Erkanli, A., & Angold, A. (2006). Is there an epidemic of child or adolescent depression? *Journal of Child Psychology and Psychiatry, 47*(12), 1263–1271.

Coyle, J., Pine, D., Charney, D., Lewis, L., Nemeroff, C., Carlson, G. Depression and Bipolar Support Alliance Consensus Development Panel. (2003). Depression and bipolar support alliance consensus statement on the unmet needs in diagnosis and treatment of mood disorders in children and adolescents. *Journal of the American Academy of Child and Adolescent Psychiatry, 42*(12), 1494–1502.

De Bolle, M., & De Fruyt, F. (2010). The tripartite model in childhood and adolescence: Future directions for developmental research. *Child Development Perspectives, 4*(3), 174–180.

Duffy, A., Alda, M., Hajek, T., & Grof, P. (2009). Early course of bipolar disorder in high-risk offspring: Prospective study. *The British Journal of Psychiatry, 195*, 457–458.

Dundon, E. (2006). Adolescent depression: A metasynthesis. *Journal of Pediatric Health Care, 20*, 384–392.

Ebner-Priemer, U., & Trull, T. (2009). Ecological momentary assessment of mood disorders and mood dysregulation. *Psychological Assessment, 21*(4), 463–475.

Eisenberg, N., Cumberland, A., Spinrad, T., Fabes, R., Shepard, S., Reiser, M., & Guthrie, I. (2001). The relations of regulation and emotionality to children's externalizing and internalizing problem behavior. *Child Development, 72*(4), 1112–1134.

Elmquist, J., Melton, T., Croarkin, P., & McClintock, S. (2010). A systematic overview of measurement-based care in the treatment of childhood and adolescent depression. *Journal of Psychiatric Practice, 16*(4), 217–234.

Emslie, G., Mayes, T., Kennard, B., & Hughes, J. (2006). Pediatric Mood Disorders. In D. Stein, D. Kupfer, & A. Schatzberg (Eds.). *The American psychiatric publishing textbook of mood disorders* (pp. 573–601). Arlington, VA: American Psychiatric Publishing, Inc.

Faulstich, M., Carey, M., Ruggiero, M., Enyart, P., & Gresham, F. (1986). Assessment of depression in childhood and adolescence: An evaluation of the center for epidemiological studies of depression scale for children (CES-DC). *American Journal of Psychiatry, 143*, 1024–1027.

Fava, G., & Tossani, E. (2007). Prodromal stage of major depression. *Early Intervention in Psychiatry, 1*, 9–18.

Fields, B., & Fristad, M. (2009). The bipolar child and the educational system: Working with schools. In R. Kowatch, M. Fristad, R. Findling, & R. Post, *Clinical manual for management of bipolar disorder in children and adolescents* (pp. 239–272). Arlington, VA: American Psychiatric Publishing, Inc.

Finkelhor, D., Ormrod, R., & Turner, H. (2007). Poly-victimization: A neglected component in child victimization trauma. *Child Abuse and Neglect, 31*, 7–26.

Gallagher, R. (2005). Evidence-based psychotherapies for depressed adolescents: A review and clinical guidelines. *Primary Psychiatry, 12*(9), 33–39.

Garber, J. (2006). Depression in children and adolescents: Linking risk research and prevention. *American Journal of Preventive Medicine, 31*, S104–S125.

Garzon, D., Nelson, J., & Figgemeier, M. (2009). Management of childhood depression. *The Clinical Advisor.* Electronic version. Retrieved from http://www.clinicaladvisor.com/Management-of-childhood-depression/PrintArticle/149979/

Geracioti, T. (2006). Identifying hypothyroidism's psychiatric presentations. *Current Psychiatry Online, 5*(11). Retrieved from http://www.currentpsychiatry.com/article_pages.asp?AID=4545&UID=Overflow

Goldstein, B., Birmaher, B., Axelson, D., Goldstein, T., Esposito-Smythers, C., Strober, M., & Keller, M. (2008). Preliminary findings regarding overweight and obesity in pediatric bipolar disorder. *Journal of Clinical Psychiatry, 69*, 1953–1959.

Hamrin, V., & Magorno, M. (2010). Assessment of adolescents for depression in the pediatric primary care setting. *Pediatric Nursing, 36*(2), 103–111.

Hamrin, V., & Pachler, M. (2007). Pediatric bipolar disorder: Evidence-based psychopharmacological treatments. *Journal of Child and Adolescent Psychiatric Nursing, 20*(1), 40–58.

Harvard Mental Health Letter. (2007). Thyroid deficiency and mental health. *Harvard Mental Health Letter, 23*(11), 4–5.

Holtmann, M., Duketis, E., Goth, K., Poustka, L., & Boelte, S. (2010). Severe affective and behavioral dysregulation in youth is associated with increased serum TSH. *Journal of Affective Disorders, 121*, 184–188.

Horowitz, J., & Marchetti, C. (2009). Mood disorders. In P. Jackson-Allen, J. Vessey, & N. Schapiro (Eds.), *Primary care of the child with a chronic condition* (5th ed.) (pp. 627–653). St. Louis, MO: Mosby Elsevier.

Howland, R. (2010). Use of endocrine hormones for treating depression. *Journal of Psychosocial Nursing, 48*(12), 13–16.

Institute of Medicine (IOM). (2009). *Preventing mental, emotional and behavioral disorders among young people: Progress and possibilities*. Washington, DC: National Academy of Sciences.

Jacobs, R., Reinecke, M., Gollan, J., & Kane, P. (2008). Empirical evidence of cognitive vulnerability for depression among children and adolescents: A cognitive science and developmental perspective. *Clinical Psychology Review, 28*, 759–782.

Jaycox, L., Stein, B., Paddock, S., Miles, J., Chandra, A., Meredith, L., Burnam, M. (2009). Impact of teen depression on academic, social, and physical functioning. *Pediatrics, 124*, e596-e605.

Jeffery, D., Sava, D., & Winters, N. (2005). Depressive disorders. In K. Cheng and K. Myers (Eds.). *Child and adolescent psychiatry: The essentials* (pp. 169–189). Philadelphia, PA: Lippincott Williams & Wilkins.

Jellinek, M., Patel, B., & Froehle, M. (Eds). (2002). Mood disorders: Depressive and bipolar disorders. *Bright futures in practice: Mental health—Volume 1. Practice guide*. Arlington, VA: National Center for Education in Maternal and Child Health.

Kessler, R., Avenevoli, S., & Merikangas, K. (2001), Mood disorders in children and adolescents: An epidemiologic perspective. *Biological Psychiatry, 49*, 1002–1014.

Kovacs, M. (1992). *Children depression inventory (CDI)*. North Tonawanda, NY: Multi-Health Systems.

Kowatch, R., Fristad, M., Birmaher, B., Wagner, K., Findling, R., Hellander, M. The Work Group Members. (2005). Treatment guidelines for children and adolescents with bipolar disorder: Child psychiatric workgroup on bipolar disorder. *Journal of the American Academy of Child and Adolescent Psychiatry, 44*(3), 213–235.

Kowatch, R., Youngstrom, E., Danielyan, A., & Findling, R. (2005). Review and meta-analysis of the phenomenology and clinical characteristics of mania in children and adolescents. *Bipolar Disorders, 7*, 483–496.

Lazaratou, H., Dikeos, D., Anagnostopoulos, D., & Soldatos, C. (2010). Depressive symptomatology in high school students: The role of age, gender, and academic pressure. *Community Mental Health Journal, 46*, 289–295.

Leibenluft, E., Charney, D., Towbin, K., Bhangoo, R., & Pine, D. (2003). Defining clinical phenotypes of juvenile mania. *American Journal of Psychiatry, 160*(3), 430–437.

Lewinsohn, P., Rohde, P., & Seely, J. (1998). Major depressive disorder in older adolescents: Prevalence, risk factors, and clinical implications. *Clinical Psychology Review, 18*(7), 765–794.

Luby, J., Belden, A., & Spitznagel, E. (2006). Risk factors for preschool depression: The mediating role of early stressful life events. *Journal of Child Psychology and Psychiatry, 47*(12), 1292–1298.

MacPhee, A., & Andrews, J. (2006). Risk factors for depression in early adolescence. *Adolescence, 41*(163), 435–466.

March, J., Silva, S., & Vitiello, B. (2006). The treatment for adolescents with depression study (TADS): Methods and message at 12 weeks. *Journal of the American Academy of Child and Adolescent Psychiatry, 45*(12), 1393–1403.

Mahon, N., & Yarcheski, A. (2001). Outcomes of depression in early adolescents. *Western Journal of Nursing Research, 23*(4), 360–375.

Mazza, J., Abbott, R., Fleming, C., Harachi, T., Cortes, R., & Park, J., et al. (2009). Early predictors of adolescent depression: A 7-year longitudinal study. *Journal of Early Adolescence, 29*, 664–692.

Merikangas, K., He, J., Burstein, M., Swanson, S., Avenevoli, S., Cui, L., & Swendsen, J. (2010). Lifetime prevalence of mental disorders in U.S. adolescents: Results from the national comorbidity survey replication adolescent supplement (NCS-A). *Journal of the American Academy of Child and Adolescent Psychiatry, 49*(10), 980–989.

Mick, E., & Faraone, S. (2009). Family and genetic association studies of bipolar disorder in children. *Child and Adolescent Psychiatric Clinics of North America, 18*, 441–453.

Moldenhauer, Z. (2006). Mood disorders. In B. Melnyk and Z. Moldenhauer (Eds.), *The KySS (Keep your children/yourself-safe and secure) guide to child and adolescent mental health screening, early and health promotion* (pp. 141–172). Cherry Hill, NJ: NAPNAP.

Mrug, S., & Windle, M. (2010). Prospective effects of violence exposure across multiple contexts on early adolescents' internalizing and externalizing problems. *Journal of Child Psychology and Psychiatry, 51*(8), 953–961.

Nemeroff, C. B., & Vale, W. W. (2005). The neurobiology of depression: Inroads to treatment and new drug discovery. *Journal of Clinical Psychiatry, 66*(Suppl 7), 5–13.

Neuroscience Educational Institute (NEI). (2009). *Understanding and managing the pieces of major depressive disorder*. Carlsbad, CA: Author.

Newman, E. (2006). Short-term play therapy for children with mood disorders. In H. Kaduson and C. Schaefer (Eds.), *Short-term play therapy for children (2nd ed.)* (pp. 71–100). New York, NY: Guilford Press.

Oland, A., & Shaw, D. (2005). Pure versus co-occurring externalizing and internalizing symptoms in children: The potential role of socio-developmental milestones. *Clinical Child and Family Psychology Review, 8*(4), 247–270.

Papolos, D., & Papolos, J. (2006). *The bipolar child: The definitive and reassuring guide to childhood's most misunderstood disorder,* (3rd ed.). New York, NY: Broadway Books.

Prager, L. (2009). Depression and suicide in children and adolescents. *Pediatrics in Review, 30*, 199–206.

Puskar, K., Bernardo, L., Fertman, C., Ren, D., & Stark, K. (2008). The relationship between weight perception, gender and depressive symptoms among rural adolescents. *Online Journal of Rural Nursing and Health Care, 8*(1), Spring.

Puskar, K., Sereika, S., & Tusaie-Mumford, K. (2003). Effect of the teaching kids to cope program on outcomes of depression and coping among rural adolescents. *Journal of Child and Adolescent Psychiatric Nursing, 16*(2), 71–80.

Radloff, L. S. (1977). The CES-D scale: A self-report depression scale for research in the general population. *Applied Psychological Measurement, 1*, 385–401.

Restifo, K., & Bogels, S. (2009). Family processes in the development of youth depression: Translating the evidence to treatment. *Clinical Psychology Review, 29*, 294–316.

Richardson, L., McCauley, E., Grossman, D., McCarty, C., Richards, J., Russo, J., & Katon, W. (2010). Evaluation of the patient health questionnnaire: 9 item for detecting major depression among adolescents. *Pediatrics, 126*, 1117–1123.

Rockhill, C., Hlastala, S., & Myers, K. (2005). Early onset bipolar disorder. In K. Cheng and K. Myers (Eds.), *Child and adolescent psychiatry: The essentials* (pp. 191–210). Philadelphia, PA: Lippincott Williams & Wilkins.

Sadock, B. J., & Sadock, V. A. (2009). *Kaplan & Sadock's concise textbook of child and adolescent psychiatry*. Philadelphia, PA: Wolters Kluwer.

Sala, R., Axelson, D., & Birmaher, B. (2009). Phenomenology, longitudinal course, and outcome of children and adolescents with bipolar spectrum disorders. *Child and Adolescent Psychiatric Clinics of North America, 18*, 273–289.

Sanci, L., Lewis, D., & Patton, G. (2010). Detecting emotional disorder in young people in primary care. *Current Opinion in Psychiatry, 23*, 318–323.

Schenkel, L., West, A., Harral, E., Patel, N., & Pavuluri, M. (2008). Parent-child interactions in pediatric bipolar disorder. *Journal of Clinical Psychology, 64,* 422–437.

Schlesinger, A. (2008). In this issue/abstract thinking: Pediatric primary care providers and depression in community settings. *Journal of the American Academy of Child & Adolescent Psychiatry, 47,* 975–976.

Siever, L.J., & Davis, K.L. (1985). Overview: toward a dysregulation hypothesis of depression. *American Journal of Psychiatry, 142,* 1017–1031.

Singh, M., Pfeifer, J., Barzman, D., Kowatch, R., & DelBello, M. (2007). Pharmacotherapy for child and adolescent mood disorder. *Psychiatric Annals, 37,* 465–476.

Stahl, S. (2008). *Stahl's essential psychopharmacology: Neuroscientific basis and practical applications* (3rd ed.). New York, NY: Cambridge University Press.

Tackett, J. (2010). Toward an externalizing spectrum in DSM-V: Incorporating developmental concerns. *Child Development Perspectives, 4*(3), 161–167.

Townsend, M. (2009). Psychopharmacology. *Psychiatric Mental Health Nursing, 6th Edition.* Philadelphia, PA: F.A. Davis Company.

U.S. Preventive Services Task Force. (2009a). *Screening for child and adolescent depression in primary care settings. A systematic evidence review.* Retrieved from http://www.uspreventiveservicestaskforce. org/uspst09/depression/chdeprat.htm

U.S. Preventive Services Task Force. (2009b). *Major depressive disorder in children and adolescents.* Rockville, MD: Agency for Healthcare Research and Quality. Retrieved from http://www.ahrq.gov/clinic/uspstf/uspschdepr.htm

Verhulst, F., Achenbach, T., Ende, J., Erol, N., Lambert, M., Leung, P., & Zubrick, S. (2003). Comparison of problems reported by youths from seven countries. *American Journal of Psychiatry, 160*(8), 1479–1485.

Vitiello, B. (2009). Treatment for adolescent depression: What we have come to know. *Depression and Anxiety, 26,* 393–395.

Watamura, S., Donzella, B., Alwin, J., & Gunnar, M. (2003). Morning-to-afternoon increases in cortisol concentrations for infants and toddlers at child care: Age differences and behavioral correlates. *Child Development, 74*(4), 1006–1020.

Weissman, M., Orvaschel, H., & Padian, N. (1980). Children's symptoms and social function self-report scales: Comparison of mothers' and children's reports. *Journal of Nervous and Mental Disease, 168,* 736–740.

West, A., Schenkel, L., & Pavuluri, M. (2008). Early childhood temperament in pediatric bipolar disorder and attention deficit hyperactivity disorder. *Journal of Clinical Psychology, 64,* 402–421.

Whooley, M., Avins, A., Miranda, J., & Browner, W. (1997). Case-finding instruments for depression: Two questions are as good as many. *Journal of General Internal Medicine, 12,* 439–445.

Wilcox, H., Field, T., Prodromidis, M., & Scafidi, F. (1998). Correlations between the BDI and CES-D in a sample of adolescent mothers. *Adolescence, 33,* 565–574.

World Health Organization (WHO). (2008). The global burden of disease: 2004 update. Geneva, Switzerland: Author.

Yackel, E., McKennan, M., & Fox-Deise, A. (2010). A nurse-facilitated depression screening program in an army primary care clinic: An evidenced-based project. *Nursing Research, 59,* S58–S65.

Yarcheski, A., & Mahon, N. (2000). A causal model of depression in early adolescents. *Western Journal of Nursing Research, 22*(8), 879–894.

Youngstrom, E., Meyers, O., Demeter, C., Youngstrom, J., Morello, L., & Piiparinen, R.L. (2005). Comparing diagnostic checklists for pediatric bipolar disorder in academic and community mental health settings. *Bipolar Disorders, 7,* 507–517.

Zuckerbrot, R., Cheung, A., Jensen, P., Stein, R., Laraque, D., & the GLAD-PC Steering Group. (2007). Guidelines for adolescent depression in primary care (GLAD-PC): I. Identification, assessment, and initial management. *Pediatrics, 120,* e1299–1312. doi:10.1542/peds.2007-1144.

10

Deliberate Self-Harm: Nonsuicidal Self-Injury and Suicide in Children and Adolescents

Edilma L. Yearwood and Eve Bosnick

Objectives

After reading this chapter, APNs will be able to

1. Differentiate between the etiologies and mental health processes involved in various deliberate self-harm behaviors such as suicidal ideation, nonsuicidal self-injury, and suicide in children and adolescents with and without a psychiatric diagnosis.
2. Identify internalizing, externalizing, and psychosocial factors that place children and adolescents at risk for engaging in a range of self-harming behaviors.
3. Describe evidence-based pharmacological and nonpharmacological care management models for use by primary care and child and adolescent psychiatric-mental health advanced practice nurses (APNs) working with youth who engage in self-harm behaviors.
4. Identify strategies for working with children and adolescents who self-harm and their families.
5. Discuss roles of the APN in the identification and care of youth who engage in self-harm behaviors.

Introduction

This chapter will focus on a variety of deliberate self-harm (DSH) behaviors, differentiate between nonsuicidal self-injury (NSSI) and suicidal self-injurious (SSI) behaviors, identify youth at risk for engaging in these behaviors, describe etiologies attributed to DSH behaviors, and present evidence-based management strategies for use when working with NSSI and suicidal youth. The accuracy of prevalence rates of NSSI in adolescents is difficult to ascertain because of the secrecy that often accompanies these behaviors. However, it is believed to range between 12% and 40% in community populations with and without a psychiatric diagnosis and between 38% and 67% in inpatient psychiatric populations (Muehlenkamp, Williams, Gutierrez, & Claes, 2009; Nixon, Cloutier, & Aggarwal, 2002; Ross & Heath, 2002).

In 2005, suicide was the third cause of death in youth and young adults ten to twenty-four years of age in the United States (U.S.) (Centers for Disease Control and Prevention [CDC], 2007). The Youth Risk Behavior Surveillance (YRBS) data on 16,410 youth in grades nine to twelve from 2008 to 2009 found that 13.8% of youth considered suicide, 10.9% had developed a plan, and 6.3% had made one or more suicidal gestures (Eaton et al., 2010). American Indian and Alaskan Native youth have the highest rates of suicide, followed by Hispanic and non-Hispanic white males (Eaton et al.). The CDC estimates that for every successful youth suicide, there are between 100 and 200 unsuccessful attempts (CDC). It is estimated that over 4,000 youth kill themselves in the U.S. and

---

Child and Adolescent Behavioral Health: A Resource for Advanced Practice Psychiatric and Primary Care Practitioners in Nursing,
First Edition. Edited by Edilma L. Yearwood, Geraldine S. Pearson, and Jamesetta A. Newland.

over 200,000 youth kill themselves worldwide annually (Wasserman, Cheng, & Jiang, 2005). Self-inflicted gunshot wounds, suffocation by hanging or use of plastic bags, and poisoning are the most frequently used methods for suicide in youth.

NSSI, also referred to as self-mutilation, self-injury, self-injurious behaviors, or para-suicide, has been analyzed and discussed in the psychiatric literature for well over sixty years. Initially, these behaviors were thought to be strongly linked to suicide. However, recent research is providing evidence that these behaviors are distinct and separate phenomena with different motivations. There are youngsters who engage in "common" NSSI behaviors with *no intent* to kill themselves, a second group of youngsters who are suicide attempters, and a third, believed to be the most pathologically entrenched group, who engage in both SSI and NSSI behaviors (Cloutier, Martin, Kennedy, Nixon, & Muehlenkamp, 2010). This chapter will describe etiologies believed to be the drivers of NSSI and SSI behaviors, factors that put youth at risk for engaging in these behaviors, clinical presentations frequently seen, assessment tools used for screening at-risk and active self-harming youth, and nursing management strategies for use with this population.

Nonsuicidal Self-Injury

To begin with, it is not uncommon for children and adolescents to experience suicidal ideation (SI), especially during stressful times when they feel that there is no good solution to their dilemma. Children should not be made to feel guilty about having SI, which is a thought or image of killing oneself. Instead, they need to recognize a range of emotions that all people experience and be taught that it is what people do with these emotions that guides the particular outcome.

Youngsters who engage in NSSI do not intend to die; they engage in the behaviors to feel better (Favazza, 1998). During the act of self-injury, the individual engages in a "socially unacceptable repetitive behavior that causes minor to moderate physical injury. When self-mutilating, the individual is in a psychologically disturbed state but is not attempting suicide or responding to a need for self-stimulation or a stereotypic behavior characteristic of mental retardation or autism" (Suyemoto, 1998, p. 532). When NSSI behaviors begin in childhood and continue throughout adolescence, these youngsters are viewed as more entrenched in the ritual and cycle of self-harming behaviors. Common descriptors used to explain the pattern of NSSI include compulsive, ritualistic, episodic, and repetitive. The level of the injury or the amount of harm to the body is usually described as mild, moderate, or extreme. Table 10.1, which was adapted from Favazza (1998), Nock (2010), and Suyemoto (1998) and Wells et al. (1998), contains a list of self-harm behaviors rated from mild to extreme. Cutting of the skin is a common act and the most common sites are the arms, legs, inner thighs, and the abdomen. Practitioners should question youth who consistently wear long-sleeve shirts and sweaters or multiple layers of clothing in warm weather and youth who are reluctant to expose certain body surface areas during physical exams. The APN needs to keep in mind that NSSI is a quick act that can occur in multiple contexts; it is usually performed in private where the individual has access to inexpensive and readily available tools.

Table 10.1 Examples of DSH behaviors

Mild to Moderate Behaviors	Extreme Behaviors
Head banging	Object insertion (risk for infection and other trauma)
Self-biting	Branding or carving words or symbols into skin
Skin picking	Deep skin cutting
Burning (first degree)	Ingesting toxic substances (poisoning)
Superficial skin cutting	Burning (second and third degree)
Trichotillomania	Severe onychophagia (nail biting that results in bleeding, infection, and mutilation)
Needle sticking	
Some forms of body piercing	
Hitting walls and objects to induce pain	
Breaking bones	
Preventing wound healing	Eye enucleation and self-castration are usually secondary to a psychotic experience

Adapted from Favazza, 1998; Nock, 2010; Suyemoto, 1998; and Wells, Haines, and Williams, 1998.

NSSI usually begins between the ages of twelve and fourteen with adolescent prevalence rates three to four times greater than adult rates (Klonsky, Oltmanns, & Turkheimer, 2003). NSSI is *deliberate, repetitive,* and *direct destruction or alteration* of body tissue that is done without conscious suicidal intent but can result in severe tissue damage (Favazza, 1998). Unfortunately, while the intent is not suicide, some who engage in NSSI inadvertently do kill themselves due to the lethality of the method chosen or the fact that they fail to access medical treatment in a timely manner. NSSI can be a culturally sanctioned behavior, a pathological act against the self to manage perceived intolerable tension, an attempt to avoid suicide (and therefore can be considered a poor coping strategy), or a drastic attempt to communicate needs and feelings to others. It is not uncommon for self-injurers to use multiple methods and more than one body location during the span of time that they engage in self-harm.

Two factors clearly evident from recent literature chronicling the development of the science about NSSI are that (1) NSSI and suicide are distinct phenomena with different intent and expected outcome and (2) NSSI in its purest form is best understood in the absence of developmental or intellectual impairment and psychosis (Favazza, 1998; Mangnall & Yurkovich, 2008). Reportedly, nearly 80% of those who engage in NSSI stop the behavior within five years (Whitlock, Eckenrode, & Silverman, 2006).

It is anticipated that *The Diagnostic and Statistical Manual for Mental Disorders-V* (DSM-V), with an expected publication date of 2013, will include NSSI as a new disorder. This is partly in response to an increase in recognition of these behaviors among adolescents and young adults and an awareness that a large percentage of those who engage in NSSI do not meet the criteria for borderline personality disorder, developmental disabilities, psychosis, or eating disorders (Peterson, Freedenthal, Sheldon, & Andersen, 2008). The proposed criteria are slated to include:

1. Engaging in self-injury five or more days with damage to the surface of the skin
2. At least two of the following: negative feelings or thoughts, preoccupation with the intended behavior, frequent urges to self-injure, or purposeful engagement in the act of self-injury
3. The act results in impairment in one or more areas of functioning and does not occur exclusively during states of psychosis, delirium, or intoxication

Two NSSI NOS (not otherwise specified) subtypes have also been proposed; in Type I, the individual engages in the act less than five times during the year, and in Type 2, the individual may actually intend to commit suicide (American Psychiatric Association [APA], 2010).

Etiology of NSSI

Several theories have been offered to explain why people engage in NSSI. These include engaging in the act to (1) change or influence negative personal affect and emotions such as anger and depression, (2) punish self, (3) influence the thoughts and behaviors of others, (4) interrupt dissociative experiences, (5) experience excitement, and (6) cope with suicidal thoughts (Klonsky, 2007). Engaging in NSSI seems to meet both intrapersonal and interpersonal needs. Risk factors include history of childhood physical or sexual abuse, perception of abandonment or isolation, low self-esteem, chronic or overwhelming stress and anxiety, poor impulse control, depression, adolescence, incarceration, living in abusive and chaotic environments, intrafamilial conflicts, and having a psychiatric disorder such as borderline personality disorder, post-traumatic stress disorder, anxiety disorder, major depression, or eating disorder (Klonsky & Muehlenkamp, 2007; Whitlock, 2010). In a sample of eighty-nine inpatient adolescents, Nock and Prinstein (2005) found that these youngsters only spent a few minutes contemplating the act before acting to self-injure. They concluded that NSSI in adolescents is an impulsive act that can occur in the absence of physical pain and in the absence of influence from alcohol and drugs. Whatever the etiology, the pattern for those who engage in NSSI is an experience of overwhelming emotions and tension; tension then increases the experience of anxiety; anxiety then increases anger or fear, which then drives the individual to isolate from others and engage in the act of self-harm.

Influencing Affect Regulation

Ample research data indicate that individuals engage in NSSI behaviors as a means of modifying negative and highly charged emotions due to their inability to tolerate these intense emotional states (Favazza, 1998; Klonsky, Oltmanns, & Turkheimer, 2003; Ross & Heath, 2003; Suyemoto, 1998). The emotions usually include anger, fear of abandonment or rejection, despair, guilt, or anxiety. Gratz and Roemer (2004) identified four components of *emotion regulation* that are precursors to understanding adaptation to emotional distress and the individual's attempts at self-regulation. First, one must be aware of and understand various emotional states commonly experienced by human beings. Second, the individual must be capable of engaging in goal-directed activities while inhibiting negative emotions experienced. Third, the individual must have the ability to use one or more strategies to manage intense or negative emotions instead of disconnecting from the emotion. Last, the individual must be willing to experience negative emotions and work through them rather than engaging in maladaptive behavioral responses. As Gratz (2007) pointed out, interventions with individuals who engage in NSSI must include teaching about a range of emotions as this may have been lacking during their formative years; promoting understanding and acceptance of different emotional states; and teaching management strategies and skills to use during emotionally charged times.

Individuals who engage in NSSI as a form of affect regulation may also be trying to externalize, through physical pain, their affective experience thereby taking control of the situation. Favazza (1998) adds that the act of self-injury temporarily relieves overwhelming anxiety in both episodic and repetitive self-injurers and meets the criteria for impulse control disorder. In a study on nearly 2,000 nonclinical military recruits, Klonsky, Oltmanns, and Turkheimer found that 4% reported engaging in self-harm behaviors and, of that group, anxiety scores were higher than scores for depression (2003).

In a sample of forty-two hospitalized NSSI adolescents, researchers found that youngsters with high levels of internalized anger endorsed more addictive behaviors associated with their self-injuring actions. These addictive features included significant preoccupation with the behavior despite associated feelings of shame and guilt, the urges themselves had been upsetting but not enough to stop the behavior, and the frequency and intensity of the behaviors had increased to achieve the same effect (Nixon, Cloutier, & Aggarwal, 2002).

As an Act of Self-punishment

Some self-injurers appear to be more self-critical and self-loathing than non–self-injurers and this schema, in combination with low self-esteem, results in NSSI as a form of self-punishment (Klonsky, 2007; Klonsky & Muehlenkamp, 2007; Ross & Heath, 2003). In a study conducted by Glassman, Weierich, Hooley, Deliberto, and Nock to see which types of childhood maltreatment were associated with NSSI, eighty-six adolescents aged twelve to nineteen years were asked to complete several self-measurement scales such as the Child Trauma Questionnaire, the Self-Rating Scale (a tool to assess self-criticism), the Self-Injurious Thoughts and Behaviors Interview, the Perceived Criticism Scale, and the Schedule for Affective Disorders and Schizophrenia for School-Aged Children–Present and Lifetime Version (K-SADS-PL). In this sample, physical neglect, sexual abuse, and emotional neglect were significantly associated with NSSI (2007). In a sample of 2,875 college students aged eighteen to twenty-four who were asked to

complete an Internet-based Survey on College Mental Health and Well-Being, 17% reported having engaged in NSSI one or more times, 40% indicated that no one was aware that they self-injure, and 53% had been victims of physical, emotional, or sexual abuse (Whitlock, Eckenrode, & Silverman, 2006).

To Influence Others

Lloyd-Richardson, Perrine, Dierker, and Kelley (2007) administered the Functional Assessment of Self-Mutilation (FASM) survey to 633 adolescents in grades nine through twelve to assess the prevalence and characteristics of NSSI in this population. Fifty-five percent of the sample indicated they had engaged in one or more acts of NSSI within the year and reported that their motivation was two-fold: to influence the behavior of others and to regulate their own emotions. More than a quarter of the total sample engaged in moderate to severe NSSI.

The function of self-injury has also been attributed to primitive attempts to manipulate others or to gain affection or attention. Klonsky and Muehlenkamp (2007) offered yet another reason for youth who engage in NSSI—to bond with peers who also self-injure. This explanation is plausible given adolescent propensity for engaging in imitative behaviors to fit in and be accepted by peers.

To Interrupt Dissociation

NSSI has also been seen as a negative coping behavior used to end dissociative experiences. Dissociation has long been associated with childhood trauma, borderline personality disorder, and severe traumatic events. The individual uses dissociation as a defense mechanism to protect against pain from trauma. During the dissociative state, the individual either feels nothing or experiences derealization or depersonalization. Experiencing a different type of pain (physical) and seeing blood is believed to interrupt the dissociative state and returns the person to a "real" or more familiar and grounded state (Klonsky, 2003; Mangnall & Yurkovich, 2008; Suyemoto, 1998). In essence, the act of self-injury serves to regulate affect.

As an Experience of Excitement

Self-injurers have also reported engaging in NSSI in order to feel "high" or obtain a sense of "excitement" from the act itself. Klonsky and Muehlenkamp (2007) point out that this group tends to engage in the act with others and report feeling an excitement comparable to that felt when bungee jumping. This is a different profile from most other self-injurers who tend to be secretive or "loners" when self-mutilating. What chronic self-injurers seem to have in common, however, is that the behavior releases neurochemical endorphins, which serve to impact or regulate their affective state (Klonsky & Muehlenkamp, 2007; Nixon, Cloutier, & Aggarwal, 2002).

To Prevent Suicide

In a self-report survey administered to 5,759 ninth-graders in Germany, nearly 11% of the sample reported engaging in DSH occasionally and 4% reported repeated engagement. Adolescent girls who smoked had a higher rate of both types of DSH, and social factors such as academic performance and health problems within the family were also triggers to NSSI. Drug use in this sample was not correlated with NSSI and the researchers concluded that the use of drugs may originally have been a factor in regulating emotions. The strongest risk factor, though, for engaging in self-harm behaviors in this sample was SI. Self-harm behaviors increased three-fold with the experience of SI in the group that engaged in self-harm occasionally and seven-fold in the group that engaged in repetitive self-harm behaviors (Brunner et al., 2007). What appears clear from the literature is that children and younger adolescents have less comorbid substance use with their NSSI than do older adolescents and adults. This may be a function of lack of access to financial resources to acquire drugs or alcohol and the availability and impulsive use of equally self-destructive strategies to cope with anxiety and emotions.

Neurochemical Influence

Research has also explored the neurochemical bases of NSSI as there appears to be a correlation between low serotonin (5-hydroxytryptamine [5-HT]) levels and depression, impulsivity, aggression, and DSH behaviors (Crowell et al., 2008). Postmortem autopsies on successful suicides revealed lower levels of serotonin in the ventral prefrontal cortex and low serotonin blood serum levels in suicide attempters (Currier & Mann, 2008; Mann, 2003). A properly functioning (adequate amount of neurotransmitters, transporter sites, and receptors) prefrontal cortex is responsible for decision-making, action, and impulse inhibition. Dysregulation of the site-specific neurotransmitter process or injury to the ventral prefrontal cortex results in disinhibition and may explain the reactive and impulsive act of self-injury. Engaging in NSSI has also been attributed to an increase in cortisol level secondary to increased stress. The increased cortisol level triggers the act of self-injury, which in turn diminishes the individual's arousal level and increases endorphin levels. This increase in endorphins leads to a calm and relaxed state (Nock & Mendes, 2008). This frequent experience of elevated endorphins after the self-harm act is thought to become addictive,

prompting the individual to repeat the act to achieve a similar calm and peaceful state.

Diagnostic and Behavioral Presentations

Rule-Out

Engaging in DSH behaviors is one criterion associated with several psychiatric disorders found in the Diagnostic and Statistical Manual of Mental Disorders (DSM-IV) (APA, 2000). Therefore, when conducting a complete assessment of these youngsters, it is important for the clinician to first rule out the following disorders, dissociative disorder, borderline personality disorder (technically diagnosed after age eighteen), and conduct or antisocial personality disorder (the latter diagnosed after age eighteen). If the youngster does not meet the criteria for any of the aforementioned disorders, NSSI must be considered. However, NSSI behaviors can co-occur with substance abuse, mood disorders, anxiety disorders, eating disorders, post-traumatic stress disorder, and dissociative and borderline personality. Youngsters who have a pervasive developmental disorder or psychosis may also exhibit self-injuring behaviors that are frequently associated with those disorders and would not meet the criteria for DSH NSSI.

Body Modifications: Culturally Endorsed Acts of Mutilation

Throughout history, cultures have engaged in body modification rituals as an expression of their beliefs, as a component of religious practices, to mark a group's identity, to indicate an individual's membership in a group, to promote healing, to identify with a spirit, or to reinforce control and social order (Favazza, 1998, 2009). Culturally endorsed body modifications can range from barbaric and painful actions such as female genital mutilation, branding, or skin scarring to more benign ritualistic acts such as piercing and tattooing. While some of these activities are self-inflicted, many are done to the individual by members of the family or cultural community as part of a rites of passage ritual. While the intent is not to contribute to the demise of the individual, physical and psychological injury can and does occur and can be more devastating to the younger the child. Culturally endorsed body modifications are not considered NSSI and do not meet the proposed DSM-V criteria.

The Internet and NSSI

The Internet can be both a positive and a negative tool for youngsters who engage in NSSI. The Internet offers anonymity and provides an avenue for social interaction for youth who engage in self-harm behaviors. They learn that they are not alone and that there are countless others out there who self-injure. Unfortunately, the Internet also contains sites that endorse and provide details on how to self-injure. Youngsters who only use the Internet to deal with their self-harm behaviors avoid working through emotions and avoid examining triggers to these behaviors (Whitlock, Lader, & Conterio, 2007).

Researchers in China surveyed 1,618 youth aged thirteen to eighteen looking at Internet addiction and self-injurious behaviors (Lam, Peng, Mai, & Jing, 2009). Approximately 11% of the participants were moderately to severely addicted to the Internet and 16% (N = 263) reported one to six or more acts of self-injury during the six months prior to the study. Internet addiction was found to be an independent risk factor of self-injurious behaviors. The researchers recommended assessing for other addictions when treating NSSI.

A study conducted by Whitlock, Powers, and Eckenrode (2006) looked at the content of Internet message boards visited by self-injurers and found both positive and negative aspects of these sites. Content analysis of 400 self-injury message boards showed that many provided informal support, gave individuals a forum to share personal stories, linked mental health disorders with self-injuring behaviors, and endorsed accessing mental health professionals for treatment. However, analysis also revealed communication about the addictive nature of self-injury, support and endorsement for concealing the behavior, and specific guidelines on how to engage in self-harm. In working with youth who self-injure and their parents, the APN should assess for use of the Internet and specific sites visited while trying to gain

understanding about the influence that this media may play in the life of the youngster. Specific sites to ask about include blogs like xanga.com, myspace. com, and facebook.com. In addition, the APN should question the sites visited on Youtube.com, whether the youth visits message boards or receives instant messages or text messages from others, and the content of those messages. Frequent bombardment with messages on "how to engage in the act" may place a vulnerable youngster at risk for following through when experiencing overwhelming emotions.

Maintenance of NSSI Behaviors

Nock (2009) constructed an integrated theoretical model that depicts how NSSI behavior develops and is maintained. The model depicted in Figure 10.1 identifies risk factors such as childhood history of physical or sexual abuse, poor impulse control, high reactivity, and parents or caretakers who are hostile and critical. Bully victimization, self-harm by peers, difficulties at school, and health problems are additional risk factors. The model also identifies vulnerabilities in the individual and in the environment that also influence behavior. When stressed, the individual engages in NSSI to regulate affect or the social situation. Nock argues that self-injuring behaviors are maintained by either positive or negative intrapersonal and interpersonal reinforcement. In assessing and working with this population, it would be important for the APN to be knowledgeable about distal or underlying behavioral drivers, youth vulnerabilities, proximal or immediate precipitating triggers, and patterns of social and affective regulation.

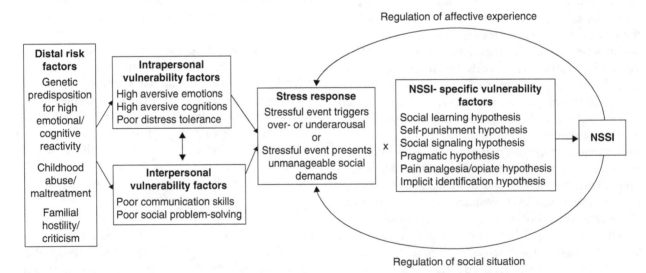

Figure 10.1 Integrated theoretical model of the development and maintenance of self-injury. Reprinted from Nock, 2009, with permission from SAGE Publications.

Assessment of Self-Injury in Primary Care

Routine assessment for NSSI behaviors should occur at all primary care health maintenance visits in conjunction with assessment for mood disorders, anxiety, depression, SI, and other psychiatric symptoms. At illness visits or episodic care, the review of systems for the chief complaint may include an assessment for psychiatric symptoms and risk for NSSI. Chief complaints that may trigger this assessment would be unexplained injuries or histories that are inconsistent with the presentation. Adolescents may present with vague complaints of headache, sleep disturbances, or other functional symptoms related to anxiety or depression. In attempting to access help, teens may present with a "hidden agenda," which may only be revealed in a confidential interview.

The APN is in the unique position of having a trusted relationship with the patient and can be the first person the patient may choose to disclose to. In accordance with the recommendations of the American Academy of Pediatrics (2008) and the Society of Adolescent Medicine (Ford, English & Sigman, 2004), a confidential history should be conducted to provide adolescents the best opportunity to disclose risk behaviors that may be injurious to them. Typically, some SI and all suicidal gestures or behaviors are exclusionary criteria to confidentiality and require that the APN inform a caretaker or parent and secure support for urgent or immediate mental health services. Differentiating between NSSI and SSI (which will be discussed later in this chapter) is essential for proper triage and management by the APN. Any patient who poses an immediate life-threatening risk requires immediate transport by police or ambulance to a psychiatric emergency center for evaluation and treatment of suicidal behavior. Those who present with an injury without suicidal intent should be sent to an emergency department for assessment and treatment of any significant wounds related to self-injury. Some patients can receive assessment and treatment in primary care and then referred to APNs in mental health for psychological counseling, treatment, and ongoing monitoring.

Most providers will screen youth routinely for concerns about troubling mood symptoms, including overwhelming anxiety and increased depressive and hopeless thoughts, or thoughts about hurting themselves or others. Youths who use NSSI to cope often experience a great deal of shame and are unwilling to disclose their behavior readily. On occasion, the provider will recognize wounds that may represent NSSI and should question the patient about them. To obtain sensitive information of this nature, APNs must use empathic and compassionate communication, active listening, and reflection. APNs should begin the assessment of NSSI by normalizing and validating the behavior in certain populations and making statements such as "Being a teenager can be a difficult time with many pressures" or "Sometimes teens may experiment with behaviors like hurting themselves to see if they can improve their moods, reduce bad feelings, or get rid of sad feelings" and "People who hurt themselves to cope with difficult times can be helped by talking to someone." Muehlenkamp (2006), Kerr, Muehlenkamp, and Turner (2010), and Nafisi and Stanley (2007) focused their interventions with self-injurers around the therapeutic relationship, validating the distress experienced prior to and during the self-harm act, helping the youngster understand the behavior in context, challenging negative beliefs, teaching new coping skills, and empowering the youngster to change the cycle of self-destructive behaviors.

"Normalizing" the youngster's behavior within the context of his or her peer group allows the youth to disclose behavior with less shame or stigma. A skilled practitioner may assess initially whether the teen knows anyone who might be using or engaging in these behaviors, including close friends, and then ask if the patient has ever tried any form of self-injury. By slowly increasing the intensity of this inquiry, patients feel more comfortable offering information from their experience. In addition, disclosure should be seen as a means to access help to deal with the patient's problems, not necessarily to stop the behavior. Kerr et al. (2010) suggest using the mnemonic STOPS FIRE (Table 10.2) as a means of assessing a patient's self-injury and to help guide referral and management strategies.

Table 10.2 STOPS FIRE Evaluation

Suicidal ideations (Assess frequency and quality)
Types (Assess types of self-injury behaviors)
Onset (When did self-injurious behaviors begin? What were precipitants?)
Place /location (What areas of the body are targeted?)
Severity of damage (Presence of bleeding, was hospitalization needed? Infection?)
Functions (What were effects of the behavior on patient and on others?)
Intensity of the urges (On a scale of 0-10, with 10 being relentless urges)
Repetition (How often is the youngster engaging in the behavior?)
Episodic frequency (How many times per day/ week/ month does youth engage in behavior?)

Reprinted from Kerr, Muehlenkamp, and Turner, 2010, with permission from the American Board of Family Medicine.

The Physical Exam

During the physical exam, the APN may notice unusual cuts, burns, nonhealing wounds, or bruises and should ask about them with respectful curiosity. A clue to self-injury is that they typically occur on the nondominant arm or hand. The extent and location of the wounds may signal the stage of addiction to the behavior. New users are more likely to use exposed areas like thighs and arms that are visible and easily accessed. The wounds of more committed users may be hidden, under arms, between the toes, and occasionally in insertions under the skin (Favazza, 1998; Nock, 2010; Whitlock, 2010). Some patients may engage in elaborate rituals that include inserting pieces of metal, wood, or plastic under the skin, which may not be immediately noticeable and are only picked up on careful palpation or radiography. The location of injury, especially if found in the genital or face region, is considered significant and would warrant earlier referral. Patients may often minimize the wounds and attempt to distract the provider from investigating them. APNs should gently interview the patient about the nature of the wounds using the above assessment. Early identification and disclosure of NSSI can prevent progression to higher levels of dependence on the behavior and result in prompt mental health referral as needed.

When a teen discloses that he or she has tried NSSI, the practitioner has a duty to assess the purpose and intent of the injury. In Figure 10.2, Williams, Daley, and Iennaco (2010) provide an algorithm for assessing the nature and extent of NSSI self-injury behavior using an approach adapted from an adolescent substance abuse assessment developed by Macdonald (1988). Table 10.3 provides an explanation for each of the stages, from 0 (no NSSI behaviors) to 4 (pervasive thinking about self-injury and engagement) (Williams et al.). Once the stage is determined, the provider can offer patient-centered messages and plans to address each stage as found in Table 10.4 (Williams et al.). Some teens may be experimenting with self-injuring behaviors as a result of peer influence and have not established a dependence or identity as real "cutters." They may be experimenting (Stage 1), trying to belong to a group of cutters, or exploring new coping mechanisms. They are not entrenched in the cycle of NSSI behavior, experience no cravings, and do not exhibit an inability to control their behavior. It would be important for the primary care APN to maintain a trusting and supportive relationship with these youths and refer to a child and adolescent mental health colleague if this youngster moves to Stage 2 (Exploration).

Early recognition and management of youngsters who engage in NSSI behaviors are important to prevent the behaviors from escalating and becoming an entrenched coping strategy. APNs in primary care are in a unique position during well- or sick-child/adolescent visits to assess for evidence of these behaviors early.

Suicide

Suicide is a serious and growing public health concern and remains the third cause of death in youth worldwide. Between 1979 and 2004, the suicide rate in children aged ten to fourteen years in the U.S. increased from 0.4 to 1.3 per 100,000 and the 2004 rate in five-to nine-year-olds was 0.01 per 100,000 (Dervic, Brent, & Oquendo, 2008). An estimated 2 million youth attempt suicide annually in the U.S. with less than 50% receiving medical treatment post attempt (American Academy of Child and Adolescent Psychiatry [AACAP], 2001). Chavira, Accurso, Garland, and Hough (2010) conducted interviews and collected questionnaire data at baseline and two years later on 1,057 youth aged eleven to eighteen in five public sector care systems (child welfare, juvenile justice, special education, alcohol and other drug treatment, and county mental health). Nearly 30% of their sample screened positive for SI and 20% had attempted it one to four or more times. Children in special education had the highest levels of SI and gestures. They strongly recommended screening and using evidence-based interventions across all public sector care environments.

Table 10.5 contains risk factors frequently attributed to those who pose the highest risk for suicide. Needless to say, youngsters with multiple risk factors and psychiatric or behavioral comorbidities should be carefully screened for immediate intervention as may be warranted. Unfortunately, what the data also show is that risk is not limited to those with a DSM-IV psychiatric diagnosis (APA,2000), as suicide is also committed by youth with subsyndromal symptoms who do not meet criteria for a diagnosis or exhibit behavioral or functional impairment.

Among youngsters, the most frequent methods in suicide attempts and completed suicides are firearms, suffocation/hanging, medication overdose (analgesics and use of multiple CNS depressants), jumping, and poisoning via ingestion of pesticides (AACAP, 2001; Dervic et al., 2008). As discussed earlier in this chapter, neurotransmitter and neuroendocrine dysregulation are also implicated as possible causes of the range of self-harm behaviors seen. Pfeffer et al. (1998) found that their prepubertal sample of children aged six to twelve who had attempted suicide had significantly lower blood levels of the enzyme tryptophan, a precursor of serotonin, than a nonsuicidal control group. Crowell et al. (2008) found lower peripheral blood levels of 5-HT in twenty

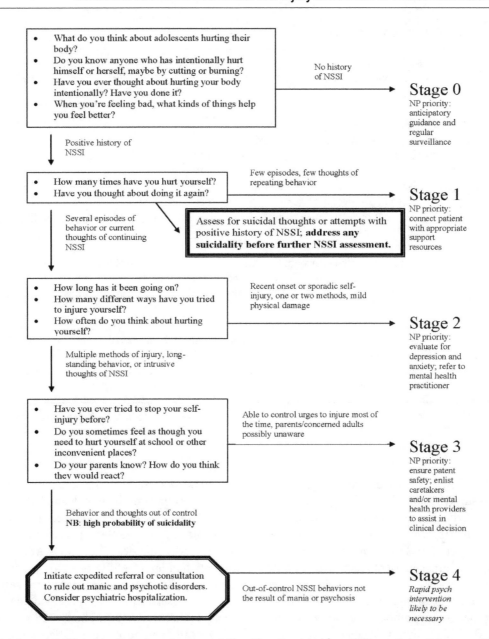

Figure 10.2 Adolescent Self-Injurious Behaviors: Assessment Algorithm. Reprinted from Williams, Daley, & Iennaco, 2010, with permission from the American Journal for Nurse Practitioners.

self-injuring adolescents compared to a matched control group. Again, low 5-HT was linked to depression, aggression, impulsivity, and self-injuring behaviors. Excessive cortisol levels due to acute stress and abnormal or hyperactive hypothalamic-pituitary-adrenal (HPA) axis functioning have also been implicated as a component of suicidal behaviors (Currier & Mann, 2008; Mann, 2003).

It is important to note that younger children who succeed in committing suicide appear to have a brief stress-suicide (impulsive) interval compared to older children and adolescents and engage in less planning with apparent lack of intent (possibly misjudging the repercussion of their behavior) (Shaffer et al., 1996). Protective factors that mitigate against suicidal behaviors include emotional well-being, religion, parent-family connectedness, school and peer connectedness, and academic achievement (Borowsky, Ireland, & Resnick, 2001).

Terminology most often used when discussing suicide includes ideation, threat, gesture, and attempt. *Ideation* refers to thinking about suicide, including being dead, when and how to carry out the act, and imagining the reaction of others to one's death. Suicidal *ideation* is a common phenomenon in youth as indicated by youth risk surveillance data (YRBS), which are collected every two years. Eaton et al. (2010) found that nearly 14% of the 16,410 youth

Table 10.3 Stages of NSSI behaviors in adolescents

Stage 0 No NSSI Behavior	• All adolescents "at risk" because of age, cultural context, and developmental level • Factors that elevate risk include family status, level of behavior in peer group, psychiatric co-morbidities, and academic performance
Stage 1 Experimentation	• Trial period of self-injury • Learns about how NSSI affects the self • Decides whether he or she likes NSSI enough to continue
Stage 2 Exploration	• Physical signs of injury more readily identified • Adolescent perceives behavior as an effective coping mechanism • Subtle signs of distress may be detected in appearance, family relationships, scholastic performance and peer group affiliation
Stage 3 Encapsulation	• Preoccupation with behavior to the clear detriment of other aspects of the adolescent's life • Urge strikes at school, in public, or at other inconvenient times • Adolescent is likely to have tried several methods of self-injury, such as cutting, scratching, burning, or self-hitting
Stage 4 Pervasive Dysfunction	• Most aspects of the adolescent's life can be considered dysfunctional • Enormity of problems leads to further escalation of NSSI behavior • Physical or psychological decompensation may ensue, with severe psychiatric symptoms or death as possible outcomes

Reprinted from Williams, Daley, and Iennaco, 2010, with permission from the American Journal for Nurse Practitioners.

from whom 2008 YRBS data were collected admitted to thinking about suicide within the previous year. Suicidal *threat* refers to verbalizing a wish to kill oneself while suicidal *gesture* is a specific behavior signaling intent (AACAP, 2001; Nock, 2010). *Threats* and *gestures* may be reactive to environmental events such as disciplinary responses from adults or discord with family and peers. Suicidal *attempt* refers to engaging in actions, which, while they may be rooted in ambivalence, have the intent of causing death (Miller, Rathus, & Linehan, 2007). The most significant predictor of a successful suicide is previous attempts. If attempts do not require medical intervention, they may be kept from the health care provider who would be unaware of this most significant risk factor. Given the troubling rates of self-harm in youth, all providers should assess for ideation, attempts, and intent using direct but gentle and supportive questioning and screening tools that are reliable, valid, and culturally and developmentally appropriate.

Suicide Screening

Examples of direct questions that should be asked include, "Did you ever feel so hopeless, sad, or upset that you wanted to die?" and "Have you ever tried to hurt yourself or spent time thinking of ways to hurt yourself?" Positive responses must be followed with an assessment

of intended method and availability, which helps the APN determine imminent risk and lethality.

There are numerous evidence-based screening tools available for the APN to use when assessing youth at risk for suicide. The Child-Adolescent Suicide Potential Index (CASPI) is a thirty-item yes/no self-report questionnaire for eight- to seventeen-year-olds that assesses for early-onset suicidal risk (Pfeffer, Jiang, & Kakuma, 2000). The CASPI was administered to 425 child and adolescent patients and nonpatients. The tool assesses three behavioral categories: anxiety-impulsivity-depression, SI and threats, and family distress. A total score of 11 or more differentiates suicidal from nonsuicidal youngsters. The Columbia Suicide Screen (CSS) for teens is a thirty-two–item tool for eleven- to eighteen-year-olds that screens for suicidal risk, ideation, and behaviors (Shaffer et al., 2004). The tool was originally developed and administered to 1,729 diverse ninth- to twelfth-graders from 1991 to 1994. Those who screened positive were then administered the Diagnostic Interview Schedule for Children (DISC) to further assess the validity of the CSS. Youngsters screen positive if they endorse any of the following: (a) SI within the past three months, (b) one or more prior suicide attempts, (c) at least three of the following are rated as bad or very bad: unhappiness,

Table 10.4 Messages to convey to self-injuring patients according to stage of NSSI behavior

These messages help balance the patient-practitioner relationship with the requirement to provide safe care. They can be conveyed verbally, through body language, or in communicating clinical decisions.

All Stages
- I don't think you're weird or crazy.
- Most people benefit from talking through their worries with a supportive person.
- I'm concerned for your well-being.
- My job is to keep you safe.

Stage 1
- We should decide together what to do about this situation.
- Your preferences are central in deciding what to do next.

Stage 2
- We should decide together what to do about this situation.
- Your preferences are central in deciding what to do next.

Stage 3
- Your preferences are important, but we need to have a plan today.
- There are programs and counselors who specialize in treating kids who harm themselves.
- We need to get your parents/caretakers involved, and I want you to be part of it.

Stage 4
- Your preferences are important, but your safety is more important.
- There are programs and counselors who specialize in treating kids who harm themselves.
- We need to get your parents/caretakers involved, and I want you to be a part of it.

Reprinted from Williams, Daley, and Iennaco, 2010, with permission from the American Journal for Nurse Practitioners.

Table 10.5 Risk factors for suicide in youth

*Mood disorders (depression and bipolar)
Psychosis
Anxiety
Perceived stressful life events
Poor impulse control
*Neurotransmitter and neuroendocrine systems dysfunction (low serotonin levels; HPA dysregulation)
Hopelessness

*Previous attempt (s)
Family history
History of victimization
LGBTQ
Multiple out of home placements (foster care, group homes, and incarceration)

Exposure to peer suicide (cluster suicides)
Substance abuse (addiction)
*Access to high lethal methods (guns, analgesics, height, pesticides)
Romantic/idealized portrayal of suicide in the media

*Older adolescent (16 years or older)
*Male
*Ethnicity (Native Americans, Hispanics, and Caucasians at highest risk)

* Increased risk.
Multiple risk-factors increase vulnerability and risk.
Adapted from AACAP (2001); Borowsky, Ireland, and Resnick (2001); and Dervic, Brent, and Oquendo (2008).

social withdrawal, irritability, anxiety, or substance abuse, and (d) expressing a desire to speak to a professional about feelings identified in item c. Additional screening with both the CASPI and the CSS has proved to be valid and reliable screening tools across youth of different ages, genders, and ethnicities.

Recent data on suicide prevention indicate that primary care APNs and other practitioners are the best hope for detecting youth at risk for suicide, educating youth and family about suicide risk factors, advocating for positive parenting and youth well-being, and initiating preventative interventions. Gardner et al. (2010) reviewed data from 1,547 youth aged eleven to twenty years who completed a computerized screening tool while waiting for their pediatric office visit appointment. The tool assessed for substance use, SI, depression, and injury risk behaviors. For the 14% (205) of youth who screened positive for SI, the primary care provider

was able to discuss SI with the youth, facilitate further triaging by social work, or make referrals for additional mental health care services at the time of the visit. In a longitudinal study conducted by Gould et al. (2009), the researchers followed 317 youth with positive SI screens for two years. At the time of the initial screen, 71% of the youth were not receiving any mental health treatment and referrals for further evaluation or treatment were made on those who met screening criteria for serious ideation or past attempts. Two years later, two-thirds of those who were referred for treatment had accessed and used treatment services. These researchers endorsed the President's New Freedom Commission on Mental Health (Department of Health and Human Services [DHHS], 2003) recommendations, which supported placing mental health screening and services within school-based health programs to reach students who would otherwise not ordinarily receive or access services.

Prevention and Assessment Tools/Strategies

APNs working with children and adolescents who self-injure are encouraged to become familiar with some of the tools available for assessment and which frequently guide the most appropriate intervention based on presenting symptoms and severity of DSH behaviors. For example, the University of Washington Behavioral Research and Therapy Clinics (http://depts.washington.edu/brtc) makes available a range of tools that practitioners can download and use to assess both NSSI and suicidal behaviors. Other tools have been included throughout this chapter.

In 2005 Mann et al. conducted a systematic review of the evidence on effective suicide prevention strategies and concluded that a combination of primary and secondary prevention efforts was most successful. Primary prevention includes educating health care providers and the community about suicide risk factors and prevention strategies and developing community programs that foster connectedness, empowerment, and positive parenting. Secondary prevention includes psychological interventions such as groups and interpersonal therapy, reducing access to lethal methods, use of medications (such as antidepressants), follow-up care post attempts, and responsible media coverage when suicides occur (Nixon & Heath, 2009).

A little-discussed prevention tool but a powerful cornerstone of psychiatric-mental health nursing is the relationship that the APN develops and builds with the children and adolescents in his or her practice. This relationship should be based on trust, honesty, caring, and advocacy. APNs in primary care often see these youngsters over a period of time in their practice and are equally involved in a long-term relationship. Attentive and reflective listening, presence, validation of contextual feelings, and respect for the youngster and his or her experiences convey a sense of caring without rushing to judge or condemn the NSSI acts. Overreactivity (shock, pity, or lecturing) may serve as a barrier in the relationship between the APN and the youth (Deiter, Nicholls, & Pearlman, 2000).

Evidence-Based Nursing Interventions

Working with self-injuring and suicidal youth is best done using an interdisciplinary or multidisciplinary approach and may require consistent or intermittent intervention over a long period of time. The treatment team may include the APN in primary care, the child and adolescent psychiatric nurse, parents, the youth, a trusted teacher or guidance counselor, and a psychiatrist or psychologist. During treatment, both the child and adolescent and the primary care APNs should anticipate relapses in self-harming behaviors secondary to the stress of working through emotions and the expectation from parents or other significant adults of healthier coping behaviors from the youngster. Minimizing frequency and severity of self-harm behaviors may be a more realistic goal than total cessation of the behaviors. Because of the more intense nature of the reparative work required with these youngsters, the primary care APN should make a referral to mental health colleagues.

There is strong evidence that cognitive-behavioral therapy (CBT) and dialectic behavioral therapy (DBT) are effective interventions for use with self-harming youth. CBT is discussed in detail in Chapter 17, and the reader is referred to that chapter for details about the method. DBT will be discussed briefly here. DBT is an intensive treatment strategy used with severe psychiatric and behavioral presentations. The initial stage of DBT involves stabilizing the individual and eliminating behavioral or environmental barriers to treatment. In stage 2, the focus is on treating any past trauma experienced. Stage 3 focuses on self-esteem development and managing problems of daily living. In stage 4, the last stage of the process, the therapist works with the individual to increase capacity for learning from new experiences. Specific skills as developed by Linehan (1993a, 1993b) include core mindfulness (increasing capacity for observation, description, and participation while increasing mindfulness); regulating emotions and increasing positive emotions; developing effective interpersonal skills; learning how to tolerate distressful emotions through distractions and self-soothing activities; and learning to walk the middle path through validation and dialectic thinking and actions. *Dialectics* is defined as change through persuasion or validation, and *mindfulness* is developing an ability to realistically (wisely) see and understand a situation or an experience without becoming overwhelmed with emotions that distort or confuse reality (Linehan; Miller et al.; Noke, 2009; Rathus & Linehan, 2007).

Extensive research has been done showing effectiveness of DBT with individuals with borderline personality disorders and with suicidal and other self-harming individuals (Fleischhaker, et al., 2011; Katz, Cox, Gunasekara, & Miller, 2004; Rathus & Miller, 2002).

James, Taylor, Winmill, and Alfoadari (2008) conducted a study in England with 16 adolescent females between the ages of fifteen and eighteen who were in treatment in an outpatient mental health clinic. Inclusion criteria included a history of six months or more of severe and persistent DSH. All participants had more than eighteen months of DSH behaviors and were not successfully treated with medications, individual therapy, or family work. The Beck Depression Inventory,

Beck Hopelessness Scale, DSM-IV Global Assessment of Functioning Scale, and Structured Clinical Interview for DSM-IV (SCID) II were used to assess all participants. DBT intervention occurred with all participants weekly in the community. DBT included skills training, individual sessions, and telephone support. The four modules of core mindfulness, distress tolerance, interpersonal effectiveness, and emotion regulation were part of the intervention. On average, participants participated in 78% of the required intervention sessions. Post treatment, there was a reduction in depression scores, hopelessness, acts of DSH, and an increase in overall functioning.

Trust and open communication will be important aspects of treatment along with exploration of stressors or triggers to self-harm behaviors. Working around increasing self-esteem, helping youngsters identify feeling states, developing tolerance for distressing feelings, improving decision-making skills, and learning alternate communication behaviors are all important components of treating self-harming youth. Parents and youth should be educated about the importance of social connectedness and participation in normal child and adolescent group activities to promote social skills, relationship building, emotional well-being, and to minimize isolation.

Medications

The use of medications must be viewed as an adjunct to other treatment modalities. Several categories of medications have been used to assist in treating self-harming youngsters. Antidepressants (specifically selective serotonin reuptake inhibitors [SSRIs]) and mood-stabilizing medications are the most frequently prescribed medications for youngsters with mood dysregulation who engage in self-harming behaviors. As noted in the chapter on psychopharmacology, there is a black box warning associated with antidepressant use in children and adolescents related to controversy over the possibility of SSRIs inducing SI and suicidal behaviors (Neuroscience Education Institute [NEI], 2009). However, reviews of the analyses conducted on large SSRI treatment trials do not support excessive concerns over the use of SSRIs with youth. Antidepressants remain the drugs of choice in managing major depression, a risk factor for engaging in self-harm behaviors. What is clear is that medications may need to be prescribed to support the success of other interventions and that failure to intervene aggressively if warranted will likely result in a poor outcome. Mood-stabilizing agents such as valproic acid (Depakote) and carbamazepine (Tegretol) may be used instead of SSRIs if there is a family history of bipolar disorder or if the mood presentation by the youngster is erratic or unusual, leading to a question about the diagnosis (AACAP, 2001; Mann et al., 2005).

Atypical antipsychotic agents such as olanzapine (Zyprexa) and risperidone (Risperdal) may be prescribed to manage impulsivity, aggression, and mood stabilization associated with NSSI. The opioid antagonist naltrexone hydrochloride (ReVia), primarily used to treat alcohol dependence by reducing craving, has also been used to treat chronic NSSI behaviors when other interventions have failed. There is *some* evidence in the literature on use of naltrexone *with autistic and intellectually disabled youngsters* to deter their self-injurious behaviors (Casner, Weinheimer, & Gualtieri, 1996; ElChaar, Maisch, Augusto, & Wehring, 2006; Sonne, Rubey, Brady, Malcolm, & Morris, 1996; Symons, Thompson, & Rodriguez, 2004). The data presented have been taken from case studies, studies with small sample sizes, and studies with varying degrees of scientific rigor. The results from these studies indicated that there was some success with the use of naltrexone in reducing frequency and intensity of self-harm behaviors. There was less evidence, however, for the use of naltrexone in reducing the craving or drive to self-injure in non–developmentally challenged populations. Additional randomized control treatment studies with large samples of nonautistic, non–developmentally delayed participants would be useful in assessing the merits of naltrexone and other medications with other populations.

APNs are advised to adhere to best practices regarding assessment, prescribing, consenting, assenting, and monitoring; when making referrals; and when engaging in collaborative practice with peers. In addition, APNs must actively engage youth and parents as partners in the treatment process to support success and to minimize risk of untoward events.

Implications for Practice, Education, and Research

APNs in practice must include an assessment of self-injurious behaviors in their work with all children and adolescents. Assessment of self-injurious behaviors can and should occur when assessing for mood and other feeling states in the youngster. Including this in the psychosocial part of a comprehensive assessment must become as commonplace as assessing for use of substances, eating patterns, and sleep history. Early case finding with these youngsters is important as early intervention can result in early treatment and a reversal of self-injury as a means of coping.

Educators teaching primary care APNs (family and pediatric nurse practitioners [FNPs, PNPs], etc.) are encouraged to inform their students about the trends regarding self-injuring behaviors in children and adolescents so that they, too, begin to incorporate this information in their assessment and primary prevention efforts with this population. In the practice setting, APNs can teach youngsters in their practice appropriate management strategies for their feelings, empower youth to talk about their feelings, and work with parents to support and promote self-esteem in their children and adolescents.

APNs are also in a unique position to conduct longitudinal research on a variety of troubling issues affecting children and adolescents. Research on NSSI and youth suicide has proliferated over the past ten years, but most of it is not being conducted by nurses. What we do know is that more research is needed on the long-term efficacy of the various treatments used with this population. APNs in primary care are in a unique position of having strong and long-lasting relationships with youngsters they see, some of whom engage in DSH behaviors. Qualitative data on the impact of the nurse-patient relationship and the course of NSSI behaviors would highlight the strength of how nurses practice and would provide needed strategies for all practitioners in primary care. In addition, as we are advocating for a collaborative practice relationship between primary care APNs and advanced practice mental health nurses, data about the prognosis of children and adolescents co-managed by these two practitioners would be useful in developing best practice treatment guidelines. One model that may work would be a treatment group for DSH youngsters led by both a primary care and a psychiatric-mental health APN. The primary care APN would bring the relational and medical expertise to the process while the psychiatric-mental health APN would bring expertise regarding knowledge of group process and knowledge of theories behind self-injuring behaviors and management strategies like CBT, among others. Other models could involve working with both the youth and parents/caretakers or conducting education campaigns in schools and communities about the prevalence of these behaviors among youth and strategies to prevent or minimize their occurrence.

Case Exemplar

A fourteen-year-old girl, Sue, presented to her primary care office with her mother for a health maintenance visit. Sue denied current medical concerns and only wanted her physical exam forms done for school. She had no past medical history and no allergies and did not take any medications regularly. With mom in the room she was aloof, and responded slowly to questions, shrugging her shoulders and making poor eye contact. She gave one-word responses and, when pressed, wouldn't elaborate regarding any other concerns about her functional health including appetite, sleep, and bowel and bladder function.

Her immunizations were up to date. Mom became easily tearful describing how Sue had been spending a lot of time in her room and wasn't going out with friends as much. She said that Sue spends a lot of time on the computer as well. Patient agreed to a confidential visit and mom was escorted to the waiting room. Mom was reassured that the provider would discuss the findings at the end of the visit. Ground rules were established for the confidential history excluding suicide, homicide, and abuse, to which the patient agreed.

Social History

Sue lived with mom and her seven-year-old brother. Mom was a hairdresser who works days and evening shifts at times. Mom and dad separated almost a year ago. Dad was living in California now and Sue denied getting to speak to him or see him very much. Mom was dating someone with whom she spent a lot of time and who had an eleven-year-old daughter whom Sue had met. Mom's boyfriend had spent the night recently. The patient said mom had "checked out." She said that means mom is just not around. She said that's OK because sometimes mom was out of control and "loses it." Sue was reluctant to explain further or provide an example of what she meant. Sue babysat her younger brother in the evenings and on the weekends, cooked his dinner and made him do homework. She reported that they fight a lot. A seventy-eight-year-old maternal grandmother lived in the next town and visited on the weekend or stayed overnight with the family from time to time. Her maternal grandmother had heart disease, arthritis, and diabetes. She also drank alcohol when she visited, got angry at times, and "screamed" at the patient when she did not answer her quickly enough. Her maternal grandfather committed suicide at age forty. Her paternal grandparents lived in Florida and were well but she had little contact with them. She denied having a close family member with whom she could confide.

Education

The patient was an A/B student and was entering high school. She did well in English and history and thought about teaching or acting in the theater some day. She belonged to the community service club and visited the elderly in a nursing home most Sundays to read to them.

Activities

Sue had a group of three or four girlfriends whom she had known over the past seven years. She said she does not have a best friend. She and her friends got together now and then and surfed social networking sites, watched movies, or went out to eat. However, she hadn't felt much like being with them for several weeks.

She used to dance and play the saxophone but since the separation from her father, she hasn't been able to due to financial constraints. She kept a diary, listened to music, and liked to spend a lot of time on the computer.

Sexual Activity

The patient denied current or past sexual activities but had been texting a guy in her neighborhood for the past week.

Substance Use

Sue denied current or past tobacco, drug, or alcohol use.

Depression

Sue denies mood swings, states "I'm fine," and denied SI or suicidal attempts.

Safety

The youngster said she feels safe in school and at home and denied current or past abuse.

Sue's physical exam revealed a slightly pale, thin, tan girl whose growth chart showed her at the 50th percentile for height and the 25th percentile for weight, which was a decrease since last year. Her vital signs were stable and her exam was normal. You noticed that she was wearing a long-sleeve tee-shirt and asked her to remove it so you can listen to her lungs. When you returned to the room, she was covering her forearms with the gown. She quickly mentioned that she was at her friend's house who has a cat and the cat scratched her left arm while she was there. You examined her forearms and notice at least twenty fine linear lacerations in various states of healing across her left forearm. She reiterated that these were caused by her friend's cat that she was holding. On further examination you noticed approximately twenty-five to thirty similar lines on her anterior thighs. The patient stated again that it was a friend's cat that scratched her when she was wearing shorts.

The APN acknowledged that some scratches from cats can look like that but that she was concerned that the patient has been experiencing a lot of pain and loneliness lately. She told Sue that some teens experiment with cutting or scratching the skin as a way to reduce bad feelings or deal with pain and loneliness. She asked the patient if she had heard of this and if she knew anyone who had tried this before. The patient acknowledged that her girlfriend had tried it using a small piece of glass and had shown her the scars on her arms. Sue then said that it had helped her with her pain when her mother was sick. The APN stated that she must have been feeling pretty bad to have tried this. The patient then admitted that she had tried "cutting using a razor blade and had cried and felt better when she saw her own blood." She said she did it about three times secretly at home and it made her

feel better each time. She said she was beginning to feel worried that she wasn't going to be able to stop. She denied wanting to die or trying to end her life and denied any previous SI. She said she just feels so bad all the time and worried and angry. The APN thanked Sue for sharing this information and praised her for being courageous, recognizing the amount of change and stress she had experienced recently. The patient began to cry and admitted that she missed her father and was so angry at her mother, that there wasn't anyone to talk to, and that she felt like her world was out of control. The APN asked the patient if she was willing to accept counseling at this time and she agreed. She stated she was worried her mother would "flip out" when they told her but the APN reassured her that she would help her disclose to her mother and get her the help she needed from a mental health counselor.

Summary

This chapter presented DSH behaviors of children and adolescents with a focus on nonsuicidal and suicidal self-injuring behaviors. Etiology of self-injury, assessment and management of these behaviors, and the roles that both the primary care and mental health APNs can have when interfacing with these youngsters were presented. In addition, the existing evidence on how best to intervene and the need for nursing research in this area were highlighted. Numerous resources are also provided to guide nursing practice with the youngsters themselves and their families.

Resources

Screening and Other Tools

The Deliberate Self-Harm Inventory (DSHI) (Gratz, 2001). A self-report 17 item questionnaire to measure nonsuicidal self-harm behaviors.

Emotion Reactivity Scale (ERS): 21 item self-report that measures emotion sensitivity, intensity and persistence. (Nock, Wedig, Holmberg & Hooley, 2008).

Ottawa Self-Injury Inventory (OSI-Clinical). (Cloutier & Nixon, 2003). A 33 item self-report questionnaire to identify clinical and psychosocial causes of self-injury.

Web-Based Injury Statistics Query and Reporting System. Available at www.cdc.gov/injury/wisqars/index.html. Accessed August 1, 2010.

Self-Injurious Thoughts and Behavior Interview (SITBI) (Nock, Holmberg, Photos, & Michel, 2007). A 72 (short form) or 169 (long form) item structured interview that assesses both NSSI and suicidal ideation and behaviors.

Self-Harm Inventory (Sansone & Sansone, 2010). A 22-item yes or no self-report questionnaire that looks at the history of self-harm in the individual. All yes responses are considered pathological and the maximum score is 22.

TeenScreen National Center for Mental Health. Retrieved from http://www.teenscreen.org/.

Common Myths about Self-Injury. Retrieved from http://www.selfinjury.

Bill of Rights for People Who Self-Harm. Retrieved from http://www.selfinjury.org/docs/brights.html

Programs or Websites

American Foundation for Suicide Prevention. Retrieved from http://www.afsp.org/.

Centers for Disease Control and Prevention.

Cornell Research Program on Self-Injurious Behavior. Retrieved from http://www.crpsib.com/whatissi.asp.

Life Signs: Self Injury Guidance and Network Support. Retrieved from http://www.lifesigns.org.uk

S.A.F.E. Alternatives. Retrieved from http://www.selfinjury.com.

References

American Academy of Child and Adolescent Psychiatry (AACAP). (2001). Practice parameters for the assessment and treatment of children and adolescents with suicidal behavior. *Journal of the American Academy of Child and Adolescent Psychiatry, 40*(7 Suppl), 24S–51S.

American Academy of Pediatrics Committee on Adolescence. (2008). Achieving Quality Health Services for Adolescents. *Pediatrics, 121*(6).

American Psychiatric Association. (2000). Diagnostic and Statistical Manual of Mental Disorders, Fourth Edition, Text Revision. Washington, DC: American Psychiatric Association.

American Psychiatric Association. (2010). Diagnostic and Statistical Manual of Psychiatric Disorders-V. Retrieved from http://www.dsm5.org/ProposedRevisions/Pages/proposedrevision.aspx?rid=443

American Psychiatric Association. (APA). (2000). Diagnostic and statistical manual of mental disorders: DSM-IV, Fourth Edition, Text Revision). Washington, DC: Author.

Borowsky, I., Ireland, M., & Resnick, M. (2001). Adolescent suicide attempts: Risk and protectors. *Pediatrics, 107*(3), 485–493.

Brunner, R., Parzer, P., Haffner, J., Steen, R., Roos, J., Klett, M., & Resch, F. (2007). Prevalence and psychological correlates of occasional and repetitive deliberate self-harm inadolescents. *Archives of Pediatric and Adolescent Medicine, 161*(7), 641–649.

Casner, J., Weinheimer, B., & Gualtieri, C. (1996). Naltrexone and self-injurious behavior: A retrospective population study. *Journal of Clinical Psychopharmacology, 16*(5), 389–394.

Castille, K., Prout, M., Marczyk, G., Shmidheiser, M., Yoder, S., & Howlett, B. (2007). The early maladaptive schemas of self-mutilators: Implications for therapy. *Journal of Cognitive Psychotherapy: An International Quarterly, 21*(1), 58–71.

Centers for Disease Control and Prevention. (2007). Suicide trends among youths and young adults aged 10–24 years—United States, 1990–2004. *MMWR, 56*(35), 905–908.

Chavira, D., Accurso, E., Garland, A., & Hough, R. (2010). Suicidal behavior among youth in five public sectors of care. *Child and Adolescent Mental Health, 15*(1), 44–51.

Cloutier, P., & Nixon, M. (2003). The Ottawa Self-Injury Inventory: A preliminary evaluation. *European Child & Adolescent Psychiatry, 12*(Suppl. 1), I/94.

Cloutier, P., Martin, J., Kennedy, A., Nixon, M., & Muehlenkamp, J. (2010). Characteristics and co-occurrence of adolescent nonsuicidal self-injury and suicidal behaviors in pediatric emergency crisis services. *Journal of Youth Adolescence, 39*, 259–269.

Crowell, S., Beauchaine, T., McCauley, E., Smith, C., Vasilev, C., & Stevens, A. (2008). Parent-child interactions, peripheral serotonin, and self-inflicted injury in adolescents. *Journal of Consulting and Clinical Psychology, 76*(1), 15–21.

Currier, D., & Mann, J. (2008). Stress, genes and the biology of suicidal behavior. *Psychiatric Clinics of North America, 31*(2), 247–269.

Deiter, P., Nicholls, S., & Pearlman, L. (2000). Self-injury and self capacities: Assisting an individual in crisis. *Journal of Clinical Psychology, 56*(9), 1173–1191.

Department of Health and Human Services (DHHS). (2003). New freedom commission on mental health, achieving the promise: Transforming mental health care in America.Rockville, MD: Author.

Dervic, K., Brent, D., & Oquendo, M. (2008). Completed suicide in childhood. *Psychiatric Clinics of North America, 31*, 271–291.

Eaton, D., Kann, L., Kinchen, S., Shanklin, S., Ross, J., Hawkins, J., et al. Centers for Disease Control and Prevention (CDC) (2010). Youth risk behavior surveillance—United States, 2009. *MMWR, 59*(SS–5), 1–10.

ElChaar, G., Maisch, N., Augusto, L., & Wehring, H. (2006). Efficacy and safety of naltrexone use in pediatric patients with autistic disorder. *The Annals of Pharmacotherapy, 40*, 1086–1095.

Favazza, A. (1998). The coming of age of self-mutilation. *Journal of Nervous & Mental Disease, 186*(5), 259–268.

Favazza, A. (2009). A cultural understanding of nonsuicidal self-injury. In M. Nock (Ed.). Understanding nonsuicidal self-injury. Washington, DC: American Psychological Association.

Fleischhaker, C., Bohme, R., Six, B., Bruck, C., Schneider, C., & Schultz, E. (2011). Dialectical behavioral therapy for adolescents (DBT-A): A clinical trial for patients with suicidal and self-injurious behavior and borderline symptoms with a one-year follow-up. *Child & Adolescent Psychiatry & Mental Health, 5*(3).

Ford, C., English, A, & Sigman, G. (2004). Confidential Health Care for Adolescents: Position Paper of the Society for Adolescent Medicine. *Journal of Adolescent Health, 35*(2), 160–167.

Gardner, W., Klima, J., Chisholm, D., Feehan, H., Bridge, J., Campo, J., Kelleher, K. (2010). Screening, triage, and referral of patients who report suicidal thought during a primary care visit. *Pediatrics, 125*(5), 945–952.

Glassman, L., Weierich, M., Hooley, J., Deliberto, T., & Nock, M. (2007). Child maltreatment, nonsuicidal self-injury, and the mediating role of self-criticism. *Behaviour Research and Therapy, 45*, 2483–2490.

Gould, M., Marrocco, F., Hoagwood, K., Kleinman, M., Amakawa, L., & Altschuler, E. (2009). Service use by at risk youths after school-based suicide screening. *Journal of the American Academy of Child and Adolescent Psychiatry, 48*(12), 1193–1201.

Grantz, KL. (2001). Measurement of deliberate self-harm: Preliminary data on the Deliberate Self-Harm Inventory. *Journal of Psychopathol Behavioral Assessment, 23*, 253–263.

Gratz, K. (2007). Targeting emotion dysregulation in the treatment of self-injury. *Journal of Clinical Psychology, 63*, 1091–1103.

Gratz, K., & Roemer, L. (2004). Multidimensional assessment of emotion regulation and dysregulation: Development, factor structure, and initial validation of the Difficulties in Emotion Regulation Scale. *Journal of Psychopathology and Behavioral Assessment, 26*, 41–54.

James, A., Taylor, A., Winmill, L., & Alfoadari, K. (2008). A preliminary community study of dialectical behavior therapy (DBT) with adolescent females demonstrating persistent, deliberate self-harm (DSH). *Child and Adolescent Mental Health, 13*(3), 148–152.

Katz, L., Cox, B., Gunasekara, S., & Miller, A. (2004). Feasibility of dialectical behavior therapy for suicidal adolescent inpatients. *Journal of the American Academy of Child & Adolescent Psychiatry, 43*(3), 276–282.

Kerr, P.L., Muehlenkamp, J.J., & Turner, J.M. (2010). Non suicidal self injury: A review of current research for family medicine and primary care physicians. *Journal of the American Board of Family Physicians. 23*(2), 240–259.

Klonsky, E., Oltmanns, T., & Turkheimer, E. (2003). Deliberate self-harm in a nonclinical population: Prevalence and psychological correlates. *American Journal of Psychiatry, 160*, 1501–1508.

Klonsky, E. (2007). The functions of deliberate self-injury, A review of the evidence. *Clinical Psychology Review, 27*, 226–239.

Klonsky, E. (2003). The functions of deliberate self-injury: A review of the evidence. *Clinical Psychology Review, 27*, 226–239.

Klonsky, E., & Muehlenkamp, J. (2007). Self-injury: A research review for the practitioner. *Journal of Clinical Psychology, 63*(11), 1045–1056.

Lam, LT., Peng, Z., Mai, J., & Jing, J. (2009). The association between Internet addiction and self-injurious behaviour among adolescents. *Injury Prevention, 15*, 403–408.

Linehan, M.M. (1993a). Cognitive behavioral treatment for borderline personality disorder. New York, NY: Guilford.

Linehan, M.M. (1993b). The skills training manual for treating borderline personality disorder. New York, NY: Guilford.

Lloyd-Richardson, E., Perrine, N., Dierker, L., & Kelley, M. (2007). Characteristics and functions of nonsuicidal self-injury in a community sample of adolescents. *Psychological Medicine, 37*(8), 1183–1192.

Macdonald, D. (1988). Substance abuse. *Pediatric Review, 10*(3), 89–95.

Mangnall, J., & Yurkovich, E. (2008). A literature review of deliberate self-harm. *Perspectives in Psychiatric Care, 44*(3), 175–184.

Mann, J. (2003). Neurobiology of suicidal behavior. *Nature Reviews-Neuroscience, 4*(10), 819–828.

Mann, J., Apter, A., Bertolote, J., Beautrais, A., Currier, D., Haas, A., & Hendin, H. (2005). Suicide prevention strategies: A systematic review. *JAMA, 294*(16), 2064–2074.

Miller, A., Rathus, J., & Linehan, M. (2007). Dialectical behavior therapy with suicidal adolescents. New York, NY: Guilford.

Muehlenkamp, J. (2006). Empirically supported treatments and general therapy guidelines for nonsuicidal self-injury. *Journal of Mental Health Counseling, 28*, 166–185.

Muehlenkamp, J., Williams, K., Gutierrez, P., & Claes, L. (2009). Rates of nonsuicidal self-injury in high school students across five years. *Archives of Suicide Research, 13*, 317–329.

Nafisi, N., & Stanley, B. (2007). Developing and maintaining the therapeutic alliance with self-injuring patients. *Journal of Clinical Psychology, 63*, 1069–1079.

Neuroscience Education Institute. (2009). Understanding and managing the pieces of major depressive disorder. Carlsbad, CA: NEI.

Nixon, M., Cloutier, P., & Aggarwal, S. (2002). Affect regulation and addictive aspects of repetitive self-injury in hospitalized adolescents. *Journal of the American Academy Child and Adolescent Psychiatry, 41*(11), 1333–1341.

Nock, M. (2010). Self-injury. *Annual Review of Clinical Psychology, 6*, 15.1–15.25.

Nock, M. (2009). Why do people hurt themselves? New insights into the nature and functions of self-injury. *Current Directions in Psychological Science, 18*(2), 78–83.

Nock, M., & Prinstein, M. (2005). Contextual features and behavioral functions of self-mutilation among adolescents. *Journal of Abnormal Psychology, 114*(1), 140–146.

Nock, M., & Mendes, W. (2008). Physiological arousal, distress tolerance, and social problem-solving deficits among adolescent self-injurers. *Journal of Consulting and Clinical Psychology, 76*(1), 28–38.

Nock, M., Wedig, M., Holmberg, E., & Hooley, J. (2008). The emotion reactivity scale: Development, evaluation, and relation to self-injurious thoughts and behaviors. *Behavior Therapy, 39*, 107–116.

Nock, M., Holmberg, E., Photos, V., & Michel, B. (2007). Self-injurious thoughts and behaviors interview: Development, reliability, and validity in an adolescent sample. *Psychological Assessment, 19*(3), 309–317.

Peterson, J., Freedenthal, S., Sheldon, C., & Andersen, R. (2008). Nonsuicidal self injury in adolescents. *Psychiatry MMC (Edgemont), 5*(11), 20–26.

Pfeffer, C., McBride, A., Anderson, G., Kakuma, T., Fensterheim, L., & Khait, V. (1998). Peripheral serotonin measures in prepubertal psychiatric inpatients and normal children: Associations with suicidal behavior and its risk factors. *Biological Psychiatry, 44*(7), 568–577.

Pfeffer, C., Jiang, H., & Kakuma, T. (2000). Child-Adolescent Suicidal Potential Index (CASPI): A screen for risk for early onset suicidal behavior. *Psychological Assessment, 12*(3), 304–318.

Rathus, J., & Miller, A. (2002). Dialectical behavior therapy adapted for suicidal adolescents. *Suicide and Life-Threatening Behavior, 32*(2), 146–157.

Ross, S., & Heath, N. (2002). A study of the frequency of self-mutilation in a community sample of adolescents. *Journal of Youth and Adolescence, 31*(1), 67–77.

Sansone, R., & Sansone, L. (2010). Measuring self-harm behavior with the self-harm inventory. *Psychiatry (Edgmont), 7*(4), 16–20.

Shaffer, D., Scott, M., Wilcox, H., Maslow, C., Hicks, R., Lucas, C., & Greenwald, S. (2004). The Columbia suicide screen: Validity and reliability of a screen for youth suicide and depression. *Journal of the American Academy of Child and Adolescent Psychiatry, 43*(1), 71–79.

Shaffer, D., Gould, M., Fisher, T., Moreau, D., Kleinman, M., & Flory, M. (1996). Psychiatric diagnosis in child and adolescent suicide. *Archives of General Psychiatry, 53*, 339–348.

Sonne, S., Rubey, R., Brady, K., Malcolm, R., & Morris, T. (1996). Naltrexone treating of self-injurious thoughts and behaviors. *Journal of Nervous and Mental Disorders, 184*(3), 192–195.

Suyemoto, K. (1998). The functions of self-mutilation. *Clinical Psychology Review, 18*(5), 531–554.

Symons, F., Thompson, A., & Rodriguez, M. (2004). Self-injurious behavior and the efficacy of naltrexone treatment: A quantitative synthesis. *Mental Retardation and Developmental Disabilities Research Reviews, 10*, 193–200.

University of Washington. Behavioral Research and Therapy Clinics [homepage]. Retrieved from http://depts.washington.edu/brtc

Wasserman, D., Cheng, Q., & Jiang, G. (2005). Global suicide rates among young people aged 15–19. *World Psychiatry, 4*(2), 114–120.

Wells, J., Haines, J., & Williams, C. (1998). Severe morbid onychophagia: The classification as self-mutilation and a proposed model of maintenance. *Australian and New Zealand Journal of Psychiatry, 32*, 534–545.

Whitlock, J. (2010). Self-injurious behavior in adolescents. *PLoS Med, 7*(5): e1000240. doi:10.1371/journal.pmed.1000240

Whitlock, J., Lader, W., & Conterio, K. (2007). The Internet and self-injury: What psychotherapists should know. *Journal of Clinical Psychology, 63*(11), 1135–1143.

Whitlock, J., Powers, J., & Eckenrode, J. (2006). The virtual cutting edge: The Internet and adolescent self-injury. *Developmental Psychology, 42*(3), 407–417.

Whitlock, J., Eckenrode, J., & Silverman, D. (2006). Self-injurious behaviors in a college population. *Pediatrics, 117*, 1939–1948.

Williams, E., Daley, M., & Iennaco, J. (2010). Assessing nonsuicidal self injurious behaviors in adolescents. *The American Journal for Nurse Practitioners, 14*(5), 18–26.

11

Perceptual Alterations Disorders

Karen G. Schepp and Eunjung Kim

Objectives

After reading this chapter, APNs will be able to

1. Describe the disorders of children and adolescents that are characterized by disturbed sensory perception and altered thought processes (psychosis not other specified and schizophrenia).
2. Identify nonspecific symptoms seen early in the prodromal phase of child and adolescent–onset psychosis and schizophrenia.
3. Demonstrate knowledge of the neurodevelopmental, neurological, genetic, and environmental factors believed to be associated with disturbed sensory perception and altered thought processes.
4. Demonstrate knowledge of the use of psychotropic medications; child, adolescent, and family education; and psychosocial supports with youth diagnosed with schizophrenia.
5. Apply theoretical knowledge about individual growth and development needs and the impact on family functioning during treatment of children and adolescents with disturbed sensory perception and altered thought processes.
6. Discuss collaborative treatment strategies that APNs in primary care and mental health can use when working with children and families affected by this disorder.

Introduction

Perceptual alterations disorders refer to conditions in which the individual experiences a change in the amount or patterning of incoming stimuli accompanied by a diminished, exaggerated, distorted, or impaired response to such stimuli (NANDA, 2007). The defining characteristics are changes in the usual response to stimuli, changes in sensory acuity, visual distortions or auditory distractions, hallucinations, change in behavior pattern or in problem-solving, poor concentration, disorientation to place, and/or altered communication pattern. Disturbed thought processes are often found with disturbed sensory perceptions. The most common disorders

that alter perceptions in children and adolescents include schizophrenia, psychosis not other specified (NOS), bipolar disorder with psychotic features, posttraumatic stress disorder (PTSD), substance abuse, and organic disorders such as brain lesions (Hlastala & McClellan, 2005). These disorders are severe and can be devastating to the child or adolescent and to the family.

Several of these disorders have nonspecific prodromal symptoms that are very similar. Specific symptoms that evolve and emerge over time include the psychotic symptoms of hallucinations or delusions. Early intervention in the management of schizophrenia and other psychotic illnesses in the child or adolescent is recognized as extremely important in preventing the transition

---

Child and Adolescent Behavioral Health: A Resource for Advanced Practice Psychiatric and Primary Care Practitioners in Nursing, First Edition. Edited by Edilma L. Yearwood, Geraldine S. Pearson, and Jamesetta A. Newland.

to psychosis, shortening the duration of the psychotic episode, and effectively managing the illness to prevent further relapse episodes with resultant degenerative neurological signs (Malla & Pelosi, 2010). To accomplish early intervention, it is important for primary care providers to be aware of the early signs and symptoms so that the child or adolescent can be referred to mental health professionals for immediate diagnostic workup and specialized treatment as needed (Emsley, 2009).

This chapter will describe the clinical symptoms associated with childhood- and adolescent-onset schizophrenia, epidemiology and etiology of the disorder, assessment tools used to assist with screening, and evidence-based management strategies for use with children, adolescents, and families. Two case exemplars will be presented to illustrate presentation, progression, and management of the disorder.

Clinical Picture

The clinical picture in perceptual alterations disorders basically involves three phases. The first phase is the premorbid phase in which there may not be obvious signs or symptoms of a disorder and the child or adolescent may seem to function quite normally even though the risk factors or vulnerabilities such as genetic makeup are still present. More recently, however, premorbid developmental impairments, including language, motor, and social deficits, are being recognized as more frequent and more pronounced in children who eventually develop childhood schizophrenia (Masi, Mucci, & Pari, 2006).

The early prodromal phase includes negative and unspecific symptoms, and the late prodromal phase or psychosis phase extends from positive but attenuated psychotic symptoms or brief and limited psychosis to full psychosis. Eventually, the psychotic phase, or first psychotic episode, as it is often called, occurs with the presence of such positive symptoms as hallucinations or delusions (Berger, Fraser, Carbone, & McGorry, 2006; Maier, Cornblatt, & Merikangas, 2003; Shioiri, Shinada, Kuwabara, & Someya, 2007). Table 11.1 shows symptoms of the disorder in progression to the psychotic episode. It is at the point of the psychotic episode that the DSM diagnostic criteria can be applied and a tentative diagnosis may be made.

Presenting Symptoms

As seen in Table 11.1, the important phase for primary care providers as well as mental health professionals is the prodromal phase where early recognition of the underlying disorder is the goal. The challenge in early recognition is the nonspecific nature of the signs and symptoms noted during this prodromal phase. *Prodromal* refers to the period of time from when the child or adolescent

Table 11.1 Symptoms in progression to psychotic episode

Premorbid Phase
Risk factors and vulnerabilities present but no noticeable change in psychosocial functioning

Early Prodromal Phase
Nonspecific and general symptoms
  Depression
  Depressed mood
  Decreased appetite
  Insomnia
  Anxiety
  Irritation
  Fear
  Autonomic symptoms
  Obsessive-compulsive–type symptoms
  Somatoform symptoms
  Eating disorder (e.g., anorexia nervosa; Kelly et al., 2004)

Late Prodromal or Psychosis Phase
  Perceptions
    Hallucinations
      Auditory (e.g., hearing voices that others do not hear)
      Visual (e.g., seeing people or figures that others do not see)
      Olfactory (e.g., smelling odors that others do not smell)
      Tactile (e.g., feeling sensations others do not feel)
    Thinking
      Delusions (e.g., grandiose, paranoid, nihilistic)
      Flight of ideas (e.g., racing thoughts, unconnected thoughts)
    Cognition
      Difficulty in concentrating
      Difficulty in retaining memory
      Difficulty in performing tasks and following instructions
    Self-awareness
      Loss of insight (e.g., denial of being ill or needing treatment)
    Affect and emotions
      Inappropriate affect
      Blunted affect
      Unable to express emotions or recognize emotions
    Behavior
      Withdrawal
      Lack of socializing
      Impaired functioning in all areas
      Strange behaviors
    Physical functioning
      Change in sleep patterns
      Change in eating behavior
      Loss of energy
      Abnormal motor activities or mannerisms

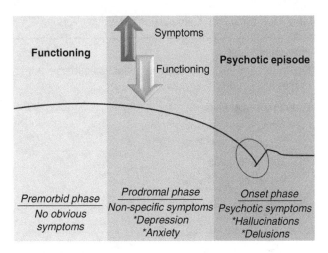

Figure 11.1 Phases, symptoms, and level of functioning leading to psychotic episode. (Reprinted from Kim, 2010, with permission from the author.)

first begins to decline in baseline level of functioning to the time that the criteria for a diagnosis of the disorder are met. The prodromal phase begins with nonspecific symptoms; gradually over time, very specific symptoms of a disorder begin to manifest including initial formation of hallucinations and/or delusions (Berger et al., 2006; McClellan, McCurry, Snell, & DuBose, 1999; White, Anjum, & Schulz, 2006). As the symptoms increase and become more specific, the child or adolescent's overall level of functioning declines. The specific symptoms are those symptoms that are commonly manifested for diagnosis of a disorder and are used as part of the diagnostic criteria for that disorder. Hallucinations and delusions are referred to as positive symptoms and are common in schizophrenia, especially auditory hallucinations and suspiciousness. Negative symptoms are also noted and include social withdrawal and inability to obtain pleasure from any activities. Specific symptoms noted in bipolar disorder include increased energy, elevated mood, and increased activity. In the manic stage of bipolar, psychotic symptoms such as hallucinations may be noted. Psychotic symptoms may also be noted in substance abuse in children and adolescents. Psychotic symptoms may be alleviated during abstinence, which would differentiate substance use from other disturbed sensory perception disorders. Symptoms may worsen in substance abuse with the use of cannabis and push the youth toward becoming at high risk for schizophrenia or other psychotic disorders (Kalapatapu & Dunn, 2010).

Figure 11.1 shows the phases and the relationship between increasing symptoms and decreasing level of functioning. Emerging evidence for schizophrenia as one perceptual alterations disorder suggests that progressive deterioration occurs from neurostructural changes and that this parallels the child's or adolescent's

functional decline (Nasrallah et al., 2009). Evidence of neurostructural changes were noted in a longitudinal study by Rapoport et al. (1999) with thirteen- to seventeen-year-olds. Those with childhood-onset schizophrenia had four times greater decrease in cortical gray matter than normal adolescents in that age group, suggesting overpruning of the cortical gray matter in those with schizophrenia. Rapoport, Addington, Frangou, and Psych (2005), using neuroimaging, reported more evidence of neurostructural changes including regional volume deficits in the frontal lobes, thalamus, and hippocampus as decline in development was noted and cognitive functioning decreased. As neurostructural changes occur, signs and symptoms of functional decline become more evident. Therefore, earlier recognition of symptoms and referral for diagnosis and treatment are the goals in order to limit or arrest developmental decline.

DSM-IV-TR Diagnostic Criteria

Since schizophrenia is the most severe form of perceptual alterations disorder, the diagnostic criteria will be presented. The diagnostic criteria for schizophrenia in adults are also used as the diagnostic criteria for children and adolescents. According to the DSM-IV-TR (APA, 2000), the diagnosis of schizophrenia is made when the symptoms include those given in Table 11.2.

There are several challenges to diagnosing perceptual alterations disorders such as schizophrenia in children or adolescents when using adult criteria. Due to the age-related characteristics, it is often difficult to determine if the child's thinking is actually psychotic or whether the child's thinking is due to an active imagination, which would be common for this age group. The duration of six months, which is one of the diagnostic criteria for schizophrenia for adults, is also challenging when evaluating a child or adolescent for schizophrenia. The symptoms may resolve before six months, especially if medication is given, so it may be difficult to know if the psychotic symptoms would be present for that length of time. Even though normal developmental behavior may at times be difficult to differentiate from pathology, the symptoms most indicative of schizophrenia in the very early onset age group are the positive symptoms such as hallucinations and delusions. The most prominent hallucination for children and adolescents is hearing voices (Masi et al., 2006).

Because of nonspecific symptoms, it is difficult to make a definitive diagnosis and not uncommon to receive a different diagnosis over time as different specific symptom patterns become evident. Also, the stigma attached to a diagnosis of schizophrenia is a factor in many cases and psychiatrists may be hesitant to label a young person with this diagnosis at such an early age.

Table 11.2 DSM-IV-TR criteria for schizophrenia

A. Characteristic symptoms: At least one month of active phase symptoms of two or more of the following with at least some signs of the disorder persisting for at least six months: (1) delusions, (2) hallucinations, (3) disorganized speech (e.g., frequent derailment or incoherence), (4) grossly disorganized or catatonic behavior, (5) negative symptoms, i.e., affective flattening, alogia, or avolition.

B. Social dysfunction: Involves dysfunction in one or more major areas of functioning or failure to achieve the expected level of functioning in the areas of: (1) interpersonal relations, (2) education, and/or (3) self-care.

C. Duration: Continuous signs of the perceptual disturbance that persists for at least 6 months with at least one month of the two or more characteristic symptoms or attenuations of those symptoms noted in Criterion A (e.g., suspiciousness, odd beliefs or unusual perceptual experiences).

D. The perceptual disturbance is not better accounted for by Schizoaffective Disorder or a Mood Disorder with psychotic features.

E. The perceptual disturbance is not due to the direct effects of physiological effects of a substance or general medical condition.

F. Relationship to Pervasive Developmental Disorder. If there is a history of Autism or other Pervasive Developmental Disorders, then the presence of delusions and hallucinations for at least one month could be indicative of schizophrenia.

Reprinted with permission from the Diagnostic and Statistical Manual of Mental Disorders, Fourth Edition, Text Revision, (Copyright © 2000). American Psychiatric Association.

Differential Diagnosis

Even though symptoms may be indicative of schizophrenia, other conditions may have similar symptomatology. Bipolar Disorder often has similar symptoms as those of schizophrenia. Approximately half of the adolescents with bipolar disorder were originally diagnosed with schizophrenia (McClellan, Werry, & Ham, 1993; Werry, McClellan, & Chard, 1991). Observing the symptom pattern over time may help to differentiate between the two disorders. Correll et al. (2007) and Frazier et al. (2007) differentiated between bipolar and schizophrenia and concluded that mania and schizophrenia prodromal characteristics overlapped considerably. However, social isolation, strange or unusual ideas, as well as impaired functioning in multiple domains were significantly more likely to be a part of the schizophrenia prodrome, while obsessions/compulsions, suicidality, difficulty thinking/

communicating clearly, depressed mood, decreased concentration/memory, tiredness/lack of energy, mood lability, and physical agitation were more likely to be a part of the mania prodrome (Correll et al.; Frazier et al.).

Organic psychosis due to substance abuse, seizure disorders, central nervous system (CNS) lesions, or infectious diseases may present with similar symptoms to schizophrenia and also need to be ruled out. Autism is seen in children less than five years of age, and although extremely rare, schizophrenia can be diagnosed in children after the age of five. Childhood disintegrative disorder and Asperger's syndrome may also resemble schizophrenia but lack the symptoms of hallucinations and delusions.

Evidence-based Data and Assessment Tools

There are basically two types of diagnostic assessment tools available for use with children and adolescents. Questionnaires are one type of tool that can be completed by the patient and/or caregiver, a parent, or a teacher. Questionnaires generally focus on broader domains of psychopathology and symptom occurrence. The Early Signs Scale (ESS) found in Table 11.3 is an example of a questionnaire used to measure prodromal symptoms of schizophrenia (Birchwood et al., 1989).

The other type of assessment tool is the structured diagnostic interview that is designed to elicit information from the child or adolescent as well as parent about the child's or adolescent's functioning and severity of symptoms for different psychiatric disorders. For the most part, the structured diagnostic interviews are administered by clinicians and, on completion, the diagnosis is made by the clinician. One diagnostic interview that is used often is the K-SADS (Schedule for Affective Disorders and Schizophrenia for School-Age Children) (Ambrosini, 2000). It is a semistructured diagnostic interview designed to assess current and past psychopathology in children and adolescents according to the DSM-IV criteria (APA, 2000). It is designed for use with children and adolescents between the ages of six to eighteen years and takes approximately seventy-five to ninety minutes to complete (Ambrosini, 2000; Calinoiu & McClellan, 2004.) It covers disruptive behavior disorders, anxiety disorders, mood disorders, eating and substance abuse disorders, and psychotic disorders including schizophrenia. The Diagnostic Interview for Children and Adolescents (DICA) is similar (Reich, 2000).

There are several scales that measure level of functioning in children and adolescents. Several have been used over long periods of time and have extensive reliability and validity estimates. The Kiddie Global Assessment Scale (K-GAS) is a clinician rating scale ranging from 1 to 9 used to rate the level of functioning (Shaffer

Table 11.3 Early Signs Scale

To Be Completed by the Individual

This questionnaire describes problems and complaints that people sometimes have. Please read it carefully. After you have done so please mark the appropriate box which best describes how much each problem has bothered you during the past week, including today. Mark only one box for each of the problems listed. When you have completed the questionnaire please return it in the stamped addressed envelope provided. Thank you very much for your help.

	Not a problem (zero times a week)	Little problem (once a week)	Moderate problem (several times a week but not daily)	Marked problem (at least once a day)
1. I talk or smile to myself				
2. I feel unable to cope				
3. I have aches and pains				
4. My speech comes out jumbled or is full of odd words				
5. I feel tired or lack energy				
6. I feel like playing tricks or pranks				
7. I am preoccupied with one or two things				
8. I feel quiet and withdrawn				
9. I feel stubborn or refuse to carry out simple requests				
10. I do not feel like eating				
11. My sleep has been restless or unsettled				
12. I lose my temper easily				
13. I feel useless or helpless				
14. I feel violent				
15. I feel dissatisfied with myself				
16. I feel as if my thoughts might be controlled				
17. Others have difficulty in following what I am saying				
18. My movements seem slow				
19. I feel depressed or low				
20. I feel very excited				
21. I feel as if I'm being laughed at or talked about				
22. I feel as if I'm being watched				
23. I feel confused				
24. I feel aggressive or pushy				
25. I think I could be someone else				
26. I feel as if my thoughts might not be my own				
27. I am open and explicit about sexual matters				
28. I feel tense, afraid, or anxious				
29. I feel forgetful or "far away"				
30. I have no interest in things				
31. I have difficulty concentrating (e.g., on TV)				
32. I behave oddly for no reason				
33. I am not bothered about my appearance or hygiene				
34. I feel irritable or quick-tempered				

Reprinted from Birchwood, Smith, MacMillan, Hogg, Prasad, Harvey, & Bering, 1989, with the permission of the authors.

et al., 1983). The Global Assessment of Functioning Scale (GAF), also clinician rated, measures the severity of symptoms and the level of functioning of youth from 1 to 100 (Endicott, Spitzer, Fleiss & Cohen, 1976). The Child and Adolescent Functional Assessment Scale (CAFAS) by Hodges (Hodges, Doucett-Gates & Liao, 1999) is completed by the clinician and measures the level of functioning of the child or adolescent in multiple domains such as role performance at home, school, and community, and behavior towards others, mood, substance use, and thinking (Hodges et al., 1999).

In schizophrenia and bipolar disorder, evidence shows many adolescents experience prodromal symptoms a year or longer before the first episode. According to Bota, Sagduyu, Filin, Bota & Munro, the prodromal symptoms may last as long as 4.3 years for males and as long as 6.7 years for females (2008). With schizophrenia, as age increases, both hallucinations and delusions become more complex and elaborate. The earlier the onset and the higher the residual level of positive and negative symptoms, the poorer the functioning and prognosis. Poor functioning is also noted in social relationships and in independent living skills (Berger et al., 2006). Corcoran et al. (2007) found that narratives by family members of patients with schizophrenia were remarkably similar: patients who were previously normal but vulnerable adolescents had social withdrawal and mood symptoms. In this premorbid phase, these adolescents were particularly nonreactive to insults by others, shy, and had social awkwardness.

Epidemiology

The prevalence of schizophrenia worldwide among adults ranges from 0.5% to 1.5% of the population. Seventy-five percent of those with schizophrenia experience the onset during adolescence and early adulthood. Rates of psychosis in children show a dramatic increase in the adolescent years and especially toward late adolescence. For schizophrenia, the rate of onset increases during adolescence and reaches the adult rate of 0.1% of new cases each year (McClellan & Werry, 1997). The disorder occurs more frequently in males at a ratio of 2:1. As age increases, more females are diagnosed with schizophrenia. The age of onset in males tends to be five years earlier than in females (McClellan & Werry,1997). In adolescents, both acute onset with symptoms occurring within the past year and insidious onset are noted (McClellan et al., 1993; Werry et al., 1991).

In early adolescence, which accounts for 15% of the population with schizophrenia, the onset is between ages thirteen and sixteen. Childhood-onset schizophrenia (COS) is between the ages of ten to thirteen and makes up 4% of the population. Very early onset schizophrenia (VEOS), which occurs before the age of ten (Mala, 2008) or before age thirteen (McClellan & Werry, 1997), accounts for 1% of the population with schizophrenia. VEOS is rare, with a prevalence rate estimated to be 1 per 10,000, and is more common in males. Eighty percent of children with VEOS report having auditory hallucinations (Mala, 2008). Of note, 75% of children diagnosed with schizophrenia have an insidious onset; only 25% have an acute onset (Masi et al., 2006).

Etiology

No single etiology has been identified for schizophrenia in children and adolescents. Most theories include both genetic and environmental factors (Rapoport et al., 2005). With the earlier onset of schizophrenia in comparison to the adolescent or adult onset, increased genetic loading or early CNS damage due to environmental stressors may be important factors in the etiology (Kalapatapu & Dunn, 2010).

Neurobiological/Neurophysiological Factors

Increasing evidence points to alterations in several neurotransmitters and pathways in the pathophysiological processes of schizophrenia. These include dopamine (DA) and glutamate (GLU) as well as gamma-aminobutyric acid (GABA), serotonin, and cholinergic and opioidergic systems. The studies that have examined the neurotransmitters and brain metabolites in children with schizophrenia report the same abnormalities as noted in adults with schizophrenia. The dopamine hypothesis maintains that hyperactivity of the dopamine system leads to an increase in positive symptoms of schizophrenia. Antipsychotics that diminish the hyperactivity of dopamine receptors decrease the positive symptoms while drugs that stimulate the dopamine receptors exacerbate psychotic symptoms. The other neurotransmitters are also involved in schizophrenia, and the impact of the newer psychotropic drugs on the abnormalities of these neurotransmitters in children and adolescents is undergoing further study (Frankenburg, 2010; Kalapatapu & Dunn, 2010).

Neurodevelopmental hypothesis maintains that the developing brain is vulnerable to genetic and environmental insults that alter the structure and function of the brain and increase the risk of psychosis later in life. Evidence points to environmental insults such as hypoxia-associated complications during pregnancy and prenatal exposures to diseases, and famine with fetal malnutrition (Dean & Murray, 2005; McClellan, Susser & King, 2006; Sharma & Harvey, 2006; Yung et al., 2007) as increasing the odds of developing earlier-onset schizophrenia. As noted above, excessive pruning of dopaminergic neurons in the brain in the period from birth to the age of twelve to fifteen years is also hypothesized to lead to the development of schizophrenia (Mala, 2008; Rapoport et al., 1999).

Brain imaging studies show consistent findings of brain tissue volume loss in schizophrenia. These findings provide evidence of a neurodegenerative process that occurs in the brains of people with schizophrenia. Gray matter volume loss in people with schizophrenia over time is associated with deterioration in overall clinical status (Nasrallah et al., 2009).

Genetic and Genomic Factors

Genetic and genomic factors are the best-established etiological determinants of schizophrenia (McClellan et al., 2008; Nasrallah et al., 2009). The best-established evidence comes from twin and family studies showing a strong genetic link to the development of schizophrenia. The results clearly indicate the heritability and genetic basis of schizophrenia but not specific genes. Monozygotic twins are shown to have 41% to 65% proband concordance rates for schizophrenia, while dizygotic twins have only 0% to 28% proband concordance rates (Cardno & Gottesman, 2000). Future trends in searching for the etiology of schizophrenia and other perceptual alterations disorders include epigenetics, which studies changes in behavior of genes and changes in the genes as a result of our own behavior (Mala, 2008).

Several chromosomal abnormalities are reported in people with schizophrenia. The 22q11 deletion on the maternal chromosome is of particular interest in the diagnosis of schizophrenia in children and adolescents. Children and adolescents with velocardiofacial syndrome have similar reduction in gray and white matter tissue volume, and the reduction is attributed to 22q11.2 nicrodeletion on the maternal chromosome (Eliez, Antonarakis, Morris, Dahoun & Reiss, 2001).

Family History

Evidence of genetic etiology in schizophrenia comes from twin and family studies. Aside from genetic factors, other family history factors are not as well established as part of the etiology of schizophrenia. In the social case history, 45% of the cases of schizophrenia were found to have a history of "broken home" with most being associated with death of a parent (Mala, 2008). Poor prognosis is found in cases where individuals with schizophrenia had a family history that includes psychosis and dysfunctional family behavior, but the evidence of these as determinants of schizophrenia due to environmental factors versus genetic factors is not well established (Mala, 2008).

Psychosocial Factors

Environmental stressors such as family or work settings that have highly expressed emotional atmospheres are known to lead to an increase in symptoms and eventual relapse for some individuals with schizophrenia. However, not all individuals exposed to such environmental stressors develop schizophrenia so the etiological evidence is weak but contributory.

Dysfunction of the "social brain" refers to deficits in social functioning and is present in many psychiatric disorders. This developmental disturbance affects the interconnections of the brain and leads to disorganization of thinking and perception, as well as inappropriate and flat affect and deficits in social functioning. This connectivity disturbance is hypothesized to be a factor in the etiology of schizophrenia (Mala, 2008).

Evidence-Based Nursing Intervention

Basically, treatment for children over age twelve and adolescents with schizophrenia is similar to the treatment for adults. The strongest evidence to date for effective treatment is the use of psychotropic medications (Kumra et al., 2007; Madaan, Dvir & Wilson 2008; Masi et al., 2006). Doses of medications are generally reduced for children and adolescents. Not all atypical psychotropic medications are shown to be safe and efficient for children. However, randomized clinical trials are under way to establish their efficacy with youth. Complications from the use of typical and atypical antipsychotics include marked weight gain, extrapyramidal symptoms, cardiometabolic risks, neuroleptic malignant syndrome, and other side effects. These effects become more obvious and problematic as more of these medications are used with children and adolescents (Correll et al., 2009; Masi et al., 2006; McClellan et al., 2007; Nasrallah et al., 2009; Varley & McClellan, 2009).

Medication adherence continues to be a major concern because so often even the parent who administers the medication to the child or adolescent is not aware of the importance of adhering to the medication schedule. Evidence of the effectiveness of visual feedback therapy to improve adherence to the medications by adults with schizophrenia has been noted (Kozuki & Schepp, 2005). At this time, little evidence exists to show the effectiveness of visual feedback therapy when used with children and adolescents. More specific detailed information about psychotropic medications and psychopharmacology with children and adolescents is presented in Chapter 6.

Strong evidence is being established that shows treatment effectiveness and cost effectiveness of involving the family in psychoeducational programs where all members of the family can learn about the disorder and symptoms along with skills to help the child or adolescent manage the illness (Breitborde, Woods & Srihari, 2009; Schepp, O'Connor & Kennedy, 2005). Different types of psychoeducational programs are being used and more evidence is becoming available about the type of program that is most effective for each age group and cultural group (Kennedy et al., 2008). Psychoeducational programs that emphasize symptom awareness and stress management skills are reported to be effective in reducing stress for the mentally ill adolescent as well as for other family members (Lee & Schepp, 2009). More detailed information is provided in Chapters 15 through 17 on treatment modalities with families and individuals.

The most promising advances in the treatment of early-onset schizophrenia are evidenced by the latest research supporting early treatment and aggressive use of psychotropic medications coupled with psychosocial family interventions. The less time between the onset of the first psychotic symptoms and the first adequate treatment, referred to as the duration of untreated psychosis (DUP), the better the short-term outcome is noted to be (Nasrallah et al., 2009; Nordentoft, Jeppesen, Petersen, Bertelsen & Thorup, 2009).

Evidence is being established that indicates it may be possible to identify, treat, and potentially improve the outcome for those who are at highest risk for developing schizophrenia. Three groups found to be at highest risk are those who have experienced (1) attenuated, positive psychotic symptoms during the past year or (2) brief intermittent episodes of frank psychotic symptoms but not lasting longer than a week and (3) those who have a relative with a psychotic disorder or who themselves have a schizotypal personality with decreased functioning over the course of the past year (Yung et al., 2007).

Evidence is beginning to be established showing CBT to be effective in the treatment of schizophrenia and in psychoeducational programs for family members (Bechdolf et al., 2005; Garety et al., 2009; Gleeson et al., 2009). Likewise, appreciative inquiry, an intervention approach derived from positive psychology, has been shown to make a significant difference in the lives of young adults with schizophrenia in their perceptions of their level of happiness and hope (Buckland, 2009). Rather than focus on deficits as so many interventions have done in the past, appreciative inquiry is an approach where strengths are emphasized and developed in young adults over a period of time as part of their treatment.

Integration with Primary Care

The roles of APNs may include (1) early detection and referral of patients who are experiencing premorbid major delay or prodromal symptoms, (2) following up the patients' conditions in annual well-child exams, (3) promoting family-centered care, (4) educating the patient and family about the disorder and management, and (5) helping adolescents and their families to make smooth transitions to care by adult primary care providers.

First, early identification of schizophrenia includes early detection and referral of patients who are experiencing premorbid major delay or prodromal symptoms. Evidence shows that 46% to 89% of affected children show premorbid major delay in one or all areas of motor, speech, and social development (Masi et al., 2006). Therefore, anyone who shows these early developmental delays should be monitored closely because these may be early manifestations of the disorder. Evidence shows that early identification of prodromal symptoms and intervention lead to appointments with primary care providers. Studies show that 75% to 90% of patients experiencing prodromal symptoms visit a physician before the onset of psychosis (Bota et al., 2008)). Early prodromal symptoms are negative symptoms and include slow changes in behaviors and mood such as social isolation, decreased school functioning, anxiety/nervousness, blunted or inappropriate affect, and anhedonia.

APNs in primary care need to distinguish whether these presentations are simply developmental or psychopathological. If it is simply developmental, the adolescents will have other symptoms. If this is psychopathological, these symptoms will not get better and may become worse to the point that they include positive symptoms. In any case, it is recommended to refer the adolescents with these symptoms to a psychiatric health care provider for further evaluation. If adolescents who had early developmental delays show the prodromal symptoms, they need to be evaluated by a specialist.

If the primary care APN is unsure about referral, help can be obtained by consulting with a child and adolescent APN in making a decision. Communications between the primary care provider and a child and adolescent APN may be different based on the care setting. If both providers are in the same building, direct communication can happen easily; this promotes continuity of care. In some hospitals, when the patient is referred to a specialist the specialist sends a summary statement of the visit to the referring service provider. In this case, the primary care providers will be kept informed about the patient's condition, allowing them to stay current with the patient, including scheduling visits as necessary. If the specialist does not send the summary of the visit, the primary care provider should ask the patient about the visit with the specialist. If there is information that the primary care provider needs from the specialist, the primary care provider should also contact the specialist directly to obtain the summary statement in order to provide safe care.

Second, if an adolescent is diagnosed with schizophrenia, a recommendation will be made to begin an antipsychotic medication. Side effects from antipsychotic medications are not uncommon and the adolescent and family need to be aware of these side effects. Patients with major mental illnesses may also have a greater risk of glucose intolerance diabetes and lipid abnormalities that seem to be present before treatment initiation (Ryan, Collins, & Thakore, 2003) and that are associated with medication effects or weight gain (Lambert, Velakoulis, & Pantelis, 2003). The use of psychotropic medication such as clozapine will require additional tests such as troponin, echocardiogram and frequent WBC and granulocyte counts. It would be important for the primary care provider to communicate with the specialist to check if he or she are monitoring for these risks. If not, it is recommended that the primary care provider closely monitor the patient at the annual exam along with a complete physical assessment. The child, adolescent, and/or parents should be told about potential side effects and what to do should they occur. It is also recommended that a full medical examination in first-episode psychosis and yearly after includes a complete blood count (CBC), lipid panel, urea and electrolytes, liver function, thyroid function, B12 and folate, random glucose, urinalysis, and creatinine clearance (Berger, Fraser, Carbone, & McGorry, 2006). Table 11.4 shows the tests that are recommended before antipsychotic medications are prescribed. In addition, it is important to check for suicidal ideation at each visit because four in ten people who suffer from schizophrenia attempt suicide and one in ten people who suffer from schizophrenia dies by suicide (Caruso, 2009). Those who are not taking their prescribed medication as directed are also at risk for symptom resurgence; therefore, it is also important to stress and assess for adherence with medication.

It would also be important for the APN to evaluate how the adolescent is doing at school and among friends. These adolescents typically have trouble with declining school performance during the prodromal stage of the disorder, and once they start psychotropic medications, the side effects could make them drowsy, interfering with their social interactions. Once the right medication and dose are found and the adolescent is taking the medication as prescribed, functioning should improve. However, the child or adolescent may con-

Table 11.4 Primary care workup prior to commencement of antipsychotic medications

Timing	Tests
Before commencement of antipsychotic medications	Full blood examination
	Lipid panel (total cholesterol, triglyceride, HDL, LDL)
	Urea and electrolytes
	Liver function (LFTs)
	Thyroid function
	B12 and folate
	Random glucose
	Urinalysis
	Creatinine clearance glucose
	LFTs with copper, heavy metal screening
	HIV/AIDS
	MRI to rule out organic etiology of psychosis
	Genetic testing (22q11 deletion syndrome)

tinue to struggle in school because of thought, language, perceptual, and motor disturbances. They may also be vulnerable because of decreased tolerance to normal stress. Adolescents may try to hide their illness from their friends, initially because of the stigma of having a mental illness. However, if the adolescents can be open and direct about their illness with friends, this may help the friends understand the illness and be supportive of them. Peer relationships are important and critical for this developmental stage.

Third, the APN needs to help families cope with the situation of having an adolescent with schizophrenia, which can be very disturbing to the family. Assessing family functioning, effect of the adolescent's illness on the family, communication, and relationship with the adolescent would be necessary. Helping the family become connected with resources in the community such as the NAMI and web sites that provide important information about schizophrenia and the medications and treatments used and recommended would be important. Providing occasional respite support to both the child and family is also critical. Respite for families may occur through in-home and out-of-home settings for various lengths of time depending on the needs of the family and available resources in the community. Primary care providers need to be familiar with local government community programs that are available for funding respite support. Respite is an important part of the continuum of services for families, which helps preserve the family unit and supports family stability (Cernoch, 1994).

Fourth, ongoing education of family members about schizophrenia would improve their coping skills and their ability to help the patient including:

- Knowledge about the illness and its symptoms
- Advantages and disadvantages of different treatment options
- Available medications and possible side effects, and signs of relapse
- Better communication with
  - The patient
  - Other family members
  - Health care providers
  - School personnel
- Availability of community services and supports including respite care
- Benefits and entitlements including how to access care
- Management of crises or bizarre and troubling behaviors
- Importance of self-care for caregivers

Last, helping the adolescent make a smooth transition to adulthood is necessary. Psychotic episodes tend to happen during stressful times when the individual feels most vulnerable such as making transitions to living away from home, going to college or going to a new job, and trying to adjust to a new environment. This means that it would be important for the APN to help the adolescent and the family find adult care providers in the area where the adolescents will now reside.

Implications for Practice, Research, and Education

Disorders with disturbed sensory perception and thought processes are difficult to diagnose. The symptom patterns tend to be nonspecific for varying lengths of time and a clear pattern of specific symptoms may not be evident for a considerable period of time, sometimes from months to years. In the meantime, families are seeking help for their child or adolescent and many times the diagnosis is not made for at least six months. Often times, mental health professionals are hesitant to give a diagnosis, especially if it is schizophrenia. Diagnosing a child or adolescent as having schizophrenia can lead to labels that are difficult to get rid of and can lead to stigma toward the individual as well as to the family. The label and stigma can be devastating especially since it can be life-long and devastating to one's self-esteem and confidence. In recent years, efforts have been made to decrease the stigma of perceptual alterations disorders such as schizophrenia so the young person can seek treatment to lessen the persistently debilitating effects of the disorder (Kalapatapu & Dunn, 2008).

As more studies yield credible evidence that can be used to guide the way for early recognition of prodromal symptoms of schizophrenia and other perception altering disorders, more interventions will become available that will be individualized to the specific needs of the child or adolescent. Genetic research will eventually lead to identification of specific genes responsible for schizophrenia and early recognition and treatment will follow. The need for early identification and early treatment prompts primary care providers to know the prodromal symptoms and refer to mental health professionals as quickly as possible so the debilitating effects of the disorder can be diminished and the disorder managed.

Research with youth with perceptual alterations disorders is challenging but the future is encouraging. More studies leading to the establishment of strong evidence-based nursing interventions for the children, adolescents, and families are being conducted. New ideas and notions that the trajectory for schizophrenia and related disorders may be altered for the good and a cure may be possible are exciting possibilities for future research. Prevention of perceptual alterations disorders is on the horizon and may one day be possible.

Since primary care providers such as pediatric nurse practitioners or family nurse practitioners are often the first health care providers to see the child or adolescent who is experiencing disturbed sensory perceptions and thought processes, these health care providers are increasingly more important as active participants of the mental health team. Their role as frontline primary care providers is crucial to early recognition and appropriate referral for those presenting with this disorder. APNs in primary care can and should remain involved with their psychiatric APN colleagues in collaborative management of children and adolescents presenting with these disorders. APNs in primary care should use educational updates on psychotropic medications, management strategies for childhood psychiatric disorders, as well as new research findings in child and adolescent psychiatry to remain current in this area.

Case Exemplar 1: Case Study of an Adolescent with Schizophrenia

John, a fifteen-year-old boy who was living at home and attending high school. He was in his sophomore year of high school. He did well during his freshmen year. He was a popular student and an athlete. His grades were As and Bs. He was active in football and other sports and was a member of the high school debate team. Although he was a sophomore, he was interested in attending college and was taking advanced placement courses. He was beginning to search for a college and planned to apply when he was a senior. John had a lot of friends. He invited fifty friends from school to his birthday party at his home six months earlier when he turned fifteen. Since then, he has become withdrawn and stays in his room most of the time when at home. He no longer has his friends over to his home. He has difficulty sleeping and remains awake most of the night pacing the floor and not sleeping. He is groggy and tired in the morning and doesn't want to go to school. His grades have dropped. He didn't do his homework. He was not eating. He said he sometimes hears voices talking to him and wonders if he is losing his mind. He said it is hard for him to talk about this and he was afraid others would find out. He didn't want his friends to know. He thought they would not accept him if they knew he was experiencing symptoms of a mental illness. He was anxious and agitated much of the time and found it difficult to relax. He had difficulty finding words to express his thoughts and feelings. He described his mind as being like a whirlwind with so many racing thoughts. He lived with his parents and sister, who was thirteen years old. He was irritable with his parents and sister and then guilty for his behavior. His maternal grandmother lived nearby and came to the house daily. He was close to his family and felt protective of them but more recently believed they were conspiring against him. He was cautious of what he said to them, especially his sister, because he thought she would tell his friends about his changing behavior.

John's appearance indicated he was not keeping up his activities of daily living (ADLs). He wore the same clothes for several days even though they were wrinkled and soiled. He didn't take a shower each morning as he was used to doing. He didn't comb his hair. He became irritable when a family member reminded him to shower and change his clothes.

John's parents made an appointment for John to see his primary care provider, family nurse practitioner, for a physical examination. In addition to performing a physical examination, she conducted a series of tests and lab work. Her aim was to rule out depression, physical illnesses, illegal drugs, and alcohol abuse. She thought he might be depressed and referred him to the family psychiatric mental health nurse practitioner (F-PMHNP) in the clinic. The F-PMHNP recognized the nonspecific symptoms (agitation, irritation) and specific attenu-

ated psychotic symptoms (conspiratory thinking) that presented in the prodromal phase and referred John for a diagnostic workup for schizophrenia. The workup included a comprehensive physical exam and a semi-structured K-SADS diagnostic interview following the APA criteria for schizophrenia. The diagnostic interview confirmed the diagnosis of schizophrenia. John began treatment with psychotropic medications. He and his family participated in a multifamily psychoeducational program to learn about his illness and how to manage it.

Case Exemplar 2: Case Study of a Seven-year-old Child with Schizophrenia

Katy, the second of two children of a middle-class family living in a suburban area of a northwest city. Katy's sister was two years older than her. Katy's mother's pregnancy was normal and Katy's birth was normal. Katy had colic the first three months and cried extensively and was difficult to comfort. After 3 months she became passive and cried very little. Her growth and development appeared to be normal. She met all the developmental milestones her first three years. She interacted normally with her sister and parents. At age four, she was in nursery school and appeared to function normally. The nursery school was a small private school with a lot of personal attention given to each child. Although shy, she made friends and liked going to nursery school. At age five, she attended kindergarten, which was in a large public school. The class was larger than she was used to in the nursery school but she appeared to adapt well. She made friends at the new school and played with the other children. She liked the classes and looked forward to going to school every day. She appeared to be progressing normally for a five-year-old.

First grade was difficult for Katy although the school was the same school she attended for kindergarten. Many of her first-grade classmates had been in her kindergarten class. Almost immediately, her behavior began to change although the change was gradual. Her attitude toward school changed. She went from liking school to not wanting to go. She began to have difficulty keeping up with her class. She had difficulty paying attention in school and following instructions. She began to have difficulty doing her school work. She was failing first grade. Her parents sought tutoring help for her but her grades didn't improve. Katy's teacher reported that Katy sat and stared into space much of the day and recommended she be evaluated for possible hearing problems. Katy's sister told her parents that she heard Katy talking to someone but no one was present. This behavior continued for several weeks while Katy became more withdrawn and less communicative with her parents and sister. By spring of first grade when she turned seven years of age, she was still attending school but her level of functioning began to decrease. She avoided the other children and hurried home after school. Her parents began to observe her talking to herself. When confronted with her behavior, she told her parents about the voices she heard. She told them how frightening the voices were and how scared she was that something might happen to her. Her parents immediately made an appointment for her to see her primary care provider. Her primary care provider conducted a thorough physical exam and referred Katy to an F-PMHNP who specialized in children and adolescents. After a thorough psychiatric history and diagnostic interview using K-SADS, Katy was diagnosed with schizophrenia. The psychiatric history revealed she had an uncle with "odd" behavior who was estranged from the family. The possibility of a family member having schizophrenia was noted. She was placed on a low dose of a neuroleptic medication, which led to partial remission of the hallucinations but she remained withdrawn. She continued in school but was placed in a special education program in her school where she was able to work at her own pace and level of functioning. Her treatment consisted of neuroleptic medication and individual counseling. In addition, she participated with her parents and sister in a psychoeducational program for families with a child with a severe mental illness.

Summary

This chapter covered child and adolescent disorders with perceptual alterations such as schizophrenia or bipolar disorder or depression with psychotic features or other conditions where psychosis is present. Since depression and bipolar disorder are covered thoroughly in other chapters, this chapter specifically focused on schizophrenia as the perceptual alterations disorder. The importance of recognizing the prodromal symptoms was emphasized so that early referral for diagnostic workup can be conducted and appropriate treatment can begin. The time factor was emphasized as important because of the neurodegenerative nature of this disorder and the need to halt or reverse the debilitating effects of the disorder as quickly as possible through the use of psychotropic medications and psychosocial interventions. The symptom patterns and phases in the manifestation of schizophrenia in children and adolescents were presented. The epidemiology and current hypotheses concerning the etiology were described. Diagnostic criteria and assessment tool were discussed. Evidence-based interventions were presented and implications for practice, research, and education were addressed. Two

actual case studies were presented. Both are examples of a perceptual alterations disorder. One was a case of an adolescent with schizophrenia and the other is the case of a seven-year-old with childhood schizophrenia. Implications for families of children and adolescents with schizophrenia or other perceptual alterations disorders were noted throughout the chapter. Finally, resources in the form of community groups, web sites, and advocacy and treatment resources were presented.

Resources on Perceptual Alterations Disorders (Community Groups, Websites, Advocacy, and Treatment Resources)

American Psychiatric Association. Practice Guideline for Treatment of Patients with Schizophrenia (2004). http://www.psych.org/research/

American Association of Child and Adolescent Psychiatry. www.aacap.org

Bazelon Center for Mental Health Law. National legal advocate for people with mental illness and intellectual disability. http://www.bazelton.org

Clinical Antipsychotic Trials of Intervention Effectiveness (CATIE). http://www.catie.unc.edu

Cochrane Database of Systematic Reviews. Excellent resource for evidence-based practice. http://www.cochrane.org/index2.htm

Expert Consensus Guidelines. Guidelines for the treatment of schizophrenia and other disorders. http://www.psychguides.com

Food and Drug Administration (FDA) Medwatch Updates regarding warnings on atypical antipsychotics. http://www.fda.gov/medwatch/safety.htm

Health Links, an evidence-based-practice search engine at the University of Washington. http://healthlinks.washington.edu/ebp

International Society of Psychiatric-Mental Health Nurses. www.ispn-psych.org

National Alliance for Research on Schizophrenia and Depression (NARSAD). Research for latest advances in schizophrenia and depression. http://www.mhsource.com/narsad.htm

National Alliance for the Mentally Ill. Information, support, and advocacy. http://www.nami.org

National Institute of Mental Health. Information on children and adolescents. www.numh.nih.gov/publicat/childmenu.cfm http://www.nimh.nih.gov/publicat/childmenu.cfm www.nimh.nih.gov/publicat/adhdmenu.cfm

National Institute of Mental Health. Information Resources and Inquiries Branch for information on research into the brain, behavior, and mental disorders. http://www.nimh.nih.gov and http://www.nimh.nih.gov/publicat/schizoph.cfm

Open the Doors. Designed to counter the stigma and distorted facts surrounding schizophrenia. The "Families and Friends" section provides several essays useful for family members and patients newly diagnosed with schizophrenia. http://www.openthedoors.com/

Mental Health Consultation Outreach for Children. Partnership Access Line (PAL). http://www.palforkids.org

Physicians Post Graduate Press, Inc. Publishes The Expert Consensus Guideline Series: Treatment of Schizophrenia http://www.psychguides.com

Psychopharmacology Algorithm Project (Harvard Medical School Department of Psychiatry). Algorithms to guide medication treatment of schizophrenia, depression, and other illnesses. http://mhc.com/Algorithms

The Reach Institute. The Resource for Advancing Children's Health. Primary Pediatric Psychopharmacology (PPP). Mini-fellowship in primary pediatric psychopharmacology, 4 day training, 6 months of biweekly phone consultation. http://www.thereachinstitute.org/ppp.html

References

Ambrosini, P.J. (2000). Historical development and present status of the schedule for affective disorders and schizophrenia for school-age children (K-SADS). *Journal of the American Academy of Child & Adolescent Psychiatry, 39,* 49–58.

APA (American Psychiatric Association). (2000). *Diagnostic and statistical manual of mental disorders,* fourth edition, text revision. Washington, DC: APA.

Bechdolf, A. Veith, V., Schwarzer, D., Schormann, M., Stamm, E., Janssen, B., Berning, J., Wagner, M., & Klosterkotter, J. (2005). Cognitive behavioral therapy in the pre-psychotic phase: an exploratory study. *Psychiatry Research, 136,* 251–255.

Berger, C., Fraser, R., Carbone, S., & McGorry, P. (2006). Emerging psychosis in young people, Part 1: Key issues for detention and assessment. *Australian Family Physicians 35*(5), 315–321.

Birchwood, M., Smith, J., MacMillian, F., Hogg, B., Prasad, R., Harvey, C., & Bering, S. (1989). Predicting relapse in schizophrenia: the development and implementation of an early signs monitoring system using patients and families as observers, a preliminary investigation. *Psychological Medicine, 19,* 649–656.

Bota, R.G., Sagduyu, K., Filin, E.E., Bota, D.A., & Munro, S. (2008). Toward a better identification and treatment of schizophrenia prodrome. *Bulletin of the Menninger Clinic, 72*(3), 210–227.

Breitborde, N.J., Woods, S.W., & Srihari, V.H. (2009). Multifamily psychoeducation for first-episode psychosis: a cost effectiveness analysis. *Psychiatric Services, 60*(11), 1477–83.

Buckland, H.T. (2009). *Young adults with schizophrenia: defining happiness, building hope.* Unpublished doctoral dissertation. Seattle, WA: University of Washington.

Calinoiu, I., & McClellan, J. (2004). Diagnostic interviews. *Current Psychiatry Reports, 6,* 88–95.

Cardno, A.G., & Gottesman, I.I. (2000). Twin studies of schizophrenia: from bow and arrow concordances to star wars Mx and functional genomics. *American Journal of Medical Genetics, 97*(1), 12–17.

Caruso, K. (2009). Schizophrenia and suicide. Retrieved from http://www.suicide.org/schizophrenia-and-suicide.html

Cernoch, J.M. (1994). Respite for children with disabilities and chronic or terminal illnesses. Retrieved from http://www.archrespite.org/archfs02.htm

Corcoran, C., Gerson, R., Sills-Shahar, R., Nickou, C., McGlashan, T., Malaspina, D., & Davidson, L. (2007). Trajectory to a first episode of psychosis: a qualitative research study with families. *Early Intervention in Psychiatry, 1,* 308–315.

Correll, C.U., Penzner, J.B., Frederickson, A.M., Richter, J.J., Auter, A.M., Smith, C.W., Kane, J.M., & Cornblatt, B.A. (2007). Differentiation in the pre-onset phases of schizophrenia and mood disorders: evidence in support of a bipolar mania prodrome. *Schizophrenia Bulletin, 33*(3), 703–714.

Correll, C.U., Manu, P., Olshansky, V., Napolitano, B., Kane, J.M., & Malhotra, A.K. (2009). Cardiometabolic risk of second-generation antipsychotic medications during first-time use in children and adolescents. *Journal of the American Medical Association, 302*(16), 1765–1773.

Dean, K., & Murray, R.M. (2005). Environmental risk factors for psychosis. *Dialogues in Clinical Neuroscience, 7*(1), 69–80.

Eliez, S., Antonarakis, S.E., Morris, M.A., Dahoun, S.P., & Reiss, A.L. (2001). Parental origin of the deletion 22q11.2 and brain development in velocardiofacial syndrome: a preliminary study. *Archives of General Psychiatry, 58,* 64–68.

Emsley, R. (2009). Editorial: Early intervention in the management of schizophrenia: introduction. *Early Intervention in Psychiatry, 3,* S1–S2.

Endicott, J., Spitzer, R.L., Fleiss, J.L., & Cohen, J. (1976). The global assessment scale. *Archives of General Psychiatry, 33,* 766–777.

Frankenburg, F.R. (2010). Schizophrenia. Emedicine. *http://emedicine.medscap.com/article/288259-print.*

Frazier J.A., McClellan, J., Findling, R.L. Vitiello, B., Anderson, R., Zablotsky, B., & Sikich, L. (2007). Treatment of early-onset schizophrenia spectrum disorders (TEOSS): Demographic and clinical characteristics. *Journal of the American Academy of Child and Adolescent Psychiatry, 46,* 979–988.

Garety, P.A., Fowler, D.G., Freeman, D., Bebbington, P., Dunn, G., & Kuipers, E. (2009). Cognitive-behavioral therapy and family intervention for relapse prevention and symptom reduction in psychosis: randomized controlled trial. *British Journal of Psychiatry, 192*(6), 412–423.

Gleeson, J.F., Cotton, S.M., Alvarez-Jimenez, M., Wade, D., Crisp, K., Newman, B., Spiliotacopoulos, D., & McGorry, P.D. (2009). Family outcomes from a randomized control trial of relapse prevention therapy in first-episode psychosis. *Journal of Clinical Psychiatry.* Epub ahead of print.

Hlastala, S.A., & McClellan, J. (2005). Phenomenology and diagnostic stability of youths with atypical psychotic symptoms. *Journal of Child and Adolescent Psychopharmacology, 15,* 497–509.

Hodges, K., Doucette-Gates, A., & Liao, Q.L. (1999). The relationship between the child and adolescent functional assessment scale (CAFAS) and indicators of functioning. *Journal of Child & Family Studies, 8*(1), 109–122.

Kalapatapu, R.K., & Dunn, D.W. (2010). Schizophrenia and other psychosis. Retrieved from http://emedicine.medscape.com/article/914840.

Kim, H.J. (Spring, 2010). Phases, symptoms & level of functioning leading to psychotic episode. Unpublished paper titled *Schizophrenia Prodrome.* University of Washington.

Kozuki, Y., & Schepp, K. (2005). Visual feedback therapy to enhance medication adherence in psychosis. *Archives of Psychiatric Nursing, 19*(2), 70–80.

Kumra, S., Oberstar, J.V., Sukich, L., Findling, R.L., McClellan, J.M., Vinogradov, S., & Schulz, C. (2007). Efficacy and tolerability of second-generation antipsychotics in children and adolescents with schizophrenia. *Schizophrenia, 34*(1), 60–71.

Lambert, T. J., Velakoulis, D., & Pantelis, C. (2003). Medical co-mobidity in schizophrenia. *Medical Journal of Australia, 178*(9), 284–289.

Lee, H., & Schepp, K. (2009). The relationships between symptoms and stress in adolescents with schizophrenia. *Issues in Mental Health Nursing, 30,* 736–744.

Madaan, V., Dvir, Y., & Wilson, D.R. (2008). Child and adolescent schizophrenia: pharmacological approaches. *Expert Opinion Pharmacotherapeutics, 9*(12), 2053–2068.

Maier, W., Cornblatt, B.A., & Merikangas, K.R. (2003). Transition to schizophrenia and related disorders: toward a taxonomy of risk. *Schizophrenia Bulletin, 29*(4), 693–701.

Mala, E. (2008). Schizophrenia in childhood and adolescence. *Neuroendocrinology Letters, 29*(6), 831–836.

Malla, A., & Pelosi, A.J. (2010). Is treating patients with first-episode psychosis cost-effective? *The Canadian Journal of Psychiatry, 55*(1), 3–8.

Masi, G., Mucci, M., & Pari, C. (2006). Children with schizophrenia: clinical picture and pharmacological treatment. *CNS Drugs 2006, 20*, 841–866.

McClellan, J.M., Werry, J.S., & Ham, M. (1993). A Follow-up study of early onset psychosis: comparison between outcome diagnosis of schizophrenia, mood disorders, and personality disorders. *Journal of Autism Developmental Disorders, 23*, 243–262.

McClellan, J.M., & Werry, J.S. (1997). Practice parameters for the assessment & treatment of children and adolescents with schizophrenia. *Journal of the American Academy of Child and Adolescent Psychiatry, 36*(Suppl 10), 177S–193S.

McClellan, J., McCurry, C., Snell, J., & DuBose, A. (1999). Early-onset psychotic disorders: Course and outcome over a 2-year period. *Journal of the American Academy of Child & Adolescent Psychiatry, 38*(11), 1380–1388.

McClellan, J.M., Susser, E., & King, M.C. (2006). Maternal famine, de novo mutations, and schizophrenia. *Journal of the American Medical Association, 296*(5), 582–584.

McClellan, J., Sikich, L., Findling, R.L., Frazier, J.A., Vitello, B., Hlastala, S.A., & Lieberman, J.A. (2007). Treatment of early-onset schizophrenia spectrum disorders (TEOSS): rationale, design, and methods. *Journal of the American Academy of Child and Adolescent Psychiatry, 46*, 969–978.

McClellan, J., Susser, E., King, M.C., Rietschel, M., Riley, B., & Zammit, S. (2008). Forum: The interplay of genes and environment in psychiatric disorders. *Psychiatry, 21*, 322–327

Nasrallah, H.A., Keshavan, M.S., Benes, F.M., Braff, D.L., Green, A.I., Gur, R.E., Kane, J.M., & Correll, C.U. (2009). Proceedings and data from the schizophrenia summit: a critical appraisal to improve the management of schizophrenia. *Journal of Clinical Psychiatry, 70*(suppl 1), 4–46.

Nordentoft, M., Jeppesen, P., Petersen, L., Bertelsen, M., & Thorup, A. (2009). The rationale for early intervention in schizophrenia and related disorders. *Early Intervention in Psychiatry, 3*, 53–57.

NANDA (North American Nursing Diagnosis Association). (2007). *Nursing diagnosis: Definition and classification, 2007–2008.* Philadelphia: Author.

Rapoport, J.L., Giedd, J.N., Blumenthal, J., Hamburger, S., Jeffries, N., Fernandez, T., Nicolson, R., & Evans, A. (1999). Progressive cortical change during adolescence in childhood-onset schizophrenia. A longitudinal magnetic resonance imaging study. *Archives of General Psychiatry, 56*(7), 649–654.

Rapoport, J.L., Addington, A.M., Frangou, S., & Psych, M.R.C. (2005). The neurodevelopmental model of schizophrenia: update 2005. *Molecular Pychiatry, 10*, 434–449.

Reich, W. (2000). Diagnostic interview for children and adolescents (DICA). *Journal of the American Academy of Child & Adolescent Psychiatry, 39*, 59–66.

Ryan, M.C., Collins, P., & Thakore, J.H. (2003). Impaired fasting glucose tolerance in first episode, drug naive patients with schizophrenia. *American Journal of Psychiatry, 160*, 284–289.

Schepp, K.G., O'Connor, F.W. & Kennedy, M. (2005). *Self-management therapy for youth with schizophrenia,* Final Report: Summary for NIMH Randomized Clinical Trial #R01-MH56580. Submitted to the National Institute of Mental health of the National Institutes of Health, Bethesda, MD.

Shaffer, D., Gould, M.S., Brasic, J., Ambrosini, J.P., Fisher, P., Bird, H., & Alushahlia, S. (1983). A children's global assessment scale (CGAS). *Archives of General Psychiatry, 40*, 1228–1231.

Sharma, T., & Harvey, P.D. (2006). *The early course of schizophrenia.* New York: Oxford University Press.

Shioiri, T., Shinada, K., Kuwabara, H., & Someya, T. (2007). Early prodromal symptoms and diagnoses before first psychotic episode in 219 inpatients with schizophrenia. *Psychiatry and Clinical Neurosciences, 61*, 348–354.

Varley, C.K., & McClellan, J.M. (2009). Implications of marked weight gain associated with atypical medications in children and adolescents. *Journal of the American Medical Association, 302*(16), 1811–1812.

Werry, J.S., McClellan, J.M., & Chard, L. (1991). Childhood and adolescent schizophrenic, bipolar and schizoaffective disorders: a clinical and outcome study. *Journal of the American Academy of Child and Adolescent Psychiatry, 30*, 457–465.

White, T., Anjum, A., & Schulz, S.C. (2006). The schizophrenia prodrome. *American Journal of Psychiatry, 163*, 376–380.

Yung, A.R., McGorry, P.D., Francey, S.M., Nelson, B., Baker, K., Phillips, L.J., Berger, G., & Amminger, G.P. (2007). PACE: a specialized service for young people at risk of psychotic disorders. *Medical Journal of Australia, 187*, S43–S46.

12

Eating Disorders in Children and Adolescents

Janiece DeSocio and Joan B. Riley

Objectives

After reading this chapter, APNs will be able to

1. Identify the signs, symptoms, medical complications, psychiatric comorbidities, and developmental differences associated with anorexia nervosa, bulimia nervosa, and binge eating disorder in children and adolescents.
2. Discuss theories of etiology associated with eating disorders, including neurobiological, genetic, family dynamics, and psychosocial factors.
3. Describe evidence-based interventions for children and adolescents diagnosed with eating disorders.
4. Differentiate roles of primary care practitioners and advanced practice psychiatric mental health nurses (PMH-APNs) in the diagnosis and treatment of children and adolescents with eating disorders.

Introduction

Results from the National Institute of Mental Health-National Comorbidity Study Replication (NIMH-NCSR) indicate that the majority of individuals with eating disorders do not receive treatment, supporting the need for increased screening in primary care (Hudson, Hiripi, Pope, & Kessler, 2007). Advanced practice nurses (APNs) working with children, adolescents, and young adults in any setting should (1) provide education about eating disorders to patients and families; (2) screen for signs and symptoms of eating disorders to promote early identification; (3) partner with patients and parents to enhance motivation and cooperation for treatment; (4) treat medical complications; (5) restore patients to a healthy weight; (6) correct maladaptive thoughts, attitudes and feelings related to food and body image; (7) improve self-esteem; (8) enhance and utilize family support; (9) treat associated and comorbid psychiatric conditions; and (10) prevent relapse or recurrence. An objective proposed for *Healthy People 2020* is "to reduce the proportion of adolescents who engage in disordered eating in an attempt to control their weight" (U.S. Department of Health and Human Services, 2009). Reducing the health consequences of eating disorders is an essential goal for all health professionals.

Many advanced nursing practice education programs do not adequately cover the recognition and management of eating disorders. This chapter provides a framework for the recognition and treatment of three eating disorder subtypes that occur during childhood and adolescence: anorexia nervosa, bulimia nervosa, and binge eating disorder.

Child and Adolescent Behavioral Health: A Resource for Advanced Practice Psychiatric and Primary Care Practitioners in Nursing,
First Edition. Edited by Edilma L. Yearwood, Geraldine S. Pearson, and Jamesetta A. Newland.
© 2012 John Wiley & Sons, Inc. Published 2012 by John Wiley & Sons, Inc.

Historical and Cultural Perspective

The documented history of eating disorders begins in the Middle Ages with accounts of early saints and martyrs who engaged in starvation and purging as expressions of asceticism. Sir William Gull is credited with the first use of the term "anorexia nervosa" to describe a condition of starvation in adolescent girls in 1874, and Gerald Russell introduced the term "bulimia nervosa" to describe a purging variant of this condition in 1979 (Gull, 1874; Halmi, 2007; Madden, 2004; Russell, 1979).

In 1978, Hilde Bruch published *The Golden Cage*, which offered a psychodynamic description of factors underlying eating disorders. Since the late twentieth century, advances in neuroscience have transformed our understanding of eating disorders. Discoveries in genetics and neurobiology have helped dispel myths about eating disorders as volitional efforts to conform to social ideals and aesthetic body types.

Sketching historical perspectives on eating disorders and their treatments, Garner and Garfinkel (1997) highlight descriptions in the literature during the mid to late twentieth century, from a comprehensive monograph on anorexia nervosa that appeared in 1960 (Bliss & Branch) to the emergence of bulimia nervosa as an identified disorder in 1979 (Russell). In the 1970s and 1980s, attention was drawn to the dangers and potential deadly consequences of anorexia nervosa by the death of singer Karen Carpenter. This attention has continued as more athletes and celebrities disclose their personal struggles with these disorders. Unfortunately, the myth that these disorders are trendy, media-driven conditions continues despite evidence that they are serious and life-threatening disorders that affect children, adolescents, and adults.

Eating disorders are commonly perceived as responses to the values and idealized body types in Western cultures. In particular, beliefs about the rarity of anorexia nervosa in non-Westernized, Third World countries continue to exist despite research evidence to the contrary. From a review of literature, Keel and Klump (2003) found evidence of anorexia nervosa in all non-Western regions of the world, including Africa, the Middle East, India, Southeast Asia, and East Asia. Cases of bulimia nervosa were reported in fewer non-Western regions, contributing to the authors' conclusions that culture may play a greater role in bulimia nervosa than in anorexia nervosa. Other factors must be considered in examining reasons for differential reporting and prevalence rates of eating disorders in Third World countries. Stigma and lack of acceptance of psychiatric disorders contribute to underdiagnosis and treatment avoidance in many countries. For example, in Middle Eastern cultures, symptoms of anorexia nervosa may be concealed from public awareness and dealt with by physical and/or verbal abuse due to fears of embarrassment and family shame (Qadan, 2009).

This historic and cross-cultural look demonstrates the battle for scientific recognition that contributes to the burden and suffering of individuals with eating disorders. In an effort to combat prevailing myths that delay recognition and treatment, Thomas Insel, director of the NIMH, redefined eating disorders as brain disorders. Regarding anorexia nervosa, he observed, "While the symptoms are behavioral, this illness has a biological core, with genetic components, and changes in brain activity and neural pathways currently under study" (correspondence, National Eating Disorders Association, October 5, 2006).

Onset and Prevalence

Eating disorders are chronic disorders that begin in childhood or adolescence and continue through adulthood. Eating disorders are the third most common chronic illness in adolescent females (Society for Adolescent Medicine, 2003). The peak onset for eating disorders is between ages fifteen and nineteen years (Bulik, Reba, Siega-Riz, & Reichborn-Kjennerud, 2005). Anorexia nervosa has a bimodal peak of onset at ages thirteen to fourteen and ages seventeen to eighteen. Authors report an increase in the incidence of anorexia nervosa in ten- to fourteen-year-olds, and cases of prepubertal anorexia nervosa have been reported in children as young as age seven years (Hoek & van Hoeken, 2003; Peebles, Wilson, & Lock, 2006). The delay in diagnosing eating disorders in children ages seven to ten years averages thirteen months, twice as long as the delay in diagnosing these disorders after age eleven (Peebles et al.).

The NIMH-NCSR identified the lifetime prevalence of anorexia nervosa as 0.9% for women and 0.3% for men, and the lifetime prevalence of bulimia nervosa as 1.5% for women and 0.5% for men (Hudson et al., 2007). At any point in time, it is estimated that between 0.3% and 0.5% of adolescent females meet diagnostic criteria for anorexia nervosa. Subthreshold or partial syndromes, defined as falling short of meeting one or more criteria for a diagnosis of anorexia nervosa, have been identified in 1.3% to 3.7% of the population (Bulik et al., 2005). Binge eating disorders occur in 1% to 2.5% of young women (Hoek & van Hoeken, 2003).

Prevalence rates for eating disorders do not fully represent the extent of body image concerns and patterns of disordered eating that can occur during adolescence. It remains unclear to what extent, if any, disordered eating relates to the brain disorders called "eating disorders." In 1999 an epidemiological study of body image and eating patterns (Project EAT) was conducted in Minnesota with over 4,500 middle school and high school students. Results from this study illuminated the number of youth who participate in a continuum of disordered eating and weight loss activities. Over 25% of girls and 17% of boys in the Project EAT study reported severe dissatisfaction with their bodies. Over 9% of girls and 13.5% of boys engaged in compensatory activities such as excessive exercise, vomiting, or laxative use to avoid weight gain. Sixteen percent of girls and over 15% of boys engaged in patterns of binge eating followed by compensatory behaviors to avoid weight gain (Ackard, Fulkerson, & Neumark-Sztainer, 2007).

Course of Illness, Remission, and Recovery

The typical course of eating disorders is marked by periods of symptom remission and exacerbation. The cognitive symptoms (e.g., obsessions about food, distorted body perceptions, obsessive drive for exercise, and fears of weight gain) usually precede the onset of restricting, bingeing, and/or purging; and cognitive symptoms; are the last to remit. Time to remission depends on the severity of symptoms at onset of treatment and the type, duration, and degree of adherence to treatment. Symptoms of restricting, bingeing, and purging can generally be extinguished within eight to twelve months of active treatment (Clausen, 2004; Couturier & Lock, 2006; Strober, Freeman, & Morrell, 1997). Research has identified the median time to full physical and cognitive/psychological remission to be shorter for patients with bulimia nervosa, averaging eleven to twenty-six months, while time to full remission for patients with anorexia nervosa can require up to six years (Clausen).

Long-term follow-up of patients with anorexia nervosa shows that approximately half of patients achieve recovery; 30% improve but retain residual symptoms; and 20% persist on a chronic disabling course. Findings for adolescents who receive treatment early in the course of illness are more optimistic, with as many as 75% achieving recovery at the ten- to fifteen-year follow-up (Herzog & Eddy, 2007).

Relapse rates over a twelve-month period are as high as 35% to 50% for patients with anorexia nervosa. Risk factors associated with relapse include failure to achieve symptom remission, greater caloric restriction at the onset of treatment, resistance to nutritional compliance, and persistence of self-evaluations focused on body size and shape (McFarlane, Olmsted, & Trottier, 2008). Normalized body weight and return of normal menses are associated with better outcomes for individuals with anorexia nervosa (Berkman, Lohr, & Bulik, 2007; Couturier & Lock, 2006). In a study of adolescents ages eleven to nineteen years who achieved weight restoration, approximately 25% required readmission to the hospital within twelve months while 75% did not. Factors that increased the risk for hospital readmission included age younger than fifteen years at time of diagnosis, achieving a lower rate of weight gain, and greater disturbances in eating attitudes (Castro, Gila, Puig, Rodriguez, & Toto, 2004). Research evidence thus points to the importance of adequate weight gain and weight restoration as minimum requirements for extended periods of remission and recovery.

The mortality rate for individuals with anorexia nervosa is estimated to be 10% over ten to twenty years of illness and is the highest mortality rate of all psychiatric disorders (Bannon, 2005). If untreated, the mortality rate increases to approximately 20% within ten years for patients with anorexia nervosa. Mortality rates for bulimia nervosa are not significantly different from the rates in age- and sex-matched populations (Berkman et al., 2007; Sokol et al., 2005). Factors associated with mortality include persistence of a very low body weight, multiple hospital admissions, use of alcohol and substances, psychiatric comorbidities, and history of suicidal behaviors (Berkman et al.). Cardiac failure and suicide are the most common causes of death (Herzog & Eddy, 2007).

Etiology

Genetic and Neurobiological Factors

Genetic and biological factors have assumed prominence in explaining the etiology of eating disorders. Twin studies estimate the heritability of these disorders to be between 50% and 83% (Klump, Bulik, Kaye, Treasure, & Tyson, 2009). Relatives of individuals with anorexia nervosa have an eleven times greater risk of developing anorexia nervosa than relatives of normal controls, and the risk of developing bulimia nervosa is four times greater among relatives of individuals with bulimia nervosa (Strober, Freeman, Lampert, Diamond, & Kaye, 2000). Additionally, there is evidence of shared genetic risk between eating disorder subtypes and other psychiatric disorders such as depression, anxiety disorders, obsessive-compulsive disorder (OCD), and Cluster C personality traits (Fairburn & Harrison, 2003; Rome et al., 2003).

Genetic studies point to polymorphisms in serotonin (5-HT) genes and brain-derived neurotrophic factors (BDNF) as biological factors that may predispose individuals to eating disorders (Klump et al., 2009). Abnormalities in 5-HT1A and 5-HT2A receptors and a reduction in cerebrospinal fluid concentrations of 5-HT metabolites have been reported in anorexia nervosa. Brain imaging studies of individuals with anorexia nervosa have identified reduced 5-HT2A receptor activity in the anterior cingulate cortex and amygdala, as well as temporal, parietal, and occipital regions of the brain (Kaye, Frank, Bailer, & Henry, 2005).

In a study of early-onset anorexia nervosa, Lask et al. (2005) used single-photon emission computed tomography (SPECT) to detect a decrease in cerebral blood flow in the left temporal region, insula, and interconnected limbic structures. This area of the brain is associated with visual-spatial perception, visual memory, and information processing as well as the regulation of appetite, emotions, and mood (Lask et al.). To date, neuroimaging studies in ill and recovered patients have not been able to definitively ascertain if the observed abnormalities are the result of preexisting brain abnormalities that increase the risk for eating disorders, or if these abnormalities are the lingering effects of brain starvation.

Altered dopamine activity in the striatum has been studied in relationship to anorexia nervosa and linked to the brain circuits involved in reward processing (Frank et al., 2005; Wagner et al., 2007). Findings implicating dopamine dysregulation include an increase in dopamine receptor binding in the striatum and a reduction in dopamine metabolites in the cerebral spinal fluid of individuals with anorexia nervosa. The dopamine circuits in the ventral tegmental area (VTA) are associated with experiences of pleasure and reward seeking behaviors. Modulation of pleasure seeking is achieved through top-down control exerted by the prefrontal cortex and mediated through the anterior cingulate cortex (ACC). Abnormalities in dopamine regulation and increased activation of top-down control may contribute to inhibition in pleasure seeking and increased focus on planning, harm avoidance, and vigilance to negative consequences in individuals with anorexia nervosa (Frank et al.; Wagner et al.).

Neuropsychological differences have been detected in individuals with anorexia nervosa, leading to theories about brain differences that affect the processing of visual-spatial information. In response to various figure-ground tests, individuals with anorexia nervosa show a bias toward details and deficits in perceiving global patterns or integrating details within larger visual gestalts. This neurocognitive deficit is referred to as "weak central coherence" and has also been observed in individuals with OCD and autism spectrum disorders. Additionally, individuals with anorexia nervosa display a deficit in "set shifting." Deficits in cognitive set shifting are associated with inflexible thinking, difficulty disengaging from tasks, and problems with transitions (Lopez, Tchanturia, Stahl, & Treasure, 2008; Treasure, 2007).

Biological Triggers

Estrogen plays a role in modulating serotonin activity. Serotonin receptor activity and serotonin gene transcription are influenced by estrogen. It has been speculated that changes in estrogen and gonadal steroids during puberty may destabilize 5-HT activity in genetically vulnerable individuals, thereby triggering the onset of eating disorder symptoms (Kaye, Guido, Bailer, & Henry, 2005; Klump & Gobrogge, 2005).

Streptococcal infections are biological triggers that have been studied in relationship to acute onset anorexia nervosa. The link between the acute onset of neuropsychiatric symptoms and streptococcal infections is referred to as PANDAS (pediatric autoimmune neuropsychiatric disorders associated with streptococcal infections). PANDAS have also been studied in relationship to the acute onset of obsessive-compulsive symptoms and stereotypical movements in prepubertal children. Case reports have linked this biological trigger to an acute onset of prepubertal anorexia nervosa, but the evidence remains inconclusive (Puxley, Midtsund, Iosif, & Lask, 2008).

Psychosocial Triggers

Psychosocial factors do not cause eating disorders but may interact with genetic and biological vulnerability to increase the risk for symptom onset and/or relapse. Certain temperament and personality styles have been associated with an increased risk for eating disorders, including personality traits of perfectionism and cognitive inflexibility. For individuals with these personality traits, change and transitions can be stressful. Certain developmental periods are recognized as times of exceptional change, including the transition from elementary school to middle school, the onset of puberty, entry into high school, and launching into independent living during late adolescence and early adulthood. These developmental transitions coincide with peak periods for onset and relapse of eating disorder symptoms.

Adolescence is second only to infancy in its rapid rate of physical growth and change. Body image concerns are common during adolescence with as many as 36% of girls and 24% of boys reporting that body image is very important to their self-esteem (Ackard et al., 2007). Participation in activities such as dance, gymnastics, and competitive sports accentuates the focus on physical attributes, and may magnify body image concerns for vulnerable adolescents. Dissatisfaction with body image can result in dieting and engaging in strenuous exercise, both of which are potential triggers for individuals who are genetically predisposed to eating disorders. There is evidence that a drop in body weight below normal levels may, in and of itself, trigger a cascade of brain changes that accelerates the development of eating disorder symptoms in vulnerable individuals. Animal research has demonstrated that restricting access to food and increasing access to running wheels in laboratory animals can induce a state of activity-based anorexia. Dieting and physical exercise are known to activate dopaminergic neurons in the mesolimbic pathway and noradrenergic neurons in the locus coeruleus, thereby inducing a focused and energized state that perpetuates the drive to exercise and interferes with food-seeking behaviors (Herzog & Eddy, 2007; Hillebrand, van Elburg, Kas, van England, & Adan, 2005; McCormick et al., 2008; Sodersten, Bergh, & Ammar, 2003).

Family Dynamics

Family characteristics have been cited as factors contributing to the risk for eating disorders. Family environments with low emotional connectedness, high parental expectations, and high parental discord have been described in the eating disorder literature (Gorwood, Kipmann, & Foulon, 2003; Tantillo, 2006). It is important to note that twin studies have found little evidence that shared environmental factors, such as familial factors, contribute to the risk for eating disorders (Bulik et al., 2006). The greatest variance in rates of eating disorders is accounted for by heritability or genetics (estimates range from 50% to 83%). Individual experiences and exposures account for as much as 38% of the variance. Only about 5% of the variance in rates of eating disorders among twins has been attributed to shared environment (Kaye et al., 2008).

The study of family environments in children and adolescents with eating disorders must take into account the amount of stress induced by having a child or adolescent with an eating disorder and the potential impact this disorder can exert on marital, parental, and family systems. The heritability of these disorders increases the likelihood that one or both parents may be affected or partially affected by an eating disorder, an anxiety or mood disorder, or personality traits that fall within the spectrum of shared genetic risk. A no-blame approach recognizes that "parents do not cause eating disorders and children do not choose them" (Kartini Clinic, n.d.-a, para. 3). Families may be affected by the genetic transmission of these disorders, but this is not something parents or children willfully choose to inflict on each other. Anxious parents may be more likely to engage in counterproductive behaviors and struggles with their children, just as anxious children may induce greater vigilance from their parents. Thus, the interactions between genetics, temperament, family dynamics, and eating disorder symptoms may be best understood as complex and multidirectional processes.

Other Risk Factors

Individuals identified at higher risk for developing eating disorders include female college students (Barker & Galambos, 2007), collegiate athletes (Greenleaf, Petrie, Carter, & Reel, 2009), young women with type 1 diabetes mellitus (Walsh, Wheat & Freund, 2000), and participants in activities that promote low body weight such as dance, wrestling, and crew. Sports that are evaluated by subjective scoring such as zure skating and gymnastics are also associated with a higher incidence of eating disorders. Less often identified risk factors include affective illness or alcoholism in first-degree relatives, a family history of eating disorders or obesity, a history of physical or sexual abuse, and restrictive parental eating behaviors, or heightened parental focus on exercise and weight control (Rome et al., 2003). Once again, these factors correlate with a greater risk for eating disorders but current evidence does not support causation.

Clinical Picture

Diagnostic Criteria

The fourth edition of the American Psychiatric Association Diagnostic and Statistical Manual of Mental Disorders (DSM-IV-TR) (American Psychiatric Association [APA], 2000) includes three broad classifications of eating disorder diagnoses: anorexia nervosa (AN) and its subtypes; bulimia nervosa (BN); and eating disorders not otherwise specified (EDNOS). Binge eating disorder (BED) is included in the EDNOS classification. The diagnostic criteria for each of these diagnoses are summarized in Table 12.1. The DSM-IV-TR characterizes anorexia nervosa by four essential criteria: (1) weight loss below 85% expected for age and height, and/or failure to gain weight during a period of growth; (2) intense fears of becoming fat; (3) disturbances in perceptions of body size and shape, which may include an exaggerated focus on body image in self-evaluations and/or denial of the seriousness of low body weight and weight loss; and (4) amenorrhea for three or more consecutive months in postmenarcheal females. In practice, the utility of the amenorrhea criterion is compromised by the ubiquitous use of oral contraceptives that artificially induce menses in postmenarcheal females, and the irrelevance of this criterion for prepubertal females and males.

Anorexia nervosa is further defined by two subtypes; the restricting subtype involves restriction of caloric intake and/or limiting the range of acceptable foods resulting in weight loss or failure to gain weight during periods of growth. In addition to these restricting symptoms, the binge/purge subtype of anorexia nervosa involves self-induced vomiting (purging) and/or the use of laxatives,

Table 12.1 DSM-IV diagnostic criteria for eating disorders

Eating Disorder	DSM-IV Criteria	Subtypes
Anorexia Nervosa (AN)	Refusal to maintain body weight at or above 85% of normal weight for age and height Intense fear of gaining weight or becoming fat, despite being underweight Disturbance in the way in which body weight or shape is experienced; undue influence on body weight or self-evaluation; or denial of the seriousness of current low body weight Amenorrhea in postmenarcheal females (missing at least 3 menstrual cycles or only having a period after administration of a hormone such as estrogen).	Restrictive type Binge-eating and purging type
Bulimia Nervosa (BN)	Recurrent episodes of binge eating in a discrete period of time involving more food than most people would eat during a similar timeframe under similar circumstances Sense of lack of control over eating during the episode Recurrent inappropriate compensatory behavior to prevent weight gain, such as self-induced vomiting, misuse of laxatives, diuretics, enemas or other medications, fasting, or excessive exercise Both binge eating and other compensatory behaviors occur on average at least twice a week for 3 months Self-evaluation is unduly influenced by body shape and weight The disturbance does not occur exclusively during episodes of anorexia nervosa	Purging type: the person regularly engages in self-induced vomiting or the misuse of laxatives or diuretics Nonpurging type: the person uses other inappropriate compensatory behaviors, such as fasting or excessive exercise, but does not regularly engage in self-induced vomiting or the misuse of laxatives or diuretics
Eating Disorder Not Otherwise Specified (EDNOS)	Disorders of eating that do not meet the criteria for any specific eating disorder. Examples include: All the AN criteria are met, except the person has regular menses All the AN criteria are met, except, despite significant weight loss, the person's current weight is in the normal range All the criteria for BN are met, except the binge eating and inappropriate compensatory mechanisms occur at a frequency of less than twice a week for less than 3 months duration Regular use of inappropriate compensatory behavior by a person of normal weight after eating a small amount of food Repeatedly chewing and spitting out, but not swallowing, large amounts of food Binge-eating disorder: recurrent episodes of binge eating in the absence of the regular use of inappropriate compensatory behaviors characteristic of BN	

diuretics, enemas, or other medications to avoid weight gain. It is important to note that both subtypes of anorexia nervosa must fulfill the essential criteria of nutritional restriction and weight loss. Nutritional restriction, weight loss, and/or failure to gain weight during periods of growth are features that distinguish anorexia nervosa, binge/purge type, from a diagnosis of bulimia nervosa (APA, 2000). In differentiating bulimia nervosa from anorexia nervosa, it is important to determine the individual's premorbid weight. A child or adolescent who is of high body weight prior to the onset of eating disorder symptoms can present for evaluation with normal or even above normal body weight; but upon further examination, a history of nutritional restriction and dramatic weight loss may be detected. In these cases, a diagnosis of anorexia nervosa is more appropriate.

Bulimia nervosa is characterized by episodes of binge eating followed by compensatory behaviors to avoid weight gain occurring at least twice a week over a three-month period. Binge episodes are defined as eating more than most people would eat in a two-hour period of time and are typically accompanied by feelings of loss of control. Compensatory behaviors most commonly used to avoid weight gain include purging and overexercising but may also include misuse of laxatives, enemas, diuretics, or emetics such as syrup of ipecac. Similar to anorexia nervosa, bulimia nervosa is characterized by an exaggerated preoccupation with body size and shape. It is distinguished from anorexia nervosa, binge/purge type, by the absence of restricting symptoms and the maintenance of normal or above normal body weight (APA, 2000).

Eating disorder, not otherwise specified (EDNOS), is the diagnostic classification used when full criteria for anorexia nervosa or bulimia nervosa are not met. Binge eating disorder is included in the EDNOS classification and is characterized by recurrent episodes of binge eating without accompanying compensatory behaviors (APA, 2000). Use of DSM-IV-TR criteria results in as many as 60% of prepubertal children with eating disorders being given the diagnosis of EDNOS (Work Group for Classification of Eating Disorders in Children and Adolescents [WCEDCA], 2007).

Developmental Variations in Symptom Presentations

The age of onset for eating disorder symptoms spans multiple developmental stages from school age through young adulthood. With symptoms emerging as young as age seven years, it is not surprising to find developmental differences in symptom presentation. DSM-IV-TR diagnostic criteria for eating disorders do not adequately address these developmental differences, with improvements expected in the proposed DSM-V as a result of workgroup recommendations (WCEDCA, 2007).

Symptoms of eating disorders in children are less common and thus more likely to evade recognition or be misdiagnosed. This is particularly troubling because of the severe impact an eating disorder can have on organ development and bone growth. Prepubertal children do not meet the amenorrhea criterion for a diagnosis of anorexia nervosa and may be less likely to verbalize fears of gaining weight or body dissatisfaction. Children and young adolescents are more likely to endorse fears of growing up or aversion to puberty, increased anxiety, and displays of a greater tendency for relentless motor activity. Determining if the child maintains 85% of expected body weight is also a moving target in the growing child. Children and young adolescents can experience a faster rate of weight loss than older adolescents and, thereby, progress more rapidly into states of medical compromise (Abbate-Daga et al., 2007; Keel et al., 2004; Peebles et al., 2006).

Medical Complications

The medical complications of eating disorders affect every body system and have the greatest impact on health and quality of life when symptoms persist during normative periods of skeletal growth and organ development. Irreversible growth stunting is one of the most emotionally and physically devastating consequences of eating disorders (Fairburn & Harrison, 2003; Katzman, 2005; Rome & Ammerman, 2003). A summary of medical complications can be found in Table 12.2.

Cardiovascular complications are among the most serious medical complications of eating disorders. It is estimated that one-third of deaths associated with eating disorders in adults are due to cardiac failure (Katzman, 2005). Cardiovascular complications can result from cardiac muscle wasting secondary to starvation in anorexia nervosa and cardiac conduction abnormalities related to electrolyte disturbances in purging subtypes. Intractable vomiting can induce metabolic alkalosis and hypokalemia, and misuse of laxatives or water loading can result in hyponatremia and metabolic acidosis (Fairburn & Harrison, 2003). Orthostatic blood pressure changes and bradycardia (daytime heart rate under 50 beats per minute or nighttime heart rate under 46 beats per minute) can be detected during physical examination. Orthostasis and bradycardia are the result of decreased basal metabolic

Table 12.2 Complications of eating disorders

Osteoporosis or osteopenia

Growth delay or stunting

Cardiac impairment

    Congestive heart failure

    Cardiac conduction abnormalities

    Mitral valve prolapse

Cognitive changes

Endocrine changes

    Oligomenorrhea or amenorrhea

Psychological dysfunction

    Depression

    Obsessive compulsive disorder

    Social phobia

    Generalized anxiety

Electrolyte abnormalities

    Hypokalemia or hyponatremia

Infertility

Dental erosion and enlarged salivary glands with purging

Liver complications

Altered gastrointestinal functioning and constipation

---

rate, increased vagal tone, and reduced cardiac contractile force and output (Katzman; Rome & Ammerman, 2003). Abnormal electrocardiogram (ECG) findings can include QTc prolongation, ST depression, and flattening of the T wave. A normal QTc interval may be observed in children and adolescents with eating disorders and is not necessarily an assurance of cardiac health (Katzman). In a state of cardiac compromise, the use of caffeine to suppress appetite and/or overexercising to avoid weight gain can induce fatal cardiac arrhythmias. Mitral valve prolapse (MVP) has been observed in over one-third of adolescents with anorexia nervosa compared to 4% of controls (Katzman). The risk for cardiac events increases during refeeding of seriously malnourished patients and is rationale for hospitalization, gradual titration of calories, and close monitoring of electrolytes and cardiac status. Congestive heart failure can occur due to shifts in fluids and electrolytes (especially phosphate) from extracellular to intracellular spaces during refeeding. Cardiac functioning is generally restored upon return to a healthy body weight but the extent to which optimal cardiac capacity is regained varies by severity of illness and the type and duration of symptoms. The misuse of syrup of ipecac to induce vomiting can cause irreversible myocarditis (Katzman; Rome & Ammerman, 2003).

Complications affecting the gastrointestinal (GI) system include a slowing of GI motility with delayed gastric emptying and constipation. These complications are the basis for common complaints about abdominal discomfort and distention following the reintroduction of food in patients with anorexia nervosa. Reassurance can be given that gastric motility usually returns to normal and constipation resolves within three weeks of resuming a balanced diet and ordered eating. Chronic misuse of laxatives may lead to persistent problems with constipation and altered GI functioning (Fairburn & Harrison, 2003; Rome & Ammerman, 2003).

Complications of the skeletal system and bone health include failure to achieve genetic height potential, osteopenia, and osteoporosis. Catch-up growth may occur if nutritional status is restored prior to the closure of epiphyseal plates. Adolescence is the peak time for bone mineralization and consolidation of bone strength. Anorexia nervosa can result in a reduction of bone mineral density (BMD) and increase the lifetime risk for fractures. In anorexia nervosa, deficiencies in dietary calcium and vitamin D are compounded by low levels of thyroid hormones, estradiol, and testosterone that affect growth factors necessary for bone mineralization and prevention of bone reabsorption. Restoring nutritional health, normalizing reproductive hormones, and prescription of appropriate weight-bearing exercise may reverse the osteopenia and osteoporosis associated with anorexia nervosa. It is important for practitioners to realize that, unlike the situation with menopausal bone loss, exogenous hormones are not useful for bone restoration in this population and should not be used (Bulik, Berkman, Brownley, Sedway, & Lohr, 2007). As many as one-third of women who recover from this disorder continue to have osteopenia of the lumbar spine (Katzman, 2005; Rome & Ammerman, 2003).

The endocrine and reproductive systems are affected by eating disorders. Malnutrition results in low levels of testosterone in males and low levels of leutenizing hormone (LH), follicle-stimulating hormone (FSH), and estradiol in females, which contributes to oligomenorrhea and amenorrhea. Evidence of higher rates of infertility, low birth weight infants, and other childbearing complications have been associated with eating disorders (Fairburn & Harrison, 2003; Favaro, Tenconi, & Santonastaso, 2006).

Compromised brain health and altered cognitive functioning occur in states of malnutrition. Cerebral atrophy with ventricular enlargement and loss of both gray matter and white matter has been observed on brain scans of patients with anorexia nervosa (Rome & Ammerman, 2003). There is some controversy over the extent to which these brain changes can be reversed; the evidence is more optimistic if symptoms are effectively treated in children and adolescents and less optimistic for adults who have a prolonged symptom course (Katzman, 2005).

Evidence of altered cognitive functioning can be detected during the mental status examination and includes cognitive latencies, flat affect, lack of emotional spontaneity, poor memory recall, inattention, and decreased concentration. Diets low in essential amino acids such as tryptophan and tyrosine can result in depletion of brain serotonin and dopamine, the neurotransmitters that regulate mood, anxiety, and attention (Kaye & Walsh, 2002). Depressed mood, irritability, and inattention often increase as eating disorder symptoms become more severe and improve in response to restored nutritional health.

Psychiatric Comorbidities

Lifetime rates of comorbid psychiatric disorders are as high as 80% in individuals with eating disorders (Anderluh, Tchanturia, Rabe-Hesketh, & Treasure, 2003; Kaye, Bulik, Thornton, Barbarich, & Masters, 2004; Keel, Klump, Miller, McGue, & Iacono, 2005; Klump et al., 2009; Wade, Bulik, Neale, & Kendler, 2000). The most common comorbid psychiatric disorders include depression, OCD, social phobia, and generalized anxiety disorder (Klump et al.).

The median age of onset for anxiety disorders is age eleven years, and the onset of an anxiety disorder often precedes the onset of eating disorder symptoms (Kaye et al.; Kessler et al., 2005). Perfectionism and Cluster C personality traits are more common in individuals with eating disorders (Anderluh et al.). The co-occurrence of anxiety and depression may be both an indication of shared genetic risk and the consequence of compromised brain nutrition that interferes with neurotransmitter synthesis. Both depression and eating disorders are associated with a greater risk for suicide (Rome et al., 2003).

Continuum of Care and Treatment

The continuum of care for eating disorder patients ranges from the least intensive care at a community outpatient level to the most intensive care in hospitals and residential treatment facilities. Outpatient treatment is often provided by physicians and APNs collaborating with therapists, nutritionists, and medical specialists. Intermediate levels of care include day treatment and partial hospitalization programs. Consultation with eating disorder specialists can assist primary care practitioners (PCPs) in making decisions about the appropriate level of care for a patient. It is important for APNs to know the criteria for various levels of care and develop a network of referral sources so that specialized evaluations and treatment can be readily initiated. Yager et al. (2006) provide practice guidelines for the treatment of patients with eating disorders. A table of the APA's Level of Care Guidelines for Eating Disorders (2010) is available online at http://www.psychiatryonline.com.

Life-threatening medical complications or suicidal thoughts and behaviors necessitate hospitalization. Common medical complications requiring hospitalization include electrolyte disturbances, weight below 85% of expected body weight, end-organ compromise, orthostatic hypotension, bradycardia, hypothermia, intractable vomiting, and/or risk of refeeding complications (Golden et al., 1997). Acute food refusal can be rationale for hospitalization, especially in children and young adolescents who are at greater risk for irreversible effects on growth (Yager et al., 2006).

Medically compromised patients who meet hospitalization criteria (American Academy of Pediatrics, 2003) are best managed by an eating disorder specialist with experience in safely initiating and monitoring the refeeding process. For severely malnourished patients who are less than 70% of ideal body weight, aggressive refeeding can cause a serious condition called *refeeding syndrome*. The goal of hospitalization is to monitor and stabilize cardiac functioning and electrolyte status while initiating refeeding. Electrolytes are monitored daily, including serum phosphorus, potassium, calcium, and magnesium. Supplements of phosphorus, magnesium, and/or potassium may be prescribed as indicated. Nasogastric feedings may be necessary to reestablish and titrate nutritional intake for patients who are unable to take sufficient nutrition by mouth. Weight gain goals during hospitalization are from 2 to 3 pounds per week. Continuous cardiac monitoring is recommended. Depending on the length and severity of illness, prolonged hospitalization may be necessary to restore cardiovascular functioning and reverse symptoms of bradycardia (especially overnight bradycardia) and orthostasis by pulse and/or blood pressure.

Outpatient goals for medical and psychiatric management of patients who do not require hospitalization (and those who return to outpatient care following hospital discharge) include continuation of weight restoration at a rate of 0.5 to 1 pound per week until a healthy weight is achieved. Other goals include normalization of eating behaviors, resumption of menses in adolescent females, and an appropriate exercise and activity plan consistent with restoration of bone health. Calcium supplements of 1200 to 1500 mg/day in three divided doses, vitamin D 400 to 1000 IU/day, and zinc 30 mg/day are recommended. Menses typically resume within six months of achieving 90% of ideal body weight. For sexually active adolescents and young adults, the risk of pregnancy may be rationale for continuing oral contraceptives, even though an important biological marker of health is disguised.

The Primary Care Practitioner Role in the Diagnosis and Management of Eating Disorders

Primary care practitioners (PCPs) and PMH-APNs have important roles in the assessment, diagnosis, and management of children and adolescents with eating disorders. Stereotypical attitudes such as the belief that only white, affluent females get eating disorders can be barriers to timely recognition of these disorders in primary care and in psychiatry. Practitioners must be aware that eating disorders affect individuals of diverse racial, ethnic, and socioeconomic backgrounds, including males and females of all body sizes and shapes.

Goals in primary care include prevention, health education for patients with identified risk factors, early symptom identification, and prompt referral to, or consultation with, eating disorder specialists for diagnostic clarification and management of the intensive phase of treatment. Identifying early signs of food and weight anxiety provides a window of opportunity to intervene before symptoms of a full-blown eating disorder develop (Rome et al., 2003; Williams et al., 2008). In order to intervene in the early stages of eating disorders, PCPs must be knowledgeable about and alert for signs and symptoms, and overcome barriers to identification. Common barriers in primary care include the infrequency of well-child visits, the busy pace of primary care practices, insufficient appointment time for in-depth exploration, and reluctance on the part of PCPs to discuss warning signs with patients and parents due to fear of inciting defensiveness (DeSocio, O'Toole, Nemirow, Lukach, & Magee, 2007).

Screening and Assessment

Most patients with eating disorders do not present to their health care providers with the complaint "I have an eating disorder." When patients with eating disorders seek health care, they typically do not voluntarily disclose their altered patterns of eating and weight control activities. The withholding of symptoms may be due to stigma, shame, or fear that discovery will interfere with their weight loss goals. Symptoms are often inadvertently discovered during routine health maintenance appointments or physical examinations for school and sports participation.

Acquiring a comprehensive health history is the most powerful tool for assessment and diagnosis of eating disorders (Pritts & Susman, 2003). Experienced APNs integrate eating disorder screening questions into interviews with all patients. The interview should include a discussion of the patient's satisfaction and perceptions of his/her body size and shape. Body weight questions focus on recent changes in weight, current weight, lowest weight, highest weight, and desired weight. Individuals with eating disorders often report unrealistically low body weight goals; others report a goal weight below a given threshold (Fairburn & Cooper, 1993).

Obtain a nutrition history and ask about eating alone and in secret, or if the patient has ever engaged in binge eating. Inquire about weight control activities including the type, frequency, and duration of exercise, restrictive patterns of eating, and any eating "rules" the patient may have. Inquire about purging behaviors, including vomiting and use of laxatives, diuretics, or diet pills. Obtain a menstrual history in female patients. Remember that primary amenorrhea may be extended beyond expected norms in nutritionally compromised adolescents, and menses may be artificially induced in females taking oral contraceptives.

While it is rare for patients to self-identify the need for treatment of their eating disorders, they may seek medical advice about symptoms associated with these disorders. Symptoms brought to the health care professional's attention may include amenorrhea, dizziness or fainting, fatigue, palpitations, hair loss or changes in hair, cold intolerance, heartburn, constipation, bloating, abdominal pain, regurgitation or rumination, and/or difficulty with sleep (Stein & Reichert, 1990).

Asking about a history of suicidal ideation and self-injurious behaviors is an essential part of the interview. Children and adolescents with eating disorders often experience feelings of self-loathing and may participate in self-injurious behaviors such as hitting or scratching themselves, punishing themselves with strenuous exercise, or using sharp objects to carve angry words on their thighs, abdomens, or body parts they consider unappealing.

The Physical Examination

The physical examination begins with a general survey of the patient's appearance. Children and adolescents with anorexia nervosa may appear lethargic and complain of feeling cold. The assessment of children and adolescents should always include identification of Tanner's stages of breast and genital development. In advanced states of malnutrition, the patient may appear cachectic with reversal or atrophy of secondary sexual development. Adolescents with bulimia may have normal body weight but display signs that raise suspicions of purging. Physical signs of purging may include enlarged parotid glands, perioral dermatitis, dental erosion, or calluses at the base of fingers (Russell sign). Essential components of the physical exam include evaluation of vital signs, which can reveal compromised cardiovascular and peripheral vascular functioning with bradycardia and orthostatic changes in blood pressure and/or pulse. Physical examination of the hair, thyroid, mouth, muscle mass, extremities, abdomen, and the neurological system may reveal signs of malnutrition. During the physical exam, scan the patient's skin for signs of self-injurious behaviors (Yager et al., 2006). Common physical exam findings are identified in Table 12.3, and differential diagnoses are included in Table 12.4.

Calculating and Plotting Height, Weight, and Body Mass Index (BMI)

Growth charts that plot height and weight over time are important tools in pediatric primary care. Routinely plotting height and weight promotes early recognition of changes in percentile patterns compared to premorbid and age-based norms. Children and adolescents with

Table 12.3 Physical exam findings of concern in patients with disordered eating

- *General appearance:* very thin, emaciated or cachectic, protuberant bony prominences (AN), overweight (BN), flat affect, sunken cheeks, grey/yellow coloring
- *Vital signs:* hypothermia, bradycardia, hypotension, orthostatic BP and/or pulse
- *Skin/hair:* dry skin, lanugo, bruising. Thinning hair, loss of hair or dry hair with loss of shine, calluses at base of fingers (Russell sign), brittle nails, acrocyanosis
- *HEENT:* dry lips, inflamed gums, loss of tooth enamel, parotitis, and sunken eyes
- *Breasts:* atrophy in postmenarche women
- *Cardiac:* bradycardia, arrhythmias, hypotension, murmurs, mitral valve prolapse
- *Extremities:* cool on palpation, peripheral edema, acrocyanosis, and Raynaud's phenomena
- *Abdomen:* scaphoid contour, epigastric tenderness (if purging by vomiting), palpable stool in bowel, abdominal masses
- *Neurological:* decreased DTRs
- *Genitourinary:* delayed puberty, inability to concentrate urine

Table 12.4 Differential diagnosis for eating disorders

- Thyroid disease
- Inflammatory bowel disease, celiac disease, or other GI diseases
- Abdominal masses causing chronic vomiting
- Cancer
- Diabetes, new onset
- Adrenal insufficiency
- Psychiatric disease: primary depression, OCD, substance abuse, psychotic conditions
- CNS disease that can cause vomiting, appetite suppression, and a depressed affect
- Chronic infections

Table 12.5 Laboratory assessment of a patient with eating disorders

- *Chemistry:* Electrolytes (K^+, Na^+, Cl^-), glucose, calcium, magnesium, phosphorus, blood urea nitrogen, creatinine (BUN and Cr important in dehydration and suspected purging), liver function
- *CBC with ESR:* Hct and Hgb
- *CK:* elevated with muscle breakdown due to overexercising or severe nutrition restriction
- *Lipid Profile:* elevated LDH (BN/binge eating), inadequate HDL
- *Thyroid function, serum prolactin, and FSH: to* evaluate amenorrhea and rule out prolactinoma, hyper- or hypothyroidism, or ovarian failure
- *Urinalysis:* to assess specific gravity for water loading to falsely elevate weight
- *Stool and urine for emetide* (byproduct of ipecac): if Ipecac use is suggested
- *Drug screen:* if indicated for a patient with possible drug use
- *Pregnancy test:* in amenorrheic females

should be adjusted for age, as parameters for healthy BMI are different for children than for adolescents and adults. Age adjusted BMI calculators are available on the Centers for Disease Control and Prevention (CDC) website and the National Library of Medicine website (http://www.nhlbisupport.com/bmi/bminojs.htm). For adults and adolescents, BMI scores below 18.5 are considered underweight; a range of 18.5 to 24.5 is considered normal body weight; above 25 is overweight; and above 30 is obese. However, it is important to realize that even a high BMI does not rule out the diagnosis of an eating disorder, including anorexia nervosa. It is the change in BMI that is critical. The high–body weight child is especially endangered by the prevailing belief that weight loss in an overweight child is always a good thing.

Laboratory Tests and Procedures

Laboratory assessment must be comprehensive when an eating disorder is suspected (Table 12.5). Common findings in the chemistry panel of the patient with bulimia nervosa include hypokalemia secondary to vomiting, decreased magnesium, and decreased chloride (Moreno & Judd, 2008). Patients with anorexia nervosa may have hypoglycemia secondary to lack of glucose precursors in the diet or low glycogen stores. Hyponatremia reflects excess water intake or poor secretion of antidiuretic hormone (ADH). An elevated blood urea nitrogen (BUN) may be due to dehydration. Hypokalemic or hypochloremic metabolic alkalosis occurs with vomiting, and acidosis may be due to laxative abuse. Minimally elevated

anorexia nervosa may fail to gain appropriate amounts of weight during periods of growth. This pattern can be visualized on the child's growth chart when the trajectory for height is not matched by a corresponding trajectory of weight gain. A weight curve that either plateaus or dips during a period of growth requires prompt evaluation.

Calculation of body mass index (BMI) is a measurement that compares height to weight and gives an objective indication of overweight, underweight, or a healthy weight for height. The formula for calculating BMI involves multiplying weight in pounds × 703 and dividing by height in inches squared. BMI calculations liver function tests are associated with a malnourished state but are not as high as seen in active hepatitis. A dramatic elevation in cholesterol is consistent with states of starvation. Other abnormal laboratory findings may include low alkaline phosphatase; extremely low sedimentation rates; low levels of FSH, LH, and estradiol and low free T_3, free T_4, and TSH. The patient may also exhibit leukopenia and thrombocytopenia (Bernstein, 2008).

An electrocardiogram should be considered to evaluate bradycardia, QTc prolongation, and cardiac conduction problems associated with electrolyte abnormalities. In addition to suicide, cardiovascular complications account for most of the morbidity and mortality associated with anorexia nervosa. A DEXA (dual energy x-ray absorptiometry) scan is indicated for males and females with six or more months of low body weight and secondary amenorrhea or prolonged primary amenorrhea in females. DEXA results must be interpreted with reference to age and sex matched populations using Z scores (not T scores). Low bone density and the associated risk for fractures can be a powerful incentive for some patients and parents to engage and commit to treatment. Conversely, normal bone density results can provide false reassurance that the problem is not medically significant.

Standardized Instruments and Assessment Tools

Information obtained through use of standardized tools can assist the practitioner in systematically evaluating symptoms and individualizing treatment plans. Examples include the Eating Disorder Examination Questionnaire (EDE-Q), the Rating of Eating Disorder Severity for Children (REDS-C), the Interview for Diagnosis of Eating Disorders, and the Yale-Brown-Cornell Eating Disorder Scale.

The EDE-Q is a self-report adaptation of a structured interview developed by Fairburn and Cooper (1993). The EDE-Q is regarded as one of the most accurate methods of assessing binge eating and is useful for tracking changes over time. Mond et al. (2008) compared the validity of the EDE-Q and the SCOFF for use in primary care (Table 12.6, SCOFF). Their results found both measures performed well in detecting cases and excluding non-cases of the most common eating disorders. Advantages of the SCOFF are its brevity and ease of use in primary care settings. It has 100% sensitivity but lower specificity with a 12.5% false-positive rate; thus, the SCOFF is best used as a screening tool rather than for diagnostic purposes (Morgan, Reid, & Lacey, 1999).

The Questionnaire for Eating Disorder Diagnoses (QEDD) is a fifty-item diagnostic instrument based on

Table 12.6 SCOFF

Do you make yourself **S**ick because you feel uncomfortably full?

Do you worry you have lost **C**ontrol over how much you eat?

Have you recently lost more than **O**ne Stone (14 pounds or 6.35 kg) in a 3-month period?

Do you believe yourself to be **F**at when others say you are too thin?

Would you say that **F**ood dominates your life?

Scoring: One point for every yes; a score of >2 indicates a likely case of AN or BN

Adapted from Morgan, Reid, and Lacey, 1999, with permission from BMJ Publishing Group Ltd.

DSM-I criteria (Mintz, O'Halloran, & Mulholland,1997). Greenleaf et al. (2009) modified this instrument for use with athletes. An instrument used to assess bulimia nervosa based on DSM-IV criteria is the thirty-six–item Bulimia Test-Revised, BULIT-R (Thelen, Mintz, & Vander Wal, 1996). The REDS-C (Rating of Eating Disorder Severity in Children) is a semistructured, clinician-administered interview to assess the severity of eating disorder symptoms in children and adolescents, aged eight to eighteen years. This diagnostic interview allows practitioners to rate child and parent responses on fourteen symptom domains and assign confidence scores to these symptom ratings. Psychometric properties of the REDS-C are in press (O'Toole, Desocio, Munoz, & Crosby, in press). Self-assessment instruments can be obtained online through Mental Health Screening, Inc. at http://www.mentalhealthscreening.org/screening/Default.aspx?&n=1. Self-assessments may be beneficial in raising self-awareness and encouraging individuals to seek care. They are appropriate for older adolescents and adults but are generally less useful for children and young adolescents.

Follow-up Care

After the intensive phase of medical stabilization and treatment, patients with eating disorders are often referred back to their PCP for follow-up care and health maintenance. The goal of the maintenance phase of treatment is to sustain symptom remission for as long as possible in order to support healthy growth and development. The PCP establishes a relationship with the patient and his/her parents to sustain their efforts toward eating disorder recovery.

Decisions about the appropriate level of care for a patient are typically ongoing and related to the patient's symptom course, which may be marked by periods of remission and exacerbation. Parents and practitioners must remain vigilant to signs of relapse. During periods of stress and transition, more frequent appointments may be warranted to monitor the patient's status. Follow-up appointments should include evaluation of vital signs with attention to changes in cardiovascular parameters that may signal relapse. The practitioner should routinely inquire about eating patterns and remain alert to reports of skipped meals or calories shaved from the meal plan as early indications of slipping back into patterns of restricting or binge eating. Weight and weight management activities should be monitored at each appointment. Urine pH may be periodically checked for alkalinity, a common sign of purging. Assessment of mood and risk for self-harm is essential and should be ongoing. It is important to realize that the patient's mood may decline during early phases of eating disorder treatment. Physical symptoms are extinguished before psychological remission occurs; it is common for patients to remain ambivalent or even resistant to treatment until psychological remission is achieved (National Collaborating Centre for Mental Health, 2004).

The Role of the PMH-APN in the Diagnosis and Management of Eating Disorders

The PMH-APN may be the first to identify an eating disorder in patients who present for evaluation of mood or anxiety symptoms. Thus, the role of the PMH-APN includes aspects of the primary care role in health education, screening, and early identification. Additionally, the PMH-APN has a role in differential psychiatric diagnosis and management of comorbid psychiatric symptoms and disorders. Both the PCP and the PMH-APN refer patients to specialized eating disorder teams for comprehensive eating disorder evaluations and the intensive phase of treatment and medical stabilization. Following the intensive phase of treatment, patients with comorbid psychiatric disorders may be referred back to the PMH-APN for ongoing management of their psychiatric needs.

Differential Psychiatric Diagnosis

In conducting a psychiatric evaluation, the PMH-APN considers other psychiatric disorders that present with changes in appetite, weight loss, and abnormal patterns of eating. In young children, a trajectory of poor growth and slow weight gain may be diagnosed as failure to thrive. Selective patterns of eating, refusal of foods because of textures or sensory sensitivities, and a narrow range of food preferences are common features in children with pervasive developmental disorders and autism spectrum disorders. Obsessive anxiety and compulsive rituals associated with order and cleanliness can make food preparation and eating a tortuous experience that contributes to weight loss in children with OCD. Food phobias and extreme fears of swallowing or choking can lead to rapid weight loss, especially in young children. Major depression may be accompanied by changes in appetite and weight, including weight loss or failure to gain weight during periods of growth. Psychomotor agitation and increased goal-directed activity occur during manic episodes and can result in weight loss due to forgetting to eat, having no time to prepare food, or taking in fewer calories than energy expended. Use of psychoactive drugs can induce appetite suppression and weight loss and is especially problematic in individuals who abuse methamphetamine or cocaine. Abnormal or bizarre eating patterns may be secondary to psychotic delusions about food, contamination, or body functions in patients with schizophrenia. In each of these conditions, an eating disorder diagnosis may be ruled out by the absence of essential features, which include fear of weight gain, an obsessive focus on calories and avoidance of foods associated with weight gain, a compulsive drive to exercise, and/or an exaggerated focus on body size and shape (Rome et al., 2003). Another important distinction is that patients with eating disorders do not experience a loss of appetite as such and are likely to be focused to the point of obsession on food, cooking elaborate meals for others, baking, reading cookbooks, or watching the Food Channel.

Differentiating a diagnosis of body dysmorphic disorder (BDD) from an eating disorder diagnosis is challenging because of the overlapping focus on body appearance. BDD usually involves a more focused preoccupation with a perceived defect in a specific body part; this focal preoccupation is a distinguishing feature that differs from the obsession with overall body weight and shape, and the weight loss goals that characterize eating disorders. A diagnosis of BDD should only be given if the patient's symptoms are not better accounted for as an eating disorder (APA, 2000).

Weight loss may also be secondary to pharmacological interventions for other disorders, such as stimulants for ADHD (attention deficit hyperactivity disorder) and topiramate for impulse control or seizure disorders. When children and adolescents present with symptoms of poor appetite and weight loss, a variety of conditions and causes should be explored, including the potential side effects of prescribed and over-the-counter medications.

The process of differential diagnosis may be complicated by the patient's reluctance or inability to report eating disorder cognitions. Young children may not be able to articulate the basis for their anxieties about food, fat, or body size. Older children and adolescents may minimize or conceal their obsessive worries and fears about food and body image because of shame, stigma, or resistance to adult interference. Extreme malnutrition and cognitive compromise can also impair the individual's insight and judgment, and make it difficult to elicit the presence or absence of eating disorder cognitions. Seeking and confirming information from parents and other sources, obtaining a nutritional history, examining trajectories of growth, and evaluating physical parameters are necessary to corroborate the presence or absence of an eating disorder (Becker, Eddy, & Perloe, 2009).

Acquiring a developmental timeline of symptom onset is crucial to rule in or rule out comorbid psychiatric disorders. Malnutrition and the resulting depletion of brain neurotransmitters may contribute to and exaggerate a host of psychiatric symptoms including depressed mood, anxiety, inattention, and hyperactivity. When these symptoms emerge subsequent to the onset of eating disorder symptoms, the effects of malnutrition on brain functioning should be suspected as the source. In such cases, psychiatric symptoms may be better accounted for as secondary to the medical condition of malnutrition.

A developmental timeline that elicits symptoms of OCD, social phobia, generalized anxiety, inattention, hyperactivity, and/or depression prior to the onset of eating disorder symptoms provides stronger support for the existence of a comorbid disorder. Failure to recognize and treat comorbid psychiatric disorders can complicate treatment of an eating disorder. Likewise, an undetected eating disorder can lead to inappropriate treatment that further compromises the patient's health. For example, without a thorough examination of eating patterns and growth, a child with an undetected eating disorder might be inappropriately diagnosed with an attention deficit disorder and started on a psychostimulant, which can suppress appetite and further compromise his/her nutritional state. Undetected eating disorders and malnutrition can interfere with the effectiveness of selective serotonin reuptake inhibitors (SSRIs) used to treat anxiety and depression. Inadequate nutrition, depletion of the brain's monoamine neurotransmitters, and low levels of estradiol should always be ruled out as potential factors contributing to treatment resistance when patients do not respond as expected to psychotropic medications.

Follow-up and Maintenance for Patients with Psychiatric Symptoms and Comorbidities

The maintenance phase of treatment for patients with eating disorders and comorbid psychiatric disorders is often co-managed by a primary care and a psychiatric provider. The stability of a patient's eating disorder symptoms is closely linked to the effective management of his/her psychiatric symptoms, requiring ongoing communication and collaboration between providers. For example, the side effects of medications such as the SSRIs may induce changes in appetite and GI symptoms that impact patient weight and meal plan compliance. Consultation between providers enables planning for more frequent medical monitoring while psychotropic medications are being initiated and adjusted. Additionally, patients managed in primary care may develop symptoms of anxiety and/or depression during the course of treatment for their eating disorders. These symptoms may represent a transitional response to coping with weight restoration and the limitations imposed by their illness. Alternatively, these symptoms may represent the emergence of a comorbid psychiatric disorder that was not previously recognized. The PCP may benefit from consultation with the PMH-APN to determine if a psychiatric evaluation is warranted for diagnostic clarification.

Engagement in self-injurious behaviors and episodes of increased suicidality are serious mental health concerns that may accompany the symptomatic course of eating disorders. PCPs who are managing patients during these periods of crisis benefit from consultation with psychiatric colleagues in evaluating patient safety and determining the need for hospitalization.

Evidence-Based Treatment for Eating Disorders

The current research evidence for efficacious interventions to treat children and adolescents with eating disorders is limited and many research findings remain inconclusive (Brownley, Berkman, Sedway, Lohr, & Bulik, 2007; Bulik et al., 2007; Mitchell, Agras, & Wonderlich, 2007; Shapiro et al., 2007). Best-practice models for treatment of children and adolescents with eating disorders are thereby guided, to a great extent, by expert consensus and exemplary programs that have achieved positive patient and family outcomes. Characteristics of programs with positive outcomes include a family-based approach and emphasis on interdisciplinary collaboration.

Family-Based Treatment

Expert consensus and research evidence support the effectiveness of family-based treatment for children and adolescents with eating disorders (Bulik et al., 2007; Keel & Haedt, 2008). The Maudsley method, which originated at the Maudsley Hospital in London, is often cited as an exemplary model of family-based treatment. Many eating disorder programs incorporate the Maudsley principles, which focus on empowering parents with a blame-free approach and helping families learn how to respond to the child or adolescent with an eating disorder.

There are other models of family-based treatment, but these models share the philosophy that parental involvement is essential and weight rehabilitation is not optional (Kartini Clinic, n.d.-b). Parents assume responsibility for implementing their child's nutrition plan, preparing meals, supervising during and after meals, monitoring their child's activities and exercise, administering medications, and meeting regularly with the treatment team. Unity of purpose between parents and the treatment team creates an environment that supports the child in relinquishing eating disorder symptoms, developing healthier attitudes and beliefs about themselves and their bodies, and learning new coping skills. As partners in all aspects of eating disorder treatment for children and adolescents, parents and families benefit from psychoeducation and therapeutic support for their essential roles. Multifamily therapy groups have been shown to strengthen interfamilial relationships and improve patient and family outcomes (Tantillo, 2006).

Psychosocial Interventions and Psychotherapy

Psychological interventions are aimed toward interrupting the patient's faulty cognitions, developing stress management and distress tolerance skills, and developing new patterns in relationships. Expert consensus and research findings support the use of individual or group cognitive-behavioral therapy (CBT) as the treatment of choice for adolescents and young adults with bulimia nervosa (Mitchell et al., 2007). Interpersonal therapy (IPT) and dialectical behavior therapy (DBT) have demonstrated promising results for adolescents and young adults with bulimia nervosa and binge eating disorder (Brownley et al., 2007; Mufson, Pollack Dorta, Moreau, & Weissman, 2004; Safer, Telch, Chen, & Linrehan, 2009; Shapiro et al., 2007). Fairburn (2008) designed a model of CBT that specifically targets faulty cognitions underlying eating disorder symptoms (CBT-E). These cognitions include an exaggerated importance placed on control of eating, shape, and weight; perfectionistic attitudes; and overreactivity to moods and interpersonal difficulties.

Psychopharmacology

Fluoxetine (Prozac) is the only medication to receive Food and Drug Administration approval for the treatment of bulimia nervosa. The best research evidence to date recommends the combined use of fluoxetine and CBT for remission of bulimia nervosa (Kaye & Walsh, 2002; Shapiro et al., 2007).

For patients with anorexia nervosa, nutrition is the best medicine and weight restoration is the foundation of treatment. Weight restoration alone may improve mood, reduce anxiety, and ameliorate the intensity of obsessions and compulsions. Research has shown promising results from the use of atypical antipsychotics, such as olanzapine, to reduce delusional thought processes, stabilize moods, and lessen anxiety associated with refeeding. Initiation of an SSRI following weight restoration to 90% of expected body weight has also been shown to extend periods of remission and reduce rates of relapse in anorexia nervosa (Couturier & Lock, 2007; Flament, Furino, & Godart, 2005; Kaye & Walsh, 2002). There is limited research evidence to guide the psychopharmacological management of eating disorders in children and adolescents. Psychotropic medications should thus be prescribed cautiously and in consultation with clinicians who specialize in treatment of children with these disorders.

Exemplary Models of Interdisciplinary Collaboration

Eating disorders affect all aspects of biological, psychological, and social functioning. Effective models of treatment thus exemplify the benefits of collaborative practice between primary care, psychiatry, eating disorder specialists, and a multidisciplinary team. Interdisciplinary roles within the eating disorder team include medical care provided by a physician or APN; psychiatric evaluations and psychotropic medications provided by a psychiatrist or PMH-APN; nutritional counseling by a nutritionist; psychotherapy provided by the psychiatric provider, a psychologist, or a clinical social worker; family education and therapy provided by a family therapist; physical therapy assessments and activity recommendations by a physical therapist; and dental care by a dentist. The APN or physician often serves as the team leader and consults with other specialists, such as cardiologists and endocrinologists, to evaluate and manage medical complications. Communication among team members is essential to establish common goals, develop and modify the treatment plan, monitor progress, and coordinate roles and responsibilities of team members (Yager et al., 2006). Clinicians at Stanford's Lucile Salter Packard Children's Hospital developed the first clinical pathway for the treatment of anorexia nervosa in adolescents. This clinical pathway can be used as a guide for the structure of the treatment plan.

Table 12.7 Resources on eating disorders

Books for Patients and Families	Bulik, C. M., & Taylor, N. (2005). *Runaway eating: The 8 point plan to conquer adult food and weight obsessions.* New York, NY: Rodale Books.
	Bryant-Waugh, R., & Lask, B. (2004). *Eating disorders: A parents' guide* (Rev. ed.). New York, NY: Brunner-Rutledge.
	Collins, L. (2005). *Eating with your anorexic: How my child recovered through family-based treatment and yours can too.* New York, NY: McGraw Hill.
	Fairburn, C. (1995). *Overcoming binge eating.* New York, NY: Guilford.
	Lock, J., & LeGrange, D. (2005). *Help your teenager beat an eating disorder.* New York, NY: Guilford.
	O'Toole, J.. (2010). *Give food a chance.* Portland, OR: PSIpress.
	Treasure, J. (2000). *Anorexia nervosa: A survival guide for families, friends, and sufferers.* Hove, UK: Psychology Press.
Nationally Recognized Facilities	Cambridge Eating Disorder Center, http://www.eatingdisordercenter.org
	University of Chicago http:// www.uchicagokidshospital.org/specialties/psychiatry/eating-disorders
	Cleveland Clinic, http://my.clevelandclinic.org/psychiatry/services/eating_disorders
	Columbia University Medical Center, http://www.columbiacenterforeatingdisorders.org
	Kartini Clinic, http://www.kartiniclinic.com
	Laureate Eating Disorders Program, http://eatingdisorders.laureate.com
	Lucile Packard Children's Hospital at Stanford, http://www.lpch.org/clinicalSpecialtiesServices/index.html
	Renfrew, http://www.renfrewcenter.com/index.asp
	Rogers Memorial Hospital, http://rogershospital.org
	Sheppard Pratt, http://www.eatingdisorder.org/
Self-Help Groups	Anorexics and Bulimics Anonymous, http://www.anorexicsandbulimicsanonymousaba.com/
	FEAST (Families Empowered And Supporting Treatment of Eating Disorders), http://www.feast-ed.org
	SEED: Students Ending Eating Disorders/Students Educating Eating Disorders or SAED: Students Against Eating Disorders (college campus groups)
	Overeaters Anonymous, http://www.oa.org/
Health Care Professional Resources	Academy for Eating Disorders (www.aedweb.org).
	Eating Disorder Referral and Information Center, www.edreferral.com
Patient, Family, and Professional Internet Resources	National Eating Disorder Association (NEDA), www.nationaleatingdisorders.org
	International Association of Eating Disorders (IAED) www.iaedp.com
	http://www.something-fishy.org/

Exemplary models of treatment offer a spectrum of services that support the patient and family through various phases of treatment. These services include eating disorder evaluations, inpatient hospitalization, day treatment or partial hospitalization, and outpatient treatment. Some programs also provide residential treatment for longer term and more intensive care. Table 12.7 includes a list of nationally recognized treatment facilities for children, adolescents, and young adults with eating disorders.

Case Exemplar

Sixteen-year-old Katie is 65 inches tall and weighed 95 pounds with a BMI of 15.8 indicating severe underweight with a BMI at the first percentile for her age. Her supine blood pressure was 90 systolic and 64 diastolic with a pulse of 38. Her standing blood pressure was 86 systolic and 68 diastolic with a pulse of 50. Her temperature was 97.6°F. She appeared cachectic and her breast development was Tanner stage 4 but atrophied. Her genital development was Tanner stage 4. She achieved menarche at age thirteen but had not had a period for eight months. Her DEXA scan showed osteopenia of the lumbar spine. Katie is a vegetarian and drinks four 32-ounce bottles of water a day. Her current weight goal is 90 pounds, but she admits that she has readjusted previous weight goals to a lower weight as soon as she achieved them. Katie participates in track and runs 5 to 7 miles a day. She stated, "The best runners are always the skinny ones." Her older sister was an accomplished athlete and Katie described herself as "much fatter than my sister" even though her sister was 1 inch taller than Katie and weighed 125 pounds. Katie's track coach encouraged her parents to seek a medical evaluation when he noticed a decline in Katie's performance. Katie has difficulty falling asleep at night, often wakes up to go to the bathroom, and has difficulty falling back to sleep. She displayed cognitive latencies and a flat affect. Katie acknowledged feeling depressed and worrying more than others her age, but in general she maintained that she did not have any problems and wished everyone would stop talking to her about her weight. Her mother reported a family history of depression and a maternal grandfather who was very tidy and orderly. A maternal aunt was diagnosed with panic attacks, and a paternal aunt had bulimia as an adolescent. Katie was hospitalized following a syncopal episode and her care was transferred to an adolescent eating disorder team. She was placed on bedrest with cardiac monitoring and a prescribed refeeding schedule. Katie was angry about being hospitalized and pleaded for discharge, accusing the team and her parents of colluding to make her fat. She secretly checked her body for any sign of weight gain by pinching and measuring folds of skin. She met with the PMH-APN on the eating disorder team, who described her diagnostic impressions as depressed mood, sleep disturbance, and cognitive latencies secondary to a primary axis I diagnosis of anorexia nervosa, restricting type. Katie also gave a history of generalized anxiety symptoms since age nine years and the PMH-APN made note to evaluate these symptoms and to consider an SSRI as Katie progressed toward weight restoration. Following hospital discharge, Katie and her parents began a family-based treatment program where Katie and her parents worked closely with an interdisciplinary team to build knowledge and coping skills to support Katie's return to health. Katie's parents took an active role in supervising Katie's meal plan and exercise until she was able to resume greater independence in maintaining healthy patterns of eating and activity. Katie benefited from group therapy with other adolescents who were experiencing similar struggles with eating disorder

cognitions and behaviors. As she progressed in treatment, her brain neurotransmitter levels were replenished and contributed to improved sleep and affect, but Katie continued to feel anxious and overexercised in an effort to control anxiety. When Katie achieved 90% of her expected weight for health, she resumed regular appointments with the PMH-APN to reevaluate symptoms of an underlying anxiety disorder. Katie and her parents agreed to a trial of an SSRI to target a reduction in anxiety and to support Katie's ability to achieve and sustain remission of eating disorder symptoms. Katie is on the path to recovery, but it will be a long road that requires ongoing monitoring and a coordinated plan for maintenance and relapse prevention that includes Katie, her parents, her eating disorder treatment team, and her primary care provider.

Implications for Prevention, Advocacy, Research, and Education

Prevention of eating disorders is a community-wide effort. APNs can be involved in education and advocacy at local, state, and national levels to promote awareness of eating disorders and the disabilities these disorders cause when they remain unrecognized and untreated. Advocacy efforts are also needed to support legislation and regulations that improve mental health benefits and provide nutritional and medical support for children and their families. Outreach to parents, teachers, coaches, club leaders, and organizers of community recreation programs is necessary to raise awareness of the signs of eating disorders and the importance of healthy nutrition and balanced physical activity. Changing our culture and overcoming the stigma and myths about eating disorders are ongoing challenges and a goal for all health professionals. Current research related to treatment of children and adolescents with eating disorders is limited. APNs are needed as research investigators and collaborators. Nursing brings a unique and valuable perspective to teams engaged in research about the etiology, symptom course, patient and family coping, and treatment of eating disorders.

Conclusion

Prevention and early detection of eating disorders should be integrated into the practice of PCPs and PMH-APNs. Early recognition can interrupt the progression of these disorders, reduce their chronic and disabling effects, and improve patient outcomes. The prognosis for patients with eating disorders is extremely variable. When symptoms persist without recognition and treatment, the prognosis is more guarded and mortality risk is higher. The PCP is in a key position to conduct health education, prevention, and routine screening for eating disorders and to support the child and family through follow-up and prevention of relapse. The PMH-APN provides primary prevention and health education about eating disorders and considers the possibility of eating disorders in processes of differential diagnosis. Specialized eating disorder teams are essential partners in managing the intensive phase of treatment and necessitate an awareness of local and regional resources for referral. Interdisciplinary collaboration is essential given the comprehensive care needs associated with managing children and adolescents with these disorders and the typical course of treatment that extends over multiple developmental transitions.

References

Abbate-Daga, G., Piero, A., Rigardetto, R., Gandione, M., Gramaglia, C., & Fassino, S. (2007). *Psychopathology, 40,* 261–268.

Ackard, D.M., Fulkerson, J.A., & Neumark-Sztainer, D. (2007). Prevalence and utility of DSM-IV eating disorder diagnostic criteria among youth. *International Journal of Eating Disorders, 40,* 409–417.

American Academy of Pediatrics (AAP), Committee on Adolescence. (2003). Policy statement: Identifying and treating eating disorders. *Pediatrics, 111,* 204–221.

American Psychiatric Association (APA). (2000). *Diagnostic and statistical manual of mental disorders, text revision, DSM-IV-TR* (4th edition). Washington, DC: Author.

Anderluh, M.B., Tchanturia, K., Rabe-Hesketh, S., & Treasure, J. (2003). Childhood obsessive compulsive personality traits in adult women with eating disorders: Defining a broader eating disorder phenotype. *American Journal of Psychiatry, 160,* 242–247.

APA. (2010). *Level of care guidelines for patients with eating disorders.* Retrieved from http://www.psychiatryonline.com/popup.aspx?aID=139471

Bannon, Y.S. (2005). Expanding clinical knowledge of eating disorders through clinical trials. *Primary Psychiatry, 12,* 32–38.

Barker, E.T., & Galambos, N.L. (2007). Body dissatisfaction, living away from parents, and poor social adjustment predict binge eating symptoms in young woman making the transition to university. *Journal of Youth and Adolescence, 36,* 904–911.

Becker, E., Eddy, K.T., & Perloe, A. (2009). Clarifying criteria for cognitive signs and symptoms for eating disorders in DSM-V. *International Journal of Eating Disorders, 42,* 611–619.

Berkman, N.D., Lohr, K.N., & Bulik, C.M. (2007). Outcomes of eating disorders: A systematic review of the literature. *International Journal of Eating Disorders, 40,* 293–309.

Bernstein, B.E. (2008). *Eating disorder: Anorexia: Differential diagnoses & workup.* Retrieved from http://emedicine.medscape.com/article/912187-diagnosis

Bliss, E.L., & Branch, C.H. (1960). *Anorexia nervosa: Its history, psychology and biology.* New York, NY: Hoeber.

Brownley, K.A., Berkman, N.D., Sedway, J.A., Lohr, K.N., & Bulik, C.M. (2007). Binge eating disorder treatment: A systematic review of randomized controlled trials. *International Journal of Eating Disorders, 40,* 337–348.

Bruch, H. (1978). *The golden cage: The enigma of anorexia nervosa.* Boston, MA: Harvard University Press.

Bryant-Waugh, R., & Lask, B. (2004). *Eating disorders: A parents' guide* (Rev. edition). New York: Brunner-Rutledge.

Bulik, C.M., Berkman, N.D., Brownley, K.A., Sedway, J.A., & Lohr, K.N. (2007). Anorexia nervosa treatment: A systematic review of randomized controlled trials. *International Journal of Eating Disorders, 40,* 310–320.

Bulik, C.M., Reba, L., Siega-Riz, A.M., and Reichborn-Kjennerud, T. (2005). Anorexia nervosa: Definition, epidemiology, and cycle of risk. *International Journal of Eating Disorders, 37,* S2-S9.

Bulik, C.M., Sullivan, P.F., Tozzi, F., Furberg, H., Lichtenstein, P., & Pedersen, N.L. (2006). Prevalence, heritability, and prospective risk factors for anorexia nervosa. *Archives of General Psychiatry, 63,* 305–312.

Bulik, C.M., & Taylor, N. (2005). *Runaway eating: The 8 point plan to conquer adult food and weight obsessions.* New York, NY: Rodale Books.

Castro, J., Gila, A., Puig, J., Rodriguez, S., & Toro, J. (2004). Predictors of rehospitalization after total weight recovery in adolescents with anorexia nervosa. *International Journal of Eating Disorders, 36,* 22–30.

Clausen, L. (2004). Time course of symptom remission in eating disorders. *International Journal of Eating Disorders, 36,* 296–306.

Collins, L. (2005). *Eating with your anorexic: How my child recovered through family-based treatment and yours can too.* New York, NY: McGraw Hill.

Couturier, J., & Lock, J. (2006). What is recovery in adolescent anorexia nervosa? *International Journal of Eatinbg Disorders, 39,* 550–555.

Couturier, J., & Lock, J. (2007). Psychopharmacology update: A review of medication use for children and adolescents with eating disorders. *Journal of the Canadian Academy of Child and Adolescent Psychiatry, 16,* 173–176.

DeSocio, J., O'Toole, J., Nemirow, S., Lukach, M., & Magee, M. (2007). Screening for childhood eating disorders in primary care. Primary care companion. *Journal of Clinical Psychiatry, 9,* 1–20.

Fairburn, C.G. (2008). *Cognitive behavior therapy and eating disorders.* New York, NY: Guilford.

Fairburn, C.G., & Cooper, Z. (1993). The eating disorder examination. In C. Fairburn & G. Wilson (Eds.), *Binge eating: Nature, assessment and treatment* (12th edition)(pp. 317–360). New York, NY: Guilford.

Fairburn, C.G., & Harrison, P.J. (2003). Eating disorders. *Lancet, 361,* 407–416.

Favaro, A., Tenconi, E., & Santonastaso, P. (2006). Perinatal factors and the risk of developing anorexia nervosa and bulimia nervosa. *Archives of General Psychiatry, 63,* 82–88.

Flament, M., Furino, C., & Godart, N. (2005). In D. Stein, B. Lerer, & S. Stahl (Eds.), *Evidence-based psychopharmacology* (pp. 204–254). New York, NY: Cambridge University Press.

Frank, G.K., Bailer, U.F., Henry, S.E., Drevets, W., Meltzer, C.C., Price, J.C., et al. (2005). Increased dopamine D2/D3 receptor binding after recovery from anorexia nervosa measured by positron emission tomography and [11C] raclopride. *Biological Psychiatry, 58,* 908–912.

Garner, D.M., & Garfinkel, P.E. (Eds.) (1997). *Handbook of treatment for eating disorders* (2nd edition). New York, NY: Guilford Press.

Golden, N.H., Jacobson, M.S., Schebendach, J., Solanto, M., Hertz, S., & Shenker, I.R. (1997). Resumption of menses in anorexia nervosa. *Archives of Pediatric and Adolescent Medicine, 151*(1), 16–21.

Gorwood, P., Kipmann, A., & Foulon, C. (2003). The human genetics of anorexia nervosa. *European Journal of Pharmacology, 480,* 163–170.

Greenleaf, C., Petrie, T. A., Carter, J., & Reel, J.J. (2009). Female collegiate athletes: Prevalence of eating disorders and disordered eating behaviors. *Journal of American College Health, 57,* 489–496.

Gull, Sir W. (1874). Anorexia nervosa. *Transactions of the Clinical Society of London, 7,* 22–28.

Halmi, K. (2007). Anorexia nervosa and bulimia nervosa. In A. Martin & F. R. Volmar, *Lewis's Child and Adolescent Psychiatry* (4th edition) (pp. 592–602). Philadelphia, PA: Lippincott Williams & Wilkins.

Herzog, D.B., & Eddy, K.T. (2007). Diagnosis, epidemiology, and clinical course of eating disorders. In J. Yager & P.S. Powers (Eds.), *Clinical Manual of Eating Disorders* (pp. 1–30). Washington, DC: American Psychiatric Publishing.

Hillebrand, J.G., van Elburg, A.A., Kas, M.J.H., van England, H., & Adan, R.A.H. (2005). Olanzapine reduces physical activity in rats exposed to activity-based anorexia: possible implications for treatment of anorexia nervosa. *Biological Psychiatry, 58*, 651–657.

Hoek, H.W., & van Hoeken, D. (2003). Review of the prevalence and incidence of eating disorders. *International Journal of Eating Disorders, 29*, 383–396.

Hudson, J.I., Hiripi, E., Pope, H.G., & Kessler, R.C. (2007). The prevalence and correlates of eating disorders in the National Comorbidity Survey Replication. *Biological Psychiatry, 61*, 348–358.

Insel, T. (2006). *Statement about eating disorders as brain disorders.* Distributed correspondence to the National Eating Disorders Association, October 5, 2006.

Kartini Clinic. (n.d.-a). *Welcome to Kartini Clinic for Disordered Eating.* Retrieved on October 12, 2009, from http://www.kartiniclinic.com

Kartini Clinic. (n.d.-b). *Solutions for eating disorders: How is Kartini Clinic different than other treatment programs?* Retrieved from http://www.kartiniclinic.com/Information-Parents/Why-Kartini-Different

Katzman, D.K. (2005). Medical complications in adolescents with anorexia nervosa: A review of the literature. *International Journal of Eating Disorders, 37*, S52-S59.

Kaye, W.H., Bulik, C.M., Plotnicov, K., Thornton, L., Devlin, B., Ficter, M.M., et al. (2008). The genetics of anorexia nervosa collaborative study: Methods and sample description. *International Journal of Eating Disorders, 41*, 289–300.

Kaye, W.H., Bulik, C.M., Thornton, L., Barbarich, N., & Masters, K. (2004). Comorbidity of anxiety disorders with anorexia and bulimia nervosa. *American Journal of Psychiatry, 161*, 2215–2221.

Kaye, W.H., Frank, G.K., Bailer, U.F., and Henry, S.E. (2005). Neurobiology of anorexia nervosa: Clinical implications of alterations of the function of serotonin and other neuronal systems. *International Journal of Eating Disorders, 37*, S15-S19. doi:10.1002/eat.20109

Kaye, W.H., & Walsh, B.T. (2002). Psychopharmacology of eating disorders. In K.L. Davis, D. Charney, J.T. Coyle, & C. Nemeroff (Eds.), *Neuropsychopharmacology: The fifth generation of progress* (pp. 1675–1683). Brentwood, TN: American College of Neuropsychopharmacology.

Keel, P.K., Fichter, M., Quadflieg, N., Bulik, C.M., Baxter, M.G., Thornton, L., et al. (2004). Application of a latent class analysis to empirically define eating disorder phenotypes. *Archives of General Psychiatry, 61*, 192–200.

Keel, P.K., & Haedt, A. (2008). Evidence based psychosocial treatments for eating problems and eating disorders. *Journal of Clinical Child and Adolescent Psychology, 37*, 39–61.

Keel, P.K., & Klump, K.L. (2003). Are eating disorders culture-bound syndromes? Implications for conceptualizing their etiology. *Psychological Bulletin, 129*(5), 747–769.

Keel, P.K., Klump, K.L., Miller, K.B., McGue, M., & Iacono, W.G. (2005). Shared transmission of eating disorders and anxiety disorders. *International Journal of Eating Disorders, 38*, 99–105.

Kessler, R.C., Berglund, P., Demler, O., Jin, R., Merikangas, K., & Walter, E. (2005). Lifetime prevalence and age-of-onset distributions of DSM IV disorders in the National Comorbidity Survey Replication. *Archives of General Psychiatry, 62*, 593–602.

Klump, K.L., Bulik, C.M., Kaye, W.H., Treasure, J., & Tyson, E. (2009). Academy for Eating disorders position paper: Eating disorders are serious mental illnesses. *International Journal of Eating Disorders, 42*, 97–103.

Klump, K.L., & Gobrogge, K.L. (2005). A review and primer of molecular genetic studies in anorexia nervosa. *International Journal of Eating Disorders, 37*, S43-S48. doi:10.1002/eat.20116

Lask, B., Gordon, I., Christie, D., Frampton, I., Chowdhury, U., & Watkins, B. (2005). Functional neuroimaging in early-onset anorexia nervosa. *International Journal of Eating Disorders, 37*, S49-S51.

Lock, J., & LeGrange, D. (2005). Help your teenager beat an eating disorder. New York, NY: Guilford.

Lopez, C., Tchanturia, K., Stahl, D., & Treasure, J. (2008). Weak central coherence in eating disorders: A step towards looking for an endophenotype of eating disorders. *Journal of Clinical and Experimental Neuropsychology, 31*, 117–125.

Madden, S. (2004). Anorexia nervosa – Still relevant in the twenty-first century? A review of William Gull's "Anorexia Nervosa". *Clinical Child Psychology and Psychiatry, 9*, 149–154.

McCormick, L.M., Keel, P.K., Brumm, M.C., Bowers, W., Swayze, V., Andersen, A., & Andreasen, N. (2008). Implications of starvation induced change in right dorsal anterior cingulated volume in anorexia nervosa. *International Journal of Eating Disorders, 41*, 602–610.

McFarlane, T., Olmsted, M.P., & Trottier, K. (2008). Timing and prediction of relapse in a transdiagnostic eating disorder sample. *International Journal of Eating Disorders, 41*, 587–593.

Mintz, L.B., O'Halloran, M.S., Mulholland, A.M., & Schneider, P.A. (1997). Questionnaire for eating disorder diagnoses: Reliability and validity of operationalized DSM-IV criteria into a self-report format. *Journal of Counseling Psychology, 44*, 63–79.

Mitchell, J. E., Agras, S., & Wonderlich, S. (2007). Treatment of bulimia nervosa: Where are we and where are we going? *International Journal of Eating Disorders, 40*, 95–101.

Mond, J.M., Myers, T., Crosby, R., Hay, P., Rodgers, B., Morgan, J., Lacey, J.H., et al. (2008). Screening for eating disorders in primary care: EDE-Q versus SCOFF. *Behaviour Research and Therapy, 46*(5), 612–622.

Moreno, M.A., & Judd, R. (2008). *Eating disorder: Bulimia: Differential diagnoses & workup.* Retrieved from http://emedicine.medscape.com/article/913721-diagnosis

Morgan, J.F., Reid, F., & Lacey, J.H. (1999). The SCOFF questionnaire: Assessment of a new screening tool for eating disorders. *British Medical Journal, 319*, 1467–1468.

Mufson, L., Pollack Dorta, K., Moreau, D., & Weissman, M.M. (2004). Interpersonal psychotherapy for depressed adolescents (2nd edition). New York, NY: Guilford Press.

National Collaborating Centre for Mental Health. (2004). *Eating disorders: Core interventions in the treatment and management of anorexia nervosa, bulimia nervosa and related eating disorders.* [Clinical guideline 9]. London, UK: National Institute for Health and Clinical Excellence. Retrieved from http://www.nice.org.uk/guidnace/CG9/niceguidance/pdf/English

O'Toole, J. (2010). *Give food a chance.* Portland, OR: PSIpress.

O'Toole, J., DeSocio, J., Munoz, D., & Crosby, R. (in press). Eating disorders in children and adolescents: Diagnostic differences and clinical challenges. In R. Striegel-Moore, S.A. Wonderlich, B.T. Walsh, & J.E. Mitchell (Eds.), *Toward an evidence based classification of eating disorders* [Monograph]. Washington, DC: American Psychiatric Association.

Peebles, R., Wilson, J.L., & Lock, J.D. (2006). How do children with eating disorders differ from adolescents with eating disorders at initial evaluation? *Journal of Adolescent Health, 39*, 800–805.

Pritts, S., & Susman, J. (2003). Diagnosis of eating disorders in primary care. *American Family Physician, 67*(2), 297–304.

Puxley, F., Midtsund, M., Iosif, A., & Lask, B. (2008). PANDAS anorexia nervosa - endangered, extinct or nonexistent. *International Journal of Eating Disorders, 41*, 15–21.

Qadan, L. (2009). Anorexia nervosa: Beyond boundaries. *International Journal of Eating Disorders, 42*, 479–481.

Rome, E.S., & Ammerman, S. (2003). Medical complications of eating disorders: An update. *Journal of Adolescent Health, 33*, 418–426.

Rome, E.S., Ammerman, S., Rosen, D.S., Keller, R.J., Lock, J., Mammel, K.A., et al. (2003). Children and adolescents with eating disorders: The state of the art. *Pediatrics, 111*, e98-e108.

Russell, G. (1979). Bulimia nervosa: An ominous variant of anorexia nervosa. *Psychological Medicine, 9*, 429–448.

Safer, D.L., Telch, C.F., Chen, E.Y., & Linehan, M.M. (2009). *Dialectical behavior therapy for binge eating and bulimia.* New York, NY: Guilford Press.

Shapiro, J.R., Berkman, N.D., Brownley, K.A., Sedway, J.A., Lohr, K.N., & Bulik, C.M. (2007). Bulimia nervosa: A systematic review of randomized controlled trials. *International Journal of Eating Disorders, 40*, 321– 336.

Society for Adolescent Medicine. (2003). Position paper: Eating disorders in adolescents. *Journal of Adolescent Health, 33*, 496–503.

Sodersten, P., Bergh, C., & Ammar, A. (2003). Anorexia nervosa: Towards a neurobiologically based therapy. *European Journal of Pharmacology, 480*, 67–74.

Sokol, M.S., Jackson, T.K., Selser, C.T., Nice, H.A., Christiansen, N.D., & Carroll, A.K. (2005). Review of clinical research in child and adolescent eating disorders. *Primary Psychiatry, 12*, 52–58.

Stein, D.M., & Reichert, P. (1990). Extreme dieting behaviors in early adolescence. *Journal of Early Adolescence, 10*, 108–121.

Strober, M., Freeman, R., Lampert, C., Diamond, J., & Kaye, W. (2000). Controlled family study of anorexia nervosa and bulimia nervosa: Evidence of shared liability and transmission of partial syndromes. *American Journal of Psychiatry, 157*, 393–401.

Strober, M., Freeman, R., & Morrell, W. (1997). The long term course of severe anorexia nervosa in adolescents: Survival analysis of recovery, relapse, and outcome predictors over 10-15 years in a prospective study. *International Journal of Eating Disorders, 22*, 339–360.

Tantillo, M. (2006). A relational approach to eating disorders multifamily therapy group: Moving from difference and disconnection to mutual connection. *Families, Systems and Health, 24*, 82–102.

Thelen, M.H., Mintz, L.B., & Vander Wal, J. (1996). The bulimia test-revised: Validation with DSM-IV criteria for bulimia nervosa. *Psychological Assessment, 8*, 219–221.

Treasure, J. (2000). *Anorexia nervosa: A survival guide for families, friends, and sufferers.* Hove, UK: Psychology Press.

Treasure, J. (2007). Getting beneath the phenotype of anorexia nervosa: The search for viable endophenotypes and genotypes. *Canadian Journal of Psychiatry, 52*, 212–219.

U.S. Department of Health and Human Services. (2009). *Healthy People 2020 Public Meetings: 2009 Draft Objectives.* Retrieved from http://www.healthypeople.gov/hp2020/Objectives/files/Draft2009Objectives.pdf

Wade, T.D., Bulik, C.M., Neale, M., & Kendler, K.S. (2000). Anorexia and major depression: Shared genetic and environmental risk factors. *American Journal of Psychiatry, 157*, 469–471.

Wagner, A., Aizenstein, H., Venkatraman, V.K., Fudge, J., May, J.C., Mazurkewicz, L., et al. (2007). Altered reward processing in women recovered from anorexia nervosa. *American Journal of Psychiatry, 164*, 1842–1849.

Walsh, J.M., Wheat, M., & Freund, K. (2000). Detection, evaluation, and treatment of eating disorders. *Journal of General Internal Medicine, 15*, 577–590.

Williams, P., Goodie, J., & Motsinger, C. (2008). Treating eating disorders in primary care. *American Family Physician, 77*, 187–195.

Workgroup for Classification of Eating Disorders in Children and Adolescents (WCEDCA). (2007). Classification of child and adolescent eating disturbances. *International Journal of Eating Disorders, 40*, S117-S122.

Yager, J., Devlin, M.J., Halmi, K.A., Herzog, D.B., Mitchell, J.E., Powers, P., & Zerbe, K.J. (2006). *Practice guidelines for the treatment of patients with eating disorders* (3rd edition). Washington, DC: American Psychiatric Association. Retrieved from http://www.psych.org/psych_pract/treatg/pg/EatingDisorder-s3ePG_04-28-06.pdf

13

Autism Spectrum Disorder

Judith Coucouvanis, Donna Hallas, and Jean Nelson Farley

Objectives

After reading this chapter, APNs will be able to

1. Describe the epidemiology and etiology of autism spectrum disorder (ASD).
2. Understand the diagnostic criteria for ASD.

3. Discuss clinical problems and evidence-based interventions for the treatment of ASD.
4. Discuss implications for practice, research, and education of APNs who care for children with ASD.

Introduction

It has been almost seventy years since child psychiatrist Leo Kanner (1943) first reported the unusual characteristics of a group of 11 children. Initially referred to as *early infantile autism* (Kanner, 1943) and now referred to as pervasive developmental disorder (PDD), this syndrome has evolved to include multiple related diagnostically detailed conditions that currently include in DSM-IV-TR: autistic disorder, Asperger's disorder, pervasive developmental disorder, not otherwise specified, childhood disintegrative disorder and Rett's disorder (American Psychiatric Association, 2000).

The U.S. Department of Health and Human Services 2010 Interagency Autism Coordinating Committee Strategic Plan for Autism Spectrum Disorder Research—January 19, 2010, reports, "Autism is now recognized as a group of syndromes denoted as autism spectrum disorder (ASD)." Autism is not a single syndrome.

Persons present with a spectrum of problems in the areas of socialization, communication, and behavior that range from mild to severely debilitating. Currently ASD is diagnosed from a combination of core behavioral characteristics that include impairment in verbal and nonverbal communication skills and social interaction and restricted, repetitive, and stereotyped patterns of behavior. Consistent with the Interagency Autism Coordinating Committee (IACC) Strategic Plan, this chapter will use the term *autism spectrum disorder* (ASD) to refer to this group of syndromes.

A rigorous national surveillance study conducted by the Centers for Disease Control and Prevention (CDC) reports approximately 1% of children are affected with ASD (Kogan et al., 2009). ASD occurs in all racial, ethnic, and socioeconomic groups, yet is four to five times more likely to occur in boys than in girls (CDC, 2010). The majority of children with ASD receive special education services and have a documented history of concerns

---

Child and Adolescent Behavioral Health: A Resource for Advanced Practice Psychiatric and Primary Care Practitioners in Nursing,
First Edition. Edited by Edilma L. Yearwood, Geraldine S. Pearson, and Jamesetta A. Newland.
© 2012 John Wiley & Sons, Inc. Published 2012 by John Wiley & Sons, Inc.

regarding development before three years of age. Cognitive impairment (i.e., IQ of 70 of less) is reported for 30% to 51% of children (CDC, 2010).

Surrounded by confusion, intrigue, and myth, ASD is one of the most complex and controversial psychiatric disorders. Each affected individual exhibits a life-long profile of unique social-communicative, cognitive, and linguistic strengths, and weaknesses, as well as sensory modulation issues. Every person with ASD is different. Individuals range from those who are nonverbal with severe challenges (classic autism) to those who are extremely intelligent, yet demonstrate markedly impaired social skills and weak perspective-taking skills (Asperger's disorder).

One of the core features of ASD is marked impairment in social functioning, regardless of intellectual or language ability (Carter, Davis, Klin, & Volkmar, 2005). Social deficits are wide-ranging and persist through adolescence and adulthood when social demands become more complex (Tantam, 2000). Developing meaningful relationships is a constant struggle for those with ASD. While typically developing children learn social skills through experience, the child with ASD must be directly taught specific skills (Bellini, 2006).

Studies have shown that there is a 50- to 100-fold increase in the rate of autism in first-degree relatives of autistic children (Filipek et al., 2000). Estimates for recurrence of ASD in siblings range anywhere from 6% to 20% (Filipek et al., 2000; Ghaziuddin, 2005). This represents a risk of over 100 times that of the general population (Ghaziuddin, 2005). No one can predict the eventual outcome for an affected child with ASD (Koegel & LaZebnik, 2004) and improvements cannot be expected to occur for all individuals even when using a specific established and evidence-based treatment.

In the past twenty years, a wealth of information has been gathered about ASD, however, no one treatment meets the needs of all children (National Institute of Mental Health [NIMH], 2008). Each child requires an individualized, systematic, and comprehensive intervention plan (Koegel & LaZebnik, 2004). Autism stories are regularly featured on Internet web sites, in talk and print media, and in mainstream magazines. Conflicting opinions regarding treatment, heated arguments about cause, and "evidence" of miracle cures are common, leaving parents confused and overwhelmed.

Parents face a daunting array of choices and decisions, often without guidance. Which interventions and treatments are best? Whom should parents trust? What will give parents hope? The estimated cost for each individual with ASD across the lifespan is $3.2 million (Ganz, 2007). Advanced practice nurses (APNs) in pediatric settings are in prime positions to guide and support parents through the myriad of decisions parents encounter daily while parenting a child with a diagnosis of ASD.

Public awareness of ASD has increased in the last decade and is likely related to closer media coverage of studies in the scientific literature related to causation and intervention. Reasons for this increase have included heightened public awareness and consequent levels of parental con\cern, development of more sophisticated screening and diagnostic tools, and improved professional proficiency in identification of children at risk. Also, changes in the DSM-IV criteria in 1994 broadened the range of disorders in the spectrum (Johnson & Myers, 2007).

Etiology

ASD is a biologically based, neurobehavioral disorder, the cause of which has continued to perplex experts in the field attempting to identify causal factors. To date, the preponderance of evidence points to multifactorial transmission (i.e., genetic susceptibility exacerbated by environmental factors). Thus, a wide range of possible etiologies have been proposed, as follows.

Disruption in Brain Structure and Function

Attempts at directly studying difference in brain structure and function in individuals with ASD has focused on use of neuroimaging techniques, such as fMRI and spectroscopy (Batshaw, Pellegrino, & Roizen, 2007; Ecker et al., 2010). Macrocephaly is frequently noted during early childhood in individuals with ASD, and some neuroimaging studies have found that this finding coincides with brain growth acceleration at about one year of age in regions of cortical white matter, as well as abnormal growth patterns in the frontal and temporal lobes and the amygdala (Levy, Mandell, & Schultz, 2009). Other studies have used neuroimaging to detect neurotransmitter activity and cortical energy utilization in high functioning adolescents with ASD. To date, these studies have identified some evidence that certain areas of the autistic brain have difficulty "networking" with other brain regions, and functional abnormalities have been noted in brain areas associated with eye gaze, processing faces, and imitation (Batshaw et al., 2007). Such difficulties often translate into a range of sensory integration and processing difficulties (Levy et al., 2009).

Parental Age

Recent research has focused on the relationship of maternal and paternal age to increased risk for ASD. A study by Reichenberg and coleagues (2006) analyzed a large Israeli military database and found that there was a significant association between advancing paternal age and risk of ASD. Another study by Shelton and cow-orkers (2010) examined a ten-year cohort of nearly five million births in California to determine if the age of mothers, fathers, or both contributes to the incidence of ASD. The results suggested that when a father was over forty and the mother was under thirty, there was a marked increase in risk.

Genetic Predisposition

In the past, autism was viewed primarily as a disorder of brain structure or function. In view of the variable phenotypes on the autism spectrum, studies are increasingly focusing on gene-environment interaction causing functional cellular changes throughout the body, such as those modulating immune response, and gastrointestinal function. A great deal of interest has surrounded identification of etiologies for autism with a strong genetic basis.

During the past few years, genetic research in ASD has been successful in identifying several vulnerability loci and a few cytogenetic abnormalities or single best mutations implicated in the causation of autism (Caglayan, 2010). The preponderance of males affected by ASD noted earlier in this chapter also suggests a genetic role in these disorders. The following three major approaches have been used to identify genetic factors linked to ASD: candidate gene studies, association with genetic disorders of known etiology, and family studies (Batshaw et al., 2007).

1. *Candidate gene studies.* This strategy targets investigation of genes thought to play a role in the neurophysiology of ASD, particularly factors affecting neuronal connectivity, such as neurotransmitters and receptor sites, cerebellar Purkinje cells, and neuronal cell adhesion (Batshaw et al., 2007; Muhle, Trentacoste, & Rapin, 2004; Hakonarson et al., 2009).

   A. *Association with genetic disorders of known etiology.* Individuals with tuberous sclerosis, an autosominal dominant disorder, and fragile X syndrome, an X-linked disorder causing intellectual disability, are at an increased risk for developing ASD. This association supports exploration of the link between known biologic anomalies and behaviors indicative of autism (Batshaw et al., 2007). Rett's syndrome is caused by a mutation of a gene that codes for the MeCP2 binding protein (Caglayan, 2010). Other genetic syndromes that are less frequently associated with development of ASD include trisomy 21, Prader Willi syndrome, Angelman syndrome, Joubert syndrome, neurofibromatosis type I,

Timothy syndrome, Williams syndrome, sex chromosome disorders, Smith-Lemli-Opitz syndrome, Cohen syndrome, PKU, Sanfillipo syndrome, Duchenne muscular systrophy, and mitochondrial disorders (Caglayan, 2010).

2. *Family studies.* Families who have multiple members with ASD undergo genetic analysis to identify the presence of any recurring DNA markers (e.g., deletions, breakages, translocations, duplications, etc.). This methodology has not yet revealed any definitive answers, but sites on chromosomes X, 2, 3, 7, 11, 15, 17, and 22 seem to be more frequently associated with an autism-linked abnormality (Johnson & Meyers, 2007). Wang and colleagues (2010) conducted genome-wide association studies on two large family cohorts of affected children of European ancestry. Their investigation identified common genetic variants at chromosome 5p14.1 that encode for neuronal cell adhesion and implicate this as a possible pathogenic basis for ASD. Monozygotic twin studies employing a broad autistic phenotype have identified between 60% and 92% concordance (Muhle, 2004). These findings strongly suggest that environmental influences on genetic makeup affect expression and severity of autistic characteristics (Inglese & Elder, 2009).

3. *Environmental influences.* Although most scientists would agree that there is a strong, genetic basis to ASD, recent debate has developed regarding the extent to which environmental factors influence the expression and severity of ASD. Thus far, no single environmental or chemical factor has been identified with development of autism, although some have shown stronger linkage. The most frequently implicated factors include the following:

   A. *Teratogens.* Several medications, when taken prenatally, have been associated with increased risk of ASD, including thalidomide, valproic acid, and mesoprostol. Some studies have investigated the role of heavy metals (mercury, lead, cadmium) on the developing fetus or newborn (Batshaw et al., 2007). To date, there are no definitive linkages or associations of specific teratogens as an etiology of ASD.

   B. There are two distinct, but linked concerns regarding *immunizations.* The first involves the measles-mumps-rubella (MMR) vaccine and the belief that its administration to genetically predisposed children causes ASD (Inglese & Elder, 2009). A systematic review for the Cochrane Database was undertaken by Demicheli, Jefferson, Rivetti, and Price (2006) to investigate possible unintended side effects and complications from MMR administration. The main finding was that MMR was an unlikely causal factor in development of autism or autism regression.

C. Another subsequent, intense debate centered on whether the sheer volume of immunizations received by children in which *thimerosal* was used as a preservative was a possible causal factor in the development of ASD. Follow-up immunization studies conducted after removal of this preservative from all vaccines failed to reveal any causal relationship (Inglese & Elder, 2009). However, despite these findings, a recent study by Freed, Clark, Butchart, Singer and Davis (2010) found that one in four parents still believe that some vaccines can cause autism in healthy children. Thus, it is crucial for pediatric health care providers to engage parents in thoughtful discussion about their concerns regarding immunizations.

D. *Viral or bacterial infections* during infancy and early childhood have also been raised as possible etiologies, especially if the infection results in severe, neurologic sequelae.

E. Also, there is no current evidence to suggest that overgrowth of *yeasts or bacteria* in the intestine is associated with increased risk of ASD (Levy & Hyman, 2005).

The Clinical Picture: Screening and Assessment

Although most children with autism can be accurately identified by an expert clinician by age three years, diagnosis of those with Asperger's syndrome and PDD–NOS often are not reliably diagnosed until late preschool age (Shattuck et al., 2009). The average age at diagnosis of autism in the United States has been estimated to range from 4.5 to 5 years of age, even though developmental concerns are often documented before three years of age (CDC, 2009; Wiggins, Baio, & Rice, 2006). The average age for identifying children with Asperger's syndrome is eight years. This delay in diagnosis may be due to a variety of professional factors, such as concerns about labeling, incorrect diagnosing, and assuming a protracted "watch and wait" attitude, under the pretext of minimizing parental worry. While parents may be the first to notice developmental problems or unusual behaviors, they may also delay reporting these concerns in hopes that their child may "grow out of it" or is just "going through a phase" (Coonrod & Stone, 2004). Some children at risk

may not have an identified "medical home" because of cultural or societal barriers, where they can receive regular health and developmental surveillance. Finally, characteristics of milder forms of ASD, or one in which lack of developmental progression is a feature, may not be as easily identifiable until a child ages and these deficits become more apparent in social and school settings.

In view of the current prevalence of ASD in this country, every advanced practice nurse (APN) who provides care to the pediatric population can expect to encounter a child with this disorder. There is clearly a mandate for APNs to establish competence in surveillance of, and screening for, ASD to facilitate early diagnosis, appropriate therapeutic interventions, and improved developmental outcomes. Although some APNs may be directly involved in the final *diagnostic* process and ongoing treatment of a child with a suspected ASD, others will continue their role as the family's "health care home" and support families in navigating their child's primary health care and developmental trajectory. Such support would include helping families access resources, engaging in ongoing collaboration with therapists, making visits to the school setting or arranging conference calls with teachers, and ensuring that the child is gaining full access to educational supports allowed by law (Lobar, Fritts, Arbide & Russell, et al., 2008).

Clinical Features

"One of the most challenging aspects in recognizing ASD is the wide heterogeneity of features in individual children" (Johnson and Myers, 2007, p. 1190). ASD shares signs and symptoms with a variety of other health and developmental problems, such as attention and adjustment disorders, anxiety, depression, sensory and cognitive deficits, or generalized developmental delays (Beauchesne and Kelley, 2004). Identifying a child with ASD is a challenging and complex process and demands astute assessment skills. There are no medical tests for diagnosing autism. Being alert to the risk factors that raise suspicion of ASD is an essential first step in developing screening proficiency. Even if the APN does not have any immediate suspicions about a possible diagnosis of ASD in a child, *any* parental concern about a child's developmental progress should be explored and serve as a compelling reason to proceed with an appropriate evaluation and screening.

Red Flags

During routine developmental surveillance, the APN should be attentive to reported or observed "red flags" that match the "core features" signifying risk for an ASD (American Psychiatric Association, 2000; Jones, Carr,

Table 13.1 Communication "red flags"

Referral Indication	Behavior
By end of 6 months	No appropriate gaze and fixation on faces, objects
	No big smiles or other warm, joyful expressions by 6 months
By 9 months	No reciprocal vocalizations between infant and caregiver
	No smiles or other facial expressions
By 12 months	No back and forth gestures, such as pointing, showing, reaching or waving bye-bye
	No babbling, such as "mama," "dada," and "baba"
By 18 months	No single words
	No simple, pretend play
By 24 months	No two-word, spontaneous meaningful phrases
	Lack of interest in other children
	Any unexplained, gradual or sudden regression of social or language skills at any age, warrants prompt referral for screening.

From Johnson and Myers, 2007; and Peacock, Hyman, and Levy, 2009.

Katelin & Klin, 2008; Phetrasuwan, Miles, & Mesibov, 2009;) (Table 13.1):

1. Significant impairment in social interaction
2. Severe delays in, or lack of, language communication skills
3. Repetitive, restricted, and stereotyped patterns of behavior, interests, and activities

Impairment in Social Interaction

The APN should be attentive to parental reports of a child who shows lack of interest in social relatedness with family and peers. The child may be described as one who prefers to be alone and shows little interest in making friends. He may be perfectly content to engage in solitary or parallel play, rather than the cooperative play that is typical of his/her age group. Depending on where a child falls on the ASD spectrum, he may be described as an "easy child," who demands little attention from caregivers. Others may be very prone to tantrums that can be easily triggered by a common sound or visual cue. The APN may find it difficult to elicit eye

contact or a social smile from the child while conducting a physical assessment or screening. Recent research indicates that early difficulties with making eye contact may be one of the strongest predictors of the eventual level of social disability in a child with ASD (Jones et al., 2008).

Delays in Language and Social Skills

Any unexplained lack of progression in language or social skill development is a compelling indication for screening and diagnostic referral for ASD. "Twenty-five to thirty percent of children with ASD develop some vocabulary words, but then stop speaking or using gestures" (Johnson & Myers, 2007, p. 1192). Other common, classic presentations of communication difficulties include delayed or absent language and engagement in "scripted speech," such as excerpts from favorite videos, songs, or TV programs. Echolalia or "parroting" may also be observed and can give a false impression of advanced language abilities. Spontaneous "pop up" words with no connection to the social context may be exhibited, as well as giant, run-on words, such as "whatisit?" or "idontknow" (Johnson & Myers, 2007, p.1192).

Repetitive and Stereotyped Patterns of Behavior and Restricted Interests

These behaviors are typically represented by engagement in a narrow repertoire of activities that are repetitive, self-stimulatory, ritualistic, and nonfunctional in nature. Such behaviors tend to be primarily manifested when the child is anxious, upset, or exposed to a novel social situation that is anxiety producing or exciting. Examples include unusual finger movements, hand flapping, head banging, rocking, bruxism, and preoccupation with an object, such as a piece of string or a wheeled toy. The child may also engage in perseverative preoccupation with a topic, game, celebrity, or TV show. Often, the initial presenting problem at a health maintenance or episodic visit may be parental and family frustration with the child's unusual adherence to habits, rituals, tantrums, and daily routines, which significantly interfere with family functioning. Some of these routines are so bizarre or entrenched that families may go to extreme lengths to adapt or acquiesce to them so as to avoid embarrassment in public places or to minimize continuous emotional upheaval in the home environment.

Once a developmental concern that may represent autism spectrum disorder is identified, there are several valid and reliable tools available that the APN can use to screen the child. These are listed in Table 13.2.

Table 13.2 Screening tools for autism in the older child

Screening Tools for Autism in the Older Child	Age Group	WWW Resource
Social Communication Questionnaire (SCQ)	> 3 years	http://wpspublish.com/
Social Responsiveness Scale (SRS)	School age	http://wpspublish.com
Screening Tool for Autism in Toddlers and Young Children (STAT)	24–36 months	http://stat.vueinnovations.com
Autism Spectrum Screening Questionnaire	6–17 years	www.springerlink.com/content/h26q7u2323251347/fulltext.pdf
Childhood Autism Spectrum Test (CAST)	5–9 years	www.autismresearchcentre.com/docs/tests/CAST_test.doc
Australian Scale for Asperger Syndrome (ASAS)	5 years and older	http://scotens.org/sen/articles/australian_scale_for_asperger.pdf
Gilliam Autism Rating Scale–2 (GARS)	3–22 years	www.pearsonassessments.com
Modified Checklist for Autism in Toddlers (M–CHAT)	16–30 months	http://firstsigns.org

Physical Assessment and Examination

When ASD is suspected and the child will be referred for further diagnostic study, the APN should compile a summary of the child's health and family history and current health status and complete an updated physical assessment. The physical exam may identify findings associated with an underlying comorbid medical condition that can accompany an ASD or represent a completely different underlying disorder.

Although there is no single or cluster of phenotypic features identified in children with an ASD, research has identified some physical findings that are more likely to be noted in the older, at-risk child. For example, dysmorphic features in a male child, such as a long face and large ears, and pubertal onset of macroorchidism, are findings that are frequently seen in fragile X syndrome (FXS), a sex chromosomal disorder. The syndrome was formerly thought to be a cause of ASD, but it is now recognized that although boys with FXS often have *symptoms* of ASD, the majority do not fully meet the criteria for actual diagnosis (Batshaw et al., 2007). Recent research indicates that only about 2% of boys with ASD also have FXS (Wassink, Piven, & Patel, 2001).

Studies have also revealed that children with autism frequently demonstrate larger head size than their peers. However, only a small percentage has frank macrocephaly (Filipek et al., 2000; Lainhart et al., 1997). Interestingly, this larger head size does not present in infancy but tends to develop later in the preschool years (Filipek et al., 2000). However, children with ASD may also exhibit microcephaly, which is associated with structural brain abnormalities, lower IQ, and seizure disorders (Miles, Hadden, & Hillman, 2000).

Careful examination of the skin is necessary to identify the presence of any hypopigmented areas (i.e., ash leaf spots) using a hand-held ultraviolet light (Wood's lamp). Such cutaneous findings are associated with tuberous sclerosis (TS), a genetic, neurocutaneous disorder. A significant number of children with TS have symptoms of autism (Batshaw et al., 2007).

On neurosensory examination, the APN should carefully evaluate for fine and gross motor delays due to hypotonia and hyporeflexia, as well as gait abnormalities and poor motor coordination, which are noted in 25% of children with an ASD. These neuromotor findings tend to be more evident in autistic children who also have cognitive impairment (Filipek et al., 1999). Those without cognitive impairment typically attain motor milestones on time. Some children in this category may even exhibit *advanced* motor skills, developed as a compensatory mechanism to obtain desired objects without using gestural or expressive language. The examiner should also observe for motor stereotypies, such as hand flapping, finger mannerisms, unusual posturing, toe walking, and rocking, which are frequently seen as motor components of ASD but do not reflect true neurological abnormalities (Filipek et al., 2000). Children with ASD usually have normal structure and function of sensory organ systems. However, they often display great difficulty in processing and integrating the sensory input, which they receive through visual, auditory, olfactory, gustatory, and proprioceptive channels. This may be manifested during physical assessment when the child is exposed to unfamiliar sights, sounds, and touch, resulting in display of unusual motor behaviors and sounds, in order to cope with heightened sensitivity to sensory input (Baranek, Boyd, Poe, Fabian, & Watson, 2007). Cuvo, Law-Reagan, Ackerlund, Huckfeldt & Kelly (2010) have outlined a full range of behavior modification techniques that can be used during the physical exam to gain fuller cooperation of the child and to enhance accuracy of the assessment findings.

The Health Care Encounter

To minimize anxiety that the child with ASD may experience in a novel and unfamiliar environment, the APN should familiarize himself/herself with techniques and strategies to smooth this transition. To deliver appropriate and effective health care, "the history, approach to the child, physical evaluation and treatment options must be considered *in the context* of the patient's diagnosis of an ASD" (Myers & Johnson, 2007, p. 1167). A variety of useful approaches cited in the literature include:

- Working closely with parents or guardians *in advance* to gather information about the child's sensory sensitivities, behavioral triggers, and preferred transitional objects that may enhance the child's level of comfort and cooperation during the visit.
- Providing the parents with a written outline of what will occur during the visit and exam before the appointment.
- Suggesting that the child and parent visit the office or clinic setting and meet staff prior to the day of the actual visit. More than one visit may be required for a child who is very easily distressed by unfamiliar experiences.
- Allowing for extra time during the visit. This provides an opportunity for the child to become familiar with the examiner and the equipment before the examiner touches the child and also allows for a slower-paced examination. A nationally representative sample found that "children with ASD spent twice as much time with the health care provider per visit compared with children in control groups" (Liptak, Stuart, & Auinger, 2006, p. 876).
- Utilizing consistent staff whenever possible.
- Instituting procedures to lessen the child's anxiety due to the unfamiliar environment and equipment, such as:
  - Using visual cues and supports, such as showing a picture of an examining tool and allowing the child to handle this equipment before attempting to use it. Providing parents with pictures or photographs ahead of time allows them to prepare at home.
  - Using an exam room that is quiet, softly lit, and free of clutter and extraneous equipment
  - Using a slow, steady pace that minimizes sudden movements or activity changes
  - Talking to the child before touching him
  - Allowing the child to handle and manipulate equipment, if appropriate and safe
  - Breaking down procedures into short, simple steps using succinct, developmentally appropriate language
  - Being honest about what is going to happen and if there will be discomfort (Inglese & Elder, 2009; Cuvo et al., 2010; Myers & Johnson, 2007).

Referral

If ASD is suspected after screening and comprehensive health assessment, the APN should refer the child and family to a professional or agency that is experienced in making this diagnosis, such as an interdisciplinary early identification program, child psychiatrist or psychologist, developmental pediatrician, speech and language pathologist, or psychiatric-mental health APN. While a screening or assessment tool provides valuable information, it is insufficient to make a diagnostic conclusion. Accurate diagnosis requires assimilating data from a variety of sources, using methods from multiple disciplines, including psychology, speech and language therapy, education, occupational therapy, etc. The end of this chapter contains referral resources that often offer services needed to evaluate a child suspected of having ASD.

Before a referral for a comprehensive diagnostic evaluation occurs, it is vital to arrange a family meeting to review assessment findings and recommendations and to discuss parents' perceptions and reactions. Such a meeting may yield a gamut of parental reactions, ranging from relief that their concerns have been validated, to denial that the child is experiencing any difficulties at all. When a parent rejects evidence of a problem with the child, it may take several interpretive sessions with the family before they are able to act on recommendations for further evaluation and intervention.

Laboratory and Diagnostic Investigations

If a full diagnostic appraisal is planned, the APN may be asked to conduct certain laboratory and diagnostic tests and forward results to the health professional that will be conducting the ASD evaluation. Although there are no specific diagnostic or laboratory procedures to definitively identify a child with ASD, certain categories of laboratory tests are generally conducted to detect disorders that may present with autism-like behaviors or are known, comorbid conditions associated with ASD. Such routine, baseline evaluations include lead screening, karyotype analysis, and molecular DNA testing for FXS. The American College of Medical Genetics also recommends testing for inborn errors of metabolism when there is a history of lethargy, recurrent vomiting, dysmorphic features, developmental regression, unknown or questionable newborn screening results, intellectual disabilities, or seizures of unknown origin (Barbaresi, Katusic & Voigt, 2006; Filipek et al., 1999). Referral to a genetic laboratory for fluorescent in situ hybridization (FISH) testing is also recommended, if comorbid intellectual disability is already identified in the child. FISH testing can help identify chromosomal abnormalities that have been linked to ASD, including chromosomes X, 2, 3, 7, 11, 15, 17, and 22 (Johnson & Myers, 2007). An electroencephalogram (EEG) should be completed if a history of seizure activity is reported. Neuroimaging studies (MRI, fMRI, SPECT, PET, and CT) are reserved as research tools in the study of autism or if there are asymmetrical or abnormal findings on neurological exam (Johnson & Myers, 2007).

Current Diagnostic Criteria

A. **Autistic Disorder:** Autistic disorder, or classic autism, is defined as a combination of language and social deficits, coupled with restricted or repetitive behavior. Children with autism usually have the most severe form of the disorder. However, some youth are referred to as "high functioning" while other youth are severely impaired. Table 13.3 gives the current diagnostic criteria for ASD (American Psychiatric Association, 2000; Batshaw et al., 2007).

B. **Asperger's Disorder:** This disorder was first described by German pediatrician Hans Asperger in 1944, when he identified a group of four children with normal IQs who demonstrated milder, autistic behaviors (Filipek, 2005). Asperger's disorder can be diagnosed if three symptoms—two related to social reciprocity and one to habitual behaviors—are present (American Psychiatric Association, 2000; Batshaw et al., 2007). The key difference between Asperger's disorder and other entities on the autism spectrum is the absence of any significant language delay. However, expressive speech of children with Asperger's disorder is frequently nonmodulated, flat, and emotionless in character. The child may have difficulty with "pragmatic" language, such as recognizing the meaning of what is said or using language appropriately in a social setting. Normal or near normal IQ is typically present, as is the ability to develop self-help and other adaptive behaviors needed to participate in activities of daily living (Inglese & Elder, 2009). Because cognitive functioning is usually within, or even above, normal ranges coupled with the lack of language delays, a diagnosis of Asperger's disorder may not be made until the child reaches school age, when social demands of the classroom setting make their functional impairments more evident.

C. **Rett's Disorder:** Rett's disorder is a neurodegenerative disorder that is seen almost exclusively in females. Developmental milestones proceed normally through early infancy, except for abnormal sleep problems. This is followed by onset of global, developmental regression between five and thirty months of age (Batshaw et al., 2007; Bienvenu et al., 2000; Phetrasuwan et al., 2009). In addition to this degeneration, other prominent features include decelerating head circumference rate, hand wringing, spasticity, breath holding, and abnormal EEG with or without clinical seizure activity. It is now possible to confirm 60% to 80% of Rett's disorder cases by conducting DNA analysis studies to identify the methyl-CpG-binding protein-2 gene (*MECP2*) on the X chromosome (Johnson & Myers, 2007; Kirby et al., 2009; Van Acker, Loncola, & Van Acker, 2005). Recent survey research suggests that the majority of women with Rett's disorder survive until middle age, "suggesting the need for careful planning for their long term care, as well as continued observation of the effects of improved clinical management on longevity" (Kirby et al., 2010, p. 138).

D. **Childhood Disintegrative Disorder:** Childhood disintegrative disorder (CDD) is a rare form of autism. It is estimated that fewer than 2 children per 100,000 with an ASD are diagnosed with CDD. It is also dominated by male prevalence at a ratio of approximately 4:1 (Filipek et al., 1999; NIMH, 2008). The disorder is distinguished by the onset of significant deterioration in social, motor, and language skills; bowel and bladder control; and intellectual function (Batshaw et al., 2007; Nash & Coury, 2003; Phetrasuwan et al., 2009). The DSM-IV-TR specifies that the onset of regression must be preceded by a period of *at least two years but not less than 10 years* of normal developmental progression (American Psychiatric Association, 2000). As developmental regression continues, the

Table 13.3 Diagnostic criteria for autistic disorder

A. A total of 6 (or more) items from the following groups:

Group 1 (At least 2 criteria)	Group 2 (At least 1 criterion)	Group 3 (At least 1 criterion)
1. Marked impairment in the use of multiple nonverbal behaviors, such as eye-to-eye gaze, facial expression, body postures and gestures to regulate social interaction	1. Delay in, or total lack of, the development of spoken language (not accompanied by an attempt to compensate through alternative modes of communication such as gesture or mime)	1. Encompassing preoccupation with one or more stereotyped and restricted patterns of interest that is abnormal either in intensity or focus
2. Failure to develop peer relationships appropriate to developmental level	3. In individuals with adequate speech, marked impairment in the ability to initiate or sustain a conversation with others	2. Apparently inflexible adherence to specific, nonfunctional routines or rituals
4. A lack of spontaneous seeking to share enjoyment, interests, or achievements with others (e.g., by lack of showing, bringing, or pointing out objects of interest)	5. Stereotyped and repetitive use of language or idiosyncratic language	3. Stereotyped and repetitive motor mannerisms (e.g., hand or finger flapping or twisting, complex whole body movements)
6. Lack of social or emotional reciprocity	7. Lack of varied, spontaneous make-believe play or social imitative play appropriate to developmental level	4. Persistent preoccupation with parts of objects.

B. Delays or abnormal functioning in at least one of the following areas with onset prior to age 3 years:
1) Social interaction
2) Language as used in social communication
3) Symbolic or imaginative play

C. The disturbance is not better accounted for by Rett's Disorder or Childhood Disintegrative Disorder

Adapted from Batshaw, Pellegrino and Roizen, 2007, with permission from Paul H. Brooks Publishing.

child also begins to exhibit the typical, core features of autism. Abnormal EEG patterns, with or without clinical seizures, are also frequently a feature of CDD. Because of the late onset of symptoms, medical evaluation should be initiated to eliminate other progressive, neurodegenerative disorders that may share features of CDD.

E. **Pervasive Developmental Disorder-Not Otherwise Specified:** PDD-NOS, often referred to as "atypical autism," is diagnosed when a child displays significant autistic symptoms but does not meet the full number or distribution of criteria needed to diagnose another entity within the autism spectrum (Batshaw et al., 2007; Phetrasuwan et al., 2009). Thus, PDD-NOS is a diagnosis of exclusion of the other entities on the autism spectrum (Filipek et al., 1999). In general, "intellectual and language skills tend to be preserved, and because of this, these children tend to be recognized by parents or professionals later than those with autistic disorder" (Volkmar & Lord, 2007, p. 8).

The diagnostic criteria for ASD will likely change with the publication of the fifth edition of the Diagnostic and Statistical Manual of Mental Disorders (DSM-V). While unclear at this writing, the changes are likely to be highly debated and controversial (http://www.dsm5.org/Proposed Revisions/Pages/InfancyChildhoodAdolescence. aspx).

Associated Conditions

Children diagnosed with ASD often display one or more associated psychiatric and/or medical conditions.

Psychiatric Comorbidities

A study conducted by Leyfer et al. (2006) using the Autism Co-morbidity Interview (ACI) identified 72% of their patient sample with at least one psychiatric disorder in addition to the primary diagnosis of autism.

1. **Intellectual Disability (ID):** Estimates of ID as a comorbidity of ASD range from 40% to 68% (Chakrabarti & Frombonne, 2001; Rice, 2009; Yeargin-Allsopp et al., 2003). IQ testing often reveals variable results, with some areas falling within normal ranges, while others are especially low (NIMH, 2008). Because some of the signs and symptoms of severe to profound intellectual disability (ID) may mimic the characteristics of ASD (e.g., stereotyped movements), careful diagnostic evaluation is needed to determine if ID is a "stand alone" diagnosis or a true comorbidity (Batshaw et al., 2007).

2. **Attention Deficit Hyperactivity Disorder (ADHD):** It is estimated that approximately 30% to 75% of children with ASD also have ADHD (Leyfer et al., 2006; Peacock et al., 2009). "Symptoms of *inattention, impulsivity and hyperactivity* observed in children with ASD are similar to those in other children with a diagnosis of only ADHD" (Posey et al., 2007, p. 538). In addition, symptoms of ASD that exacerbate the hallmark criteria of ADHD include poor reading of social cues, reduced ability to use "self-talk" to work through problems, and a diminished sense of self-awareness. Thus, when children cannot stay focused on situations that they do not understand, they will develop a short attention span. Inattention is usually twice as frequent as combined inattention-hyperactivity in the ASD population. As in children with *only* ADHD, the autistic child who has this comorbidity can perseverate on a preferred activity. However, there has been some disagreement as to whether this diagnosis can be ascribed "when the characteristic criteria outlined in the DSM-IV only occur in the context of an ASD" (Posey, 2007, p. 538). Although debate about this diagnostic rule continues and it is likely to change in DSM-V, there can be no doubt that these behaviors are some of the most disruptive and frequently reported by parents and teachers (Posey et al., 2007).

3. **Mood Disorders:** Comorbid mood disorders are estimated to occur in 25% to 40% of older children diagnosed with ASD (Peacock, Hyman, & Levy, 2009). Such disorders include, but are not limited to, major depression, bipolar illness, and anxiety disorders. Identification of such disorders is most readily apparent in children and adolescents who have sufficient language skills and insight to permit standard application of diagnostic criteria for these diagnoses (Batshaw et al., 2007). As these children grow older and confront increasing difficulties with social interaction and communication, it is understandable that they develop anxiety, avoid peers, favor a rigid adherence to sameness, and have a relative preference for *things* that are predictable, rather than *people* (Kutscher, 2006).

As Reaven (2009) notes: "Individuals with developmental disabilities are at increased risk for developing a variety of co-occurring mental health conditions, compared to children with a history of typical development … children with high-functioning autism and Asperger's Disorder are at even greater risk for developing psychiatric symptoms, particularly anxiety symptoms" (p. 193).

It can be quite challenging to identify psychiatric symptoms in a normally developing child, and more so in a child with a developmental disorder when "psychosocial masking" makes it difficult for a child to report psychiatric symptoms because of his/her cognitive and/or language impairments (Reaven, 2009). In an effort to address this issue, Leyfer et al. (2006) modified the Kiddie Schedule for Affective Disorders and Schizophrenia (K-SADS) by adding screening questions and revising coding options to better indicate common psychiatric symptoms in the ASD population. The modified instrument, the Autism Co-Morbidity Interview-Present and Lifetime Version (ACI-PL), was found to be a valid and reliable semistructured interview tool to identify psychiatric conditions in older children and adolescents with ASD.

4. **Depression:** In a study of 109 children with ASD aged five to seventeen conducted by Leyfer et al. (2006), almost 25% of the sample met lifetime diagnostic criteria for a depressive episode significant enough to impair daily functioning.

5. **Anxiety Disorders:** Various types of anxiety disorders are thought to be so common in ASD that there has been some consideration by autism experts that this should be included as a defining characteristic for the diagnosis (Leyfer et al., 2006). Subtypes of anxiety disorders that most frequently occur in older children with ASD include generalized anxiety disorder, separation anxiety, specific or social phobias, and obsessive-compulsive disorder (Reaven, 2009). Reported rates of occurrence of at least one of these types of anxiety disorder have ranged from 17% to 84% (Leyfer et al., 2006). Leyfer et al. (2006) attribute such wide variation in incidence to the use of different evaluation tools, employment of lay interviewers in some studies, and differences in the characteristics of the children who were studied. Symptoms associated with anxiety can significantly interfere with the child's functioning at home, at school, and in the community and exacerbate the core deficits of the primary ASD diagnosis (Reaven, 2009). Clues

that an anxiety disorder may coexist with an ASD include fears and worries that are out of proportion to a situation; symptoms that increase in frequency, duration, and intensity over time; and symptoms that are not responsive to normal reassurances (Reaven, 2009).

6. **Obsessive-Compulsive Disorder (OCD):** Although symptoms of generalized anxiety disorder, social phobia, and separation anxiety tend to be similar, the symptoms associated with OCD are felt to be qualitatively different. An individual with OCD has persistent, illogical, and obsessive thoughts and ideas that cannot be suppressed and that are often associated with repetitive behaviors or mental acts, such as checking and rechecking, counting, hoarding, and maintaining symmetry and order within the environment. Leyfer et al. (2006) note that in reviewed studies, the rate of OCD in children with ASD ranged from 1.5% to 81%.

7. **Phobias:** The development of irrational fears in children with ASD is a common finding. Specific phobias occur more frequently than social phobias, and prevalence has been estimated to range from 44% to 64% of children with autism (Leyfer et al., 2006). Fear of loud sounds is one of the most frequently noted phobias in the ASD population (Leyfer et al., 2006).

8. **Challenging Behaviors:** Challenging behaviors in children with ASD often include physical aggression, property destruction, defiance, tantrums including head banging, self-injurious behaviors (SIB), pica, and attention deficit (Horner, Carr, Strain, Todd, & Reed, 2002; Horner, Diemer, & Brazeau, 1992; Ospina et al., 2008; Reichele, 1990). Although these behaviors may not meet diagnostic criteria for a specific disorder, children who present with one or more of these challenging behaviors negatively impact the relationship with their parents, siblings, peers, and adversely impact their ability to attend to learning in classroom and home environments. A functional assessment includes an interview, direct observation, and functional analysis of behavior. This assessment is used to determine the relationship between the environmental events and occurrence of specific challenging behaviors and should occur prior to beginning any intervention (Horner et al. 2002).

Medical Comorbidities

1. **Sleep Disturbances:** Sleep disturbances are a frequently reported problem in children with ASD at all levels of functioning. Prevalence estimates range from 44% to 83% and include difficulties with prolonged sleep latency, restless sleep, insistence on co-sleeping, and frequent awakenings (Wiggs & Stores, 2004; Williams, Sears, & Allard, 2004). Research evidence supports screening all children with ASD for sleep disturbances during each annual and episodic visit. Children with suspected sleep apnea warrant additional testing and should be referred to a sleep specialist for polysomnography (Ivanenko & Johnson, 2008). Positive screening results should lead to a clinical diagnosis of a functional sleep disorder and formulation of an individualized treatment plan. Interventions to restore more normal sleep patterns in the child with an ASD are crucial, as sleep deprivation and disruption inevitably contribute an added stressor to already stressed families (Doo & Wing, 2006).

2. **Fragile X Syndrome:** FXS is an X-linked disorder that is the most common inherited cause of intellectual disabilities. The term "fragile" was assigned to this condition because of the appearance of an easily broken site at the distal end of the long arm of the X chromosome on karyotype analysis. It is estimated that FXS is a comorbidity in 5% of individuals with autism (Caglayan, 2010). Caglayan (2010) further reports that it has been estimated that approximately 90% of males with FXS "exhibit one or more of the three major characteristics of autism, such as difficulties with social interaction, lack of eye contact, social anxiety and avoidance, perseverative speech, stereotypic behavior, hypersensitivity to sensory stimuli, impulsive aggression or self injurious behavior" (p. 131).

3. **Tuberous Sclerosis:** TS is an autosomal dominant, neurocutaneous disorder caused by the *TSC1* and *TSC2* genes on chromosome 16 that code for the protein tuberin. It is estimated that 1% to 4% of individuals with ASD have TS (Batshaw et al., 2007). Affected children display a range of features, depending on the penetrance of the gene, including adenoma sebaceum, hypopigmented skin lesions (ash leaf spots), seizures, and benign growths or *tubers*, which can affect the brain, skin, and major organs. Mild to moderate intellectual disability often accompanies this disorder when tuberous growths develop in the brain.

4. **Epilepsy:** The reported prevalence of seizures in children diagnosed with ASD varies widely in the literature, ranging from 11% to 39% (Barbaresi et al., 2006; Myers & Johnson, 2007; Peacock et al., 2009). Barbaresi et al. (2006) report that onset of

seizures in individuals with autism peaks in early childhood and adolescence. Although all classifications of seizure types may be seen, complex partial seizures with a temporal lobe focus seem to be most prevalent. There is also increased likelihood of a child with ASD demonstrating an abnormal EEG pattern without the occurrence of clinical seizure activity (Batshaw et al., 2007).

5. **Tic Disorders:** Up to 9% of children with ASD also have motor or vocal tics (Ringman & Jankovic, 2000). If tic behavior persists for at least one year, an associated diagnosis of Tourette's syndrome can be ascribed to the child. The co-occurrence of tic disorders in children with diagnosed ASD has also been linked to an increased risk of developing more complex psychiatric symptomatology (Gadow & DeVincent, 2005).

Interventions and Plan

The ideal intervention for youth with ASD is individualized and treats each child's complex and unique set of communicative, behavioral, sensory, and cognitive characteristics. There is no cure, but intervention can improve quality of life and bring about substantial improvement in symptoms. Treatment must be intensive and may involve a multidisciplinary team of professionals and therapists. Most health professionals agree that the earlier the intervention, the better is the prognosis. Unfortunately, the nature of the disorder has attracted many controversial and unproven treatments and parents should use caution before adopting such approaches. APNs are in prime positions to help parents evaluate potential treatments and develop a treatment plan.

Interventions for Speech and Language Development

If a child is not diagnosed with ASD prior to the age of four or five, the prekindergarten physical examination or the pre–kindergarten school screening test may be the first time that a differential diagnosis of ASD is considered by the primary care APN. If the child received a possible diagnosis of ASD in the preschool years, the parents may have been hopeful that early intervention services would prepare the child for regular kindergarten. If the child is physically well, most often the child only has primary care visits annually beginning at the age of three; thus the primary care APN may suddenly be confronted with parents who are baffled with the educational system and are questioning what may happen to the child. The primary care APN may be assessing the child for the first time in the pediatric office as the child

may be a new patient or a child who has just entered the foster care system.

The primary care APN will make referrals to the school system if the child is over three years old; the children then receive special services within the school system. The APN may also refer the child for a neurodevelopmental examination with a pediatric developmental specialist and/or a psychiatrist or psychiatric APN. Specific interventions for the child will be based on the assessment findings and the specific diagnosis.

It is imperative for parents to understand that acquisition of useful spoken language by children with a diagnosis of Asperger's or within the ASD requires intensive and lengthy educational processes that often have less-than-optimal outcomes (Goldstein, 2002; Howlin & Rutter 1989). Children with a diagnosis of Asperger's may have higher IQs and understandable language; however, the child's language skills may not "fit" normal conversation patterns and may not be socially acceptable. Speech patterns and language development for a child with a diagnosis of ASD also vary significantly as the child may use a few words or gestures or may have a severe deficit and no spoken language.

Since language proficiency and IQ have been shown to be related to the outcomes for children with ASD (Venter, Lord, & Schopler, 1992), a significant amount of research has focused on acquisition of spoken language (Rogers et al., 2006). However, results of long-term outcome studies conducted in the late 1980s and 1990s in children with a classic diagnosis of autism have estimated that between one-third and two-thirds of children with ASD never acquire spoken language (Charlop & Haynes, 1994; Frankel, Leary, & Kilman, 1987; Weitz, Dexter, & Moore, 1997) and that 80% of children with a diagnosis of autism have no spoken language or only exhibit self-stimulatory or echolalic utterances when they enter kindergarten (Bondy & Frost, 1994a; Kraijer, 1999). These studies are the underpinnings of the treatment for children with a diagnosis of ASD after the 1990s, when interventions for children with ASD have intensively focused on helping children acquire language skills (Rogers et al., 2006). Thus, both primary care and mental health APNs are confronted with helping parents cope with a child who has ubiquitous speech problems. It is helpful for APNs to understand the types of interventions that have been tested in children with a diagnosis of ASD and those that lend evidence of success; today, parents are Internet savvy and may raise questions about programs that may or may not be available or applicable to their child, and the parents will need guidance from the APN to understand the current best available evidence to help their child.

Early models for speech development focused on applying learning theory principles within a behavioral developmental context (Rogers et al., 2006). The "discrete trial teaching" described in 1964 used adult-delivered instruction in massed trials in which the children were taught to respond to simple instructions from the adult through the imitation of manual, oral motor, and vocal behavior and then to imitate speech (Wolf, Risely, Mees, & Risely, 1964). A second developmental model described in 1968 (Hart & Risley, 1968; Prizant & Wetherby, 1998) used a child-initiated behavior followed by adult response of providing the child with the child-requested object which was viewed as a "natural reinforcer." Both of these developmental approaches to speech acquisition have been found to be effective in a number of independent replications (Goldstein, 2002; Koegel, 2000). However, both of these approaches required a minimum of one year of treatment involving twenty-five to forty hours of intervention each week in both educational and home settings.

The need to study more efficient ways to help children acquire spoken language resulted in researchers designing and testing methods that use language within the context of social interactions. An example of this approach is the Picture Exchange Communication System (PECS) (Frost & Bondy, 2002). Children were taught to approach a picture of a desired item, then to give the picture to a communication partner in exchange for receiving the item. In an experimentally controlled study, Carr and Felce (2007) investigated the effect of implementing PECS as a teaching strategy. After fifteen hours of PECS training over a period of four to five weeks, five of twenty-four children in the treatment group showed increases in speech production either in initiating communication or responding to staff or in both communicating and responding.

The Denver Model (Rogers, Hall, Osaki, Reaven, & Herbison, 2000) is an individualized developmental approach supported by the massed trial and naturalistic behavioral teaching but integrates the concepts of establishing an interpersonal relationship with speech acquisition. Children have a combination of once-weekly fifty-minute therapy sessions and daily home review by the parent. Teaching strategies include motivating social games, teaching imitation of actions on objects, focus on receptive understanding, object associations, increasing verbal approximations of target words, and including reinforcement at each stage of learning (Rogers et al., 2000, 2006).

Other researchers have suggested that part of the mechanism involving speech impairment in children with autism includes an oral motor dysfunction (Adams, 1998; Page & Boucher, 1998). The PROMPT model was designed based on the interrelationships of developing speech motor control with integration of sensory modalities and the enhancement of social-emotional interactions.

Rogers et al. (2006) investigated the effectiveness of the Denver Model and the PROMPT model on speech acquisition in ten nonverbal children with a diagnosis of autism that were matched in pairs and randomized to treatment. At the end of twelve weeks in which the children received one-hour weekly sessions of therapy and daily one-hour home interventions from the parents, eight of the ten children used five or more functional words spontaneously and spoke multiple times per hour by the end of the treatment program.

APNs must relay to the parents the significance of daily parental involvement in the home environment. Research evidence suggests that parents who work closely with the classroom teachers and speech therapists by continuing the educational curriculum for speech development at home on a daily basis see greater improvements in language acquisition for their children (Rogers et al., 2000).

Interventions for Social Skill Development

In the past decade there has been a significant increase in the amount of research on social skills interventions for those with ASD (Reichow & Volkmar, 2008). Comparisons of the efficacy of different training strategies are beginning (Reichow & Volkmar, 2008; Wang & Spillane, 2009; White, Keonig, & Scahill, 2007). However, which intervention is most effective for which children remains unknown (Wang & Spillane, 2009). Social skill interventions should be individualized and focused on the unique characteristics of the specific child (Bellini & Peters, 2008). Common social skill interventions include the following:

Direct Instruction

Individual and group instruction programs are child specific and typically focus on developing basic interpersonal skills, conversational dialogue, play and friendship skills, social problem solving, and emotion processing (Bellini, 2006; Coucouvanis, 2005; Krasny, Williams, Provencal, & Ozonoff, 2003). Strategies include prompting, coaching, role modeling, role play, scripting, structured teaching, guided activities, and feedback. While promising, these strategies and programs require further study to determine treatment efficacy (Reichow & Volkmar, 2008).

Video Modeling

An emerging strategy is video modeling (Bellini & Akullian, 2007). Using the child or other designated models, including commercially prepared videos, the child learns by observing and imitating social behaviors of those depicted in the video. This approach has promise as a highly effective intervention (Wang & Spillane, 2009).

Use of a Social Story™

A Social Story™ (Gray, 2000) describes a situation, skill, or concept in narrative format. It includes a clear description of the situation, the perspective of others in that same situation, and a statement of desired social response from the child. Social Stories™ require more study of treatment effectiveness (Wang & Spillane, 2009).

Peer-Mediated Intervention

Peer-mediated intervention strategies train nondisabled peers as buddies, mentors, and playmates. Usually classmates, trained peers initiate interactions and respond appropriately to children with ASD in structured and natural environments (Bellini, 2006). This intervention has support and should be considered a recommended practice for all individuals with autism (Reichow & Volkmar, 2008).

Interventions for Challenging Behaviors

A recent systematic review of the literature on interventions for challenging behaviors showed that studies tended to be methodologically weak, with few participants, and reported results for short-term follow-up only. Thus, the value of the behavioral interventions toward impacting challenging behaviors provided limited clinical evidence (Ospina et al. 2008). As a result, the current trend is to identify and recommend individualized treatment plans for each child based on the presenting symptoms and the assessment of the child's individualized responses to the behavioral interventions.

Environmental engineering is a strategy that has shown success in altering the future likelihood of challenging behaviors (Horner et al., 2002). Strategies include changing the physical characteristics of the environment in which the child plays, learns, and interacts with others, altering schedules, reorganizing social groups at home and school, and using curricula adjustment to meet the individual needs of the child (Carr, Langdon, & Yarbrough, 1999; Carr et al., 1994).

Structured teaching using the Treatment and Education of Autistic and related Communication-handicapped Children (TEACCH) method (Mesibov, 1997; Mesibov, Shea, & Schopler, 2005) has shown promise although the reports of success are not from controlled studies. Elements of structured teaching include organizing the physical environment, predictable sequences of activities, and visually structured

activities (Myers, Johnson, & the Council on Children with Disabilities, 2007).

Positive behavior support (PBS) has been studied with a small number of participants and has been shown to be an effective strategy for reducing challenging behaviors. PBS emphasizes person-centered values, lifestyle change, and a comprehensive approach to the challenging behaviors (Buschbacher & Fox, 2003). Similarly, a meta-analysis by Ospina et al. (2008) concluded that the Lovass technique, which is a behavioral intervention treatment based on applied behavioral analysis and uses discrete trial teaching, was superior to other interventions (Lovass, 1987).

An acute exacerbation of aggressive behaviors should be investigated by the APN for possible medical causes such as infections and conditions that cause pain, such as otitis media, pharyngitis, dental abscesses, urinary tract infections, or onset of menstrual cycle in an adolescent (Myers et al., 2007).

Interventions for Sleep Problems

Individualized treatment plans are formulated based on the child's presenting sleep disturbance, the length of time the sleep disturbance has persisted, the pattern of the disturbance, the sleep environment, the effect on parents and all household members, previous treatments, and their impact on the problem. Treatment plans may include behavioral interventions, medication, herbal treatments, massage therapy, or a combination of two or more of these modalities (Ivaneko & Johnson, 2008; Polimeni, Richdale, & Francis, 2005). Reports of treatment success or failure are limited since the majority of the studies on treatment outcomes for sleep disturbances in children with ASD and especially autism are limited by sample size or individual case reports (Escalona, Field, Singer-Strunck, Cullen, & Hartshorn, 2001; Ivaneko & Johnson, 2008; Polimeni et al., 2005; Weiskop, Matthews, & Richdale, 2001; Weiskop, Richdale, & Matthews, 2005).

Behavioral interventions may focus on a gradual reduction of previously established excessive bedtime rituals, strategies to reduce and eliminate tantrums, consistent reinforcement and appropriate rewards, calming parental behaviors (i.e., speaking calmly), and a calm environment (calm background music) at least one-half hour before the established bedtime (Escalona et al., 2001; Ivaneko & Johnson, 2008; Polimeni et al., 2005; Weiskop et al., 2001; Weiskop et al., 2005). More recent biological research on sleep-wake cycles has the potential to contribute to affective interventions for children with ASD. Future research studies that investigate the establishment of a new pattern for sleep through activation of the suprachiasmatic nucleus

Table 13.4 Communication interventions

Intervention	Description	Investigators/Reviewers
Sign language stand alone	Not effective: multiple studies revealed a diminished likelihood of speech development	Reviewed: Goldstein, 2002
Total communication	Speech plus sign provided limited evidence. However, this strategy may be a beginning point for early vocabulary learning	Reviewed: Goldstein, 2002
Discrete-trial training formats	Language production and comprehension have been shown to be primarily effective in the behaviors of interest but limited evidence for functioning on everyday activities	Reviewed: Goldstein, 2002
Time delay and correction procedures	Delay is imposed between a stimulus and a prompt with modeling to imitate the expected response	Charlop, Schreibman, and Thibodeau, 1985
Milieu language	Uses child's desires and interests to encourage speech Lacks strong evidence of effectiveness	Hart and Risley, 1975

(SCN) (Fuller, Gooley, & Saper, 2006)—for example, by dimming lights prior to sleep followed by exposure to bright light immediately after awakening—may hold promise for changing the physiological mechanisms of the sleep-wake cycle in children. Medications for treatment of insomnia may be prescribed and reevaluated one and three months after the initiation (see Chapter 6).

Psychopharmacology Interventions Specific to ASD Population

Seventy percent of children with ASD eight years and older receive psychiatric medication, often treated under the ASD diagnosis, even though the target symptoms may be commonly associated with other disorders (Oswald & Sonenklar, 2007). Psychopharmacology agents are used to treat severe and sustained behaviors that are negatively impacting a child's ability to participate in daily activities. They may also be used when other treatment approaches have failed to adequately improve symptoms or to treat coexisting psychiatric disorders, such as ADHD, OCD or Tourette's. In ASD, psychiatric medications are matched to the individual patient's presenting symptoms.

Typical reasons for prescribing medication include irritability, aggression, temper outbursts, self-injurious behavior, hyperactivity, poor attention span, poor impulse control, anxiety, fears, obsessive phenomena, rituals, compulsions, tics, depressed mood, and sleep problems (Findling, 2005).

Medications are not used to treat core deficits of autism but to treat symptoms. The response to medications is often different than for typically developing children, requiring lower dosages and slower titration (Table 13.4). More controlled and randomized medication trials in children and youth with ASD are needed.

To initiate medication treatment, the APN should carefully identify and assess the specific problem or symptom to be treated and the degree of interference with daily functioning. If the presenting problem is within the APN's scope of practice, the next step is to determine the frequency, intensity, and duration of the problem, and any exacerbating factors, such as illness, setting, time of day, recurrent event, or coexisting condition. The response to previously tried behavioral intervention should be reviewed and a system to monitor the target behavior and adverse events at baseline and at regular intervals developed (see Chapter 6).

Atypical Antipsychotic Agents

The Food and Drug Administration has approved risperidone and aripiprazole for the symptomatic treatment of irritability in children and teens with autism ages six to seventeen. Risperidone has been found effective in decreasing severe tantrums, aggression and self-injurious behavior (Scahill, Koenig, Carroll, & Pachler, 2007). Aripiprazole is used to treat similar behaviors.

In addition to the risk of dyskinesia, one of the principal safety concerns with atypical antipsychotic medication is severely increased appetite and weight gain (McCracken, 2005). Children taking risperidone can become markedly obese. Prior to beginning medication management, the APN should assess the child's height, weight, and body mass index (BMI) and determine the total caloric intake needed to maintain a normal growth pattern. The APN must evaluate the child's diet and lifestyle to identify needed changes, while also monitoring height, weight, and abdominal girth at every visit. Monitoring also includes fasting plasma glucose, fasting lipid panel, blood pressure, and pulse at baseline, three months, and every six months (Correll, 2008).

Dietary modifications frequently include the following: replace sugar-containing drinks with water, dilute fruit juice, replace soft drinks with sparkling water mixed with a small amount of juice, increase fresh fruits, vegetables, and fiber whenever possible, choose low-fat products, and monitor serving sizes and portions. Finally, reduce and preferably eliminate the consumption of sugared candy and treats. Lifestyle modifications include increasing exercise such as jumping on a trampoline, swimming, walking, riding bikes, or playing chase games while reducing time spent in sedentary activities.

Another side effect of risperidone is an elevated prolactin level. Hyperprolactinemia may cause gynecomastia, galactorrhea, irregular menses, amenorrhea, sexual dysfunction, and reduced fertility (Roke, van Harten, Boot, & Buitelaar, 2009). Serum prolactin levels should be monitored every six months. Antipsychotic-induced hyperprolactinemia can be treated by reducing the dose or switching to a prolactin-sparing antipsychotic, such as quetiapine or ziprasidone (Roke et al., 2009).

Selective Serotonin Reuptake Inhibitors (SSRIs)

SSRIs are commonly used off label in children with ASD. Open-label and retrospective studies suggest improvement in overall global functioning and in a wide range of symptoms (anxiety, aggression, repetitive behavior), but a recent analysis found no evidence that SSRIs are effective in treating autism (Williams, Wheeler, Silove, & Hazell, 2010).

A major concern in treating children and teens with SSRIs is the risk of activation. Activation events include irritability, anger outbursts, excitability, manic symptoms, hyperactivity, agitation, nervousness, sleep disturbance lability, and hostility. Mood must be monitored very closely and it may take up to eight to ten weeks to achieve moderate total daily doses. Mood lability, difficulty settling at night, irritability, and mild agitation may be signs of an activation syndrome (McCracken, 2005). The decision to treat conditions that accompany ASD, such as OCD or depression, with an SSRI should be made on an individual basis (Williams et al., 2010). The best responders may be those with ASD who do not have high levels of agitation or mood cycling at baseline. If activation occurs, reduce the dose and slow further titration.

Stimulants

Stimulants are used in children with ASD to treat symptoms of hyperactivity, poor attention span, and poor impulse control. Clinical studies with methylphenidate suggest that 50% of children with ASD show a positive response versus 75% of typical children with ADHD. The mean improvement is 20% to 25% versus 50% in typical children with ADHD (Scahill & Pachler, 2007). There are no data on long-term treatment with stimulants in children with ASD.

The major concern with stimulants is loss of appetite, increased agitation and irritability, tic onset, and sleep disturbance. To improve tolerance, use lower doses, longer titration periods, and extended release preparations (McCracken, 2005).

Complementary and Alternative Medicine Interventions

Complementary and alternative medicine (CAM) interventions encompass a broad range of practices and treatments (Table 13.5). Parental use of CAM in children with ASD is significantly increased when such children experience ID or global developmental delays in addition to ASD (Hanson et al., 2007). Many parents believe CAM is safer than more conventional medicine and that it treats the underlying cause of ASD (Hanson et al., 2007). Despite the lack of treatment efficacy, CAM is reported by parents and some professionals to improve behavior, speech, learning, sleep, eye contact, and social interaction.

One of the most popular CAM treatments is the gluten-free/casein-free (GFCF) diet. Gastrointestinal (GI) problems impact some people with autism and reports in the lay literature indicate children on this specialized diet show improved attention, focus, language, and social skills. Gluten is found in the seeds of various plants—wheat, oat, rye, and barley—and casein is the principal protein in cow's milk. It has been hypothesized that these proteins are absorbed differently in children with autism and act like opiates in the brain (Levy & Hyman, 2005).

It is prudent for the APN to monitor the child's GI health. If a child presents with recurrent abdominal pain, diarrhea, constipation, bloating, reflux, or related issues (including a significant behavior change), it is reasonable to evaluate the GI tract. If a problem is suspected, the APN can take a comprehensive diet and GI history and consider referring the child to a pediatric gastroenterologist.

Adherence to the GFCF diet is difficult, expensive, and time-consuming and is not recommended as a standard treatment for ASD (Millward, Ferriter, Calver, & Connell-Jones, 2009). Other common CAM treatments for children with ASD are listed in Table 13.5.

Because of the pervasive use of CAM there is a need for more rigorous research into efficacy. Presently there is

Table 13.5 Psychopharmacology and ASD

Drug	Target Behavior(s)	Dosing	Adverse Effects
Antipsychotics			
*risperidone	Irritability (aggression, agitation, temper outbursts, self-injurious behavior)	Initiation dose 0.25 mg daily Expected range 0.5–3 mg daily	Weight gain. Note: Provide healthy lifestyle instruction at every visit
SSRIs			
**fluoxetine	Major depression, OCD anxiety	Initiation dose Child: 2.5–5 mg daily Teen: 5 mg daily Initial target Child: 10–20 mg Teen: 10–20 mg Expected range Child: 5–40 mg Teen: 10–60 mg	Activation: agitation, insomnia, increased activity, increased anxiety, mood lability To avoid activation: Initiate with very low starting doses Titrate very gradually, much slower than for a typical child/adult Nausea, vomiting sedation
**sertraline	OCD anxiety	Initiation dose Child: 10–25 mg Teen: 25–50 mg Initial target Child: 50 mg Teen: 50 mg Expected range Child: 50–150 mg Teen: 50–200 mg Increase doses at 1–2 week intervals	Be aware of CAM use
**fluvoxamine	OCD anxiety	Initiation dose Child: 25 mg Teen: 25–50 mg Initial target Child: 150 mg Teen: 200 mg Expected range Child: 50–200 mg Teen: 100–300 mg Divide doses >50 mg Increase by 25 mg every 1–2 weeks	
Stimulants			
***methylphenidate	Hyperactivity Impulsivity Inattention		Higher than expected rate of adverse events (10% vs. < 2% in typical kids). Irritability, increased aggression, insomnia, anorexia, increased stereotypic behavior

*FDA approved for children with autism ages 5–17.
**FDA approved for children with major depression/OCD.
***FDA approved for children with ADHD.
From Gleason et al., 2007; and McCracken, 2005.

Table 13.6 Common CAM treatments for ASD

Biologically Based Treatment	Purpose	Method
Special diets	To treat GI problems that are believed to cause autism	Gluten free, casein free, sugar free Specific carbohydrate and yeast free
Antifungal agents, probiotics, digestive enzymes	Reduce presumed fungal infections in the intestine	Tablet, powder
Antiviral agents, intravenous immunoglobulins	Modulate the immune system	Intravenous
Chelation therapy	Remove heavy metals from the body	Intravenous
Hyperbaric oxygen therapy	Increase oxygen levels in the brain	High pressure chamber
Vitamin and mineral supplement: B6 (pyridoxine) and magnesium, B12, DMG (dimethylglycine), C and D, fish oil/essential fatty acids	Modulate neurotransmitter production/ brain development/ presumed deficiency to improve behavior, speech, learning and eye contact	Tablet, pill, powder, cream, liquid, gel, injection
Non–biologically Based Treatments		
Auditory integration training	Treat sound sensitivity	Exposure to sound via earphones
Vision therapy	Affect visual scrutiny	Eye exercises, prism lens
Sensory integration therapy	Facilitate the nervous system's ability to process and modulate sensory input	Brushing, weighted vest, swinging, jumping, body sock, massage, joint compression
Animal therapy	Improve social and relationship skills	Interacting with animals

From Hanson et al., 2007; Levy and Hyman, 2005; and Association for Science in Autism Treatment website: http://www.asatonline.org/intervention/treatments.desc.htm

insufficient empirical data supporting or refuting claims of "cure" or even improvement (Myers & Johnson, 2007). Currently the available data are inadequate to guide treatment recommendations (Myers & Johnson, 2007).

APN best practices include the following:

- Be aware that families will use CAM.
- Inquire what treatments are being used.
- Provide unbiased information and advice.
- Identify risks and potential harmful effects.
- Maintain open communication.
- Critically evaluate the scientific merits of treatments and share the information with parents.

Integration with Primary Care

ASDs are pervasive, chronic conditions that do not remit with the passage of time. There is no known cure. Treatment requires multimodal collaboration from numerous professionals, including those in medical, educational, mental health, and specialty-based settings.

Consumers report confidence and trust in the care provided by nurses and nurses are cited as the most trusted health professionals (http://www.medicalnewstoday.com/articles/173627.php). Historically, APNs are essential professionals in the management of chronic conditions. They are likely to comprehend the context within which a child and family live, thus lending an understanding of their specific needs and how to address them. A partnership between psychiatric and pediatric advanced practice nurses can offer considerable leadership and guidance to the family struggling with ASD. Such a team of APNs is in a unique position to provide counseling, support, ongoing education, recommendations, referrals, advocacy, and case management throughout the life span of the individual with ASD.

Implications for Practice, Research, and Education

With 1 in 110 children affected by ASD, all APNs need to be prepared for the unique challenges and great diversity of these children. Parents and professionals are faced with difficult decisions when choosing treatments. There are no well-established clinical practice guidelines for treatment of ASD. Most professionals agree that early intervention is crucial and that most individuals respond favorably to highly structured behavioral programs. There is a growing body of empirical evidence that supports the use of behavioral/psychoeducational interventions and some medications for treatment of specific symptoms. However, for the numerous interventions currently in use, little scientific evidence from randomized controlled trials supports their efficacy. Many families use complementary and alternative treatments. Engaging families in open and honest discussions about the purpose, means, and desired treatment outcome(s) of any intervention option is essential for all practitioners.

Safe, effective, and personalized interventions are needed across the life span. In 2009, the Interagency Autism Coordinating Committee Strategic Plan for ASD Research reported: "Rigorous scientific studies are needed to develop and safely test the efficacy of comprehensive interventions, and to identify which elements are most effective in reducing or ameliorating symptoms for which persons" (http://iacc.hhs.gov/reports/2009/iacc-strategic-plan-for-autism-spectrum-disorder-research-jan26.shtml). Parents, caregivers, educators, and service providers must have this critical information when making treatment decisions. Intervention research requires large-scale studies that include randomized controlled trials. Evidence-based practice has become the standard in the field of health care. This standard of practice is needed in the treatment of ASD. Special attention is needed to treat co-occurring medical and psychiatric conditions as well as clinical trials of widely used interventions, such as CAM. While the body of research examining the efficacy of various treatments for ASD continues to grow, outcome studies of the effectiveness of behavioral, developmental, and cognitive therapies and approaches are also needed.

Based on the complexities of the diagnosis and management of children with ASD and the potential for comorbid conditions, and the number of children with these diagnosis that are seen in primary care centers, it is time to consider changes in the educational preparation of APNs. Pediatric advanced practice nursing students would benefit from a rotation in a behavioral management setting in which educational outcomes emphasize direct experiences in the assessment, diagnosis, and treatment of children with mental health disorders. Outcomes should also focus on the family dynamics and psychosocial support needed by the parents to help their child achieve his or her potential.

Likewise, rotations in child and adolescent mental health centers should be mandatory for psychiatric mental health providers who are now being educated within a family-based framework that may not offer specific child and adolescent rotations. Psychiatric APNs must understand the neuropsychiatric processes that influence the cognitive growth and development of children and adolescents to effectively treat children and help them become functional adults.

Case Exemplar

An eight-year-old girl, Susan, presented to her APN in primary care. She was diagnosed with ASD at age twenty-one months by a developmental pediatrician and had minimal communication skills, attended special education classes each day, and had been medically well. The child was not receiving any medication at this time and parents had been reluctant to consider this treatment intervention. Mother reported increasing irritability and disruptive behavior at home and school of a two-week duration. Despite a specialized behavior plan at school and home, the youngster had become more aggressive, hitting peers at school and siblings at home.

The APN, using an evidence-based practice model and the information presented by the parents and school, developed a clinical decision-making plan to better manage the problematic behaviors.

Clinical question: For an eight-year old child with a diagnosis of ASD who presents with new-onset irritability and disruptive behaviors, is the use of atypical antipsychotics or adding additional therapy sessions more effective in the management of new-onset disruptive behaviors?

A PubMed search at http://www.ncbi.nlm.nih.gov/ revealed two reports that assisted in planning care:

Pharmacotherapy of irritability in pervasive developmental disorders.

Stigler KA, McDougle CJ. Child Adolesc Psychiatr Clin N Am. 2008 Oct;17(4):739–52, vii–viii. Review. PMID: 18775367 [PubMed - indexed for MEDLINE]

Scott LJ, Dhillon S.

Risperidone: a review of its use in the treatment of irritability associated with autistic disorder in children and adolescents. Paediatr Drugs. 2007;9(5):343–54. Review. PMID: 17927305 [PubMed - indexed for MEDLINE]

A recommended plan of care was developed, based on the evidence from this search of the clinical question, the APNs knowledge (expert opinion) of ASD, and consideration of parent preferences. The APN began a discussion with parents on the merits of a trial of risperdone to better manage the child's aggressive and disruptive behaviors. The APN carefully explored the parental attitudes and beliefs about medication management and reviewed risks, benefits, side effects, and other treatment options. The APN discovered that the parents viewed needing medication as a marker that their daughter was "worse" and not likely to make developmental gains. The realities of this were explored with parents and they agreed to a trial of risperdone. She was started on risperdone 0.25 mg twice a day and showed a 50% improvement in disruptive behaviors at home and school.

Summary

ASDs are life-long developmental neuropsychiatric disorders that exist on a continuum from mild to severe. Each affected individual presents with a distinct set of characteristics that include behavioral, communication, and social impairments. Comorbid psychiatric and medical conditions are common. Due to the pervasiveness, complexity, and uniqueness of these characteristics, it is essential that treatment be individualized. APNs are in unique positions to partner with each other, family members, and other treatment providers to facilitate collaboration and optimize treatment outcomes for the child. Such working partnerships can continue to address challenges as the child transitions into adulthood.

Resources

Research Journals

The Journal of Autism and Developmental Disorders (JADD). Published by Springer

FOCUS on Autism and Other Developmental Disorders. Published by Hammill Institute on Disabilities and Sage

Autism Research. Published by Wiley InterScience

Autism – The International Journal of Research and Practice. Published in the U.K. by Sage Publications

Information and Resources

Association for Science in Autism Treatment: www.asatonline.org: The mission is to share accurate, scientifically sound information about autism and treatments for autism

Autism Science Foundation: www.autismsciencefoundation.org

Autism Science Foundation's mission is to support the autism research and to provide information about autism to the general public and increase awareness of autism spectrum disorders and the needs of individuals and families affected by autism.

Autism Society: www.autism-society.org: The Autism Society exists to improve the lives of those affected by autism, to provide public awareness about the day-to-day issues faced by people on the spec-

trum, advocate for appropriate services for individuals across the lifespan, and provide the latest information regarding treatment, education, research and advocacy.

Autism Source: www.autismsource.org: an on-line referral data base to find local resources, providers, services and support

Autism Speaks: www.autismspeaks.org: The mission of Autism Speaks is to facilitate global research into the causes, treatments, prevention and an eventual cure for autism, to raise public awareness about autism and its effects on individuals, families, and society, and to provide information and resources to improve the outcome of children, adolescents, and adults affected by autism.

Autism Watch: www.autism-watch.org: The purpose of Autism Watch is to provide basic information about autism, offer scientific analysis of autism therapies, discuss the merits of the many proposed causes of autism, identify reliable sources of help and information, report improper actions to regulatory agencies, and help people seek legal redress if they have been victimized.

Centers for Disease Control and Prevention: www.cdc.gov/ncbddd/autism: Information for families, people with ASD, health care providers, educators and policy makers, including facts, screening and diagnosis, treatment, data and statistics, research, links, etc.

First Signs: www.firstsigns.org: First Signs is dedicated to educating parents and professionals about autism and related disorders. The First Signs website provides information on a range of issues: from monitoring development, to concerns about a child; from the screening and referral process, to sharing concerns.

Interactive Autism Network: www.iancommunity.org: IAN was established at Kennedy Krieger Institute and is funded by a grant from Autism Speaks. IAN's goal is to facilitate research that will lead to advancements in understanding and treating autism spectrum disorders.

National Autism Center: www.nationalautismcenter.org: The National Autism Center is dedicated to serving children and adolescents with Autism Spectrum Disorders by providing reliable information, promoting best practices, and offering comprehensive resources for families, practitioners, and communities.

Quackwatch: www.quackwatch.com : a nonprofit corporation whose purpose is to combat health-related frauds, myths, fads, and fallacies. Information on quackery, questionable therapies.

TEACCH: Treatment and Education of Autism and related Communication-handicapped CHildren: www.teacch.com: an evidence-based service, training, and research program for individuals of all ages and skill levels with autism spectrum disorder

100 Useful Sites, Networks, and Resources for Parents of Autistic Children: www.mastersinhealthcare.com/blog/2009/100-useful-sites-networks-and-resources-for-parents-of-autistic-children/

Publishers That Specialize in ASD and Related Disabilities

Autism Asperger Publishing Company: www.asperger.net

Future Horizons: www.fhautism.com

Woodbine Publishing House: www.woodbinehouse.com

Brookes Publishing: www.brookespublishing.com

Jessica Kingsley Publishers:www.jkp.com

References

Adams, L. (1998). Oral-motor and motor-speech characteristics of children with autism. *Focus on Autism and Other Developmental Disabilities, 13*, 108–112. doi:10.1177/108835769801300207

American Psychiatric Association. (2000). *Diagnostic and statistical manual of mental disorders* (4th ed., Text Revision). Washington, DC: Author.

Baranek, G., Boyd, B., Poe, M., Fabian, D., & Watson, L., (2007). Hyperresponsive sensory patterns in young children with autism, developmental delay and typical development. *American Journal on Mental Retardation, 112*(4), 233–245.

Barbaresi, W., Katusic, S., & Voigt, R. (2006). Autism: A review of the state of the science for pediatric primary health care providers. *Archives of Pediatrics and Adolescent Medicine, 160*, 1167–1175.

Batshaw, M., Pellegrino, L., & Roizen, N. (2007). *Children with disabilities*. (6th ed.), Baltimore, MD: Paul H.Brooks Publishing.

Beauchesne, M., & Kelley, B. (2004). Evidence to support parental concerns as an early childhood indicator of autism in children. *Pediatric Nursing, 30*(1), 57–67.

Bellini, S. (2006). *Building social relationships: A systematic approach to teaching social interaction skills to children and adolescents with autism spectrum disorders and other social difficulties*. Shawnee Mission, KS: Autism Asperger Publishing Company.

Bellini, S. & Akullian, J. (2007). A meta-analysis of video modeling and video self-modeling interventions for children and adolescents with autism spectrum disorders. *Exceptional Children, 73*(3), 264–287.

Bellini, S., & Peters, J. (2008). Social skills training for youth with autism spectrum disorders. *Child and Adolescent Psychiatric Clinics of North America, 17*(4), 857–873.

Bienvenu, T., Carrie, A., deRoux, N., Vinet, P., Couvert, L., Arzimanoglou, A., & Chelly, J. (2000). MECP2 mutations account for most cases of typical forms of Rett Syndrome. *Human Molecular Genetics, 9*(9), 1377–1384.

Bondy, A.S., & Frost, L.A. (1994). The Delaware Autistic Program. In S.L. Harris, & J.S. Handleman (Eds.). *Preschool education programs for children with autism*. Austin, TX: Pro-Ed.

Buschbacher, P. W., & Fox, L. (2003). Understanding and intervening with the challenging behavior of young children with autism spectrum disorder. *Language, Speech, and Hearing Services in Schools, 34*, 217–227. Retrieved from http://lshss.asha.org/cgi/reprint/34/3/217

Caglayan, A. (2010). Genetic causes of syndromic and non-syndromic autism. *Developmental Medicine and Child Neurology, 52*, 130–138. doi: 10.1111/j.1469-8749.2009.03523.x

Carr, D., & Felce, J. (2007). Brief report: Increase in production of spoken words in some children with autism after PECS teaching to Phase III. *Journal of Autism and Developmental Disorders, 37*, 780–787.

Carr, E.G., Levin, L., McConnachie, G., Carlson, J.I., Kemp, D.C., & Smith, C.E. (1994). *Communication based intervention for problem behavior: A user's guide for producing positive change*. Baltimore, MD: Paul H. Brookes.

Carr, E.G., Langdon, N.A., & Yarbrough, S. (1999). Hypothesis-based intervention for severe problem behavior. In A.C. Repp & R.H. Horner (Eds.). *Functional analysis of problem behavior: From effective assessment to effective support*. Belmont, CA: Wadsworth Publishing.

Carter, A.S. Davis, N.O. Klin, A., & Volkmar, F.R. (2005). Social development in autism. In F.R. Volkmar, R. Paul, A. Klin, & D. Cohen (Eds.) *Handbook of autism and pervasive developmental disorders: Vol. 1, Diagnosis, development, neurobiology, and behavior*. Hoboken, NJ: John Wiley & Sons.

Centers for Disease Control. (2010). Autism and Developmental Disability Monitoring Network. Retrieved from http://www,cdc.gov/ncbddd/autism/addm.html.

Chakrabarti, S., & Fombonne, E. (2001). Pervasive developmental disorders in preschool children. *JAMA, 285*(24), 3093–3099.

Charlop, M.H., & Haymes, L.K. (1994). Speech and language acquisition and intervention: behavioral approaches. In J.L. Matson (Ed.), *Autism in children and adults: Etiology, assessment and intervention*. Pacific Grove, CA: Brooks/Cole.

Charlop, M.H., Schreibman, L., & Thibodeau, M.G. (1985). Increasing spontaneous verbal responding in autistic children using a time delay procedure. *Journal of Applied Behavior Analysis, 18*(2), 155–166.

Coonrod, E., & Stone, W. (2004). Early concerns of parents of children with autistic and nonautistic disorders. *Infants and Young Children, 17*(3), 258–268.

Correll, C. (2008). Antipsychotic use in children and adolescents: Minimizing adverse effects to maximize outcomes. *Journal of the American Academy of Child & Adolescent Psychiatry, 47*(1), 9–20.

Coucouvanis, J. (2005). *Superskills: A social skills group program for children with Asperger Syndrome, high functioning autism and related challenges*. Mission, KS: Autism Asperger Publishing Company.

Cuvo, A., Law-Reagan, A., Ackerlund, J., Huckfeldt, R., & Kelly, C. (2010). Training children with autism spectrum disorders to be compliant with a physical exam. *Research in Autism Spectrum Disorders, 4*, 168–185. doi:10.1016/j.rasd.2009.09.001

Demicheli, V., Jefferson, T., Rivetti, A., & Price, D. (2006). Vaccines for measles, mumps and rubella in children. *Cochrane Database of Systematic Reviews, 4*, Art. No.: CD004407. doi:10.1002/14651858.CD004407.pub2

Doo, S., & Wing, Y. (2006). Sleep problems of children with pervasive developmental disorders: Correlation with parental stress. *Developmental Medicine and Child Neurology, 48*, 650–655. doi:10.1111/j.1469-8749.2006.tb01334.x

Ecker, C., Marquand, A., Mourao-Miranda, J., Johnston, P., Daly, E., Brammer, M., & Murphy, D. (2010) Describing the brain in autism in five dimensions: Magnetic resonance imaging-assisted diagnosis of autism spectrum disorder using a multiparameter classification approach. *The Journal of Neuroscience, 30*(32), 10612–10623. doi: 10.1523/JNEUROSCI.5413-09.2010

Escalona, A., Field, T., Singer-Strunk, R., Cullen, C., Hartshorn, K. (2001). Brief report: Improvements in the behavior of children with autism following massage therapy. *Journal of Autism and Developmental Disorders. 31*, 513–516. doi:10.1023/A1012273110194

Filipek, P.A., Accardo, P.J., Baranek, G., Cook, E.H., Dawson, G., Gordon, B., & Volkmar, F.R. (1999). The screening and diagnosis of autism spectrum disorders. *Journal of Autism and Developmental Disorders, 29*(6), 439–484.

Filipek, P.A., Accardo, P.J., Ashwal, S., Baranek, G.T., Cook, E.H., Dawson, G., & Volkmar, F. R. (2000). Practice parameter: Screening and diagnosis of autism: Report of the quality standards subcommittee of the American Academy of Neurology and the Child Neurology Society. *Neurology, 55*(4), 468–479.

Filipek, P. (2005). The medical aspects of autism. In F. Volkmar, R. Paul, A. Klin & D. Cohen (Eds.), *Handbook of autism and pervasive developmental disorders* (3rd edition; pp. 534–578). Hoboken, NJ: John Wiley & Sons.

Findling, R.L. (2005). Pharmacologic treatment of behavioral symptoms in autism and pervasive developmental disorders. *The Journal of Clinical Psychiatry, 66*(Suppl. 10), 26–31.

Frankel, R., Leary, M., & Kilman, B. (1987). Building social skills through pragmatic analysis: Assessment and treatment implications for children with autism. In D. Cohen, O. Donellan, & R. Paul (Eds.). *Handbook of autism and pervasive developmental disorders*. New York: Wiley.

Freed, G., Clark, S., Butchart, Am., Singer, D., & Davis, M. 2010. Parental vaccine safety concerns in 2009. *Pediatrics, 125*(4), 654–659. doi:10.1542/peds.2009-1962

Frost, L.A., & Bondy, A.S. (2002). *PECS: The picture exchange communication system training manual* (2nd edition). Newark, DE: Pyramid Educational Products Inc.

Fuller, P.M., Gooley, J., & Saper, C.B. (2006). Neurobiology of the sleepwake cycle: Sleep architecture, circadian regulation and regulatory feedback. *Journal of Biological Rhythms, 26,* 482–493. doi:10.1177/0748730406294627

Gadow, K., & DeVincent, C. (2005). Clinical significance of tics and attention deficit hyperactivity disorder in children with pervasive developmental disorder. *Journal of Childhood Neurology, 20,* 481–488.

Ganz, M.L. (2007). The lifetime distribution of the incremental societal costs of autism. *Archives of Pediatric Adolescence Medicine, 161*(4), 343–349.

Ghaziuddin, M. (2005). A family history study of Asperger syndrome. *Journal of Autism and Developmental Disorders, 35*(2), 177–182.

Gleason, M.M., Egger, H.L., Emslie, G.J., Greenhill, L.L., Kowatch, R.A., Lieberman, A.F., Luby, & Zeanah, C.H. (2007). Psychopharmacological treatment for very young children: contexts and guidelines. *Journal of the American Academy of Child and Adolescent Psychiatry, 46,* 1532–1572.

Goldstein, H. (2002). Communication intervention for children with autism: a review of treatment efficacy. *Journal of Autism and Developmental Disorders, 32,* 373–396. doi:10.1023/A:1020589821992

Gray, C. (2000). *The new social story book: illustrated edition.* Arlington, TX: Future Horizons.

Hakonarson, H., Schellenberg, G., Pericak-Vance, M., Geschwind, D., Grant, S., Dawson, G., & Wang, K., (2009). Common genetic variants on 5p14.1 associate with autism spectrum disorders. *Nature, 459,* 528–533. doi: 10.1038/nature07999

Hanson, E., Kalish, L.A., Bunce, E. Curtis, C., McDaniel, S.Ware, J., & Petry, J. (2007). Use of complementary and alternative medicine among children diagnosed with autism spectrum disorder. *Journal of Autism and Developmental Disorders, 37,* 628–636.

Hart, B., & Risley, T.R. (1980). In vivo language intervention. Unanticipated general effects. *Journal of Applied Behavior Analysis, 13,* 407–432. doi:10.1901/jaba.1980.13-407

Horner, R.H., Diemer, S.M., & Brazeau, K.C. (1992). Educational support for students with severe problem behaviors in Oregon: A descriptive analysis from the 1987–88 school year. *Journal of the Association for Persons with Severe Handicaps, 17,* 165–169.

Horner, R.H., Carr, E.G., Strain, P.S., Todd, A.W., & Reed, H.K. (2002). Problem behavior interventions for young children with autism: A research synthesis. *Journal of Autism and Developmental Disorders, 32,* 423–446.

Howlin, P., & Rutter, M. (1989). Mother's speech to autistic children: A preliminary causal analysis. *Journal of Child Psychology and Psychiatry, 30,* 819–843.

Inglese, M., & Elder, J. (2009). Caring for children with autism spectrum disorder, Part I: Prevalence, etiology and core features. *Journal of Pediatric Nursing, 24*(1), 41–48.

Ivanenko, A., & Johnson, K. (2008). Sleep disturbances in children psychiatric disorders. *Seminars in Pediatric Neurology, 15,* 70–78.

Johnson, C., & Myers, S. (2007). Identification and evaluation of children with autism spectrum disorders. *Pediatrics, 120*(5), 1183–1215.

Jones, W., Carr, K., Katelin, B., & Klin, A. (2008). Absence of preferential looking to the eyes of approaching adults predicts level of social disability in 2 year old toddlers with autism spectrum disorder. *Archives of General Psychiatry, 65*(8), 946–954.

Kanner, L. (1943). Autistic disturbances of affective contact. *Nervous Child, 2,* 217–250.

Kirby, R., Lane, J., Childers, J., Skinner, S., Annese, F., Barrish, J., & Percy, A. (2010). Longevity in Rett Sydrome: Analysis of the North American database. *The Journal of Pediatrics, 156*(1), 135–138.

Koegel, L.K. (2000). Interventions to facilitate communication in autism. *Journal of Autism and Developmental Disorders, 30,* 383–391. doi:10.10.1023/A:1005539220932

Koegel, L.K., & LaZebnik, C. (2004). *Overcoming autism: Finding the answers, strategies and hope that can transform a child's life.* New York, NY: Penguin Books.

Kogan, M.D., Blumberg, S.J., Schieve, L.A., Boyle, C.A., Perrin, J.M., Ghandour, R.M., & van Dyck, P.C. (2009). Prevalence of parent-reported diagnosis of autism spectrum disorder among children in the US, 2007. *Pediatrics, 124,* 1395–1403. doi:peds.2009-1522v1-peds.2009-1522

Kraijer, D.W. (1999). Autism and autistic like conditions in mental retardation. *Journal of Disability Research, 43,* 342–343.

Krasny, L., Williams, B.J., Provencal, S., & Ozonoff, S. (2003). Social skills interventions for the autism spectrum: essential ingredients and a model curriculum. *Child and Adolescent Psychiatric Clinics of North America, 12*(1), 107–122.

Kutscher, M. (2006). *Autism spectrum disorders* (Monograph). Retrieved from http://pediatricneurology.com/autism.htm

Lainhart, J., Piven, J., Wzorket, J., Landa, R., Santangelo, S., Coon H., & Folstein, S., (1997). Macrocephaly in children and adults with autism. *Journal of the American Academy of Child and Adolescent Psychiatry, 36,* 282–290.

Levy, S., & Hyman, S. (2005). Novel treatments for autism spectrum disorders. *Mental Retardation and Developmental Disabilities Research Reviews, 11*(2), 131–142.

Levy, S., Mandell, D., & Schultz, R. (2009). Autism. *The Lancet, 374,* 1627–1638. doi:10.1016/S01406736(09)61376-3

Leyfer, O., Folstein, S., Bacalman, S., Davis, N., Dinh, E., Morgan, J., & Lainhart, J. (2006). Co-morbid psychiatric disorders in children with autism: Interview development and rates of disorders. *Journal of Autism and Developmental Disorders, 36*(7), 849–861. doi: 10.1007/s10803-006-0123-0

Liptak, G., Stuart, T., & Auinger, P. (2006). Health care utilization and expenditures for children with autism: Data from a US national sample. *Journal of Autism & Developmental Disorders, 36*(7), 871–879.

Lobar, S., Fritts, M., Arbide, Z., & Russell, D. (2008). The role of the nurse practitioner in an individualized education plan and coordination of care for the child with Asperger's syndrome. *Journal of Pediatric Health Care, 22*(2), 111–119. doi:10.1016/j.pedhc.2007.04.001

Lovaas, O.I. (1987). Behavioral treatment and normal educational and intellectual functioning in young autistic children. *Journal of Consulting and Clinical Psychology, 55,* 3–9. Retrieved from http://www.chicagobehaviordevelopment.com/cbd/wp-content/uploads/2010/08/Lovaas-1987.pdf

McCracken, J.T. (2005). Safety issues with drug therapies for autism spectrum disorders. *The Journal of Clinical Psychiatry, 66*(Suppl 10), 32–37.

Mesibov, G.B., Shea, V., & Schopler, F. (2005). *The TEACCH Approach to Autism spectrum disorders.* New York, NY: Kluwer Academic/Plenum.

Mesibov, G.B. (1997). Formal and informal measures on the effectiveness or the TEACCH programme. *Autism, 1,* 25–35. doi:10.1177/1362361397011005

Meyers, S.M., Johnson, C.P., & the Council on Children with Disabilities. (2007). Management of children with autism spectrum disorder. *Pediatrics, 120,* 1160–1182. Retrieved from http://www.pediatrics.org/cgi/content/full/120/5/1162

Miles, J., Hadden, T., & Hillman, R. (2000). Head circumference is an independent clinical finding associated with autism. *American Journal of Medical Genetics, 95,* 339–350. doi:10.1002/1096-8628(20001211)954<339:AID-AJMG9>3.0CO;2-B

Millward, C., Ferriter, M., Calver, S.J., & Connell-Jones, G.G. (2008). Gluten- and casein-free diets for autistic spectrum disorder. *Cochrane Database of Systematic Reviews, 2*, CD003498. doi:10.1002/14651858.CD003498.pub3

Muhle, R., Trentacoste, S., & Rapin, I. (2004). The genetics of autism. *Pediatrics, 113*, e472–e486. doi:10.1542/peds.113.5.e472

Myers, S., Johnson, C., & Council on Children with Disabilities. (2007). Management of children with autism spectrum disorders. *Pediatrics, 120*, 1162–1182. doi:10.1542/peds.2007-2362

Nash, P., & Coury, D. (2003). Screening tools assist with diagnosis of autism spectrum disorders. *Pediatric Annals, 32*(10), 664–670.

National Institute of Mental Health [NIMH]. (2008). *Autism spectrum disorders*. No. 08-5511. Washington, DC: U.S. Department of Health and Human Services.

Ospina, M. B., Seida, J.K., Clark, B., Karhaneh, M., Hartling, L., Tjosvold, L., Vandermermeer, B., & Smith, V. (2008). Behavioural and developmental interventions for autism spectrum disorder: a clinical systematic review. *Plos One, 3*(11), e3755. doi:10.1371/journal.pone.0003755

Oswald, D.P., & Sonenklar, N.A. (2007). Medication use among children with autism-spectrum disorders. *Journal of Child and Adolescent Psychopharmacology, 17*(3), 348–355.

Page, J., & Boucher, J. (1998). Motor impairments in children with autistic disorder. *Child Language Teaching and Therapy, 14*, 253–259. doi:10.1177/026565909801400301

Peacock, G., Hyman, S., & Levy, S. (2009, July 22). National Center of Medical Home Initiatives for Children with Special Needs. Autism identification and management webinar. Webinar presented by the American Academy of Pediatrics and the National Center of Medical Home Initiatives. American Academy of Pediatrics. Retrieved from http://www.medicalhomeinfo.org/downloads/ppts/asdwebinar.ppt

Phetrasuwan, S., Miles, M., & Mesibov, G. (2009). Defining autism spectrum disorders. *Journal of the Society of Pediatric Nurses, 14*(3), 206–209.

Polimeni, M.A., Richdale, A.L., & Francis, A.J. (2005). A survey of sleep problems in autism, Asperger's disorder and typically developing children. *Journal of Intellectual Disability Research, 49*(4), 260–268.

Posey, D.J., Aman, M.G., McCracken, J.T., Scahill, L., Tierney, E., Arnold, L.E., & McDougle, C.J. (2007). Positive effects of methylphenidate on inattention and hyperactivity in pervasive developmental disorders: an analysis of secondary measures. *Biological Psychiatry, 61*, 538–544.

Prizant, B.M., & Wetherby, A.M. (1998). Communication intent: A framework for understanding social communicative behavior in autism. *Journal of the American Academy of Child and Adolescent Psychiatry, 26*, 472–479.

Reaven, J. (2009). Children with high functioning autism spectrum disorders and co-occurring anxiety symptoms: Implications for assessment and treatment. *Journal of the Society of Pediatric Nurses, 14*(3), 192–199.

Reichele, J. (1990). *National working conference on positive approaches to the management of excess behavior: Final report and recommendations*. Minneapolis, MN: Institute on Community Integration, University of Minnesota.

Reichenberg, A., Gross, R., Weiser, M., Bresnahan, M., Silverman, J., Harlap, S., & Susser, E. (2006). Advancing paternal age and autism. *Archives of General Psychiatry, 63*(9), 1026–1032.

Reichow, B., & Volkmar, F.R. (2008). Social skills interventions for individuals with autism: Evaluation for evidence-based practices within a best evidence synthesis framework. *Journal of Autism and Developmental Disorders, 38*, 1311–1318.

Rice, C. (2009, December). Prevalence of autism spectrum disorders: Autism and developmental disabilities monitoring network. *Morbidity and Mortality Weekly Report, 58*(SS10), 1–20.

Ringman, J., & Jankovic, J. (2000). Occurrence of tics in Asperger syndrome and autistic disorder. *Journal of Child Neurology, 15*(6), 394–400.

Rogers, S.J., Hayden, D., Hepburn, S., Charlifue-Smith, R., Hall, T., & Hayes, A. (2006). Teaching young nonverbal children with autism useful speech: A pilot study of the Denver Model and PROMPT interventions. *Journal of Autism and Developmental Disorders, 3*, 1007–1024. doi:10.1007/s10803-006-0142-x

Rogers, S.J., Hall, T., Osaki, D., Reaven, J., & Herbison, J. (2000). A comprehensive, integrated, educational approach to young children with autism and their families. In S.L. Harris & J.S. Handleman (Eds.), *Preschool education programs for children with autism* (2nd edition). Austin, TX: Pro-Ed.

Roke, Y., van Harten, P.N., Boot, A.M., & Buitelaar, J.K. (2009). Antipsychotic medication in children and adolescents: a descriptive review of the effects on prolactin level and associated side effects. *Journal of Child and Adolescent Psychopharmacology, 19*, 403–414.

Scahill, L., & Pachler, M. (2007). Treatment of hyperactivity in children with pervasive developmental disorders. *Journal of Child and Adolescent Psychiatric Nursing, 20*(1), 59–62.

Scahill, L., Koenig, K., Carroll, D., & Pachler, M. (2007). Risperidone approved for the treatment of serious behavioral problems in children with autism. *Journal of Child and Adolescent Psychiatric Nursing 20*(3), 188–190.

Shattuck, P.T., Durkin, M., Maenner, M., Newschaffer, C., Mandell, D.S., Wiggins, L., & Cuniff, C. (2009). Timing of identification among children with an autism spectrum disorder: Findings from a population-based surveillance study. *Journal of the American Academy of Child and Adolescent Psychiatry, 48*(5), 474–483.

Shelton, J., Tancredi, D., & Hertz-Picciotto, I. (2010). Independent and dependent contributions of advanced maternal and paternal ages to autism risk. *Autism Research, 3*(1), 30–39. doi:10.1002/aur.118

Tantam, D. (2000). Adolescence and adulthood of individuals with Asperger syndrome. In A. Klin, F.R. Klin, & S.S. Sparrow (Eds.) *Asperger Syndrome*. New York, NY: The Guilford Press.

U.S. Department of Health and Human Services.(January 26, 2009). The Interagency Autism Coordinating Committee Strategic Plan for Autism Spectrum Disorder Research. Retrieved from http://iacc.hhs.gov/reports/2009/iacc-strategic-plan-for-autism-spectrum-disorder-research-jan26.shtml

Van Acker, R., Loncola, J., & Van Acker, E. (2005). Rett syndrome: A pervasive developmental disorder. In R. Volkmar, R. Paul, A. Klin, & D. Cohen (Eds.), *Handbook of autism and pervasive developmental disorders, Vol. 1.* (pp. 126–164). Hoboken, NJ: John Wiley & Sons.

Venter, A., Lord, C., & Schopler, E. (1992). A follow-up study of high-functioning autistic children. *Journal of Child Psychology and Psychiatry, 33*, 489–507. Retrieved from http://www.ncbi.nlm.nih.gov/pubmed/1577895

Volkmar, F., & Lord, C. (2007). Diagnosis and definition of autism and other autism spectrum disorders. In Volkmar, F. (Ed.), *Autism and Pervasive Developmental Disorders* (2nd edition, pp. 1–31). Cambridge: Cambridge University Press.

Wang, P., & Spillane, A. (2009). Evidence-based social skills interventions for children with autism: A meta-analysis. *Education and Training in Developmental Disabilities, 44*(3), 318–342.

Wang, K., Zhang, H., Dequiong, M., Bucan, M., Glessner, J., Abrahams, B., & Hakonarson, H. (2010). Common gene variants on 5p14.1 associated with autism spectrum disorders. *Nature, 459*, 528–533. doi:10.1038/nature/07999

Wassink, T., Piven, J., & Patil, S., (2001). Chromosomal abnormalities in a clinic sample of individuals with autistic disorder. *Psychiatric Genetics, 11*, 57–63.

Weiskop, S., Matthews, J., & Richdale, A. (2001). Treatment of sleep problems in a 5-year old boy with autism using behavioural principles. *Autism, 5*, 209–221.

Weiskop, S., Richdale, A., & Matthews, J. (2005). Behavioural treatment to reduce sleep problems in children with autism or fragile X syndrome. *Developmental Medicine & Child Neurology, 47*, 94–104. doi:10.1111/j.1469-8749.2005.tb01097.x

Weitz, C., Dexter, M., & Moore, J. (1997). AAC and children with developmental disabilities. In S. Glenn & D.C. Decoste (Eds.), *Handbook of augmentative and alternative communication.* San Diego, CA: Singular Publishing.

White, S., Koenig, K., & Scahill, L. (2007). Social skills development in children with autism spectrum disorders: A review of the intervention research. *Journal of Autism and Developmental Disorders, 37*, 1858–1868.

Wiggins, L., Baio, J., & Rice, C. (2006). Examination of the time between first evaluation and first autism spectrum diagnosis in a population-based sample. *Journal of Developmental and Behavioral Pediatrics, 27*(2), S79–S87.

Wiggs, L., & Stores, G. (2004). Sleep patterns and sleep disorders in children with autism spectrum disorders: Insights using parent report and actigraphy. *Developmental Medicine and Child Neurology, 46*(6), 372–380. doi:10.1017/S0012/62204000611

Williams, K., Wheeler, D.M., Silove, N., & Hazell, P. (2010). Selective serotonin reuptake inhibitors (SSRIs) for autism spectrum disorders (ASD). *Cochrane Database of Systematic Reviews, 8*, CD004677. doi:10.1002/14651858.CD004677.pub2

Williams, P., Sears, L., & Allard, A. (2004). Sleep problems in children with autism. *Journal of Sleep Research, 13*, 265–268.

Wolf, M., Risley, T., & Mees, H. (1964). Application of operant conditioning procedures to the behaviour problems of an autistic child. *Behaviour Research and Therapy, 1*, 305–312. Retrieved from http://www.garfield.library.upenn.edu/classics1983/A1983RG31100001.pdf

Yeargin-Allsopp, M., Rice, C., Karapurkar, T., Doernberg, N., Boyle, C., & Murphy, C. (2003). Prevalence of autism in a US metropolitan area. *Journal of the American Medical Association, 289*(1), 49–55.

14

Learning and Intellectual Disabilities

Linda M. Finke and Patricia Ryan-Krause

Objectives

After reading this chapter, APNs will be able to

1. Discuss assessment and identification of learning and intellectual disabilities.
2. Discuss the impact of diagnosis of learning or intellectual disability on the family and child.
3. Identify strategies to help families with a child with a learning or intellectual disability cope and navigate the complex systems of health care, schools, and community resources.
4. Describe how advanced practice nurses (APNs) can work collaboratively to provide services to children and adolescents with learning and intellectual disabilities.

Introduction

It is estimated that from 5% to 15% of school-aged children have a learning or intellectual disability (Hendriksen et al., 2007; Lagae, 2008). In part, the number of children affected is difficult to determine because the terms used to describe and diagnose children with learning or intellectual disabilities vary. Prevalence data of learning disabilities also suggest that males are affected more frequently than females, with a range of 2.8–4.8 to 1 (Grizzle & Simms, 2005). Learning disabilities in children refer to problems in the skills needed for reading, written and spoken language, and math, while children who are diagnosed with an intellectual disability are delayed in overall development including life skills and may have a lower intellectual level than children of the same chronological age. Children with intellectual disabilities may have previously been labeled with the diagnoses of mental retarded, developmentally delayed, or intellectually challenged.

There are frequent overlaps in characteristics and concepts when discussing intellectual and learning disabilities and youngsters with these challenges often have one or more comorbidities. Definitions the reader should be aware of include the following:

1. The American Association of Intellectual and Developmental Disabilities (AAIDD) defines an *intellectual disability* as a significant limitation in intellectual functioning such as the ability to reason, learn, and problem solve along with limitations in adaptive skills including conceptual, social, and practical skills beginning before the age of eighteen (n.d.).
2. The Individuals with Disabilities Education Improvement Act (IDEA) of 2004 defines a *learning*

Child and Adolescent Behavioral Health: A Resource for Advanced Practice Psychiatric and Primary Care Practitioners in Nursing,
First Edition. Edited by Edilma L. Yearwood, Geraldine S. Pearson, and Jamesetta A. Newland.
© 2012 John Wiley & Sons, Inc. Published 2012 by John Wiley & Sons, Inc.

disability as a "disorder in one or more of the basic psychological processes involved in understanding or in using language, spoken or written, that may manifest itself in an imperfect ability to listen, think, speak, read, write, spell, or do mathematical calculations, including conditions such as perceptual disabilities, brain injury, minimal brain dysfunction, dyslexia and developmental aphasia" (pp. 2657–2658).

This chapter will differentiate between intellectual and learning disabilities, describe the types of disabilities most frequently seen, provide screening information that can be used in primary care, describe evidence-based interventions used with this population, and present a case study highlighting the experience of a youngster with a learning disability.

Intellectual Disabilities

The American Psychiatric Association is poised to replace the diagnostic label of mental retardation with intellectual disabilities in the next Diagnostic and Statistical Manual of Mental Disorders (DSM-V) (APA, 2010). The proposed change will state that the diagnosis of intellectual disabilities is made on the basis of intellectual and adaptive functioning deficits and not on intellectual quotient (IQ). Nevertheless, it is often difficult to diagnose intellectual disabilities because there is no accurate test, and symptoms, best described as behaviors, vary greatly. Intelligence testing is highly inaccurate in these children because of their delayed development and delayed ability to communicate, read, write, and perform tasks of daily living. Often their comprehension level is higher than is demonstrated by their verbal and writing skills.

While there are several identified causes of intellectual disabilities, 40% of those diagnosed cannot be connected with an identified cause. Chromosomal abnormalities are found in about 7% of children with intellectual disability (Knight et al., 1999). These abnormalities include Down syndrome (twenty-one chromosomes) and fragile X syndrome (changed *FMR1* gene on X chromosome). Fragile X syndrome is the leading cause of an inherited intellectual disability (Schwarte, 2008). The disability is two times more common in boys than in girls with the diagnoses affecting 1 in 4000 boys. Fragile X syndrome is caused by the loss of expression of the *FMR1* gene. The *FMR1* gene is necessary for normal learning and memory development in the brain. Other identified causes of an intellectual disability include fetal alcohol syndrome, poor prenatal care or prenatal injury, and toxic environmental exposures during formative developmental periods. Readers are referred to Chapter 13 in this text for a comprehensive description of the needs of children with an autism spectrum disorder as they, too, can present with learning and intellectual disability challenges.

To complicate matters more, the prevalence of other disabilities often co-occurs with intellectual disabilities. Physical disabilities such as cerebral palsy and other brain injuries may also be present. These children may have cardiac disorders, seizure disorders, or attention deficit hyperactivity disorder (ADHD). They also may present with self-injurious behavior such as hand biting, hair pulling, head banging, or picking at clothing or skin. Children with intellectual disabilities are at a 40% higher prevalence of psychiatric disorders than other children (Emerson & Hatton, 2007; Faust & Scior, 2007). Again, the assessment of mental health problems in children with an intellectual disability is difficult because with this population, invalidated methods (i.e., methods not standardized for use with children with intellectual disabilities) are used to determine the presence of a mental health problem (Kaptein, Jansen, Vogels, & Reijneveld, 2007). The clinical picture may be further complicated by medications the child is taking because of physical or mental health concerns.

Intellectual Disabilities Associated with Learning

One example of a learning disability is a learning disorder. A learning disorder/disability is "an unexpected, specific and persistent failure to acquire efficient academic skills despite conventional instruction, *adequate intelligence* and socio-cultural opportunity" (Lague, 2008 p. 1261). In the past, the issue of discrepancy between a child's IQ and academic performance was often used as part of the diagnostic criteria for learning disabilities. In 2004 the revisions to IDEA indicated "the criteria adopted by the State must not require the use of a severe discrepancy between intellectual ability and achievement for determining whether a child has a specific learning disability, as defined in 34 CFR 300.8(c)(10)" (U.S. Department of Education, n.d., & para; 2). Research has also minimized the use of discrepancy since specific learning disabilities can occur with any IQ level (Shaywitz & Shaywitz, 2003).

Etiology of Learning Disorders

Recent literature suggests a genetic component to learning disabilities. Factors potentially associated with learning disabilities are prematurity, chronic medical conditions like epilepsy, cerebral palsy, exposure to environmental toxins, and developmental delays (Lagae, 2008). Some research suggests lower socioeconomic status, parental substance abuse, poor prenatal care and nutrition, poverty, and less literacy exposure may also contribute to learning disabilities (Sices, Taylor, Freebairn, Hansen, & Lewis, 2007). The American Academy of Pediatrics (AAP) recently stated that "about 40% of siblings, children, or parents of an affected individual will have dyslexia, but conversely some individuals may have dyslexia without any family history of this or related learning disorders" (2009, p. 838). The genetic foundation of learning disorders may be formed not by isolated genes but rather by a combination of genes and the pathways that these genes regulate. The genetic basis of learning disabilities is quite complex but it may eventually be possible to identify children who are at risk for disabilities so that early interventions might be developed (Friend, DeFries, & Olson, 2008).

Types of Learning Disabilities

Reading Disability (Dyslexia)

The most common type of learning disability relates to language usage in reading, spelling, and writing (Lagae, 2008). Reading disability is often used synonymously with dyslexia (Vellutino, Fletcher, Snowling, & Scanlon, 2004). About 80% of individuals diagnosed with a learning disability have a disorder of reading (Shaywitz & Shaywitz, 2003). Reading disorders involve poor phonological awareness or difficulty in recognizing the unique sound patterns made by different letters and combinations of letters. This makes rapid decoding of the written word very difficult and results in difficulty with sight word recognition, trouble with syllabication, and poor fluency (AAP, 2009).

Rhyming is an early demonstration of phonological awareness. This is a skill developed by 80% of children between three and four years of age but it must progress to blending sounds, segmenting words, and deleting and replacing letters to form new words (Grizzle & Simms, 2005). Another early indicator of reading disorders is lack of print-concept knowledge. This is an important component of preliteracy and refers to the understanding of left-to-right directionality, uppercase and lowercase alphabet recognition, and principles of writing (Sices, Taylor, Freebairn, Hansen, & Lewis, 2007). If careful assessment of language development is performed periodically in early childhood, it may be possible to identify many children at high risk for reading difficulties.

Math Disability (Dyscalculia)

The second most common type of learning disability is dyscalculia. There may be signs in early childhood such as difficulty understanding concepts such as "more" and "less," difficulty with sorting objects into groups by size, difficulty recognizing patterns, and difficulty comparing and contrasting concepts like "smaller/bigger" or "taller/shorter." Counting, number recognition, and matching numbers with amounts can also be difficult for these children (Kadosh & Walsh, 2007).

School-aged children with dyscalculia may have difficulty with basic mathematical operations. Memory issues make it difficult to master math facts and to hold basic information in short-term memory while manipulating other information in the given problem. Language issues make it difficult to read and comprehend the content of word problems. Problems with visuospatial relationships may contribute to math disorders. These problems can interfere with the ability to learn from material presented on a white board, computer screen, or projector. Children can have difficulty organizing written math information on a page so it then becomes impossible to correctly compute the answer. These children may also find it difficult to visualize patterns and successfully move through sequential operations.

Writing Disability (Dysgraphia)

The third common type of learning disability is a disorder of written expression. There are no specific early signs of disorders of written expression that may accurately identify a child at a very young age. However, individuals with dysgraphia are often found to have difficulties with sequencing information and may have fine motor difficulties, which make getting a thought onto paper a very difficult task. These individuals often have excellent verbal skills and can accurately relate information and ideas. However, they have great difficulty in combining the demands of abstract thinking with the fine motor tasks of using a writing implement and sequencing letters and words into meaningful written expression. Children with dysgraphia often produce very limited written work with little elaboration in their writing.

Intellectual Disabilities: Clinical Picture

Early diagnosis of an intellectual disability is important so children and their families can begin working toward meeting the child's potential. However, reaching an early diagnosis is complicated as has previously been discussed. Presenting problems indicating an intellectual disability are usually as simple as the child not meeting expected developmental milestones such as sitting up, rolling over, crawling and walking, or, for an older child, talking. The parent often brings this delay in developmental milestones to the health care provider's attention during routine well-child checks or the

Table 14.1 Difficulties that may be associated with learning disabilities

- Following directions.
- Getting and staying organized at home and school.
- Understanding verbal directions.
- Learning facts and remembering information.
- Learning subjects taught in school (for example, math, reading, or spelling) but seeming smart in other things.
- Fitting in with peers or communicating with others.
- Sounding words out and reading or spelling.
- Writing clearly (may have poor handwriting).
- Concentrating and finishing schoolwork (may daydream a lot).
- Explaining information clearly with speech or in writing.

From the American Academy of Pediatrics, 2010.

health care provider notes the lack of development. A complete physical exam might detect physical and congenital abnormalities such as large ears, an elongated face, prominent jaw line, macrocephaly, macro-orchidism, a narrow and high-arched palate, and hyperextensible joints associated with fragile X syndrome. A round face with eyes that slant upward, low muscle tone, a palm crease (simian line), and a protruding tongue may be associated with Down syndrome.

Genetic testing would be necessary to confirm the diagnosis. Various diagnostic tests may need to be conducted to rule out a variety of disorders including neurological abnormalities, endocrine disorders, or hearing problems. Adaptive skills assessment is essential for children with a suspected intellectual disability. Common tools used are the Vineland Adaptive Behavior Scales or the Bayley III (Finke & Greenberg, 2009). APNs can be trained to administer either test. Both tests are questionnaires that can be completed while working with the child's parents and observing the child. A functional level can be determined from the tests, which can serve as the baseline for interventions to improve the child's level of functioning.

Since some of the etiologies and risk factors for intellectual and learning disabilities are understood, it is possible to identify and intervene early with these children, making routine early pediatric screening in primary care essential. Early detection, a full assessment by a trained provider, and early interventions may ameliorate some of the actual developmental problems associated with disabilities and subsequently decrease the negative emotional effects associated with these challenges (Byrd, 2005). The AAP recommends that information from the child/teen and parent be gathered about intellectual and learning-related abilities during routine visits. See Table 14.1 for a list of learning abilities to screen for.

A major role for the APN is to prepare the parents and child for any needed diagnostic testing and to explain the results of completed tests. Researchers have determined that children with intellectual disabilities suffer from pain more than their peers (Breau & Burkitt, 2009). Limited communication skills and maladaptive behavior often make any kind of diagnostic testing stressful for these youngsters. Decreased comprehension by the child and an inability to express herself or himself may lead to frustration and acting out behaviors. In an advocacy role, the APN should work with other health care providers to prepare for the child's procedure and to suggest changes in the normal routine that may facilitate testing and its outcomes. For example, changes in the routine such as allowing parents to stay in the room with the child, medicating the child, and breaking the procedure into smaller segments may be helpful.

Parents or caretakers may also express concerns about the impact of the intellectual disability on the child's self-concept. Donohue, Wise, Romski, Henrich, and Sevcik (2010) conducted a study on thirty-eight children, ages seven to thirteen, classified by their school district as having mild intellectual disabilities. All children were referred to the study by their classroom teachers because of their difficulty with learning to read or with language skills. The researchers wanted to examine the appropriateness of two self-concept measures for use with this population, the multidimensionality of self-concept in children with mild intellectual disabilities, and to understand the relationship between the self-concept measures and reading achievement.

The measures used were the Harter Pictorial Scale of Perceived Competence and Social Acceptance for Children and the Self Description Questionnaire Individual Administration, which elicited their response to statements read to them. The Harter Pictorial Scale proved to be the better measure to use with the children in the sample because it was a shorter tool. In addition, findings indicated that, similar to other developing children, self-concept in children with mild intellectual disabilities matures during the elementary school years affecting the child's academic achievement (including language and reading skills). Researchers recommended that teachers and parents focus on maximizing self-concept in this population as early as possible in order to support healthy social and emotional development and maximize academic performance (Donohue et al., 2010). Nurses can help parents focus on the child's strengths, praise accomplishments, and engage the child in activities in which they can succeed. In addition, referral to activities and groups that focus on skill development and self-concept enhancement may be helpful.

Table 14.2 Selected developmental screening tools

Name of Tool	Screening Domains	Ages	Source
Parent Report Tools			
Ages & Stages Questionnaires (ASQ)	Communication, fine and gross motor, problem solving, personal adaptive skills Pass / Fail score for each domain	4–60 months	Squires, J., Potter, L., & Bricker, D. (1999). *The ASQ User's Guide* (2nd ed.). Baltimore, MD: Paul H. Brookes
Parents' Evaluation of Developmental Status (PEDS)	Development and behavior Useful for surveillance	Ages 0–8	Glascoe, F.P. (1999). Toward a model for an evidenced-based approach to developmental/ behavioral surveillance, promotion and patient education. *Ambulatory Child Health, 5,* 197–208
Child Development Inventory (CDI)	Social, self-help, motor, language, and general development skills	18 months to 6 years	Ireton, H. (1992). *Child Development Inventory Manual.* Minneapolis, MN: Behavior Science Systems Inc. Doig, K.B., Macias, M.M., Saylor, C.F., Craver, J.R., & Ingram, P.E. (1999). The child development inventory: A developmental outcome measure for follow-up of the high risk infant. *Journal of Pediatrics, 135,* 358–362
Child Performance Tools			
Battelle Developmental Inventory Screening Tool, (2nd ed.). (BDI-ST)	Personal-social, adaptive, motor, communication, and cognitive development Scoring is pass/fail	0–95 months	Newborg J. (2004). *Battelle Developmental Inventory* (2nd edition). Itasca, IL: Riverside Publishing
Bayley Infant Neurodevelopmental Screen (BINS)	Neurologic functions, auditory, visual and tactile receptive function, expressive function & cognitive processing	3–24 months	Aylward, G.P. (1995). *Bayley Infant Neurodevelopmental Screener.* San Antonio, TX: Psychological Corp. Aylward, G.P., Verhulst, S.J., & Bell, S. (2000). Predictive utility of the BSID-II Infant neurodevelopmental screener (BINS) risk status classifications: clinical interpretation and application. *Dev Med Child Neurol, 42,* 25–31
Brigance Screens-II	Articulation, expressive and receptive language, gross & fine motor skills, general knowledge, social skills, and pre-academic skills	0–90 months 0–23 months use parent report tool	Glascoe F.P. (2005). *Technical Report for the Brigance Screens.* North Billerica, MA: Curriculum Associates Inc. Glascoe, F.P. (2002). The Brigance Infant-Toddler Screen (BITS): Standardization and validation. *J Dev Behav Pediatr, 23,* 145–150
Denver-II Developmental Screening Test	Expressive & receptive language, gross & fine motor skills, personal-social skills Scoring: Normal, questionable, and abnormal	0–6 years	Frankenburg, W.K., Camp, B.W., & Van Natta, P.A. (1971). Validity of the Denver Developmental Screening Test. *Child Dev, 42,* 475–485 Frankenburg, W.K., Dodds, J., Archer, P., Shapiro, H., & Bresnick, B. (1992). The Denver II: A major revision and restandardization of the Denver Developmental Screening Test. *Pediatrics, 89*(1), 91–97 Denver Developmental Materials Inc., P.O. Box 371075, Denver, CO

Nursing Interventions

Children with an intellectual disability will have the same childhood illnesses, such as otitis media, that all children experience. The difference may be the difficulty in pinpointing the problem due to the lack of communication skills and low tolerance of pain. For the APN, diagnosing the problem may take on a "explore and discover mission" when the child presents with an elevated temperature or pain. An assessment of the child would need to be more extensive and perhaps at a different pace than if the child could communicate symptoms in an age-appropriate fashion.

Medication management is also important for these youngsters. As mentioned earlier, a child with an intellectual disability may be on a number of medications including anticonvulsants (for a seizure disorder or to regulate mood), stimulants (to manage symptoms of attention deficit hyperactivity disorder), selective serotonin reuptake inhibitors (SSRIs) (Food and Drug Administration approved for treatment of pediatric depression), or other psychotropic medications to treat comorbid disorders. They and their parents/caregivers will need to be taught the importance of taking their medications as prescribed and the symptoms the medication targets. For example, a stimulant medication like methylphenidate (Ritalin) may be prescribed to assist the child with tasks requiring attention. Optimal attention skills are needed to facilitate the learning process, which may already pose a difficulty for this youngster.

Ruling out the presence of an underlying hearing deficit is a critical first step in the assessment process for children with an intellectual disability or learning disabilities. The findings from auditory screening may highlight the need for further testing and may explain the reason behind behavioral acting out by the youngster. Regardless, screening provides the APN with information to guide appropriate supportive interventions. Although newborn screening protocols vary from state to state, it is essential that normal newborn hearing screening results be confirmed and reevaluated periodically. If timely appointments for extensive hearing evaluations are unavailable, the APN should advocate for the child and family with the appropriate agency responsible for such evaluations. In addition, receiving results of comprehensive hearing evaluations in a timely manner is equally important. Despite a previous finding of normal newborn hearing screening, it is always important to acknowledge parental concerns about hearing difficulties at any age and to perform routine office screening. Patients should be referred to a pediatric audiologist for diagnostic evaluation following abnormal or inconclusive screening results.

In addition to hearing assessments, all children should be routinely screened for deficits in vision and referred for complete ophthalmologic evaluations if there are any issues discovered during screening procedures. Office and school screenings do not identify near-vision problems such as convergence or accommodative insufficiency and significant deficits in close vision. Any child suspected of an intellectual or learning disability should be referred to a pediatric ophthalmologist for evaluation and further treatment if needed (AAP, 2009).

Primary Care Screening

Developmental surveillance at all well-child visits is imperative. The longitudinal process of surveillance allows the APN to look at the child in context and gather important developmental information over time to facilitate early case-finding and engage in preventive interventions (Glascoe & Robertshaw, 2007). Careful questioning of parents about the child's current developmental achievements at each visit provides the APN with valuable information about the progression of milestones in each developmental domain. At regular intervals (nine, eighteen, and twenty-four or thirty months), the AAP (2009) recommends the use of standardized screening tools. The AAP statement offers a variety of appropriate screening tools to use at these specific intervals. Some tools depend on parental report of developmental abilities while other tools require the child to perform a variety of developmental activities. An extensive list of recommended screening tools to be used at the recommended intervals of nine, eighteen, and thirty months are found in Table 14.2.

In addition to screening, it is important to discuss linguistic skills that should be emerging in the preschool years with the parents or caregivers. These include rhyming, recitation of nursery rhymes, letter recognition, auditory comprehension of multiple-step directions, and an awareness of print literacy (Grizzle & Simms, 2005). These activities can be easily incorporated into preschool well-child visits.

Conducting a careful history of the preschool child's participation and progress in preschool, Head Start, or structured day care settings provides important clues about the child's overall language development and exposure to verbal and print activities. Since language issues may impact social and emotional development, family and peer interactions are important to assess at routine primary care visits. Concerns voiced by parents or professionals in these settings merit a referral to the local school system for a complete speech and language evaluation and, if warranted by history, a complete psychoeducational and social-emotional evaluation. APNs must be aware of community services and resources for preschool learning needs. These include services provided by the local school system, community playgroups, library literacy programs, social skills groups, or lists of professionals who provide individual services.

Although worrisome symptoms may be present in early childhood, it is often not until school age that specific concerns about learning or intellectual abilities are raised by parents and school personnel (Byrd, 2005). APNs continue to be important participants in the evaluation and referral processes since they know the family and social history as well as the child's past medical and developmental history. APNs know medical conditions such as iron deficiency, lead poisoning, seizures, and asthma as well as genetic conditions such as fragile X syndrome that may impact learning and academic performance. Medications for already identified chronic conditions such as seizures and asthma may impact learning potential by causing drowsiness or overactive behavior, which should be explained to the parents and school personnel as warranted.

Even in children without previously identified medical or learning problems, surveillance and screening of school progress are essential in the primary care setting and questions about school adjustment and achievements are critical components in a complete review of systems. For school-aged children, the APN can review report cards, encourage the child to read brief passages of grade-appropriate books recommended by local schools, and engage the child in memory, spelling, and math games during the health assessment visit.

Several screening tools are useful in the early assessment of school problems. These tools help to discriminate if the cause of poor school performance may be a learning issue, a mental health issue, or a behavioral issue. The *Pediatric Symptom Checklist* (Jellinek, Murphy, & Little, 1999) is an easy-to-use tool that screens children from four through eighteen years of age for cognitive, emotional, and behavioral issues. After the general area of concern is identified, other disorder-specific tools are available to further assess concerns. Positive results on any of these tools require further assessment and management by the primary care provider, mental health specialist, and school or education personnel. Since intellectual disabilities are complex disorders often with comorbid mental health issues, a collaborative effort among all professionals is most effective. See Table 14.3 for additional behavioral, learning, and mental health screening tools.

It is not uncommon for parents of high school–aged children to raise concerns about their adolescent's academic progress. Lack of motivation, failing grades, oppositional behavior, and poor self-esteem are frequently reported. Undiagnosed learning disabilities may contribute to an adolescent's downward spiral. To sort out potentially multifaceted issues, joint and separate interviews with parents and the adolescent must be conducted and a confidentiality agreement clearly established. Obtaining releases for health care providers to speak with school personnel is also useful since exchange of academic, behavioral, and medical information may help define the components of school difficulties.

Additional tools to elucidate learning problems from preschool through adolescence are available for use in primary care settings. The Aggregate Neurobehavioral Student Health and Educational Review (ANSER) system gathers concise information about a child's health, development, attention, family, and social history as well as current academic functioning (Levine, 1980, n.d.-a). ANSER forms are completed by parents and teachers and suggest further evaluation for learning disabilities, attention, and emotional and/or behavioral problems. For a list of these neurodevelopmental tools, see Table 14.4.

Extensive manuals come with these tools so that APNs may administer them after careful review and practice. Results of these evaluations are best combined with teacher and parent reports and help to define the learning profile and needs of the child. Current Procedural Terminology (CPT) codes are available for the billing of these services.

Postscreening Assessment and Treatment Planning

After a positive screening for learning issues at any age, a specialized and focused multidisciplinary evaluation should be conducted by a Birth to Three program, local school system, or other professionals trained in intellectual or learning disabilities assessment. A complete list of community and professional resources with contact information is helpful to give to parents. Once a child turns three years of age, the local public school is responsible by federal law for the evaluation and provision of services if a disability is detected (IDEA, n.d.).

A written parental request for a school evaluation is often effective in starting the evaluation process. Individual state regulations determine the length of time allowed between request for evaluation and completion of evaluation. Assessment of school-aged children and teens includes IQ testing (Weschler, 1991) to measure cognitive abilities and achievement tests such as the Woodcock-Johnson (McGrew & Woodcock, 2001) or the Wide Range Achievement Test (Wilkinson & Robertson, 2006) to evaluate grade-level progress in academic areas of reading, writing, and math. Additional assessments may include speech and language, gross motor, visual-fine motor, auditory processing, visual and auditory acuity, and mental health evaluation. School or clinical

Table 14.3 Selected developmental screening tools

Name and Authors	Age Group	Number of Items	Description
Center for Epidemiological Studies Depression Scale for Children (Faulstich, Carey, Ruggiero, Enyart, & Gresham, 1986)	Children Adolescents	20-item self-report	The Center for Epidemiological Studies Depression Scale for Children (CES-DC) is a depression inventory with possible scores ranging from 0–60. Higher scores indicate increasing levels of depression with a score of 15 as suggestive of depressive symptoms in children and adolescents.
Columbia DISC Depression Scale (Shaffer, Fisher, & Lucas, 2003) [Diagnostic Interview Schedule for Children is now the *CDS-Columbia Depression Scale*.]	11 and older	22-question surveys for teens and parents	The Columbia DISC Depression Scale is to be completed separately by both the teen and a parent. (no=0, yes=1). Assesses chances of depression.
Screen for Child Anxiety Related Disorders (Birmaher, Khetarpal, Cully, Brent, & McKenzie, 1995)	9- to 18-year-olds	41-item self-report	The Screen for Child Anxiety Related Disorders (SCARED) is a survey to be completed by the child and parent separately. A total score of ≥ 25 may indicate the presence of an anxiety disorder. Scores higher that 30 are more specific to the type of anxiety disorder.
Vanderbilt Scales (Wolraich, Hannah, Pinnock, Baumgaertel & Brown, 1996)	6- to 12-year-olds	55 items	The Vanderbilt ADHD Rating Scale-Parent (VADPRS) is a reliable, cost-effective assessment for ADHD in clinical and research settings. Evaluates for ADHD and other comorbid conditions. It takes 10 minutes or less to complete. The VADPRS has two components: symptom assessment and impairment of performance at home, in school, and in social settings. The automated feedback report provides instant scoring and item analysis.
Conners' Rating Scales (Conners, 1990)	3- to 17-year-olds		Screening tool for ADHD. Parent and teacher versions of the tool. Tool has been revised several times, number of items is version dependent.

psychologists and speech and language specialists will frequently be the health care providers completing most of the assessment at this level of evaluation.

Once the evaluations are completed, a joint meeting of parents and all involved professionals should be convened. The purpose of this meeting would be to review the evaluation results, determine if the child meets the diagnostic criteria of specific intellectual or learning disability, and develop an Individual Education Plan (IEP) to meet the specific learning needs of the child. IEP meetings are held periodically or at least annually to review student progress and determine need for change in services. The IEP specifically describes goals, objectives, and the means to achieve them in measurable terms. This is a legal document to which the school is obliged to adhere (IDEA, n.d.). Students with a diagnosis of a specific learning or intellectual disability may receive a variety of services to remediate the challenges the youngster faces. These services may include but are not limited to:

1. One-on-one tutoring or personal aide, resource room with a special education teacher, individual psychological therapy, resource support in the regular classroom, speech and language services, occupational therapy services, social work

Table 14.4 Neurodevelopmental screening tools developed by Levine

Name	Age Group	Number of Items	Description
Pediatric Extended Evaluation at Three (PEET)	3-year-olds	Assesses 28 tasks in 5 basic areas of development: gross motor, language, visual-fine motor, memory, and intersensory integration.	Following assessment of these developmental tasks using the PEET, the examiner rates the child's selective attention, processing efficiency, and adaptation to the examination on the Assessment of Behavior Rating Scale. The child's overall language skills can be recorded on the Global Language Rating Scale, and the results of a physical examination on the general health assessment.
Pediatric Evaluation of Educational Readiness (PEER)	4- to 6-year-olds	Assesses 29 tasks in 6 different areas of development: orientation, gross motor, visual-fine motor, sequential, linguistic, and pre-academic learning.	PEER is a combined neurodevelopmental, behavioral, and health assessment. It is intended to generate a profile of a child's developmental and behavioral strengths and weaknesses that may be helpful in planning integrated health, educational, and developmental services. The child is also rated on 10 dimensions of selective attention and activity, processing efficiency, and adaptation.
Pediatric Early Elementary Examination (PEEX2)	6- to 9-year-olds	Assesses 31 tasks in 5 different areas of development: fine motor/ graphomotor function, language function, gross motor function, memory function, and visual processing function.	After assessment with the PEEX 2, children are also rated on selective attention and behavior at 3 points throughout the exam.
Pediatric Evaluation of Educational Readiness at Middle Childhood (PEERAMID)	9- to 15-year-olds	Assesses 35 tasks. PEERAMID 2 assesses a child's performance on 35 tasks in 5 different areas of development: fine motor/ graphomotor function, language function, gross motor function, memory function, and visual processing function.	PEERAMID 2 now contains tasks that tape the higher language abilities needed for success in secondary school, including the interpretation of ambiguous sentences and the ability to draw verbal inferences.

Compiled from Blackman et al., 1983; Coleman & Levine, 1988; Levine, 1983, 1985, n.d.-b; Levine, Meltzer, et al., 1983; and Levine, Oberklaid, et al., 1980.

services, assistive technology such as personal computers, tablets and recording devices.

2. If a child is determined to have educational needs that can be met in the regular classroom a 504 documented plan is developed. Section 504 of the Rehabilitation Act of 1973 grants accommodations in the classroom that will eliminate barriers and enhance learning through use of reasonable accommodations.

Specific Federal Acts Protecting Those with Disabilities

Health care providers must be knowledgeable about federal legislation and how each state interprets and implements these regulations. The IDEA and the Americans with Disabilities Act (ADA) (http://www.ada.gov) are both federal statutes that mandate services to ensure education services for children with disabilities

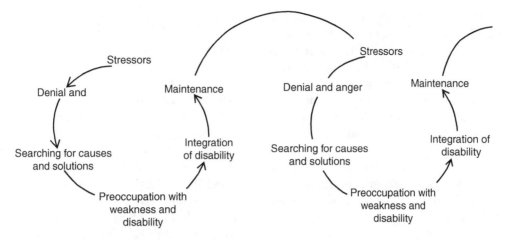

Figure 14.1 The Typology Model of Family Adjustment and Adaptation. (Reprinted from Finke, 1995, with permission from Lippincott Williams & Wilkins.)

to support their success. IDEA mandates that children with disabilities up to twenty-one years are identified, evaluated by an interdisciplinary team, and educated in the least restrictive environment and that parents have the right to due process to secure the most appropriate educational services.

These statutes provide for accommodations to include but are not limited to preferential seating, modified assignments, human and technical assistance to support learning, extended time on assignments, and in-class and standardized tests. The IDEA requires that a written individualized IEP be developed stipulating the services needed by the child with the disability. IEPs are to be reevaluated every three years. It also mandates the school district to provide the revenue and or human resources to execute the plan.

Section 504 of the Rehabilitation Act of 1973 is a civil rights law that requires schools to eliminate barriers that would prevent students from participating in programs and services offered in a general curriculum. Reasonable accommodations must be made for the child with a disability and the 504 plan should be reevaluated annually (National Center for Learning Disabilities [NCLD], n.d.).

Assisting with Family Coping

Parents are of course usually worried and anxious about the child and the identified delays or learning problems. The parents often feel guilty or responsible for the child's problems and will move through a grief cycle that begins as most grief with denial and disbelief (Finke, 1995). Parents may have difficulty accepting the diagnoses. Their denial is compounded by the fact that an exact cause frequently cannot be determined and a prediction of the child's future developmental level also cannot be

predetermined. Families move to the next stage which is anger followed by a searching for causes and solutions. Frequently no cause is identified so families move from searching for a cause to preoccupation with the weaknesses and disability. Families cycle through the various stages of grieving and coping over and over and health care providers often only see the family when there is a crisis, illness, or behavioral issue (Finke). It is important to view the process as a cycle so the APN can intervene and facilitate the move to the acceptance stage. Family members may move through the stages at different paces, which can also add to the stress on the family system (Figure 14.1).

The APN needs to assist the family in each stage of grief by working with the child's strengths to support reaching the child's potential. Families can best assist their child if they focus on strengths and build on achievements to help the child reach her or his highest level. Families should also focus on the child's individual successes and not make comparisons to normal or appropriate milestones based on chronological age. The child's progress should be based only on his or her developmental achievements.

For adolescents with intellectual disabilities, this can be a particularly difficult time because the lack of social skills may be more noticeable to family members, peers, and the adolescent. It is also frequently at the beginning of adolescence that children with intellectual disabilities become increasingly aware of the differences between themselves and other individuals their age. Adolescence is a time for more independence and activities such as driving a car, which may not be possible for an individual who has an intellectual disability.

The APN should also be mindful of the impact of having a brother or sister who is different on the other children in the family. Siblings are often placed in the position to watch over their brother or sister who may be chronologically older or they may find themselves defending their sibling in social situations with their own peers or others. The fact is that as the family matures, siblings will gain more responsibility for the brother or sister with an intellectual or developmental disability. Families need to plan and discuss strategies early in the process and not wait until there is a family crisis such as an illness or death of a parent.

Older children and families may be even more stressed. Co-occurring problems and difficulty in pinpointing a cause may be more frustrating especially if mental health problems are part of the clinical picture (Faust & Scior, 2007). Parents worry about the strain on their child, who does not understand what they are feeling. Parents also feel they are alone in finding answers and appropriate interventions to assist their child. It is important for the APN to remain family focused and view the family as an essential part of the treatment team. Of course, the family knows the child best and must incorporate the child's needs and behavior into their activities and daily life. Children with an intellectual disability often have difficulty with disruptions in routines. Assessment of the family and family behavior patterns should be continuous. Behavior of family members may induce the child's difficult behaviors, resulting in development and maintenance of a circular pattern of negative behaviors (Wright & Leahy, 2009).

Over the life span of the child, diagnostic labels may change. Parents and the child often struggle with labels and parents may resist a child being given a diagnosis at all. APNs need to point out to parents and older children that without a diagnosis, the child will not qualify for any additional assistance at school or from social agencies. Funding follows diagnosis. Families who focus on the child's needs and not the title will be able to seek the most appropriate resources to help their child move forward.

Teachers and other school personnel are also important members of the treatment team. Their observations and goals need to be incorporated into the treatment plan. The APN may also find herself or himself in the advocacy role for the family with the school. Individual needs may take a backseat to larger school or classroom goals, and the APN will need to facilitate the child's and family's needs being heard and met by the school. Parents may need coaching concerning assertiveness and advocacy so they can be more effective in navigating the health care system and the school system. If social services are involved such as Medicaid, even more coordination and advocacy may be needed to combine efforts and work toward mutual goals that are in the child's best interest.

Resiliency Model

The use of the resiliency model of family stress, adjustment, and adaptation is a useful approach to assist families with children who have a disability and help them connect to community resources. The resiliency model builds on the work of McCubbin and Patterson (1983) and their *Typology Model of Family Adjustment and Adaptation* (McCubbin, 1995). The Typology Model of Family Adjustment and Adaptation is a collaborative model that enhances the connection of the family to the community and available resources to assist them in meeting the child's needs. All families cope with stresses over time and those experiences affect the family's perceptions over time. Families with a child who has a disability face even more stresses as they interact with the health care system, the school system, and community systems. Stressors build up but so do coping strategies used by the family. McCubbin and Patterson labeled the adjustment of the family to stressors as adaptation. During adaption, families try to use their usual patterns of coping and those often do not work or do not work for long due to the high level of stress. For the family to move to a more effective level of functioning, they must make changes in patterns of interaction and roles that meet the needs of the child with the disability and those of other family members (Kosciulik, McCubbin, & McCubbin, 1993).

Families learn with the assistance of the APN to use their strengths and resources within the extended family and to connect to resources in the community (Early & Glenmays, 2000). Social support and hardiness have been found to be predictors of successful adaptation by families (Weiss, 2002). Using a strengths perspective, the APN forms a collaborative partnership with the family to assist them in meeting their goals. The APN can activate community resources such as respite care, funding sources, occupational or physical therapy, and transportation (Finke, 2006). The APN should serve as advocate for the family and as problem solver with the school system to find solutions to best meet the needs of the child and his or her family. As the child develops new problems, situations will arise that will need new interventions. Research has shown that the child, especially in adolescence, can be a reliable source to determine personal strengths and difficulties (Emerson, 2005).

Tools such as genograms (pedigree) and ecomaps can provide the APN with the information needed to assist families in reaching out to resources (Wright & Leahey, 2009). A genogram is a picture of the family tree that includes genetic connections, family events such as marriages, births of children, deaths, and health conditions. The genogram is an illustration of the family resources as well as possible connections and sources of assistance such as respite relief. The genogram can also be an important diagnostic tool to identify possible genetic causes of disabilities. The ecomap is an illustration of the community systems that influence each family member and again may be turned into resources. For example, the school would be part of the ecomap as would health care providers and community agencies. The ecomap starts with a circle around the family with lines drawn to community systems that impact each family member. Lines can be doubled and tripled to note positive relationships, and train track lines can be drawn to demonstrate negative influences. The ecomap can be used by the APN and family to identify possible sources for assistance such as a community agency that provides transportation or recreational activities.

The first step is always helping the family determine their own goals and not take on the goals of the APN or other social agencies. For example, some services may push respite care away from the child's home. Some children and families may find respite care in their own home more comfortable, or the other way around. Family belief systems, finances, community resources, and extended family are just a few of the pieces that may determine what is best for the child and family.

Parents should be discouraged from spending money on unproved approaches. Other alternative approaches such as movement and auditory therapies, chiropractic manipulation, nutritional supplements, and brain mapping have not been proved to be effective through evidence-based research (Kemper, Vohra, & Walls, 2008). APNs must be respectful of parents' quest for a cure and seek to educate families about accepted and proven therapies and treatments for disabilities while cautioning them about the potential dangers of unproven approaches. Parents and children, when old enough, should be encouraged to reach out to others with similar issues and participate in support groups. There are many online resources such as the web sites, such as Arc of the United States (TheArcLink.org), which is an organization that advocates for the rights of children and adults with developmental delays. There are state and local chapters as well. The Arc web site has a wealth of information and links to resources about special education, education information about specific diagnoses, and financial resources. The National Center for Learning Disabilities (NCLD.org) has information about specific learning disabilities and links to other resources as well. A similar organization is the Learning Disabilities Association of America (www.ldaamerica.org). Talking with other family members and people with similar issues can be a great comfort and provide support and a wealth of information. Parents need to be referred to educational sessions early about their child's right to a "free and appropriate education" governed by federal and state regulations. The rights begin for children at birth and extend to twenty-one years of age, so parents need to be well informed early in the process.

Community resources vary across states and regions. Parents need to be connected to resources in their community to assist with education, health needs, social supports, financial resources, respite care, etc. APNs can be a direct link to these resources.

Conclusion

After the discovery of an intellectual or learning disability, coping is a major lifelong challenge for the child and the entire family. APNs can provide the needed screening, interventions, and continued support to families to help their family member reach his or her potential. The APN works with the family to progress to the highest potential for all family members. The family is assessed, connected to resources, and assisted through the continuing cycle of coping and building on strengths as the family climbs the ladder of optimal development.

Case Exemplar

Kenneth was a full-term infant born by repeat cesarean section following his mother's healthy pregnancy. He was the second B+ child born to his O− mother. No neonatal issues of jaundice, hypothermia, or neurological issues were noted. Early development was marked by advanced motor abilities including a steady gait and upright stair climbing by ten months of age. Early language skills were adequate, but there was little interest in word play, rhyming, or listening to stories despite daily efforts to engage him in these activities. At three years of age, he sustained a closed head injury, which resulted in a transient loss of vision. Vision returned within an hour, and skull films and a computed tomography scan were normal after this event.

The preschool years were marked by numerous misarticulations. No other issues were noted during his kindergarten readiness evaluation so Kenneth was determined "ready" and entered kindergarten at the age of five years 3 months. In kindergarten it was noted that he was bright and engaging but had limited interest in letter recognition or letter-sound identification. Social skills, behavior, and attention were appropriate and Kenneth was promoted to first grade despite parental concerns about reading readiness.

In the fall of first grade, he was identified by his experienced teacher as not meeting grade expectations for reading so he was placed in a reading support group with other similarly functioning first graders. This group was removed from the regular classroom daily for these additional services. Progress was adequate and promotion followed.

Second grade found Kenneth falling further behind with reading acquisition. When his parents expressed their concerns, they were assured by school authorities that Kenneth was "just not like his brother," who had been a gifted reader since age four, and that Kenneth was making acceptable progress. Separate out-of-classroom reading support continued; no formal assessments were conducted because "it was too early"; promotion followed.

During the summer following second grade, Kenneth was evaluated at a university center for learning and attention disorders. He was found to have an IQ of 126 with a significant discrepancy between his verbal and performance scores and a deficit in phonological awareness. This evaluation gave him the diagnosis of specific learning disability and entitled him to an IEP with daily resource room intervention, reading support in the classroom, and individual speech therapy.

Similar services continued through fifth grade despite Kenneth's increasing objections to being removed from this class and growing resentment at being labeled. Negative and oppositional behaviors developed only at home and sessions of family counseling ensued.

A triennial review prior to middle school revealed that Kenneth had made progress but still required additional time to complete reading assignments due to slow processing resulting from phonological deficits. Some disorders of written output were identified by Kenneth relating excellent ideas but having great difficulty in getting complex thoughts down on paper. Instead of an IEP, a 504 plan was developed, which gave him additional time on reading and writing assignments and separate testing situations for routine and standardized testing. He no longer qualified for an IEP because he no longer demonstrated significant delays or discrepancies between verbal and performance IQ scores.

High school was academically and emotionally challenging. Kenneth insisted he participate in college and honors courses despite the increasing volume of reading and extensive time required for test preparation. Several teachers recognized his difficulties with test-taking and offered oral tests, which he found much easier.

He excelled as a state champion track athlete and student government president but all was not accomplished without high stress and extreme anxiety as he sought to overcome his disabilities by achieving in other areas.

The disability label granted Kenneth additional time on his college board examinations. This allowed him to better demonstrate his abilities. An Ivy League education was Kenneth's dream despite the enormous effort that academics required of him. His dream was fulfilled by an acceptance but the struggles continued. He was expected to participate in huge core classes, taking exams from fast-moving slide presentations using a clicker to respond after trying to commit massive amounts of information to memory. With parents and insightful teachers no longer available to advocate for him, Kenneth learned to become his own advocate, requesting oral examinations, alternative assignments, and other ways to demonstrate his mastery of class material. Kenneth participated as a varsity runner three seasons each year and graduated with honors from an Ivy League institution, dealing with his learning issues every day.

This exemplar demonstrates many themes common to individuals with learning disabilities:

- Early language difficulties
- Possibility of head trauma as contributing factor
- School refusal to take parental concerns seriously and moving children through the system without examining the total child
- Need for additional evaluations outside of school
- Emotional impact of being labeled and perceived as different from peers and sibs
- Value of developing affinities and importance of experiencing success in other areas
- Need for ongoing evaluation and redesigning of academic supports
- Need for advocacy (parental, medical, educational, self)
- Possibility of success and fulfillment.

References

American Academy of Pediatrics (AAP). (2009). Learning disabilities, dyslexia, and vision. *Pediatrics, 124,* 837–844.

American Academy of Pediatrics (AAP). (2010). *Common learning disabilities.* Retrieved from http://www.healthychildren.org/English/health-issues/conditions/learning-disabilities/pages/Common-Learning-Disabilities.aspx

American Association on Intellectual and Developmental Disabilities (AAIDD). (n.d.). Intellectual disabilities. Retrieved from http://www.aaidd.org

American Psychiatric Association. (2010). *Diagnostic and Statistical Manual of Mental Disorders* (fifth edition). Washington, DC: Author.

Aylward, G.P. (1995). *Bayley infant neurodevelopmental screener.* San Antonio, TX: Psychological Corp.

Aylward, G.P., Verhulst, S.J., & Bell, S. (2000). Predictive utility of the BSID-II infant neurodevelopmental screener (BINS) risk status classifications: Clinical interpretation and application. *Dev Med Child Neurol, 42,* 25–31.

Birmaher, B., Khetarpal, S., Cully, M., Brent, D.A., & McKenzie, S. (1995). *Screen for child anxiety related disorders (SCARED).* Pittsburgh, PA: University of Pittsburgh, Western Psychiatric Institute and Clinic.

Blackman, J.A., Levine, M.D., Markowitz, M.T., & Aufseeser, C.L. (1983). The pediatric extended examination at three: A system for diagnostic clarification of problematic three-year-olds. *Journal of Developmental Behavioral Pediatrics, 4,* 143–150.

Breau, L.M., & Burkitt, C. (2009). Assessing pain in children with intellectual disabilities. *Pain Research Management, 14*, 116–120.

Byrd, R. (2005). School failure: Assessment, intervention and prevention in primary care pediatric care. *Pediatrics in Review, 26*, 233–243.

Coleman, W.L., & Levine, M.D. (1988). Attention deficits in adolescence: Description, evaluation, and management. *Pediatrics in Review, 9*, 287–298. doi:10.1542/pir.9-9-287

Conners, C.K. (1990). *Conners' rating scales.* North Tonawanda, NY: Multi-Health Systems, Inc.

Doig, K.B., Macias, M.M., Saylor, C.F., Craver, J.R., & Ingram, P.E. (1999). The child development inventory: A developmental outcome measure for follow-up of the high risk infant. *Journal of Pediatrics, 135*, 358–362.

Donohue, D., Wise, J., Romski, M., Henrich, C. & Sevcik, R. (2010). Self-concept development and measurement in children with mild intellectual disabilities. *Developmental Neurorehabilitation, 13*, 322–334.

Early, T., & GlenMaye, L. (2000). Valuing families: Social work practice with families from a strengths perspective. *Social Work, 45*, 118–130.

Emerson, E. (2005). Use of strengths and difficulties questionnaire to assess the mental health needs of children and adolescents with intellectual disabilities. *Journal of Intellectual and Developmental Disabilities, 30*, 14–23.

Emerson, E., & Hatton, C. (2007). Mental health of children and adolescents with intellectual disabilities in Britain. *British Journal of Psychiatry, 191*, 493–499.

Faulstich, M.E., Carey, M.P., Ruggiero, L., Enyart, P., & Gresham, F. (1986). Assessment of depression in childhood and adolescence: An evaluation of the center for epidemiological studies depression scale for children (CES-DC). *Am J Psychiatry, 143*, 1024–1027.

Faust, H., & Scior, K. (2008). Mental health problems in young people with intellectual disabilities: The impact on parents. *Journal of Applied Research in Intellectual Disabilities, 21*, 414–424.

Finke, L., & Greenberg, C. (2009). The child with a developmental disability. In V. Bowden & C. Greenberg (Eds.), *Children and their families: The continuum of care.* Philadelphia, PA: Lippincott, Williams and Wilkins.

Finke, L. (2006). Family therapies. In W. Mohr (Ed.), *Psychiatric-mental health nursing.* Philadelphia, PA: Lippincott, Williams & Wilkins.

Finke, L. (1995). Mental retardation. In B. Johnson (Ed.), *Child and adolescent family psychiatric nursing.* Philadelphia, PA: J.B. Lippincott.

Frankenburg, W.K., Camp, B.W., & Van Natta, P.A. (1971). Validity of the Denver developmental screening test. *Child Dev, 42*, 475–485.

Frankenburg, W.K., Dodds, J., Archer, P., Shapiro, H., & Bresnick, B. (1992). The Denver II: A major revision and restandardization of the Denver developmental screening test. *Pediatrics, 89*, 91–97.

Friend, A., DeFries, J., & Olson. K. (2008). Parental education moderates genetic influences on reading disability. *Psychological Science, 19*, 1124–1130.

Glascoe, F.P. (1999). Toward a model for an evidenced-based approach to developmental/behavioral surveillance, promotion and patient education. *Ambulatory Child Health, 5*, 197–208.

Glascoe, F.P. (2005). *Technical report for the Brigance screens.* North Billerica, MA: Curriculum Associates Inc.

Glascoe, F.P. (2002). The Brigance infant-toddler screen (BITS): Standardization and validation. *J Dev Behav Pediatr, 23*, 145–150.

Glascoe, F., & Robertshaw, N. (2007). New AAP policy on detecting and addressing developmental and behavioral problems. *Journal of Pediatric Health Care, 21*, 407–412.

Grizzle, K., & Simms, M. (2005). Early language development and language learning disabilities. *Pediatrics in Review, 26*, 268–22.

Hendriksen, J., Keulers, E., Feron, F., Wassenberg R., Jolles, J., & Vles, J. (2007). Subtype of learning disabilities, *European Child and Adolescent Psychiatry, 16*, 517–524.

Individuals with Disability Education Improvement Act of 2004. Pub. L. No. 108–446. 118 Stat. 2647 (2004).

Individuals with Disability Education Improvement Act (IDEA). (n.d.). *Learning disabilities.* Retrieved from www2.ed.gov/policy/speced/guid/idea/idea2004.html http://www.copyright.gov/legislation/pl108-446.pdf

Ireton, H. (1992). *Child development inventory manual.* Minneapolis, MN: Behavior Science Systems Inc.

Jellinek, M,. Murphy J., & Little, M. (1999). Use of the pediatric symptom checklist (PSC) to screen for psychosocial problems in pediatric primary care: A national feasibility study. *Archives of Pediatric and Adolescent Medicine, 153*, 254–260.

Kadosh, R., & Walsh, V. (2007). Dyscalculia. *Current Biology, 17*, 946–947.

Kaptein, S., Jansen, D.E.M.C., Vogels, A.G.C., & Reijneveld, S.A. (2007). Mental health problems in children with intellectual disability: Use of the strengths and difficulties questionnaire. *Journal of Intellectual Disability Research, 52*, 125–131.

Kemper, K.J., Vohra, S., & Walls, R. (2008). American Academy of Pediatrics, Task Force on Complementary and Alternative Medicine, Provisional Section on Complementary, Holistic, and Integrative Medicine: The use of complementary and alternative medicine in pediatrics. *Pediatrics, 122*, 1374–1386.

Knight, S., Regan, R., Nicod, A., Horsley, S., Homfray, T., Winter, & Flint, J. (1999). Subtle chromosomal rearrangements in children with unexplained mental retardation. *Lancet, 354*, 1676–1681.

Kosiulek, J., McCubbin, M., & McCubbin, H. (1993). A theoretical framework for family adaptation to head injury. *Journal of Rehabilitation, 59*, 40–45.

Lagae, L. (2008). Learning disabilities: Definitions, epidemiology, diagnosis, and intervention strategies. *Pediatric Clinics of North America, 55*, 1259–1268.

Levine, M.D. (1980). *The Anser system parent questionnaire: Form 2P.* Cambridge, MA: Educators Publishing Service Inc.

Levine, M.D. (1983). *The pediatric early elementary examination.* Cambridge, MA: Educators Publishing Service Inc.

Levine, M.D. (1985). *Examiners manual, PEERAMID: Pediatric examination of educational readiness at middle childhood* Cambridge, MA: Educators Publishing Service Inc.

Levine, M.D. (n.d.-a). *The ANSER system: Grades Pre-K-6.* Available at http://eps.schoolspecialty.com/products/details.cfm?seriesonly=1762m

Levine, M.D. (n.d.-b). *Neurodevelopmental examinations (PEET, PEER, PEEX 2, PEERAMID).* Available at http://eps.schoolspecialty.com/cs/how_to_order.cfm

Levine, M.D., Meltzer, L.J., Busch, B., Palfrey, J., & Sullivan, M. (1983). The pediatric early elementary examination: Studies of a neurodevelopmental examination for 7- to 9-year old children. *Pediatrics, 71*, 894–903.

Levine, M.D., Oberklaid, F., Ferb, T.E., Hanson, M.A., Palfrey, J.S.m & Aufseeser, D.L. (1980). The pediatric examination of educational readiness: Validation of an extended observation procedure. *Pediatrics, 66*, 341–349.

McCubbin, M. (1995). The typology model of adjustment and adaptation: A family stress model. *Counseling and Guidance, 10*(4), 31–37.

McCubbin, M., & Patterson, J. (1983). The family stress process: The double ABCX model of adjustment and adaptation. In

H. McCubbin, M. Sussman, & J. Patterson (Eds.), *Social stress and the family: Advances and development in family stress theory and research* (pp. 7–37). New York, NY: Haworth Press.

McGrew, K.S., & Woodcock, R. (2001). *Woodcock-Johnson III technical manual.* Chicago, IL: Riverside Publishing.

National Center for Learning Disabilities (NCLD). (n.d.). *Section 504 and IDEA comparison chart.* Retrieved from http://www.ncld.org/at-school/your-childs-rights/iep-aamp-504-plan/section-504-and-idea-...

Newborg, J. (2004). *Battelle developmental inventory* (second edition). Itasca, IL: Riverside Publishing.

Rehabilitation Act of 1973, Pub. L. No. 93–112 (1973).

Shaywitz, S., & Shaywitz, B. (2003). Dyslexia (specific learning disability). *Pediatrics in Review, 34,* 147–152.

Schwarte, A. (2008). Fragile X syndrome. *School Psychology Quarterly, 23,* 290–300.

Shaffer, D., Fisher, P., & Lucas, C. (2003). The diagnostic interview schedule for children (DISC). In M.J. Hilsenroth, D.L. Segal, & M. Hersen (Eds.), *Comprehensive handbook of psychological assessment* (Vol 2) (pp. 256–270). New York, NY: Wiley.

Sices, L., Taylor, H., Freebairn, L., Hansen, A., & Lewis, B. (2007). Relationship between speech-sound disorders and early literacy skills in preschool-age children: Impact of comorbid language impairment. *Journal of Developmental and Behavioral Pediatrics, 28,* 438–447.

Squires, J., Potter, L., & Bricker, D. (1999). *The ASQ user's guide* (second edition). Baltimore, MD: Paul H. Brookes Publishing.

U.S. Department of Education Office of Special Education Programs. (n.d.). *Identification of specific learning disabilities.* Retrieved from http://idea.ed.gov/explore/view/p/%2Croot%2Cdynamic%2CTopicalBrief%2C23%2C

Vellutino, F., Fletcher, J., Snowling, M., & Scanlon, D. (2004). Specific reading disability (dyslexia): What have we learned in the past four decades? *Journal of Child Psychology and Psychiatry, 45,* 2–40.

Weiss, M.J. (2002). Hardiness and social support as predictors of stress in mothers of typical children, children with autism, and children with mental retardation. *Autism, 6,* 115–130.

Wechsler, D. (1991). *The Wechsler intelligence scale for children* (third edition). San Antonio, TX: The Psychological Corporation.

Wilkinson, G.S., & Robertson, G.J. (2006). *Wide range achievement test: fourth edition.* Lutz, FL: Psychological Assessment Resources.

Wolraich, M.L., Hannah, J.N., Pinnock, T.Y., Baumgaertel, A., & Brown, J. (1996). Comparison of diagnostic criteria for attention-deficit hyperactivity disorder in a county-wide sample. *Journal of the American Academy of Child and Adolescent Psychiatry, 35,* 319–324.

Wright, L., & Leahey, M. (2009). *Nurses and families: A guide to family assessment and intervention* (fifth edition). Philadelphia, PA: F.A. Davis.

15

Nonpharmacological Treatment Modalities: Play and Group Therapies

Judith Hirsh and Edilma L. Yearwood

Objectives

After reading this chapter, APNs will be able to

1. Understand the historical, theoretical, conceptual, and treatment processes associated with play and group therapies.
2. Identify diagnostic and behavioral symptom clusters that can be addressed through use of play or group therapy techniques.
3. Critique the evidence on effectiveness of specific play and group therapy techniques with children and adolescents.
4. Identify how APNs can use play and group therapy techniques in their primary care and mental health practices.

Introduction

Nonpharmacological treatment of children with mental and behavioral health concerns includes the treatment modalities of play and group therapies. Play therapy is a complex modality and includes techniques such as child-centered, prescriptive or directive, bibliotherapy, expressive play, cognitive-behavioral therapy, projective and symbolic play, filial therapy, and group therapy. Group therapy interventions with children and adolescents strive to educate, facilitate relationships, and provide youngsters with corrective emotional experiences.

Therapists (psychiatric-mental health [PMH] nurse practitioners or clinical nurse specialists who are referred to as advanced practice nurses [APNs], psychologists, psychiatrists, or social workers) incorporate a variety of toys and media during *play therapy* sessions to guide the child to better communicate with others, become self-aware, express feelings and thoughts (catharsis), and learn new or enhanced ways of relating and interacting in the world. The therapist ensures that there is safe, psychological distance from problematic issues and facilitates developmentally appropriate expression of thoughts, feelings, and behaviors (Association for Play Therapy [APT], 2001; Bonner, 2004; Gil, 2004; Johnson, Pedro-Carroll, & Demanchik, 2005; Kot & Tyndall-Lind, 2005; Schaefer & Reid 1986; Terr 2003). Play therapy is defined by the APT as the "systematic use of a theoretical model to establish an interpersonal process in which trained play therapists use the therapeutic powers of play to help clients prevent or resolve psychosocial difficulties and achieve optimal growth and development" (APT, n.d., para. 2).

Thus, play therapy conducted by APN therapists has scientific underpinnings and mounting clinical evidence

Child and Adolescent Behavioral Health: A Resource for Advanced Practice Psychiatric and Primary Care Practitioners in Nursing, First Edition. Edited by Edilma L. Yearwood, Geraldine S. Pearson, and Jamesetta A. Newland.
© 2012 John Wiley & Sons, Inc. Published 2012 by John Wiley & Sons, Inc.

for support as a treatment modality. Likewise, the "art" of developmentally appropriate play is a skill set that can be taught to pediatric/family nurse practitioners for use during assessment of children and adolescents to help reduce anxiety and successfully engage young children and adolescents in a meaningful interaction during a physical examination. The art of play includes such strategies as asking the child to blow bubbles while listening to chest sounds, making a finger "become magical" by lighting up the tip of the finger with the otoscope before examining the child's ear, and role playing with school-age children and adolescents to reduce the potential for engaging in high-risk behaviors. Thus, play and play therapy are an integral part of the assessment and intervention processes in pediatric health care.

Group therapy involves a collection of individuals, having something in common, who meet together to work with one or more therapists or counselors toward some element of change. Change can occur at the individual, interpersonal, or group level. Group participation and effectiveness rely on dynamics and interactions within the group to increase knowledge, understanding, and insight while also improving social skills and promoting behavioral change (American Group Psychotherapy Association, 2007).

This chapter will address the importance and evidence-based benefits of play and group therapies, highlight research on neurobiological impact from use of these modalities, and describe the significance of these interventions in promoting healthy child and adolescent growth and development. Theoretical foundations on which these modalities are based are also briefly discussed. Evidence exists for using these therapeutic modalities for specific symptom clusters, behaviors, genders, and age groups. This chapter provides an introductory overview and encourages the APN in primary care to (a) seek further education and skills in basic play and group therapy techniques for use with common behavioral presentations; (b) refer children and adolescents to child and adolescent PMH APNs trained and certified in these treatment modalities; and (c) work collaboratively with PMH APNs to meet both the medical and behavioral/mental health needs of the pediatric population.

Play Therapy

The Importance of Play

Play has been shown to be an essential factor in healthy cognitive, physical, and emotional development. Unfortunately, recent studies and surveys reveal a decline in free play in children beginning in preschool (American Academy of Pediatrics 2006; Wenner, 2009). A recent article in *Scientific American* discussed the importance of free play citing it as essential to developing healthy social skills, effectively solving problems, coping with stress, and building cognitive skills (Wenner). Free play affords children the opportunity to use imagination and creativity, enhance communication skills, and master new skills. Playing with peers in unstructured ways affords the development of interpersonal skills, including sharing, learning to be fair, compromising, and taking turns. Through play, frustration tolerance develops, as well as motivation and persistence to achieve a desired goal.

In 2007 Ginsburg et al. published the American Academy of Pediatrics position paper on play, which emphasized the need for an appropriate individualized balance between scheduled organized adult-supervised activities and family/parent-child interactions related to play. The balance as related to play also included child-centered activities with peers, consideration of the child's temperament, academic needs, and environmental and family needs. This balance is believed to offer protective factors and builds resilience during stages of child development. Play recommendations included (a) the use of toys to promote childhood imagination and fantasy, (b) education of parents on the value of being supportive and nurturing during play activities, and (c) the need to encourage parents to involve themselves in their children's creative play while discouraging passive play. An example of passive play is time alone with computers and television.

Neurobiology of Play

The brain structures shown by researchers to be involved in play behaviors are the cerebellum, cortex, prefrontal cortex, and thalamus. Scientists studying human development and play conclude that play contributes to neurological growth, particularly in complex, socially skilled, and cognitively adaptable developing brains (Frost, 1998; Henig, 2008).

The brainstem has the primary function of regulating core physiology and primary sensory processing. Play activity with infants and toddlers include peak-a-boo and tactile sensory play. Rhythmic and patterned sensory play with an attuned and responsive caregiver promotes attachment, state regulation, and resilience. Beginning in infancy through childhood, games that promote development of the midbrain also incorporate motor control and secondary sensory processing. Examples include listening to and playing music, singing, engaging in gross and fine motor games, and repeating rhymes, poems, and stories. During the period from early childhood through puberty the limbic system develops. Learning to appropriately interpret nonverbal communication; accurately reading social cues; and expressing creativity through art, music, and drama are all believed to enhance limbic system development (Gaskill, 2004, 2010). Engaging in games that facilitate social skills is thought to improve sharing, taking turns, and frustration tolerance. Participating in play groups has been attributed to improved memory, emotional regulation, attachment, affiliation, affect regulation, and primary sensory integration.

Another brain region, the (neo) cortex develops during childhood and is believed to be responsible for reasoning, problem-solving, abstraction, socioemotional integration, and secondary sensory integration. Overall, emotional and cognitive growth in children is promoted by the use of humor, language, art, and games with rules or strategy that supports exploration, critical thinking, problem solving, and storytelling/story creation (Gaskill, 2004, 2010; Perry 2006).

Historical Development of Play Therapy
Theoretical Frameworks of Play

There are a variety of theoretical styles for conducting play therapy. One predominant framework is a child-centered approach, in which the child chooses the activity and paces the therapy. It is based on humanistic philosophies offered by Carl Rogers (Johnson et al., 2005; O'Connor, 2000; Rogers, 1951) and Axline (1978). Children control their own growth toward maturity, self-actualization, and healing. The child's perception of his reality is most important; therefore, it is expressed without the therapist's interpretation or confrontation. In this method, the therapist must learn to trust the process. Treatment is not specific to any issue or identified problem (Table 15.1).

The other predominant framework is directive or prescriptive therapy. Here the therapist chooses the therapeutic activity and paces the sessions. This approach can be shorter or time-limited, attaining goals more quickly than the child-centered approach. It is flexible in that the therapist matches the technique or intervention with the presenting symptoms. The principles of prescriptive play therapy include using various play methods during a session to address identified issues or problems. Without a strict adherence to a particular technique, the treatment is customized for that particular child. It is multimodal, multicomponent, and multilayered, using scientific evidence as a guide for effectively intervening, including published practice guidelines and manuals (National Institute for Play, 2009; Schaefer, 2001).

In cognitive-behavioral play therapy (CBPT), Knell (1998) incorporated Beck's cognitive-behavioral therapy with therapeutic play. CBPT can be used with preschool children and relies on flexibility and a decreased need for verbalization. Therapists model improved behavior, using metaphor or other indirect expression of change via play techniques. CBPT matches the child's developmental level with an appropriate therapeutic behavioral intervention. For example, Cohen and Deblinger (2004) used dolls and puppets to cognitively reframe and gradually expose children and adolescents to trauma issues. When used, this method is directive, time-limited, structured, and problem-oriented. This intervention is considered successful if thoughts, feelings, and beliefs of the child or adolescent are changed (Shelby & Felix, 2005). For example, a sexually abused child or teen enters treatment feeling responsible and guilty for the abuse. The treatment process produces a change in which the child or teen can place responsibility and guilt with the adult or abuser for the abuse.

Adlerian play therapy is based on Adler's individual psychology, which includes beliefs that humans have an inherent need to belong, feel connected to others, are goal-directed, and want to feel adequate and valued and that all behavior has a purpose (Kottman, 2001). Theraplay was developed by Ann Jernberg in the late 1960s. Using this method, treatment is a directive, short-term structured intervention promoting the early healthy bond between child and caregiver. It involves nurturing physical contact between child and parent and/or child and therapist using all the senses as part of the modality, but touch is most often the primary intervention (Munns, 2000).

Ecosystemic play therapy incorporates elements of analytic, child-centered, cognitive-behavioral, and theraplay into a humanistic, phenomenological, theory-dependent approach. The goal is to help children get their needs met in ways that do not interfere with the needs of others. Building attachment is a priority. The therapist uses interpretations, corrective experiences, goal setting, and advocacy as part of the therapeutic process (O'Connor, 2001).

Filial therapy, developed in the 1960s by Louise and Bernard Guerney, is an intensive, structured, time-limited (twenty to twenty-four sessions) technique in which parents are taught to be more therapeutically involved with their child. Through weekly didactic group training, homework, role play, and supervision in the outpatient setting and then at home, parents are taught basic child-centered play therapy principles. They learn to convey empathy, acceptance, and encouragement as well as appropriate limit setting and consequences. The intervention is deemed successful when positive changes are noted in the parent-child relationship, family environment, decreased levels of parental stress, increased self-esteem in the child, child adjustment, and improved behavior (Rennie & Landreth, 2000; VanFleet, 2005; VanFleet, Ryan, & Smith, 2005).

Table 15.1 Historical development of play therapy

Time Frame	Theorist/Milestone
1900s	**S. Freud** (1909): Applied theory of instinctual drives to child psychotherapy. Bibliotherapy was used as an educational tool to provide information.
1920s	**C. Jung**: Developed analytic model of psychotherapy and interpretation (use of symbols, metaphors and archetypes) **M. Lowenfeld**: Used sand and miniature objects to uncover unconscious issues **A. Freud**: Developed the child psychotherapy model
1940s	**C. Rogers:** Client-centered therapy **V. Axline**: Developed the principles of child-centered treatment. Wrote Dibs in Search of Self.
1950s–1960s	**M. Klein**: Equated play with free association used in adult therapy. **E. Erikson**: Developed the 8 stages of psychosocial development needed for emotional health. **J. Piaget**: Credited with the Cognitive Development Model which stated that children develop intelligence by doing, imitating, observing, and interpreting. Play was viewed as a continuous organization and re-organization of experiences that begin in infancy. **J. Bowlby**: Attachment Theory: Wrote about the importance of object relations (trust, protection, limits, and meeting needs) and understanding transitional objects. **A. Jernberg**: Developed the Theraplay Model at Head Start in Chicago.

1970s–1980s	**R. Gardner**: Created psychotherapeutic games for use with resistant children ages 4–15. Examples:
	  Mutual Storytelling Game(1971)
	  Talking, Feeling & Doing Game (1973)
	  Storytelling Game (1988)
	O'Connor & Schaefer: Started the Association of Play Therapy (APT)
	Bowlby & Ainsworth (1988): Described healthy and pathological coping styles based on quality of parent-child attachment

1990s	**Decade of the Brain**: An increase in research led to increased knowledge and understanding of neurobiology and neurophysiology. **Benedict (1997)**: Conducted research on play themes of safety, anger, loss, constancy, and nurturance. Developed Thematic Play Therapy
2000	**Ray, Bratton, Rhine & Jones** (2001) conducted meta-analysis of studies from 1940–2000 on effectiveness of play therapy.

Table created from information found in "A History of Play Therapy" from the British Association of Play Therapists.

In summary, PMH APNs most often use child-centered and/or prescriptive models to gather assessment data and continue using these models, perhaps alternating them during the treatment process. CBPT, theraplay, and filial therapy models require specialized training and supervision. They are also time intensive. The Alderian and ecosystemic models reflect more of the basic nursing principles of care; therefore, elements of these models (the need to belong, need to have value, be goal-directed, experience attachment, and a corrective experience of interaction) are used by PMH APNs. These techniques can also be learned by APNs who practice in pediatric primary care settings as part of brief office-based interventions to begin the process of changing unacceptable behaviors. Intradisciplinary referrals would have the advantage of APNs using the same techniques to begin the change process.

Play Therapy as Evidence-Based Practice

Evidence-based practice reviews of child play therapy are limited in number compared to those found in psychotherapy with adult populations. Saunders, Berliner, and Hanson (2004) conducted an extensive review of the literature and developed twenty-four treatment-specific guidelines for primary psychotherapeutic interventions with child abuse victims and families. Each protocol met the criteria of having a sound theoretical base, clinical anecdotal literature, high acceptance among practitioners, low risk of harm, and empirical support for their utility. The twenty-four protocols were organized into child-focused, parent, parent-child, and family-focused interventions. Offender-focused interventions comprised the third section.

The researchers cited only one treatment protocol, trauma-focused play therapy, as meeting the highest standard for effective treatment. Trauma-focused play therapy met the criteria by having a sound theoretical base, substantial clinical or anecdotal literature review, and acceptance as a clinical practice that posed little risk when used. Behavioral parent training met a lower ranked category of criteria, yet was evaluated as supported and acceptable treatment. It is often used with other populations efficaciously and has been researched in randomized controlled studies (Saunders et al., 2004).

Research-supported treatments were found to be based on cognitive-behavioral approaches using behavioral as well as cognitive techniques and to be targeted at both the individual child and the parent or family system. They were goal-directed, structured, and built on consecutive skill levels until the goal of treatment was reached. They emphasized skill building by role-play, homework and management of emotional distress (self-regulation), and repetition of skills at the therapy site and at home.

Meta-analysis of six decades of research (Bratton & Ray, 2000) identified eighty experimental research studies from 1942 to 2000, examining the efficacy of play therapy as a treatment modality. Most of the research was conducted in the 1970s (N = 23), 1980s (N = 16), and 1990s (N = 17). Participants ranged in age from three to seven years and were placed into nondirective or child-centered play therapy on average for twelve sessions. Reviewing problem areas that had at least eight empirical studies, they concluded that positive outcomes were noted across all areas reviewed. But the most significant finding about the efficacy of play therapy was in improved self-concept, behavioral and emotional adjustment, social skills, intelligence, and reduction of anxiety and fear.

Ray, Bratton, Rhine, and Jones (2001) conducted a meta-analysis of ninety-four studies that included 3,263 subjects. They showed play therapy (N = 70) to be an effective modality, filial therapy (N = 28) to also be effective, and a combination of the two (N = 3) to be most effective. Therapy style was most often child-centered (N = 74) and behavioral or directive (N = 12). The meta-analysis supported prior research, although on a small sample size (N = 23), as to the duration of play therapy treatment. The mean number of sessions for the combined intervention was 16.5 and filial therapy was 14.5 sessions. They found that in the solo play therapy group, treatment effectiveness grew with an increased number of sessions, culminating at a peak of thirty-five to forty-five sessions and then leveling off. Davenport and Bourgeois's 2008 review of the literature validated the 2000 and 2001 meta-analyses regarding the significance of involving the family or parent in their own parallel treatment. They noted the improved quality of parent-child interactions as being a focus in effective play-based interventions particularly with aggressive young children.

Symptom Clusters

Play therapy is most often used for symptoms identified as either internalizing (emotional) or externalizing (disruptive, aggressive). Internalizing symptoms reflect all the anxiety disorders; the affective or mood disorders including suicidal ideation; psychosis, including hallucinations; and somatic disorders. The externalizing disorders include attention deficit hyperactivity disorder, rule-breaking disorders such as conduct disorder and oppositional defiant disorder, personality disorders, Tourette's, and attachment disorders (Achenbach, 1966; Achenbach & Rescorla, 2001; Eisenberg et al., 2001; Tackett, 2010). There is some overlap in the two clusters with behaviors characteristic of eating disorders, substance abuse, schizophrenia, and autism spectrum disorders.

Play Techniques for Assessment and Treatment

Providing quality care involves a thorough and comprehensive assessment of the child and family. Gathering data about risk factors, mental status assessment, peer and family interactions, developmental milestones of the child and family, and environmental factors all contributes to successful treatment during the play therapy process. Assessment and treatment are conducted in part by using the expressive play therapies (art, stories, and sandplay).

Play Therapy Toolkit

Art

Using the medium of art, the PMH APN asks a child/adolescent to draw a picture that may explain his/her feelings about an event. Likewise, during primary care visits, the primary care APN often asks a child to draw a picture as part of a developmental assessment. Assessing artwork includes the use of colors, shading, spatial aspects including symmetry and use of background and foreground, developmental expectations of skill, objects included or excluded, and imagery. Art is quite effective as a mode of expression for children's emotional issues (trauma, illness, and feelings). While PMH APNs learn to assess artwork for therapeutic interventions, primary care APNs are taught to view the artwork from a developmental perspective. However, the primary care APN must be cognizant of "normal" versus "abnormal" drawings and make an appropriate referral for the child whose artwork is outside the norm. For example, primary care APNs have and should continue to refer children whose drawings are suggestive of sexual or physical abuse to PMH APNs or other mental health practitioners (Figure 15.1).

When given free choice of art supplies, this youngster drew on black construction paper (mood), in appropriate crayon colors. He added a jumping frog in deep water smiling (activity level and inappropriate affect), with rain, clouds, and sun occurring simultaneously.

Sandplay

As a therapeutic modality, the technique of sandplay has evolved from its origins, which were based on Jung's theories (1968) and then incorporated Lowenfeld's concepts (1999). Jung saw play as a process in which the child's unconscious "bubbles up" with no control such as when daydreaming. He viewed toys as symbols that could be used to activate the unconscious. A central concept in Jung's work was the idea of the need for balance in order to have psychic health. Jung thought that symptoms were symbols of conflict. He viewed imagination and creative fantasy as important in the therapeutic process.

The archetypes (instinctual representations and metaphor) are potentially positive or negative. Jung thought that the self was the central organizing archetype which served to heal and which sought balance by restoring equilibrium. The role of the therapist in this technique is to use knowledge of healing archetypes and symbols to validate, support, contain, and help make meanings and connections for the child or adolescent to examine (Carey, 1999).

The therapist using Lowenfeld's technique has the child or adolescent use sand, landscape symbols, and animals to create a "picture." The therapist then helps the child or adolescent examine recurring themes, objects, and archetypes in order to help the youngster understand issues, which were perhaps not clear when they created the "picture" (Lowenfeld, 1999).

Kalff's (2003) model of sandplay incorporates Jung's and Lowenfeld's models. When using Kalff's model, therapists are silent observers. Stages of psychological development are considered when evaluating a tray for how objects are placed in the sand, overall symmetry and image produced, the use of animals and vegetation, conflict between good and evil, and a balance of opposites (Carey, 1999; Kalff, 2003).

Puppets

Using expressive therapy techniques such as puppets to tell stories allows children to externalize their conflicts, distress, and concerns. Puppet characters effectively provide psychological distance from the issue or fantasy. Puppet shows may be used to present psychoeducational material, role play, and support cognitive change. A variety of puppet types promote symbolic expression of feelings or events (Figure 15.2). Assessment techniques have been developed that use puppets in gathering data

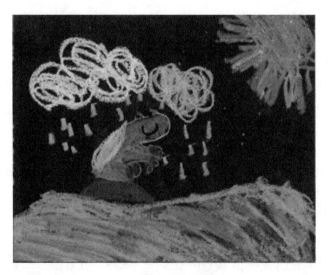

Figure 15.1 Drawing by a 7-year-old depicting bipolar experience.

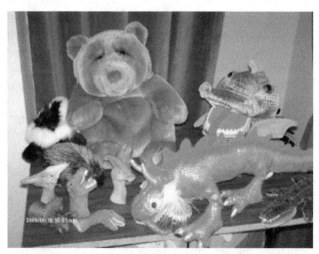

Figure 15.2 Examples of puppets used in play therapy.

about child and family experiences (Knell & Beck, 2000; Depa & Astramovich, 2008).

Bibliotherapy

Since the early 1900s, bibliotherapy has developed into a prescriptive play intervention in which the therapist selects a story that matches the client's conflict with healthier resolution offered than the one already chosen. It may be used as part of CBPT or as an assessment technique. The process promotes growth by being centered on the guided discussions after the story is told. Hynes and Hynes-Berry (1986) defined bibliotherapy as a four-step interactive process that may take place individually or in groups. The process includes (1) recognizing the subjective value of the story (catharsis), (2) exploring the meaning of who, what, when, where, and why, (3) examining new connections in thoughts, and (4) applying new insights or creating new solutions. The results are evident in improved self-esteem, awareness of feelings, empathy, and assimilation of psychological or social values into the participant's behavior and personality (Hynes & Hynes-Berry).

The use of metaphor is important to mention here as it is evident not only in stories and puppet play but in other expressive modalities. A metaphor is an externalized symbolic representation of something or someone from one's own experience which allows for catharsis, insight, growth and change. Goal-oriented metaphors have been developed into stories for therapeutic use (Lankton & Lankton, 1989; Mills & Crowley, 1986).

Games

Gardner's psychotherapeutic games *Talking, Feeling and Doing* (2001) and *Storytelling* (1975) are based on his mutual storytelling technique (1975). The technique originally attempted to have uncooperative or resistant children verbalize their fantasies and, with the assistance of the therapist, analyze them. The children received chips and small prizes for their cooperation. The therapist would present stories based on the children's issues, using their characters and settings but offering healthier resolutions or adaptations. These "games" are still widely used by trained play therapists (Bellinson, 2002; Gardner, 2001).

"Themed" card decks were developed for the *Talking, Feeling and Doing* game and are useful in promoting expression of feelings about issues such as anger, divorce, good behavior, shyness, and teasing. Other card games that elicit data about thoughts and feelings can also be useful during the assessment and treatment process and are most popular with adolescents (Arneson, 2003; Crary & Katayama, 2004). Structured games can be used as assessment tools in gathering data on social skills, self-discipline, cooperation, socioflexibility, leadership, emotional control, tolerance, and problem solving. Structured games are recognized by behaviorists as having therapeutic value in changing maladaptive behavior by developing new skills (Bellinson, 2002; Swank, 2008). Assessment tools have been developed that gather data on development, facilitate psychiatric diagnosis, and examine parent-child interactions and family systems, peer interactions, and projective play (Carey, 1999; Gitlin-Weiner, Sandgrund & Schaefer, 2000; Landreth, 2001).

Group Therapy

The use of group therapy with adults has a long and rich history. While group work with children has been documented for over seventy years, much less group therapy research and publications are available for this population. Moreno is credited with coining the term *group therapy* in 1932, and Slavson was called the Father of Group Psychotherapy in the 1940s. Early theorists who used group therapy in their work with children and adolescents included Moreno, Slavson, Fraiberg, Bettelheim, Redl, and Durkin (Kraft, 1996). A good historical summary of group work can be found in a review by Barlow, Burlingame, and Fuhriman (2000). The power of groups as a therapeutic intervention lies in their cost-effectiveness compared to individual interpersonal therapy, their ability to be focused and time-limited, and the fact that group work as a treatment modality fostered relationship building.

More recently, Yalom (1995) has been credited with what we know about curative group factors and functions of groups. The major strengths of groups as described by Yalom include the power of the here and now interactions between group members, opportunity for development of self-awareness secondary to repeated interactions and actions in the group, and the opportunity the group offers for corrective emotional experiences. Yalom identified 11 essential curative factors within groups that support behavioral change in group members. These include instillation of hope, universality, catharsis, imparting information, family recapitulation, altruism, socializing techniques, interpersonal learning, cohesiveness, existential factors, and imitative behaviors. Research with youth on their perceptions of the most helpful group factors include group cohesiveness (relationships), catharsis, universality, hope, interpersonal learning, and support (Fuhriman, Burlingame, Seaman, & Barlow, 1999; Mishna, 2004; Shechtman & Gluk, 2005).

Group Characteristics

Most group experiences for children and adolescents occur in settings that they frequent. Schools account for approximately 79% of group activities followed by community agencies, hospitals, and clinics (Kulic, Horne, & Dagley, 2004). Most of the group work occurring in schools has a preventative focus. Group work has been conducted by a variety of individuals with various levels of training, comfort, and skills. The type and purpose of the group will often dictate who conducts the group. To be most effective, however, groups should be conducted by appropriately trained and supervised individuals.

Groups are most successful if members are motivated to participate in the process, are able to commit to appropriate group behaviors (nonaggressive, able to take turns, able to listen to others), and can maintain group confidentiality as warranted. Groups can vary in the number of times they meet (once to ten times or more), the length of the session (i.e., thirty to ninety minutes), and where they meet (an office, conference room, classroom, or group room). Groups can vary in size depending on the function of the group. In order to be more effective and support member participation, counseling and therapy groups function better if size is limited to six to ten members. Psychoeducation groups, however, can be larger but should not be so large that they overwhelm the leader, distract, or inhibit member participation.

It is generally recognized that most groups, including child and adolescent groups, go through stages in their development and work. These stages are frequently referred to as initial or beginning, working, and termination. Group members are usually unsure of what to do or say during the initial phase and will either take the behavioral lead from the group leader, resist participation, or challenge and question the purpose or group process. During the working phase, the members are engaged, provide feedback, and usually do most of the work with the leader serving as a supportive resource or catalyst to steer the group in a particular direction. In the termination phase, group members may regress to earlier behaviors due to fear about their personal capabilities in the absence of the group. Some may express anger towards the leader or fellow group members based on fear of abandonment while others may voice uncertainty about how to fill the void in time, structure, and relationships that mark the upcoming end of the group.

There are four common types of groups as identified by the Association for Specialists in Group Work (ASGW) (1991). Each requires specific training based on professional standards:

1. *Task or work groups:* Focus is on specific activities that the group develops or works to accomplish within a designated time frame. Examples include an art project, creating information manuals, or building a tree house.

2. *Psychoeducation groups:* Groups use a teaching format to impart information, skills, or knowledge about specific content area to affected and/or unaffected individuals (primary or secondary prevention). Examples include social skills development, obesity prevention, managing transitions, and learning about the effects of medications.

3. *Counseling groups:* Focus is on making positive adjustments to interpersonal or behavioral problems of group members. The process involves in-depth cognitive exploration of experiences, emotional catharsis, and ego strengthening. Development of personal competencies is often a goal of counseling groups. Examples include bereavement/loss and grief, anger management, addictions, and depression management groups.

4. *Therapy groups:* Groups use traditional psychotherapy techniques to focus on more ingrained and long standing personality and interpersonal problems. The goal is to remediate psychological problems (ASGW). Examples include groups for individuals with eating disorders, those with borderline personality, and those who self-harm.

Counseling and therapy groups have a different theoretical foundation than CBT groups, which tend to focus on cognitive changes as discussed in Chapter 17. The framework for counseling and therapy groups is primarily humanistic, with the leader encouraging communication that fosters self-disclosure and affective exploration to support insight into personal behaviors (Shechtman, 2007).

Groups are usually considered open or closed to additional members. Closed groups do not allow new members into the group once the group begins its work because of the potential to disrupt the process of the group when new members are added. Membership in a closed group is set for the duration of the group to enhance the effectiveness of the group work. Open groups are groups that allow members to join at any point in the trajectory of the group. An example of an open group would be an Alateen support group for adolescents in the community.

Group content usually refers to what is said in the group while process refers to what happens in the group (behaviors, alliances, omissions, activities, rituals, etc.). It is important for the group leader to establish basic group norms at the beginning of any group that is formed and to invite members to add additional "rules" or behavioral expectations to the list. Common norms include getting to group on time, treating others with respect, maintaining the confidentiality of all group members (what happens in group stays in group), and no hitting or intimidation of others. In counseling and therapy groups, leaders also discourage members from developing intimate relationships with each other as this would pose a distraction and interfere with the work of the group. This issue can be particularly problematic in adolescent and early adult aged groups where participants may also be struggling with isolation and yearning for intimate relationships.

Who Is Best Suited for Groups?

The use of groups as a treatment modality is effective with most youngsters including those traumatized, learning disabled, bullying victims, substance abusers, those with low self-esteem, younger children, and older adolescents. There are differing opinions about groups for conduct disordered children. These are usually difficult groups to conduct because of the amount of resistance and testing of the leader that occur and may be more effective with the use of two group leaders. Ang and Hughes (2001) conducted a meta-analysis of social skills groups with conduct-disordered youth and concluded that homogeneous groups of conduct-disordered youth should be discouraged because they appear to result in escalation of antisocial behaviors. Gifford-Smith, Dodge, Dishion, and McCord (2005), on the other hand, thought that group characteristics can be mediated to avoid a negative outcome. Mediating factors include a skilled group therapist, groups with younger children, and group leader attention to a more heterogeneous group composition. However, the use of gender-specific groups for sensitive topics and certain developmental ages has been effective (Avinger & Jones, 2007).

Shechtman (2007) reported on data that show that among the three attachment styles of secure, anxious, and avoidant, avoidant children tend to resist self-disclosure, are less motivated to participate, and are more disruptive in groups. She recommends, however, that most children should be tried in groups and that it is the responsibility of the group leader to monitor and set limits on negative member behaviors as they occur. Repeated negativistic and disruptive behavior should not be tolerated and would indicate that the particular group member is not ready for a group experience. It is counterproductive to maintain a disruptive member in any group.

Effective Group Leader Characteristics

It is the responsibility of the group leader to set the tone of the group experience, ensure safety of group members, and protect the boundaries within the group and between the group and external entities. The climate or tone of the group as set by the leader and maintained by all group members can either impede or support group outcomes (Kivlighan & Tarrant, 2001). It is the responsibility of the group leader to provide information, use reflection to promote communication, pose thoughtful questions, model prosocial behaviors, and gently guide the group toward its goal.

Horne, Stoddard, and Bell (2007) identified nine characteristics of group leaders that make them more effective in accomplishing the goals of the group. These included an ability to demonstrate empathy; an ability to build relationships; skills around respectful communication; ability to maintain positive expectations for change within the group; a sense of humor; ability to maintain structure, limits, rules, and the group focus; ability to work with resistance from group members; good teaching skills; and skills to empower group members.

PMH APNs receive training and supervision in this treatment modality and in their clinical practice become skilled in the dynamics and processes of group therapy. Primary care APNs may study group therapy in their educational preparation but most have limited experiences as group therapy leaders. However, this may be an excellent opportunity for a collaborative practice model between the two APN specialties. For example, children with diagnoses that require behavioral changes such as asthma, attention deficit hyperactivity disorder (ADHD), and obesity in a primary care practice may be considered for their own group-specific concern with parental consent and child assent to participate. The group could be co-led by the primary care and PMH APNs. The group could be time limited and focus on emotional adjustment to a specific condition; for example, the relationship between obesity and health status and group education around safe, healthy lifestyle modifications such as exercise and healthy eating. Such office-based group strategies are an ideal forum for intradisciplinary partnerships between primary care and PMH APNs to meet the total health care needs of both the child and family.

Further Evidence for Groups

Hetzel-Riggin, Brausch, and Montgomery (2007) conducted a meta-analysis of English-language studies on sexual abuse treatment outcomes for children conducted between 1975 and 2004. Twenty-eight studies met the inclusion criteria of youth aged three to eighteen years who had been sexually abused for which there was documented treatment outcomes. They concluded that benefit from specific types of treatment was related to the child's secondary behavioral presentation or symptoms. Play therapy was most effective for children with poor social functioning while group therapy was most effective for youth with low self-concept post abuse. This evidence is particularly important for primary care APNs to aid in making appropriate referrals. For example, children who are determined to have poor social functioning on routine office-based screening tools (i.e., DDST II: Ages and Stages Questionnaire: Brigance Screen) should be referred for evaluation to a PMH APN or therapist who performs play therapy. For those experiencing acute distress, CBT along with individual therapy may be most effective as Hetzel-Riggin and colleagues concluded.

In another study, records from 1997 to 2005 of 617 sexually abused and reactive children were reviewed for recidivism (re-abused or who abused other children) and non-recidivism during that time period. Records of children receiving group therapy and whose parents were also in treatment were compared to those who did not receive group treatment. The goals of the group therapy sessions were to reduce trauma symptoms and prevent future re-victimization and sexual reactivity. Findings indicated that children who attended at least five group therapy sessions were less likely to be victimized again or to victimize other children, indicating that group therapy was an effective prevention treatment modality with this population (Duffany & Panos, 2009).

SuperKids is a therapeutic social and art skills group therapy strategy developed in 1999 for use with autistic children and adolescents. The groups of six children and a group leader met weekly for an hour for the entire school year. Social skills taught included conversation skills, identifying and expressing feelings, eye contact, environmental awareness, modulating voice, and emotions. In 2004, data were collected from parents and teachers of forty-four primary and secondary school children enrolled in the afterschool SuperKids strategy. The questionnaire measures assessed for social skills and problem behaviors. The researchers found that there was significant improvement in child assertion scores along with decreased behavioral, hyperactivity, and internalizing problem scores in the sample (Epp, 2008).

Kulic et al. (2004) reviewed studies conducted from 1974 to 1997 to determine the effectiveness of prevention-based groups for two- to eighteen-year-olds. From the fifty-six outcome studies that met inclusion criteria, the researchers concluded that the average child receiving treatment using a group modality was better off (positive outcome) than 73% of the controls who had not received group intervention. Other researchers conducted a randomized clinical trial (RCT) to determine the efficacy of a brief manual-based anger management group therapy for adolescents. Fifty hospitalized participants were randomly assigned to a four-session (forty-five to fifty minute) anger management intervention or to a control group that viewed psychoeducational videos for forty-five to fifty minutes. Preintervention and postintervention self-report and standardized scales were used to assess anger and antisocial behavior. In addition, classroom and unit observation of behaviors were also collected and analyzed. Researchers found that the anger scores in the experimental group decreased even with the use of a short duration anger management group intervention, again supporting the view that brief group therapy intervention was more effective than no intervention (Snyder, Kymissis, & Kessler, 1999).

Last, the Bully Busters Program developed by Horne, Batolomucci, and Newman-Carlson (2003) used a group psychoeducation approach to educate teachers and students about the prevalence of bullying and equipped them with skills to prevent and manage bullying behaviors in school. Data collected to date from the program indicate that it is having a positive impact on management of school bullying.

Practice, Education, and Research Implications

The number of children seen today in primary care offices for routine health care who have a mental health diagnosis is staggering. In any one office day, the primary care provider may have over one-half of the children present with oppositonal defiant disorder, ADHD, an autism spectrum disorder, anxiety, or depression. As such, it is time to examine the curriculum content of advanced practice programs, in particular, pediatric nurse practitioner (PNP) programs, to include more content on these disorders and a clinical rotation in a pediatric psychiatric outpatient setting to become more comfortable with assessment of these disorders in primary care. The Pediatric Nursing Certification Board (PNCB) (www.pncb.org) and the National Association of Pediatric Nurse Practitioners (NAPNAP) (www.napnap.org) have begun to address this issue. The PNCB, beginning in 2011, will offer an examination for PNPs and FNPs that will include content on prevention, screening, early intervention, referral to trained mental health practitioners, and collaborative follow-up of common mental and behavioral health presentations. Melnyk and Moldenhauer (2006) developed the *Keep your children and yourself Safe and Secure (KySS) Guide to Child and Adolescent Mental Health Screening, Early Intervention and Health Promotion.* KySS, an initiative of NAPNAP, serves as an excellent resource of assessment/screening tools for use by all APNs working with children and adolescents with behavioral and emotional concerns.

Research on play and group therapy modalities has primarily been conducted by psychologists, social workers, and other social scientists. APNs in child and adolescent mental health and primary care practices are in a unique position to conduct collaborative research with each other to develop a body of knowledge that is nursing specific in these areas. Topics might include conducting longitudinal inquiries on outcomes for children who participate in different treatment modalities; longitudinal outcomes of specific preventative psychoeducational groups, RCTs on outcomes related to group leader style or group leader discipline, effectiveness of play or group modalities in immigrant versus nonimmigrant groups and across ages and gender, and effectiveness of various combined modalities for specific behavioral or diagnostic disorders. Research conducted to date on play and group modalities has been criticized for not having large enough sample sizes; therefore, large-scale quantitative inquiries addressing this issue would be a significant contribution to nursing science and treatment modality effectiveness.

Summary

Play and group therapies can remediate most risk factors of mental illness and behavioral difficulties and are effective and evidenced-based psychotherapeutic interventions for a variety of emotional conditions in children and adolescents. The importance of play and ability to function appropriately in group situations have been noted by child therapists, researchers, counselors, teachers, parents, and children themselves. The relationship-oriented, family-system, strength-based techniques characteristic of play and group therapies are synergistic to the scientific yet humanistic foundation of nursing, which also incorporates these principles into practice (Delaney, 2008).

APNs without specialty education in child and adolescent mental health treatment are encouraged to seek continuing education and /or training about the specialized modalities of play and group therapies. This knowledge would enhance their practice and add additional assessment skills and interaction techniques for use with a variety of children and adolescents presenting with common diagnosable and undiagnosed behaviors in primary care (Association for Play Therapy, 2005; Saunders et al., 2004). APNs in both specialties should keep in mind that these modalities are efficacious interventions when used with multiple child and adolescent diagnostic and behavioral presentations.

Case Exemplar

Mona is a 9-year-old Caucasian girl who entered treatment at age seven for complaints of anxiety and fears, extended emotional outbursts, bedtime issues, and aggressive physical tantrums toward her mother. She was referred by her pediatric primary care provider, a PNP. This collaborative relationship between PNP and psychiatric-mental health nurse practitioner (PMH NP) continues with updates (results of blood work, height, weight, psychiatric medication management) to each provider as needed. Ongoing communication was consented to by her mother. Some states in the United States regard this as best practice, in addition to HIPAA guidelines. Mona had no friends, was more comfortable with adults than peers, and made grandiose and provocative comments and physical movements (kicking, judo moves) while interacting with peers and some adults. Her parents separated when she was three years old and she has regular visits with her father. There is family history of emotional disturbance on both sides of her family. Mona's parents also fit criteria for diagnosable disorders (Figure 15.3).

Emotional outbursts were common to both parents especially when they interacted with each other, often in front of Mona. Parenting styles of her parents were polar opposites. Father was inconsistent and controlling. His boundaries were poor. He exhibited provocative behavior during interactions not only with family members but treatment professionals.

Mother has learned to set consistent and firm limits, to clarify boundaries, and to offer choice and reward or consequence. Mom remains overwhelmed by violent extended outbursts. She feels unsupported by (ex) husband, her family, and the school system as Mona's behavioral outbursts do not occur at school or with other family members but were observed in the treatment area in mom's presence.

Treatment with Mona over two years by a PMH NP has included an inpatient psychiatric hospitalization after becoming suicidal when she began to hear voices telling her to hurt herself. Medications were started, were effective, and continued. Parents were encouraged to seek their own individual psychotherapy and psychoeducation related to growth and development, special needs children, and discipline.

Mona engaged in a variety of nonpharmacological, child-centered treatments on a weekly basis. There was a period when she insisted on dividing the session time for directive play therapy and child-centered activity. She expressed her anger and learned skills to better manage anger and frustrations with peers and her parents through playing psychotherapeutic board games, using a bop-bag to direct anger at specific targets, and using art as a tool to express herself while managing her fears,

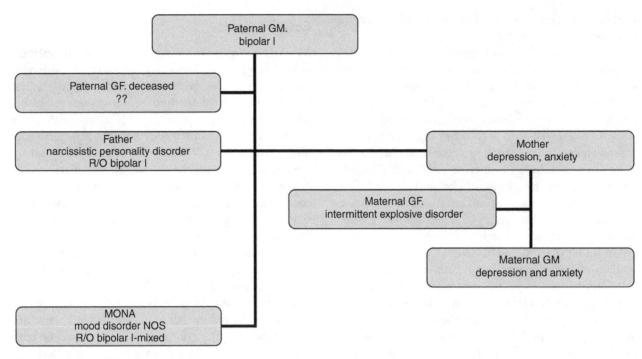

Figure 15.3 Mona's family genogram.

anxiety, and anger. She often used sandplay to express, process, and understand her unconscious and conscious daily worries and experience. Over time, sessions were decreased to twice per month. Social skills continued to be lacking, frequently demonstrated at school and after-school program. Social skills programs on CD-ROM were utilized with her. She demonstrated knowledge but lacked the ability to apply skills. Mona was referred to a ten-week social skills group conducted at a psychiatric hospital by a social worker and psychologist. Mona was able to learn to apply what she learned and has enhanced her social skills abilities and knowing when to ask for adult help. She made friends in the group and was socially more comfortable with peers. This was demonstrated by going to sleep-away camp for a short time over the summer. To date, she continues to socialize with peers from camp and her social skills group. She continues in play therapy treatment twice per month to monitor her fears, anxieties, and sadness. She is monitored for recurrence of any sleep disturbances, recurrence of any symptoms requiring hospitalization or medication adjustment, or frustration with parents and peers that may lead to recurrence of acting-out behaviors.

Resources

American Group Psychotherapy Association Practice Guidelines for Group Psychotherapy, Science to Service Task Force. http://www.agpa.org

American Psychological Association (APA, Washington DC). Publishers of Magination Press, children's books on mental health issues, http://www.maginationpress.com

Association for Play Therapy Inc. Clovis, CA., national and local chapter information and CEU's, regional training centers and distance learning programs, www.a4pt.org

Association for Specialists in Group Work (ASGW). A Division of the American Counseling Association. The purpose of ASGW is to establish standards for professional and ethical practice, support research knowledge development and dissemination, and provide professional leadership in the field of group work, http://www.asgw.org

University of North Texas, Center for Play Therapy, library and education programs, http://cpt.unt.edu

References

Achenbach, T. (1966). The classification of children's psychiatric symptoms. *Psychological Monographs, 80*(615).

Achenbach, T., & Rescorla, L. (2001). *Manual for the ASEBA school-age forms and profiles*. Burlington, VT: University of Vermont Research Center for Children, Youth & Families.

American Academy of Pediatrics. (2006). *The importance of play in promoting healthy child development and maintaining strong parent-child bonds* [Clinical report]. Retrieved from http://www.aap.org

American Group Psychotherapy Association. (2007). Practice guidelines for group psychotherapy. Retrieved from http://www.agpa.org/guidelines/AGPA%20Practice%20Guidelines%202007-PDF.pdf

Ang, R., & Hughes, J. (2001). Differential benefits of skills training with antisocial youth based on group composition: A meta-analytic investigation. *School Psychology Review, 31*, 164–185.

Arneson, L. (2003). *Thoughts and feelings: A sentence completion card game*. Rancho Santa Fe, CA: Bright Spots. Available at www.brightspotsgames.com

Association for Play Therapy. (n.d.). About play therapy overview. Retrieved from http//www.a4pt.org/ps.playtherapy.cfm?ID-1158

Association for Play Therapy. (2005). *Sample syllabus: Introductory graduate play therapy course*. Clovis, CA: Author.

Association for Play Therapy. (2001). Why play therapy? [Video] Available at About Play Therapy from http://www.a4pt.org.

Association for Specialists in Group Work. (ASGW). (2001). Professional standards for the training of group workers. In G. Gazda, E. Ginter, & A. Horne (Eds.), *Group counseling and therapy* (pp. 363–388). Boston, MA: Allyn & Bacon.

Avinger, K., & Jones, R. (2007). Group treatment of sexually abused adolescent girls: A review of outcome studies. *American Journal of Family Therapy, 35*, 315–326.

Axline, V. (1978). *Play therapy*. New York: Ballantine Books, Inc.

Barlow, S., Burlingame, G., & Fuhriman, A. (2000). Therapeutic application of groups: From Pratt's "Thought control classes" to modern group psychotherapy. *Group Dynamics: Theory, Research, and Practice, 4*, 115–134.

Bellinson, J. (2002). *Children's use of board games in psychotherapy*. Northvale, NJ: Jason Aronson.

Benedict, H., & Mongovern, L. (1997). Thematic play therapy: An approach to treatment of attachment disorders in young children. In H. Kaduson, D. Cangelosi & C. Schaefer (Eds.), *The playing cure: Individualized play therapy for specific childhood problems* (pp. 277–315). Northvale, NJ: Jason Aronson.

Bonner, B. (2004). Cognitive-behavioral and dynamic play therapy for children with sexual behavior problems and their caregivers. In B.E. Saunders, L. Berliner, & R. F. Hanson (Eds.), *Child physical and sexual abuse: Guidelines for treatment* (pp. 34–36). Charleston, SC: National Crime Victims Research and Treatment Center.

Bowlby, J. (1988). *A secure base: Parent-child attachment and healthy human development*. New York: Basic Books, Inc.

Bratton, S., & Ray, D. (2000). What the research shows about play therapy. *International Journal of Play Therapy, 9*(1), 47–88.

British Association of Play Therapists. History of play therapy. Retrieved from http://www.bapt.info/historyofpt.htm

Carey, L. (1999). *Sandplay therapy with children and families*. Northvale, NJ: Jason Aronson.

Crary, E., & Katayama, M. (2004). *The self-calming card deck*. Seattle, WA: The Parenting Press. Retrieved from www.ParentingPress.com

Cohen, J., & Deblinger, E. (2004). Trauma-focused cognitive behavioral therapy. In B.E. Saunders, L. Berlinger, & R.F. Hanson (Eds.), *Child physical and sexual abuse: Guidelines for treatment* (pp. 49–51). Charleston, SC: National Crime Victims Research and Treatment Center.

Davenport, B., & Bourgeois, N. (2008). Play, aggression, the preschool child and the family: A review of the literature to guide empirically informed play therapy with aggressive preschool children. *International Journal of Play Therapy, 17*(1), 2–23.

Delaney, K. (2008). Psychotherapy with children. In K. Wheeler (Ed.), *Psychotherapy for the advanced practice psychiatric nurse* (pp. 330–352). St. Louis, MO: Mosby.

Depa, M., & Astramovich, R. (2008). Puppetwork with victims of sexual abuse. *Play Therapy, 3*(2), 10–13.

Duffany, A., & Panos, P. (2009). Outcome evaluation of a group treatment of sexually abused and reactive children. *Research on Social Work Practice, 19*, 291–303.

Eisenber, N., Cumberland, T., Fabes, R., Shepard, S., Reiser, M., Murphy, B., & Guthrie, I. (2001). The relations of regulation and emotionality to children's externalizing and internalizing problem behavior. *Child Development, 72*, 1112–1134.

Epp, K. (2008). Outcome-based evaluation of a social skills program using art therapy and group therapy on the autism spectrum. *Children & Schools, 30*(1), 27–36.

Erikson, E. (1980). *Identity and the life cycle*. New York, NY: W.W. Norton & Co., Inc.

Frost, J. (1998, June). Neuroscience, play and child development. Presentation at the IPA/USA Triennial National Conference, Longmont, CO.

Gardner, R. (1975). The mutual storytelling technique. In R.A. Gardner (Ed.), *Psychotherapeutic approaches to the resistant child* (pp. 101–140). New York, NY: J. Aronson.

Gardner, R. (2001). The talking, feeling and doing game. In C.E. Schaefer & S.E. Reid (Eds.), *Game play* (pp. 78–108). New York, NY: John Wiley & Sons.

Gaskill, R. (2010). Neurobiology of play therapy. *Play Therapy, 5*(4), 18–22.

Gaskill, R. (2004). Neurosequential development and experiential play therapy with traumatized children. Paper presented at the Association for Play Therapy Annual Conference. October, Denver, CO.

Gifford-Smith, M., Dodge, K., Dishion, T., & McCord, J.(2005). Peer influence in children and adolescence: Crossing the bridge from development to intervention science. *Journal of Abnormal Child Psychology, 33*(3), 255–265.

Gil, E. (2004). Trauma-focused play therapy. In B.E. Saunders, L. Berlinger, & R. F. Hanson (Eds.), *Child physical and sexual abuse: Guidelines for treatment* (pp. 54–55). Charleston, SC: National Crime Victims Research and Treatment Center.

Ginsburg et al. (2007). The importance of play in promoting healthy child development and maintaining strong parent-child bonds. *Pediatrics, 119*, 182–191.

Gitlin-Weiner, K., Sandgrund, A., & Schaefer, C. (Eds.). (2000). *Play diagnosis and assessment* (second edition). New York, NY: John Wiley & Sons.

Henig, R. (2008). Taking play seriously. Retrieved from http://www.nytimes.com/2008/02/17/magazine/17play.html

Hetzel-Riggin, M., Brausch, A., & Montgomery, B. (2007). A meta-analytic investigation of therapy modality outcomes for sexually abused children and adolescents: An exploratory study. *Child Abuse & Neglect, 31*, 125–141.

Horne, A., Stoddard, J., & Bell, C. (2007). Group approaches to reducing aggression and bullying in school. *Group Dynamics: Theory, Research, and Practice, 11*, 262–271.

Horne, A., Bartolomucci, C., & Newman-Carlson, D. (2003). *Bully Busters: A teacher's manual for helping bullies, victims, and bystanders (Grades K-5)*. Champaign, IL: Research Press.

Hynes, A., & Hynes-Berry, M. (1986). *Biblio / poetry therapy: The interactive process: A handbook*. Boulder, CO: Westview Press.

Johnson, D., Pedro-Carroll, J., & Demanchik, S. (2005). The primary mental health project: A play intervention for school-aged children. In L.A. Reddy, T.M. Files-Hall, & C.E. Schaefer (Eds.), *Empirically based play interventions for children* (pp. 13–30). Washington, DC: American Psychological Association.

Jung, C. (Ed.). (1968). *Man and his symbols*. New York, NY: Dell Books.

Kalff, D. (2003). *Sandplay: A psychotherapeutic approach to the psyche*. Cloverdale, CA: Temenos Press.

Kivlighan, D., & Tarrant, J. (2001). Does group climate mediate the group leadership-group member outcome relationship? A test of Yalom's hypotheses about leadership priorities. *Group Dynamics: Theory, Research, and Practice, 5*(3), 220–234.

Knell, S. (1998). Cognitive-behavioral play therapy. *Journal of Clinical Child Psychology, 27,* 28–34.

Knell, S., & Beck, K. (2000). The puppet sentence completion task. In K. Gitlin-Weiner, A. Sandgrund, & C.E. Schaefer (Eds.), *Play diagnosis and assessment* (second edition) (pp. 704–721). New York, NY: John Wiley & Sons.

Kot, S., & Tyndall-Lind, A. (2005). Intensive play therapy with child witnesses of domestic violence. In L.A. Reddy, T.M. Files-Hall, & C.E. Schaefer (Eds.), *Empirically based play interventions for children* (pp. 31–49). Washington, DC: American Psychological Association.

Kottman, T. (2001). Adlerian play therapy. *International Journal of Play Therapy, 10*(2), 1–12.

Kraft, I. (1996). History. In P. Kymissis & D. Halperin (Eds.), *Group therapy with children and adolescents.* Washington, DC: American Psychiatric Press.

Kulic, K., Horne, A., & Dagley, J. (2004). A comprehensive review of prevention groups for children and adolescents. *Group Dynamics: Theory, Research, and Practice, 8,* 139–151.

Landreth, G. (Ed.). (2001). *Innovations in play therapy: Issues, process and special populations.* Philadelphia, PA: Brunner Routledge.

Lankton, C., & Lankton, S. (1989). *Tales of enchantment: Goal oriented metaphors for adults and children in therapy.* New York, NY: Brunner Mazel.

Lowenfeld, M. (1999). *Understanding children's sandplay: Lowenfeld's world technique.* Cambridge, MA: Margaret Lowenfeld Trust.

Melnyk, B., & Moldenhauer, Z. (2006). *The KySS Guide to child and adolescent mental health screening, early intervention and health promotion.* Cherry Hill, NJ: National Association of Pediatric Nurse Practitioners.

Mills, J., & Crowley, R. (1986). *Therapeutic metaphors for children and the child within.* New York, NY: Brunner Mazel.

Mishna, F., & Muskat, B. (2004). "I'm not the only one!" Group therapy with older children and adolescents who have learning disabilities. *International Journal of Group Psychotherapy, 54,* 455–476.

Munns, E. (Ed.). (2000). *Theraplay: Innovations in attachment-enhancing play therapy.* Northvale, NJ: Jason Aronson.

National Institute for Play Therapy. (2009). Play science: The seven patterns of play. Retrieved from http://nifplay.org

Newman-Carlson, D., & Horne, A. (2004). Bully Busters: A psychoeducational intervention for reducing bullying behavior in middle school students. *Journal of Counseling and Development, 82,* 259–268.

O'Connor, K.J. (2000). *The play therapy primer* (pp. 3–58). New York, NY: John Wiley.

O'Connor, K. (2001). Ecosystemic play therapy. *International Journal of Play Therapy, 10*(2), 33–44.

Perry, B. (2006). Applying principles of neurodevelopment to clinical work with maltreated and traumatized children: The neurosequential model of therapeutics. In N.B. Webb (Ed.), *Working with traumatized youth in child welfare* (Ch. 3). New York, NY: Guilford Press.

Ray, D., Bratton, S., Rhine, T., & Jones, L. (2001). The effectiveness of play therapy: Responding to the critics. *International Journal of Play Therapy, 10*(1), 85–108.

Rennie, R., & Landreth, G. (2000). Effects of filial therapy on parent and child behaviors. *International Journal of Play Therapy, 9*(2), 19–37.

Rogers, C. (1951). *Client-centered therapy.* Boston, MA: Houghton Mifflin.

Saunders, B., Berliner, L., and Hanson, R.F. (Eds.). (2004). *Child physical and sexual abuse: Guidelines for treatment.* Charleston, SC: National Crime Victims Research and Treatment Center.

Schaefer, C. (2001). Prescriptive play therapy. *International Journal of Play Therapy, 10*(2), 57–73.

Schaefer, C., & Reid, S. (1986). *Game play: Therapeutic use of childhood games.* New York, NY: John Wiley.

Shechtman, Z. (2007). How does group process research inform leaders of counseling and psychotherapy groups? *Group Dynamics: Theory, Research, and Practice, 11*(4), 293–304.

Shechtman, Z., & Gluk, O. (2005). An investigation of therapeutic factors in children's groups. *Group Dynamics: Theory, Research, and Practice, 9*(2), 127–134.

Shelby, J., & Felix, E. (2005). Posttraumatic play therapy: The need for an integrated model of directive and non-directive approaches. In L. Reddy, T.M. Files-Hall, & C.E. Schaefer (Eds.), *Empirically based play interventions for children* (pp. 79–103). Washington, DC: American Psychological Association.

Snyder, K., Kymissis, P., & Kessler, K. (1999). Anger management for adolescents: Efficacy of brief group therapy. *Journal of the American Academy of Child and Adolescent Psychiatry, 38,* 1409–1416.

Swank, J. (2008). The use of games: A therapeutic tool with children and families. *International Journal of Play Therapy, 17,* 154–167.

Tackett, J. (2010). Toward an externalizing spectrum in DSM-V: Incorporating developmental concerns. *Child Development Perspectives, 4*(3), 161–167.

Terr, L.(2003). Wild child: How three principles of healing organized 12 years of psychotherapy. *Journal of the American Academy of Child & Adolescent Psychiatry, 42,* 1401–1409.

VanFleet, R. (2005). *Filial therapy: Strengthening parent-child relationships through play* (second edition). Sarasota, FL: Professional Resource Press.

VanFleet, R., Ryan, S., & Smith, S. (2005). Filial therapy: A critical review. In L.A. Reddy, T.M. Files-Hall, & C.E. Schaefer (Eds.), *Empirically based play interventions for children* (pp. 241–264). Washington, DC: American Psychological Association.

Wenner, M. (2009). The serious need for play. *Scientific American.*

Yalom, I. (1995). *The theory and practice of group psychotherapy* (fourth edition). New York, NY: Basic Books.

16

Individual and Family Therapies

Kathleen Scharer

Objectives

After reading this chapter, APNs will be able to

1. Identify different types of therapies that would be appropriate for a particular child and /or family.
2. Discuss the evidence base for each therapy presented.

3. Determine which treatments might be provided within the advanced practice nurse's (APN) setting and what qualifications would be needed to provide the treatment.
4. Make an informed decision about the mental health treatment referral needs of children and adolescents.

Introduction

The purpose of this chapter is to discuss the major types of individual and family therapies useful for children and adolescents, the evidence of their effectiveness, and any particular problems for which they have been proven effective. This allows the primary care advanced practice nurse (APN) to make an informed selection of treatments and providers when making referrals for their patients. Psychotherapy involves using planned interventions or counseling designed to reduce maladaptive behavior, reduce stress, or enhance adaptive behaviors. There are various forms of therapy that are developmentally appropriate for children and adolescents and for particular types of problems; selecting the best form and type of evidence-based intervention is an important factor in the success of the therapy. Most therapies involve some type of interpersonal interactions, that is, talk between patient and therapist or with others in

the session. For children, talk is important but may be supplemented with play, rewarding certain behaviors, behavioral rehearsal, games, stories, or other activities that allow the child to express and/or practice certain emotions or behaviors. Elsewhere in this book, chapters have been devoted to important types of therapies such as play therapy, group therapy, and cognitive-behavioral therapy (CBT). This chapter will address other types of evidence-based therapies that are useful to children and their families.

Generally, the primary goal of therapy is to help individuals change problematic behavior. In many types of therapy, with adults and adolescents, this is believed to occur through interpretations the therapist makes and shares with the patient. These interpretations help patients develop a new understanding of themselves and their behavior to enable them to make a change. Interpretations only work if the child can comprehend the interpretation and is cognitively mature enough to

---

Child and Adolescent Behavioral Health: A Resource for Advanced Practice Psychiatric and Primary Care Practitioners in Nursing,
First Edition. Edited by Edilma L. Yearwood, Geraldine S. Pearson, and Jamesetta A. Newland.
© 2012 John Wiley & Sons, Inc. Published 2012 by John Wiley & Sons, Inc.

incorporate this understanding. Behavioral treatments do not rely on making interpretations but are focused on the belief that if behavior changes, the emotional and cognitive processes will also change. Some points to consider in selecting a therapy are related to the child's developmental stage. Therapies that involve mature cognition for success are not likely to be effective with young children.

Several factors about children must be taken into account when making a choice of therapy for younger children. For example, the young child believes that the world revolves around himself or herself. As the child matures, this omnipotence diminishes and other causes for problems can be understood by the child. We know that this omnipotent stance can remain for highly emotionally charged issues into adolescence, long beyond when it disappears for routine things. It is not uncommon for even early adolescents to feel responsible for their parents divorcing when the adolescent had no real responsibility for the problems of the parents. Additionally, young children have trouble linking past events and emotions to the present because their sense of time is not yet developed. An example of this undeveloped sense of time is the frequent question of young children when traveling: "Are we there yet?" Preadolescent and younger children also have difficulty understanding conscious versus unconscious motivations for behavior. Explanations that a behavior has some unconscious motivation would typically be rejected by the child in favor of a conscious explanation; this is not resistance on the child's part but an effect of normal cognitive development. Abstract reasoning does not develop until formal operations develop in adolescence so the child cannot always see the perspective of others. Selecting an intervention that relies on how a younger child's behavior affects another is not likely to be effective.

One of the most difficult decisions in psychotherapy is determining what type of therapy and which therapist are most appropriate for a particular child and family. In many cases, children and their families are referred to a mental health provider because the referring practitioner knows the mental health provider or the referral is to a mental health system or office, rather than to a specific therapist. This may not result in the best choice of therapy for the child or family. There are multiple types of therapies; some have a greater base of evidence than others and some are more suited to particular types of problems. Not every practitioner is an expert in all types of therapy; in reality, most practices use one or two types of therapy with perhaps some aspects of others mixed into their practice. By understanding the various types of therapies, the primary care APN can make the best selection for youth who need assistance.

Individual Therapy

Individual therapy for children and adolescent is typically provided within a developmental framework. What would work for a five-year-old is hardly appropriate for a sixteen-year-old. In addition, behavior that would be considered "normal" for one age group would raise grave concerns for another. For example, imaginary playmates are common in young children but would be considered questionable in an adolescent. Some therapies, such as play therapy, which is being discussed elsewhere in this book (see Chapter 15), are only appropriate for younger children; the typical adolescent would be offended if offered a sand tray and puppets or other similar toys for therapy. Even within a developmental phase, what one child needs may be quite different from what another child needs.

Younger children may also have more difficulty interpreting and/or reporting events that occur, so their reporting of events must be often validated with parents and, in school-aged children, with teachers. In most therapy sessions, the therapist spends at least a little time with the parents of young children. Most adolescents are very concerned about what an individual therapist might say to their parents and do not want their therapist to speak with their parents unless the teen is present. Respecting the privacy of the child of any age must be carefully balanced with the needs of the parent to understand the therapeutic process and the progress of the child in therapy. In the following material, the word "child" is used to mean individuals up to eighteen years of age, unless distinctions between adolescents and children need to be specifically made.

Cognitive-Behavioral Therapy

CBT has the most extensive research base of any psychotherapy. It has been widely used with children with good effects. Because of the amount of evidence available on CBT, it will be addressed on its own in Chapter 17.

Psychodynamic Psychotherapy

The term "psychodynamic psychotherapy" covers a broad spectrum of interventions that can range from child psychoanalysis to once-a-week sessions with the therapist. Psychodynamic therapies are an outgrowth of the work of Sigmund Freud with the modification and input from many other therapists including Melanie Klein, Anna Freud, Heinz Kohut, Donald Winnicott, Otto Kernberg, Margaret Mahler, and John Bowlby (Fonagy, 1999).

What Is It?

Some psychodynamic therapies are very expressive in nature while others are more supportive. However, the commonality in these approaches is the belief that the problems that bring the child to therapy stem from the stress of a conflicting motivational states. This form of therapy is believed to be therapeutic because it helps individuals build on their own inherent capacities for understanding and emotional responsiveness. Therapists aid in this process by communicating an understanding of a child's conflicting motivations and the responses to these motivations. While there are differences in the way psychodynamic psychotherapy can be operationalized, there are some commonalities in beliefs about the treatment. The therapist sees the problem as the child's reaction to the external world as based on past representations of events. This is the notion of psychological causation. The therapist believes that there are unconscious mental processes that affect the child's reaction to the external world. The therapist also believes that the child has mental representations of events with others that form the basis of interactions with others. In the therapist's view, the child has experienced intrapsychic conflict and uses defenses to protect against these conflicts. Psychodynamic psychotherapists also believe that a child's symptoms have several layers of meaning and the job of the therapist is to interpret and explain these to the child. The therapist has the assumption that transference will occur and is the child's displacement of unresolved issues from previous relationships, usually with parents, onto the therapist. The relational aspects of the therapy relationship are also seen as beneficial to the child's functioning (Fonagy, 1999).

For Whom Does It Work?

Psychodynamic psychotherapy by its nature requires that the child or adolescent have good verbal skills and the ability to think of behavior as influenced by thoughts and feelings. The child or adolescent needs to be able to tolerate some anxiety and conflicts, especially around issues previously not allowed into consciousness without experiencing increased disorganization. The parents, or care givers in another milieu in which the child is residing, need to be able to support the child in a long-term therapeutic relationship and encourage the child's commitment to the therapeutic process. A basic assumption is that the child's problem is due to some internal conflict. Children have to be developmentally age appropriate unless the developmental deficits are the result of the internal conflict requiring therapy. Children also need to be able to sustain a long-term relationship and be able to trust the therapist. Children must have developed the understanding that they have a responsibility for their problems and behaviors (Fonagy, 1999). Generally speaking, psychodynamic psychotherapy is useful for children who are considered neurotic rather than more severely disturbed children.

What Happens in Therapy?

In psychodynamic psychotherapy, the therapist attempts to understand and create a model of the child's thoughts and feelings through what the child reports, through nonverbal play, through any dreams that are reported, or through other behaviors. Additional information may be obtained from parents, teachers, and others in contact with the child. Using the model, the therapist tries to help the child understand his inappropriate or irrational feelings and beliefs. Some techniques are often used in the therapeutic process. Supportive interventions are used to reduce anxiety or increase the child's sense of mastery. This can be done through suggesting ideas to the child, reassuring the child about fears or concerns, providing information as needed, or being empathetic to the child's situation. Therapists also clarify the children's affect and verbalization to help the child understand and may make direct comments about repeated behaviors as a way of directing the child's attention to these. Sometimes summarizing or paraphrasing things the child says can help the child continue to discuss things with the therapist. Interpretations are used to describe ideas or beliefs of which the child may not be consciously aware and to which the child may not be ready to listen. It is imperative then that the therapist time interpretations carefully and select those for which the evidence is fairly conclusive (Fonagy, 1999).

What Is the Evidence Base for This Therapy?

The research on psychodynamic psychotherapy is somewhat limited because it is not a therapy that is easily manualized; it must be adapted to every child. For a long time there was a dearth of studies supporting the approach as Fonagy noted in 1999. However, research in other fields has led to a recent upsurge in research on psychodynamic psychotherapy. For example, support for unconscious processes has come from a group of German scientists (Soon, Brass, Jochen Heinz, & Haynes, 2008) who have demonstrated with functional magnetic resonance images (MRIs) that unconscious processes precede awareness by seven to ten seconds when making a decision. Other work on subliminal perception has shown that an unconscious prime (subliminal message) with a positive direction can be a powerful motivation to act (Aarts, Custers, & Marien, 2008). Efforts to understand neurobiology have led to an understanding of how important emotions are in motivation. Panskeep (1998) demonstrated that emotions arising in the limbic system link to the prefrontal cortex and temporal lobes though the hypothalamus to affect motivations. Blair et al. (2007) have shown the impact of emotion on cognitive processes and the reverse process of cognitive effects on emotion. Defense mechanisms have been documented through neuroimaging techniques (Anderson et al., 2004; Depue, Curran, & Banich, 2007). The vast literature on attachment theory has helped explicate the importance of therapist-client attachment for the therapeutic process in psychodynamic psychotherapy. With these foundations, research on psychodynamic psychotherapy has been increasing. Some research findings have demonstrated the positive effects of psychodynamic psychotherapy continuing to increase after the therapy has ended (Shedler, 2010).

A meta-analysis of twenty-three studies for a total of 1,365 adult depressed subjects was conducted on short-term psychodynamic psychotherapy (Driessen et al., 2010). The meta-analysis concluded that short-term psychodynamic psychotherapy was effective for this population. The treatment effective sizes were large and were maintained for up to a year post treatment. Additionally, measures of the level of depression showed a significant decrease from the subjects in the control groups. However, when compared to results of other therapies, such as CBT or interpersonal psychotherapy (IPT) for depression, psychodynamic psychotherapy was slightly less effective over time but the trend was not significant (Driessen et al., 2010). A 2007 meta-analysis of treatment for children and adolescents looked at psychotherapy, including CBT, psychodynamic psychotherapy, and various other psychotherapies compared to treatment as usual (Watanabe, Hunot, Omori, Churchill, & Furukawa, 2007). The researchers found that while psychotherapy of all types had an advantage over treatment as usual, this advantage did not persist beyond six months.

Less research has been done on psychodynamic psychotherapy for children and adolescents. Trowell et al. (2007) conducted a randomized controlled trial of seventy-two patients aged nine to fifteen with moderate to severe depression. They compared psychodynamic individual psychotherapy and family therapy. Each group received therapy over nine months. Approximately 75% of the patients in each group were not clinically depressed following treatment, and 100% of the children receiving the individual psychodynamic psychotherapy showed no depression six months after treatment; while of the family therapy group, 81% were no longer clinically depressed. In another study, the short- and long-term effects of time-limited psychodynamic psychotherapy were tested (Muratori, Picchi, Bruni, Patarnello, & Romagnoli, 2003). Fifty-eight children

from 6.3 to 10.9 years of age were included in the study. The group receiving the individual psychodynamic psychotherapy had major improvements. Major improvements for the experimental group were found on both the Child Global Adjustment Scale and the Child Behavior Checklist (CBCL). After two years there were major improvements on the CBCL, including on the externalizing disorders scales. However, since this study did not use randomized assignment, the results must be viewed with caution (Muratori et al.).

Thus, while more research on psychodynamic psychotherapy has been done with adults, the research on its efficacy with children and adolescents is scarce. The research that has been done has mixed results. Therefore, psychodynamic psychotherapy should be used with caution.

How to Become a Psychodynamic Therapist

Typically learning to be a competent psychodynamic therapist involves advanced training in psychiatry, psychology, psychiatric nursing, social work, or counseling with a focus on this method and often postgraduate training. It is important to have close supervision by a competent psychodynamic therapist to learn how to make appropriate interpretations. Sometimes individual psychodynamic therapy for the therapist is also recommended. The Psychoanalytic Institute of New York University offers postgraduate training programs. For information visit their website: http://www.med.nyu.edu/psa/education/PTY/psychotherapy.html. No professional organization specifically for psychodynamic therapists was found.

Interpersonal Psychotherapy

IPT is based on the interpersonal theory of Harry Stack Sullivan who believed that personality is developed from the reflected appraisals of others. Sullivan believed that mental illnesses developed in the context of social relationships that were not effective. Sullivan met Alfred Meyer during his education in psychotherapy and was introduced to Meyer's theory that psychological disorder developed from the individual's struggle to deal with his social environment. Sullivan applied these ideas to the treatment of schizophrenia (New World Encyclopedia contributors, 2008). Later his ideas became the basis for IPT. IPT is also based on attachment theory of John Bowlby (Mufson & Sills, 2006).

What Is It?

As currently practiced, IPT was developed by Gerald Klerman and Myrna Weissman (International Society for Interpersonal Psychotherapy, 2010). The patient's interpersonal interactions are examined in relationship to the patient's depressive symptoms. IPT recognizes the significance of the current interpersonal world of the client in symptom development and maintenance. IPT is directive and active, with an explicit focus for the client and therapist. There are three components of depression in the IPT model of depression: (1) symptom formation, (2) social functioning, and (3) personality contributions.

For Whom Does It Work?

IPT was initially developed to treat major depression in short-term therapy in about twelve to sixteen sessions. It has subsequently been modified and researched in a number of different age groups and with a wide variety of diagnoses, such as anorexia nervosa (Rieger et al., 2010), substance misuse, bulimia nervosa (Arcelus et al., 2009; Fairburn, Jones, Peveler, Hope, & O'Connor, 1993), dysthymia, post traumatic stress disorder (PTSD), somatization disorder, and some anxiety disorders with adults (Cyranowski et al., 2005). It is a manualized therapy, and for each adaptation for depression the manuals are used but different components are emphasized (International Society for Interpersonal Psychotherapy, 2010). A specific manual for adolescent depression, called IPT-A, has been developed and tested (Mufson & Sills, 2006).

What Happens in Therapy?

There are certain theoretical assumptions underpinning IPT. First, IPT does not consider that psychological problems come only from the interpersonal realm—psychological problems all occur in an interpersonal context. This interpersonal context is interdependent with the psychological problems. Therefore, IPT aims to intervene in this interpersonal context to achieve some symptom relief. The therapist presents as warm and in a collaborative relationship to the patient; however, there is strict adherence to the manual. In this short-term therapy, regression is discouraged by a focus within every session on the upcoming termination.

Sessions are usually weekly for an hour. In the first session, an assessment is done of the patient's illness and social context. The illness is explained to the patient in interpersonal terms. The process of the sessions in IPT is described to the patient. An "interpersonal inventory" is completed which depicts and categorizes the important relationships in the patient's life into the four components of depression: role transitions, grief, interpersonal disputes, and interpersonal deficits.

The remaining sessions, except the last two, deal with the problematic relationships in the patient's life; little emphasis is placed on the illness, except to ask about the severity of the symptoms. The final two sessions focus on termination, which is presented as a loss experience

from which the patient can learn more about the response to loss and how well IPT has helped in modulating responses to loss. The therapist uses active listening and clarification to help demonstrate to the patient any biases. For interpersonal disputes role-playing and communication analysis can be helpful in resolving the disputes. Within the safety of the session, encouragement of affect allows the patient to experience emotions that might be considered unpleasant, such as the sadness from loss. The patients are encouraged to generate problem solutions as much on their own as possible, thus gradually phasing out the need for a therapist. It is this process of patients learning to initiate their own changes that accounts for the symptomatic improvement peaking around three to six months after treatment is terminated.

What Is the Evidence Base for This Therapy?

IPT has been studied for many years. Several large-scale, randomized, controlled trials with adults have been conducted which support the efficacy of IPT. In 1973 a study by the New Haven-Boston Collaborative began testing IPT against amitriptyline and in combination. IPT was found to be as effective as the drug and, when used in combination, had an additive effect to the drug (Weissman, Prusoff, & DiMascio, 1979). A larger NIMH-funded randomized study compared CBT, IPT, imipramine, and usual care. IPT, CBT, and imipramine were equally efficacious in treating depression. Those patients with the higher scores on the Hamilton Rating Scale who were considered to be severely depressed responded as well to IPT as to imipramine while CBT was not as efficacious with this more severely depressed group of patients (Elkin et al., 1989). The University of Pittsburg Group led by Kruper and Frank has studied the effects of long-term maintenance therapy on depression. They had three-year results demonstrating that a combination of imipramine and monthly maintenance IPT successfully prevented the recurrence of depression (Frank et al., 1990).

Studies about IPT-A have been conducted over the past eleven years (Bearsley-Smith et al., 2007; Gunlicks-Stoessel, Mufson, Jekal, & Turner, 2010; Mufson, Weissman, Moreau, & Garfinkel, 1999; Tang, Jou, Ko, Huang, & Yen, 2010). Mufson, Dorta, et al. (2004) reported on a clinical trial of IPT-A in a school-based setting and compared it with treatment as usual. The results of the study showed that not only was ITP-A statistically significantly better, it was also clinically better than treatment as usual.

Young, Mufson, and Gallop (2010) evaluated the efficacy of a prevention program for depression in fifty-seven adolescents randomized to either usual school counseling or IPT with an adolescent skills training model (IPT-AST), which was a modification of IPT-A. At the end of the intervention the adolescents in the IPT-AST group reported significantly greater improvement in symptom level and overall functioning at post intervention but during the remainder of the eighteen months, rates of change slowed for the IPT-AST group while the school counseling group continued to improve so that the changes were no longer significant. However, IPT-AST has the benefit of returning the adolescents to school work and other activities sooner.

The combined use of IPT and antidepressant medication for adolescents has not been studied in a clinical trial to date. Several studies with adults have combined IPT and antidepressants with positive results but in adolescence, most researchers have promoted the use of IPT-A as a stand-alone intervention because of the black box warnings on many antidepressants recommending that they be used with care in this age group.

How Do You Become a Therapist?

The International Society for Interpersonal Psychotherapy (ISIP) website (International Society for Interpersonal Psychotherapy, 2010) describes the training for those interested in becoming IPT therapists. The first requirement is that potential trainees have a clinical background with a sound understanding of mood disorders. The trainees read the IPT manual and attend a two- to four-day training course. This is followed by supervision with a supervisor registered through the ISIP or the United Kingdom Interpersonal Therapy's organization, known as UKIPTSIG. The first case seen by the trainee must be a patient with a major depressive disorder, and the second case must be a person with dysthymia, adolescent depression, or eating disorder. The minimum amount of supervision is on two cases. All sessions must be tape recorded. The supervisor selects a minimum of three sessions to review and rate on the IPT competency scale. After the supervisor deems the trainee has meet the competencies on two cases, the training is considered to be finished (ISIP, 2010). The ISIP can be accessed online at: http://www.interpersonalpsychotherapy.com/index.cfm?ID=71

Multisystemic Therapy

Multisystemic therapy (MST) was developed specifically to salvage children and adolescents who have demonstrated serious antisocial behavior. The program focuses on the entire world of the youth including families, friends, schools, teachers, and even the neighborhood. It is an individual therapy integrated with family therapy and environmental therapy.

What Is It?

MST is targeted for the toughest offenders, male and female, between twelve and seventeen years of age. The treatment program is based on the theory of social ecology, which considers the determinants of the child's behavior to be multilayered, like an onion, with the child being the central core and family, friends, teachers, school, and neighborhood making up the additional layers. The child's behavior is influenced by the interaction among all of these groups with the child. To effectively treat the youth's antisocial behavior, MST must be able to address all of aspects of the child's life in order to change the youth's problem behavior. The ultimate aim of MST is to surround the youth with layers of people who promote prosocial behavior rather than antisocial behavior (Henggler, Schoenwald, Bourduin, Rowland, & Cunningham, 2009).

For Whom Does It Work?

MST was developed specifically to treat antisocial youths. However, it has been adapted to other types of children and youth. For example it is being tried as a treatment for youth with severe type 1 diabetes (Ellis et al., 2005, 2007; Ellis, Weiss, Han, & Gallop, 2010), asthma management (Naar-King, Ellis, Kolmodin, Cunningham, & Secord, 2009), serious emotional disturbances (Rowland et al., 2005), adolescent substance abuse (Randall, Henggeler, Cunningham, Rowland, & Swenson, 2001) and youth psychiatric emergencies (Henggeler, et al., 1999), and child abuse families (Brunk, Henggeler, & Whelan, 1987). These many adaptations of the original program speak to its strength as a treatment when a strong supportive environment is needed to encourage the youth's healthy development.

What Happens in Therapy?

MST is multifaceted treatment as its name implies. Increasing the parenting skills of the child's caregivers and changing the behavior of the antisocial youth are at the core of the treatment process, but MST is not delivered in an office on a once-a-week or once-a-month basis; rather the therapist goes to where the youth hangs out, to school, and to the home. Therapists often see the members of the youth's ecological system more than once a week since all of these individuals have affected the youth. These meetings are not conducted strictly during standard business hours. The MST team members are on call twenty-four hours a day and every day of the week. Naturally this requires that the therapist have quite limited caseloads. Dropouts are also reduced by this process because barriers to getting the youth to a therapy session are avoided.

Family-focused therapy is intensive; goals include increasing parenting skills, improving all relationships within the family, involving the youth with peers who do not engage in antisocial behaviors, helping the youth to achieve academically or vocationally, helping the youth find positive activities in which to engage such as sports, and creating a support network of extended family, friends, and neighbors who will aid the caregivers in maintaining change (Henggeler, Schoenwald, et al., 2009). To achieve these goals, family members collaborate with MST team members to develop the treatment plan that makes sense to the family and builds on their strengths. This collaboration increases the likelihood of the success of the treatment plan.

What Is the Evidence Base for This Therapy?

The evidence base for MST is extensive. The first publications began in 1986, which labeled the treatment as multisystemic and described the effects on the youth and family (Henggeler, Rodick, et al., 1986). Studies have demonstrated efficacy (Borduin, Cone, et al., 1995; Borduin, Henggeler, et al., 1990; Brunk et al., 1987) of the intervention. Next came effectiveness trials conducted in real world situations with less control and oversight by the original researchers (Henggeler, Melton, Brondino, Scherer, & Hanley, 1997; Henggeler, Melton, & Smith, 1992). Also as the success in helping antisocial youths with substance abuse problems became apparent, mixed efficacy-effectiveness trials were conducted (Brown et al., 1997; Henggeler, Clingempeel, Brondino, & Pickrel, 2002; Rowland, Chapman, & Henggeler, 2008). Other studies targeted implementation to different types of problems as detailed earlier.

How Do You Become a Therapist?

Four types of training are used in the MST model to maintain quality. Since MST is delivered by a team, the team trains together. First the professional attends a five-day training session. Therapists are asked to read the MST manual prior to training, which includes both didactic and experiential learning. Therapists who are conducting MST also participate in quarterly booster training, which is an onsite, 1.5 days of training, used to enhance the team's knowledge and skills. Onsite supervision is also provided weekly and there is weekly expert consultation for the team. Supervision of MST therapists is also manualized and supervisors must also undergo training in MST. The expert consultant works with the supervisors to help them develop their supervisory skills in MST. For online information about MST go to: http://www.mstservices.com/index.php/training/training

Eye Movement Desensitization and Reprocessing

Eye movement desensitization and reprocessing (EMDR) is a scientifically validated, psychotherapeutic approach. The theory behind EMDR is that many psychological problems are caused by traumatic experiences or disturbing life events. These traumatic or disturbing events impair the person's processing abilities and the ability to integrate experiences in the central nervous system. EMDR seems to have a direct effect on the way that the brain processes information. Normal information processing is resumed, so following a successful EMDR session a person no longer relives the strong negative images, sounds, and feelings when the event is brought to mind.

What Is It?

EMDR was developed in 1987 by Dr. Francine Shapiro, who made a chance observation that eye movements could reduce disturbing thoughts in certain situations. The combination of remembering the traumatic event, describing the negative feelings, and the multisaccadic eye movements done in sets can desensitize the patient to the traumatic event in as little as one session. EMDR can be viewed as a physiologically based therapy that allows a person to see previously disturbing material in a new and less distressing way. EMDR has standard protocols and has helped many people since its development (Rodenburg, Benjamin, de Roos, Meijer, & Stams, 2009).

For Whom Does It Work?

The patients most likely to benefit from EMDR are those individuals who have experienced traumatic events. These can be accidents, war trauma, rape, child abuse, domestic violence, or any other event that leaves strong negative images or feelings that recur and bother the person (Ahmad, Larsson, & Sundelin-Wahlsten, 2007).

What Happens in Therapy?

The amount of time required to complete EMDR will vary according to the history of the patient. The protocol targets three areas: past memories, present disturbances, and future actions. The aim of therapy is to help patients process all of the experiences that are causing the problem, thus resolving the symptoms of the patient (Shapiro, 1989).

The therapist completes a thorough history and assessment to identify the specific targets for therapy. Next, the therapist teaches the client certain skills that will be necessary for the actual treatment, including establishing a trusting relationship, and calming techniques. In the third phase of treatment, the patient begins the process of selecting a particular scene from the target event that most clearly represents the target event, identifies a negative self-statement associated with the event like, "I am helpless," and develops a statement describing a more positive belief such as, "I am in control" (EMDR International Association [EMDRIA], 2003).

Reprocessing takes about three sessions. In this phase the rapid eye movements or taps or tones are used along with verbalizing the negative self-statement and recalling the target picture. Phase four involves the desensitization processes. This phase works with all of the patient's emotions as well as others that may arise during the sessions. (EMDRIA, 2003). In phase five, the goals are to increase the strengths of the patient's positive belief. In the sixth phase, the patient is asked to recall the disturbing event and to assess if there is any residual tension left in the body. If so, reprocessing is repeated. Calming techniques learned by the patient can be used to achieve a sense of calmness. The final phase is reevaluation, which actually occurs at the beginning of every session. In this phase, the therapist evaluates how the patient is doing, identifies any new problems that need to be resolved, and plans for this. The patient is also educated about using the techniques in the future (EMDRIA, 2003).

What Is the Evidence Base for This Therapy?

The clinical efficacy of EMDR in post-traumatic stress disorder treatment for adults has been tested and has been well established in a meta-analysis (Bisson et al., 2007). At least twenty studies have shown EMDR to be efficacious in trauma applications. Several meta-analyses have been done (Bradley, Greene, Russ, Dutra, & Westen, 2005; Davidson & Parker, 2001; Rodenburg et al., 2009; Seidler & Wagner, 2006). From these meta-analytic reviews, EMDR could be regarded as an effective trauma therapy among other established trauma therapies. However, only Rodenburg et al. (2009) focused on studies of children receiving EMDR. This meta-analysis reported on seven studies; the combined number of children in the studies was 206, about half of whom were in the control group. Findings in these children showed that EMDR was efficacious in treating the symptoms associated with PTSD, and these researchers were able to demonstrate incremental efficacy of EMDR when it was used along with other established treatments. No other published meta-analyses of EMDR with children were found. In addition, only one new study written in English was available upon search (Kemp, Drummond, & McDermott, 2010).

More recently, general research on EMDR has been directed toward identifying the mechanisms of why bilateral stimulation seems to be effective in desensitizing patients who have experienced trauma (Christman,

Propper, & Dion, 2004; Gunter & Bodner, 2008; Shapiro, 2007). New evidence generated on the neurobiological processes underlying the effectiveness of EMDR will strengthen belief of the results found in non-physiological studies. In summary, there is good evidence to show that EMDR can be a valuable therapy in situations of trauma.

How Do You Become a Therapist?

Qualifications for licensed mental health professionals vary by discipline. Medical doctors must have specialist training in psychiatry and be licensed. Registered nurses must have a master's degree in psychiatric nursing and be registered by their state board of nursing. Other mental health clinicians must have completed a master's level or doctorate level graduate program with a focus in the mental health field (social work, counseling, marriage and family therapy, or psychology) *and* must be licensed or certified through their state or national credentialing board. Some limited licenses in some states (including LLP (limited liability partnership in Michigan) meet this requirement. Clinicians who completed degrees in art therapy and drug and alcohol counseling must first submit information to EMDRIA about their program to determine if they qualify for training. Training can occur throughout the course of a semester for a university program or be tailored to fit the needs of the trainees if offered in some other arrangement (EMDRIA, 2003). Consult the EMDRIA website for further information (http://www.emdria.org/).

Family Therapy

Family therapy is often used in the treatment of a child's mental health problems because the child's problem affects the entire family unit. For many years families were believed to be the major source of childhood mental health problems; now we recognize that while families may unwittingly contribute to the child's problems, many childhood mental health problems have a neurobiological basis. Even when the problem is primarily neurobiological, the child's behavior affects the family, which in turn affects the child. Helping families sort through these issues is critical in helping the child. In some cases young children may be excluded from family therapy sessions even when they are the presenting problem for the family; this is much less true for adolescents. Sometimes this is an appropriate decision, if the child is very young or very disruptive. If some cases marital issues seem to be negatively influencing the child's behavior and sessions with just parents are needed. There is no one model that works for all families. What is important to know is the rationale of the therapist in making the decision to include or exclude children in family session. In one study by Johnson (1995), half of the therapists responding to a survey did not include children in family therapy because they were not comfortable working with children due to a lack of training. Yet children want to be included in family sessions, sometimes by talking and at other times with activities (Stith, Rosen, McCollum, Coleman, & Herman, 1996) Therefore, it is important to ask the family therapist about the inclusion of children in family sessions and how that decision is made. Family therapies can be divided into two major groups: systemic therapies that are at least loosely based on systems theory and behavioral family therapies that use primarily behavioral techniques to reduce problems within the family. Behavioral therapy and CBT are described in Chapter 17 and will not be included here. The principles described in Chapter 17 are the same when applied in the context of family therapy.

Evidence for specific types of family therapy other than CBT can be difficult to find. Research on therapies other than CBT decreased significantly in 1980s (Durlak & McGlinchey, 1999) and sometimes the evidence available for a particular therapy is quite weak. Many of the articles about research on family therapy for children and adolescents discuss family therapy as one method without specifying a particular type or even combining types. Table 16.1 shows various forms of systemic family therapies, what they are, for whom they are effective, and the extant evidence. Systems theory therapies are typically taught to mental health professionals either during their graduate education or through workshops. Supervision in the techniques is considered necessary at least until the professional becomes competent in the new techniques. Unlike many of the individual therapies, there are not web sites or organizations for the various forms of family therapy. Rather, the American Association for Marriage and Family Therapy is the professional association for this group of professionals (http://www.aamft.org/). There are chapters or divisions in some states that also have websites. Additionally, there is an international organization for family therapy (http://www.ifta-familytherapy.org/index.html).

Parent and Teacher Training

Directly working with parents about parenting issues is another way to influence a child's mental health. Some childhood problems do appear to be related to parenting approaches. The work of Gerald Patterson (1982) showed that different parenting styles affected the child's behavior. By helping parents learn different parenting approaches, the child's behavior can be corrected before

it becomes a major problem. The parenting programs discussed here are all evidence-based, many with years of research behind them. The programs are built on social learning theory.

Triple P-Positive Parenting Program

The Triple P-Positive Parenting Program is a public health approach to parenting (Sanders, 2003). It aims to prevent more serious problems in children and adolescents by delivering services to parents at five different levels, depending upon need.

What Is It?

Universal Triple P is delivered via media such as radio and television. The goal of Universal Triple P is to use mass media to reach many parents and provide information about common problems, such as shopping with young children (Prinz & Sanders, 2007; Sanders & Prinz, 2008). Level two is single-session interaction with parents around a particular short-term problem. Level three is designed to be a four-session intervention delivered in the context of brief sessions, approximately twenty minutes each. One reason for the shortness of these sessions was to allow the delivery by primary health care providers. The case exemplar provides an example of how a pediatric nurse practitioner might apply Primary Care Triple P in practice. Parents identify a specific problematic behavior of their child such as not following requests or being rude and within the sessions are taught how to monitor the behavior, develop a behavioral plan, implement it, and assess the results (Sanders, Tully, Turner, Maher, & McAuliffe, 2003). Level four Triple P is an eight- to ten-session program designed to help parents manage their children's more serious problems, such as conduct disorders or attention deficit hyperactivity disorder (ADHD) (Bodenmann, Cina, Ledermann, & Sanders, 2008). Level four Triple P is more in depth and includes some parent-child sessions with the provider. Parents are taught fifteen parenting behaviors, which they implement to help their child. Level five Triple P is essentially an add-on to level four and is used when more serious problems are identified (Hoath & Sanders, 2002). There have been various modifications of the Triple P programs for use with different groups and problems.

Case Exemplar

This case illustrates implementation of Primary Care Triple P by a pediatric nurse practitioner. Mrs. Jones brought her eight-year-old son, Timmy, to the pediatric nurse practitioner (PNP) for a routine health care

Table 16.1 Comparison of different systemic therapies

Type	What is it?	For whom does it work?	What happens in therapy?	What is the evidence base?
Attachment-focused	Based on Bowlby's attachment theory, attachment-focused therapy is used to provide a secure base from which the individual can learn and grow. In this safe environment, the family can explore problems and find better ways to interact	Depressed adolescent males (Diamond, Reis, Diamond, Siqueland, & Issacs, 2002); young children with attachment disorders; others with attachment problems, such as abused children	Each family member must have a solid attachment to the therapist. This is created by the therapist being accepting of all family members, and by being non-judgmental, demonstrating relaxed engagement, playfulness, curiosity, and empathy. The therapist seeks to know each family member well and reflects that understanding through empathy. Information about child development, family processes, attachment, and intersubjectivity are shared to the extent needed. Within this environment, problems in the family are discussed and understood related to attachment and intersubjectivity. Family members' affect intentions and awareness are tracked, verbalized, and new meanings are co-created (Hughes, 2007)	Diamond and colleagues (2002) studied 32 adolescents with a major depressive disorder in a randomized controlled trial over two years. The youth received either 12 weeks of Attachment Based Family Therapy (ABFT) or waitlist control group for 6 weeks. Eighty-one percent of the youth in ABFT arm of the trial were no longer depressed and had reduced anxiety while only 47% of the control arm had improved. Family conflict also improved with ABFT
Experiential	In experiential family therapy, the family is involved in various activities as a family that are used to depict the family problems while encouraging family members to openly express how they are feeling. Behavior problems are believed to emanate from the smothering of emotions. The task of therapy is to unblock defenses and release people's innate vitality. This therapy stems from the work of Carl Whitaker	This therapy has been used primarily for treating depression, based on the studies in the literature	The experience the family had is discussed and emotions are explored (Nichols & Schwartz, 2004). A type of activity that might be used in experiential therapy is role reversal in which family members play each other during some situation. This provides the individual an opportunity to experience the emotional reactions the other experiences during the real situation. This role reversal can be helpful in changing long standing interaction patterns within a family. Other techniques can include family sculpting, family art therapy, family puppet interviews, and Gestalt empty chair exercise	Evidence for experiential therapy is fairly recent. Some studies have been testing the efficacy of the therapy (Carryer & Greenberg, 2010; Ellison, Greenberg, Goldman, & Angus, 2009; Greenberg & Watson, 1998; Pos, Greenberg, & Warwar, 2009). Generally, the studies have shown some success with experiential therapy
Multidimensional (MDFT)	MDFT is similar to Multisystem Therapy (MST) in that it uses an integrative, systems oriented approach. The youth, the family, and the community are all involved in this therapy. Treatment can be provided in any number of settings, including	MDFT is aimed at treating adolescents with drug abuse and related behavior problems but has also been used for children with foster home placement behavior problems (Chamberlain,	Treatment can be provided in any number of settings, including foster care. The family develops competency in collaborating with any social systems in which the youth is involved including school, juvenile justice system, or recreational activities. Therapies are individualized to the needs of the children (Liddle, 2010)	There is strong evidence of the effectiveness of this approach in various settings, including an international trial (Chamberlain et al., 2007; Chamberlain et al., 2008; Henderson, Dakof, Greenbaum, & Liddle, 2010; Liddle et al., 2001; Liddle, Dakof, Turner, Henderson, &

Approach	Description	Population / References	Technique	Evidence
	foster care. The family develops competency in collaborating with any social systems in which the youth is involved including school, juvenile justice system, or recreational activities	Leve, & DeGarmo, 2007; Leve, Fisher, & Chamberlain, 2009)		Greenbaum, 2008; Marvel, Rowe, Colon-Perez, Diclemente, & Liddle, 2009; Rigter et al., 2010; Shelef, Diamond, Diamond, & Liddle, 2005)
Narrative	In narrative therapy the focus is on using a comparison for learning. Each individual has a personal narrative which can include different versions of the self, some of which are problematic. Families also develop narratives about themselves. Individuals and families tend to judge themselves by the narratives of the society in which they live (Nichols & Schwartz, 2004). The therapist uses a technique for externalizing the problem story so the family can consider times when it is and is not a problem	Parent-child conflicts (Besa, 1994). Obsessive-compulsive disorders (McLuckie, 2006). Blended families with role conflicts (Shalay & Brownlee, 2007)	When a family comes in to therapy, there are problem-laden narratives among the family members. These problem stories are often kept active because of their connection to others. The therapist seeks to help the family members redevelop these stories with more positive outcomes, to help them look at what is stopping them from behaving in more successful ways. As a more positive account of the person develops, the problems fade into the background (White & Epston, 1990). Therapists may use between session tasks to help families re-author their narratives (Besa, 1994)	Besa's study (1994) demonstrated effectiveness in changing parent-child conflicts with narrative therapy
Solution-focused	Brief therapy focused on developing solutions to problems the family already uses. The idea behind solution-focused therapy is to focus on the family's goals and reaching their goals. Strengths and solutions are focused on what is used when the problem is not occurring. Focus is on doing more of what is working	Children with oppositional defiant disorder (ODD) (Conoley et al., 2003) or with other behavior problems	Attention is not paid to family structure or rules. The therapist, assuming an approach of curiosity, and in the role of non-expert collaborator, helps the family construct solutions to their problems. Family sets a joint goal. Therapist poses the miracle question: "If a miracle happened tonight and removed the problem we just discussed, how would things be different?" Then family members state willingness to make it happen and confidence it could (Conoley et al., 2003). Berg and Steiner (2003) offer many suggestions on creative ways to engage children in solution-focused family therapy, e.g., puppet play. Children may feel safe discussing difficult issues through puppets when they would not feel safe talking directly about the issues. Another child friendly activity is to ask the child to state three wishes. This allows the child to fantasize about the future and think about how life could be different	Conoley et al. (2003) conducted a carefully controlled study of three families with children with ODD, using a treatment manual and validated measures

(continued)

Table 16.1 (*cont'd*)

Type	What is it?	For whom does it work?	What happens in therapy?	What is the evidence base?
Strategic	Problems in families develop because of a lack of alternatives or an unhelpful way of linking explanations and behaviors. Emphasis is on the therapist being curious about the relationship between the beliefs and behaviors of family members. An assumption of Brief Strategic Family Therapy (BSFT) is that if the therapist alters the family and extended family, they become a continuous positive influence on the youth (Santisteban et al., 1997)	Adolescents with substance abuse problems or conduct problems. Adolescents with anxiety disorders	There are three major parts of the BSFT model: (1) Joining, (2) Family Pattern Diagnosis, and (3) Restructuring. Joining with the family results in an effective collaboration and minimizes dropping-out or resisting change. The therapist becomes the family leader. Family pattern diagnosis involves identifying the maladaptive family behavior patterns that are perpetuating the problem. This identification allows restructuring, which is the process of modifying the family patterns of interaction and helping the family reorganize and modify family roles. The result is to reduce the potential for drug abuse by the adolescent (Santisteban et al., 1997)	Coatsworth and colleagues (2001) demonstrated that brief strategic family therapy was more effective in retaining and treating conduct disordered and anxious teens than in a community clinic. Brief strategic therapy is being compared to treatment as usual in a large NIH multi-site study (Santisteban et al., 1997). The NIDA study is also approximating the implementation of BSFT as a real world therapy with success (Santisteban et al., 2003)
Structural	Problems develop from inappropriate family structure or organization. Therapy focuses on reestablishing appropriate boundaries between parents and child(ren) and family and extended family (Minuchin, Auerswald, King, & Rabinowitz, 1964). The goal of therapy is to redesign the family structure to be more positive	Children with conduct problems, psychosomatic problems such as intractable asthma, anorexia nervosa, brittle diabetes	Therapist takes command of sessions, takes responsibility for moving the family in the desired direction. The therapist Is very active in sessions and may redirect family members in seating arrangements or to whom each is speaking. Family may be directed to enact the problem behavior or change interactional patterns (Cottrell & Boston, 2002). Sometimes play activities can be used to unbalance the non-adaptive system in which the child has too much control and to reinforce the executive role of the parents (Sori, 1995)	In multiple cases, structural family therapy was effective with psychosomatic illness (Liebman, Minuchin, & Baker, 1974)

appointment. During the visit, Mrs. Jones mentioned that Timmy was playing on a Little League baseball team but was having trouble being a good sport. The PNP inquired about Timmy's behavior in other arenas and Mrs. Jones reported that he wasn't a problem at home or at school. Further investigation revealed Little League to be the main activity in which Timmy had to compete with other children. The PNP, who had been trained to deliver Primary Care Triple P, asked the mother if she would like some help with this problem to prevent it from becoming a more ingrained behavior. The mother gratefully replied that she would. The PNP explained that Triple P was designed to help the parent learn skills that can be used to manage children's behavior such as Timmy was displaying. She explained that the mother would need to attend four sessions of about twenty minutes each with the PNP and do some at-home activities in between sessions. The PNP suggested they have the first session immediately. They discussed the behavior in detail. She asked Mrs. Jones if she attended the games and to describe her behavior as well as that of the coach and other parents. The PNP requested that Mrs. Jones monitor the specific behavior during the first week but not make any changes in what she was currently doing. She also provided Mrs. Jones with a parenting booklet and lent her a DVD to watch over the coming week. Mrs. Jones also had to complete some questionnaires about influences on children's behavior and a Parenting Experiences Scale.

In session two, the PNP reviewed all of the data with Mrs. Jones in a guided participation manner, helping the mother to identify whether she was accidently reinforcing the poor sportsmanship and how much she had worked with Timmy on competition; together they developed a parenting plan based on a Triple P Tip Sheet on Sport and used parenting strategies discussed in the DVD. The tip sheet provided both information and suggestions for managing the behavior. Mrs. Jones was encouraged to select management strategies from the tip sheet and to write out the plan. Specific behavioral goals were set. Monitoring during the coming week continued.

In session three, the PNP and Mrs. Jones reviewed the monitoring and refined the parenting plan. Mrs. Jones was asked to evaluate what went well with the plan, what did not go well, and to problem solve to improve the plan. Typically, monitoring showed only minimal improvement at this point but the mother was encouraged to continue the monitoring.

In session four, which was usually two to four weeks after session three, the mother reviewed the monitoring of the problem behavior and again progress was discussed. The plan may be further refined if needed but typically the behavior has improved. Generalization of the steps to other situations was discussed as is planning ahead for

high risk situations. Mrs. Jones was encouraged to use the model in the future but to feel free to ask for further sessions if she had trouble or needed more help.

Because the sessions are only about twenty minutes long, the PNP felt comfortable delivering Primary Care Triple P in the practice setting. Her experience with Primary Care Triple P is that it is an effective method for helping parents learn techniques that are going to be most effective in helping their child learn important life skills and to deal with specific problems before they become more serious or influence the child's overall mental health.

For Whom Does It Work?

Because there are both preventative and treatment aspects to the interventions, Triple P is a universal approach to parenting. It has been used to decrease the amount of child abuse in a community (Prinz, Sanders, Shapiro, Whitaker, & Lutzker, 2009), for helping families with a disabled or autistic child (Sanders, Mazzucchelli, & Studman, 2004; Whittingham, Sofronoff, Sheffield, & Sanders, 2009), for helping teens transition to high school (Ralph & Sanders, 2003; Ralph, Stallman, & Sanders, 2004), for externalizing disorders such as disruptive behaviors and ADHD (Connell, Sanders, & Markie-Dadds, 1997), for children with developmental disabilities (Plant & Sanders, 2007), for preventing drug abuse (Sanders, 2000), for lifestyles changes with obese children (West, Sanders, Cleghorn, & Davies, 2010), and even for families with gifted children (Morawska & Sanders, 2008). Triple P has been used in large urban areas, in rural counties, with indigenous peoples, and in many different countries. It has been delivered in person, in groups, via television or other mass media, by Internet, and even self-directed. It is indeed a universal program for parents.

What Happens in Therapy?

The Triple P programs are built on a framework of self-regulation. Parents are taught self-regulations skills with the goal of building their self-regulation capacities and then modeling and teaching these to their children (Sanders, 2008). Parents are helped to change their parenting strategies through increasing self-efficacy and parental self-efficacy, using self-management tools, promoting personal agency, and developing sound problem solving skills. The program is built on five principles of positive parenting: a safe and engaging environment, a positive learning environment, assertive and consistent discipline, realistic expectations, and taking care of oneself as a parent (Sanders & Ralph, 2001). Parents identify specific goals they would like to accomplish with their children based on an assessment and then in a guided participation model (Sanders & Lawton, 1993) with the therapist, work on a plan to accomplish the goal. Parents are taught specific skills that enhance their relationship with their child, encourage children's desirable behaviors, manage misbehaviors, anticipate and plan for risky behaviors, coach their children in learning new behaviors and skills, learn self-regulations skills, manage their own moods, and increase their coping skills and partner support skills (Sanders & Ralph, 2001).

What Is the Evidence Base for This Therapy?

The research base for the Triple P program is extensive with over 100 studies completed since the early 1980s. The program has been implemented and studied internationally. It was developed in Queensland, Australia, by Dr. Mathew Sanders and has been widely implemented in Australia, Europe, Asia, and the United States (US). Studies have been conducted in many of these countries (Leung, Sanders, Leung, Mak, & Lau, 2003) and Triple P has been the subject of several meta-analyses, which have demonstrated effectiveness (de Graaf, Speetjens, Smit, de Wolff, & Tavecchio, 2008a; de Graaf, Speetjens, Smit, de Wolff, & Tavecchio, 2008b; Nowak & Heinrichs, 2008; Thomas & Zimmer-Gembeck, 2007). Many of the previously cited articles also contribute to the evidence for this program.

How Do You Become a Therapist?

The Triple P program is tightly controlled to ensure treatment fidelity; all practitioners must undergo training for each specific type of Triple P they provide. Regular supervision or consultation is recommended and specific forms, teaching materials, and information sheets for parents must be purchased through the Triple P program. Checklists are used to help the practitioner maintain treatment fidelity. Each provider is accredited through an additional day of skills demonstration. Primary care providers or child psychiatric nurses could become trained in providing various levels of this intervention and use it in their practices. In the US, training and certification are available through Triple P America (http://www.triplep-america.com/index.html). Outside of the US, please check the Triple P International Website (http://www.triplep.net/). Training can either be provided through open enrollment wherever Triple P is holding training or training for a group of individuals can be arranged through Triple P America.

The Incredible Years

The Incredible Years (IY) Training Series is an approach to providing training for parents, teachers, and even young children with conduct problems,

including ODD and conduct disorders. Many parents identify conduct problems in preschoolers that do not meet all of the criteria for a diagnosis of either conduct disorder or ODD. Children who display ODD symptoms in the preschool years have two to three times the risk of becoming violent and chronic juvenile delinquents (Loeber et al., 1993; Patterson, Capaldi, & Bank, 1991). These disorders have been discussed in depth in other chapters in this book and the reader is referred to them for a more complete description of the problems.

What Is It?

The IY Training Series was developed by Carolyn Webster-Stratton, a nurse and a psychologist, to reduce conduct problems in young children. It was built on social learning theory. There are training programs for parents, teachers, and even for the children themselves to help learn skills to react in more socially expected ways (Webster-Stratton & Reid, 2010).

For Whom Does It Work?

The underpinning of the program is that as conduct problems continue they become more entrenched and are harder to treat in older children and adolescents. By modifying family and child components of the behaviors problems early, the children are able to develop healthier behaviors. Most recently, the program has been implemented and evaluated with eight- to twelve-year-old children and has shown that children can improve their behaviors even at that age (Webster-Stratton & Reid, 2010).

What Happens in Therapy?

There are three separate training programs for parents, teachers, and children. The parent training programs were begun in 1980 and have been recently updated to cover four age ranges: infancy, toddler, preschool, and school age up to age thirteen. The length of the programs varies by the age of the child with the program for infancy lasting eight to nine weeks and increasing up to eighteen weeks for the preschool and school-age parents. A series of videotaped vignettes are used by the therapist to promote discussion, problem solving, and collaborative learning (Webster-Stratton & Reid, 2010, p. 196). Parents learn a series of nonviolent strategies for managing their child's behavior. Parents are taught self-control related to anger management and using positive self-talk to deal with more negative self-messages. Parents are also taught how to teach problem solving skills to their child. The programs use a parent handbook to supplement the sessions with the therapist (Webster-Stratton & Reid, 2010).

The teacher training program is a six-day program that focuses on improving the teacher's classroom management skills, increasing the teacher's use of effective discipline strategies, helping the teacher learn to collaborate with parents, increasing the teacher's ability to foster social competence among the students, and strengthening the teacher's use of coaching for academic, social emotional, and persistence skills of the child. Teachers are taught to monitor closely for aggressive behaviors and to intervene appropriately. There is also a book for teachers to use along with their training program (Webster-Stratton & Reid, 2010).

Because children contribute to their problems of conduct, a training program for children using video vignettes was developed. The training consists of twenty-two sessions that teach children problem solving and social skills with the children meeting in small groups of six. The goals of this program are to strengthen social skills and appropriate play skills, help children recognize and label their emotions, increase their empathy, boost academic skills, reduce aggression and defiance, promote compliance with others, and increase self-confidence and self-esteem.

What Is the Evidence Base for This Therapy?

The IY parent programs have been well studied for effectiveness. There have been many randomized controlled trials that have shown that the program makes a significant difference in parenting behaviors including reductions in harsh discipline compared to the wait-list control group (Gross et al., 2003; Lavigne et al., 2008; Reid, Webster-Stratton, & Hammond, 2007; Webster-Stratton, 1984; 1990, 1998). Research has shown that the teacher and child training are also helpful especially when combined with parent training (Webster-Stratton & Hammond, 1997).

While the program has been provided primarily through the University of Washington Parenting Clinic, the program has been implemented by five investigators in mental health clinics with families of children with conduct problems and by four investigators with high risk families living in poverty. Two of the replications were conducted in the United Kingdom and one was done in Norway with the remaining being conducted in the US.

How Do You Become a Therapist?

To provide the Incredible Years Training Series, group leaders need to be certified through training for each component of the program either in Seattle or through onsite training within the community. Individuals seeking certification can come from a variety of disciplines such as nursing, psychology, social work, counseling, education, or psychiatry and should have received training in group work, behavior management, and child development. After the training, certification must be obtained by completing at least two groups and having these reviewed by a supervisor or mentor. Also, feedback from participants must be obtained. These processes help ensure that the program is delivered as intended (Incredible Years, 2010). When referring a family to the Incredible Years Program, it is important to know the therapist has been certified in the appropriate training needed by the family. Information about training and certification can be obtained by going to the Incredible Years website (http://www.incredibleyears.com/).

Parent Management Training—the Oregon Model

The Parent Management Training—Oregon Model (PMTO™) is designed to treat or prevent antisocial behavior problems in children and adolescents. It was developed at the Oregon Social Learning Center (OSLC) over more than four decades through research on children and their families.

What Is It?

As the OSLC's name suggests, the theoretical underpinnings of PMTO™ are based on social learning, social interaction, and behavioral theories. Social learning and behavioral theories are used to examine how behavior patterns become entrenched, while the social interaction theory is used to understand the connections among family members and friends that lead to various behavior patterns that contribute to mental health or problems (Forgatch & Patterson, 2010).

For Whom Does It Work?

Antisocial behavior is seen as a continuum that begins with relatively minor problems such as temper tantrums, biting, hitting, or noncompliance in young children that parents often accidentally negatively reinforce. In some children, the behaviors stop, while in others covert antisocial behaviors such as lying, stealing, fire setting, animal cruelty, or truancy develop as the child gets older if parental discipline is harsh. These behaviors may also be reinforced through peer behaviors. Parents are seen as an important early factor in serious antisocial behavior in a child. Patterson demonstrated the cycle of coercive behavior that can develop in families in which one person starts a cycle of coercion and that is responded to with negative reciprocity; it ends when one of the players ends the cycle with a negative behavior, thus winning that round. In families with a clinical level of problem, the cycles occur quite frequently, as often as four times an hour and can begin as early as two years of age (Patterson, 1982). Thus, children with disruptive behaviors and their families are the primary users for this program.

What Happens in Therapy?

PMTO™ can be delivered in single family or group sessions. Family sessions usually run sixty minutes long and twenty-five to thirty sessions are the norm; group treatment runs for fourteen sessions for ninety minutes. In individual sessions, children may be involved to some degree depending upon the family's and therapist's preferences. Treatment sessions are generally highly structured and consist of a warm-up activity, then review of assigned homework, the introduction and practicing of new concepts or skills, and then end with a new assignment for homework. Midweek calls are used to promote the success of the treatment (Forgatch & Patterson, 2010).

Forgatch and Patterson (2010) described the treatment as having five dimensions including scaffolding (breaking down complex behaviors into more manageable steps while using positive reinforcement to teach children more prosocial behavior), monitoring behavior by parents, limit setting, problem-solving skills, and positive involvement of parents with children. The goal of PMTO™ treatment is to empower parents to use positive parenting practices rather than coercive or harsh discipline. One important component is teaching parents emotional regulation though role-play. Strategies used for face-to-face issues such as fighting are time-outs. For behaviors such as lying or stealing, extra chores are used or possibly fines with privilege removal being used for time-out refusal or refusing to do assigned chores.

What Is the Evidence Base for This Therapy?

There is a significant body of research supporting PMTO™; over twenty-five studies have demonstrated the efficacy of the model (e.g., Chamberlain, Leve, et al., 2007, 2008; DeGarmo & Forgatch, 2007; DeGarmo, Patterson, & Forgatch, 2004; Forgatch & DeGarmo, 1999; Forgatch, Patterson, Degarmo, & Beldavs, 2009; Ogden, Forgatch, Askeland, Patterson, & Bullock, 2005; Patterson, Chamberlain, & Reid, 1982). Many other studies are available that describe effectiveness implementations or variations on the program.

How Do You Become a Therapist?

In 1997, the materials, policies, and procedures for training others to provide PMTO™ were developed to implement the training in Norway (Forgatch & Patterson, 2010). Training was accomplished through six workshops each lasting three days and then coaching, which

was done from videotaped therapy sessions. Trainees each had to see five families. Two of these families were seen for certification. Since then, Implementation Scientists International, Inc. was developed at OSLC to provide training in PMTO. The group works with the community or group to ensure that the intervention will be delivered with fidelity to the core dimensions of the program. The goal is to have a sustainable implementation with a long-term commitment to PTMO™ and future generations of PTMO™ therapists trained by local PTMO™ coaches. Further information on resources for PMTO™ can be obtained from the OSLC web site http://www.oslc.org/resources/clinician-books.html or for training information from the Implementation Scientists International, Inc. website http://www.isii.net/website.isii/NewFiles/training.html.

Parent-Child Interaction Therapy

Parent-Child Interaction Therapy (PCIT) was developed by Shelia Eyberg et al. (2001) to treat young children with disruptive behaviors. It is designed to help parents learn to be more warm and nurturing while establishing firm controls (Pincus, Santucci, Ehrenreich, & Eyberg 2008).

What Is It?

The goal of PCIT is to teach parents an authoritative style of parenting (Zisser & Eyberg, 2010). The authoritative style of parenting has been demonstrated in various studies to be the most effective of the four identified styles of parenting— authoritative, authoritarian, neglectful, and permissive (e.g., Baumrind, 1971; Boveja, 1998; Glasgow, Dornbusch, Troyer, Steinberg, & Ritter, 1997; Querido, Warner, & Eyberg, 2002). In PCIT, parents are taught to interrupt the negative coercive relationship that develops between parent and child when the child has disruptive behavior problems. Parent and child are seen together in this model of parenting therapy (Zisser & Eyberg, 2010).

For Whom Does It Work?

It is effective for families engaged in the coercive cycle of parenting that often evolves in families when children have a disruptive behavior problem. It is more effective for younger children since the disruptive patterns are less entrenched in younger children.

What Happens in Therapy?

In therapy, each session has a teaching component in which the therapist explains and models or role-plays certain skills; then the parent works with the child, practicing the skills while the therapist acts as coach (Zisser &

Eyberg, 2010). Skills include those that are child-directed interaction skills such as letting the child lead an activity, showing approval, reflection of the child's behavior and parent-directed interaction skills which include making commands that are specific, age appropriate, and positively stated. Initially the child-directed interactional skills are the focus as parents learn to give positive attention and ignore negative behaviors, unless they are aggressive or destructive. In this case the parent tells the child their special time has ended and to disengage until a later time when the child is calm.

During parent-directed interactions, parents learn when to give explanations, how not to argue with the child, and specific steps to follow after giving a command to the child. These steps begin with a warning and then time-out with the parent establishing the specific time-out length if the warning is insufficient. If the child leaves the time-out chair, a time-out room is used. Parents are coached about how to manage any escalation of behavior that may occur early in this process as the child learns to follow direction. Progress in therapy is measured by observation and coding of the parent's skill development and by completing the intensity scale of the Eyberg Child Behavior Inventory (Zisser & Eyberg, 2010).

What Is the Evidence Base for This Therapy?

The evidence base for PCIT is strong. It has been in use since the 1980s and various studies have been done testing PCIT with other populations besides families with children with disruptive behavior disorders such as those with intellectual disability, autism spectrum disorders, or problems related to prematurity (Bagner & Eyberg, 2007; Choate, Pincus, Eyberg, & Barlow, 2005; Matos, Bauermeister, & Bernal, 2009; Pincus et al., 2008; Solomon, Ono, Timmer, & Goodlin-Jones, 2008), in different ethnic, cultural, or racial groups (Leung, Tsang, et al., 2009; Matos et al., 2009; McCabe & Yeh, 2009; Phillips, Morgan, Cawthorne, & Barnett, 2008), for families where child maltreatment has occurred (Chaffin et al., 2004; Timmer, Urquiza, et al., 2006), or in different settings or modalities (Funderburk, Ware, Altshuler, & Chaffin, 2008; Lyon & Budd, 2010; Lyon et al., 2009; Niec, Hemme, Yopp, & Brestan, 2005; Timmer, Zebell, Culver, & Urquiza, 2010). In addition, several studies have tested the efficacy of the intervention (Bagner & Eyberg, 2007; Boggs et al., 2004; Eyberg et al., 2001; Funderburk, Eyberg et al., 1998).

How Do You Become a Therapist?

Training to conduct PCIT requires that the therapist have a minimum of a master's degree in an appropriate discipline, complete forty hours of face to face contact with a certified PCIT trainer that includes theoretical content, coding practice, case observations, and guided coaching with families to develop the needed skill set. This is followed in two to six months with advanced training with actual cases. Then the trainee must complete at least two PCIT cases and be in regular contact with their trainer for about a year. Trainees must have a skill review via some observation—live, videotape, or teleconferencing. Further information about training requirements is available on the PCIT website (http://www.pcit.org/guidelines.php).

Summary

Many types of therapies are available for helping children and their families with mental health problems. Individual therapies and parent training programs have a broader evidence-base than do family therapies. While other types of therapies exist, the therapies presented in this chapter have the most evidence and are among the best known for children.

References

Aarts, H., Custers, R., & Marien, H. (2008). Preparing and motivating behavior outside of awareness. *Science, 319*, 1639–1610. doi. 10.1126/science.1150432

Ahmad, A., Larsson, B., & Sundelin-Wahlsten, V. (2007). EMDR treatment for children with PTSD: Results of a randomized controlled trial. *Nordic Journal of Psychiatry, 61*, 349–354. doi:10.1080/08039480701643464

Anderson, M.C., Ochsner, K.N., Kuhl, B., Cooper, J., Robertson, E., Gabrieli, S.W., & Gabrieli, J.D. E. (2004). Neural systems underlying the suppression of unwanted memories. *Science, 303*, 232–235.

Arcelus, J., Whight, D., Langham, C., Baggott, J., McGrain, L., Meadows, L., & Meyer, C. (2009). A case series evaluation of the modified version of interpersonal psychotherapy (IPT) for the treatment of bulimic eating disorders: A pilot study. *European Eating Disorders Review, 17*, 260–268. doi:10.1002/(ISSN)1099-096810.1002/erv.v17:410.1002/erv.932

Bagner, D.M., & Eyberg, S.M. (2007). Parent-child interaction therapy for disruptive behavior in children with mental retardation: A Randomized controlled trial. *Journal of Clinical Child and Adolescent Psychology, 36*, 418–429.

Baumrind, D. (1971). Current patterns of parental authority. *Developmental Psychology Monograph, 4*, 1–103.

Bearsley-Smith, C., Browne, M.O., Sellick, K., Villanueva, E.V., Chesters, J., Francis, K., & Reddy, P (2007). Does interpersonal psychotherapy improve clinical care for adolescents with depression attending a rural child and adolescent mental health service? Study protocol for a cluster randomised feasibility trial. *BMC Psychiatry 7*, 53–59. doi. 10.1186/1471-244X-7-53

Berg, I.K., & Steiner, T. (2003). *Children's solutions work.* New York, NY: Norton.

Besa, D. (1994). Evaluating narrative family therapy using single-system research designs. *Research on Social Work Practice, 4*, 309–325. doi. 10.1177/104973159400400303

Bisson, J.I., Ehlers, A., Matthews, R., Pilling, S., Richards, D., & Turner, S. (2007). Psychological treatments for chronic post-traumatic stress disorder, Systematic review and meta-analysis. *British Journal of Psychiatry, 190*, 97–104.doi. 10.1192/bjp.bp.106.021402

Blair, K.S., Smith, B.W., Mitchell, D.G.V., Morton, J., Vythilingam, M., Pessoa, L., & Blair, R.J.R (2007). Modulation of emotion by cognition and cognition by emotion. *Neuroimage, 35*(1), 430–440. doi:10.1016/j.neuroimage.2006.11.048

Bodenmann, G., Cina, A., Ledermann, T., & Sanders, M.R. (2008). The efficacy of the Triple P-Positive Parenting Program in improving parenting and child behavior: A comparison with two other treatment conditions. *Behaviour Research and Therapy, 46*, 411–427. doi:10.1016/j.brat.2008.01.001

Boggs, S.R., Eyberg, S.M., Edwards, D.L., Rayfield, A., Jacobs, J., Bagner, D., & Hood, K.K.(2004). Outcomes of parent-child interaction therapy: A comparison of treatment completers and study dropouts one to three years later. *Child & Family Behavior Therapy, 26*, 1–22. doi. 10.1300/J019v26n04_01

Borduin, C.M., Cone, L.T., Mann, B.J., Henggeler, S.W., Fucci, B.R., Blaske, D.M., & Williams, R.A. (1995). Multisystemic treatment of serious juvenile-offenders - Long-term prevention of criminality and violence. *Journal of Consulting and Clinical Psychology, 63*(4), 569–578.

Borduin, C.M., Henggeler, S.W., Blaske, D.M., & Stein, R. (1990). Multisystemic treatment of adolescent sexual offenders. *International Journal of Offender Therapy and Comparative Criminology, 35*, 105–114.

Boveja, M.E. (1998). Parenting styles and adolescents' learning strategies in the urban community. *Journal of Multicultural Counseling and Development, 26*(2), 110–119.

Bradley, R., Greene, J., Russ, E., Dutra, L., & Westen, D. (2005). A multidimensional meta-analysis of psychotherapy for PTSD, *American Journal of Psychiatry, 162*(2), 214–227.

Brown, T.L., Swenson, C.C., Cunningham, P.B., Henggeler, S.W., Schoenwald, S.K., & Rowland, M.D. (1997). Multisystemic treatment of violent and chronic juvenile offenders: Bridging the gap between research and practice. *Administration and Policy in Mental Health, 25*(2), 221–238.

Brunk, M., Henggeler, S.W., & Whelan, J.P. (1987). A comparison of multisystemic therapy and parent training in the brief treatment of child abuse and neglect. *Journal of Consulting and Clinical Psychology, 55*, 311–318.

Carryer, J.R., & Greenberg, L.S. (2010). Optimal levels of emotional arousal in experiential therapy of depression. *Journal of Consulting and Clinical Psychology, 78*(2), 190–199. doi:10.1037/a0018401

Chaffin, M., Silovsky, J.F., Funderburk, B., Valle, L.A., Brestan, E.V., Balachova, T., & Bonner, B.L. (2004). Parent-child interaction therapy with physically abusive parents: Efficacy for reducing future abuse reports. *Journal of Consulting and Clinical Psychology, 72*(3), 500–510. doi:10.1037/0022-006x.72.3.500

Chamberlain, P., Leve, L.D., & DeGarmo, D.S. (2007). Multidimensional treatment foster care for girls in the juvenile justice system: 2-year follow-up of a randomized clinical trial. *Journal of Consulting and Clinical Psychology, 75*(1), 187–193. doi:10.1037/0022-006x.75.1.187

Chamberlain, P., Price, J., Leve, L.D., Laurent, H., Landsverk, J.A., & Reid, J.B. (2008). Prevention of behavior problems for children in foster care: Outcomes and mediation effects. *Prevention Science, 9*(1), 17–27. doi:10.1007/s11121-007-0080-7

Choate, M.L., Pincus, D.B., Eyberg, S.M., & Barlow, D.H. (2005). Parent-child interaction therapy for treatment of separation anxiety disorder in young children: A pilot study. *Cognitive and Behavioral Practice, 12*(1), 126–135.

Christman, S.D., Propper, R.E., & Dion, A. (2004). Increased interhemispheric interaction is associated with decreased false memories in a verbal converging semantic stress associates paradigm. *Brain & Cognition, 56*, 313–319. doi:10.1016/j.bandc.2004.08.005

Coatsworth, J.D., Santisteban, D.A., McBride, C.K., & Szapocznik, J. (2001). Brief strategic family therapy versus community control: Engagement, retention, and an exploration of the moderating role of adolescent symptom severity. *Family Process, 40*(3), 313–332.

Connell, S., Sanders, M.R., & Markie-Dadds, C. (1997). Self-directed behavioral family intervention for parents of oppositional children in rural and remote areas. *Behavior Modification, 21*, 379–408.

Conoley, C.W., Graham, J.M., Neu, T., Craig, M.C., O'Pry, A., Cardin, S.A., & Parker, R.I. (2003). Solution-focused family therapy with three aggressive and oppositional-acting children: an N=1 empirical study. *Family Process, 42*(3), 361–374.

Cottrell, D., & Boston, P. (2002). Practitioner review: The effectiveness of systemic family therapy for children and adolescents. *Journal of Child Psychology & Psychiatry & Allied Disciplines, 43*(5), 573–586.

Cyranowski, J.M., Frank, E., Shear, M.K., Swartz, H., Fagiolini, A., Scott, A.M., & Kupfer, D.J. (2005). Interpersonal psychotherapy for depression with panic spectrum symptoms: A pilot study. *Depression and Anxiety, 21*, 140–142. DOI: 10.1002/da.20069

Davidson, P.R., & Parker, K. (2001). Eye movement desensitization and reprocessing (EMDR): A meta-analysis. *Journal of Consulting and Clinical Psychology 69*, 305–316.

de Graaf, I., Speetjens, P., Smit, F., de Wolff, M., & Tavecchio, L. (2008a). Effectiveness of the Triple P Positive Parenting Program on behavioral problems in children A meta-analysis. *Behavior Modification 32*(5), 714–735. doi:10.1177/0145445508317134

de Graaf, I., Speetjens, P., Smit, F., de Wolff, M., & Tavecchio, L. (2008b). Effectiveness of the Triple P-Positive Parenting Program on parenting: A Meta-analysis. *Family Relations, 57*, 553–566. doi:10.1111/j.1741-3729.2008.00522.x

DeGarmo, D.S., & Forgatch, M.S. (2007). Efficacy of parent training for stepfathers: From playful spectator and polite stranger to effective stepfathering. *Parenting-Science and Practice, 7*(4), 331–355.

DeGarmo, D.S., Patterson, G.R., & Forgatch, M.S. (2004). How do outcomes in a specified parent training intervention maintain or wane over time? *Prevention Science, 5*(2), 73–89.

Depue, B.E., Curran, T., & Banich, M.T. (2007). Prefrontal regions orchestrate suppression of emotional memories via a two-phase process. *Science, 317*(5835), 215–219. doi:10.1126/science.1139560

Diamond, G.S., Reis, B.F., Diamond, G.M., Siqueland, L., & Issacs, L. (2002). Attachment-based family therapy for depressed adolescents: A treatment development study. *Journal of the American Academy of Child and Adolescent Psychiatry, 41*, 1190–1196. doi:10.1097/01.CHI.0000024836.94814.08

Driessen, E., Cuijpers, P., de Maat, S.C.M., Abbass, A.A., de Jonghe, F., & Dekker, J.J.M. (2010). The efficacy of short-term psychodynamic psychotherapy for depression: A meta-analysis. *Clinical Psychology Review 30*(1), 25–36. doi:10.1111/j.1600-0447.2009.01526.x

Durlak, J.A., & McGlinchey, K.A. (1999). Child therapy outcome research. Current status and some future priorities. In E. Russ & T.H. Ollendick (Eds.), *Handbook of psychotherapies with children and families* New York: Kluwer Academic/Plenum Publishers.

Elkin, I., Shea, M.T., Watkins, J.T., Imber, D.M., Sotsky, S.M., Collins, J.F., & Parloff, M.B. (1989). National Institute of Mental Health Treatment of Depression Collaborative Research Program: General effectiveness of treatments. *Archives of General Psychiatry, 46*, 971–982.

Ellis, D.A., Frey, M.A., Naar-King, S., Templin, T., Cunningham, P., & Cakan, N. (2005). Use of multisystemic therapy to improve regimen adherence among adolescents with type 1 diabetes in chronic poor metabolic control - A randomized controlled trial. *Diabetes Care, 28*(7), 1604–1610. doi:10.1089/apc.2006.20.112

Ellis, D.A., Templin, T., Naar-King, S., Frey, M.A., Cunningham, P.B., Podolski, C.L., & Cakan, N. (2007). Multisystemic therapy for adolescents with poorly controlled type 1 diabetes: Stability of treatment effects in a randomized controlled trial. *Journal of Consulting and Clinical Psychology, 75*(1), 168–174. doi:10.1037/0022-006x.75.1.168

Ellis, M.L., Weiss, B., Han, S., & Gallop, R. (2010). The influence of parental factors on therapist adherence in multi-systemic therapy. *Journal of Abnormal Child Psychology, 38*(6), 857–868.doi:10.1007/s10802-010-9407-0

Ellison, J.A., Greenberg, L.S., Goldman, R.N., & Angus, L. (2009). Maintenance of gains following experiential therapies for depression. *Journal of Consulting and Clinical Psychology, 77*(1), 103–112. doi:10.1037/a0014653

EMDR International Association. (2003, 10/25/09). Definition of EMDR. Retrieved from http://www.emdria.org/associations/5581/files/Website%20EMDRIA%20Definition%20of%20EMDR%20Revised%20102509.pdf

Eyberg, S.M., Funderburk, B.W., Hembree-Kigin, T.L., McNeil, C.B., Querido, J.G., & Hood, K.K. (2001). Parent-child interaction therapy with behavior problem children: One and two year maintenance of treatment effects in the family. *Child & Family Behavior Therapy, 23*(4), 1–20.

Fairburn, C.G., Jones, R., Peveler, R.C., Hope, R.A., & O'Connor, M. (1993). Psychotherapy and bulimia nervosa: Longer-term effects of interpersonal psychotherapy, behavior therapy, and cognitive behavior therapy. *Arch Gen Psychiatry, 50*(6), 419–428. doi:10.1001/archpsyc.1993.01820180009001

Fonagy, P. (1999). Psychodynamic psychotherapy. In S.W. Russ & T.H. Ollendick (Eds.), *Handbook of psychotherapies with children and families* (1st ed., pp. 87–106). New York: Kluwer Academic/Plenum Publishers.

Forgatch, M.S., & DeGarmo, D.S. (1999). Parenting through change: An effective prevention program for single mothers. *Journal of Consulting and Clinical Psychology, 67*(5), 711–724.

Forgatch, M.S., & Patterson, G.R. (2010). Parent Management Training–Oregon Model. In J.R. Weisz & A.E. Kazdin (Eds.), *Evidence-based psychotherapies for children and adolescents* (second ed., pp. 159–178). New York: Guilford Press.

Forgatch, M.S., Patterson, G.R., Degarmo, D.S., & Beldavs, Z.G. (2009). Testing the Oregon delinquency model with 9-year follow-up of the Oregon Divorce Study. *Development and Psychopathology, 21*(2), 637–660. doi:10.1017/s0954579409000340

Frank, E., Kupfer, D.J., Perel, J.M., Cornes, C., Jarrett, D.B., Mallinger, A.G., & Grochocinski, V.J. (1990). Three-Year outcomes for maintenance therapies in recurrent depression. *Arch Gen Psychiatry, 47*(12), 1093–1099. doi:10.1001/archpsyc.1990.01810240013002

Funderburk, B.W., Eyberg, S.M., Newcomb, K., McNeil, C.B., Hembree-Kigin, T., & Capage, L. (1998). Parent-child interaction therapy with behavior problem children: Maintenance of treatment effects in the school setting. *Child & Family Behavior Therapy, 20*(2), 17–38.

Funderburk, B.W., Ware, L.M., Altshuler, E., & Chaffin, M. (2008). Use and feasibility of telemedicine technology in the dissemination of Parent-Child Interaction Therapy. *Child Maltreatment, 13*(4), 377–382. doi:10.1177/1077559508321483

Glasgow, K.L., Dornbusch, S.M., Troyer, L., Steinberg, L., & Ritter, P.L. (1997). Parenting styles, adolescents' attributions, and educational outcomes in nine heterogeneous high schools. *Child Development, 68*(3), 507–529.

Greenberg, L., & Watson, J. (1998). Experiential therapy of depression: differential effects of client-centered relationship conditions and process experiential interventions. *Psychotherapy Research, 8*(2), 210–224.

Gross, D., Fogg, L., Webster-Stratton, C., Garvey, C., Julion, W., & Grady, J. (2003). Parent training of toddlers in day care in low-income urban communities. *Journal of Consulting and Clinical Psychology, 71*(2), 261–278. doi:10.1037/0022-006x.71.2.261

Gunlicks-Stoessel, M., Mufson, L., Jekal, A., & Turner, J.B. (2010). The impact of perceived interpersonal functioning on treatment for adolescent depression: IPT-A versus treatment as usual in school-based health clinics. *Journal of Consulting and Clinical Psychology, 78*(2), 260–267. doi:10.1037/a0018935

Gunter, R.W., & Bodner, G.E. (2008). How eye movements affect unpleasant memories: Support for a working-memory account. *Behaviour Research and Therapy 46*(8), 913–931.doi:10.1016/j.brat.2008.04.006

Henderson, C.E., Dakof, G.A., Greenbaum, P.E., & Liddle, H.A. (2010). Effectiveness of multidimensional family therapy with higher severity substance-abusing adolescents: Report from two randomized controlled trials. *Journal of Consulting and Clinical Psychology.*

Henggeler, S.W., Clingempeel, W.G., Brondino, M.J., & Pickrel, S.G. (2002). Four-year follow-up of multisystemic therapy with substance-abusing and substance-dependent juvenile offenders. *Journal of the American Academy of Child and Adolescent Psychiatry, 41*(7).

Henggeler, S.W., Melton, G.B., Brondino, M.J., Scherer, D.G., & Hanley, J.H. (1997). Multisystemic therapy with violent and chronic juvenile offenders and their families: The role of treatment fidelity in successful dissemination. *Journal of Consulting and Clinical Psychology, 65*(5), 821–833.

Henggeler, S.W., Melton, G.B., & Smith, L.A. (1992). Family preservation using multisystemic therapy - An effective alternative to incarcerating serious juvenile-offenders. *Journal of Consulting and Clinical Psychology, 60*(6), 953–961.

Henggeler, S.W., Rodick, J.D., Borduin, C.A., Hanson, C.L., Watson, S.M., & Urey, J.R. (1986). Multisystemic treatment of juvenile offenders: Effects on adolescent behavior and family interactions. *Developmental Psychology, 22*, 132–141.

Henggeler, S.W., Rowland, M.D., Randall, J., Ward, D.M., Pickrel, S.G., Cunningham, P.B., & Santos, A.B. (1999). Home-based multisystemic therapy as an alternative to the hospitalization of youths in psychiatric crisis: Clinical outcomes. *Journal of the American Academy of Child and Adolescent Psychiatry, 38*(11), 1331–1339.

Henggler, S.W., Schoenwald, S.K., Bourduin, C., Rowland, M.D., & Cunningham, P.B. & (2009). *Multisystemic therapy for antisocial behavior in children and adolescents* (second ed.). New York: Guilford Press.

Hoath, F.E., & Sanders, M.R. (2002). A feasibility study of Enhanced Group Triple P - Positive Parenting Program for parents of children with attention-deficit/hyperactivity disorder. *Behaviour Change, 19*(4), 191–206.

Hughes, D.J. (2007). *Attachment-focused family therapy.* New York W. W. Norton, Publishers.

Incredible Years. (2010). About Incredible Years certification/accreditation and the process. Retrieved from http://www.incredibleyears.com/Certification/about.asp

International Society for Interpersonal Psychotherapy. (2010). Interpersonal psychotherapy–An overview. 2010. Retrieved from http://www.interpersonalpsychotherapy.org/

Johnson, L.M. (1995). *The inclusion of children in the process of family therapy.* Purdue, Purdue IN.

Kemp, M., Drummond, P., & McDermott, B. (2010). A wait-list controlled pilot study of eye movement desensitization and reprocessing (EMDR) for children with post-traumatic stress disorder (PTSD) symptoms from motor vehicle accidents. *Clinical Child Psychology and Psychiatry, 15*(1), 5–25. doi:10.1177/1359104509339086

Lavigne, J.V., LeBailly, S.A., Gouze, K.R., Cicchetti, C., Pochyly, J., Arend, R., Binns, H.J. (2008). Treating oppositional defiant disorder in primary care: A comparison of three models. *Journal of Pediatric Psychology, 33*(5), 449–461.doi:10.1093/jpepsy/jsm074

Leung, C., Sanders, M.R., Leung, S., Mak, R., & Lau, J. (2003). An outcome evaluation of the. implementation of the Triple P-Positive Parenting Program in Hong Kong. *Family Process, 42*(4), 531–544.

Leung, C., Tsang, S., Heung, K., & Yiu, I. (2009). Effectiveness of Parent-Child Interaction Therapy (PCIT) among Chinese families. *Research on Social Work Practice, 19*(3), 304–313. doi:10.1177/1049731508321713

Leve, L.D., Fisher, P.A., & Chamberlain, P. (2009). Multidimensional treatment foster care as a preventive intervention to promote resiliency among youth in the child welfare system. *Journal of Personality, 77*(6), 1869–1902.doi:10.1111/j.1467-6494.2009.00603.x

Liddle, H.A. (2010). Multidimensional Family Therapy: A science-based treatment system. *Australian & New Zealand Journal of Family Therapy, 31*(2), 133–148.

Liddle, H.A., Dakof, G.A., Parker, K., Diamond, G.S., Barrett, K., & Tejeda, M. (2001). Multidimensional family therapy for adolescent drug abuse: Results of a randomized clinical trial. *American Journal of Drug and Alcohol Abuse, 27*(4), 651–688.

Liddle, H.A., Dakof, G.A., Turner, R.M., Henderson, C.E., & Greenbaum, P.E. (2008). Treating adolescent drug abuse: a randomized trial comparing multidimensional family therapy and cognitive behavior therapy. *Addiction, 103*(10), 1660–1670. doi:10.1111/j.1360-0443.2008.02274.x

Liebman, R., Minuchin, S., & Baker, L. (1974). The use of structural family therapy in the treatment of intractable asthma. *Am J Psychiatry, 131*(5), 535–540. doi:10.1176/appi.ajp.131.5.535

Loeber, R., Wung, P., Keenan, K., Giroux, B., Stouthamerloeber, M., Vankammen, W.B., & Maughan, B. (1993). Developmental pathways in disruptive child-behavior. *Development and Psychopathology, 5*(1–2), 103–133.

Lyon, A.R., & Budd, K.S. (2010). A community mental health implementation of Parent-Child Interaction Therapy (PCIT). *Journal of Child and Family Studies, 19*(5), 654–668. doi:10.1007/s10826-010-9353-z

Lyon, A.R., Gershenson, R.A., Farahmand, F.K., Thaxter, P.J., Behling, S., & Budd, K.S. (2009). Effectiveness of Teacher-Child Interaction Training (TCIT) in a preschool setting. *Behavior Modification, 33*(6), 855–884. doi:10.1177/0145445509344215

Marvel, F., Rowe, C.L., Colon-Perez, L., Diclemente, R.J., & Liddle, H.A. (2009). Multidimensional Family Therapy HIV/STD Risk-Reduction Intervention: An integrative family-based model for drug-involved juvenile offenders. *Family Process, 48*(1), 69–84.

Matos, M., Bauermeister, J.J., & Bernal, G. (2009). Parent-Child Interaction Therapy for Puerto Rican preschool children with ADHD and behavior problems: A pilot efficacy study. *Family Process, 48*(2), 232–252. doi:10.1111/j.1545-5300.2009.01279.x

McCabe, K., & Yeh, M. (2009). Parent-Child Interaction Therapy for Mexican Americans: A randomized clinical trial. *Journal of Clinical Child and Adolescent Psychology, 38*(5), 753–759. doi:10.1080/15374410903103544

McLuckie, A. (2006). Narrative family therapy for paediatric obsessive compulsive disorder. *Journal of Family Psychotherapy, 16*(4), 83–106.

Minuchin, S., Auerswald, E., King, C., & Rabinowitz, C. (1964). The study and treatment of families that produce multiple acting-out boys. *American Journal of Orthopsychiatry, 34*, 125–134.

Morawska, A., & Sanders, M.R. (2008). Parenting gifted and talented children: what are the key child behaviour and parenting issues? *Australian and New Zealand Journal of Psychiatry, 42*(9), 819–827. doi:10.1080/00048670802277271

Mufson, L., Dorta, K.P., Wickramaratne, P., Nomura, Y., Olfson, M., & Weissman, M.M. (2004). A randomized effectiveness trial of interpersonal psychotherapy for depressed adolescents. *Archives of General Psychiatry, 61*, 577–584.

Mufson, L., & Sills, R. (2006). Interpersonal Psychotherapy for depressed adolescents (IPT-A): An overview. *Nordic Journal of Psychiatry 2006;60:. 60*, 431–437. doi:1080/08039480601022397

Mufson, L., Weissman, M.M., Moreau, D., & Garfinkel, R. (1999). Efficacy of Interpersonal Psychotherapy for Depressed Adolescents. *Arch Gen Psychiatry, 56*(6), 573–579. doi:10.1001/archpsyc.56.6.573

Muratori, F., Picchi, L., Bruni, G., Patarnello, M., & Romagnoli, G. (2003). A two-year follow-up of psychodynamic psychotherapy for internalizing disorders in children. *Journal of the American Academy of Child and Adolescent Psychiatry 42*(3), 331–339. doi:10.1097/01.CHI.0000037033.04952.7F

Naar-King, S., Ellis, D., Kolmodin, K., Cunningham, P., & Secord, E. (2009). Feasibility of adapting multisystemic therapy to improve illness management behaviors and reduce asthma morbidity in high risk African American youth: A case series. *Journal of Child and Family Studies, 18*(5), 564–573. doi:10.1007/s10826-009-9259-9

New World Encyclopedia contributors. (2008). Harry Stack Sullivan [Electronic Version]. *New World Encyclopedia*. Retrieved from http://www.newworldencyclopedia.org/entry/Harry_Stack_Sullivan?oldid=687861.

Nichols, M.P., & Schwartz, R.C. (2004). *Family therapy: Concepts and methods* (6th ed.). New York: Allyn & Bacon.

Niec, L.N., Hemme, J.M., Yopp, J.M., & Brestan, E.V. (2005). Parent-child interaction therapy: The rewards and challenges of a group format. *Cognitive and Behavioral Practice, 12*(1), 113–125.

Nowak, C., & Heinrichs, N. (2008). A comprehensive meta-analysis of Triple P-Positive Parenting Program using hierarchical linear modeling: Effectiveness and moderating variables. *Clinical Child and Family Psychology Review, 11*, 114–144. doi:10.1007/s10567-008-0033-0

Ogden, T., Forgatch, M.S., Askeland, E., Patterson, G.R., & Bullock, B.M. (2005). Implementation of parent management training at the national level: The case of Norway. *Journal of Social Work Practice, 19*(3), 317–329. doi:10.1080/02650530500291518

Panksepp, J. (1998). *Affective neuroscience*. New York: Oxford University Press.

Patterson, G., Capaldi, D., & Bank, L. (1991). An early starter model for predicting delinquency. In D.J. Pepler & K.H. Rubun (Eds.), *The development and treatment of childhood aggression* (pp. 139–168). Hillsdale, NJ: Erlbaum.

Patterson, G.R. (1982). *Coercive family processes*. Eugene, OR: Castalia.

Patterson, G.R., Chamberlain, P., & Reid, J.B. (1982). A comparative evaluation of a parent training program. *Behavior Therapy, 13*(5), 638–650.

Phillips, J., Morgan, S., Cawthorne, K., & Barnett, B. (2008). Pilot evaluation of parent-child interaction therapy delivered in an Australian community early childhood clinic setting. *Australian and New Zealand Journal of Psychiatry, 42*(8), 712–719.

Pincus, D.B., Santucci, L.C., Ehrenreich, J.T., & Eyberg, S.M. (2008). The implementation of modified Parent-Child Interaction Therapy for youth with separation anxiety disorder. *Cognitive and Behavioral Practice, 15*(2), 118–125. doi:10.1016/j.cbpra.2007.08.002

Plant, K.M., & Sanders, M.R. (2007). Reducing problem behavior during care-giving in families of preschool-aged children with developmental disabilities. *Research in Developmental Disabilities, 28*(4), 362–385. doi:10.1016/j.ridd.2006.02.009

Pos, A.E., Greenberg, L.S., & Warwar, S.H. (2009). Testing a model of change in the experiential treatment of depression. *Journal of Consulting and Clinical Psychology, 77*(6), 1055–1066. doi:10.1037/a0017059

Prinz, R., Sanders, M., Shapiro, C., Whitaker, D., & Lutzker, J. (2009). Population-based prevention of child maltreatment: The U.S. Triple P System population trial. *Prevention Science, e pub ahead of print 1/22/2009.*

Prinz, R.J., & Sanders, M.R. (2007). Adopting a population-level approach to parenting and family support interventions. *Clinical Psychology Review, 27*(6), 739–749.

Querido, J.G., Warner, T.D., & Eyberg, S.M. (2002). Parenting styles and child behavior in African American families of preschool children. *Journal of Clinical Child and Adolescent Psychology, 31*(2), 272–277.

Ralph, A., & Sanders, M.R. (2003). Preliminary evaluation of Group Ten Triple P program for parents of teenagers making the transition to high school. *Australian e-Journal for the Advancement of Mental Health, 2*(3), 1–10.

Ralph, A., Stallman, H., & Sanders, M.R. (2004). Teen Triple P: A universal approach to reducing risk factors for behavioural and emotional problems in adolescents at the transition to high school. *Australian Journal of Psychology, 56* (3 Supplement S), 217–217.

Randall, J., Henggeler, S.N., Cunningham, P.B., Rowland, M.D., & Swenson, C.C. (2001). Adapting multisystemic therapy to treat adolescent substance abuse more effectively. *Cognitive and Behavioral Practice, 8*(4), 359–366. doi:10.1016/j.addbeh.2003.08.045

Reid, M.J., Webster-Stratton, C., & Hammond, M. (2007). Enhancing a classroom social competence and problem-solving curriculum by offering parent training to families of moderate- to high-risk elementary school children. *Journal of Clinical Child and Adolescent Psychology, 36*(4), 605–620.

Rieger, R., Van Buren, D.J., Bishop, M., Tanofsky-Kraff, M., Welch, R., & Wilfleyb, D.E. (2010). An eating disorder-specific model of interpersonal psychotherapy (IPT-ED): Causal pathways and treatment implications. *Clinical Psychology Review 30*(4), 400–410. doi:10.1016/j.cpr.2010.02.001

Rigter, H., Pelc, I., Tossmann, P., Phan, O., Grichting, E., Hendriks, V., et al. (2010). INCANT: A transnational randomized trial of Multidimensional Family Therapy versus treatment as usual for adolescents with cannabis use disorder. *BMC Psychiatry, 10.* 1–8. doi:10.1186/1471-244X-10-28

Rodenburg, R., Benjamin, A., de Roos, C., Meijer, A.M., & Stams, G.J. (2009). Efficacy of EMDR in children: A meta-analysis. *Clinical Psychology Review, 29*(7), 599–606. doi:10.1016/j.cpr.2009.06.008

Rowland, M.D., Chapman, J.E., & Henggeler, S.W. (2008). Sibling outcomes from a randomized trial of evidence-based treatments with substance abusing juvenile offenders. *Journal of Child & Adolescent Substance Abuse, 17*(3), 11–26. doi:10.1080/15470650802071622

Rowland, M.D., Halliday-Boykins, C.A., Henggeler, S.W., Cunningham, P.B., Lee, T.G., Kruesi, M.J.P., et al. (2005). A randomized trial of multisystemic therapy with Hawaii's Felix Class Youths. *Journal of Emotional and Behavioral Disorders, 13*(1), 13–23.

Sanders, M. (2003). Triple P - Positive Parenting Program: A population approach to promoting competent parenting. *Australian e-Journal for the Advancement of Mental Health (AeJAMH), 2*(3).

Sanders, M.R. (2000). Community-based parenting and family support interventions and the preventing of drug abuse. *Addictive Behaviors, 25*(6), 929–942.

Sanders, M.R. (2008). Triple P-Positive Parenting Program as a public health approach to strengthening parenting. *Journal of Family Psychology, 22*(4), 506–517. doi:10.1037/0893-3200.22.3.506

Sanders, M.R., & Lawton, J. (1993). Therapeutic process issues in the assessment of family problems: The guided participation model of information transfer. *Child & Family Behavior Therapy, 15*(2), 5–35.

Sanders, M.R., Mazzucchelli, T.G., & Studman, L.J. (2004). Stepping Stones Triple P: The theoretical basis and development of an evidenced-based postive parenting program for families with a child who has a disability. *Journal of Intellectual and Developmental Disability, 29*(3), 265–283. doi:10.1080/13668250412331285127

Sanders, M.R., & Prinz, R.J. (2008). Ethical and professional issues in the implementation of population-level parenting interventions. *Clinical Psychology-Science and Practice, 15*(2), 130–136.

Sanders, M.R., & Ralph, A. (2001). *Practitioner's manual for primary care Teen Triple-P.* Milton, Queensland, Australia: Families International Publishing.

Sanders, M.R., Tully, L., Turner, K.M., Maher, C., & McAuliffe, C. (2003). Training GPs in parent consultation skills. An evaluation of training for the Triple P-Positive Parenting Program. *Australian Family Physician, 32*(9), 763–768.

Santisteban, D.A., Coatsworth, J.D., Perez-Vidal, A., Kurtines, W.M., Schwartz, S.J., LaPerriere, A., & Szapocznik, J. (2003). Efficacy of brief strategic family therapy in modifying Hispanic adolescent behavior problems and substance use. *Journal of Family Psychology, 17*(1), 121–133. doi:10.1037/0893-3200.17.1.121

Santisteban, D.A., Coatsworth, J.D., Perez-Vidal, A., Mitrani, V., JeanGilles, M., & Szapocznik, J. (1997). Brief structural/strategic family therapy with African American and Hispanic high-risk youth. *Journal of Community Psychology, 25*(5), 453–471.

Seidler, G.H., & Wagner, F.E. (2006). Comparing the efficacy of EMDR and trauma-focused cognitive-behavioral therapy in the treatment of PTSD: A meta-analytic study. *Psychological Medicine, 36*(11), 1515–1522. doi:10.1017/S0033291706007963

Shalay, N., & Brownlee, K. (2007). Narrative Family Therapy with blended families. *Journal of Family Psychotherapy, 18*(2), 17–30.

Shapiro, F. (1989). Eye movement desensitization: a new treatment for post-traumatic stress disorder. *Journal of Behavior Therapy and Experimental Psychiatry, 20*(3), 211–217.

Shapiro, F. (2007). EMDR and case conceptualization from an adaptive information processing perspective. In F. Shapiro, F.W. Kaslow & L. Maxfield (Eds.), *Handbook of EMDR and family therapy processes* (pp. 3–34). Hoboken, NJ: John Wiley & Sons Inc,.

Shedler, J. (2010). The efficacy of psychodynamic psychotherapy. *American Psychologist, 65*(2), 98–109. doi:10.1037/a0018378

Shelef, K., Diamond, G.M., Diamond, G.S., & Liddle, H.A. (2005). Adolescent and parent alliance and treatment outcome in multidimensional family therapy. *Journal of Consulting and Clinical Psychology, 73*(4), 689–698. doi:10.1037/0022-006x.73.4.689

Solomon, M., Ono, M., Timmer, S., & Goodlin-Jones, B. (2008). The effectiveness of Parent-Child Interaction Therapy for families of children on the autism spectrum. *Journal of Autism and Developmental Disorders, 38*(9), 1767–1776. doi:10.1007/s10803-008-0567-5

Soon, C.S., Brass, M., Jochen Heinze, H., &c, & Haynes, J.D. (2008). Unconscious determinants of free decisions in the human brain. *Nature Neuroscience, 11*, 543–545.

Sori, C.F. (1995). The "art" of restructuring. *Journal of Family Psychotherapy, 6* (2), 13–31.

Stith, S.M., Rosen, K.H., McCollum, E.E., Coleman, J.U., & Herman, S.A. (1996). The voices of children: Pre-adolescent children's experiences in family therapy. *Journal of Marital and Family Therapy, 22*(1), 69–86.

Tang, T.-C., Jou, S.-H., Ko, C.-H., Huang, S.-Y., & Yen, C.-F. (2010). Randomized study of school-based intensive interpersonal psychotherapy for depressed adolescents with suicidal risk and parasuicide behaviors. *Psychiatry and Clinical Neurosciences 2009; 63: 463–470.* doi:doi:10.1111/j.1440-1819.2009.019

Thomas, R., & Zimmer-Gembeck, M. (2007). Behavioral outcomes of parent-child interaction therapy and Triple P—Positive Parenting Program: A review and meta-analysis. *Journal of Abnormal Child Psychology, 35*, 475–495. doi:10.1007/s10802-007-9104-9

Timmer, S.G., Urquiza, A.J., Herschell, A.D., McGrath, J.M., Zebell, N.M., Porter, A.L., & Vargas, E.C. (2006). Parent-child interaction therapy: Application of an empirically supported treatment to maltreated children in foster care. *Child Welfare, 85*(6), 919–939.

Timmer, S.G., Zebell, N.M., Culver, M.A., & Urquiza, A.J. (2010). Efficacy of adjunct in-home coaching to improve outcomes in Parent-Child Interaction Therapy. *Research on Social Work Practice, 20*(1), 36–45. doi:10.1177/1049731509332842

Trowell, J., Joffe, I., Campbell, J., Clemente, C., Almqvist, F., Soininen, M., & Tsiantis, J (2007). Childhood depression: a place for psychotherapy. An outcome study comparing individual psychodynamic psychotherapy and family therapy. *European Child and Adolescent Psychiatry 16*(3), 157–167. doi:10.1007/s00787-006-0584-x

Watanabe, N., Hunot, V., Omori, I.M., Churchill, R., & Furukawa, T.A. (2007). Psychotherapy for depression among children and adolescents: a systematic review. *Acta Psychiatrica Scandinavica, 116*(2), 84–95. doi:10.1111/j.1600-0447.2007.01018.x

Webster-Stratton, C. (1984). Randomized trial of two parent-training programs for families with conduct- disordered children. *Journal of Consulting and Clinical Psychology, 52*(4), 666–678.

Webster-Stratton, C. (1990). Enhancing the effectiveness of self-administered videotape parent training for families with conduct-problem children. *Journal of Abnormal Child Psychology, 18*, 479–492.

Webster-Stratton, C. (1998). Preventing conduct problems in Head Start children: Strengthening parenting competencies. *Journal of Consulting and Clinical Psychology, 66*(5), 715–730.

Webster-Stratton, C., & Hammond, M. (1997). Treating children with early-onset conduct problems: A comparison of child and parenting interventions. *Journal of Consulting and Clinical Psychology, 65*(1), 93–109.

Webster-Stratton, C., & Reid, M.J. (2010). The Incredible Years parent, teachers and children training series. In J. R. Weisz & A. E. Kazdin (Eds.), *Evidenced-based psychotherapies for children and adolescents* (2nd ed., pp. 194–210). New York: Guilford Press.

Weissman, M.M., Prusoff, B.A., & DiMascio, A. (1979). The efficacy of drugs and psychotherapy in the treatment of acute depressive episodes. *American Journal of Psychiatry, 136*, 555–558.

West, F., Sanders, M.R., Cleghorn, G., & Davies, P.S.W. (2010). Randomised clinical trial of a family-based lifestyle intervention for childhood obesity involving parents as the exclusive agents of change. *Behaviour Research and Therapy, 48*, 1170–1179. doi:10.1016/j.brat.2010.08.008

White, M., & Epston, D. (1990). *Narrative means to therapeutic ends.* New York: Norton.

Whittingham, K., Sofronoff, K., Sheffield, J., & Sanders, M.R. (2009). Stepping Stones Triple P: An RCT of a parenting program with parents of a child diagnosed with an autism spectrum disorder. *Journal of Abnormal Child Psychology, 37*(4), 469–480. doi:10.1007/s10802-008-9285-x

Young, J.F., Mufson, L., & Gallop, R. (2010). Preventing depression: A randomized trial of interpersonal psychotherapy-adolescent skills training. *Depression and Anxiety, 27*(5), 426–433. doi:10.1002/da.20664

Zisser, A., & Eyberg, S.M. (2010). Parent-Child Interaction Therapy and the treatment of disruptive behavior. In J.R. Weisz & A.E. Kazdin (Eds.), *Evidence-based psychotherapies for children and adolescents* (2nd ed., pp. 179–193). New York: The Guilford press.

17

Cognitive and Behavioral Approaches in Child and Adolescent Mental Health Treatment

Kathleen R. Delaney and Elizabeth Hawkins-Walsh

Objectives

After reading this chapter, APNs will be able to

1. Identify evidence-based cognitive and behavioral interventions appropriate for children and adolescents with serious emotional disorders.
2. Understand the proposed mechanism of action for specific cognitive and behavioral interventions designed for children and adolescents.
3. Apply the principles of cognitive and behavioral interventions to pediatric primary care.

4. Describe select cognitive and behavioral interventions that target the parents of children and adolescents who are exhibiting disruptive and anxious behaviors.
5. Describe how primary care and psychiatric-mental health APNs can work collaboratively to provide a range of preventive, acute, and long-term behavioral health care to children, adolescents, and their families.

Introduction

Numerous efficacious treatments exist for the mental health problems that children and adolescents experience. In fact, Hibbs (2001) estimated that there are approximately 450 child/adolescent psychotherapeutic modalities. With such a broad array of available therapies, it is critical that child/adolescent providers use techniques that are efficacious, appropriate to presentation, and consistent with the parents' and child's preference. The consumer also expects that the provider has the training to implement the intervention.

This chapter focuses on both cognitive and behavioral psychotherapeutic approaches—ones that have proved effective for particular child/adolescent mental health disorders. Chapters in this text dealing with specific disorders have also included discussion of cognitive or

other behavioral approaches. Here we seek an in-depth understanding of these interventions, particularly the evidence base that supports their use, principles underlying why they should work, and the neuroscience that clarifies their mechanism of action for a given disorder.

It is quite common to see the therapies assigned the label cognitive-behavioral therapy (CBT), a merger of the two schools that occurred when cognitive therapies began to employ behavioral techniques, particularly in the treatment of panic disorder (Rachman, 1997). Some of the treatments discussed here will be labeled CBT, meaning the cognitive intervention that targets thoughts/thinking as well as the behaviors; it is common that the same intervention effects thoughts as well as behaviors. Indeed it is often difficult to separate the two since changes in thinking will foster behavior change and improved behaviors will influence thinking (Knapp & Beck, 2008). However, treatments with a predominantly cognitive-behavioral approach will be discussed separately from those that operate *solely* on behavioral principles. This somewhat artificial division will be used to make clear an intervention's underlying mechanism of action.

Another distinction is between cognitive-behavioral interventions and cognitive-behavioral *therapy*. In conducting cognitive therapy, the therapist builds a cognitive conceptualization of the person's difficulties and therapy follows a cognitive model; problems and issues are translated into cognitive terms (Beck, 2001). While there have been adoptions of this traditional cognitive therapy model for children (Friedberg & McClure, 2002), cognitive-behavioral interventions in child therapies do not necessarily aim to arrive at and operate from a cognitive conceptualization of the child's difficulties. Rather, particularly in a nursing approach, therapeutic interventions target specific behaviors that are troublesome to the child, particularly those the family views as impeding development/ functioning (Selekman, 1997). The broad aim of therapy is to help the child achieve regulation of thoughts, affects, or behaviors (Delaney, 2008).

The chapter begins with an explanation of cognitive and behavioral treatments and their basic mechanisms of action. Next, specific CBT techniques will be explained and organized as interventions known to be efficacious for specific mental health issues of children. In both primary and specialty mental health care, nurses aim to help children and their parents change behaviors/thoughts that are causing distress or limiting functioning. Pediatric primary care is an ideal site for focused CBT or behavioral interventions because of the collaborative nature of the relationship between the pediatric nurse practitioner (PNP) and the patient, the use of defined goal setting and monitoring, the directive active approach, and the focus on the here and now rather than the past.

As a general rule, the intensity of services should match the intensity of the child's needs. Indicators for when a child's mental health issue may require specialty mental health care have been discussed throughout this book. For most of this chapter, interventions are delineated for particular behaviors and childhood disorders without consideration of where they are used, be it primary or specialty mental health care. However, a set of interventions that will be delineated by "site" are techniques for common child behavior issues that are more likely to be addressed in primary care.

Cognitive Techniques

While Beck is sometimes thought of as the father of cognitive therapy, other important theories emerged in the twentieth century that laid the groundwork for Beck's innovations. For instance, social learning theorists led the way for cognitive approaches when they detoured from psychology's prevailing behaviorist approach and declared explanations for human behaviors were more than stimulus-response sequences. They maintained that we learn how to think about social situations by *observing* how others think and behave (Bandura, 1977). One of the fathers of social learning theory was Albert Bandura, who detailed the process of observational learning in what he termed social cognitive theory (Bandura, 1989).

In his theory, Bandura stressed the importance of particular psychological processes that were involved in observational learning. Briefly, they involve attention processes, particularly how one directs attention and arousal, and retention processes, meaning the observer's ability to take in, encode, and retain what they have observed. Observational learning is also influenced by motivation and arousal. In considering cognitive-behavioral techniques it is useful to remember these basic psychological processes (attention, arousal, motivation, retention) because they will influence how children respond to proposed cognitive techniques.

Cognitive therapy assumes that much of a client's problems rest with the way they take in and process information. When Beck introduced cognitive therapies, he hypothesized that at the core of psychiatric syndromes such as anxiety and depression was a systematic bias in thinking, particularly the way situations were interpreted (Beck, 1964). He found that by helping patients uncover these biases and practice alternative ways to thinking, patients' symptoms improved and, with training in the skills, the improvements were sustained. Illnesses such as depression and anxiety also often involve automatic, negative thoughts, and self-defeating core beliefs. In cognitive therapy, this faulty thinking is explored and replaced with alternative positive ways to interpret a situation (Beck, 1995).

In cognitive therapy, the therapist works with clients to raise their awareness of the cognitions, perceptions, beliefs, and attributions that arise in response to particular stimuli (Beck, 1995). To accomplish this, clients are often instructed to write down thoughts around a particular situation or record what they were thinking when a particular mood overtook them. Here the individual gains practice in bringing thoughts (and the accompanying assumptions and beliefs) into awareness and how thoughts are related to a mood or emotional response (Greenberg & Padesky, 1995). This systematic approach to uncovering the relationship between thoughts and emotional responses is also a component of child cognitive interventions (Friedberg & McClure, 2002; Kendall & Grosch, 1994).

Sometimes one's thoughts seem to *automatically* move to a negative assumption about presenting stimuli or events. In cognitive work, the individual challenges the "evidence" that supports these negative assumptions and formulates refuting evidence that would discount them. The client is guided to understand how the thoughts and emotions affect subsequent behavior (Beck, 1995). Cognitive therapy improves anxious and depressive behaviors via challenging negative thoughts, then practicing alternative, more positive thinking (Beck, 2001). Generally, cognitive interventions with children have proved to be effective and reduced symptoms, particularly for anxiety and depressive disorders (Munoz-Solomando, Kendall, & Whittington 2008; Weisz, Hawley & Doss, 2004).

Cognitive therapy is by nature a structured process. While cognitive work with children does not exactly mirror the process of adult therapy, several of the basic principles hold. Uncovering the relationship between thoughts, emotions, and behavior remains a foundation of the work (Kendall, 2006b). Guided exercises are developed to help children and adolescents develop alternative behavioral and cognitive responses to troublesome situations (Friedberg & McClure, 2002). In child therapy, the concept of "cognitions" broadens to include the way information is processed and stored in memory (Reinecke, Dattilio, & Freeman, 2004). Accordingly, treatment is aimed at the development of an array of cognitive skills such as problem solving and development of focused coping strategies and affect regulation skills. The CBT programs described here are aimed at both the development of a cognitive skill (to address a cognitive deficiency) and of techniques that increase awareness of the maladaptive relationship of emotions, thoughts, and behaviors (to address a cognitive distortion) (Kendall, 2006b).

Cognitive Techniques Used with Children

There are numerous summaries of the cognitive therapy programs that have proved to be effective with children identified with particular disorders. They are indexed in books (Hibbs & Jensen, 1999; Kazdin & Weisz, 2003; Kendall, 2006a; Steele, Elkins, & Roberts, 2008) and scholarly articles (e.g., Burns, 2003; Rzepski & Jarasek, 2005). The Substance Abuse and Mental Health Services Administration (SAMHSA) also catalogs evidence-based therapies on its National Registry of Evidence-Based Programs (NREEP, n.d.). Evidence-based treatments (including CBT interventions) have also been organized via a system devised by the Child and Adolescent Health Division (CAMHD) of the Hawaii Department of Health (CAMHD, 2007). Here treatments are categorized by how they address a targeted behavior (e.g., anxious/avoidant

behaviors) and then evaluated according to the strength of supporting evidence (for each particular behavior). Treatments are also broken down by the frequency of a particular practice element. For instance, in the eighty-three studies that support interventions for anxious or avoidant behaviors, exposure therapy is a practice element approximately 75% of the time (CAMHD, 2007). Thus, the CAMHD system provides the most prevalent practice elements used in the various evidence-based programs that are designed to address a particular disorder.

In this review of cognitive and behavioral techniques, we will discuss both specific interventions and the accompanying, most prevalent practice element of the programs. As previously discussed, many of the interventions discussed in this section utilize a CBT approach, meaning their active elements address both thought and behavior. These interventions often combine principles of behavior therapy (e.g., reinforcement) and cognitive techniques (e.g., self-talk) to build what Kendall (2006b) calls a "coping template." While many of these techniques cross over several childhood diagnoses, for clarity, specific techniques will be considered under particular diagnostic categories.

Cognitive and Cognitive-Behavioral Approaches for Anxious Behaviors

Anxiety in children is one of the most pervasive of childhood disorders, effecting 10% to 15% of children (Costello et al., 2003). The types of anxiety are varied as is the underlying neurobiology (Engel, Bandelow, & Gruber, 2009). The focus here is on the group of anxiety disorders that begin to appear in childhood (separation anxiety disorder, social phobia, and generalized anxiety disorder) (Pine, 2007). While specific anxiety disorders and their treatments may be discussed as separate entities, comorbidity, particularly with other anxiety disorders, is ubiquitous (Saaverda & Silverman, 2002).

National treatment guidelines as well as meta-analyses of anxiety treatment research endorse CBTs as efficacious for a variety of anxiety disorders (Connolly, Bernstein, & Workgroup on Quality Issues, 2007; Silverman, Pina, & Viswesvaran, 2008). One of the most researched CBT approaches is Philip Kendall's program, Coping Cat (Flannery-Schroeder & Kendall, 2000; Kendall, 1994; Kendall et al., 1997). Kendall's innovative program targets several areas of anxious behavior with slightly different interventions. Anxious feelings, thoughts, and attributions are addressed with cognitive techniques (to increase awareness and challenge unrealistic cognitions); anxious self-talk is replaced with coping self-talk and a coping plan. When the child succeeds at these new coping strategies, they are provided with a self-reward (behavioral component).

This CBT model operates on the theory that children exhibiting early signs of anxiety have developed a pattern of responding with fear to particular stimuli. This in turn affects how they pay attention to the event and the attributions they form about the cause of the event (Kendall, 2006b). Repeated experiences of apprehension establish a cognitive template (or filter), which then influences how the child allocates attention (i.e., they have difficulty switching attention away from anxiety-provoking events) (Muris, Meesters, & Rompelberg, 2006; Pine, 2007; Roy et al., 2008). In the CBT framework, the child learns first to recognize anxious feelings, then examines the accompanying attributions, and finally practices alternative ways of thinking about the situation (Kendall& Suveg, 2006). Via this reappraisal of anxious thoughts, the child is building a new, more adaptive cognitive template around particular events.

Other successful variations of CBT for anxiety are programs using a group format (Barrett, 1998) and curricula that involve the parents of anxious children, a particularly important component of treatment of this population (Silverman et al., 2008). Many of these programs need additional testing with diverse populations to build data supporting their efficacy across cultures. However, based on two studies, group format CBT for anxiety has proved probably efficacious for Hispanic/Latino and African American youth (Huey & Polo, 2008).

Currently there are only isolated imaging studies on how cognitive therapy effects neural tracks believed to be involved in anxiety disorders. Existing data suggest that CBT may dampen an overactive amygdala, which has been conditioned to respond too quickly with a fearful response to any variety of stimuli (Porto et al., 2009). Theoretically, a therapeutic correction occurs with CBT because thinking patterns (such as reappraisal) strengthen the slower cortical processing circuits that interpret stimuli, circuits that in turn dampen amygdala activation (Cozolino, 2002). Additional study of the neural circuitry of anxiety in children will help clarify the exact mechanisms that need to be targeted in therapy, particularly modifying the ventral lateral prefrontal cortext, which allocates attention to potential threat (Pine, 2007).

CBT programs for specific child/adolescent anxiety disorders often have additional components that address particular aspects of the syndrome. For instance, social phobia involves a complex cascade where a child's lack of success in social situations leads to the expectancy of failure and negative anticipations of future social performance (Spence, 2003). These negative attributions/expectancies generate both anxiety and avoidance of social situations, which begins a cycle of social skills deficits, poor social outcomes, negative cognitions, and avoidance (Spence, Donovan, & Brechman-Toussaint, 2000). Thus, social phobia is viewed as a complex phenomenon where poor social performance becomes intertwined with anxiety symptoms and negative attributions (Spence, 2003). For this reason, cognitive interventions tailored to social phobia (social anxiety disorder) also include social skills or social effectiveness training.

One probably efficacious program for social phobia combines CBT with a skill-based curriculum aimed at improving social fluency (Spence et al., 2000). In this program children are taught micro-level (e.g., eye contact) and macro-level social skills (e.g., conversation skills) as well as social problem solving. In the CBT component of the program, participants examine and challenge the evidence supporting their anxious perceptions. This intervention successfully reduced the level of social anxiety in treatment groups and research participants were less likely to retain the diagnosis of social phobia (Spence et al., 2000).

Intervention programs for childhood obsessive-compulsive disorder (OCD) also have a slightly different emphasis. In the cognitive model of OCD, compulsions are seen as a response to anxious sensations (usually arising from an obsessive fear). In line with this theory, performing the compulsive behavior actually helps children reduce their anxious feelings and the subsequent relief reinforces their compulsions. A pattern then develops: when such children encounter an anxiolytic stimulus, their response involves a focus on the related compulsions. This focus on compulsions prevents normal habituation and realistic appraisal of the fearful stimuli (Flament, Gettler, Irak, & Blier, 2007). The treatments for OCD involve CBT techniques but rely heavily on exposure and response prevention (ERP). With this intervention the youth is slowly exposed to stimuli that would normally illicit obsessive fears, but they are taught to resist engaging in compulsive behaviors (Barrett et al., 2008).

This intervention maps on the pathophysiology of OCD, which is increasingly seen to involve the cortical-striatal-thalamic track, particularly the interplay of the orbitofrontal cortex (OFC), caudate nucleus, thalamus, and anterior cingulate cortex (ACC) (MacMaster, O'Neill, &Rosenberg, 2008). Speaking to adult OCD, Carter (1994) explains the interplay of these neural structures in the following manner: when persons with OCD encounter situations that raise unease, a loop of neuronal activity begins from the caudate (the urge to do something about it), to the OFC that registers the feeling that something is wrong, and then back through the ACC, which keeps attention fixed on the feeling of unease. An ERP approach breaks this cycle by exposing the child (gradually) to feared situations while simultaneously reducing the compulsive behavior (Flament et al., 2007).

The two sets of studies that follow this format and are rated as Type I studies given their design and replication are the Pediatric Obsessive Compulsive Treatment Study (POTS) (Franklin, March, & Foa, 2001) and several studies by Barrett and colleagues (e.g., Barrett, Healy-Farrell, & March, 2004). Both of these groups of controlled studies involve several treatment conditions (family participation and medication) as well as manualized CBT with an ERP emphasis (see review in Barrett et al., 2008). The POTS protocol also includes psychoeducation, cognitive training, mapping OCD behaviors, and ERP (Franklin, Foa, & March, 2003).

The cognitive component of this intervention incorporates positive self-talk, cognitive restructuring, and cultivating a dampened response to rising anxious thoughts. The cognitive work is seen to increase a youth's sense of personal efficacy, predictability, and controllability (March et al., 2001). Nurses intervening with children struggling with OCD behaviors should familiarize themselves with these programs, particularly the accompanying explanatory models, which provide a theory for why the intervention components lead to outcomes. Such understanding is important not only for increasing treatment fidelity but also for educating the family/child on the theory of the therapy.

Cognitive and Cognitive-Behavioral Approaches for Depressed Behaviors

Depression in youth carries a high prevalence (2 million youth, or 8.3% of population ages twelve to seventeen) and significantly impacts on important areas of functioning (SAMSHA, 2009). CBTs have proved effective for the treatment and prevention of child and adolescent depression (Cuijpers et al., 2008; Horowitz & Garber, 2006). The three CBT programs highlighted here are ones that are probably most efficacious for children (self-control therapy), for adolescents (Coping with Depression-Adolescent [CWD-A]), and for children and adolescents (the Penn Prevention Program, also known as the Penn Resiliency Program [PRP]) (David-Ferdon & Kaslow, 2008). We begin with a review of the shared elements of these efficacious programs and highlight how they address core elements of youth depression.

All of the programs (PRP, CWD-A, and self-control therapy) operate on a CBT model and contain practice elements that involve recognition of negative thinking and reappraisal. For instance, in the PRP, youth are taught the linkages between how they think, feel, and behave as well as problem-solving skills. Using a CBT approach, they learn how to challenge negative thinking, that is, evaluate the accuracy of the thought, the evidence to support it, and then devise an alternate, more positive response. This program has been implemented in a variety of settings, including schools (Gillham, Reivich, & Frères, 2007) and primary care (Gillham, Hamilton, & Freres, 2006). While there has been some question as to

its effectiveness with diverse populations, it has proved effective with children of Latino and Asian cultures but less so with teens of African American descent (Cardemil et al., 2007; Yu & Seligman, 2002).

A program identified by the acronym ACTION also uses CBT reframing but is tailored for younger children and based on self-control therapy (Stark, Hargraves, & Sander, 2006). A particular focus of ACTION is teaching children how to recognize emotions and become more aware of their moods and responses. The program also addresses cognitive deficiencies, particularly problem solving. Via these strategies, children learn that they can deal with negative moods; which in turn builds their confidence in their ability to take action to improve their mood. When tested with a population of European children, results continued to improve over a one-year period, leading the investigators to conclude that time and practice are needed for the young child to integrate CBT thinking into daily life (De Cuyper et al., 2004). They also concluded that programs such as ACTION have successfully adjusted CBT techniques to demands that are age-appropriate for eight- to twelve-year-old children.

These programs theoretically dampen depressive symptoms for several reasons. According to a basic theory of CBT, depressed adolescents have developed a pattern of pessimistic thoughts and negative attributions that create and maintain a depressed mood (Asarnow, Jaycox, & Tompson, 2001). With CBT, youth learn how to substitute a more adaptive and positive attribution style, which in turn changes behaviors (Asarnow et al., 2001). A CBT approach is the foundation of Treatment for Adolescents with Depression (TADS), a multisite, national research project that tested and compared the efficacy of treatment combinations for depression (Rhode, Feeny, & Robins, 2005).

In studies conducted largely with adults, using neuroimaging techniques, researchers have investigated why CBT dampens depression. Basically, reappraisal of negative thoughts and mood is thought to change patterns of brain activity (Dichter, Felder, & Smoski, 2008). With CBT there is an increased activity in the dorsal-lateral side (DLPFC) and ventromedial parts of the PFC and decreased activity in the amygdala and orbitofrontal area (Roffman, et al., 2005). In effect, the working memory (DLPFC) is helping to dampen an established pattern of negative affective response that has become patterned in the amygdala. It is believed that as individuals exercise a different (more positive) thinking pattern, growth occurs at the synaptic level, and, via this neural plasticity, the circuitry supporting this new thinking pattern is strengthened (Tryon, 2009).

While an exciting innovation, CBT may not sufficiently address all the aspects of youth depression. Recently, Miller (2007) suggested that there are several fundamental components to child and adolescent depression: hedonic capacity, stress sensitivity, attention impairments, and ruminative self-focus. In a similar view, Asarnow and colleagues (2001) suggest teens are particularly vulnerable to the stressors they face and that depressive cycles often begin as a response to stress (Asarnow et al., 2001). Finally, the stress vulnerability theory posits that depressed youth often view stressful events as overwhelming, a perception that provokes a hopeless response (Haeffel & Grigorenko, 2007). These theories (stress vulnerability and Miller's core components) provide a framework for advanced practice nurses (APNs) in choosing interventions for depressed teens (i.e., how the program speaks to a youth's loss of interest and lack of pleasure [hedonic capacity], how it boosts resilience in response to stress-provoking events, or how the intervention works at the level of a teen's ruminative negative self-focus). The goal is to empower youth to deal with stress via problem solving, self-control therapy, and building resiliency.

When discussing treatment options with the youth and his/her parent, it is important to highlight the relationship between stress sensitivity, negative ruminations, and lack of involvement in pleasurable activity. This is the approach in the CWD-A program. CWD-A has a cognitive component but also asks the teen to engage in pleasant activity-scheduling to address the typical loss of interest and lack of pleasure (hedonic capacity) (e.g., Clarke et al., 1995). CWD-A includes conflict-reduction techniques, which should help teens deal with the stressful situations they encounter as adolescents. The CWD-A has been extensively researched and guided the development of the TADS protocol (David-Ferdon & Kaslow, 2008). We know that teens may resist mental health treatment because of their mistrust in mental health professionals' ability to understand their situation and the stigma that mental illness carries (Draucker, 2003). When nurses encounter teens in distress, they should directly address the depression but keep in mind these developmental concerns and expect the teens to normalize their behaviors/symptoms.

Other Child/Adolescent Disorders Addressed with CBT Interventions

Evidence-based cognitive interventions have been developed for children and adolescents coping with a variety of mental health issues. Here we discuss evidence-based approaches for three conditions: trauma-focused CBT for traumatized children, anger management for children displaying disruptive behavior problems, and CB self-care for older adolescents dealing with binge eating. Since the basic mechanisms of CBT have been explained

in detail, highlighted are components of these three programs that have been designed to address the specific presentation of the disorder.

Trauma-focused CBT (TF-CBT) is a well-established therapy for children and adolescents exposed to traumatic events (Silverman et al., 2008). TF-CBT programs use cognitive techniques and include education about abuse and healthy sexuality, relaxation techniques, and a behavioral component of gradual exposure using narrative or creative materials (Silverman et al., 2008). The TF-CBT program developed by Cohen and Mannarino (1996) follows an intentional progression of interventions where the child is first educated on abuse and normal sexuality, and then taught relaxation techniques, coping strategies, and affect regulation, skills that gradually prepare the child to think about and discuss their trauma. It is only toward the end of the therapy, now equipped with tools to handle the accompanying emotional arousal, that the child creates a trauma narrative. TF-CBT has an accessible training protocol that is available both in live sessions and online (Medical College of South Carolina, 2005).

CBT approaches to disruptive behaviors disorders. Disruptive behavior problems (DBP) in children manifest as noncompliance, aggression, and negative emotionality. Although a degree of controversy surrounds the DBP classification, particularly with preschool children, it has become clear that symptoms of DBP can be isolated and that screening tools do differentiate youth referred for problem behavior from nonreferred preschool children (Keenan & Wakschlag, 2004). Aggression and noncompliance of young children are frequent issues in both pediatric primary care and mental health clinics. Here we will review both a CBT approach and later a family-based behavioral approach (behavioral parent training) (Breitenstein, Hill, & Gross, 2009).

In a review of research targeting children exhibiting disruptive behaviors, Eyberg, Nelson, and Bog (2008) determine that two child-based CBT interventions are probably efficacious: anger control training and group assertiveness training. Eyberg and her colleagues (2008) note that anger control training is based on the social information processing model of anger, which maps how children take in and organize social information (Crick & Dodge, 1994). Children with disruptive behaviors have been found to use more action-oriented, nonverbal solutions to social problems, mislabel arousal as anger, and distort others' motives in social situations; their bias is to perceive threat even in benign interactions (Dodge & Crick, 1990).

Since much of their anger/aggression generates from this perceived threat, one component of anger control therapy is examining vignettes of social encounters and discussing the possible motives of participants

(Lochman, Barry, & Pardini, 2003). In this anger management program students practice a stop–think method to decrease impulsive responses and consider alternative solutions to social situations. Here, children are also learning the problem-solving process. Three years postintervention, the now teenage research participants demonstrated decreased drug involvement as well as improvements in moderator variables (self-esteem, approach to problem situations) (Lochman et al., 1993).

Group assertiveness training has also been identified as a probably efficacious treatment for children displaying disruptive behaviors (Eyberg et al., 2008). As the name suggests, the intervention focuses on teaching an aggressive teen effective relationship skills, particularly communicating and relating to others on the basis of mutual respect (Huey & Rank, 1984). The intervention demonstrated that teens taught an assertive response, a forthright one where they stand up for their rights without threat, led to decreased levels of anger. Unfortunately, this approach has not been extensively replicated.

Cognitive interventions for eating disorders. The cognitive model for eating disorders depicts a complex interrelationship of psychological risk factors that lead a youth into negative affect states-tensions, ones that are relieved by restrictive eating or binging/purging (Williamson et al., 2004). As the youth's cognitive map around eating and thinness progresses, Williamson and colleagues (2004) believe that distortions around body image form along with an extreme desire for thinness and selective attention to food cues/body messages. The bulk of evidence-based interventions for eating problems are family based (Keel & Haedt, 2008), but one cognitive-based individual approach that is possibly efficacious is CBT guided self-care (Schmidt et al., 2007). Here adolescents are initially taught to monitor thoughts and feeling and attempt to uncover their connection to bulimic behavior. Information is provided on how bulimic symptoms are maintained. In a workbook-type format, they are also taught problem solving and behavioral techniques to interrupt cycles of disordered behavior. In a test of the model against traditional family approaches, the CBT self-care model performed better, reducing both binge eating and vomiting (Schmidt et al., 2007).

Cognitive Interventions in Primary Care

Many of the interventions just described are also used in primary care (Box 17.1). To begin we highlight cognitive reframing because it lies at the heart of many clinician-parent interactions. It has long been recognized that parents' perceptions of their children, how they see their children compared to other children, may be a powerful determinant in a child's future well-being. Elsie Broussard's early work with the Neonatal Perception

---

Box 17.1 Cognitive-behavioral techniques useful in primary care for children with problems of mild anxiety and/or depression

Relaxation plans
Deep breathing
Progressive relaxation
Fear hierarchies constructing anxiety ladders
Planning gradual exposures
Recognition of cognitive distortions
ABC mediational model
Use of positive self-talk
Identifying and eliminating negative self-talk
Review and encouragement of healthy sleep/physical
    activity/diet
Behavioral activation–ensuring pleasurable activities

Inventory (1976), Green and Solnit's descriptions of vulnerable children (1964), and Levy's descriptions of parental overuse of medical care for children seen as "at risk" (1980) have played a powerful role in shaping pediatric clinicians' awareness of the need to nurture parents' healthy perceptions of their children.

Cognitive reframing with an infant: Mrs. T, the mother of two-week-old, Lacy, arrived at the clinic looking exhausted. Lacy was her second baby who weighed 9 lb at birth; she was a vigorous newborn who had already regained birth weight and more. Her mother reported that Lacy screamed loudly when she was hungry, "ate all night" and she was concerned that she was going to be "fat." Upon further questioning, the practitioner learned that her first child, Sarah, arrived six weeks early, weighed less than 5 lbs, slept for long periods of time, and had to be awoken to eat. At the age of three Sarah was a well-developed, but thin child with an easy going, quiet disposition. Further questioning revealed that Mrs. T's husband had been able to stay at home for three weeks when Sarah was born but now had a new job which required him to leave the house first thing in the morning and return late at night. Mrs. T was worried about disturbing his sleep at night and wondered why Lacy was eating so often. Mrs. T also mentioned that she "used to be fat" and hoped "that Lacy wouldn't take after my side of the family."

Cognitive reframing with a toddler: Mr. and Mrs. J brought four-year-old Joey in for a preschool check-up. Joey's past medical history, physical examination, and developmental assessment were normal. As part of her history taking, the practitioner asked the parents what Joey was particularly good at. Mrs. J immediately responded that he was good at putting together puzzles and working with his small cars. When they were asked, "What are the most difficult things for Joey?" she responded that Joey was shy and always found it difficult to enter new situations.

The practitioner asked Mr. J if he had any ideas why this was. Mr. J responded, "No, that is just how he has always been – kind of a "scaredy cat really. He doesn't get that from me!" Further history revealed that Joey had always been slow to warm up to new people and places. Joey had one good friend with whom he played happily and at whose house he was comfortable. Mrs. J sheepishly admitted she had always wondered if he had developed this way because she had been hospitalized when he was a baby and she had had to leave him with an aunt for two weeks. Even though the aunt was a warm and mothering type, Mrs. J had always worried that Joey had been affected by her absence.

Example of active monitoring: Jack, a four-year-old boy, was brought in with a new-onset stutter. Jack's father reported that he was not concerned since his older brother had had a stutter that was temporary and had not returned. However Jack's mother was worried. Jack had just begun a new preschool and she was fearful that the other children would make fun of him. *Was this a developmentally normal stutter which could be expected to resolve without intervention within a few months? Or was it likely to persist over time and worsen, becoming a chronic stutter?* The APN obtained a history including family history, other changes in behavior, new stressors, coping skills, parents' knowledge about stuttering, their level of concern, details of how the family was currently responding to the stutter, as well as the child's reactions. If the age, history, and presentation all lead the provider to expect a normal developmental resolution, the pediatric provider should spend a few moments explaining what is known about developmental stuttering (*Psychoeducation);* what is believed to be the best approach/response to the child (*Ignoring*); how long it is reasonable to merely follow it, and when to consider a referral. In addition, the APN should acknowledge parental concerns and understands that some parents immediately request a referral to a speech therapist. However, the APN should also help the parents understand that if a child detects that his stuttering makes a parent anxious, it may increase the child's own anxiety.

Jack's parents decided to delay initiating a referral. His mother seemed reassured and believed she could "ignore" his stuttering for a trial period. They agreed to follow-up with the provider in four weeks. If the stuttering worsened before then, they would call. The four week follow-up appointment (visit or call) was scheduled that day. (If the parent cancels the appointment or fails to call, the provider should initiate a follow-up.) When the mother returned with Jack four weeks later, she reported that the stuttering still occured at times but she was more optimistic about its transience. She wondered if it was related to his new classroom. She agreed to use a daily record sheet to record the frequency of stuttering provided by the clinician (*Monitoring*). The sheet provides columns that identified specifics regarding when the stuttering occurred, evidence of stress in the child, and responses to the child. At the next visit (telephone call), the parents reported that the stuttering was much better, and that they had noticed with the use of the monitoring sheets that the stuttering was worse in the mornings before leaving for school. But as Jack became more comfortable with his new classmates and teacher, and had more stories about friends at school, it lessened. It only occasionally reoccurred now on Monday mornings before school. *The worksheet became an important tool for parents to monitor whether or not the problem was increasing or decreasing, what environment appeared to be most problematic, and any noticeable triggers or consequences.* Similarly, if the problem had continued beyond the time when the provider and or parent were comfortable with the behavior and a referral was made, the worksheet would provide valuable information to the specialty colleague about the early onset and nature of the problem.

The first case example of a mother and her infant reveals many potential avenues for primary mental health interventions, including use of a screening tool for possible postpartum depression and a review of social supports available to this mother. It also illustrates how a parent may form faulty perceptions of a newborn; one colored by lack of information, situational stressors, or previous experiences. As in this vignette, skilled clinicians will realize a primary consideration is the parents need for support and, in this instance, sleep. They will also recognize the opportunity to educate new parents about the wide range of normal newborn behaviors, variations in temperament, and expected differences in term and premature infant's sleep and growth. As illustrated in this case example, the goal in primary care is to assist new parents in developing a more favorable appraisal of their infant's behaviors by helping the parent "reframe" any sense that there is something wrong with a baby displaying normal developmental behaviors.

The second case in this vignette illustrates how reframing of behaviors might occur with the parent of a toddler. In this vignette, a major task for the pediatric provider was helping the parents to understand the role of temperament as an innate style of reacting; a style that is neither good nor bad. Further discussions and readings about temperament allowed Mr. and Mrs. J to form a "*new cognitive appraisal*" of who their son was, and what it meant (and didn't mean) to have a child with a slow-to-warm-up temperament. In this case example, over time a "goodness of fit" was achieved, and his parents were able to provide support when their child encountered normal challenges with change. Mrs. J no longer worried that she had caused him to develop this way with her absence. And Mr. J was able to begin to see the strengths that often accompany a slow-to-warm-up temperament."

Behavioral Interventions

Pediatric Primary Care as a Natural Setting for Behavioral Care

The practice of pediatrics in this country is unique in providing twenty-three regularly scheduled well-child visits for children from birth through adolescence. The purpose of these visits is to promote and protect the health and development of the child and to allow time for parents to address issues of concern with a pediatric health care provider. Pediatric and health policy advocates have repeatedly urged pediatric health care providers to become more attentive and better skilled at identifying and responding to behavioral and mental health concerns during these well-child visits (Schor & Elfenbein, 2004). Rigorous studies examining the effectiveness of cognitive and behavioral approaches delivered by primary care providers are still lacking. However, primary care–based behavioral interventions are likely to be effective techniques for addressing some of the more common behavioral issues that providers encounter (Stein, Zitner, & Jensen, 2006).

Pediatric health care providers have long recognized the important role of providing guidance and counseling to parents. While clinicians may not immediately think of the term "behavioral intervention," they know the importance of coaching parents through the steps of a reward chart and the use of stickers for a child with enuresis. Similarly, during a sports physical, it is quite natural to brainstorm with an adolescent on the football team who is failing chemistry, an intervention that may not be formally viewed as problem solving. The growing support for the role of the primary care provider in preventive mental health is based upon the realization that early interventions with problem behavior may eliminate the progression of more serious and persistent mental health concerns (Institute of Medicine, 2009).

Reframing the Well-Child Visit

At the first visit to the pediatric practice, whether it is prenatal or at a few days of age, parents benefit by being introduced to the concept of a health care home for their newborn, one that will routinely include screening and discussions of all the potential risks to health and well-being. Parents should learn that the major threats to their child's well-being will come not from disease but rather from unsafe environments and behaviors. Parents who are prepared to expect routine discussion of development, individual temperament, discipline, and behavioral patterns at regularly scheduled visits (along with nutrition, sleep, and immunizations) are more likely to be attuned to early concerns. They will also come to know that the pediatric health care home is a place to address these issues early on.

This proactive approach on the part of providers will also dispel the confusion that still exists among many parents about the real purpose of well-child visits (Radecki, et al. 2009). It has been suggested that the failure on the part of some pediatric clinicians to address ongoing behavioral issues has led some families to mistakenly think of these appointments as "visits for shots" or "school physicals." The well-child visit traditionally includes components of prevention, screening, and anticipatory guidance. Assuring that these components include attention to mental health is critical.

Preventive Mental Health

Increasing recognition of the *persistence* of unattended early behavior problems in children (Kessler et al., 2005) further supports the need for pediatric primary care providers to engage in early mental health prevention. For many years early childhood behavior problems were perceived to be fleeting and not likely to persist or predict later mental health problems. While developmental variations continue to be appreciated, studies are beginning to reveal the persistence of behavior problems that first may be seen in the preschool years. Indeed, national epidemiological studies reveal half of all cases of mental illness reveal themselves before the age of fourteen (Kessler et al., 2005).

A pediatric health care provider is usually regarded by parents as the "expert" in the early behaviors of infants and young children. Parents bring problems or concerns with sleeping, eating, crying, or elimination to the pediatric office from the earliest days of life. The mother of a four-month-old does not hesitate to bring worries to the pediatric health care provider about why her daughter is not sleeping, is disinterested in eating, or will not stop crying. Similarly, mothers will bring questions about why a child screams when approached by strangers at nine months or clings to a mother's dress on the first day of school. These behaviors are seen by a pediatric clinician as "normal" and most clinicians will provide appropriate education and anticipatory counseling to the parent.

But what about the child whose early demonstration of difficulty is not fleeting? What about the child whose intense behaviors are persistent or cause unusual distress to the child or parent? Is this a normal variant or is it a harbinger of problems to come? The answer is likely unknown and may not be appreciated for several months or years. Yet the pediatric provider with enhanced knowledge in preventive behavioral health, who has served in a collaborative partnership with the family and a child and adolescent mental health APN, is likely to be the ideal person to support and guide parents as they engage in the challenges of parenting a child with troubling behaviors. Thus the pediatric health care home becomes the natural place for early recognition and early intervention to take place. In this model of care, families are provided needed support around parenting children with difficult behaviors, while avoiding the risks of premature labeling or over-diagnosis.

Researchers have also documented the effectiveness of *indicated* prevention in primary care. A unique study in Western Australia demonstrated long-term effectiveness of a brief, thirty-minute counseling intervention with parents of preschool children around behavior problems by a single general pediatrician (Cullen & Cullen, 1996). Beardslee and colleagues (2003) used the primary care arena to conduct an efficacy trial of a manual-based preventive intervention for children of depressed parents. The intervention was created to be used by clinicians from a variety of backgrounds (nurses, pediatricians, and mental health clinicians). In Beardslee's research, one group received six to eleven sessions of treatment, while the other, more limited intervention group only received two "lecture condition" meetings with parents. As expected, more change was reported in the heavier intervention group but, impressively, parents in both groups reported significant change in child-related behaviors and attitudes. This study demonstrates that even a brief, simple intervention had an enduring effect on the families' abilities to problem solve.

Behavioral Interventions in Primary Care: Brief Interventions

In the past, clinicians might have taken a "wait and see" approach to behaviors of concern. Today, they are more likely to approach such conditions with active support and focused monitoring. The Guidelines for Adolescent Depression in Primary Care (GLAD-PC) delineate the components of this active approach when dealing with adolescents with mild depression (Cheung et al., 2007). Early intervention in primary care may involve a range of activities including psychoeducation, supportive counseling, facilitating self-management, behavioral activation, regular monitoring of symptoms, and possibly referral for peer or parent support group or classes.

In this and other instances, the provider may be unsure whether the behavior is developmentally a nor-mal variant, will likely disappear without intervention, or will respond well to active support. Active monitoring alone may include the use of monitoring or screening tools that help the provider and family follow how the child is doing and whether the problem behavior is improving or getting worse. Active support and monitoring are particularly helpful in those conditions/situations where a diagnosis can only be made in hindsight. The additional use of contracts, checklists, goal setting, and rewards provides tools that may assist in changing the behavior itself.

Overview of Behavioral Techniques Used in Both Specialty and Primary Care

The therapeutic interventions discussed in this section will be based on theories of classic conditioning, operant conditioning, or observational learning. The notion of classic conditioning has its origins in Pavlov's experiments where he demonstrated that there are aspects of a species' response system that are more or less innate and that response systems could be manipulated so as to illicit a response with a novel stimuli (Tamminga 2006). For instance, it is natural for humans and animals to begin to salivate at the sight of food. Pavlov demonstrated in his experiments with dogs that if food was repeatedly paired with a bell (conditioned stimuli), eventually the dog will salivate to the sound of a bell. In such an experimental condition, food is termed an unconditioned stimuli. Salivating to a bell is termed a conditioned response. A conditioned response can be extinguished. Repeatedly presented with the bell and no food, eventually the dog will stop salivating. In this instance, the animal has formed a new memory (and a new association to the bell), one that does not involve a food link. This new learning is called extinction and the process used to create new stimulus response learning is called extinction training (Bouton, 2004).

Research has demonstrated that humans also form conditioned responses to situations or stimuli. The process is extremely important to understanding anxiety where in essence, a stimulus (that under most circumstances would be seen as benign) becomes associated with fear and triggers an anxious response. It has been suggested that humans are born with few fears but acquire numerous conditioned fears over the course of their lifetime (Davis, 2004). For example, individuals can come to respond to a stimulus (say the sight of a dog) with a conditioned response (apprehension). Perhaps at one time the individual had been involved in a fearful incident with a dog; now just the sight of a dog generates apprehension. This is an example of classic conditioning—behaviors that appear due to an antecedent condition.

Operant conditioning deals with how a behavior is modified by the response to that behavior. One of the simplest distinctions between classic and operant conditioning is that classic conditioning is dealing with an association that has formed between two stimuli; operant conditioning concerns the associations that form between a behavior and a consequence. In the United States, operant conditioning is associated with the work of B.F. Skinner. Operant conditioning begins with the assumption that the consequences of a particular behavior, particularly how others respond to that behavior, will influence the future occurrence of that behavior. For example, if following a behavior the child is praised (a positive effect), this praise (a reinforcer) will increase the likelihood that the child will repeat this behavior in the future. In operant conditioning, there are four conditions of interest: ones involving the addition of a reinforcer (positive reinforcement or punishment) and ones involving the removal of a stimulus (negative reinforcement or punishment).

Negative reinforcement can often perpetuate a child's noncompliance. For instance, if by arguing the child avoids cleaning his room (the parent gives up on the request), the parent has inadvertently reinforced (negatively) the child's arguing; that is, following the arguing, the adverse stimulus (the request to clean the room) was removed. The next time the child is asked to tidy his room, it is more likely he will argue, a behavior in which he has found success in avoiding a task he viewed as distressing. Operant conditioning is the umbrella for a wide variety of techniques such as ones used in token economies and behavioral parent training (Spiegler & Guevremont, 2003). There are also behavioral techniques that rely on extinction of a conditioned response, such as systematic desensitization or exposure therapy.

Using the CAMHD framework, evidence-based *behavior* therapies are presented. Several interventions for childhood/adolescent disorders, such as psychoeducation or relaxation techniques, do not strictly fall into behavioral or cognitive categories. These are extremely useful therapies, but, for the purpose of this chapter, the discussion focuses on behavioral techniques, ones designed to impact on observed behavior by altering reinforcement patterns or by extinction of conditioned responses. Also included in this section are behavioral approaches for childhood disorders that are aimed to improve the child's behavior by altering the way parents respond to the behaviors and behavioral approaches used in primary care for common childhood behavior problems.

Behavioral Approaches for Anxious Behaviors

Several behavioral approaches are probably efficacious in the treatment of childhood anxiety disorders, particularly exposure therapy in the treatment for specific phobias (Silverman et al., 2008) and exposure-based CBT for the treatment of OCD (Barrett et al., 2008). In exposure therapy the child is exposed to stimuli that in the past have triggered obsessive fears or phobic responses. In the case of OCD, during exposure to the stimuli, the child is encouraged to resist engaging in compulsive behaviors (Barrett et al., 2008). In the treatment of specific phobias, the child is exposed to anxiolytic stimuli but remains in the situation long enough for the anxiety to substantially decrease.

With children, this therapy is frequently designed in a gradual exposure program. In this format, the therapist, in collaboration with the child/parent, draws up a list of feared stimuli, ordered according to the intensity of the associated fear. The exposure begins with the least feared stimuli, and as the child successfully stays with that situation until the anxiety dissipates, he or she is exposed to increasingly more intense stimuli (Friedman, Munir, & Erickson, 2008). The child habituates to the anxiety because theoretically anxiety attenuates after a prolonged contact with the feared stimulus (March et al., 2001). Along with adequate exposure, the child must be encouraged not to engage in any ritual or avoidance behavior, the response prevention component to the intervention.

Two variations of exposure therapy involve the use of exposure with contingency management (CM) and self-control (SC) procedures. With CM the exposure is accompanied by contingencies, reinforcers the child identifies as rewarding; with SC the child is taught how to use self-regulation skills to control phobic avoidance behaviors (Silverman et al. 1999). In a trial of the two methods, against a controlled condition, Silverman and colleagues demonstrated that CM and SC procedures were equally effective in treating phobic children. CM procedures are more in line with an operant behavioral approach since they use positive reinforcement to increase the appearance of the desired targeted behavior.

Parent Training

Another approach to anxiety treatment targets families, particularly parents who had a current or lifetime diagnosis of anxiety and a child between the ages of seven and twelve (Ginsburg, 2009). The program was designed to address several modifiable risk factors; it teaches parents how to reduce parental overprotection and how to avoid modeling anxious responses. Also presented are instructions on cognitive restructuring and building children's problems-solving skills. Via this program, Ginsburg successfully reduced the expression of anxiety symptoms in children in a treatment group. Modeling adaptive nonanxious responses is a form of social learning; here the child observes and gradually replicates the response of parents. While modeling has not been tested as extensively as exposure techniques, it has intuitive appeal as a method for promoting positive coping.

Behavioral Approaches for Attention Deficit Hyperactivity Disorder

In comparison to the considerable literature on the use of stimulant medication in the treatment of attention deficit hyperactivity disorder (ADHD), there has been less research into a broad range of behavioral interventions. Behavioral treatment implemented in parent training programs and schools has been found to be efficacious (Chronis, Jones, & Raggi, 2006; Pelham & Fabiano, 2008; Pelham, Wheeler, & Chronis, 1998). Efficacious interventions for ADHD include intensive behavioral peer interventions delivered in a summer camp setting (Pelham & Fabiano, 2008; Pelham & Hoza, 1996). The CAMHD analysis of treatment notes that combined behavioral and pharmacological intervention, as evidenced particularly in the Multimodal Treatment Study of Children with ADHD (MTA), demonstrated the largest effect size of all treatments in the best support category (CAMHD, 2007).

In the CAMHD report, behavioral parent training (BPT) or parent management training (PMT) demonstrated a good effect size and is supported by a large evidence base of use (Chronis et al., 2004; Pelham & Fabiano, 2008). One of the most widely distributed BPT programs is the Incredible Years Program (IYP) developed by Carolyn Webster-Stratton (1998), which uses group discussion of videotaped parent-child interactions to develop a parent's problem solving, positive parenting approaches, and effective limit setting. PMT relies heavily on increasing a parent's use of positive reinforcement (particularly praise and positive attention) to increase the output of desired behaviors. Critiques of the program have noted that some BPT programs lack methodological rigor and have limited social validation (Wiese, 2006). Innovations in the BPT methodology are emerging, such as in the Chicago Parent Program, which uses traditional BPT methods but has revised the intervention so that it is congruent with the parental challenges across cultures and socioeconomic groups (Gross, Garvey, Julion, & Fogg, 2009).

The neurobiology of ADHD is increasingly understood as a manifestation of poorly performing prefrontal cortex (PFC) neural tracks that influence attention, reading reward salience, and response inhibition (Arnsten, Berridge, & McCracken, 2009). Though largely confined to animal and adult models, investigators are also clarifying how stimulants enhance PFC tracks (Berridge, 2006). One interesting line of neurobiological research directly bears on the use of positive reinforcement in ADHD interventions. It involves how children with ADHD recall and anticipate positive reinforcement (Tripp & Wickens, 2009). The investigations suggest that these children have problems with anticipation of reinforcement due to a dopamine transfer deficit (Tripp & Wickens, 2008). If additional research confirms this process, it could explain some of children's issues with reward-based decision making and motivation and may lead to novel, effective behavioral interventions.

Behavioral Approaches for Autistic Spectrum

Behavioral approaches for children with autism have, over the past forty years, taken several shifts in emphasis from initial attempts to shape imitation of social behaviors to the current pivotal response interventions (Koegel, Koegel, & McNerney, 2001). Isolating highly effective behavioral approaches is complicated by methodological issues including the heterogeneity of the samples, variability in teaching approaches, and lack of randomized controlled studies (Rogers & Vismara, 2008). A behavioral method that has the best support (CAMHD, 2007) and meets criteria for a probably efficacious intervention is intensive behavioral intervention (IBI) (Rogers & Vismara, 2008).

Investigations included under the umbrella of IBI share basic principles though they do not necessarily follow the same protocol (Ramey & Ramey, 1998). Starting from an individualized assessment of each child's skills and deficits, teaching methods and reinforcers are individualized. The focus is on skill development and use of positive reinforcement to build skills. The programs also aim at increasing motivation to respond so that the child eventually self-initiates social interactions (Koegel et al., 2001). In some programs, the teaching proceeds in stages: first the teaching relationship is established by choosing tasks that the child is likely to perform, thus optimizing the child's success (Lovaas & Smit, 2003). Here the therapist is attempting to reinforce success, withhold reinforcement for avoidance behaviors, and increase the child's motivation. The Lovaas method moves through five additional stages where communication and interactions skills become increasingly more complex and challenging.

While the method differs slightly, pivotal response therapy (PRT) is also structured to increase the child's motivation to respond via positive reinforcement procedures (Koegel, Koegel, & Brookman, 2003). Both of these interventions are designed as intensive interventions that occur throughout the day and delivered by professionals specially trained in the methods. Koegel and colleagues (2003) demonstrated that parents could be trained to use PRT interventions to further daily, in-home learning opportunities. They also provided support for individual components of the PRT program. As this research expands, APNs might draw upon interventions contained in IBI programs for both treatment planning and parent education.

Behavioral Approaches for Disruptive Behaviors

The CAMHD review of interventions targeting children who display disruptive behaviors organized 173 interventions into thirty-four treatment families. From these groups, the behavioral therapies with good support were PMT and contingency management; those with good support include problem solving and combination of PMT and skills training (CAMHD, 2007). These findings mirror a review of psychosocial interventions with children with DBP, which named two behavioral treatments as probably efficacious: PMT and problem-solving training (Eyberg et al., 2008).

Using PMT methods, several programs have demonstrated success at helping parents successfully deal with their child's disruptive and noncompliant behaviors. The IYP includes components for family/parent, child, and school/teacher. Outcomes of the program include strengthening students' social-emotional competence, increasing self-control behaviors, and reducing aggression and associated behaviors (Webster-Stratton, 1998). Theoretically, the program succeeds by effective use of operant conditioning, both increasing positive reinforcement for desired behaviors and teaching parents effective discipline strategies.

Other PMT programs (Triple P-Positive Parenting Program, Parent Child Interaction Therapy) operate within a similar theoretical framework (Eyberg et al., 2008). Two PMT programs (Helping the Noncompliant Child, Parent Management Training Oregon Model) include operant conditioning techniques but emphasize behavior modification and techniques to interrupt the coercive cycle of parent-child interaction (Eyberg et al., 2008). The coercive cycle is an explanatory model that maps how escalating tense interactions between parent and child negatively reinforce a child's noncompliance (Patterson & Reid, 1984). It is a useful theory for APNs as they work with parents who have moved into counterproductive patterns of dealing with their child's noncompliance. Contingency management, where children are rewarded for desired behavior, is a technique used to modify a range of behavior particularly aggression and

noncompliance (Hoagwood et al., 2001). It is often used in classroom settings, where it has been found to be highly effective in reducing negative behaviors and increasing prosocial skills (Barkley et al., 2000). Contingency management operates on principles of operant conditioning; desired behaviors are reinforced usually with a tangible reward. The planning and implementation of such programs require that parents understand the theory of action. There are many varieties of token systems and the structure of the program should fit the behavior the parent is attempting to modify (Barkley, 1997).

Behavior Change Strategies with Young Children in Primary Care

Most pediatric clinicians have an assortment of favorite behavioral strategies that they use in counseling parents about behavior management (Box 17.2). The majority of early behavioral concerns in young children that parents experience consist of difficulties in compliance. Providers can anticipate this natural stage and begin early to assist parents by helping them understand the concept of discipline. Contrary to many parents' understanding, discipline is a method of *teaching* a child how to live comfortably and successfully in a world that will make requests, have rules, and have expectations. Following the long tradition of anticipatory guidance, before the situation actually presents itself, many providers introduce the topic of discipline by the nine-month well-child visit.

A useful concept for explaining discipline is the discipline triangle. One side of the triad represents the toddler's natural desire to please and is grounded in a strong and loving relationship with parents. A second side represents the positive reinforcement parents provide that naturally encourage desired behaviors. The third and smaller side represents the negative reinforcements that are used when needed to discourage behaviors that are unwanted. The triangle reinforces the view that toddler

---

Box 17.2 Behavioral strategies useful in primary care

Checklists/monitoring
Antecedent behavior consequence chart
Diaries/journals
Reward charts
Special times
Planned ignoring
Time-ins and time-outs
Logical consequences
Goal-setting/target behaviors
Positive and negative reinforcements
Differential reinforcement of incompatible behaviors

behavior is a function of social learning and interaction but is also shaped by behavioral approaches. These processes are the basis of learned behaviors, but when problem behaviors arise, it is helpful to use the triangle to see where changes could be made to improve behavior.

Case Exemplar

Use of the discipline triad: Mrs. M called the office to talk about two-year-old Mark, who was "driving her crazy." She reported that ever since two-month-old Jenny was born, Mark had been "getting worse" every day. She stated that Mark was having more and more "meltdowns." He got into things he shouldn't or pretended to hurt himself and cried and screamed until she puts Jenny down and attended to him. The APN asked Mrs. M to use a behavior worksheet to keep track of the antecedents and consequences of Mark's "meltdowns." On the chart Mrs. M recorded the antecedents to "melt downs," the subsequent behavior, and the consequences of the behavior. When Mrs. M arrived for her appointment she brought her chart with her. Before the APN sat down she had already announced that she could see when Mark was having his "meltdowns." "He was fine whenever anyone else was in the house. He played with his toys or talked to her sister or husband. But the minute it was just us—me and the baby and him, he was terrible, especially in the afternoons." When asked how she responded to his behavior, she reported that "sometimes I don't have any choice … I try to ignore him but usually I have to put the baby back in bed and send him to his room. He won't go on his own so I have to take him. He doesn't even seem to mind that so I am not sure what good it does. He stops screaming as soon as I put the baby down."

The APN reminded Mrs. M that many two-year-olds seek some sort of parental response (a word or smile or pat) every few minutes. They also discussed the need to be sure when she asked her son not to do something that he have something to do in its place and has the skills to do it. Using the visual diagram of the discipline triangle, Mrs. M and the clinician were able to discuss the likely influences on Mark's new tantrums. Mrs. M already understood how a new baby in the family may be seen by a two-year-old as a threat to his special relationship with his mother (bottom of triangle). She also realized Mark's "meltdowns" were being reinforced by exactly what he probably wanted – his mother put the baby down and picked Mark up to take him to his room. Even getting negative attention from his mother felt better than being "ignored." Mrs. M was able to strategize on new approaches to Mark's behavior. She and the PNP discussed the principle of extinction that suggested she remove the reinforcement that was keeping the problem behavior going. She understood that ignoring was probably the best response to his tantrums whenever possible. The practitioner reminded her of the likelihood of an initial response burst in which Mark would seem to get worse and have more tantrums than before, so the approach would require patience. Finally, they discussed the line of the triangle representing the positive reinforcements that shape behavior. Mrs. M was able to identify some new ways that she could remember to pay attention to Mark's good behavior such as "catching him being good" and remembering to offer frequent positive statements, praise, and hugs throughout the day.

Critical to addressing behavioral problems in primary care is the manner in which behavioral issues are approached and discussed and how follow-up is planned. In a study that explored the perceptions of parents of preschool-aged children regarding the helpfulness of their pediatrician regarding behavioral concerns (Hawkins-Walsh, 1999), several parents expressed ambivalence about whether their pediatricians really wanted to be used as resources for behavioral issues. Some parents reported that when they asked about how to handle a problem, they were usually offered a "suggestion" as to how to cope; however, it was done in an unconvincing and offhand way as if to suggest that it might or might not work. When the strategy did not work, they believed they would be bothering the pediatrician to ask again for another approach. These parents failed to perceive that attending to behavioral and mental health concerns was a legitimate part of the pediatric clinician's role. An office that is equipped with prepared screening tools, handouts, appropriate videos, and structured follow-up leaves no doubt with parents that the clinician is committed to the "whole" child and his or her family. In addition, following up with parents about the effectiveness of a particular approach provides the clinician with the necessary feedback about what worked and what did not.

Conclusion

The future direction of behavioral and cognitive-behavioral science will likely proceed in several ways. With the increasing interest in affective neuroscience, one would anticipate that more affect regulation strategies will enter into CBT packages of treatment. Of course, indirectly, CBT does help a child control affects, particularly negative and anxious emotions. But the future may hold a more concentrated effort to help children achieve regulation (Izard et al., 2008). There is need for CBT and behavioral interventions for several serious emotional disorders of childhood, such as pediatric bipolar disorder, where only a few promising programs currently exist (Pavuluri, 2004). There is also a tremendous need for evidence-based treatments for ethnic minority youth (Huey & Polo, 2008).

The future will likely hold the development of additional computer-based CBT programs specifically for youth. Such programs already exist for several childhood disorders, such as encopresis. There is also emerging evidence that computer-delivered CBT is superior to wait list control in helping children manage anxiety symptoms (March, Spence, & Donovan, 2009). Such programs hold particular promise for child psychiatry where the maldistribution of child mental health providers makes access to treatment a serious issue.

With increased understanding of the neurobiology of illness, novel therapies will emerge that directly address the putative neural track underlying the psychological process key to the expression of the disorder. For instance, researchers are increasingly interested in the ventral lateral PFC and its role in sustaining attention to anxiolytic stimuli and its overactivity in anxious teens (Pine, 2007). Pine suggests that the future may hold intervention directly aimed at attention training with anxious teens.

The near future also holds models of collaborative care where mental health specialists are co-located within the pediatric primary care home. The concept of a health care home that integrates mental and physical health care for children is grounded in the belief that the pediatric provider recognizes the unique developmental trajectory that provides children and families with both opportunity and risk as their child grows. The pediatric primary health care home is also family focused and recognizes that the seeds of behavioral problems and their likely solutions lie within the family. The richness of the special relationship that can develop over time between families and a trusted APN in pediatrics, family, or mental health sets the stage for successful behavioral intervention.

To maximize this opportunity, the pediatric nurse practitioner must take an active role in helping parents to "reframe" their understanding of the well-child visit from one with a focus on physical well-being to one that addresses the comprehensive set of factors that are likely to threaten a child's health (Melnyk & Moldenhauer, 2005). These include a contextual approach including the child's genetic endowment, temperament, environment, early child care, the school setting, family structure, and community safety (Hagan, Shaw, & Duncan, 2008).

Many APNs are seeking additional training in cognitive and behavioral skills to enhance their effectiveness in supporting families (Hawkins-Walsh et al., 2010; Reach Institute, n.d.; Schor & Elfenbein, 2004). Some practitioners may decide to seek advanced training in specific therapy schools while other clinicians will choose a more limited role incorporating CBT and behavioral approaches within the well-child and office visits. While many pediatric providers may not identify themselves as "therapists," the literature increasingly supports the importance of even limited psychosocial interventions in affecting behavior and cognitive changes (Lemanek, Kamps, & Chung, 2001). The question of how extensive a role the primary care provider should play in the management of common behavioral problems will continue to be addressed as changes occur within the financing and reimbursement of health care, the availability of mental health specialists, the changes in primary care training, and the research demonstrating the effectiveness of mental health screening by pediatric primary care providers.

Resources

National Association of Pediatric Nurse Practitioners (n.d.) About KYSS, accessed December 1, 2010, http://www.napnap.org/Programs AndInitiatives/KySS/AboutKySS.aspx

Penn Resiliency Project. Retrieved from http://www.ppc.sas.upenn. edu/prplessons.pdf

References

Asarnow, J.R., Jaycox, L.H. & Thompson, M.C. (2001). Depression in youth: Psychosocial interventions. *Journal of Clinical Child Psychology, 3*, 33–47.

Bandura, A. (1989). Social cognitive theory. In R. Vasta (Ed.), *Annals of child development. Vol 6. Six theories of child development* (pp. 1–60). Greenwich, CT: JAI Press.

Bandura, A. (1977). *Social learning theory.* New York: General Learning Press.

Barkley, R.A. (1997). *Defiant children: A clinician's manual for assessment and parents training.* New York: Guilford Press.

Barkley, R.A., Shelton, T.L., Crosswait, C., Moorehouse, M., Fletcher, K., Barrett, S., Jenkins, L., & Metevia, L. (2000). Multimethod psycho-educational intervention for preschool children with disruptive disorder: Preliminary results at post-treatment. *Journal of Child Psychology and Psychiatry, 42*, 319–332.

Barrett, P.M. (1998). Evaluation of cognitive-behavioral group treatments for childhood anxiety disorders. *Journal of Clinical Child Psychology, 27*, 459–468.

Barrett, P.M., Farrell, L., Pina, A.A., Peris, T.S., & Piacentini, J. (2008). Evidence-based psychosocial treatments for child and adolescent obsessive compulsive disorder. *Journal of Clinical Child and Adolescent Psychology, 37*, 131–155.

Barrett, P.M., Healy-Farrell, L., & March, J.S. (2004). Cognitive-behavioral family treatment of child obsessive-compulsive disorder. A controlled trial. *Journal of the American Academy of Child and Adolescent Psychiatry, 32*, 430–441.

Beardslee, W.R., Gladstone, T.R., Wright, E.J., & Cooper, A.B. (2003). A family-based approach to prevention of depressive symptoms in children at risk: Evidence of parental and child change. *Pediatrics, 112*, e119–e131. Retrieved from www.pediatrics.org/cgi/content/full/112/2/e119

Beck, A.T. (1964). Thinking and depression, II: Theory and therapy. *Archives of General Psychiatry, 10*, 561–571.

Beck, J.S. (1995). *Cognitive therapy: Basics and beyond.* New York: Guilford Press.

Beck, J.S. (2001). Why distinguish between cognitive therapy and cognitive behavior therapy? *Beck Institute Newsletter,* February 2001. Retrieved from http://www.beckinstitute.org/Library/Info Manage/Zoom.asp?InfoID=150&RedirectPath=Add1&FolderID=177&SessionID={941A3C8E-FF76-4552-BA57-EBB89177D81E}&InfoGroup=Main&InfoType=Article&SP=2

Berridge, C.W., Devilbiss, D.M., Andrzejewski, M.E., & Arnsten, A.F. (2006). Methylphenidate preferentially increases catecholamine neurotransmission within the prefrontal cortex at low doses that enhance cognitive function. *Biological Psychiatry, 60,* 1111–1120.

Bouton, M.E. (2004). Context and behavioral processes in extinction. *Learning and Memory*, 11, 485–494.

Breitenstein, S.M., Hill, C., & Gross, D. (2009). Understanding disruptive behavior problems in preschool children. *Journal of Pediatric Nursing,* 24, 3–12.

Broussard, E. (1976). Neonatal predictors and outcomes at 10/11 years. *Child Psychiatry and Human Development,* 7, 85–93.

Burns, B. (2004). Children and evidence-based practice. *Psychiatric Clinics of North America, 26,* 955–970.

Cardemil, E.V., Reivich, K.J., Beevers, C.G., Seligman, M.E., & James, J. (2007). The prevention of depressive symptoms in low income, minority children: Two-year follow-up. *Behaviour Research and Therapy, 45,* 313–27.

Carter, R. (1994). *Mapping the mind.* Berkley, CA: University of California Press.

Cheung, A., Zuckerbrot, R., Jensen, P., Ghalib, K., Laraque, D., Stein, R. & GLAD-PC Steering Group (2007). Guidelines for adolescent depression in primary care (GLAD-PC): II. Treatment and ongoing management. *Pediatrics,* 120(5), e1313–e1326.

Child and Adolescent Mental Health Division (CAMHD). (2007). *2007 Biennial Report: Effective psychosocial interventions for youth with behavioral and emotional needs.* Retrieved from http://oregon.gov/DHS/mentalhealth/ebp/reports/biennial07effective-hawaii.pdf

Chronis, A.M., Chacko, A., Fabiano, G.A., Wymbs, B.T., & Pelham, W.E. (2004). Enhancements to the standard behavioral parent training paradigm for families of children with ADHD: Review and future directions. *Clinical Child and Family Psychology Review,* 7, 1–27.

Chronis, A.M., Jones, H.A., & Raggi, V.L. (2006). Evidence-based psychosocial treatments for children and adolescents with attention-deficit/hyperactivity disorder. *Clinical Psychology Review,* 26, 486–502.

Chronis, A.M., Chacko, A., Fabiano, G.A., Wymbs, B.T., & Pelham, W.E. (2004). Enhancements to the standard behavioral parent training paradigm for families of children with ADHD: Review and future directions. *Clinical Child and Family Psychology Review,* 7, 1–27.

Cohen, J.A., & Mannarino, A.P. (1996). A treatment outcome study for sexually abused preschool children. *Journal of the American Academy of Child and Adolescent Psychiatry,* 24, 42–50.

Connolly, S.D., Bernstein, G.A., & Workgroup on Quality Issues. (2007). Practice parameters for the assessment and treatment of children and adolescents with anxiety disorders. *Journal of the American Academy of Child and Adolescent Psychiatry,* 46, 267–283.

Costello, E.J., Mustillo, S., Erkanli, A., Keeler, G., & Angold, A. (2003). Prevalence and development of psychiatric disorders in childhood and adolescents. *Archives of General Psychiatry,* 60, 837–844.

Cozolino, L.J. (2002). *The neuroscience of psychotherapy.* New York: W.W. Norton.

Crick, N.R., & Dodge, K.A. (1994). A review and reformulation of social-information-processing mechanisms in children's development. *Psychological Bulletin, 115,* 74–101.

Cuijpers, P., van Straten, A., Smit, F., Mihalopoulos, C., & Beekman, A. (2008). Preventing the onset of depressive disorders: A meta-analytic review of psychological interventions. *American Journal of Psychiatry, 165,* 1272–80.

Cullen, K.J., & Culllen, A.M. (1996). Long-term follow-up of the Busselton six-year controlled trial of prevention of children's behavior disorders. *Journal of Pediatrics, 129,* 136–139.

David-Ferdon, C., & Kaslow, N.J. (2008). Evidence-based psychosocial treatments for child and adolescent depression. *Journal of Clinical Child and Adolescent Psychology, 37,* 62–104.

Davis, M. (2004). Functional neuroanatomy of anxiety and fear. In D. Charney & E.J. Nestler (Eds.), *Neurobiology of mental illness, second edition* (pp. 584–604). New York: Oxford Press.

De Cuyper, S., Timbremont, B., De Braet, V, & Wullaert, T. (2004). Treating depressive symptoms in schoolchildren: A pilot study. *European Child and Adolescent Psychiatry, 13,* 105–114.

Delaney, K.R. (2008). Psychotherapy with children. In K. Wheeler (Ed.), *Psychotherapy for the advanced practice nurse* (pp. 330–352). St. Louis: Mosby.

Dichter, G.S., Felder, J.N., & Smoski, M. (2008). Treatment resistant depression: Effects of psychotherapy on brain function. *Psychiatric Times, 25,* 10.

Dodge, K.A., & Crick, N.R. (1990). Social information-processing bases of aggressive behavior in children. *Personality and Social Psychology Bulletin, 16,* 8–22.

Draucker, C.B. (2005). Processes of mental health service use by adolescents with depression. *Journal of Nursing Scholarship, 37,* 155–162.

Engel, K., Bandelow, B., & Gruber, O. (2009). Neuroimaging in anxiety disorders. *Journal of Neural Transmission, 116,* 703–716.

Eyeberg, S.M., Nelson, M.M., & Boggs, S.R. (2008). Evidenced-based psychosocial treatments for children and adolescents with disruptive behavior. *Journal of Clinical Child and Adolescent Psychology, 37,* 215–237.

Flament, M.F., Geller, D., Irak, M., & Blier, P. (2007). Specificities of treatment in pediatric obsessive-compulsive disorder. *CNS Spectrum, 12,* 43–57.

Flannery-Schroeder, E.C., & Kendall, P.C. (2000). Group and individual cognitive-behavioral treatments for youth with anxiety disorders: A randomized clinical trial. *Cognitive Therapy and Research, 24,* 251–278.

Franklin, M., Foa, E., & March, J.S. (2003). The pediatric obsessive-compulsive disorder treatment study: Rationale, design and methods. *Journal of Child and Adolescent Psychopharmacology, 13,* s39–s51.

Friedberg, R.D., & McClure, J.M. (2002). *Clinical practice of cognitive therapy with children and adolescents.* New York: Guilford Press.

Friedman, S.L., Munir, K.M., & Erickson, M.T. (2008). Anxiety disorder, specific phobia: Treatment and medication. Retrieved from http://emedicine.medscape.com/article/917056-treatment.

Gillham, J.E., Hamilton, J., & Freres, D.R. (2006). Preventing depression among early adolescents in the primary care setting: A randomized controlled study of the Penn Resiliency Program. *Journal of Abnormal Child Psychology, 34,* 203–19.

Gillham, J.E., Reivich, K.J., & Freres, D.R. (2007). School-based prevention of depressive symptoms: A randomized controlled study of the effectiveness and specificity of the Penn Resiliency Program. *Journal of Consulting and Clinical Psychology, 75,* 9–19.

Ginsburg, G.S. (2009). The child anxiety prevention study: Intervention model and primary outcomes. *Journal of Consulting and Clinical Psychology, 77,* 580–587.

Green, M., & Solnit. A. (1964). Reactions to the threatened loss of a child: A vulnerable child syndrome. *Pediatrics, 34,* 58–66.

Greenberg, D., & Padesky, C.A. (1995). *Mind over mood: Change how you feel by changing how you think*. New York: Guilford Press.

Gross, D., Garvey, C., Julion, W., Fogg, L., Tucker, S., & Mokros, H. (2009). Efficacy of the Chicago parent program with low-income African American and Latino parents of young children. *Prevention Science, 10,* 54–65.

Haeffel, G.J., & Grigorenko, E.L. (2007). Cognitive vulnerability to depression: Exploring risk and resilience. *Child and Adolescent Clinics of North America, 16,* 435–48.

Hagan, J.F., Shaw, J.S., & Duncan, P.M. (Eds.) (2008). *Bright futures: guidelines for health supervision of infants, children, and adolescents* (third edition). Elk Grove Village, IL: American Academy of Pediatrics.

Hawkins-Walsh, E. (1999). Parental attitudes toward pediatric primary care providers as resources for behavioral care during well child visits. *Dissertation Abstracts International: Section B; The Science and Engineering, 60*(4-B), 1530.

Hawkins-Walsh, E., Crowley, A., Melnyk, B., Beauchesne, M., Brandt, P., & O'Haver, J. (2011). Improving healthcare quality through an AFPNP national nursing education collaborative to strengthen PNP curriculum in mental/behavioral health and evidence-based practice. *Journal of Professional Nursing, 27,* 10–18.

Hibbs, E.D. (2001). Evaluating empirically based psychotherapy research for children and adolescents. *European Child and Adolescent Psychiatry, 10,* 3–11.

Hibbs, E.D., & Jensen, P. (Eds.). (1996). *Psychosocial treatments for children and adolescent disorders: Empirically based strategies for clinical practice*. Washington, D.C.: American Psychological Association.

Hoagwood, K., Burns, B.J., Kiser, L., Ringeisen, H., & Schoenwald, S.K. (2001). Evidence-based practice in child and adolescent mental health services. *Psychiatric Services, 52,* 1179–1189.

Horowitz, J.L., & Garber, J. (2006). The prevention of depressive symptoms in children and adolescents: A meta-analytic review. *Journal of Consulting and Clinical Psychology, 74,* 401–415.

Huey, S.J., & Polo, A.J. (2008). Evidence-based therapies for ethnic minority youth. *Journal of Clinical Child and Adolescent Psychology, 27,* 262–301.

Institute of Medicine. (2009). Preventing mental, emotional, and behavioral disorders among young people: progress and possibilities. Retrieved from http://www.iom.edu/en/Reports/2009/Preventing-Mental-Emotional-and-Behavioral-Disorders-Among-Young-People-Progress-and-Possibilities.aspx.

Izard, C.E., King, K.A., Trentacosta, C.J., Morgan, J.K., Laurenceau, J.P., Krauthamer-Ewing, E., & Finlon, K.J. (2008). Accelerating the development of emotion competence in Head Start children: Effects on adaptive and maladaptive behavior. *Development and Psychopathology, 20,* 369–397.

Kazdin, A.E., & Weisz, J.R. (Eds.). (2003). *Evidence-based psychotherapies for children and adolescents*. New York: Guilford Press.

Keel, P.K., & Haedt, A. (2008). Evidence-based psychosocial treatments for eating problems and eating disorders. *Journal of Clinical Child and Adolescent Psychology, 37,* 39–61.

Keenan, K., & Wakschlag, L.S. (2004). Are oppositional defiant and conduct disorder symptoms normative behaviors in preschoolers? A comparison of referred and non-referred children. *American Journal of Psychiatry, 161,* 356–8.

Kendall, P.C. (1994). Treatment of anxiety disorders in children: A randomized clinical trial. *Journal of Consulting and Clinical Psychology, 62,* 100–110.

Kendall, P.C. (Ed.). (2006a). *Child and adolescent therapy: Cognitive-behavioral procedures, third edition*. New York: Guilford Press.

Kendall, P.C. (2006b). Guiding theory for therapy with children and adolescents. In P.C. Kendall (Ed.), *Child and adolescent therapy: Cognitive-behavioral procedures,* (third edition) (pp. 3–30). New York: Guilford Press.

Kendall, P.C., Flannery-Schroeder, E., Panichelli-Mindel, S.M., Southam-Gerow, M., Henin A., & Warman, M. (1997). Therapy for youths with anxiety disorders: a second randomized clinical trial. *Journal of Consulting and Clinical Psychology, 65,* 366–380.

Kendall, P.C., & Grosch, E.A., (1994). Cognitive-behavioral interventions. In T. H. Ollendick, N., King, J., & W. Yule (Eds.), *International handbook of phobic and anxiety disorders in children and adolescents* (pp. 415–438). New York: Plenum Press.

Kendall, P.C., & Suveg, C. (2006). Treating anxiety disorders in youth. In P.C. Kendall (Ed.), *Child and adolescent therapy: Cognitive-behavioral procedures* (third edition) (pp. 243–294). New York: Guilford Press.

Kessler, R.C., Berglund, P., Demler, O., Jin, R., Merikangas K.R., & Walters, E.E. (2005). Lifetime prevalence and age of onset distributions of DSM-IV disorders in the National Comorbidity Survey Replication. *Archives of General Psychiatry, 62,* 593–602.

Knapp, P., & Beck, A.T. (2009). Cognitive therapy: Foundations, conceptual models, applications and research. *Review of Brazilian Psychiatry, 20,* S54–S64.

Koegel, R.L., Koegel, L.K., & McNerney, E.K. (2001). Pivotal areas in intervention for autism. *Journal of Clinical Child Psychology, 30,* 19–32.

Koegel, R.L., Koegel, L.K., & Brookman, L.I. (2003). Empirically supported pivotal response interventions for children with autism. In A.E. Kazdin & J.R. Weisz (Eds.), *Evidence-based psychotherapies for children and adolescents* (pp. 341–357). New York: Guilford Press.

Lemanek, L., Kamps, J., & Chung, N.B. (2001). Empirically supported treatments in pediatric psychology: regimen adherence. *Journal of Pediatric Psychology, 26,* 253–375.

Levy, J. (1980). Vulnerable children: Parents' perspectives and use of medical care. *Pediatrics, 65,* 956–963.

Lochman, J.E., Barry, T.D., & Pardini, D.A. (2003). Anger control training for aggressive youth. In A.E. Kazdin & J.R Weisz (Eds.). *Evidence-based psychotherapies for children and adolescents* (pp. 263–281). New York: Guilford Press.

Lochman, J.E., Wayland, K.K., & White, K.J. (1993). Social goals: Relationship to adolescent adjustment and to social problem solving. *Journal of Abnormal Child Psychology, 21,* 135–151.

Lovaas, O.I., & Smith, T. (2003). Early and intensive behavioral intervention in autism. In A.E. Kazdin & J.R. Weisz (Eds.), *Evidence-based psychotherapies for children and adolescents* (pp. 325–340). New York: Guilford Press.

March, J.S., Franklin, M., Nelson, A., & Foa, E. (2001). Cognitive-behavioral psychotherapy for pediatric obsessive-compulsive disorder. *Journal of Clinical Child Psychology, 30,* 8–18.

March, S., Spence, S., & Donovan, C.L. (2009). The efficacy of an internet-based cognitive behavioral therapy intervention for child anxiety disorders. *Journal of Pediatric Psychology, 34,* 474–487.

MacMaster, F.P., O'Neill, J., & Rosenberg, D.R. (2008). Brain imaging in pediatric obsessive-compulsive disorder. *Journal of the American Academy of Child and Adolescent Psychiatry, 47,* 1262–1272.

Medical College of South Carolina. (2005). TF-CBT Web. Retrieved from http://tfcbt.musc.edu/

Melnyk, B., & Moldenhaurer, Z. (2005). *The KYSS Guide to Child and Adolescent Mental Health Screening, Early Intervention and Health Promotion*. Cherry Hill, N.J.: NAPNAP

Miller, A. (2007). Social neuroscience of child and adolescent depression. *Brain and Cognition, 65,* 47–68.

Munoz-Solomando, A., Kendall, T., & Whittington, C.J. (2008). Cognitive-behavioral therapy for children and adolescents. *Current Opinion in Psychiatry, 21*, 332–337.

Muris, P., Meesters, C., & Rompelberg, L. (2006). Attention control in middle childhood: Relations to psychopathological symptoms and threat perception distortions. *Behavior Research and Therapy, 45*, 997–1010.

National Registry of Evidence Based Programs and Practices (NREPP). (n.d.). *SAMHSA's National Registry for Evidence Based Programs and Practices.* Retrieved from http://www.nrepp.samhsa.gov/index.asp

Patterson, G.R., & Reid, J.B. (1984). Social interaction processes within the family: The study of the moment-to-moment transactions in which human social development is embedded. *Journal of Applied Developmental Psychology, 5*, 237–262.

Pavuluri, M.N., Grayczyk, P., Carbray, J., Heidenreich, J., Henry, D., & Miklowitz, D. (2004). Child and family focused cognitive behavior therapy in pediatric bipolar disorder. *Journal of the American Academy of Child and Adolescent Psychiatry, 43*, 528–537.

Pelham, W.E., & Fabiano, G.A. (2008). Evidence-based psychosocial treatments for attention-deficit/hyperactivity disorder. *Journal of Clinical Child and Adolescent Psychology, 37*, 184–214.

Pelham, W.E., & Hoza, B. (1996). Intensive treatment: a summer treatment program for children with ADHD. In E. D Hibbs & P. Jensen (Eds.), *Psychosocial treatments for children and adolescent disorders: Empirically based strategies for clinical practice* (pp. 311–340). Washington, D.C.: American Psychological Association.

Pelham, W.E., Wheeler, T., & Chronis, A. (1998). Empirically supported psychosocial treatments for attention deficit disorder. *Journal of Clinical Child Psychology, 27*, 190–205.

Pine, D.S. (2007). Research review: A neuroscience framework for pediatric anxiety disorders. *Journal of Child Psychology and Psychiatry, 48*, 631–648.

Porto, P.R., Oliveira, L., Mari, J., Volchan, E., Figueira, I., & Ventura, P. (2009). Does cognitive behavioral therapy change the brain? A systematic review of neuroimaging in anxiety disorders. *Journal of Neuropsychiatry and Clinical Neuroscience, 21*, 114–125.

Rachman, S. (1997). The evolution of cognitive behaviour therapy. In D. Clark, C.G. Fairburn, & M. G. Gelder (Eds.), *Science and practice of cognitive behaviour therapy* (pp. 1–26). Oxford: Oxford University Press.

Radecki, L., Olson, L., Frinter, M., Tanner, L., & Stein, M. (2009). What do families want from well-child care? Including parents in the rethinking discussion. *Pediatrics, 124*, 858–865.

Ramey, C.T., & Ramey, S.L. (1998). Early intervention and early experience. *American Psychologist, 53*, 109–120.

Reach Institute. Retrieved from http://www.thereachinstitute.org/primary-care-professionals.html

Reinecke, M.A., Dattilio, F.M., & Freeman, A. (2004). What makes for an effective treatment. In M.A. Reinecke, F.M. Dattilio, & A. Freeman (Eds.), *Cognitive therapy with children and adolescents: Second edition: A casebook for clinical practice* (pp. 1–18). New York: Guilford Press.

Rohde, P., Feeney, N.C., & Robins, M. (2005). Characteristics and components of the TADS CBT approach. *Cognitive Behavioral Practice, 12*, 186–197.

Roffman, J.L., Marci, C.D., Glick, D.M., Dougherty, D.D., & Rauch, S.L. (2005). Neuroimaging and the functional neuroanatomy of psychotherapy. *Psychological Medicine, 35*, 1385–1398.

Rogers, S.J., & Vismara, L.A. (2008). Evidence-based comprehensive treatment for early autism. *Journal of Clinical Child and Adolescent Psychology, 37*, 8–38.

Roy, A.K., Vasa, R.A., Bruck, M., Mogg, K., Bradley, B.P., Sweeney, M., Bergman, R.L., McClure-Tone E.B., Pine, D.S., & CAMS Team. (2008). Attention bias toward threat in pediatric anxiety disorders. *Journal of the American Academy of Child and Adolescent Psychiatry, 47*, 1189–1196.

Rzepski, B., & Jarasek, N. (2005). An overview of evidence-based psychotherapy for children and adolescents. *Connecticut Medicine, 69*, 553–559.

Saavedra, L.M., & Silberman, W.K. (2002). Classification of anxiety disorders in children: What a difference two decades make. *International Review of Psychiatry, 14*, 87–101.

Schmidt, U., Lee, S., Beecham, J., Perkins, S., Treasure, J.T., Yi, I., Winn, S., & Eisler, I. (2007). A randomized controlled trial of family therapy and cognitive behavior therapy guided self-care for adolescents with bulimia nervosa and related disorders. *American Journal of Psychiatry, 164*, 591–598.

Schor, E., & Elfenbein, C. (2004). A need for faculty development in developmental and behavioral pediatrics. *Issue Brief (Commonwealth Fund), Oct*(785):1–8.

Selekman, M.D. (1997). *Solution-focused therapy with children: Harnessing family strengths for systematic change.* New York: Guilford Press.

Silverman, W.K., Ortiz, C.D., Viswesvaran, C., Burns, B.J., Kolko, D.J., Putnam, F.W., & Amaya-Jackson, L. (2008). Evidence-based psychosocial treatments for children and adolescents exposed to traumatic events. *Journal of Clinical Child and Adolescent Psychology, 37*, 156–183.

Silverman, W.K., Pina, A.A., & Viswesvaran, C. (2008). Evidence-based psychosocial treatments for phobic and anxiety disorders in children and adolescents. *Journal of Clinical Child and Adolescent Psychiatry, 37*, 105–130.

Spiegler, M.D., & Guevremont, D.D. (2003). *Contemporary behavior therapy.* Belmont, CA: Wadsworth.

Spence, S.H., Donovan, C., & Brechman-Toussaint, M. (2000). The treatment of childhood social phobia: The effectiveness of a social skills-training-based, cognitive-behavioral intervention with and without parental involvement. *Journal of Child Psychology and Psychiatry, 41*, 713–726.

Spence, S.H. (2003). Social skills training with children and young people: Theory, evidence and practice. *Child and Adolescent Mental Health, 8*, 84–96.

Stark, K.D., Hargraves, J., & Sander J. (2006). Treatment of childhood depression: The ACTION treatment program. In P.C. Kendall (Ed.), *Child and adolescent therapies: Cognitive-behavioral procedures* (third edition; pp. 162–216). New York: Guilford Press.

Steele, R.G., Elkins, T.D., & Roberts, M.C. (Eds.). (2008). *Handbook of evidenced-based therapies for children and adolescents.* New York: Springer.

Stein, R., Zitner, L, & Jensen, P. (2006). Interventions for adolescent depression in primary care. *Pediatrics, 118*, 669–682.

Substance Abuse and Mental Health Services Administration. (2009). *Results from the 2008 National Survey on Drug Use and Health: National Findings* (Office of Applied Studies, NSDUH Series H-36, HHS Publication No. SMA 09-4434). Rockville, MD.

Tamminga, C.A. (2006). The anatomy of fear extinction. *American Journal of Psychiatry 163*, 6.

Tripp, G., & Wickens, J.R. (2008). Research review: Dopamine transfer deficit: a neurobiological theory of altered reinforcement mechanisms in ADHD. *Journal of Child Psychology and Psychiatry, 49*, 691–704.

Tripp, G., & Wickens, J.R. (2009). Neurobiology of ADHD. *Neuropharmacology, 57*, 579–589.

Tryon, W.W. (2009). Cognitive processes in cognitive and pharmacological therapies. *Cognitive Therapy Research, 33*, 570–584.

Webster-Stratton C. (1998). Prevention of conduct problems in Head Start children: Strengthening parenting competencies. *Journal of Consulting and Clinical Psychology, 66,* 715–730.

Wiese, M.R.R. (2006). A critical review of parent training research. *Psychology in the Schools, 29,* 229–236.

Weisz, J.R., Hawley, K.M., & Doss, A.J. (2004). Empirically tested psychotherapies for youth internalizing and externalizing problems and disorders. *Child and Adolescent Psychiatric Clinics of North America, 13,* 729–815.

Williamson, D.A., White, M.A., York-Crowe, E., & Stewart. T. M. (2004). Cognitive-behavioral theories of eating disorders. *Behavior Modification, 28,* 711–738.

Yu, D.L., & Seligman, M.E.P. (2002). Preventing depressive symptoms in Chinese children. *Prevention and Treatment, 5,* art id 9.

SECTION 3
Special Populations

18

Disorders Specific to Infants and Young Children

Sandra J. Weiss and Cathy Quides

Objectives

After reading this chapter, APNs will be able to

1. Identify major mental health problems experienced by infants, toddlers, and preschool children.
2. Describe varied methods for assessing mental health problems of young children.

3. Identify approaches to intervention that consider specific symptoms, developmental issues, and family context.

Introduction

Over the last twenty years, awareness has increased regarding the existence and importance of mental health problems experienced by infants, toddlers, and preschool children. These problems are typically not transient syndromes but become chronic, recurring problems (Briggs-Gowan & Carter, 2008; Luby, Si, Belden, Tandon, & Spitznagel, 2009). In fact, evidence has grown to suggest that the origins of many psychiatric illnesses in adulthood stem from biological and developmental disruptions early in life (Shonkoff, Boyce, & McEwen, 2009). It is essential, then, that clinicians learn to recognize signs and symptoms associated with emotional and behavioral problems during the first few years of life. Early intervention can prevent development of more severe problems or have implications for a better prognosis (Carter, Briggs-Gowan, & Davis, 2004).

Prevalence of Mental Health Problems

Few studies have examined the prevalence of mental health problems in children six years of age or younger. Available studies conducted in community or primary care settings with children who were two to five years old indicate that rates of mental illness for young children (i.e., having at least one mental disorder) ranged from 14% to 26.4% based on classifications in the Diagnostic and Statistical Manual of Mental Disorders (DSM-IV-TR) (American Psychiatric Association, 2000; Egger & Angold, 2006). Among those diagnosed, comorbidity was common, with dysfunction across multiple systems. Many children also were found to have "subthreshold" symptoms, suggesting that they were at high risk of developing a mental disorder in the future.

Diagnoses for mental health problems in children tend to differ by age. A review of research data specific

Child and Adolescent Behavioral Health: A Resource for Advanced Practice Psychiatric and Primary Care Practitioners in Nursing,
First Edition. Edited by Edilma L. Yearwood, Geraldine S. Pearson, and Jamesetta A. Newland.
© 2012 John Wiley & Sons, Inc. Published 2012 by John Wiley & Sons, Inc.

to infants and toddlers referred to a community mental health clinic found that regulation disorders, developmental disorders, and adjustment difficulties were the most common diagnoses (Wright, Holmes, Stader, Penny, & Wieduwilt, 2004). Problems in the parent-child relationship are also prevalent. Studies of preschoolers—of both community samples and those referred for mental health services—have shown that they are more likely to be diagnosed with an externalizing than an internalizing disorder (Lavigne, LeBailly, Hopkins, Gouze, & Binns, 2009; Wilens et al., 2002). For instance, Wilens et al. found that 86% of children at mental health clinics had attention deficit hyperactivity disorder (ADHD), and 61% had oppositional defiant disorder (ODD). Some studies suggested that boys were more likely to have an ODD diagnosis than were girls. These findings may reflect greater difficulty in assessing emotional or internalizing symptoms in young children because of their developmental limitations in describing their inner experience and their caregivers' trouble recognizing inner fears or sadness in contrast to external behaviors.

Existing research highlights the importance of ongoing mental health assessment and focused treatment for young children rather than assuming that problems will be "outgrown" or adopting a "wait and see" attitude. Yet studies show that only 3.3% to 25% of children diagnosed with a mental health problem were referred for any mental health evaluation or treatment (Egger & Angold, 2006; Lavigne et al., 2009).

The Nature of Mental Health Problems in Early Childhood

Etiology

Most mental disorders of young children are viewed within the context of a stress diathesis model (Hankin & Abela, 2005). Specific genetic, structural, neurophysiological/chemical vulnerabilities interact with environmental adversities such as biological stressors/toxins, deprivation, or abuse to bring about mental disorders. Psychopathology that involves difficulty regulating sensory perception and behavior or developmental impairments that cut across systems appear to be caused primarily by neurobiological risk factors, although the nature of a child's social environment can either exacerbate or reduce the effect of the neurobiological vulnerability (Cicchetti & Curtis, 2006).

Disorders that involve posttraumatic stress, depression, or other affective problems may be influenced more substantially by caregiving environments, losses, and exposure to major life stress. But even for these disorders, genetic predisposition or neurobiological deficits/dysfunction can leave a child significantly more vulnerable to environmental adversity (Blandon, Calkins, Keane, & O'Brien, 2008; Boyce & Ellis, 2005). More in-depth discussion of the etiology of specific disorders can be found in relevant chapters throughout this book.

A Diagnostic Classification System for Young Children (Zero to Three)

Traditionally, concerns have been voiced about diagnostic systems for young children in light of rapid developmental changes and the risk of stigmatizing labels. More current views emphasize the importance of early identification of specific problems for focused treatment and the necessity of a diagnosis for services to be reimbursed. However, many mental health professionals have expressed concern about the adequacy of the DSM-IV-TR for assessing the very young child's unique situation.

To address these concerns, a multidisciplinary group affiliated with the National Center for Infants, Toddlers and Families developed a new diagnostic system, the Diagnostic Classification of Mental Health and Developmental Disorders of Infancy and Early Childhood (DC:0-3) (Zero to Three, 1994), which has undergone one revision (DC:0-3R) (Zero to Three, 2005). Although originally developed for children ages three years and under, it has become a useful diagnostic system for considering mental disorders of all young children, including those of preschool age. Diagnoses using the DC:0-3R system consider a child's maturational and environmental changes over time and remain open to modification based upon these changes. Similar to the DSM-IV-TR, the DC:0-3R is multiaxial but has a more significant focus on developmental and relational issues (Table 18.1).

Although the nosology of mental health disorders for young children is still in development, studies have supported the validity and utility of the DC:0-3 diagnostic system (Cordeiro, Caldeira da Silva, & Goldschmidt, 2003; Guedeney et al., 2003). It has been noted that DC:0-3 is superior for assessment of young children in certain problem areas and provides important classifications that are not available in the DSM-IV-TR (Scheeringa, Peebles, Cook, & Zeanah, 2001). For classifications shared by both systems, there is good agreement in diagnosing young children (Frankel, Boyum, & Harmon, 2004; Thomas & Guskin, 2001). Because the DC:0-3R appears to be the best classification system for young children to date, this chapter will be organized according to its diagnoses. Related diagnostic classifications from DSM-IV-TR are shown in Table 18.2.

Table 18.1 Multi-axial assessment within two classification systems

Axis	DC:0-3R	DSM-IV-TR
I	Primary Diagnostic Categories (see Table 4.2) [Includes a decision tree to prioritize diagnostic classification for comorbid disorders]	Primary Diagnostic Categories (see Table 4.2)
II	Relationship Disorders between Child and Parent/Caregiver: • Over- or underinvolved • Anxious/tense • Angry/hostile • Abusive (verbally, physically, or sexually) • Mixed [Includes a Parent-Infant Global Assessment Scale and a Relationships Problems Checklist]	Personality Disorders
III	Medical and Developmental Disorders and Conditions	Medical Conditions
IV	Psychosocial and Environmental Stressors [Includes a checklist to assess stressors and environmental challenges specific to young children (e.g. educational and child care environments; trauma-related exposure)]	Psychosocial and Environmental Stressors
V	Emotional and Social Functioning [Includes a rating scale to assess specific age-appropriate capacities in areas such as: • Attention and regulation • Early problem-solving • Use of symbols in communication and thought • Engagement with others	Global Assessment of Overall Functioning and Ability to Carry Out Activities of Daily Living [Includes a rating scale to assess psychological, social, and occupational functioning]

Posttraumatic Stress Disorder

In posttraumatic stress disorder (PTSD), a child has experienced a single event, series of connected events, or chronic, enduring stress that elicits symptoms of traumatic stress. Symptoms generally parallel those found for older children. However, reexperiencing of the event(s) is likely to occur during play via reenactment that appears compulsive and fails to relieve anxiety, through repeated statements or questions about the event, or through repeated nightmares about the event(s). Numbing of responsiveness may be indicated by interference with developmental momentum after the event. For example, a child may show increased social withdrawal, temporary loss of previous skills such as toilet training or language, or a decrease in play. Arousal may be exhibited by night wakening and terrors, bedtime protest, significant attentional difficulties, and hypervigilance or exaggerated startle. Fears, aggression, or other problems that were not present before the event(s) may emerge, such as separation anxiety, fear of the dark, aggression toward animals or peers, and inappropriate sexual behavior.

Deprivation/Maltreatment Disorder

This disorder is a type of PTSD associated with the caregiving environment and may show some of the symptoms described earlier. However, the child will have experienced (1) intense and persistent physical or psychological neglect or abuse by a caregiver, (2) frequent changes in, or the inconsistent availability of, the primary caregiver, or (3) other types of neglect or maltreatment that compromise appropriate care of the child. These situations often undermine the child's basic sense of security or prevent stable attachments. Specific symptoms include a failure to initiate or respond appropriately in social interactions or the manifestation of ambivalent or contradictory social

Table 18.2 Diagnostic classifications for mental health and developmental disorders of infancy and early childhood

DC:0-3R Diagnosis	DSM-IV-TR Diagnosis
Posttraumatic Stress Disorder	Posttraumatic Stress Disorder
Deprivation/Maltreatment Disorder	Reactive Attachment Disorder
Disorders of Affect	
• Prolonged Bereavement/Grief Reaction	
• Anxiety Disorders	
◦ Separation Anxiety Disorder	Separation Anxiety Disorder
◦ Specific Phobia	Specific Phobia
◦ Social Anxiety Disorder	Social Phobia
◦ Generalized Anxiety Disorder	Generalized Anxiety Disorder
◦ Anxiety Disorder NOS	Anxiety Disorder NOS
• Depression	
◦ Type I: Major Depression	Major Depressive Disorder
◦ Type II: Depressive Disorder NOS	Depressive Disorder NOS
• Mixed Disorder of Emotional Expressiveness	Mood Disorder NOS
Adjustment Disorder	Adjustment Disorder
Regulation Disorders of Sensory Processing	
• Hypersensitive Type A: Fearful/Cautious	Anxiety Disorder NOS
• Hypersensitive Type B: Negative/Defiant	Disruptive Behavior Disorder NOS
• Hyposensitive/Underresponsive	
• Sensory Stimulation-Seeking/Impulsive	Attention-Deficit/Hyperactivity Disorder
	Impulse Control Disorder
	Oppositional Defiant Disorder
Sleep Behavior Disorder	
• Sleep-Onset Disorder	Primary Insomnia
	Circadian Rhythm Sleep Disorder
• Night-Waking Disorder	Sleep Terror Disorder
	Sleepwalking Disorder
Feeding Behavior Disorders	Feeding Disorder of Infancy or Early Childhood
• Feeding Disorder of State Regulation	
• Feeding Disorder of Caregiver-Infant Reciprocity	
• Infantile Anorexia	
• Sensory Food Aversion	
• Feeding Disorder associated with a Medical Condition	
• Feeding Disorder associated with GI Insults	
	Pica
	Rumination
Disorders of Relating and Communicating	
• Multisystem Developmental Disorder	Autistic Disorder
	Pervasive Developmental Disorder NOS
	Asperger's Disorder
	Childhood Disintegrative Disorder
	Rett's Disorder

responses such as approach-avoidance. A child may also show extreme vigilance or excessively inhibited responses to caregivers or others. Alternatively, the child may show indiscriminant social behavior such as excessive affection toward relative strangers or lack of selectivity in attachment figures.

Disorders of Affect

Disorders of affect are the largest diagnostic category for young children, including grief reactions, anxiety disorders, depressive disorders, and a mixed disorder of emotional expressiveness. For young children, affect disorders often involve relationship problems between caregiver and child. However, the child's affective and behavioral difficulties must be evident in interactions beyond a single caregiver or context for any of the diagnoses to be appropriate.

Prolonged Bereavement/Grief Reactions

This disorder can occur when a young child loses a primary caregiver. Young children do not usually have the emotional and cognitive capacity to handle a major loss and other caregivers may not be available to provide the necessary support. The child may show symptoms associated with protest, despair, or detachment. These symptoms can include (1) crying, calling, or searching for a lost caregiver while refusing others' attempts to comfort, (2) emotional withdrawal, along with lethargy, sad facial expression, and lack of interest in usual activities, (3) disruption of eating and sleeping, (4) regression or loss of previously achieved developmental milestones (e.g., reverting to bed wetting or baby talk), (5) constricted range of affect, (6) detachment from reminders of the lost caregiver such as seeming indifferent or not recognizing photographs or the mentioning of a caregiver's name, or (7) extreme sensitivity to reminders of the lost caregiver, involving acute distress when the caregiver's possessions are touched by others or taken away. The child may also react strongly to any changes in customary objects or situations in the household.

Anxiety Disorders of Infancy and Early Childhood

An anxiety disorder involves evidence of excessive anxiety or fear that persists for at least two weeks and interferes with play, speech, sleep, relationships, or other functioning. The child's specific symptoms may indicate one of the following anxiety disorders in young children: separation anxiety disorder, specific phobia, social anxiety disorder, generalized anxiety disorder, or another anxiety disorder not specified. See Chapter 8 for further information about these disorders. In addition to standard anxiety symptoms in children, anxiety disorders at this age may be observed as uncontrollable crying or screaming, sleeping and eating disturbances, or recklessness.

Depression of Infancy and Early Childhood

In the DC:0-3R, depression may be diagnosed as major depression or a depressive disorder not otherwise specified. Depression is addressed in detail in Chapter 9. For very young children, key symptoms include sadness, little interest in play or eating favorite foods, diminished capacity to protest in situations where protest would be typical of the child, excessive whining or irritability, and diminished social interaction or attempts to engage with others.

Mixed Disorder of Emotional Expressiveness

In this disorder, children have an ongoing difficulty expressing emotions that would be appropriate for their stage of development. These difficulties are thought to reflect pervasive problems in their affective development and experiences. The disorder may manifest in a number of ways (thus the label "Mixed"). In one type of presentation, the child may have an absence of, or a constricted range of expression in, one or more specific emotions or types of affect that are developmentally expected such as joy, anger, fear, empathy, or sadness. For instance, a child may show no fear or anxiety in situations where fear may serve an adaptive or protective function. Or the preschooler may have no apparent concern for another child whom he hits with a rock. In contrast, excessive emotional intensity may be observed, usually accompanied by poor modulation of emotional expression. For example, a child may be unable to control his anger, resulting in violent, persistent tantrums. Last, a disorder of emotional expressiveness may involve reversal of the particular affect appropriate to a situation such as a child's laughing when sad or angry. It has been suggested that problems with emotional expressiveness in young children may be precursors to varied types of later psychopathology (e.g., personality disorders, bipolar disorder). Whether initial problems in expressiveness persist and grow into other mental disorders over time may depend on the nature of the caregiving received by the child and his/her exposure to other risk or protective factors.

Adjustment Disorder

This disorder is described in both DC:0-3R and DSM-IV-TR as mild, transient, situational symptoms that are tied to an event or change such as the illness of a mother, parental separation, or placement at a new day care facility. The particular symptoms shown by a child may be varied, reflecting unique temperament, developmental age, and circumstances faced by the child. For instance, the child may withdraw and be more subdued, become more oppositional and angry, or regress in toilet training. However, to be labeled as an adjustment disorder, the child's symptoms should not be explainable by other diagnoses and must last from only a few days to no longer than four months. Symptoms that persist beyond that point usually indicate an enduring disorder of a different type.

Regulation Disorders of Sensory Processing

Regulatory disorders are one of the most unique diagnostic areas for young children. The three types of regulation disorder are hypersensitivity, hyposensitivity, and sensory stimulation-seeking. Children who are hypersensitive may be very fearful and cautious or negative and defiant. These behaviors are the child's way of responding to excessive overreactivity to stimulation such as touch, noise, or lights. Children who are hyposensitive are underresponsive to stimulation such as sounds or movement. They may appear withdrawn or difficult to engage or be self-absorbed with their own sensations (e.g., picking at their skin or repeating the same sound over and over) rather than communicating with others. In the third type, a child seems to crave sensory stimulation and is typically impulsive in his/her behavior. For instance, a child might not be able to wait his turn to roll on a ball that is located in a circle of children. He might push other children down to get to the ball, use it in a more aggressive and vigorous way than expected, and appear fearless or reckless in his movements. Regulatory problems can be seen in a variety of symptoms, including physiological reactivity (irregular breathing, startles), motor activity (jerky movements, constant movement), attention (inability to focus or perseveration on a small detail), or behavioral organization (aggression or impulsivity).

Children of the sensory stimulation-seeking type of regulation disorder may be classified as having ADHD in the DSM classification system. ADHD is fully discussed in Chapter 7, but it is important to know that hyperactive-impulsive symptoms are prominent in preschool years, in contrast to attention problems that emerge later in school-aged children (Steinhoff et al., 2006). A decision to diagnose ADHD in young children must be made with consideration for the norms of expected behavior in preschool children who are still developing their abilities to pay attention and "sit still" upon request.

Regulation disorders that involve sensory stimulation-seeking (as well as those involving negativity and defiance in response to hypersensitivity) may also be diagnosed as ODD using the DSM (see Chapter 9). Angry, argumentative, and noncompliant behaviors associated with ODD are a frequent reason for referral of preschool children to mental health professionals (Rockhill, Collett, McClellan, & Speltz, 2006). For a preschool child, some of these behaviors are generally more common because of the child's less-developed abilities in managing emotions and behavior. As a result, any diagnosis must consider whether a child's symptoms are more frequent and intense or last longer than would be expected for children of that age. In the proposed edition of DSM-V (American Psychiatric Association, 2010), a disorder called "temper regulation disorder" is being added. This newly proposed disorder is congruent with a regulation disorder of sensory processing (hypersensitivity of the negative/defiant type) in the DC:0-3R.

Sleep Behavior Disorder

When a young child has no symptoms indicative of affective disorder, a regulation disorder of sensory processing, or posttraumatic stress disorder but does experience sleep disturbance, a sleep behavior disorder is possible. A common sleep problem in young children involves trouble settling into sleep or having difficulty returning to sleep once awake. These symptoms would be indicative of a sleep-onset disorder. A second major type of sleep behavior disorder for young children is night-waking disorder. In this type, a child may have trouble maintaining sleep without waking up or have night terrors that wake the child. In both types of sleep disorder, children often show excessive sleepiness or difficulties developing a predictable sleep-wake schedule.

Feeding and Eating Disorders

There are six different types of feeding disorder. A child may have a feeding behavior disorder (1) of state regulation, (2) of caregiver-infant reciprocity, (3) associated with a concurrent medical condition, (4) associated with insults to the gastrointestinal tract, involving (5) infantile anorexia, or (6) sensory food aversions. Each type of feeding disorder reflects the causative factors involved in the feeding problems and difficulty establishing regular feeding patterns with adequate or appropriate food intake. Feeding disorders in which there are problems with state regulation or caregiver-infant reciprocity may involve either lack of adequate food intake or overeating, where the child does not regulate eating based upon feelings of hunger or fullness. A diagnosis of feeding disorder would not be made if feeding problems are only one aspect of a more generalized response that is more reflective of posttraumatic stress, regulation disorder of sensory processing, affective disorder, or adjustment disorder.

The DSM-IV-TR also specifies pica and rumination as eating disorders in early childhood. Pica involves the eating of non-nutritive substances such as feces or paint while rumination is the repeated regurgitation and re-chewing of food. Both of these disorders are usually time limited and disappear after a short period of time. However, rumination can create enduring problems in the relationship between caregiver and infant. Pica can lead to impairment of cognition or physical health problems if toxic substances are ingested.

Disorders of Relating and Communicating

Young children who experience these disorders have severe difficulties in their communication and ability to relate to others. The DC:0-3R system classifies these difficulties as multisystem developmental disorder (MSDD). All children with this disorder have significant impairments in verbal and nonverbal communication (including preverbal gestural problems). They also experience significant dysfunction in perception and comprehension of auditory stimuli, difficulty planning and organizing their movements, and hyperreactivity and or hyporeactivity to touch, movement, visual, and other sensations. However, some of these children have the ability to engage their primary caregiver in a relationship and show potential for intimacy and closeness in relating while others do not. Three patterns of MSDD have been identified based upon severity of the child's symptoms. In Pattern A, children are socially unrelated and aimless most of the time, with severe difficulty in organizing their motor behavior. For example, simple gestures are difficult. In Pattern B, children are intermittently related and capable of simple intentional gestures after nine months of age. In Pattern C, children over fifteen months of age have the capacity for consistent relatedness to others. Even when they are generally avoidant or rigid in their interactions, they have periods of warm pleasurable affect and use social gestures such as reaching, vocalizing, or exchanging objects with the caregiver. They are also capable of more complex interactive behavior such as walking a parent to the door when they are leaving. The closest DSM-IV-TR classifications for these problems are the pervasive developmental disorders discussed in Chapter 13.

Mental Health Assessment of Infants and Young Children

Practice parameters for assessment of mental disorders experienced by children and adolescents have been published by the American Academy of Child and Adolescent Psychiatry (AACAP, 1997a). A number of AACAP publications address the assessment of specific problems that are relevant to preschool and older children. Reference to these parameters can be found in the resource section at the end of this chapter. In addition, the AACAP has developed specific Practice Parameters for Psychiatric Assessment of Infants and Toddlers (AACAP, 1997b; Thomas, 1998). These guidelines recommend that assessment of young children should include a developmental, relational, and multidimensional approach. Considerations related to each of these factors are raised in the discussion that follows.

A Developmental Approach to Assessment

Since "abnormal" behavior can only be defined in comparison to expected developmental capabilities, a developmental assessment of young children is essential. A valid assessment depends on knowledge of developmental norms for children from birth to six years of age; thus, a child development handbook is an essential reference for any child mental health practitioner or primary care provider (Davies, 2004). Practitioners must also be sensitive to the fact that developmental changes occur more rapidly in early childhood than they do for older children. The developmental assessment provides descriptive information that may help to explain any contributions of a child's constitutional endowment or maturational forces to his/her mental health problems. The assessment includes information regarding communication (including speech and language for toddlers and preschool children), motor control and coordination, adaptive behavior, regulatory and coping strategies, and social engagement/socialization.

The Brazelton Neonatal Behavioral Assessment Scale–2 (Brazelton & Nugent, 1995) is still a widely used developmental assessment for neonates, measuring habituation, motor tone and activity, self-regulation, stress response, and alertness/interactive capacity. The Bayley Scales of Infant Development (Bayley, 2000) are the most widely used for infants and toddlers (ages one to forty-two months). These scales assess cognition, language, socioemotional, motor, and adaptive behavior domains. However, the Mullen Scales of Early Learning (Mullen, 1995) are preferred by many developmental psychologists for use with young children (birth to sixty-eight months) because of their focus on more complex processes associated with auditory, visual, and language development as well their utility in following children from early infancy through preschool age. The Battelle Developmental Inventory (Newborg, 2004) is also used for children ages six months through six years to assess domains such as personal-social, motor, and communication. Administration time for the full inventory is lengthier than others although it does have a shortened screening version. Its diagnostic accuracy has been questioned by some clinicians (Gilliam & Mayes, 2000). All of these assessments require training, usually in the form of a one-day workshop.

In addition to clinician-administered tests, questionnaires completed by a parent or caregiver are available to screen for developmental issues, including the Vineland Adaptive Behavior Scales (Sparrow, Cicchetti, & Balla,

2005), the Ages and Stages Questionnaire (Squires & Bricker, 2009), and three separate development inventories created for infants, young children, and preschool children by Ireton (1992). All of these questionnaires are completed by parents or other caregivers. They do not require extensive training and provide manuals with specific guidelines for administration and scoring. As a result, they are practical options for primary care and psychiatric practitioners.

Developmental capacities and limitations affect a child's participation in a mental health evaluation. Instruments and approaches must be sensitive to the developmental abilities and challenges facing the child. Assessment tools must also be normed and tested specifically with the age group of the child who is being evaluated.

A Relational Approach to Assessment

A young child's environment is inextricably linked to his/her mental health. For preschool children and younger, the primary caregiver (usually the parent) is a central attachment figure and has a significant influence over the way in which the child experiences the world. Assessment of the child's interaction with this caregiver/parent is essential. However, assessment of relationship with both parents is the ideal when possible. A number of measures have been developed for assessing interactions of young children and their parents or primary caregivers. Those that have utility for clinical practice are highlighted in Table 18.3 and will be described here.

Assessment of Parent-Child Interaction Based on Parental Report

The Parenting Stress Index (PSI and PSI/Short Form) (Abidin, 1995) is a commonly used questionnaire completed by the parent or caregiver regarding her perceptions of stress affecting the parent-child relationship, including stress specifically associated with the child. The full assessment has domains for both parent and child characteristics. The child domain assesses aspects of temperament as well as acceptability of the child to the parent and the child's reinforcement of the parent. The parent domain assesses factors such as attachment to the child, perceived competence in the parent role, and varied risk and protective factors associated with the parent's health and environment. The short form has subscales for difficult child temperament, dysfunctional parent-child interaction, and parental distress as well as total stress.

The Parental Acceptance-Rejection Questionnaire (Rohner, 2005) is an assessment of general acceptance versus maltreatment of the child by the caregiver, based on parental report of their specific attitudes and behaviors. It provides a score for overall rejection of the child as well as subscales for warmth, neglect, aggression/

Table 18.3 Assessments of the parent-child relationship

Parent Report Assessments	Domains Assessed
Parenting Stress Index	Parental Stress Parent-Child Dysfunctional Interaction Difficulty of Child
Parental Acceptance-Rejection Questionnaire	Acceptance Generalized Rejection Aggression/Hostility Neglect
Parent-Child Conflict Tactics Scales	Corporal Punishment Physical Abuse Psychological Aggression Neglect Nonviolent Discipline

Observational Assessments	Domains Assessed
Parent-Child Interaction Scales	Parent: Sensitivity Responsiveness to Distress Growth-Fostering Behavior - Cognitive - Socioemotional Infant: Clarity of Cues Responsiveness
Parent-Infant Relationship Global Assessment Scales	Adaptation versus Impairment (Abuse, Anger/Hostility, Anxious/Tense, Overinvolvement, Underinvolvement)

hostility, and generalized rejection. The Parent-Child Conflict Tactics Scales (Straus, Hamby, Finkelhor, Moore & Runyan, 1998; Straus & Mattingly, 2007) also assesses child maltreatment. This parent self-report tool consists of subscales for nonviolent discipline, psychological aggression, physical abuse, corporal punishment, and neglect. It has both a long and a short version. Assessments that use parent report can acquire detailed information about the typical child-parent interaction that could not otherwise be identified. However, all parent reports have some inherent bias.

Observational Assessments of Parent-Child Interaction

Use of observational methods avoids the bias from parental reports, but observational measures often require more extensive training and certification before using them. The Parent-Child Interaction Teaching and Feeding Scales (Sumner & Spietz, 1994) is a frequently used assessment for parent-child interactions involving children who are infants through three years of age. The subscales are used to rate caregiver sensitivity, responsiveness to the child's distress, and growth-fostering behavior toward the child during typical feeding and a semistructured teaching situation. The scales also assess the child's clarity of cues and responsiveness in these interactions with the caregiver. Videotapes of parent and child during the teaching and feeding situations facilitate rating of the interactions but are not essential. Training is required for use of this assessment.

The Parent-Infant Relationship Global Assessment Scale (PIR-GAS) is a rating scale that is part of the DC:0-3R, Axis II evaluation of disturbances in a parent-child relationship (Zero to Three, 2005). It captures general strengths versus problems in relationships ranging on a scale from well adapted to grossly impaired, with documentation of maltreatment. Ratings in the bottom third of the scale are assessed further for specific relationship disorders, including abuse (verbal, physical, or sexual), anger/hostility, anxiety/tension, overinvolvement, and underinvolvement. A Relationship Problems Checklist is available to help document the likelihood of a specific relationship disorder. Ratings on the PIR-GAS should be based on as many observations of the child and parent as possible to ensure reliability of the clinician's evaluation. A comprehensive clinical interview with the parent is also important to understand her views of the child and the dyadic relationship.

Many other observational measures with psychometric support are available to measure parent-child interaction but most require videotaping, have multiple episodes that must be evaluated, or involve home visits. Thus, they are better suited for research or when a very comprehensive assessment of the dyad is needed.

A Multidimensional Approach to Assessment

A multidimensional approach to assessment entails the use of varied components and methods rather than reliance on one brief clinical encounter with the young child and family (Egger, 2009). When mental health assessment of young children is based upon limited information, important signs or symptoms may go unrecognized and certain behavior or input may be misconstrued or overgeneralized. Economic pressures to constrict the assessment process can lead to an inaccurate or missed diagnosis, resulting in lack of essential or appropriate treatment or in unnecessary treatment that may have potentially harmful consequences for the child.

Essential components of any assessment with young children include (1) an interview with and other input from the primary caregiver/parent, (2) observation during the clinician's interaction with the child, and (3) observation of the child-caregiver dyad (discussed previously under "A Relational Approach to Assessment"). Input from other informants, such as additional family members or child care providers, is also helpful whenever possible. It is common for discrepant or conflicting impressions to emerge in an assessment of a young child. For instance, family members may differ in their views or a clinician's observations may offer findings that do not support a parent's reports obtained through an interview or questionnaire. These discrepancies can provide a better understanding of the challenges faced by the child if they are carefully considered. In addition, assessment needs to be an ongoing process, not dependent upon one session with the child or family. It is also important to remember that observations in a clinic or hospital environment may not generalize to other times and settings.

Input from the Parents or Primary Caregiver

Parental involvement in the assessment process is critical, although not sufficient. For some young children, parents may be the only adults who can reliably comment on their child's behavior. They can also facilitate their child's comfort with aspects of the assessment that include play or developmental tests. Last, their involvement can increase their understanding of important issues for discussion with the clinician and how they can support the child's progress as any intervention is planned. It is important to note, however, that parents may have only modest accuracy in identifying their child's emotional and behavioral problems, typically reporting fewer symptoms than children actually experience (Jensen et al., 1999). In fact, meta-analyses of correlations between children's self-ratings of their own problems and ratings by adults raise important questions regarding the validity of parent reports in key symptom areas (Achenbach, Krukowski, Dumenci, & Ivanova, 2005; Renk & Phares, 2004).

A very useful method for structuring a parent/caregiver interview is the Preschool Age Psychiatric Assessment (PAPA) (Egger, Ascher, & Angold, 1999; Egger & Angold, 2006). The PAPA has been developed for use with a child ages two through five years, although most aspects of the interview have relevance to slightly younger and older children as well. The interview examines all DSM-IV-TR criteria that are relevant to younger children, diagnoses addressed in DC:0-3R, and certain symptoms and behaviors not currently in any of the diagnostic systems. It also provides for assessment of family environment, family psychosocial problems, life events, and disability related to symptoms. The PAPA takes about two hours to complete and is available in both English and Spanish. A number of questionnaires are also available for assessing mental health problems in young children (Table 18.4). These are usually completed by the parent(s) or primary caregiver.

The most widely used and well tested assessment is Achenbach and Rescorla's (2000) Child Behavior Checklist (CBCL), completed by a parent/primary caregiver, and Caregiver-Teacher Report Form, typically

Table 18.4 Assessments of mental health in early childhood

Assessment	Domains Assessed	Age of Child
Child Behavior Checklist	Clinical Scales: Emotional Reactivity Anxiety/Depression Somatic Problems Withdrawal Attention Problems Aggressive Behavior Sleep Problems DSM Scales: Affectivity Anxiety Oppositional Defiant Pervasive Developmental Attention-Deficit/Hyperactivity	1½ to 5 years
Early Childhood Screening Assessment	Overall Problem Risk	1½ to 5 years
Infant-Toddler Social and Emotional Assessment I	ITSEA (Full Version): Internalizing Externalizing Dysregulation Competence BITSEA (Brief Version): Total Problems Total Competence	1 to 3 years
Toddler Behavior Screening Inventory	Total Problems Frequency of Problems	1 to 3½ years
Behavior Assessment System for Children	Adaptive Scales: Adaptability Functional Communication Social Skills Activities of Daily Living Clinical Scales: Aggression Anxiety Attention Problems Atypicality Depression Hyperactivity Somatization Withdrawal	2 to 5 years
Pediatric Symptom Checklist	Psychosocial Impairment	3 to 6+ years

Note. ITSEA: Infant-Toddler Social and Emotional Assessment
BITSEA: Brief Infant-Toddler Social and Emotional Assessment

completed by a child care provider or preschool teacher. The versions of these forms for ages 1½ to 5 years assess seven syndromes (e.g.. anxious/depressed, attention problems, aggressive behavior) that can also provide information on overall problems of either an internalizing or externalizing nature. In addition, the assessment can be used to identify a child's risk for five DSM-related diagnoses: affective problems (depression and dysthymia), anxiety (generalized and separation anxiety as well as specific phobias), ADHD, pervasive developmental problems (autism and Asperger's), and oppositional defiant problems. The different parent and teacher scales allow the clinician to acquire assessments of the child's functioning both at home and in other environments (such as child care or preschool). A briefer, but more limited, measure for the same age group is the Early Childhood Screening Assessment (Gleason, Zeanah, & Dickstein, 2010), developed specifically for primary care settings. This one-page parent questionnaire assesses the child's overall clinical risk for mental health problems and allows parents to indicate—for each item on the questionnaire—whether they have concerns about that aspect of their child's behavior. A unique feature of this measure is the inclusion of four items assessing parental depression and distress.

For children ages one to three years, there are two other useful assessments that can be completed by parents. One is the Infant-Toddler Social and Emotional Assessment (ITSEA), which comes in both a full form and a brief (BITSEA) sixty-item version (Briggs-Gowan et al., 2004; Carter, Briggs-Gowan, Jones, & Little, 2003). Like the CBCL, the ITSEA examines externalizing and internalizing problems as well as dysregulation and an assessment of competencies. The brief screening version (BITSEA) provides only a general index of potential problem severity and competency, with little attention to the specific nature of the problems. Another general screening tool for number and frequency of problems is the Toddler Behavior Screening Inventory (McCain, Kelley, & Fishbein, 1999; Mouton-Simien, McCain, & Kelley, 1997). It lacks testing with ethnically and socioeconomically diverse families in contrast to the other assessments.

For children ages 2½ to 5 or 6 years, the Behavior Assessment System for Children (BASC) (Reynolds & Kamphaus, 1992, 2002), the Early Childhood Symptom Inventory (ECSI) (Gadow & Sprafkin, 2000; Sprafkin, Volpe, Gadow, Nolan, & Kelly, 2002), and the Pediatric Symptom Checklist (PSC) (Jellinek et al., 1988; Jellinek & Murphy, 1990) are also available. All of these are easy to administer and provide cut-off scores or norms for general psychosocial impairment. Like the CBCL, the BASC and the ECSI allow for a fairly comprehensive

assessment of specific types of problems. The BASC provides a detailed differentiation of externalizing and internalizing problems as well as adaptive skills; it is also available in Spanish. The ECSI identifies problems related to specific DSM-IV diagnoses. In contrast, the PSC is a general screen for overall psychosocial impairment but does not provide scores for specific problem areas.

The assessments just given provide general measures of psychiatric symptoms in early childhood. There are also screening tools as well as detailed assessments for specific psychiatric disorders of young children. These can be used when a specific problem is suspected or once a child has been referred for a comprehensive workup by more specialized clinicians.

Observation and Interaction with the Child

Direct observation of young children's behavior is always necessary, both with the caregiver and separate from the caregiver. There is potential variability of behavior and experience across conditions so it is important to gather information about responses in different settings, at different times, and from varied people. The assessment environment can influence the child's response, especially the degree of structure in the assessment procedures, the complexity of the physical layout of the room, a child's familiarity with the environment, and adults who are interacting with the child. These factors should be considered in planning an assessment that is most useful for each particular child and allows for the best evaluation of specific functions or behaviors. Usually, some combination of a structured and unstructured format yields the most meaningful information, allowing children to show their strengths and limitations in the fullest way. Factors such as time of day and the child's resulting degree of fatigue or hunger can also influence a child's responses substantially so clinical observations and tests should be scheduled accordingly.

The Infant and Toddler Mental Status Exam (ITMSE) (Benham, 2000) is widely recognized for its usefulness in assessing the mental status of children from birth to five years. It was originally published by the American Academy of Child and Adolescent Psychiatry as part of the Practice Parameters for Assessment of Infants and Toddlers (AACAP, 1997b). The ITMSE provides a structure for examining traditional domains of the mental status exam but with modifications appropriate to young children. The ITMSE is useful in organizing observational data from a variety of sources. Instructions and guidelines for the examiner are provided. The domains examined with the ITMSE are shown in Table 18.5.

Table 18.5 Dimensions assessed with the Infant-Toddler Mental Status Exam

Appearance

Reaction to the Situation

Self-Regulation

Motor Coordination

Speech and Language

Thought

Affect and Mood

Structure and Content of Play

Cognition

Relatedness

For children as young as two or three years, many play-based methods can be used to gather information. Examples include the Berkeley Puppet Interview (Measelle, Ablow, Cowan, & Cowan, 1998) and the story stem technique (Gaensbauer & Kelsay, 2008; Warren, Emde & Sroufe, 2000). The puppet interview helps children express their feelings by projecting them onto the puppets. It has nine subscales that assess most of the DSM-IV-TR disorders. In the story stem technique, the clinician begins a story around specific toys that are put in front of the child and asks the child to complete the story by showing or telling the clinician what happens next. In addition to these approaches, a variety of helpful aids are available such as pictures and books of doll faces or animals showing different emotions or situations from which children can choose. Resources for assessment are referenced at the end of the chapter.

Evidence-Based Intervention

Five types of intervention are most commonly used to treat mental health problems in early childhood. These include behavioral therapies, play therapy, child-parent therapy, use of psychotropic agents, and ecosystemic interventions that address risk factors in the child's environment. Because few studies have been conducted to evaluate interventions for young children, there is simply less evidence available than for older children or adults. Reasons for the lack of studies include (1) minimal appreciation previously of the profound importance of early sensitive periods in neurobiological development and their role in later mental health outcomes and (2) the absence of appropriate measures to assess outcomes for young children. However, researchers have begun to address these problems within the last decade. Each of the interventions discussed here has shown effectiveness for various mental health problems experienced by young children, as evidenced by research, reviews of data from case studies, or expert consensus (Burns & Hoagwood, 2005; Zimmer-Gembeck, 2007). Table 18.6 presents the major interventions used with young children, along with their most common rationale for use and the typical age range of children with whom they are used.

Behavioral Therapies

Behaviorally based interventions build upon operant and classic conditioning theories and are used when the goal is to increase adaptive behavior for the child or reduce problematic behavior. Behavioral intervention involves approaches such as shaping, prompting, and reinforcement (Goodman & Scott, 2005; Koegel, Koegel, & Brookman, 2003). For preschool children, these approaches are widely used to enhance behaviors associated with relating and communicating in disorders such as autism or to address aggressive or impulsive behaviors that may stem from regulation disorders of sensory processing (Tamm et al., 2005; Webster-Stratton, Reid, & Hammond, 2004). Parent training in behavioral therapies can be effective to help parents manage problem behaviors through use of prompts and praise as well as token systems that pair reinforcers such as food or toys with tokens such as marbles (Morawska & Sanders, 2006). Parent training also involves teaching them to give clear, concise directions to enhance the child's compliance.

In addition, systematic desensitization (a classic conditioning technique) may help a young child to overcome a specific phobia or address avoidance of certain situations or stimuli that a child associates with previous traumatic stress. These and basic cognitive-behavioral approaches have shown much promise in treating sexually abused preschool children, indicating that children as young as three years of age can understand and benefit from cognitive-behavioral approaches such as relaxation techniques, creation of a stimulus hierarchy of fears, and graded exposure to achieve engagement with a trauma memory or feared object (Deblinger, Stauffer, & Steer, 2001; Scheeringa et al., 2007). These latter approaches become effective when cognitive abilities such as abstract reasoning and a beginning understanding of causal relationships emerge around thirty-six months of age. See Chapter 17 for further discussion of behavioral therapies.

Play Therapy

Beginning at about two years of age, a child develops the capacity for imagery and symbolism. Fantasy play is a central feature of development that begins at about

Table 18.6 Indications for various types of intervention with young children

Type of Intervention	Rationale for Use	Typical Age Range
Behavioral Therapy	Child's problematic behaviors need to be reduced and more adaptive ones developed	1 to 6 years
Play Therapy	Child's emotions need to be expressed and/or worked through	2 to 6 years
Parent-Child Therapy	Improvement in parent's attitudes or in the parent-child relationship is needed	6 months to 6 years
Medication	A neurochemical imbalance or deficit needs to be addressed	3 to 6 years
Environmental Intervention	Stressors in the physical or psychosocial environment need to be resolved or decreased	Birth to 6 years

3 years of age. Also, between 2 and 3 years of age, a child starts to use very brief sentences consisting of a few words and can answer simple questions. All of these capacities allow a child to participate in representational play, including symbolization, enactment of situations, and storytelling. Children also can begin to report their life experiences as they relate to the play and develop a narrative about their life with some understanding of its continuity over time. Lastly, emotional competence is developing during preschool years, including skills in the understanding, expression, and regulation of emotional states. Play therapy for toddlers and preschool children capitalizes on these emerging capabilities using both psychodynamic and client-centered underpinnings as a theoretical base (Chethik, 2000; Landreth, 2002a, 2002b; Schaefer, Kelly-Zion, McCormick, & Ohnogi, 2008).

In addition to being a window to the young child's inner world, play therapy is a comfortable, age-appropriate way for the child to approach needed change. Play therapy can assist in both expression of the child's emotions and experiences as well as in the building of emotion-based skills such as coping and self-regulation. These two components have been described as expressive and formative aspects of play therapy (Benham & Slotnik, 2006; Russ, 2004). Through the expressive component, a child can explore a variety of feelings through both play activities and accompanying verbalization. Through the formative component, a child can acquire new capacities for impulse control, frustration tolerance, sublimation, and other affect management strategies. Depending on particular needs of a child, clinicians can work solely with the child or in conjunction with a parent/caregiver, sometimes called filial therapy (Landreth & Bratton, 2006). However, the focus of the therapy

is still on the child, with the clinician helping parents enhance their child's mental health through play techniques. See Chapter 15 for a more detailed discussion of play therapy.

Child-Parent Therapy

Child-parent therapy involves dyadic psychotherapy for a young child and his/her primary caregiver. It typically involves a combination of developmental guidance, insight-oriented psychotherapy, emotional support, and practical help for the parent/caregiver (Lieberman, 2004; Lieberman & Van Horn, 2009). The relationship is the focus of the intervention, with the goal being enhanced ability of the caregiver to provide responsive, therapeutic care to the young child. The interaction between child and parent during play sessions is the basis for observation and discussion with the caregiver, serving as a stimulus for examination of his/her own emotional issues and challenges. Current problems in the child-parent relationship are related to the caregiver's past and present difficulties. The caregiver is helped to separate these issues from his/her care of the child and to modify any detrimental approaches the caregiver may be using in caring for the child. This type of intervention has been especially successful with young high-risk children who have been traumatized and with mothers and children who are living in violent situations (Lieberman, Ghosh-Ippen, & Van Horn, 2005).

Child-parent therapy has been used most frequently to work with parents of infants and toddlers. Packaged programs are available to assist practitioners, such as the "Circle of Security" (Marvin, Cooper, Hoffman, & Powell, 2002) and "Watch, Wait and Wonder" (Muir, Lojkasek, & Cohen, 1999). Similarly, a technique called "interaction guidance" helps parents develop an understanding of their own and their infant/toddler's behavior (McDonough, 2004). In each of these approaches, discussion of videotapes of interactive play sessions are used to highlight and reinforce a parent's positive interactions with a child and to offer suggested changes to more troublesome interactions.

Child-parent therapies most frequently build on theoretical foundations having psychodynamic traditions, including object relations and attachment theories (Bienenfeld, 2006; Cassidy & Shaver, 2008). Studies support the value of such interventions in improving caregiving behavior, reducing parental stress and child behavior problems, and enhancing adaptive behaviors for young children (Bakermans-Kranenburg, van IJzendoorn, & Juffer, 2003; Lieberman, Ghosh-Ippen, & Van Horn, 2006).

Psychopharmacology

While the safety and efficacy of using psychotropic medications with older children are more accepted, prescribing these medications to preschool-aged children or younger elicits some degree of apprehension in clinicians and families alike. In addition, guidelines addressing use of psychotropic medications for treating mental health problems in this younger age group are limited. The impact of early exposure to psychotropic agents is poorly understood, including effects on the brain during the rapid neurodevelopmental changes occurring in the first six years of life. However, research efforts are in place to build a body of knowledge that can inform and guide clinical practice (Greenhill et al., 2003).

Thus, the APN must approach the use of psychotropic medications in this age group carefully, conservatively, and with ample consideration given to potential benefits and costs of their use in each individual situation. Psychotherapeutic interventions should be the first line of treatment and ideally continued, even after addition of medication. Consensus among some experts is that persistence of symptoms and functional impairment at a moderate to severe level warrants implementation of a trial of medication, whereas medication is not indicated when symptoms and functional impairment are mild (Fanton & Gleason, 2009; Gleason et al., 2007). Adequate time must be given to families for discussion of expected benefits and potential side effects. Part of this discussion, when applicable, should include informing the family about off-label use of medications.

There are currently only four medications that are Food and Drug Administration (FDA) approved for psychiatric treatment in children younger than six years: chlorpromazine, haloperidol, and risperidone for severe behavioral problems, and dextroamphetamines for ADHD. This means that when decisions about medication choice need to be made the APN may face the reality of recommending medication for off-label use. An important point to bear in mind for both the clinician and the family is that off-label does not necessarily mean lack of efficacy, only that the FDA has not given approval for the medication to be used for a specific purpose in a particular age group. There are algorithms that have been developed from research and case reports that can guide clinicians in making decisions about off-label use for young children who have ADHD, disruptive behavior disorders, anxiety disorders, mood disorders, pervasive developmental disorders, and sleep disorders (Gleason et al., 2007). Off-label medications that are often recommended include methylphenidate for ADHD, fluoxetine for depression or anxiety disorders, and clonidine as a second-line agent for ADHD. There has also been limited success with use of clonidine to address aggression, hypervigilance, and generalized anxiety associated with PTSD (Harmon & Riggs, 1996).

Once the family has been fully informed and agrees to a trial of psychotropic medication, a plan for monitoring benefits and side effects needs to be developed. There should be agreement as to what symptoms and behaviors are to be the focus of treatment. Input from beyond the family (e.g., from therapists or preschool teachers) is essential. Ongoing communication with the primary care provider is important. Initial contact with the family should be frequent in the interest of nurturing a trusting nurse practitioner–family relationship, as the family's anxiety level is likely to be high in the beginning. Practical challenges need to be addressed early on, such as side effects of the medication and how it is formulated to ensure that the child will take it. As the child and family settle into a maintenance phase, contact can be less frequent, though it will remain important for the nurse practitioner to be available and supportive throughout treatment. Once all involved agree that the child has been stable for awhile, a medication discontinuation trial can be attempted. During this phase of treatment, more frequent contact is recommended.

There have been concerns expressed about the growing number of preschool children receiving psychotropic medication as treatment (Debar, Lynch, Powell, & Gale, 2003; Zito & Safer, 2005). However, use of psychotropic medication in children preschool age and younger can be an effective option when psychotherapy or other interventions have not brought about adequate relief of symptoms. Used conscientiously and in a planned way, with parent/caretaker's understanding and support, these agents can allow very young children to develop and engage in their world at a more optimal level.

Environmental Intervention

Environmental interventions are those that identify and address environmental needs and problems that may place the mental health of children at risk or preclude their benefiting from other interventions. Ecosystemic models of care consider relationships within families, their immediate communities, and the wider culture. Thus, addressing problems in the child's environment may target a variety of areas, including (1) the need for parent therapy that attends to a parent's own psychological symptoms, (2) family therapy to reduce conflict/violence and enhance the cohesion, adaptability, or coping among members of the family, and (3) larger social interventions to deal with problems in foster/child care, in the preschool setting, or socioeconomic constraints. These interventions build upon general system theories that recognize the impact of exposure to multiple stressors from multiple contexts on the young child's mental health (Bronfenbrenner, 1989; Cowan & Cowan, 2006). Environmental interventions often are used in conjunction with other types of intervention such as play therapy or child-parent therapy (Ammen & Limberg, 2005; Limberg & Ammen, 2008).

Environmental interventions are responsive to a "systems of care model" recommended by the Surgeon General's Commission on Mental Health of Children (U.S. Public Health Service, 2000), whereby the child and family have access to a wide range of services that address multiple needs. This approach requires collaboration between service agencies and providers to coordinate and create integrative care. Environmental approaches show evidence of great potential to improve outcomes for very young children and their families (Olds, Sadler, & Kitzman, 2007; Pulleyblank, 2004).

Collaboration between Primary Care and Child Psychiatry

Early signs of potential mental health problems are typically identified by the pediatric nurse practitioner (PNP), pediatrician, or other primary care provider (PCP) during routine well-baby/child visits. Parents or caregivers may raise specific concerns or the PCP may observe certain behaviors of the child during her/his general assessment, suggesting the need for further screening. In some agencies, the PCP might perform more focused assessments of specific mental health concerns if screening is warranted. In most agencies, the child is then referred by a PCP to professionals who have specialized preparation in child mental health. This individual may be an advanced practice child or family psychiatric nurse or other mental health professional. Rather than a direct referral, the PCP may use a telephone/email consultation or bring in the mental health professional for an on-site consultation. Based on this more thorough discussion, a plan can then be developed for further screening or intervention in the primary care setting or for more detailed assessment or treatment at a mental health clinic/agency in complex cases.

In integrated practice environments, mental health professionals and pediatric practitioners may be housed in the same facility. Such environments can reduce any stigma and a family's fears regarding seeing a mental health professional because the family is familiar with seeing their PCP at the same site. The integrated environment can enhance coordination between primary care and behavioral health as well as a family's awareness of the availability and importance of mental health services (Weiss, Haber, Horowitz, Wolfe, & Stuart, 2009).

Case Exemplar

Jacob is a 3½-year-old boy referred for a mental health evaluation by his PNP. The referral has been made to an early childhood mental health agency. A family psychiatric nurse practitioner (FPNP) at the agency conducted a telephone interview with Jacob's PNP, who had become concerned about his mental health based on observations during primary care visits, as well as family history and family dynamics that put him at risk. In addition, he had scored below the norm in the area of communication on an Ages and Stages Questionnaire (ASQ). Jacob's general health is good with the exception of wheezing with upper respiratory infections that has been responsive to bronchodilator treatment.

Jacob lives with his parents and two maternal half-brothers (ages six and eight years) in a small two-bedroom apartment. His mother has a history of bipolar disorder, substance abuse, and learning disabilities. She was abandoned by her single mother and entered the foster care system as a teenager. His father has a history of ADHD, depression, and substance abuse. One half-brother was being treated for anxiety and depression; the other, for ADHD.

Jacob was exposed in utero to tobacco, alcohol, and methamphetamine. He was delivered vaginally at term with a positive toxicology screen for amphetamines but no other perinatal or neonatal complications. Both parents were in their twenties at the time of his birth. Child Protective Services was involved until he was eighteen months of age. During that period the family had access to many services and did relatively well; but once these services ended, the family's life became increasingly chaotic. The parents are caring but overwhelmed. Jacob's father has a part-time job at a supermarket; his mother has not been employed for several years.

The FPNP brought Jacob and his family in for an observational interview using the Infant and Toddler Mental Status Exam (ITMSE). Jacob played with his back to his brothers, as if guarding his toys. With the FPNP he was reluctant to interact and kept his eyes downcast, though with gentle encouragement he would engage briefly in reciprocal play with a ball. He was mostly mute, offering occasional softly spoken one-word responses to questions. At times he appeared to not understand simple instructions, behavior that his parents interpreted as defiance. The session was filled with bickering among the brothers interspersed with loud bursts of crying and screaming from Jacob when one of his brothers grabbed a toy from him. The parents attempted to manage the boys' behavior with varying degrees of patience and frustration and were successful only sometimes.

The FPNP next conducted a diagnostic interview with Jacob's parents using the PAPA. His parents also completed a CBCL. Based on information gathered through interviews, observations and the CBCL, a diagnosis of *mixed disorder of emotional expressiveness* was made, with indications that he was at risk of developing an anxiety disorder. Concern about his communication skills that arose from completion of the ASQ was also incorporated into the treatment plan, as communication delays could be affecting Jacob's emotional reactivity. The FPNP engaged Jacob's parents in a discussion of the many factors impacting his behavior and mental health, and together they formulated a treatment plan:

1. Enrollment in a therapeutic nursery school (TNS), including play therapy with the FPNP
2. Family therapy and psychoeducation
3. Wrap-around services for assistance with practical needs
4. Case management by the FPNP for care coordination
5. Use of psychotropic medication put on hold initially until the effects of other interventions are assessed; hypervigilance and anxiety around children in the TNS resulted in the FPNP later prescribing clonidine in consultation with the psychiatrist.
6. Referral for a speech/language evaluation
7. Monitoring by the PNP of wheezing episodes and the impact of illness/medications on Jacob's behavior
8. Ongoing mutual consultation between the FPNP and PNP

Implications for Research and Education

There is an urgent need for increased research in the field of early childhood mental health. Because of the problems associated with self-report by young children, researchers often choose to study mental health problems in older groups of children or adolescents. However, the foundations of many disorders emerge in early childhood, and it is essential to understand early markers of later problems and the course of particular problems from birth into school age and beyond. The DC:0-3R classification system has advanced the ability to appropriately diagnose mental health problems of young children. However, there is still a need to clarify how signs and symptoms of various disorders may differ in infants, toddlers, and preschool-age children. Improved understanding of symptoms in the first two years of life is particularly critical. There should also be eventual congruence between the DC:0-3 and DSM classification systems. In addition, there is the need for continued development and refinement of psychometrically sound mental health assessments for children ages six and under. Lack of assessments for initial problems during the first year of life is especially problematic. Development of screening tools for identification of specific mental disorders is also essential, especially internalizing disorders that are more difficult to assess in young children. The high incidence of diagnoses for ADHD and ODD in children under six years of age may be due, to some extent, to less difficulty identifying externalizing problems in children, combined with the availability of specific screening tools to assess these disorders in this age group. Last, continued attention must be given to the evaluation of both preventive and treatment interventions for young children. This last decade has seen significant advances in the evidence base to support the efficacy of a variety of interventions for this age group. Larger studies are now needed to demonstrate their effectiveness when used in practice environments with diverse populations of children and families.

There is also a need for improved education in the assessment and treatment of young children's mental health problems. Because of the broad range of age groups that must be covered in pediatric and child psychiatric specialty education, most of the focus is often on school-aged children and adolescents. In addition, faculty members with expertise in the mental health problems of young children are frequently unavailable. These deficits are even more likely in education for medical or psychiatric family practice where coursework and clinical experience have a life span focus. However, inadequate content about mental health problems of young children and lack of clinical experience with this population are unacceptable in any educational program whose graduates will have responsibility for child or family health. If necessary, experts from the community, from other disciplines, or from other universities should be used as consultants or adjunct faculty to provide content about mental health assessment and treatment for children from birth to six years of age.

Resources

Websites

American Academy of Child and Adolescent Psychiatry. http://www.aacap.org/

American Academy of Pediatrics, Bright Futures Initiative. http://brightfutures.aap.org/

Center for Play Therapy. http://cpt.unt.edu

Head Start Programs, U.S. Department of Health and Human Services, Administration for Children and Families. www.acf.hhs.gov/programs/ohs

National Center for Infant and Early Childhood Health Policy at UCLA, www.healthychild.ucla.edu

National Institute of Mental Health (NIMH), Medication Resource List. http://www.nimh.nih.gov/health/publications/mental-health-medications/alphabetical-list-of-medications.shtml

Research Diagnostic Criteria – Preschool Age (RDC-PA). www.infantinstitute.org/RDC-PA.htm

Zero to Three: Center for Infants, Toddlers and Families. http://www.zerotothree.org/site/PageServer?pagename=homepage

Reference Books

Buysse, V., & Wesley, P. (2006). *Evidence-based practice in the early childhood field*. Washington, D.C.: National Center for Infants, Toddlers, and Families.

DelCarmen-Wiggins, R., & Carter, A. (Eds,). (2004). *Handbook of infant, toddler and preschool mental health assessment*. New York, NY: Oxford University Press.

Finello, K. (2005). *Handbook of training and practice in infant and preschool mental health*. New York, NY: Josssey Bass.

Guedeney, A., & Maestro, S. (Eds.). (2003). The use of the diagnostic classification 0-3. *Infant Mental Health Journal, 24*(3)[Special Issue].

Keilty, B. (Ed.). (2009). *The early intervention guidebook for families and professionals: Partnering for success*. New York, NY: Teachers College Press.

Lieberman, A., Wieder, S., & Fenichel, E. (1997). *DC:0-3 casebook: A guide to the use of zero to three's "diagnostic classification of mental health and developmental disorders of infancy and early childhood" in assessment and treatment planning*. Washington, DC: National Center for Infants, Toddlers, and Families.

Luby, J.L. (2006). *Handbook of preschool mental health: Development, disorders and treatment*. New York, NY: Guilford Press.

Maldonado-Duran, J.M. (2002). *Infant and toddler mental health: Models of clinical intervention with infants and their families*. Washington, DC: American Psychiatric Publishing, Inc.

Papousek, M., Schieche, M.. & Wurmser, H. (2007). *Disorders of behavioral and emotional regulation in the first years of life: Early risks and intervention in the developing parent-infant relationship*. Washington, DC: National Center for Infants, Toddlers, and Families.

Parlakian, R. (2004). *How culture shapes social-emotional development: Implications for practice in infant-family programs*. Washington, DC: National Center for Infants, Toddlers, and Families.

Sameroff, A.T., McDonough, S.C., & Rosenblum, K.L. (Eds.). (2005). *Treating parent-infant relationship problems: Strategies for intervention*. New York, NY: Guilford Press.

Shonkoff, J., & Meisels, S.J. (Eds.). (2000). *Handbook of early childhood intervention*. Cambridge, UK: Cambridge University Press.

Shonkoff, J., & Phillips, D. (2000). *From neurons to neighborhoods: The science of early childhood development*. Washington, D.C.: National Academies Press.

Zeanah, C. (2009). *Handbook of infant mental health* (third edition). New York, NY: Guilford Press.

Zeanah, P., Stafford, B., & Zeanah, C. (2005). *Clinical interventions to enhance infant mental health: A selective review*. Los Angeles, CA: National Center for Infant and Early Childhood Health Policy at University of California Los Angeles.

Zero to Three. (2005). *Diagnostic classification of mental health and developmental disorders of infancy and early childhood (DC: 0-3R)*. Revised Edition. Washington, D.C.: National Center for Infants, Toddlers and Families.

References

Abidin, R.R. (1995). *Parenting stress index: Manual*. Charlottesville, VA: University of Virginia, Pediatric Psychology Press.

Achenbach, T., & Rescorla, L.A. (2000). *Manual for the ASEBA preschool forms and profiles: An integrated system of multi-informant assessment*. Burlingon, VT: University of Vermont Department of Psychiatry.

Achenbach, T., Krukowski, R., Dumenci, L., & Ivanova, M. (2005). Assessment of adult psychopathology: Meta-analyses and implications of cross-informant correlations. *Psychological Bulletin, 131*, 361–382.

American Academy of Child and Adolescent Psychiatry. (1997a). Practice parameters for the psychiatric assessment of children and adolescents. *Journal of the American Academy of Child and Adolescent Psychiatry 36*(10 suppl), 4s–20s.

American Academy of Child and Adolescent Psychiatry. (1997b). Practice parameters for the psychiatric assessment of infants and toddlers (0-36 months). *Journal of the American Academy of Child and Adolescent Psychiatry 36*(10 suppl), 21s–36s.

American Psychiatric Association. (2000). *Diagnostic and statistical manual of mental disorders* (fourth edition, text revision). Washington, D.C.: American Psychiatric Press.

American Psychiatric Association. (2010). *Proposed draft revisions to DSM disorders and criteria*. Retrieved from ww.dsm5.org/ProposedRevisions/Pages/Default.aspx

Ammen, S., & Limberg, B. (2005). Play therapy with preschoolers using the ecosystemic model. In K. Finello (Ed.), *Handbook of training and practice in infant and preschool mental health* (pp. 207–232). New York, NY: Jossey Bass.

Bakermans-Kranenburg, M., Van IJzendoorn, M., & Juffer, F. (2003). Less is more: Meta-analysis of sensitivity and attachment interventions in early childhood. *Psychological Bulletin, 129*, 195–215.

Bayley, N. (2000). *Bayley scales of infant development* (third edition). San Antonio, TX: Psychological Corporation.

Benham, A. L. (2000). The observation and assessment of young children including use of the infant-toddler mental status exam. In C.H. Zeanah (Ed.), *Handbook of infant mental health* (second edition) (pp. 249–266). New York, NY: The Guilford Press.

Benham, A.L., & Slotnick, C.F. (2006). Play therapy: Integrating clinical and developmental perspectives. In J.L. Luby (Ed.), *Handbook of preschool mental health* (pp. 331–371). New York, NY: Guilford Press.

Bienenfeld, D. (2006). *Psychodynamic theory for clinicians.* Philadelphia, PA: Lippincott, Williams & Wilkins.

Blandon, A., Calkins, S., Keane, S., & O'Brien, M. (2008). Individual differences in trajectories of emotion regulation processes: The effects of maternal depressive symptomatology and children's physiological regulation. *Developmental Psychology, 44*, 1110–1123.

Boyce, W.T., & Ellis, B. (2005). Biological sensitivity to context: An evolutionary developmental theory of the origins and functions of stress reactivity. *Development and Psychopathology, 17*, 271–301.

Brazelton, T.B., & Nugent, K. (1995). *The neonatal behavioral assessment scale.* Cambridge, MA: MacKeith Press.

Briggs-Gowan, M.J., & Carter, A.S. (2008). Social-emotional screening status in early childhood predicts elementary school outcomes. *Pediatrics, 121*, 957–962.

Briggs-Gowan,M.J.,Carter,A.S.,Irwin,I.R.,Wachtel,K.,&Cicchetti,D.V. (2004). The brief infant-toddler social emotional assessment: Screening for social-emotional problems and delays in competence. *Journal of Pediatric Psychology, 29*, 143–155.

Bronfenbrenner, U. (1989). Ecological systems theory. In R. Vasta (Ed.), *Annals of child development* (pp. 187–248). Greenwich, CT: JAI.

Burns, B., & Hoagwood, K. (Eds.). (2005). Evidence-based practice, part II: Effecting change [Special Issue]. *Child and Adolescent Psychiatric Clinics of North America, 14*(2).

Carter, A., Briggs-Gowan, M.J., Jones, S., & Little, T.D. (2003). The infant-toddler socio-emotional assessment: Factor structure, reliability, and validity. *Journal of Abnormal Child Psychology, 31*, 495–514.

Carter, A., Briggs-Gowan, M.J, & Davis, N. (2004). Assessment of young children's social-emotional development and psychopathology: Recent advances and recommendations for practice. *Journal of Child Psychology and Psychiatry, 45*, 109–134.

Cassidy, J., & Shaver, P.R. (Eds.). (2008). *Handbook of attachment: Theory, research and clinical applications.* New York, NY: Guilford Press.

Chethik, M. (2000). *Techniques of child therapy: Psychodynamic strategies* (second edition). New York, NY: Guilford Press.

Cicchetti, D., & Curtis, W.J. (2006). The developing brain and neural plasticity: Implications for normality, psychopathology and resilience. In D. Cicchetti & D. Cohen (Eds.), *Developmental psychopathology: Theory and method* (Vol. 2) (pp. 26–33). Hoboken, NJ: John Wiley & Sons.

Cordeiro, M., Caldeira da Silva, P., & Goldschmidt, T. (2003). Diagnostic classification: Results from a clinical experience of three years with DC:0-3. *Infant Mental Health Journal, 24*, 349–364.

Cowan, P., & Cowan, C. (2006). Developmental psychopathology from family systems and family risk factors perspectives: Implications for family research, practice and policy. In D. Cicchetti & D. Cohen (Eds.), *Developmental psychopathology: Theory and Method* (pp. 530–587). Hoboken, NJ: John Wiley & Sons.

Davies, D. (2004). *Child development: A practitioner's guide* (second edtion). New York, NY: Guilford Press.

DeBar, L.L., Lynch, F., Powell, J., & Gale, J. (2003). Use of psychotropic agents in preschool children: Associated symptoms, diagnoses and health care services in a health maintenance organization. *Archives of Pediatrics and Adolescent Medicine, 157*, 150–157.

Deblinger, E., Stauffer, L., & Steer, R. (2001). Comparative efficacies of supportive and cognitive behavioral group therapies for young children who have been sexually abused and their non-offending mothers. *Child Maltreatment, 6*, 332–343.

Egger, H. (2009). Psychiatric assessment of young children. *Child and Adolescent Psychiatric Clinics of North America, 18*, 559–580.

Egger, H., & Angold, A. (2006). Common emotional and behavioral disorders in preschool children: Presentation, nosology, and epidemiology. *Journal of Child Psychology and Psychiatry, 47*, 313–337.

Egger, H.L., Ascher, B.H., & Angold, A. (1999). *The preschool age psychiatric assessment: Version I.I.* Unpublished interview schedule. Durham, NC: Center for Developmental Epidemiology, Department of Psychiatry and Behavior Sciences, Duke University Medical Center.

Fanton, J.F., & Gleason, M.M. (2009). Psychopharmacology and preschoolers: A critical review of current conditions. *Child and Adolescent Psychiatric Clinics of North America, 18*, 753–771.

Frankel, K.A., Boyum, L.A., & Harmon, R.J. (2004). Diagnoses and presenting symptoms in an infant psychiatry clinic: Comparison of two diagnostic systems. *Journal of the American Academy of Child and Adolescent Psychiatry, 43*, 578–587.

Gadow, K.D., & Sprafkin, J. (2000). *Early childhood symptom inventory–4. Screening manual.* Stonybrook, NY: Checkmate Plus.

Gaensbauer, T.J., & Kelsay, K. (2008). Situational and story-stem scaffolding in psychodynamic play therapy with very young children. In C.E. Schaefer, S. Kelly-Zion, J. McCormick, & A. Ohnogi (Eds.), *Play therapy for very young children* (pp. 173–198). Lanham, MD: Jason Aronson.

Gilliam, W.S., & Mayes, L.C. (2000). Developmental assessment of infants and toddlers. In C.H. Zeanah, Jr. (Ed.), *Handbook of infant mental health* (pp. 236–248). New York, NY: Guilford.

Gleason,M.M.,Egger,H.L.,Emslie,G.J.,Greenhill,L.L.,Kowatch,R.A., Lieberman, A.F., & Zeanah, C.H. (2007). Psychopharmacological treatment for very young children: Contexts and guidelines. *Journal of the American Academy of Child and Adolescent Psychiatry, 46*, 1532–1572.

Gleason, M.M., Zeanah, C.H., & Dickstein, S. (2010). Recognizing young children in need of mental health assessment: Development and preliminary validity of the early childhood screen assessment. *Infant Mental Health Journal, 31*, 335–357.

Goodman, R., & Scott, S. (2005). Behaviorally-based treatments. In R. Goodman & S. Scott (Eds.), *Child psychiatry* (pp. 273–280). Oxford, UK: Blackwell Publishing.

Greenhill, L., Jensen, P., Abikoff, H., Blumer, J., Deveaugh-Geiss, J., Fisher, C., & Zeanah, C. (2003). Developing strategies for psychopharmacological studies in preschool children. *Journal of the American Academy of Child and Adolescent Psychiatry, 42*, 406–414.

Guedeney, N., Guedeney, A., Rabouam, C., Mintz, A, Danon, G., Huet, M., & Jacqueman, F. (2003). The zero to three diagnostic classification: A contribution to the validation of this classification from a sample of 85 under-threes. *Infant Mental Health Journal, 24*, 313–336.

Hankin, B., & Abela, F. (2005). *Development of psychopathology.* Thousand Oaks, CA: Sage Publications.

Harmon, R.J., & Riggs, P.D. (1996). Clonidine for posttraumatic stress disorder in preschool children. *Journal of the American Academy of Child and Adolescent Psychiatry, 35*, 1247–1249.

Ireton, H.R. (1992). *Child development inventories.* Minneapolis, MN: Behavior Science Systems.

Jellinek, M.S., & Murphy, J.M. (1990). The recognition of psychosocial disorders in pediatric office practice: The current status of the pediatric symptom checklist. *Journal of Developmental and Behavioral Pediatrics, 11*, 273–278.

Jellinek, M.S., Murphy, J.M., Robinson, J., Feins, A., Lamb, S., & Fenton, T. (1988). Pediatric symptom checklist: Screening school-age children for psychosocial dysfunction. *Pediatrics, 112*, 201–209.

Jensen, P.S., Rubio-Stipec, M., Canino, G., Bird, H.R., Dulcan, M.K., Schwab-Stone, M.E., & Lahey, B.B. (1999). Parent and child contributions to diagnosis of mental disorder: Are both informants always necessary? *Journal of the American Academy of Child and Adolescent Psychiatry, 38*, 1560–1579.

Koegel, R., Koegel, L., & Brookman, L. (2003). Empirically supported pivotal response interventions for children with autism. In A.E. Kazdin (Ed.), *Evidence-based psychotherapies for children and adolescents* (pp. 341–357). New York, NY: Guilford Press.

Landreth, G. (2002a). *Play therapy: The art of the relationship.* New York, NY: Brunner-Routledge.

Landreth, G. (2002b). *Innovations in play therapy.* New York, NY: Brunner-Routledge.

Landreth, G., & Bratton, S. (2006). *Child-parent relationship therapy.* New York, NY: Routledge.

Lavigne, J.V., LeBailly, S.A., Hopkins, J., Gouze, K.R., & Binns, H.J. (2009). The prevalence of ADHD, ODD, depression, and anxiety in a community sample of 4 year-olds. *Journal of Clinical Child & Adolescent Psychology, 38*, 315–328.

Lieberman, A.F. (2004). Child-parent psychotherapy. In A. Sameroff, S. McDonough, & K. Rosenblum (Eds.), *Treatment of infant-parent relationship disturbances* (pp. 97–122). New York, NY: Guilford Press.

Lieberman, A.F., Ghosh-Ippen, C., & Van Horn, P. (2006). Child-parent psychotherapy: 6 month follow up of a randomized controlled trial. *Journal of the American Academy of Child and Adolescent Psychiatry, 45*, 913–918.

Lieberman, A.F., & Van Horn, P. (2009). Giving voice to the unsayable: Repairing the effects of trauma in infancy and early childhood. *Child and Adolescent Psychiatric Clinics of North America, 18*, 707–720.

Lieberman, A.F., Van Horn, P., & Ghosh-Ippen, C. (2005). Toward evidence-based treatment: Child-parent psychotherapy with preschoolers exposed to marital violence. *Journal of the American Academy of Child and Adolescent Psychiatry, 44*, 1241–1248.

Limberg, B., & Ammen, S. (2008). Ecosystemic play therapy with infants, toddlers and their families. In C. Schaefer, P. Kelly-Zion, & J. McCormick (Eds.), *Play therapy for very young children* (pp. 103–124). New York, NY: Jason Aronson.

Luby, J., Si, X., Belden, A., Tandon, M., & Spitznagel, E. (2009). Preschool depression: Homotypic continuity and course over 24 months. *Archives of General Psychiatry, 66*(8): 897–905.

Marvin, R., Cooper, G., Hoffman, K., & Powell, B. (2002). The circle of security project: Attachment-based intervention with caregiver-preschool child dyads. *Attachment and Human Development, 4*, 107–124.

McCain, A., Kelley, M., & Fishbein, J. (1999). Behavioral screening in well-child care: Validation of the toddler behavior screening inventory. *Journal of Pediatric Psychology, 24*, 415–422.

McDonough, S.C. (2004). Interaction guidance: Promoting and guiding the caregiving relationship. In A. Sameroff, S. McDonough, & K. Rosenblum (Eds.), *Treating parent-infant relationship problems: Strategies for intervention* (pp. 79–96). New York, NY: Guilford Press.

Measelle, J.R., Ablow, J.C., Cowan, P.A., & Cowan, C.P. (1998). Assessing young children's views of their academic social and emotional lives: An evaluation of the self-perception scales of the Berkeley Puppet Interview. *Child Development, 69*, 1556–1576.

Morawska, A., & Sanders, M.R. (2006). Self-administered behavioral family intervention for parents of toddlers: Part I. Efficacy. *Journal of Consulting and Clinical Psychology, 74*, 10–19.

Mouton-Simien, P., McCain, A.P., & Kelley, M.L. (1997). The development of the toddler behavior screening inventory. *Journal of the Abnormal Child Psychology, 2*, 59–61.

Muir, E., Lojkasek, M., & Cohen, N. (1999). *Watch, wait and wonder.* Toronto, ON: Hincks-Dellcrest Institute.

Mullen, E.M. (1995). *Mullen scales of early learning.* Circle Pines, MN: American Guidance Service.

Newborg, J. (2004). *Battelle developmental inventory* (second edition). Itasca, IL: Riverside Publishing.

Olds, D., Sadler, L., & Kitzman, H. (2007). Programs for parents of infants and toddlers: Recent evidence from randomized trials. *Journal of Child Psychology and Psychiatry, 48*, 355–391.

Pulleyblank, C.E. (2004). The heart of the matter: Integration of ecosystemic family therapy practices with systems of care mental health services for children and families. *Family Process, 43*, 161–173.

Renk, K., & Phares, V. (2004). Cross-informant ratings of social competence in children and adults. *Clinical Psychology Review, 24*, 239–254.

Reynolds, C.R., & Kamphaus, R.W. (1992). *Behavior assessment system for children: Manual.* Circle Pines, MN: American Guidance Service.

Reynolds, C.R., & Kamphaus, R.W. (2002). *The clinician's guide to the behavior assessment system for children.* Paris, France: Laviosier.

Rockhill, C.M., Collett, B.R., McLellan, J.M., & Speltz, M.L. (2006). Oppositional defiant disorder. In J. Luby (Ed.), *Handbook of preschool mental health* (pp. 80–114). New York, NY: Guilford Press.

Rohner, R. (2005). *Handbook for the study of parental acceptance and rejection: The parental acceptance-rejection test manual.* Storrs, CT: University of Connecticut Press.

Russ, S.W. (2004). *Play in child development and psychotherapy: Toward empirically supported practice.* Mahwah, NJ: Erlbaum.

Schaefer, C.E., Kelly-Zion, P., McCormick, J., & Ohnogi, A. (Eds.). (2008). *Play therapy for very young children.* New York, NY: Jason Aronson.

Scheeringa, M.S., Peebles, C.C., Cook, C.A., & Zeanah, C.H. (2001). Toward establishing procedural, criterion, and discriminant validity for PTSD in early childhood. *Journal of the American Academy of Child and Adolescent Psychiatry, 40*, 52–60.

Scheeringa, M.S., Salloum, A., Arnberger, R., Weems, C., Amaya-Jackson, L., & Cohen, J. (2007). Feasibility and effectiveness of cognitive-behavioral therapy for PTSD in preschool children: Two case reports. *Journal of Traumatic Stress, 20*, 631–636.

Shonkoff, J.P., Boyce, W.T., & McEwen, B.S. (2009). Neuroscience, molecular biology, and the childhood roots of health disparities: Building a new framework for health promotion and disease prevention. *Journal of the American Medical Association, 301*, 2252–2259.

Sparrow, S.S., Cicchetti, D. V., & Balla, D. (2005). *Vineland adaptive behavior scales* (second edition). Circle Pines, MN: American Guidance Service.

Sprafkin, J., Volpe, R., Gadow, K., Nolan, E., & Kelly, K. (2002). A DSM-IV referenced screening instrument for preschool children: The early childhood symptom inventory. *Journal of the American Academy of Child and Adolescent Psychiatry, 41*, 604–612.

Squires, J., & Bricker, D. (2009). *Ages and stages questionnaire: Users guide.* Baltimore, MD: Paul H. Brookes Publishing.

Steinhoff, K., Lerner, M., Kapilinsky, A., Kotkin, R., Wigal, S., Steinberg-Epstein, R., & Swanson, J. (2006). Attention-deficit/hyperactivity disorder. In J. Luby (Ed.), *Handbook of preschool mental health* (pp. 63–79). New York, NY: Guilford Press.

Straus, M., Hamby, S., Finkelhor, D., Moore, D., & Runyan, D. (1998). Identification of child maltreatment with the parent-child conflict tactics scales: Development and psychometric data for a national sample of American parents. *Child Abuse and Neglect, 22*, 249–270.

Straus, M., & Mattingly, M. (2007). *A short form and severity level types for the parent-child conflict tactics scales.* Durham, NH: Family

Research Laboratory, University of New Hampshire. Retrieved on December 1, 2010, from http://unhinfo.unh.edu/fri

Summner, S., & Spietz, A. (1994). *NCAST: Caregiver/parent interaction feeding and teaching scales.* Seattle, WA: University of Washington.

Tamm, L., Swanson, J., Lerner, M., Childress, C., Patterson, B., Lakes, K., & Cunningham, C. (2005). Intervention for preschoolers at risk for attention-deficit hyperactivity disorder (ADHD): Service before diagnosis. *Clinical Neuroscience Research, 5,* 247–253.

Thomas, J., & Guskin, K. (2001). Disruptive behavior in young children: What does it mean? *Journal of the American Academy of Child and Adolescent Psychiatry, 40,* 44–51.

Thomas, J. (1998). Summary of the practice parameters for the psychiatric assessment of infants and toddlers (0–36 months). *Journal of the American Academy of Child and Adolescent Psychiatry, 37,* 127–132.

U. S. Public Health Service. (2000). *Report of the surgeon general's conference on children's mental health.* Washington, DC: Author.

Warren, S.L., Emde, R.N., & Sroufe, L.A. (2000). Internal representations: Predicting anxiety from children's plan narratives. *Journal of the American Academy of Child and Adolescent Psychiatry, 39,* 100–107.

Webster-Stratton, C., Reid, M., & Hammond, M. (2004). Treating children with early onset conduct problems: Intervention outcomes for parent, child and teacher training. *Journal of Clinical Child and Adolescent Psychology, 33,* 105–124.

Weiss, S., Haber, J., Horowitz, J., Stuart, G., & Wolfe, B. (2009). The inextricable nature of mental and physical health: Implications for integrative care. *Journal of the American Psychiatric Nurses Association, 15,* 371–382.

Wilens, T.E., Biederman, J., Brown, S., Monuteaux, M., Prince, J., & Spencer, T.J. (2002). Patterns of psychopathology and dysfunction in clinically referred preschoolers. *Journal of Developmental and Behavioral Pediatrics, 23,* S31–S36.

Wright, H., Holmes, G., Stader, S., Penny, R., & Wieduwilt, K. (2004). Psychiatric diagnoses of infants and toddlers referred to a community mental health system. *Psychological Reports, 95,* 495–503.

Zero to Three. (1994). Diagnostic classification of mental health and developmental disorders of infancy and early childhood (DC:0-3). Washington, D.C.: National Center for Infants, Toddlers and Families.

Zero to Three. (2005). Diagnostic classification of mental health and developmental disorders of infancy and early childhood. Revised Edition (DC:0-3R). Washington, D.C.: National Center for Infants, Toddlers and Families.

Zimmer-Gembeck, T.R. (2007). Behavioral outcomes of parent-child interaction therapy and triple p-positive parenting program: A review and meta-analysis. *Journal of Abnormal Child Psychology, 35,* 475–495.

Zito, J., & Safer, D. (2005). Recent child pharmacoepidemiological findings. *Journal of Child and Adolescent Psychopharmacology, 15,* 5–9.

19

Juvenile Justice Populations

Deborah Shelton and Elizabeth Bonham

Objectives

After reading this chapter, APNs will be able to

1. Identify the political and social issues influencing health care for juvenile justice populations.
2. List the clinical profile of the young offender.
3. Understand the roles of the mental health and primary care APN who is providing care to this population.

Introduction

More than 2.2 million youths are arrested each year in the United States, with more than 110,000 youth incarcerated in juvenile correctional facilities (Snyder & Sickmund, 2006). Once incarcerated, these youths are at an increased risk of committing future crimes (Bullis, Yovanoff, Mueller, & Havel, 2002; Doren, Bullis, & Benz, 1996) and are at additional risk of becoming unhealthy and unproductive adults. A life trajectory that continues to include criminality jeopardizes future employment; career; and living options, while straining social, legal, and health resources and putting undue burden on both families and victims (Unrah, Gau, & Waintrup, 2009). Costs are difficult to contain when the average rate of recidivism at twelve months post-release for youthful offenders is nearly 55% (Snyder & Sickmund).

Nationally, delinquency cases are estimated to be more than 31 million youths under juvenile court jurisdiction in 2005. Of these youths, 80% were between the ages of ten and fifteen years, 12% were age sixteen, and 8%

were age seventeen. Although the juvenile courts processed 53.8 delinquency cases for every 1,000 juveniles in the population, the delinquency case rate declined by 15% from 1997 to 2005. Interestingly, between 1985 and 2005, case rates more than doubled for drug law violations, public order offenses (disorderly conduct, breach of peace), and person offenses (assault, robbery, rape, and homicide), while property offenses (burglary, larceny, theft, arson, vandalism, trespassing, stolen property) declined (Puzzanchera & Sickmund, 2008).

A policy statement by the American Academy of Pediatrics (AAP) Committee on Adolescence (2001) entitled "Health Care for Children and Adolescents in the Juvenile Correctional Care System" reported that a growing body of evidence showed that young people in juvenile systems were at a considerably higher risk for health, mental health, social, family, substance abuse, and other problems. For all youthful offenders, the most significant health problems noted were substance abuse problems (Horgan, Skwara, & Strickler, 2001) that led to justice system involvement. Sadly, proven treatment

---

Child and Adolescent Behavioral Health: A Resource for Advanced Practice Psychiatric and Primary Care Practitioners in Nursing,
First Edition. Edited by Edilma L. Yearwood, Geraldine S. Pearson, and Jamesetta A. Newland.

options were underutilized (Ericson, 2001). Despite this, some improvements in outcomes have been seen with regard to youthful offenders. Rates for juvenile violent crime arrests dropped over the previous eight years (Snyder, 2004), and the racial disparity in juvenile arrest rates for violent crimes declined between the years of 1980 and 2002 (Snyder). Yet, youth who became involved with juvenile justice systems continued to be those who were challenged by a myriad of adverse environmental experiences, which critically influenced poor psychosocial adjustment (Kiriakidis, 2008).

Many factors are operating in adolescents' offending behavior. A combination of various risk factors with additive and/or interactional effects (Farrington, 1995) confronts the advanced practice nurse (APN) in practice. The challenges are striking. This chapter will provide an overview of the contemporary issues with a focus on key topics pertinent to the management of behavioral presentations. These include the significance of maintaining a developmental perspective; assessment of risk and amenability to treatment; and supportive and treatment-focused interventions for youth who often live in crisis and require a focus on community, cultural, and gender-specific needs. Issues involve the difficult work of engaging families; and, of course, how "public" safety and security, the priority of justice systems, alter the landscape of care. The chapter will also review the role of the pediatric APN treating physical health issues in the population and identifying health risks specific to a juvenile justice population.

A Developmental Perspective

One factor complicating care of young offenders is society's ambivalence regarding how they view the adolescent offender. The range of perceptions varies from immature children who should not be punished for their misdeeds to fully mature individuals who should be held to the same standards of responsibility as adults. The debate over at what age this change occurs, carries, too, the debate of whether to treat or to punish the individual. While some U.S. states do not have a legally defined age of criminal responsibility (minimum age of arrest) for young offenders or have different definitions, a common law definition sets the minimum age at seven years (Griffin, Torbert, & Szymanski, 1998; Wiig, 2001). The minimum age varies from age six in North Carolina to age ten in Mississippi, Colorado, Kansas, Pennsylvania, and Wisconsin.

A study group convened by the Office of Juvenile Justice and Delinquency Prevention defined "child delinquents" as juveniles between the ages of seven and twelve years who had committed a delinquent act or an act that would be a crime if committed by an adult. The arrest rate of child delinquents changed between 1988 and 1997 with arrests for violent crimes increasing by 45% and drug abuse violations increasing by 156% (Snyder, Espiritu, Huizinga, Loeber, & Petechuk, 2003). The total volume of child delinquency cases handled in the juvenile courts is large. In 1997, it was estimated that over 181,000 youths were younger than thirteen years at the time of court intake (Snyder, 2001). Snyder et al. (2003) have shown that youth referred to a court for a delinquency offense for the first time before the age of thirteen were far more likely to become chronic juvenile offenders than were youth first referred to court at an older age. The upper age of juvenile court jurisdiction generally is seventeen years; older first-time delinquents have fewer years of opportunity to develop into chronic juvenile offenders.

Other behavior exhibited as a recurrent pattern of negativistic, defiant, disobedient, and hostile behavior toward others lasting at least six months during childhood and adolescence (American Psychiatric Association, 1994) was classified as disruptive but non-delinquent behavior. It is important to note that youth who deviate from the accepted community norm and commit an illegal act are not automatically labeled "delinquent." Isolated single incidents are usually tolerated by the community or neighborhood. This changes when the number of incidents or the severity of the acts is of such a nature they cannot be ignored. Juvenile delinquent acts then can be separated into two general classifications: criminal offenses and status offenses (Roberts, 2004). Criminal offenses are considered illegal whether committed by an adult or youth and include crimes against persons and property such as assault, arson, robbery, theft, and drug-related crimes. Status offenses are those misbehaviors that would not be considered a crime if committed by an adult, and include such acts as truancy, curfew violations, and elopement.

Professionals agree that no single risk factor leads a young child to delinquency (Loeber & Farrington, 2001; McCord, Spatz-Windom, & Crowell, 2001), and when a very young child engages in delinquent acts, the likelihood of extended juvenile offending over time increases as the number of risk factors and the risk factor domains increases (Burns et al., 2003) without effective intervention.

The challenge lies in understanding that while there are some risk factors found to be common among youth who commit delinquent acts, the patterns and particular combination of risk factors are unique to that child and the context in which that child lives (family and community). It is known that the most important risks in early childhood stem from some combination of individual factors and family factors. A child with lead exposure, hyperactive and temperamental, and with substance-abusing parents who are inconsistent in their child-rearing practices and may from time to time be involved themselves with the criminal justice system is at risk for interface with the juvenile justice system without intervention.

Voisin et al. (2007) studied 554 incarcerated youths between the ages of fourteen and eighteen years and found a lack of familial social support and community monitoring were associated with prevalence rates for sexual-risk, suicidal threats, and drug, alcohol, and tobacco use that were markedly higher in the two months prior to detention than rates for the general adolescent population. Slightly more than 76% of these youths were exposed to one or more types of violence in their community. Moving into school age and adolescence, new risk factors related to influences from school, peers, and the community played a larger role. Youth gang data examined over a fifteen-year period revealed that gang membership was most prevalent between the ages of fifteen to seventeen years and becoming more prominent among females. It is interesting to note that since 1991, Caucasians comprised the predominant group, followed by African Americans. Previous to this time, Hispanic youth were the predominant group in gangs (Howell, Egley, & Gleason, 2002).

The Community Context

"Community" evokes the notion of a geographic location containing rituals and traditions that contribute to a sense of connection and belonging. Community includes *membership*, the feeling of belonging; *influence*, a sense of mattering; *integration and fulfillment of needs*, having individual needs met through community resources; and *shared emotional connection*, the belief that members share the similarities of their community experience (McMillan & Chavis, 1986). Further defining elements include culture and developmental niche. A developmental niche is composed of physical and social settings, historical customs, and child-rearing practices of the caretakers (Super & Harkness, 2002). Additionally, a developmental niche is a physical, emotional, and social place where youths becomes aware of their world and their place in it.

Communities, or neighborhoods, provide protective factors and normative influences that contribute to a high level of collective efficacy (Sampson, Raudenbush, & Earls, 1997). This community has informal and formal social controls such as monitoring and supervising youth that the collective community mutually and willingly uses for the common good. The community can be identified by low rates of homicide, violence, and social disorder, for example. In contrast, a disadvantaged community poses environmental risk factors that imperil youth interaction with the developmental niche. A disadvantaged community has a high proportion of single-parent families headed by females, poverty, and unemployment, which when all are combined create a socioeconomic challenge that contributes to delinquency and youth victimization. Adolescents who grow up in disadvantaged communities are at particularly high risk for unhealthy psychological and physical development (Mohr & Tulman, 2000). In terms of juvenile delinquency, Howell (1995) noted that community risk factors included availability of drugs, firearms, laws that were not enforced, media portrayals of violence, transitions and mobility, and low neighborhood attachment.

An adolescent's attachment to a community is based on the interactions with the community and neighborhood. Much of an adolescent's misbehavior is due to environmental issues rather than biological factors (Steinberg & Schwartz, 2000). A youth's neighborhood is an environment where influential interactions take place. For example, one neighborhood influence is to exert both formal and informal social controls. Informal social controls are for the common good of the neighborhood members and are demonstrated through appropriate behaviors known as social authority. In a neighborhood that is disadvantaged by having few resources and members who are either unable or unwilling to monitor youth activities, a youth's first observation of social authority may be the corrections officer in juvenile detention. Because youth are developmentally and deeply affected by events that occur during adolescence (Arredondo, 2003; Steinberg & Schwartz), what happens in the home community as well as in the detention community affects how the youth later views social authority.

Community is contextually and developmentally significant to the adolescent's own ecological landscape. For example, a youth's neighborhood provides a significant community contextual factor. Examples of other contextual factors are the rules that a youth learns through the socialization process and the presence or absence of economic opportunities. Developmental contexts of the youth include physical and mental illness, IQ, and level of functioning. Characteristics of individual family members such as chronic physical or mental illness, criminal record, substance abuse, and level of involvement with the youth (Preski & Shelton, 2001) also contribute to the ecological community landscape. These all in turn contribute to an adolescent's view of neighborhood and community.

Medical and Mental Health Needs of Incarcerated Youth

Research conducted over the past ten years has expanded our understanding of the nature and prevalence of mental health disorders among the juvenile justice population. It is known that youth who are in the juvenile justice system experience substantially higher rates of mental disorder than youth in the general population (Skowyra & Cocozza, 2007). Studies have consistently found that among youth who are placed in juvenile justice placements, 70% have at least one diagnosable mental disorder (Shufelt & Cocozza, 2006). Skowyra and Cocozza further specified that among males, 66.8% had a mental disorder; with disruptive disorders (44.9%) most prevalent, followed by substance use disorders (43.2%), anxiety disorders (26.4%), and mood disorders (14.3%). Females had higher rates for any disorder (81%) with anxiety disorders (56%) most prevalent; followed by substance use disorders (55.1%), disruptive disorder (51.3%), and mood disorder (29%). For many youths, their mental health status was complicated by the presence of more than one disorder (79%). Approximately 60% of those who met criteria for a mental health diagnosis were also diagnosed with a co-occurring substance use disorder (Shufelt & Cocozza). Co-occurring substance use disorders were most common for youth with a diagnosis of disruptive disorder (70.4%), but 53.2% had anxiety disorders and 61.3% had mood disorders.

In addition of the prevalence of mental illness and substance abuse among youth who become involved in juvenile justice systems, a pattern of more complex health problems is also evidenced, adding to challenges in clinical management and increased health care costs. Some of the risks leading to their involvement with justice systems, such as disorganized and poor family supports, also impact their health status (Shelton, 2000). More than half of the families of adolescents with a preexisting medical problem seemed to be unable or unwilling to assist in ensuring that the adolescent receives proper medical care after release (Feinstein et al., 1998). These youths come to juvenile justice systems with previously unattended chronic medical conditions, such as dental, dermatological, orthopedic, nutritional, and respiratory problems (American Academy of Pediatrics, 2001; Anderson & Farrow, 1998). Numerous studies confirmed that approximately 46% of all youths entering juvenile justice systems had documented medical conditions (Anderson, Vostanis, & Spencer, 2004; Hein et al., 1980; Shelton, 2000), including conditions found commonly in adolescence, such as asthma, hypertension, acne, and diabetes.

Conditions occurring at a greater rate in incarcerated youth than youth who were not incarcerated included a 7% prevalence of tuberculosis confirmed by positive skin testing (Hein et al., 1980) and a 90% prevalence of dental caries or missing, fractured, or infected teeth (Matson, Bretl, & Wolf, 2000). Drug use, initiation of sexual intercourse at a young age, having multiple sexual partners, and inconsistent use of condoms put juvenile detainees at lifetime risk for developing HIV infection or AIDS (Morris et al., 1995). In a study of 901 adolescent offenders, Matson et al. found African American youth reporting higher rates of sexual activity (84%) compared to Caucasian (74%) and Hispanic (73%) youth. Seven percent of detained youths reported history of a sexually transmitted disease (STD); 24% were females and 7% were males. Gonorrhea was the most common infection (44%), followed by *Chlamydia* (42%), *Trichomonas* (25%), herpes (4%), and venereal warts (8%). Griel and Loeb (2009), in a literature review of physical health issues in incarcerated youth, cited high risk of chronic illness, such as hepatitis C and obesity. Figure 19.1 illustrates a checklist for use with youth in placement. Developed by an APN who treats youth in detention settings, it offers a brief screen to identify areas requiring further assessment by the nurse.

As the number of females entering the juvenile justice system increases, the numbers of those who are pregnant increases. A national survey involving juvenile facilities found that approximately two-thirds of 261 correctional facilities housed between one and five pregnant adolescents on any given day (Breuner & Farrow, 1995). Nesmith, Klerman, Oh, and Feinstein (1997) reported that 25% of juvenile male detainees were fathers. These youth perceived fathering a child to be desirable, that they were capable of being a father to a child, and that they could be responsible for the child and mother. In a second study, Feinstein et al. (1998) reported that parents and their friends would be pleased if adolescent detainee males were to father a child. This held true for black youth over non-Hispanic whites.

Youth who become incarcerated appear to have a tendency toward injury. Nearly 20% of incarcerated youths had previously been hospitalized, 50% for non–athletic-related trauma such as stab wounds (Feinstein et al., 1998). Shelton (2005) reported in a study of 290 detained youths that 20% had physical injuries including burns, sprains, broken bones, and head injuries. Twelve percent of these youths reported that they had not received treatment for their injuries. In a survey of 192 young detainees, of the 21 (11%) reporting a history of head injury requiring some medical attention, half had sustained loss of consciousness (Dolan, Holloway, Bailey, & Smith, 1999). It is not unusual for incarcerated youths to have incidents requiring medical attention while incarcerated.

Figure 19.1

CHECKLIST FOR YOUTH IN PLACEMENT

- ❏ Social service contact _____
- ❏ Original PCP contacted Y / N

    Name _____ Contact number _____
- ❏ Primary care records

    Requested **Y / N** Received **Y / N**
- ❏ Subspecialist(s) Identified **Y / N** _____
- ❏ Hospitalizations
- ❏ Allergies _____
- ❏ Medications _____
- ❏ Immunizations UTD
- ❏ Infectious disease exposure _____
- ❏ Injuries / Violence

    LOC _____
- ❏ Safety perception
- ❏ Dental health
- ❏ Vision
- ❏ Hearing
- ❏ Nutrition
- ❏ Pulmonary
- ❏ Cardiac
- ❏ GI
- ❏ GU
- ❏ Neurologic / Behavioral
- ❏ Musculoskeletal
- ❏ Substance use

Developed and reprinted courtesy of Paula Deaun Jackson.

Mental Illness and Juvenile Offending

There is no doubt that the prevalence of mental illness is much greater among juvenile offenders than in the general population, but the reasons for this overlap are many. Related to an elevated risk for criminal behavior are mental illnesses that involve difficulties in emotion regulation or impulse control, and aggression. A study by Cropsey, Weaver, and Dupre (2008) examined predictors of involvement in a juvenile justice system for 636 hospitalized psychiatric adolescent patients. A logistic regression analysis was conducted to determine predictors of juvenile justice involvement. Significant predictors of juvenile justice involvement included being male, having a parent with a history of legal involvement, having a family history of substance use, having a diagnosis of childhood disruptive disorder, using cocaine, being sexually active, and having a history of aggression. These were all significant independent predictors of juvenile justice involvement. Both cocaine use and a history of aggression more than doubled an adolescent's odds of juvenile justice involvement. A second study by Preski and Shelton (2001) reviewed a random sample of 355 detained and committed youths and examined individual, family, and community characteristics to predict child maltreatment in a juvenile delinquent population. This model found that youths were three to four times more likely to commit a serious offense when exposed to community violence; when the mother had a mental illness; when the youth was a substance user and had a father and siblings who were substance users; and/or when siblings and family members were involved in criminal justice systems. Both studies point to the overlap among substance use, violence, and disruptive behaviors. Community environments favorable toward drug use and crime support violent lifestyles, which spill over into the lives of youth.

Teplin et al. (2006) examined rates of mental disorders by gender, race, and ethnicity. In a comparison of six studies, they concluded that among youth with major mental disorders (n = 305), more than half of females and nearly three-quarters of males had any substance use disorder. Differences between females and males (and the corresponding odds ratios), however, were not statistically significant. Among females with major mental disorders, significantly more non-Hispanic whites (50%) and Hispanics (43.3%) had drug and alcohol use disorders than did African Americans (21.3%). Significantly more Hispanic females (52.5%) had alcohol use disorders than did African Americans (26.6%). Among males with major mental disorders, no significant differences existed relative to race and ethnicity. Among females with major mental disorders,

no significant differences existed by age. Among males, nearly 90% of those age sixteen years and older with a major mental disorder also had a substance use disorder; this was significantly more than in males aged ten to thirteen (55.2%) and fourteen to fifteen (60.6%). Teplin et al. also noted that for youth with drug and alcohol use disorders that 34.9% of females and 34.3% of males had a major mental disorder. There were no significant differences by gender, race/ethnicity, or age.

Substance Abusing Youth and Juvenile Offending

The link between adolescent substance abuse and juvenile criminal offending and substance use disorders has been well established. The overlap between substance abuse and offending differs from that between offending and other forms of mental illness because adolescent substance use is in itself an illegal behavior. The National Institute on Drug Abuse (NIDA, 2006) reported that among adolescents detained for criminal offending in 2000, 56% of boys and 40% of girls tested positive for drug use. Substance Abuse and Mental Health Services Administration (SAMSHA, 2004) reported the substance use disorder rate among adolescents aged twelve to seventeen years who had ever been in jail or detention was 23.8%, nearly triple the 8% rate for youth in that age range who had never been jailed or detained. National data showed that the criminal justice system accounted for 55% of male admissions and 39% of female admissions to publicly funded substance abuse treatment programs. These statistics make the criminal justice system the nation's major referral source for adolescent substance users, causing some to conclude that it had become the de facto drug treatment system in the United States (SAMSHA, 2007).

It is important to distinguish between substance use and clinical substance use disorders. *Clinical substance use disorders* reflect a more problematic pattern of use and are associated with impaired functioning. Rates of substance use disorders among juvenile offenders vary substantially depending both on the criteria used to define the disorder and on the settings (such as juvenile detention, secure confinement, intake, or community) that are sampled. Detained adolescents show high rates of substance use disorders. Chassin (2008) noted that although juvenile offenders had higher rates of substance use disorders than the general adolescent population, in most samples the majority of young offenders did not have a clinical diagnosis. However, with rates varying between 25% and 67%, the prevalence of substance abuse disorder was substantial, suggesting that the treatment need was significant. Treatment was more appropriate for those youths with clinical substance use disorders (NIDA, 2006). Identifying young offenders with such disorders requires screening, and for those who screen positive, a thorough diagnostic evaluation. These evaluations help determine if detoxification is necessary, how intensive treatment should be, and the location or placement for treatment (community, residential, or secure). Screening and assessment pose several challenges. Most standardized measures and structured interviews rely on self-report data, which require comprehension of complex questions as well as accurate and honest reports. Because substance use is illegal, adolescents may be unwilling to disclose their use. In a study of juvenile detainees, McClelland, Teplin, and Abram (2004) found that at least half of adolescent cocaine users denied recently using cocaine and concluded that self-reports may thus be more accurate for past use than for current use. NIDA (2006) recommends monitoring drug use through urinalysis or other objective methods. Currently, assessment of substance use disorders requires characterizing substance use-related social consequences, dependence symptoms, and the associated impairment using the standard American Psychiatric Association criteria (Martin, Chung, Kirisci, & Langenbucher, 2006). Martin et al. note that adolescents fall short of diagnostic thresholds, making treatment decisions difficult.

Assessing Risk and Amenability to Treatment

In 2005 the American Academy of Child and Adolescent Psychiatry recommended that all youth referred to correctional settings be evaluated for risk of violent behavior. The evaluation necessitates that two key determinations be made: the risk of future harm to the community posed by an adolescent and how likely that adolescent was to benefit from interventions. Decisions weighing risk and amenability to treatment are made throughout the justice process; determinations are rooted in judgments about how much risk an adolescent poses to the community and what available services might move him/her back along a positive path. Although the two determinations are interrelated, assessing risk and amenability are somewhat distinct clinical tasks. Risk for future offending is based on the nature and severity of the offense as well as the number of past offenses and whether the offenses were violent, against a person, willful, and premeditated (Salekin, Yff, Neumann, Leistico, & Zalot, 2002). Amenability to interventions and sanctions is related to the adolescent's offense history, environmental and personality characteristics, willingness to engage in treatment, past treatments, availability of services, and age. Mulvey and Reppucci (1984) noted that

the organizational characteristics of the juvenile justice system, such as the limited availability of services and the competence of service providers, also influenced assessment of risk and amenability determinations.

Because the juvenile justice system is charged not only with punishing the guilty and protecting the public but also with rehabilitating young offenders, clinicians working with the juvenile justice system must make judgments about offenders' risk of future violence and their likely amenability to treatment. Literature concludes that combining clinical and actuarial decision making is in fact a reasonable approach to assessment. Clinicians need to be aware that within both of these realms, instruments and methods vary tremendously in their effectiveness (Kettles, 2004). The actuarial approach involves formal algorithmic procedures. These are highly predictive in suggesting the likelihood of a specified event happening in the future using a consistent and systematic method for collecting and combining information. Most commonly, such an approach is to assign points to particular characteristics of an individual and combine these points to obtain an overall score (Hart, 1998; Kraemer et al., 1997). The clinical approach (Grove & Meehl, 1996), by contrast, relies on human impression by reaching a judgment about the likelihood of an event happening after considering how different characteristics of an individual and his situation increase or decrease the chances that an adverse event will occur. Interestingly, Monahan (1981) found this approach to be approximately 33% accurate.

The systematic integration of actuarial and clinical information, referred to as structured clinical judgment by Webster, Hucker, and Bloom (2002), is a process where a trained clinician with the appropriate expertise follows objective guidelines for collecting information consistently (either scores on assessment tools or ratings based on clinical impressions across a set of predetermined domains) and then combines this information the same way across each case. The actuarial instrument acts as an anchor from which the clinician can justify a higher or lower assessment of the probability of future violence. Structured clinical judgment provides a more consistent evaluation of the information regarding a case and more reliable judgments across the set of cases seen. Edens, Campbell, and Weir (2007) conducted a meta-analysis of psychopathy measures and found structuring clinical judgments to improve clinical methods placed them on nearly equal footing with actuarial methods. However, a fourth method was proposed by Woods, Reed, and Robinson (1999) that goes beyond the structured clinical judgment method. The Normative Approach (Woods et al.) offers a development process for the individual that is empirically grounded and based on clinically relevant norm-based ordinal scales. The developmental focus of this approach may be most significant for assessment of the younger population. The authors suggested that the model offered a more objective and interpretable means of comparing intervention results, processing data for comparison with recidivism data, and was useful for longitudinal evaluation of specific treatment goals and, therefore, effectiveness of treatment.

A comprehensive approach to assessment, the combined risk-and-need approach, goes beyond calculating a single score of how likely a juvenile might be to re-offend to include an assessment of protective factors or treatment needs (Hoge, 2002; Lewis & Webster, 2004). With this approach, risk is not treated as a stable characteristic of the adolescent, assuming that risk may be lowered by a targeted intervention in the community. For example, an adolescent with a drug or alcohol problem who has a poor school attendance record may be at higher risk for re-offending but may also be a good candidate for positive community adjustment if that problem could be addressed effectively. In this way, the risk-and-need assessment strategy goes beyond simply sorting youth into risk groups by providing information about how targeted interventions may reduce their risk. This strategy allows the clinician to use results from the assessment to identify treatment interventions specific to an individual's needs.

Among the mental health interview and rating systems available, the Massachusetts Youth Screening Instrument-Second Version (MAYSI-2) (Grisso & Barnum, 2006) was developed as a mental health screening tool for use in juvenile justice settings. A brief fifty-two–item standardized self-report form, the MAYSI-2 evaluates seven domains: (1) alcohol/drug use, (2) angry-irritable, (3) depressed-anxious, (4) somatic complaints, (5) suicide ideation, (6) thought disturbance (males only), and (7) trauma experiences. Vincent, Grisso, and Terry (2005) reported that the MAYSI-2 had been adopted for use in forty-eight states; thirty-five states used the screener statewide. Several studies reported that girls scored higher on the MAYSI-2 and that subsets of items may better predict severe mental illness (Cruise, Dandreaux, Marsee, & Deprato, 2008; Ford, Chapman, Pearson, Borum, & Wolpaw, 2007). Vincent, Grisso, Terry, and Banks (2008) conducted a national meta-analysis of a sample of 70,423 youths from 283 juvenile justice probation, detention, or corrections programs and found that girls were on average 1.8 (95% confidence interval [CI], 0.98–1.10) to 2.4 (95% CI, 2.38–2.48)

times as likely as boys to have clinical elevations on all applicable MAYSI-2 scales except the Alcohol/Drug Use Scale. On the Alcohol/Drug Use Scale, a sex effect existed, but only among younger youths. Whites were more likely to have clinical elevations than blacks or Hispanics, but disparities varied across mental health categories and across sites. Researchers concluded that at the aggregate level, 72% of girls and 63% of boys had a clinical elevation on at least one MAYSI-2 scale. While race differences were considered small, whites were more likely to have alcohol, drug problems, and suicide ideation than blacks or Hispanics, but not more likely to have symptoms of depression, anxiety, or thought disturbance compared to these same subgroups.

A systematic method for assessing the future risk of violence with acceptable predictive accuracy has been met with some success with the Structured Assessment of Violence Risk in Youth (SAVRY) (Borum, Bartel, & Forth, 2005; Webster, Muller-Isberner, & Fransson, 2002). The SAVRY taps three risk domains (historical risk factors, social/contextual risk factors, and individual/clinical factors), drawn from existing research and the professional literature on adolescent development as well as on violence and aggression in youth. Each of the twenty-four risk items is rated from low to high; six protective factor items are rated as either present or absent. The SAVRY is useful in the assessment of either males or females between the ages of twelve and eighteen years. Based on the structured clinical judgment model, the SAVRY assists in structuring an assessment so that the important factors will not be missed and, thus, will be emphasized when formulating a final professional judgment about a youth's level of risk. A prospective study of sixty-six male adolescents referred to a Dutch juvenile correctional and treatment facility found interrater reliability of the SAVRY scores was good (Lodewijks, Doreleijers, Ruiter, & Borum, 2008). The predictive validity of the SAVRY for physical violence against persons was excellent. The SAVRY also had good predictive validity for violence against objects, verbal threats, and violations of rules but not for verbal abuse. The results of this study provided strong support for the structured professional judgment model of risk assessment in general and for the SAVRY in particular. Duits, Doreleijers, and van den Brink (2008) found twenty-four of thirty SAVRY items could be extracted from at least 90% of the pretrial mental evaluation files. These authors found that individual items, specifically "negative attitudes" and "psychopathic traits," were the most powerful clinical predictors of high risk of violent recidivism. The SAVRY items are useful as a "checklist" in the evaluation and pretrial assessment, and along with clinical judgment, the scale is useful for daily practice.

Among self-report measures related to risk of future violence, the Antisocial Process Screening Device (APSD) has been reported as predictive of antisocial behavior and the likelihood of successful involvement in treatment (Falkenbach, Poythress, & Heide, 2003; Frick & Hare, 2001; Spain, Douglas, Poythress, & Epstein, 2004). This twenty-item measure is designed for youth ages six to thirteen years and is to be completed by parents or teachers. In a study by Spain et al. (2004), the APSD was compared with a second self-report measure, the modified Childhood Psychopathy Scale (mCPS), and a clinician-administered measure, the Hare Psychopathy Checklist: Youth Version (PCL:YV). Authors found that the self-report measures were more consistent and strongly related to treatment progress compared with the clinician-rated PCL:YV. These findings indicated a relationship between psychopathic features in youth and criminal justice outcomes, but the authors cautioned that this relationship might be measure dependent; meaning that in any given study the conclusions that are drawn may depend in part on the measure that is used. They concluded that the best way to avoid this problem was to follow the old adage of using multiple measures and multiple methods of assessment.

Mulvey and Islen (2008) reported that there is no self-report measure of treatment amenability but that measures of motivation to change may act as a proxy for treatment amenability. The University of Rhode Island Change Assessment (URICA) (McConnaughy, DiClemente, Prochaska, & Velicer, 1989) has variable predictive ability, although very few studies have examined motivation to change in young offender populations. Cohen, Glaser, Calhoun, and Petrocelli (2005) conducted a pilot test of the URICA with a sample of 131 male adolescents (59.5% African American, 32.8% Caucasian American, 7.6% Hispanic American) ranging in age from thirteen to seventeen years (mean = 15.3 years, SD = 1.27 years), who were incarcerated in a juvenile detention facility. In comparison to a psychiatric sample of inpatient adolescents, the present sample followed a somewhat similar pattern of subscale scores but reported statistically significant higher mean scores on Precontemplation and statistically significant lower mean scores on Contemplation and Maintenance, suggesting that the young offenders were less prepared to make changes with regard to interpersonal problems than inpatient adolescents. The authors suggested that it was possible that the differences were due, at least in part, to the types of problems experienced by each sample (i.e., internalizing and externalizing behavior problems). Regarding psychometric properties, the internal consistency coefficients (alphas) for scores from three (Contemplation, Action, and Maintenance) of the four subscales were judged to be adequate. However, the internal consistency estimate for the Precontemplation subscale scores was below .70 and thus deemed insufficient, requiring additional consideration when administered to adolescent offenders.

One interview-based rating system for assessing treatment amenability, the Risk, Sophistication-Maturity, and Treatment Amenability-instrument (RST-i) (Salekin, 2001), has demonstrated reliability and validity in a study of 126 male young offenders between the ages of twelve to seventeen years (mean = 15.28 years, SD = 1.19). The sample consisted of fifty-eight African Americans (46%), fifty-two Caucasians (41%), six Hispanics (5%), and ten individuals of other ethnicities (8%). Preliminary data showed that the RST-i was predictive of important juvenile justice and clinical outcomes, such as treatment compliance (Leistico & Salekin, 2003). The scale, however, was relatively new, and more research on its predictive validity, especially in comparison with other risk-and-need measures, was recommended.

Page and Scalora (2003) suggested that assessment of locus of control (LOC) may be another way to determine treatment amenability. Through a review of the LOC literature, these authors found that an internal orientation had been found to relate to increased treatment participation, help-seeking behaviors, and positive treatment outcomes. Further, an external orientation had been found to be related to poorer treatment participation and outcomes. Generally, LOC scales target individual beliefs about internal versus external influences in a variety of settings. Although, the majority of LOC instruments developed for children and adolescents focus on issues associated with academic achievement, the Nowicki–Strickland Children's Locus of Control Scale (NS-LOC) (Nowicki & Strickland, 1973) and the Rotter Internal–External Control of Reinforcement Scale (Rotter I-E) (Rotter, 1966) have been reported as the most frequently used in research with young offender populations. White (2001) studied LOC of thirty-four African American incarcerated youth aged fifteen to eighteen years compared with a community norm. The NS-LOC scale mean for the sample was 40.75 (SD, 0.537) compared to the mean of 32 (SD, 2.5) for the national sample (t = 3.468, p = .001). This suggested that the sample of young offenders was significantly more internal in their LOC orientation than other children in their age range nationally. White concluded that the findings suggested that these young offenders held stronger than normal beliefs in the efficacy of self and reliance on their own efforts toward advancement. White went on to say that the youths' attempts to attain wealth and the amenities of life were a bit misguided and described the sample as having the "raw materials for success except the guidance, maturity, and training to focus their immense potential" (p. 86). The dynamic quality of LOC may be helpful in assessing juvenile offenders' response to treatment interventions. Using this approach, appropriate progress in therapy would be demonstrated by a shift from a more external orientation to a more internal orientation monitored and assessed over time.

Disproportionate Minority Confinement/Contact

It is unfortunate that many youths who come before juvenile courts are in need of mental health and other health treatment. Systematic assessment of health status and deficits is recommended for every incarcerated youth. This includes family history, trauma exposure, immunization status, health history, past hospitalizations, chronic untreated health problems, and dental and sexual health. Table 19.1 offers a sample checklist for systematically assessing these issues in incarcerated youth. Each area of the assessment should be explored in depth if problems are identified for the youth. This might involve obtaining past medical records, interviewing parental caregivers, or speaking with probation staff who might have additional information. For some youths, an appearance before the juvenile court initiates formal specialized interventions to ameliorate these problems. For incarcerated youth, the APN in the juvenile justice system has the opportunity to act as a gatekeeper for specialized social service and health interventions that otherwise would not have been accessed.

For other youths, an appearance before the juvenile court is the latest link in a chain of social service interventions that began in non–justice service sectors like primary care, community mental health, substance abuse, education, or child welfare. For these youths, ongoing delinquency may reflect a failure of community-based service interventions or alternatively may reflect the intensity of social service needs that remain unmet (Shelton, 2005).

One reason practitioners came to favor the use of actuarial approaches to dispositional decision making is the consensus that the use of subjective approaches has led to disparities in the treatment of minority and nonminority youth. What began as a concern about disproportionate minority confinement, where juveniles of color were more likely to be locked up than were white juveniles with similar criminal records, has evolved to a concern about disproportionate minority contact or

Table 19.1 Sample assessment checklist for incarcerated youth

- General health
  - Nutrition and eating habits, dental condition & history of care
  - Physical fitness, hygiene, and sleep patterns
  - Normal growth and development
  - Sexual behaviors, childbearing, and parenting
- Treated and untreated conditions
  - Acute and chronic illnesses, injuries, or bedwetting
  - Self-care strategies
- Mental health
  - Anxiety, depression, suicide potential, and other vulnerabilities/precautions
  - Anger, aggression, and other behavioral symptoms
  - Substance use: tobacco, drugs, alcohol, and over-the-counter products
  - Abuse, exposure to violence, and neglect
  - Perception of delinquency history, date of first offense
- Cognitive and learning capabilities
  - Decision-making and planning capabilities
  - Intellectual level and learning disabilities
- Family history
  - Family members with history of incarceration
  - Past and current caregivers
  - Household membership
- Treatment service utilization
  - Hospitalizations, community-based services
  - Special accommodations
- Supports/strengths
  - Peer, school, and family relationships, community supports
  - Social skills, coping strategies
  - Skills, talents, wishes, and dreams

a discovery that minority and nonminority youths are treated differentially at all points in the system.

The juvenile courts have a variety of disposition alternatives at their disposal to meet mandates to promote public safety, to hold youthful offenders accountable for their delinquent behavior, and to promote youth development. Probation is the most commonly used disposition (Schwalbe, Hatcher, & Maschi, 2009). Generally, probation programs combine monitoring and enforcement functions with case management functions. However, these programs vary in the relative emphasis between these functions and in intensity. An array of dispositional alternatives or graduated sanctions (Howell, 1995) run along a continuum ranging from least restrictive (diversion programming) to most restrictive (intensive probation or institutional commitment). This system of graduated sanctions holds youths accountable for their past misconduct and protects the public from future delinquency. Placement on the graduated sanctions continuum is determined by such legal factors as offense severity, offense history, and risk of future delinquency. Graduated sanctions are distinct from identified treatment needs. This distinction suggests that offense characteristics should govern judicial decisions regarding disposition severity, whereas health and mental health needs should govern judicial decisions regarding intervention types (Howard, 1995). Research suggests that this distinction has not always been clear, resulting in the system biases now seen.

Several studies have found that alcohol and drug abuse predicted more severe dispositions (Campbell & Schmidt, 2000; Fader, Harris, Jones, & Poulin, 2001) and showed that an additive effect was found for family factors, such as poor parenting or supervision and parental substance abuse. Prior involvement with child protective services predicted secure confinement of the youth (Campbell & Schmidt). Fader et al. found specific family-level factors, maternal substance abuse, history of family violence, and history of dependency referrals to have an effect on disposition severity, particularly when combined with juveniles with substance abuse and parental substance abuse histories. A study conducted by Schwalbe et al. (2009) found that prior participation in select social services influenced the judicial decision-making process so that youths whose delinquency was not prevented by early service involvement were less likely to receive community-based sanctions. Alternatively, youths whose first formal agency contact was with the juvenile justice system were more likely to receive community-based sanctions. This finding was consistent with earlier research conducted by Lyons, Baerger, Quigley, Erlich, and Griffin (2001) and Sanborn (1996). Schwalbe et al. concluded that the results of this study showed that the most prominent influences on disposition severity were treatment needs. Youths with more serious drug use and school-related problems tended to have more severe dispositions, and youths with more family-based problems tended to have less severe dispositions. They also noted that these effects varied with gender, citing the "judicial double-standard" hypothesis advanced by Chesney-Lind and Sheldon (2003), which references the historical paternalism of the juvenile justice system toward female offenders resulting in harsher sanctions upon male offenders.

Individualized Treatment Programming

As clinicians, the importance of treatment programming designed for individual needs is easily understood but may be more difficult to achieve for youth in community settings within juvenile justice systems given mandates and limitations of the child and adolescent treatment system. Two examples are presented to demonstrate the application of individualized treatment programming: first, the example of youth who are sexual offenders; and second, an examination of disruptive and delinquent adolescent females.

Youthful Sex Offenders

It was not until the 1980s that research focused upon youth who committed sex offenses. Previously, their behavior was often explained as normal experimentation or developmental curiosity, whereas the focus of investigation of deviant sexual behavior was on the adult sexual offender (Veneziano & Veneziano, 2002). Although these numbers are believed to be underreported, adolescents are known to commit a substantial number of sex offenses, including 20% of all arrests for sex offenses and approximately 33% of all sex offenses against other children (National Center on Sexual Behavior of Youth, 2008; Worling & Curwin, 2000). The research literature indicates that juvenile sexual offenders are a heterogeneous population with diverse characteristics and treatment needs. This group of young offenders vary with respect to the onset of these offending behaviors (some at puberty and others at very young ages) and in terms of the ages of their victims and whether their offenses involve psychological coercion or violence (Righthand & Welch, 2001). Even when considering differences in methodologies in various studies conducted on this population, the following characteristics of adolescent sexual offenders have been repeatedly described across the literature: a history of severe family problems; separation from parents and placement away from home; experience of sexual abuse, neglect, or physical abuse; social awkwardness or isolation; academic and behavioral problems at school; and psychopathology (van Wijk et al., 2006; Veneziano & Veneziano).

Because of the nature of their offenses, the treatment of juvenile sex offenders must address both the needs of the individual and the needs of the community. Until recently, the majority of treatment programs had been modeled after adult programming and was residential and long term in nature. Many treatment programs for juveniles who have committed sex offenses use cognitive-behavioral techniques conducted in groups (Fanniff & Becker, 2006). Components of these programs address reductions in cognitive distortions and deviant sexual arousal, resolving traumatic consequences associated with being victimized, and enhancing management of emotions increasing empathy, while enhancing problem-solving skills and age-appropriate social skills, including dating skills. Community-based clinicians face difficult circumstances that may jeopardize treatment progress and youth engagement, although they have the unique opportunity of treating these adolescents within the context of their families, schools, and communities. These clinicians have the advantage of accessing the multiple information sources that can provide insight into the world of the youth and his or her family. Caution is needed, however, as one maneuvers through the system, conscientiously avoiding any splitting between youth, families, and agencies as a result of the chaotic lifestyles and demands of these high risk youth. The inaccessibility of adolescents due to their involvement in other activities or avoidant behavior, defiance, and the testing of limits, in combination with the known barriers to keeping appointments, challenge even the most skilled community-based clinician. Working with these youths in the community, however, provides a living laboratory for teaching and observing the newly acquired skills of the youth, monitoring of targeted risks and overall functioning. APNs effectively implement behavior modification plans by being familiar with the multiple systems within which the youth is involved. Kolko, Noel, Thomas, and Torres (2004) emphasize the importance of creating opportunities for the adolescent to make healthy choices about mental and physical health that foster a sense of control and contribution.

Delinquent and Disruptive Female Offenders

Individualized treatment is key in a juvenile justice system that has over the years been designed primarily for the largely male population it serves. It is clear that adolescent females are strikingly different than their male counterparts. Among these differences is the likelihood of girls to engage in relational forms of aggression (Hipwell & Loeber, 2006) and for their aggressive behaviors to increase with age compared to boys (Odgers & Moretti, 2002). Aggression is most often indirect rather than overt physical aggression (Vaillancourt et al., 2002). It is interesting to note that although lower prevalence rates for conduct disorder (CD) are noted among females, Webster-Stratton (1996) noted that girls portrayed more severe behavior problems than boys. Loeber and Keenan (1994) coined the phrase "gender paradox" to describe the phenomenon whereby few girls meet the diagnostic criteria for CD. This is in part because current diagnostic nosology, measurement tools, and developmental models were developed for boys with CD and do not address female behavior problems well or they are just being overlooked by clinicians. Poor assessment and diagnosis impact access to appropriate services.

Appropriate gender-specific programming for females needs to address the numerous risk factors including suboptimal parenting practices, family dysfunction, maltreatment, and involvement with deviant peers. There is some evidence to suggest that these risk factors are especially salient for girls due to their higher levels of investment in interpersonal relationships (Hipwell & Loeber, 2006). Girls, for example, are more likely to be rejected by their prosocial peers for their behavioral problems. They are also more at risk for developing affiliations with older, deviant partners, which may increase their risk for relationship difficulties and antisocial behaviors. Authors suggest that antisocial girls may be exposed to a greater number or accumulation of risks within the family as well, such as poor parenting, family conflict, and sexual maltreatment (Henggeler, Edwards, & Borduin, 1987).

Case Exemplar

Charlotte was a 13-year-old, mixed race (Caucasian/ Native American) girl who was adjudicated to the local detention center because of probation violation. She was in the sixth grade but said, "I have a hard time concentrating and don't know much." She was the youngest of four female siblings and currently lived with her paternal aunt on an Native American reservation.

In her initial health assessment interview with the APN in detention, Charlotte said it had been a long time since she saw a health care provider. She carried an inhaler with an expired date of use for her occasional asthmatic events. She last saw her mother when she was nine years old and had never met her biological father. Charlotte and her extended family were well known to the county welfare and legal enforcement agencies due to numerous reports of school truancy, running away, and domestic violence. As a latency-aged child, Charlotte was sexually abused by her uncle and lived with her paternal aunt. She was twelve weeks pregnant by her fourteen-year-old boyfriend, had been to one prenatal appointment, and was ambivalent about having a baby. She reported she started using marijuana when she was seven years old because her cousins, whom she admired, did so. She admitted to liking the way "weed" made her feel ("I'm not so tense") and denied using alcohol or any other substances.

No primary care records were obtained as Charlotte had no knowledge of previous providers. She was able to give the name of the clinic where she received one prenatal assessment; the APN contacted this setting, with Charlotte's and her aunt's written permission. No other subspecialists were involved in her care.

After physical examination, it was identified that Charlotte was 65 inches tall and weighed 120 lb. She had no known allergies and was not taking any medication other than her inhaler. Her immunizations were not up to date according to her aunt. She had no infectious disease exposure. She had five small healed scars on her back that appeared to be old cigarette burns. She denied knowing what caused these scars. Her vision and hearing screens were within normal limits. Her pulmonary, cardiac, and gastrointestinal systems were negative. She was, at the time of evaluation, experiencing symptoms of a urinary tract infection with burning on urination. Her neurologic and musculoskeletal systems were within normal limits. A complete blood count (CBC) done at admission showed mild anemia. She had not received dental care in several years and appeared to have dental caries. She smoked marijuana three days before coming to detention and no other substances were evident in her urine toxicology screen.

At the behavioral health screen done at intake in the juvenile detention center, Charlotte was assigned to a juvenile justice specialist, who performed an assessment and evaluation using the MAYSI-2 for mental health screening, SAVRY for risk assessment, URICA for treatment amenability, and NS-LOC for treatment response. Charlotte's MAYSI-2 score indicated clinical elevation on Alcohol/Drug, Depressed-Anxious, and Trauma Experiences domains. SAVRY scores did not indicate a negative attitude or psychopathic traits so Charlotte was assessed as not at risk for future violence. Her URICA score was high in Precontemplation consistent with her developmental and chronological age. Her NS-LOC score suggested an internal LOC substantiated by Charlotte's unsolicited, recurring theme of "I am in charge of me."

Disposition: Charlotte was admitted to the girls' detention unit for forty-five days. Prenatal care was arranged through a community partnership the detention center has with the local health department's Adolescent Parent Child Clinic. Prior to this appointment, the detention APN sent her urine for assessment and began treating her urinary tract infection. At the first appointment with the prenatal clinic, occurring a week after coming to detention, she was started on prenatal vitamins; health teaching about pregnancy choices was done with Charlotte and her aunt, who visited her regularly. She received a dental check-up in detention and follow-up for the dental caries. Charlotte participated in the classes offered in detention about nutrition, exercise, trauma, and anger management. While initially hesitant to involve herself with staff or peers, she seemed to make use of the information. Charlotte decided, while in detention, to keep her baby.

Upon discharge, at the end of forty-five days, Charlotte was reevaluated with the MAYSI-2 and found to be a good candidate for an intensive, family-based treatment approach. She was discharged to the community-based Family Support Services Program and assigned to an APN who was certified in child and adolescent psychiatric mental health nursing as well as case management and functional family therapy. The treatment plan formulated with Charlotte, her aunt, the probation officer, the school counselor, and the APN included individual and family therapy with an emphasis on symptom and medication management, resolving traumatic sequelae, learning problem-solving and social skills, and mitigating educational deficits. Charlotte also began working with a community agency focused on helping teen mothers deal with their pregnancy and neonates. She remained in her aunt's care while receiving services. The APN coordinated her first appointment at a primary care clinic close to the Native American reservation where Charlotte resided.

Evidence-Based Practice

According to the Coalition for Juvenile Justice (2000), there are nine components of effective treatment for juvenile offenders: (1) highly structured, intensive programs focusing on changing specific behaviors; (2) development of basic social skills; (3) individual counseling directly addressing behavior, attitudes, and perceptions; (4) sensitivity to race, culture, gender, and sexual orientation; (5) family involvement in the treatment and rehabilitation of their children; (6) community-based, rather than institution-based, treatment; (7) services, support, and supervision that "wrap around" a child and family in an individualized way; (8) recognition that youth think and feel differently than adults, especially under stress; and (9) a strong aftercare treatment component. While only a few examples of evidence-based practices are presented here, excellent additional information can be obtained regarding model and promising programs from sites such as the Center for the Study and Prevention of Violence (2009; *Blueprints for Violence Prevention*) and the Center on AIDS and Community Health (2009; *Diffusion of Effective Behavioral Interventions*).

In an analysis comparing the effectiveness of clinical interventions, Hipwell and Loeber (2006) found Parent Management Training (PMT)(Nock, 2003) to be the best documented and evaluated treatment for preadolescent children's conduct problems. An evidence-based treatment for preadolescent children with oppositional defiant behavior and CD problems, PMT is based on social-learning principles and evidence that maladaptive parent-child interactions play a central role in the development and maintenance of children's behavior problems. PMT aims to improve the quality and frequency of positive parenting skills and thereby improve child behavior (Nock). PMT is manualized, including parent and teacher training, child treatment, and a website for both parents and clinicians.

Functional family therapy (FFT) has thirty years of clinical and research evidence supporting its application across the United States and other countries (Sexton &

Alexander, 2000). Designed for youth between the ages of eleven and eighteen years, from diverse racial and ethnic groups, FFT is a short-term intervention (eight to twelve sessions with thirty hours of direct service added for more challenging cases) spread over a three-month period. The primary focus of intervention is the family and reflects an understanding that positive and negative behaviors both influence and are influenced by multiple relational systems. As family members work to resolve their own issues, the outcomes of greater self-sufficiency, fewer total treatment needs, and lower costs are realized as recidivism rates are reduced. At the level of clinical practice, FFT includes an intervention map that forms the basis for clinical decisions. This map provides the clinician flexible structure by identifying treatment strategies with a high probability of success and facilitates clinical options. Three intervention phases are specified: engagement and motivation, behavior change, and generalization. Each intervention phase addresses different risk and protective factors and requires particular skills from the clinician providing treatment. The map helps the clinician to remain focused within a family structure, which often involves disruption.

Multisystemic therapy (MST) is an intensive, family-based treatment approach developed in the 1970s for improving the antisocial behavior of serious juvenile offenders (Henggeler et al., 1991). MST seeks to reduce youth criminal activity and other kinds of negative behavior by limiting the need for incarceration or other types of out-of-home placement. MST is based on the belief that youth behavior is determined by multiple factors (individual, family, peer, or community) that can be targeted to promote positive behavioral change. Individualizing the intervention to the needs of the youth and the family, MST treatment may aim to improve a caregiver's discipline practices, decrease the youth's interaction with deviant peers, improve the youth's school performance, or aim to produce other positive results. MST treatment is conducted in the natural environment to assist in functioning. The intervention involves several hours of contact per week, generally for about four months. MST is different than other family approaches in that considerable attention is paid to breaking social networks that are linked with antisocial behavior, removing barriers to service, and providing more intensive than traditional family therapies.

Nursing's Contributions to the Field

Several developing nursing interventions have been designed and are undergoing testing to demonstrate their effectiveness by nurses for youthful offender populations. The HomeCare Program (Pearson, 2009),

first started in 2003, targets youth between the ages of eleven and sixteen years in the juvenile justice system who are leaving detention centers and are in need of referral to a longer-term psychiatric care provider. The model, conceptualized as a "bridging service," was developed on the premise that a child/adolescent psychiatric APN and a child psychiatrist team would treat children and adolescents in the federally qualified health care (FQHC) system, integrating care with child psychiatric staff in that environment. Designed for APNs with prescriptive authority, the clinician team conducts evaluations and provides medication management services. Case management is provided by APNs with referrals from probation or parole officers or the child welfare worker. The program was developed to provide a resource for detention-involved youths who require psychotropic medication as a condition of their release and return to the community. The average length of time from referral to intake is fourteen days. Of 900 referrals received, 17% are referred again for services after discharge from HomeCare. Over the years, program eligibility has broadened to include any youth aged sixteen to eighteen years involved with juvenile justice, juvenile parole, or adult probation or those dually involved with the child welfare system and juvenile justice. As youth leave HomeCare, they are assigned a therapist in the FQHC system and are offered a "medical home." A program manual is in process, and outcome data around re-arrest patterns are being analyzed.

A second developing evidence-based practice designed as a prevention program uses expressive arts as a medium for middle school–aged minority youth in high-risk neighborhoods. Developed by Shelton (2009), LEAD (Leadership, Education, Achievement and Development) is a fourteen-week, two to three times–per–week contact program that utilizes a community partnership for program delivery. This program, designed to explore concepts about self, self and family, self and school, self and community, and self and the world uses music, art, literature, drumming, journaling, and dance to teach relaxation, communication and anger management skills to assist youth to express, grieve, and communicate about their lives. The intervention has flexibility and has been modified and tested with Latino adolescent females on probation and is currently being tested as a linking program, beginning during incarceration and following youth into the community. Outcomes have demonstrated improved self-esteem, resilience, perceived anger control, improved relationships with their community mentors, and no contacts with police while in the program. Longitudinal and continued study is needed.

An interesting one-day traffic offender program (TOP), designed as an injury prevention program, began in 1990 for youthful alcohol or drug traffic offenders between the ages of sixteen and twenty-five years (Byrd, 1997). The aim of the program was to educate these high-risk drivers regarding the possible consequences of their poor driving behaviors. This APN-driven intervention is a collaborative effort between a hospital and community traffic safety and law enforcement agencies. Two area judges enroll the offenders in the program as part of their sentence. Limited to an enrollment of seven persons per class, these offenders are sentenced to one day in the hospital. On this day they visit different areas where care to trauma victims is provided, talk to staff, go to the bedside, and, where possible in critical care and the neuroscience units, hear reports about the patients' conditions and care required. Confidentiality forms are signed and rarely do patients or families refuse participation. In fact, families of head injury victims have requested to talk with the group. The day includes role-playing and active participation to reenact crashes, life with disabilities, and simulated activities involving memory loss. A visit to rehabilitation therapy and a frank discussion with a traffic accident victim from the community who sustained a head injury complete the day. Evaluation of this intervention was based on pre–post test reports of improved knowledge and limited by lack of follow-up to ascertain true changes in behavior.

Conclusion

The history of treating youth in juvenile justice systems is still fairly young, gaining much attention following a decade of rising youth violence between 1983 and 1993. These rates of youth violence have since peaked and even made a slight decline. Yet the number of youths in need of treatment services remanded to juvenile justice systems has not declined. Highlighted as a national crisis in the call to the nation in the 1999 "Report of the Surgeon General's Conference on Children's Mental Health: A National Action Agenda" (U.S. Department of Health and Human Services), the failure to appropriately treat youth and families with complex and challenging problems was noted. Long-standing stigma that surrounds mental illness, a fragmented and poorly financed service system, and limited capacity to treat contribute toward this ongoing trend of serving youth in a service system that was never designed to provide these types of clinical services.

The physical health needs of a juvenile justice population are equally as important as the behavioral health issues they present. The primary care APN in the detention center is in a unique position to begin assessing and treating the myriad of physical health needs presented by this population. Both aspects require assessment,

treatment, and case management to ensure that this vulnerable population gets care.

This chapter has briefly explored the factors contributing to youthful offending behaviors. As has been seen, these youths are at risk for psychiatric and substance abuse disorders that contribute to their offending behaviors. The physical health needs of juvenile offenders are often ignored and unmet. Detailed assessment of risk and determining their amenability to treatment are critical for determining placement and for advocating on behalf of youth for the least restrictive placement. Topics specific to juvenile systems, such as overrepresentation of minorities in the system and the lack of gender-specific treatment services, were discussed; several evidence-based treatment programs that have been found to be effective with young offenders and their families were highlighted. The few examples of nurse-designed and -led interventions have been noted. APNs in any setting where they are likely to encounter youth involved in the juvenile justice system can make use of the information presented here regarding physical health vulnerabilities and behavioral health problems.

APNs, as leaders, can reach beyond their roles of clinical excellence by being knowledgeable of their professional association's actions to advocate and protect these youths and their families (Delaney, Shelton, Bonham, Pearson, & Thomas, 2008). Nurses have a long history of working with many vulnerable populations, yet many programs that nurses implement on a daily basis do work but their evidence is poorly documented and poorly disseminated. The role of the APN in today's world reaches beyond that of the practitioner to include advocate and researcher—or at least to include collaboration with other nurses (psychiatric and primary care) who have these special skills to create nursing teams that pose nursing solutions.

Websites/Resources

The Center for Children & Youth Justice http://www.ccyj.org/

The National Juvenile Justice Network http://www.njjn.org/issues.html

Center for the Promotion of Mental Health in Juvenile Justice http://www.promotementalhealth.org/

Center for the Study and Prevention of Violence (CSPV) www.colorado.edu/cspv

National Center for Juvenile Justice www.ncjj.org

National Center for Mental Health and Juvenile Justice www.ncmhjj.org

Office of Juvenile Justice and Delinquency Prevention www.ojjdp.gov

References

American Academy of Child and Adolescent Psychiatry. (2005). Practice parameter for the assessment and treatment of youth in juvenile detention and correctional facilities. *Journal of the American Academy of Child & Adolescent Psychiatry, 44,* 1085–1098.

American Academy of Pediatrics, Committee on Adolescent Health. (2001). Health care for children and adolescents in the juvenile correctional care system. *Pediatrics, 107,* 799–803.

American Psychiatric Association. (1994). *Diagnostic and statistical manual of mental disorders* (fourth edition). Washington, D.C.: American Psychiatric Association Press.

Anderson, B., & Farrow, J.A. (1998). Incarcerated adolescents in Washington State health services and utilization. *Journal of Adolescent Health, 22,* 363–367.

Anderson, L., Vostanis, P., & Spencer, N. (2004). Health needs of young offenders. *Journal of Child Health Care, 8,* 149–164.

Arredondo, D.E. (2003). Child development, children's mental health and the juvenile justice system. *Stanford Law and Policy Review, 14,* 13–28.

Borum, R., Bartel, P., & Forth, A. (2005). Structured assessment of violence risk in youth (SAVRY). In T. Grisso, G. Vincent, & D. Seagrave (Eds.), *Mental health screening and assessment in juvenile justice* (pp. 311–323). New York, NY: Guilford.

Breuner, C.C., & Farrow, J.A. (1995). Pregnant teens in prison: Prevalence, management, and consequences. *Western Journal of Medicine,162,* 328–330.

Bullis, M., Yovanoff, P., Mueller, G., & Havel, E. (2002). Life on the "outs"—examination of the facility-to-community transition of incarcerated youth. *Exceptional Children, 69,* 7–22.

Burns, B.J., Howell, J.C., Wiig, J.K., Augimeri, L.K., Welsh, B.C., Loeber, R.L., & Petechuk, D. (2003). Treatment, services, and intervention programs for child delinquents. Bulletin Series: Child Delinquency, (NCJ 193410). Washington, D.C.: Office of Juvenile Justice and Delinquency Prevention, U.S. Department of Justice.

Byrd, C. (1997). Injury prevention program for youthful traffic offenders. *Journal of Emergency Nursing, 23*(4), 326–329.

Campbell, M.A., & Schmidt, F. (2000). Comparison of mental health and legal factors in the disposition outcome of young offenders. *Criminal Justice and Behavior, 21,* 688–715.

Center on AIDS & Community Health. (2009). *Diffusion of effective behavioral interventions (DEBIs).* Retrieved from http://www. effectiveinterventions.org/

Center for the Study and Prevention of Violence. (2009). *Blueprints for violence prevention.* Retrieved from http://www.colorado.edu/ cspv/blueprints/

Chassin, L. (2008). Juvenile justice and substance use. *The Future of Children, 18*(2), 165–183.

Chesney-Lind, M., & Sheldon, R.G. (2003). *Girls, delinquency, and juvenile justice* (3rd ed.). Belmont, CA: Wadsworth.

Coalition for Juvenile Justice. (2000). Handle with care: Serving the mental health needs of young offenders. Coalition for Juvenile Justice 2000 Annual Report. The Sixteenth Annual Report to the President, the Congress, and the Administrator of the Office of Juvenile Justice and Delinquency Prevention. Retrieved from http:// www.eric.ed.gov/ERICWebPortal/custom/portlets/recordDetails/ detailmini.jsp?_nf pb=true&_&ERICExtSearch_SearchValue_0=E D453465&ERICExtSearch_SearchType_0=no&accno=ED453465

Cohen, P.J., Glaser, B.A., Calhoun, G.B., & Petrocelli, J.V. (2005). Examining readiness for change: A preliminary evaluation of the University of Rhode Island Change Assessment (URICA) with incarcerated adolescents. *Measurement & Evaluation in Counseling & Development, 38*(1), 45–62.

Cropsey, K.L., Weaver, M.F., & Dupre, M.A. (2008). Predictors of involvement in the juvenile justice system among psychiatric hospitalized adolescents. *Addictive Behaviors, 33*(7), 942–948.

Cruise, K.R., Dandreaux, D.M., Marsee, M.A., & Deprato, D.K. (2008). Identification of critical items on the Massachusetts Youth Screening Instrument-2 (MAYSI-2) in incarceration. *International Journal of Forensic Mental Health,7*(2), 121–132.

Delaney, K.R., Shelton, D., Bonham, B., Pearson, G., & Thomas, J. (2008). Meeting the mental health needs of youth in juvenile justice: the nurses' role. *Journal of Child and Adolescent Psychiatric Nursing, 21*(2), 116–117.

Dolan, M., Holloway, J., Bailey, S., & Smith, C. (1999). Health status of juvenile offenders. A survey of young offenders appearing before the juvenile courts. *Journal of Adolescence, 22,* 137–144.

Doren, B., Bullis, M., & Benz, M.R. (1996). Predicting the arrest status of adolescents with disabilities in transition. *The Journal of Special Education, 29,* 363–380.

Duits, N., Doreleijers, T.A.H., & van den Brink, W. (2008). Assessment of violence risk in youth for juvenile court: Relevant factors for clinical judgment. *International Journal of Law & Psychiatry, 31*(3), 236–240.

Edens, J.F., Campbell, J.S., & Weir, J.M. (2007). Youth psychopathy and criminal recidivism: A meta-analysis of the psychopathy checklist measures. *Law and Human Behavior, 31*(1), 53–75.

Ericson, N. (2001). *Substance abuse: The nation's number one health problem.* OJJDP Fact Sheet. (FS-200117) Washington, D.C.: U.S. Department of Justice, Office of Justice Programs, Office of Juvenile Justice and Delinquency Prevention.

Fader, J.J., Harris, P.W., Jones, P.R., & Poulin, M.E. (2001). Factors involved in decisions on commitment to delinquency programs for first-time juvenile offenders. *Justice Quarterly, 18,* 323–341.

Falkenbach, D., Poythress, N.G., & Heide, K.M. (2003). Psychopathic features in a juvenile diversion population: Reliability and predictive validity of two self-report measures. *Behavioral Sciences and the Law, 21,* 787–805.

Fanniff, A.M., & Becker, J.V. (2006). Specialized assessment and treatment of adolescent sex offenders. *Aggression and Violent Behavior, 11*(3), 265–282.

Farrington, D.P. (1995). The development of offending and antisocial behavior from childhood: Key findings from the Cambridge study in delinquent development. *Journal of Child Psychology and Psychiatry, 36,* 929–964.

Feinstein, R.A., Lampkin, A., Lorish, C.D., Klerman, L.V., Maisiak, R., & Oh, M.K. (1998). Medical status of adolescents at time of admission to a juvenile detention center. *Journal of Adolescent Health, 22,* 190–196.

Ford, J.D., Chapman, J.F., Pearson, G., Borum, R., & Wolpaw, J.M. (2008). Psychometric status and clinical utility of the MAYSI-2 with girls and boys in juvenile detention. *Journal of Psychopathology and Behavioral Assessment, 30,* 87–99.

Frick, P.J., & Hare, R.D. (2001). *The Antisocial Process Screening Device.* Toronto, Ontario: Multi-Health Systems.

Griel, L.C., & Loeb, S.J. (2009). Health issues faced by adolescents incarcerated in the juvenile justice system. *Journal of Forensic Nursing, 5,* 162–179.

Griffin, P., Torbert, P., & Szymanski, L. (1998). *Trying Juveniles as Adults in Criminal Court: An Analysis of State Transfer Provisions.* Report. Washington, D.C.: U.S. Department of Justice, Office of Justice Programs, Office of Juvenile Justice and Delinquency Prevention.

Grisso, T., & Barnum, R. (2006). *Massachusetts Youth Screening Instrument-2: User's manual and technical report.* Sarasota, FL: Professional Resource Press.

Grove, W., & Meehl, P. (1996) Comparative efficiency of informal (subjective and impressionistic) and formal (mechanical, algorithmic) prediction procedures: The clinical–statistical controversy. *Psychology, Public Policy and Law, 2,* 293–323.

Hart, S.D. (1998). The role of psychopathy in assessing risk for violence: conceptual and methodological issues. *Legal and Criminal Psychology, 3,* 121–137.

Hein, K., Cohen, M.I., Lit, I.F., Schonberg, S.K., Meyer, M.R., Marks, A., & Sheehy, A.J. (1980). Juvenile detention: Another boundary issue for physicians. *Pediatrics, 66,* 239–245.

Henggeler, S., Borduin, C., Melton, G., Mann, B., Smith L., Hall, J., Fucci, B. (1991). Effects of Multisystemic Therapy on drug use and abuse in serious juvenile offenders: A progress report from two outcome studies. *Family Dynamics of Addiction Quarterly, 1*(3) 40–51.

Henggeler, S., Edwards, J., & Borduin, C. (1987). The family relations of female juvenile delinquents. *Journal of Abnormal Child Psychology 15:* 199–209.

Hipwell, A.E., & Loeber, R. (2006). Do we know which interventions are effective for disruptive and delinquent girls? *Clinical Child and Family Psychology Review, 9*(3/4), 221–255.

Hoge, R.D. (2002). Standardizing instruments for assessing risk and need in youthful offenders. *Criminal Justice and Behavior, 29*(4), 380–396.

Horgan, C., Skwara, K.C., & Strickler, G. (2001). Substance abuse: The nation's number one health problem. Princeton, NJ: Robert Wood Johnson Foundation. Retrieved from http://www.rwjf.org/files/publications/other/SubstanceAbuseChartbook.pdf

Howell, J.C. (1995). (Ed.). Guide for implementing the comprehensive strategy for serious, violent, and chronic juvenile offenders. (NCJ 153571). Washington, D.C.: U.S. Department of Justice, Office of Justice Programs, Office of Juvenile Justice and Delinquency Prevention.

Howell, J.C., Egley, A., & Gleason, D.K. (2002). *Modern-day youth gangs.* Juvenile Justice Bulletin (NCJ 191524). Washington, D.C.: U.S. Department of Justice, Office of Justice Programs, Office of Juvenile Justice and Delinquency Prevention.

Kettles, A.M. (2004). A concept analysis of forensic risk. *Journal of Psychiatric and Mental Health Nursing, 11,* 484–493

Kiriakidis, S.P. (2008). Moral disengagement: Relation to delinquency and independence from indices of social dysfunction. *International Journal of Offender Therapy and Comparative Criminology, 52*(5), 571–583.

Kolko, D.J., Noel, C., Thomas, G., & Torres, E. (2004). Cognitive-behavioral treatment for adolescents who sexually offend and their families: Individual and family applications in a collaborative outpatient program. *Journal of Child Sexual Abuse, 13*(3/4), 157–192.

Kraemer H., Kazdin A., Offord D., Kesler R., Jensen P., & Kupfer, D. (1997). Coming to terms with the terms of risk. *Archives of General Psychiatry, 54,* 337–343.

Leistico, A.M., & Salekin, R.T. (2003). Testing the reliability and validity of the risk, sophistication-maturity, and treatment amenability instrument (RST-i): An assessment tool for juvenile offenders. *International Journal of Forensic Mental Health, 2*(2), 101–117.

Lewis, A.H.O., & Webster, C.D. (2004). General instruments for risk assessment. *Current Opinion in Psychiatry, 17*(5), 401–405.

Lodewijks, H.P.B., Doreleijers, T.A.H., de Ruiter, C., & Borum, R. (2008). Predictive validity of the Structured Assessment of Violence Risk in Youth (*SAVRY*) during residential treatment. *International Journal of Law & Psychiatry, 31*(3), 263–271.

Loeber, R., & Farrington, D. P. (Eds.). (2001). *Child delinquents: Development, intervention and service needs.* Thousand Oaks, CA: Sage.

Loeber, R., & Keenan, K. (1994). The interaction of conduct disorder and its comorbid conditions: Effects of age and gender. *Clinical Psychology Review, 14,* 497–523.

Lyons, J., Baerger, Q., Quigley, P., Erlich, J., & Griffin, E. (2001). Mental health service needs of juvenile offenders: A comparison of detention, incarceration, and treatment settings. *Children's Services: Social Policy, Research, and Practice, 4,* 69–85.

Martin, C.S., Chung, T., Kirisci, L., & Langenbucher, J.W. (2006). Item response theory analysis of diagnostic criteria for alcohol and cannabis use disorders in adolescents: Implications for DSM-V. *Journal of Abnormal Psychology, 115*(4), 807–814.

Matson, S.C., Bretl, D., & Wolf, K. (2000). Health care needs of detained youth. *Journal of Correctional Health Care, 7,* 245–261.

McConnaughy, E.I., DiClemente. C.C., Prochaska, J.O., & Velicer, W.F. (1989). Stages of change in psychotherapy: A follow-up report. *Psychotherapy, 26,* 494 503.

McClelland, G., Teplin, L.A., & Abram, K. (2004). *Detection and prevalence of substance use among juvenile detainees.* (NCJ 203934). OJJDP Juvenile Justice Bulletin. Washington, D.C.: Office of Juvenile Justice and Delinquency Prevention, Office of Justice Programs, U.S. Department of Justice.

McCord, J., Spatz-Windom, C., & Crowell, N.A. (Eds.). (2001). *Juvenile crime: Juvenile justice.* Washington, D.C.: National Academies Press. Retrieved from http://books.nap.edu/openbook.php?record_id=9747&page=R1

McMillan, D., & Chavis, D. (1986). Sense of community: a definition and theory. *Journal of Community Psychology, 14,* 6–23.

Mohr, W.K., & Tulman, L. J. (2000). Children exposed to violence: Measurement considerations within an ecological framework. *Advances in Nursing Science, 23*(1), 59–68.

Monahan, J. (1981). *Predicting violent behaviour.* Beverly Hills, CA: Sage Library of Social Research.

Morris, R.E., Harrison, E.A., Knox, G.W., Tromanhauser, E., Marquis, D.K., & Watts, L.L. (1995). Health risk behavioral survey from 39 juvenile correctional facilities in the United States. *Journal of Adolescent Health, 17,* 334–344.

Mulvey, E.P., & Iselin. A.M.R. (2008). Improving professional judgments of risk and amenability in juvenile justice. *The Future of Children, 18*(2), 35–57.

Mulvey, E.P., & Reppucci, N.D. (1984). Perceptions of appropriate services for juvenile offenders. *Criminal Justice and Behavior, 11*(4), 401–422.

National Center on Sexual Behavior of Youth. (2008). *Frequently asked questions about Adolescent Sex Offenders (ASOs).* Retrieved from http://www.juvenilelaw.org/Articles/2008/McLaughlinNCSBYFAQs.pdf

National Institute on Drug Abuse. (2006). *Principles of drug abuse treatment for criminal justice populations: A research-based guide.* (NIH Pub. No. 06-5316). Bethesda, MD: National Institutes of Health. Retrieved from http://www.drugabuse.gov/PODAT_CJ/principles/

Nesmith, J.D., Klerman, L.V., Oh, M.K., & Feinstein, R.A. (1997). Procreative experiences and orientations toward paternity held by incarcerated males. *Journal of Adolescent Health, 20,* 198–203.

Nock, M.K. (2003). Progress review of the psychosocial treatment of child conduct problems. *Clinical Psychology: Science & Practice, 10,* 1–28.

Nowicki, S., & Strickland, B.R. (1973). A locus of control scale for children. *Journal of Consulting and Clinical Psychology, 40,* 148–150.

Odgers, C.L., & Moretti, M.M. (2002). Aggressive and antisocial girls: Research update and future challenges. *International Journal of Forensic and Mental Health, 2,* 17–33.

Page, G.L., & Scalora, M.J. (2003). The utility of locus of control for assessing juvenile amenability to treatment. *Aggression and Violent Behavior, 9*(5), 523–534.

Pearson, G. (2009). Getting juvenile justice clients home: A primary care bridging service. Frontline Reports. *Psychiatric Services, 60*(12), 1691.

Preski, S., & Shelton, D. (2001). Modeling the role of contextual, child, and parental factors in predicting criminal outcomes in adolescence. *Issues in Mental Health Nursing, 22*(2), 197–206.

Puzzanchera, C., & Sickmund, M. (2008). *Juvenile Court Statistics 2005.* Pittsburgh, PA: National Center for Juvenile Justice.

Righthand, S., & Welch, C. (2001). *Juveniles who have sexually offended.* Washington, D.C.: Office of Juvenile Justice and Delinquency Prevention.

Roberts, A.R. (2004). An overview of juvenile justice and juvenile delinquency. In A.R. Roberts (Ed.), *Juvenile justice sourcebook: Past, present and future.* New York, NY: Oxford Press, Inc.

Rotter, J.B. (1966). Generalized expectancies for internal versus external control of reinforcement. *Psychological Monographs, 80,* 1–28.

Salekin, R.T. (2001). *A manual for risk, sophistication-maturity, and treatment amenability-instrument (RST-i).* Odessa, FL: Psychological Assessment Resources.

Salekin, R.T., Yff, R.M.A., Neumann, C.S., Leistico, A.M.R., & Zalot, A.A. (2002). Juvenile transfer to adult courts: A look at the prototypes for dangerousness sophistication-maturity and amenability to treatment through a legal lens. *Psychology, Public Policy, and Law, 8*(4), 373–410.

Sampson, R.J., Raudenbush, S.W., & Earls, F. (1997). Neighborhoods and violent crime: a multilevel study of collective efficacy. *Science, 277,* 918–924.

Sanborn, J.B. (1996). Factors perceived to affect delinquent dispositions in juvenile court: Putting the sentencing decision into context. *Crime & Delinquency, 42,* 99–113.

Schwalbe, C., Hatcher, S., & Maschi, T. (2009). The effects of treatment needs and prior social services use on juvenile court decision making. *Social Work Research, 33*(1), 31–40.

Sexton, T.L., & Alexander, J.F. (2000). *Functional Family Therapy.* Juvenile Justice Bulletin (NCJ 184743). Washington, D.C.: U.S. Department of Justice, Office of Justice Programs, Office of Juvenile Justice and Delinquency Prevention. Retrieved from http://www.ncjrs.gov/pdffiles1/ojjdp/184743.pdf

Shelton, D. (2009). Leadership, education, achievement, and development: A nursing intervention for prevention of youthful offending behavior. [Special issue: Violence, crime, and mental health]. *Journal of the American Psychiatric Nurses Association, 14*(6), 429–441.

Shelton, D. (2005). Patterns of treatment services and costs for young offenders with mental disorders. *Journal of Child & Adolescent Psychiatric Nursing, 18*(3), 103–112.

Shelton, D. (2000). Health status of young offenders and their families. *Journal of Nursing Scholarship, 32*(2), 173–178.

Shufelt, J.L., & Cocozza, J.J. (2006). Youth with mental health disorders in the juvenile justice system: Results from a multi-state prevalence study. *Research and Program Briefs.* Delmar, NY: Center for Mental Health and Juvenile Justice. Retrieved from http://www.ncmhjj.com/pdfs/publications/PrevalenceRPB.pdf

Skowyra, K.R., & Cocozza, J.J. (2007). *Blueprint for change: A comprehensive model for the identification and treatment of youth with mental health needs in contact with the juvenile justice system.* (#2001-BR-JX-0001). Delmar, NY: Policy Research Associates, Inc. Retrieved from http://www.ncmhjj.com/Blueprint/pdfs/Blueprint.pdf

Snyder, H.N. (2004*). Juvenile arrests, 2002.* Juvenile Justice Bulletin (# 1999-JN-FX-K002). Washington, D.C.: U.S. Department of Justice Programs Office of Juvenile Justice and Delinquency Prevention.

Snyder, H.N. (2001). Epidemiology of official offending. In R. Loeber and D. P. Farrington (Eds.), *Child delinquents: Development, intervention, and service needs* (pp. 25–46). Thousand Oaks, CA: Sage Publications, Inc.

Snyder, H.N., Espiritu, R.C., Huizinga, D., Loeber, R., & Petechuk, D. (2003). *Prevalence and development of child delinquency.* Child Delinquency: Bulletin Series. (# 95-JD-FX-0018). Washington, D.C.: U.S. Department of Justice: Department of Justice Programs, Office of Juvenile Justice and Delinquency Prevention.

Snyder, H.N., & Sickmund, M. (2006). *Juvenile offenders and victims: 2006 national report.* Washington, D.C.: U.S. Department of Justice: Department of Justice Programs, Office of Juvenile Justice and Delinquency Prevention. Retrieved from http://www.ncmhjj.com/Blueprint/pdfs/Blueprint.pdf

Spain, S.E., Douglas, K.S., Poythress, N.G., & Epstein, M. (2004). The relationship between psychopathic features, violence and treatment outcome: The comparison of three youth measures of psychopathic features. *Behavioral Sciences & the Law, 22*(1), 85–102.

Steinberg, L., & Schwartz, R.G. (2000). Developmental psychology goes to court. In T. Grisso & R.G. Schwartz (Eds.), *Youth on trial: A developmental perspective on juvenile justice* (pp. 9–31). Chicago, IL: The University of Chicago Press.

Substance Abuse and Mental Health Services Administration. (2004). *Substance use, abuse, and dependence among youths who have been in jail or a detention center.* National Survey on Drug Use and Health Report. Rockville, MD: Office of Applied Studies. Retrieved from http://www.oas.samhsa.gov/nhsda/2k3nsduh/2k3Results.htm

Super, C.M., & Harkness, S. (2002). Culture structures the environment for development. *Human Development, 45,* 270–274.

Teplin, L.A., Abram, K.M., McClelland, G.M., Mericle, A.A., Dulcan, M.K., & Washburn, J.J. (2006). *Psychiatric Disorders of Youth in Detention.* (Pub. No. NCJ 210331). Washington, D.C.: Office of Juvenile Justice and Delinquency Prevention, U.S. Department of Justice, Office of Justice Programs. Retrieved November 11, 2009, from http://www.ncjrs.gov/pdffiles1/ojjdp/210331.pdf

Unrah, D.K., Gau, J.M., & Waintrup, M.G. (2009). An exploration of factors reducing recidivism rates of formerly incarcerated youth with disabilities participating in a re-entry intervention. *Journal of Child and Family Studies, 18,* 284–293.

U.S. Department of Health and Human Services. (1999). *Mental Health: A Report of the Surgeon General—Executive Summary.* Rockville, MD: Author.

Vaillancourt, T., Cote, S., Farhat, A., Boulerice, B., Boivin, M., & Tremblay, R. (2002). *The development of indirect aggression among Canadian children.* Paper Presented at 15th World Meeting, International Society for Research on Aggression. Montreal, Canada. Abstract retrieved from http://www.israsociety.com/xv/index.html

Van Wijk, A., Vermeiren, R., Loeber, R., T Hart-Kerkhoffs, L., Doreleijers, T., & Bullens, R. (2006). Juvenile sex offenders compared to non-sex offenders: A review of the literature 1995–2005. *Trauma, Violence, & Abuse, 7*(4), 227–243.

Veneziano, C., & Veneziano, L. (2002). Adolescent sex offenders: A review of the literature. *Trauma, Violence & Abuse, 3*(4), 247–260.

Vincent, G.M., Grisso, T., Terry, A., & Banks, S. (2008). Sex and race differences in mental health symptoms in juvenile justice: The MAYSI-2 national meta-analysis. *Journal of the American Academy of Child and Adolescent Psychiatry, 47*(3), 282–290.

Vincent, G.M., Grisso, T., & Terry, A. (2005). *The MAYSI-2 national norm study: A new approach to norming tests.* Paper presented at the annual meeting of the American Psychology Law Society, La Jolla, CA. Retrieved from http://www.maysiware.com/NationalNormsChapter.pdf

Voisin, D.R., Salazar, L.F., Crosby, R., DiClemente, R.J., Yarber, W.L., & Staples-Horne, M. (2007). Witnessing community violence and health-risk behaviors among detained adolescents. *American Journal of Orthopsychiatry, 77*(4), 506–513.

Webster, C.D., Hucker, S.J., & Bloom, H. (2002). Transcending the actuarial versus clinical polemic in assessing risk for violence. *Criminal Justice and Behavior, 29*(5), 659–665.

Webster, C.D., Muller-Isberner, R., & Fransson, G. (2002). Violence risk assessment: Using structured clinical guides professionally. *International Journal of Forensic Mental Health, 1*(2), 185–193.

Webster-Stratton, C. (1996). Early-onset conduct problems: Does gender make a difference? *Journal of Consulting and Clinical Psychology, 64*, 540–551.

White, D.W. (2001). *Self-concept and locus of control among recidivist juvenile offenders* (Doctoral dissertation). Retrieved from Dissertations & Theses: Full Text. (Pub. No. AAT 3026530).

Widom, C. (2001). Child abuse and neglect. In S. White (Ed.), *Handbook of youth and justice* (pp. 31–47). Dordrecht, The Netherlands: Kluwer Academic Publishers.

Wiig, J.K. (2001). Legal issues. In R. Loeber & D.P. Farrington (Eds.), *Child delinquents: Development, intervention, and service need* (pp. 323–338). Thousand Oaks, CA: Sage Publications, Inc.

Woods, P., Reed, V., & Robinson, D. (1999). The behavioral status index: Therapeutic assessment of risk, insight, communication and social skills. *Journal of Psychiatric and Mental Health Nursing, 6*, 79–90.

Worling, J.R., & Curwin, T. (2000). Adolescent sexual offender recidivism: Success of specialized treatment and implications for risk prediction. *Child Abuse and Neglect, 24*, 965–982.

20

Substance Use

Maureen Reed Killeen, Caroline R. McKinnon, and Judith Hirsh

Objectives

After reading this chapter, APNs will be able to

1. Identify developmental patterns and consequences of substance use, abuse, and dependence in children and adolescents.
2. Recognize common tools used to assess substance use.

3. Describe the continuum of substance use conditions.
4. Discuss evidence-based interventions and treatments for selected substance use conditions.
5. Describe implications for advanced practice nurses (APNs).

Introduction

In the United States and other high-income countries, tobacco and alcohol dependence are among the top causes of disease burden (Mokdad, Marks, Stroup, & Gerberding, 2004). In 2000, alcohol and illegal drugs were estimated to cause 30.6% of deaths of fifteen- to twenty-nine-year-olds in developed countries and contribute to 23.3% of the total global burden of disease for the same age group (Toumbourou et al., 2007). While rates of illicit drug use have been slowly decreasing since the late 1990s, misuse of prescription drugs has increased over the past five years (National Institute on Drug Abuse [NIDA], 2010a). Prescription opioid analgesics now account for more deaths than heroin and cocaine (Centers for Disease Control and Prevention [CDC], 2010).

This chapter will examine early use of substances including alcohol, tobacco, and illicit drugs and the misuse of prescription and over-the-counter (OTC) drugs and other psychoactive substances. A developmental lens

will be used to examine patterns of adolescent alcohol and other drug (AOD) use, the trajectory of substance use conditions, and the effects of substance use on the developing adolescent. Risk and protective factors for substance use disorders (SUDs) will be examined and linked to screening, assessment, diagnosis, and treatment. These include evidence-based interventions that can be delivered by APNs in primary care settings and criteria to use when referring for specialty treatment. This chapter concludes with implications for advanced practice nursing and a case exemplar illustrating the principles discussed in the chapter.

Terminology

Table 20.1 summarizes terms that have been used to describe patterns of substance use, acute intervention, and failed outcome. The World Health Organization (WHO) (1992, 1994/2006, 2011) also publishes a lexicon of alcohol and drug terms.

Child and Adolescent Behavioral Health: A Resource for Advanced Practice Psychiatric and Primary Care Practitioners in Nursing,
First Edition. Edited by Edilma L. Yearwood, Geraldine S. Pearson, and Jamesetta A. Newland.
© 2012 John Wiley & Sons, Inc. Published 2012 by John Wiley & Sons, Inc.

Table 20.1 Terminology for patterns of substance use

Term	Description	Reference
Substance use disorders (SUDs)	Includes severe abuse and dependence of specific substances with impairments/ Overlaps with harmful use and addiction.	NIDA, 2010c
Experimentation	Social use of alcohol, tobacco, inhalants, and marijuana with little or no adverse consequences or change in behavior.	American Academy of Pediatrics (AAP), 2008; Levy, Vaughn, & Knight 2002
Harmful use/problem use	Recurrent pattern of psychoactive use that causes actual damage to physical or mental health including legal, social, school and career, interpersonal problems. Use may include multiple substances.	WHO, 1992
Regular use/abuse	Engaging in increased frequency including binges with friends. Psychoactive substance use which causes actual damage to physical or mental health including legal, social, school and vocational problems, interpersonal problems, risky or dangerous behaviors.	Moritsugu & Li, 2008; WHO, 1992
Dependence	Multiple problems, loss of control over use, preoccupation with use, tolerance and withdrawal. Isolation from social, occupational and recreational activity.	AAP, 2008; Levy et al., 2002
Addiction	Multiple problems, loss of control over use, preoccupation with use, tolerance and withdrawal. Experiences cravings, tolerance and withdrawal. Brain circuits are changed related to resisting reward, motivation, memory, and internal control.	NIDA, 2010c
Detox	First step toward treatment; not considered treatment. For adolescents, usually not indicated except for opiate addiction.	Woody et al., 2008
Relapse	Viewed as complex, dynamic interaction among risks and situational determinants wherein the individual returns to substance use after a period of abstinence. Occurs often in more than half of adolescent users within 3 months, two-thirds within 6 months of completing treatment. Multiple causes include polydrug use, peer relationships, and persistent smokers. Boys more likely than girls. African Americans more likely than whites.	Ciesla, 2010, Ciesla, Valle, & Spear, 2008; DeDios, Vaughn, Stanton, & Niaura, 2009; Witkiewitz & Marlatt, 2004

Trends in Substance Use During Childhood and Adolescence

Trends in reports of substance use by adolescents are mixed (Johnston, O'Malley, Bachman, & Schulenberg, 2010). Smoking tobacco is now at the lowest point since surveys of high school students began in 1975 and alcohol use and binge-drinking among twelve- to twenty-year-olds have been steadily declining. Use of illicit drugs including methamphetamine, cocaine, heroin, and hallucinogens has declined since the late 1990s and continued to decrease from 2004 to 2009. Despite these improvements, when looking at the data closer, other trends are less hopeful.

In 2009, 27% of youths between twelve and twenty years old reported drinking alcohol, including 3.5% of twelve- to thirteen-year-olds, 13.1% of fourteen- to fifteen-year-olds, 26.3% of sixteen- to seventeen-year-olds, and almost half of eighteen- to twenty-year-olds. Binge drinking was reported by 18% of twelve- to seventeen-year-olds with 5.4% reporting being heavy drinkers. In addition, 10% of youths aged twelve to seventeen years were current illicit drug users, and 23% were current tobacco users (Substance Abuse and Mental Health Services Administration [SAMHSA], 2010). Results from the NIDA Monitoring the Future Survey on Adolescent Drug Use indicated that marijuana use in eighth, tenth, and twelfth graders increased by 10% between 2009 and 2010, surpassing smoking of cigarettes in this age group. In addition, the use of ecstasy (MDMA), a synthetic psycho-stimulant that is similar to methamphetamine and the hallucinogen mescaline, is rising at an alarming and significant rate in eighth and tenth graders (NIDA, 2010a).

Use of smokeless tobacco increased among tenth grade students, and there has been a major increase in the number of high school students who misuse prescription and nonprescription drugs. Nearly 1 in 10 twelfth grade students misused hydrocodone in the past year and 1 in 20 misused oxycodone (NIDA, 2010a). Use of specific substances in specific age groups continues to be a concern.

Rates of SUD with illicit drug abuse and dependence declined while rates of alcohol abuse and dependence remained steady (SAMHSA, 2010). SUDs are increasingly viewed as developmental in nature. Adults with SUD typically began using substances in adolescence or late childhood. Evidence is accumulating that the emergence and progression of SUD is influenced by development, that early use affects development, and that efforts to prevent and treat SUDs must take into account developmental issues in order to be successful (Masten, Faden, Zucker, & Spear, 2008; Wagner, 2008). Substance use in adolescence progresses through a series of stages (American Academy of Pediatrics [AAP], 2000; Levy, Vaugh, & Knight, 2002) with teens first going from abstinence to a period of *experimentation*. Some teens then progress from experimentation to a pattern of *regular use* and then to *problem or harmful use*.

Statistics Related to Substances of Abuse by Youth

Alcohol

Alcohol is the most widely used substance of abuse among youth. Although some begin drinking in elementary school, alcohol use typically begins in early adolescence.

Rates of alcohol use increase sharply between twelve and twenty-one years of age. Almost 50% of eighth graders and over 76% of high school seniors reported having used alcohol at least once in their lives (Felgus, Caldwell, & Hesselbrock, 2009) with 18% of twelve- to seventeen-year-olds reporting drinking monthly (SAMHSA Center for Substance Abuse Treatment [CSAT], 2006). Among twelfth graders, over half reported having been drunk, 30% reported binge drinking, and 3% reported daily drinking (Johnston, O'Malley, Bachman, & Schulenberg, 2009). All levels of drinking from use to binge drinking (five or more drinks per occasion) to heavy drinking (five or more drinks on five or more occasions within the past month) increased with age during adolescence (SAMHSA/CSAT).

Drinking *patterns* also vary by age. Adolescents drink less frequently than young adults, but drink more per occasion, frequently engaging in binge drinking. The number of binge drinking days increases during adolescence until age twenty, levels off, and then decreases markedly throughout the 20s and during each succeeding decade (Masten et al., 2008; SAMHSA/CSAT, 2006). Such high-risk drinking patterns make adolescents more vulnerable to the development of alcohol dependence. The earlier the onset of drinking, the higher is the risk of developing dependence. The incidence of alcohol dependence begins near age eleven years, peaks at eighteen, and declines rapidly from eighteen to twenty-five years (Gelhorn et al., 2008). The highest prevalence of alcohol dependence in the United States is among eighteen- to twenty-year-olds (Masten et al., 2008; Moritsugu & Li, 2008).

Adolescents may be more susceptible than adults to alcohol-induced brain damage with repeated and excessive use of alcohol. Chronic heavy drinking during adolescent development is associated with cognitive deficits and alterations in brain activity and structure. Use also affects growth and reproductive hormones and increases liver enzymes indicative of liver damage (Tapert, Caldwell, & Burke, 2004/2005). Despite only a few years of excessive drinking, adolescents meeting criteria for an alcohol use disorder exhibit cognitive deficits associated with reductions in the volumes of the hippocampus and prefrontal cortex (Nixon & McClain, 2010). Although rare in adolescents, abrupt cessation of drinking in alcohol-dependent individuals can produce signs of withdrawal and an abstinence syndrome with increased risk of seizures.

Tobacco

Tobacco is the most addictive substance of abuse besides heroin (Kandel, Hu, Griesler, & Schaffran, 2007). Nicotine dependence symptoms occur early in the experience of young smokers, often beginning within days to weeks of the first inhaled cigarette, long before they smoke daily and after exposure to only low doses of nicotine. Among sixth graders followed for four years, 10% lost autonomy over their smoking within two days, 25% within thirty days of first inhaling, and 50% by the time they were smoking seven cigarettes per month. Half of those who met diagnostic criteria for dependence did so by the time they were smoking forty-six cigarettes per month (DiFranza et al., 2007). In addition to the long-term health effects of tobacco use, adolescent smoking is associated with early use of alcohol and other drugs and with higher rates of relapse following treatment for AOD dependence (deDios, Vaughn, Stanton, & Niaura, 2009).

Illicit Drug Use

The usual pattern for drug abuse typically begins in early adolescence with legal substances such as alcohol and tobacco and progresses to inhalants and more easily accessible drugs such as marijuana and prescription drugs. In 2009, the proportions of the nation's eighth, tenth, and twelfth graders who reported any illicit drug use in the past year were 15%, 29%, and 37%, respectively (Johnston et al., 2010).

Marijuana

Marijuana remains the most commonly used illicit substance by adolescents. Following years of declining use, self-reported marijuana use among American adolescents has been increasing slowly but steadily since 2007 (Johnston et al., 2010). Marijuana use in 2009 among eighth, tenth, and twelfth graders combined was between 12% and 14% (Johnston et al., 2009; SAMSHA/OAS, 2009b). Approximately 9% to 10% of seventeen-to eighteen-year-olds met diagnostic criteria for marijuana abuse, and almost 8% met criteria for marijuana dependence.

Marijuana dependence is similar to other substance dependence disorders, but typically is less severe. Marijuana dependence typically includes a long-standing pattern of daily use with significant consequences in terms of relationships, finances, and productivity. Most users have made numerous attempts to quit and view themselves as being unable to stop. When a marijuana dependent person stops use, withdrawal occurs within twenty-four to forty-eight hours, peaks within four to six days, and lasts one to three weeks (Budney, Hughes, Moore, & Vandrey, 2004; Budney, Roffman, Stephens, & Walker, 2007).

Stimulants

Cocaine use has declined markedly over the past ten years to approximately 1.5% of twelfth graders and approximately 1% of tenth and eighth graders reporting cocaine use during a thirty-day period. Methamphetamine is another powerful stimulant that is addictive. Rates of methamphetamine use among adolescents have declined from 4.7% of twelfth grade students in 1999 to 1.2% in 2009 (Johnston et al., 2010). This information is collected in the annual Monitoring the Future Survey on Adolescent Drug Use. The stimulants that are most likely to be misused by adolescents are prescription drugs prescribed for attention deficit hyperactivity disorder (ADHD). Immediate-release methylphenidate or dexamphetamine can be crushed and snorted to produce a more intense "rush" than oral ingestion produces. Over the past several years, long-acting stimulants with absorption methods designed to prevent misuse by crushing and inhaling have been prescribed yet have not prevented adolescents from diverting their prescribed stimulants to other adolescents (Fournier & Levy, 2006).

Opioids

Opioids or narcotics include prescription pain relievers (morphine, codeine, oxycodone) and illicit drugs such as heroin. Although opioid withdrawal is very uncomfortable and patients feel terribly ill, it is not dangerous if the individual is otherwise healthy (NIDA, 2005; SAMHSA/CSAT, 2006). The current prevalence of use of narcotics other than heroin is 9.2% among twelfth grade students. There has been an increased use of two prescription pain relievers, oxycontin and vicodan, since 2002. In 2009, prevalence rates in grades eight, ten, and twelve were 2.5%, 8.1%, and 9.7%, respectively. Prescription pain reliever misuse is not only prevalent; it is severe. From 1998 to 2008, the number of admissions for substance abuse treatment who reported any pain reliever abuse increased fourfold across all age groups. Among twelve- to seventeen-year-olds, the increase was almost 10-fold from 0.6% of admissions to 5.2% (SAMHSA, 2010).

Heroin, a highly addictive, rapid-acting, illegal opiate derived from morphine, is the most abused opiate. It can be snorted or injected into muscles, but most heroin-dependent users inject intravenously, which produces a surge of pleasure within seconds. In addition to the risks of death due to overdose, heroin users are at greater risk of developing a number of physical health problems. Withdrawal symptoms often occur within a few hours of the last dose. Heroin's withdrawal symptoms peak between forty-eight and seventy-two hours after the last dose and typically gradually decrease over the course of one week. Following acute withdrawal, a longer-term abstinence syndrome persists with cravings and general malaise (NIDA, 2010b). Most new users of heroin are over eighteen years of age. Reported heroin use peaked in 1996 among eighth grade students at 1.6%, and in 2000 for twelfth graders at 1.5%. Since then, heroin use has declined to a prevalence of 0.7% to 0.9% (Johnston et al, 2010).

Prescription and Nonprescription Drug Use

Seven of the top ten drugs abused by twelfth grade students were prescription or OTC drugs. Commonly, nonmedical use (NMU) of prescription drugs involves opiates, stimulants, sedatives, and anxiety and sleep medications (McCabe, Boyd, & Young, 2007). In 2008, 15.4% of twelfth graders reported NMU of a prescription drug in the past year (Johnston et al., 2009). Recently, misuse of OTC medications such as cold preparations containing dextromethorphan has increased (Johnston et al., 2010).

Inhalants

Inhalant use is deliberately inhaling volatile substances such as glue, shoe polish, or toluene to produce a psychoactive effect. Inhalants are inexpensive, accessible, and addictive. Inhalents are quite toxic and can be lethal at any time, including the first use. Inhalant use tends to occur primarily among younger teens and decreases in older age groups. Inhalants are the most frequently reported substances used by twelve- and thirteen-year-olds (SAMHSA/OAS, 2009b).

Neurobiology

Adolescents differ from adults in their response to alcohol and other drugs in ways that increase the likelihood that they will engage in high-risk patterns of use and will increase their risk of subsequently developing AOD dependence. Two models of the effects of AOD have been used to explain the development of drug dependence: incentive sensitization and hedonic allostasis (Wand, 2008). For some individuals, casual AOD use sensitizes the mesolimbic reward system so that the person becomes extremely motivated to use AODs again to obtain the rewarding effects. With hedonic allostasis, chronic AOD use results in down-regulation and reduced activity of positive reward circuits, which generates a chronic internal stress situation characterized by withdrawal symptoms, sadness, and anxiety. This negative effect drives craving, not to seek pleasure but to avoid the negative effect state (Wand).

During early stages of AOD use, positive reinforcement typically motivates repeated use. Chronic exposure to AOD results in neuroadaptation, leading to development of tolerance. Increased doses of the substance are required to obtain rewarding effects. Once neuroadaptation occurs, removal of the substance leads to withdrawal symptoms (Gilpin & Koob, 2008; NIDA, 2008; NIDA, 2010c). The transition to dependence is affected by patterns of AOD use and by stress. Binge drinking with its high blood levels of alcohol followed by frequent withdrawals is a particularly high-risk pattern. During late stages of alcohol dependence neurodegeneration occurs with decreased stem cell neurogenesis and decreased survival of neurons produced during the binge. Neurodegeneration affects the prefrontal cortex (PFC) and orbitofrontal cortex (OFC), leading to impaired executive function, increased impulsivity, and impaired inhibition. Alcohol-induced changes to the dopamine (DA) system are associated with increased alcohol-seeking and consumption in animal models (Gilpin & Koob).

Adolescents require a larger dose of alcohol to reach the same blood alcohol level as adults. Adolescents are more sensitive to the rewarding effects of alcohol, but are less sensitive to negative intoxicating effects such as sedation and motor impairment that serve as cues to regulate intake. As a result, adolescents are more likely to engage in binge drinking, a pattern that is associated with development of alcohol dependence, and with neurodegenerative effects. Active brain development in adolescence makes areas serving cognitive, emotional, and behavioral regulation particularly vulnerable to the adverse effects of alcohol (Clark, Thatcher, & Tapert, 2008). As a result, adolescents have a physiological propensity toward excessive drinking while at the same time, they are even more susceptible to the neurodegenerative effects of drinking that can lead to addiction.

Several of the mechanisms underlying the development of alcohol dependence are also evident in development of nicotine dependence. Nicotine enhances DA release in the nucleus accumbens (NAc) by activating nicotinic cholinergic receptors on presynaptic glutamate neurons and postsynaptic DA neurons in the ventral tegmental area (VTA), and desensitizing postsynaptic receptors on GABA interneurons in the VTA. Alpha-4 beta-2 nicotinic cholinergic receptors on DA neurons in the VTA become desensitized by the time a cigarette is finished. As they resensitize to their resting state, the smoker experiences craving and withdrawal (Stahl, 2008). Adolescent brains experience enhanced short-term positive effects and reduced adverse effects of nicotine, and these differing effects correspond with significant age changes in cortical regions during early adolescence (Leslie et al., 2004).

In summary, all substances of abuse directly or indirectly enhance release of DA in the mesolimbic reward centers. Adolescents are particularly vulnerable to development of SUDs due to their propensity for binging (a pattern of use that accelerates the transition to dependence), their vulnerability to neurodegenerative effects of alcohol and other substances, and their stage of brain maturation.

Etiology

Risk and Protective Factors

Accumulating evidence suggests that adolescent SUDs are the result of complex transactions among genetic and environmental influences. Moreover, studies of genetic and environmental risk factors point to common mechanisms underlying the development of dependence on alcohol and other drugs of abuse (Dick & Agrawal, 2008; Thatcher & Clark, 2008).

The presence of an SUD in a parent is a consistent risk factor for adolescent substance use and SUDs (Thatcher & Clark, 2008) and the first clue that these risks may be heritable. Genes contribute significantly to AOD dependence, with heritability estimates ranging from 0.50 to 0.60 for alcohol dependence and from 0.45 to 0.79 for illicit drugs (Dick & Agrawal, 2008). Genes that have been identified as conferring risk for AOD disorders include genes that encode proteins involved in alcohol metabolism, neurotransmission involving gamma-aminobutyric acid (GABA) receptors, acetylcholine, endogenous cannabinoids and endogenous opioids, and the dopamine system (Dick & Agrawal, 2008; Peterson, 2004/2005).

Problem use of alcohol in adolescence has been found to be more heritable than initiation of use. Alcohol initiation and use are associated with family and peer environments, while problem use has high heritability and is influenced by peers and accessibility of alcohol, with only a small contribution by the family environment (Rose & Dick, 2004/2005).

Developmental processes are among the most consistent nonspecific predictors of SUDs in adolescence and adulthood. Individual differences in preschool children's abilities to modulate expression of emotions, to sustain attention, and to regulate their behavior are evident early and are stable aspects of temperament across childhood and adolescence. Difficulties in self-regulation in cognitive, behavioral, and emotional domains limit children's successful adaptation to environmental demands. Childhood *psychological dysregulation* (also called *behavioral dysregulation*) is a behavioral phenotype (observable characteristics resulting from interactions between genotype, environmental influences, and random variations) that is associated with AOD problems later in adolescence (Thatcher & Clark, 2008). Psychological dysregulation strongly predicts AOD initiation and use, acceleration of AOD use, and related problems during adolescence (Thatcher & Clark). Early aggression and other externalizing symptoms in early childhood predict SUD outcomes fifteen to twenty years later. Moreover, those who show the greatest continuity in externalizing problems are the most likely to develop the more chronic and more severe forms of SUDs as adults (Zucker, Donovan, Masten, Mattson, & Moss, 2008).

Environmental risk and protective factors include parental and peer influences. Despite the stability of genetic and temperamental characteristics, child-rearing environments are important in modulating the risks associated with dysregulation. Child rearing environments characterized by warmth, consistent, moderate discipline and less stress are most effective in lowering levels of externalizing behaviors and drug involvement in adolescence. Parents who are responsive to their children's needs actually increase the child's capacity for self-regulation (Zucker et al., 2008).

Conversely, child maltreatment, neglectful parenting, and lack of parental supervision are associated with increased risk of substance use. Maltreated children are seven times more likely to report alcohol use by age twelve and, on average, report use of alcohol two years earlier than controls (Thatcher & Clark, 2008). Families in which a parent has an SUD are especially risky because of the increased genetic risk for children, the affected parent's modeling substance use and shaping alcohol-related expectancies, and the effects of disrupted parenting due to the parent's SUD. Nonalcohol-specific risk factors include coexisting psychiatric disorders or cognitive dysfunction in parents, low socioeconomic status, and increased family aggression and violence.

Early substance use itself is a risk factor for progression to more severe substance use and polysubstance use in adolescence and SUDs in adulthood. Individuals who initiate alcohol use prior to age fourteen are more likely to use other drugs and to develop SUD in adulthood than are those who start to drink at a later age (Hingson, Heeren, & Edwards, 2008; Hingson, Heeren & Winter, 2006). The risks for initiation of use differ from those that contribute to progression from initial use to SUDs. Environmental factors, especially peers and availability of alcohol, are more influential for timing of initial use, while genetic factors are more influential for accelerating progression from initiation to heavier use (Thatcher & Clark, 2008). In addition, stress influences the transition from AOD use to dependence and addiction (Wand, 2008).

Children with multiple risks, such as having parents with SUDs, high levels of psychological dysregulation, and early use of one or two substances, demonstrate significantly earlier use and problems with tobacco, alcohol, marijuana, and cocaine (Clark, Cornelius, Kirisci, & Tarter, 2005). In addition, genetic and environmental risk factors not only have additive effects, they also influence each other. In order for some genes to encode abnormal proteins, certain environmental inputs must "turn them on," and the environments to which adolescents are exposed are frequently the result of adolescents being attracted to certain environments because of genetic influences.

Clinical Presentation

Clinical presentation depends on where the adolescent is on the continuum between experimentation and dependence. The severity of SUD is defined by the extent of drug or alcohol involvement, whether multiple substances are used, and the severity of the consequences experienced as a result of substance use. Tobacco has the highest mortality risk and disease burden of all substances of abuse; the effects of tobacco dependence are typically not evident until later in life (Rehm, Taylor, & Room, 2006). Substance use is associated with all three leading causes of death among adolescents and young adults: accidental injury, homicide, and suicide (Newbury-Birch et al., 2009).

Youth with identified substance use problems are also more likely to have an earlier age of onset of sexual activity, more sexual partners, higher rates of sexually transmitted infections, and higher rates of pregnancy (Tapert, Aarons, Sedlar, & Brown, 2001). Despite the numerous negative consequences of substance use, many young people are unaware of the risks associated with substance use. Only 40% of adolescents perceived great risk from having five or more drinks once or twice a week, and only 34.2% perceived great risk from monthly marijuana use (SAMHSA Office of Applied Studies [OAS], 2009a). Substance using adolescents frequently have inflated estimates of the extent to which drinking or drug use is a "normal" adolescent behavior. They may also engage in other risky behaviors such as sexual activity, driving while intoxicated, riding with an intoxicated driver, and other impulsive behaviors that pose harm to themselves or others (Feldstein & Miller, 2006).

Table 20.2 provides an overview of drugs of abuse, signs and symptoms of intoxication and withdrawal, and potential physical and mental health effects of which all APNs working with this population should be aware.

Screening, Brief Intervention, Referral, and Treatment (SBIRT)

Screening

The purpose of screening is to identify those who may be at increased risk for developing a substance use disorder so that preventive interventions can be implemented (O'Connell, Boat, & Warner, 2009). Screening also can identify adolescents whose pattern of substance involvement requires further assessment. In primary care settings, SUD screening questions are embedded in checklists that ask about family history or list symptoms in the personal history. Pediatric practices often include questions about child-rearing, children's academic performance, relationships with peers, and any behavior problems. Screening young children for behavioral and emotional dysregulation can identify those at increased risk for later substance use problems in adolescence (Zucker et al., 2008).

Screening children and adolescents for substance use conditions is a critical intervention in the prevention and early detection of more serious levels of illness. Since earlier initiation of substance use is associated with the development of higher comorbidity and increased difficulty in quitting (Palmer et al., 2009; Patton et al., 2007; Winters & Lee, 2008), screening promotes early recognition of hazardous use of substances that might progress to an SUD. Substance use is progressive, both in terms of progressing from tobacco to alcohol to illicit drugs or to polysubstance use, but also in terms of frequency and severity (e.g., progressing from experimentation to regular use to problem use, abuse, and dependence). The APN's early recognition of high-risk behaviors can help prevent the negative physical and mental health consequences associated with persistent substance use (Maggs, Patrick, & Feinstein, 2008; Tingen, Andrews, & Stevenson, 2009).

Practice guidelines for pediatricians, pediatric nurses, and child psychiatrists recommend routine screening of all adolescents for use of tobacco, alcohol, and illicit drugs and misuse of prescription and nonprescription drugs at every routine health care visit (AAP, 2008; American Academy of Child & Adolescent Psychiatry [AACAP], 2005; Fournier & Levy, 2006; Kulig & Committee on Substance Abuse, 2005; National Association of Pediatric Nurse Practitioners [NAPNAP], 2009; National Institute on Alcohol Abuse and Alcoholism [NIAAA], 2005). Knight et al. (1999) recommended screening adolescents whenever the opportunity arose, such as during sports and school entrance physical examinations and illness or injury-related office visits.

Evidence-Based Assessment Tools

Screening

Screening for substance use begins by asking questions about lifetime or recent use of psychoactive substances. Several well-validated self-report instruments are available for screening for alcohol and other substances and can be found in Table 20.3. However, the strength of the psychometric data of these tools when used for adolescents varies (Knight, Sherritt, Harris, Gates, & Chang, 2003; Shields, Campfield, Howell, Wallace, & Weiss, 2008).

Table 20.2 Selected drugs of abuse, signs of intoxication and withdrawal, and potential health consequences

Substance: Category and Name	Examples of Street Names	DEA Schedule/ Method(s) of Ingestion	Signs of Intoxication/Withdrawal	Potential Health Consequences
Cannabinoids				
Hashish	Boom, chronic, gangster, hash, hash oil, hemp	I/swallowed, smoked	Conjunctivitis, appetite stimulation, euphoria, slowed thinking and reaction time, confusion, impaired balance and coordination	Cough, frequent respiratory infections, impaired memory and learning, increased heart rate, anxiety, panic attacks, acute psychotic symptoms (auditory and visual hallucinations, paranoid delusions, confusion, and amnesia)
Marijuana (Cannabis)	Grass, weed, pot, herb, dope, hash, blunt, joint, Mary Jane	I/swallowed, smoked	*Withdrawal: restlessness, irritability, insomnia, loss of appetite*	
CNS Depressants				
Alcohol	Booze, drinks, firewater, highballs, moonshine, white lightning	Not scheduled/ swallowed	Disinhibition, mood lability, impaired judgment, slurred speech, incoordination, unsteady gait, nystagmus, flushed face *Withdrawal: Tremors, nausea/vomiting, tachycardia, sweating, elevated blood pressure, depressed mood, irritability, transient hallucinations or illusions, headache, insomnia, seizures, delirium*	Impaired memory and learning, impaired judgment, elevated liver enzymes, liver disease, disruption of hormones needed for normal organ, muscle, and bone development during puberty, peripheral neuropathy, Wernicke's encephalopathy, psychosis, cardiomyopathy, risk for fetal alcohol syndrome
Barbiturates	Barbs, reds, red birds, phennies, tooies, yellows, yellow jackets	II,II,V/ injected, swallowed	Reduced anxiety, feeling of well-being, lowered inhibitions, slowed pulse and breathing, lowered blood pressure, poor concentration	Fatigue; confusion; impaired coordination, memory, and judgment Barbiturates: depression, slurred speech, irritability, dizziness, life-threatening withdrawal
Benzodiazepines (other than flunitrazepam)	Candy, downers, sleeping pills, tranks	IV/ swallowed, injected	Barbiturates and benzodiazepines: sedation, drowsiness	Benzodiazepines: dizziness
Flunitrazepam (Rohypnol)	Forget-me-pill, Mexican Valium, R2, Roche, roofies, roofinol, rope, rophies	IV/ swallowed, snorted	GHB: drowsiness, nausea Methaqualone: euphoria	Flunitrazepam: visual and GI distrubances, urinary retention, memory loss for the time of drug's effects
GHB (Gamma-hydroxybutyrate)*	G, Georgia homeboy, grievous bodily harm, liquid ecstasy	I/ swallowed	*Withdrawal: nausea/vomiting, malaise, weakness, tachycardia, sweating, anxiety, irritability, orthostatic hypotension, tremor, insomnia, seizures*	GHB: Headache, loss of consciousness, loss of reflexes, seizures, coma, death *Associated with risk of sexual assault
Methaqualone	Ludes, mandrex, quad, quay	I/ injected, swallowed		Methaqualone: poor reflexes, slurred speech, coma

(continued)

381

Table 20.2 (cont'd)

Substance: Category and Name	Examples of Street Names	DEA Schedule/ Method(s) of Ingestion	Signs of Intoxication/*Withdrawal*	Potential Health Consequences
Dissociative Anesthetics				
Ketamine	Cat, K, Special K, vitamin K	III/ injected, snorted, smoked	Increased heart rate and blood pressure, impaired motor function	Memory loss; numbness, nausea/vomiting, seizures, coma, death (greatest risk at high doses and/or when used with other CNS depressants)
PCP and analogs	Angel dust, boat, hog, love boat, peace pill	I, II/ injected, swallowed, smoked	Ketamine: delirium, depression, respiratory depression/arrest (at high doses) PCP: Decreased blood pressure and heart rate, panic, aggression, violence, suicidal ideation	
Hallucinogens				
LSD	Acid, blotter, boomers, cubes, microdot, yellow sunshine	I/ swallowed, absorbed through mouth tissues	Altered states of perception and feeling, nausea, sensitivity to light and sound LSD and mescaline: increased body temperature, heart rate, blood pressure; loss of appetite, sleeplessness, numbness, weakness, tremors	Persisting perception disorder (flashbacks)
Mescaline (Peyote)	Buttons, cactus, mesc, peyote	I/ swallowed, smoked	Psilocybin: nervousness, paranoia	
Psilocybin	Magic mushroom, shrooms, purple passion	I/ swallowed		
Opioids and Morphine Derivatives				
Codeine	Captain Cody, Cody, schoolboy, doors & fours, loads, pancakes & syrup	II, III, IV, V/ injected, swallowed	Pain relief, euphoria, drowsiness, pupil constriction (or dilation due to anoxia from severe overdose), impaired attention and memory	Nausea/vomiting, confusion, sedation, respiratory depression/arrest, unconsciousness, coma, death Injectables: additional risks for HIV/AIDS, hepatitis B & C
Fentanyl and analogs	Apache, China girl, China white, dance fever, friend, goodfella, jackpot, murder 8, TNT	I, II/ injected, smoked, snorted	Heroin: staggering gait *Withdrawal: craving, dysphoric mood, nausea/vomiting, muscle aches, lacrimation or rhinorrhea, papillary dilation, piloerection, sweating, abdominal cramping, diarrhea, yawning, fever, insomnia*	
Heroin	Brown sugar, dope, H, horse, junk, smack, white horse	I/ injected, smoked, snorted		
Morphine	M, Miss Emma, monkey, white stuff	II,III/ injected, swallowed, smoked		

			Intoxication effects	Potential health consequences
Opium	Big O, black stuff, block, gum, hop	II, III, V/ swallowed, smoked		
Oxycodone HCL	Oxy, O.C., killer	II/ swallowed, snorted, injected		
Hydrocodone bitartrate, acetaminophen	Vike, Watson-387	II/ swallowed		
Stimulants				
Amphetamine	Bennies, black beauties, crosses, hearts, speed, uppers	II/ injected, swallowed, smoked, snorted	Increased heart rate, blood pressure, temperature, feelings of exhilaration, increased mental alertness	Rapid/irregular heartbeat, reduced appetite, weight loss, heart failure, nervousness, insomnia, malnutrition, headaches, panic attacks, nausea, abdominal pain chest pain, respiratory failure, stroke, seizure
Cocaine	Blow, bump, C, crack, coke, rock, snow, toot	II/ injected, swallowed, smoked, snorted	Amphetamine: rapid breathing Cocaine: increased temperature	Amphetamine: Loss of coordination, irritability, anxiousness, delirium, panic, psychosis, impulsive behaviors, aggressiveness
Methylendioxy-methamphetamine (MDMA)	Adam, clarity, ecstasy, Eve, lover's speed, peace, STP, X, XTC	I/ swallowed,	MDMA: mild hallucinogenic effects, euphoria, bruxism, increased tactile sensitivity	Cocaine: Chest pain, respiratory failure, nausea, stroke, seizure, headache, malnutrition, panic attacks
Methamphetamine	Chalk, crank, crystal, fire, glass, go fast, ice, meth, speed	II/ injected, swallowed, smoked, snorted	Methamphetamine: aggression violence, psychotic behavior	MDMA: Impaired memory and learning, hyperthermia, cardiac toxicity, renal failure, liver toxicity
Methylphenidate	JIF, MPH, R-ball, Skippy, the smart drug, vitamin R	II/ injected, swallowed, snorted	Nicotine: Increased heart rate, blood pressure, metabolism, rapid/irregular heartbeat, heart failure, nervousness	Methamphetamine: Memory loss, cardiac and neurological damage, impaired memory and learning
Nicotine	Cigarettes, cigars, smokeless tobacco, snuff, spit, bidis, chew	Not scheduled/ smoked, snorted, taken in snuff and spit tobacco	*Withdrawal from amphetamines and cocaine: craving, dysphoria, fatigue, vivid & unpleasant dreams, insomnia or hypersomnia, increased appetite, psychomotor retardation or agitation, severe depression, suicidal and/or paranoid ideation* *Withdrawal from nicotine: craving, dysphoria, depressed mood, insomnia, irritability, frustration, anxiety, difficulty concentrating, decreased heart rate, increased appetite/weight gain*	Nicotine: Adverse pregnancy outcomes, chronic lung disease, cardiovascular disease, stroke, cancer, tolerance, addiction

(continued)

383

Table 20.2 *(cont'd)*.

Substance: Category and Name	Examples of Street Names	DEA Schedule/ Method(s) of Ingestion	Signs of Intoxication/*Withdrawal*	Potential Health Consequences
Other Compounds				
Anabolic steroids	Arnolds, gym candy, juice, pumpers, shot gunning, stackers, roids	III/ injected, swallowed, applied to skin	*Withdrawal: mood swings, fatigue, restlessness, loss of appetite, insomnia, reduced sex drive, cravings, depression, suicidal ideation, attempts*	Hostility/aggression, acne, premature growth stoppage, prostate cancer, reduced sperm production, shrunken testicles, breast enlargement, menstrual irregularities, masculine characteristics, hypertension, blood clotting, cholesterol changes, liver cysts and cancer, kidney cancer
Dextromethorphan (DMX)	Candy, dex, robotripping, Robo, skittling, Triple C	Not scheduled/ swallowed	Dissociative effects, distorted visual perceptions	At higher doses, similar to dissociative anesthetic drugs
Inhalants	Laughing gas, poppers, snappers, whippets	Not scheduled/ inhaled through mouth or nose	Stimulation, loss of inhibition, headache, nausea, vomiting, slurred speech, loss of motor coordination	Wheezing/unconsciousness, cramps, weight loss, muscle weakness, depression, memory impairment, damage to cardiovascular and nervous systems, sudden death, hearing loss, bone marrow damage, liver and kidney damage, increased risk of contracting and spreading infectious disease due to association with unsafe sexual practices

Adapted from National Institute on Drug Abuse (NIDA) www.drugabuse.gov

Table 20.3 Selected screening tools for adolescent substance use problems

Instrument	Reference	Items	Brief Description
Alcohol Use Disorders Identification Test (AUDIT)	Bohn & Babor, 1995	10	Focuses on identifying hazardous alcohol consumption prior to dependence
CRAFFT	Knight et al., 1999	6	Brief screen of AOD use and consequences Suitable for primary care
Drug Abuse Screening Test for Adolescents (DAST-A)	Martino, Grilo, & Fehon, 2000	27	Predicts DSM-IV substance-related disorders
Hooked on Nicotine Checklist (HONC)	Wheeler et al., 2004	10	Self-report or interview measure of nicotine dependence and severity
Modified Fagerström Tolerance Questionnaire (mFTQ)	Prokhorov, Koehly, Pallonen, & Hudmon, 1998	7	Emphasizes behavioral aspects of nicotine dependence
Nicotine Dependence Scale for Adolescents (NDSA)	Nonnemaker, et al., 2004	6	Self-report measure of withdrawal avoidance and craving experience
Nicotine Dependence Syndrome Scale (NDSS)	Shiffman, Waters, & Hickcox, 2004	19	Measures five factors: drive, priority, tolerance, stereotypy, and continuity

The CRAFFT found in Box 20.1 is a six-item screening tool that is preceded by three opening questions: *During the past twelve months did you drink any alcohol (more than a few sips)? Smoke any marijuana or hashish? Use anything else to get high?* If the answer to all three questions is no, only the first CRAAFT question is asked. If any of the three opening questions are endorsed, the adolescent is asked to answer the six CRAAFT questions. Positive responses to two or more questions suggest the need for further assessment by a specialist (Knight et al., 1999, 2002).

Brief Interventions

Often brief interventions include five common elements: (1) assessment and direct feedback; (2) negotiation and goal setting; (3) behavioral modification techniques; (4) self-help bibliotherapy; and (5) follow-up and reinforcement (Babor, Higgins-Biddle, Saunders, & Monteiro, 2001; Levy & Knight, 2008; Levy, Vaughn, et al., 2002). Screening and immediate brief interventions in primary care settings with APNs who have a relationship with the child or adolescent can promote significant reductions in tobacco and alcohol use. For example, if the adolescent has a positive screen for substance use when administered the CRAFFT, further assessment is warranted and a referral should be made. The APN must determine level of severity of the adolescent's substance use and whether the adolescent meets criteria for a diagnosis of substance abuse or dependence. Adolescents should also be screened for mental health problems at the same time. At least 64% of adolescents with SUD in inpatient and residential programs also meet criteria for a comorbid psychiatric diagnosis (Jaycox, Morral, & Juvonen, 2003). Mental health disorders commonly associated with substance use include

---

Box 20.1 CRAFFT: Questions to identify adolescents with substance abuse problems

C Have you ever ridden in a **car** driven by someone (including yourself) that was "high" or had been using alcohol or drugs?

R Do you ever use alcohol or drugs to **relax,** feel better about yourself, or fit in?

A Do you ever use alcohol or drugs while you are by yourself or **alone**?

F Do you ever **forget** things you did while using alcohol or drugs?

F Does your **family** or **friends** ever tell you that you should cut down on your drinking or drug use?

T Have you ever gotten in **trouble** while you were using alcohol or drugs?

ADHD, conduct disorder, mood disorders, and trauma related symptoms (Chan, Dennis, & Funk, 2008).

Adolescents who have experimented should be provided a risk reduction intervention, such as *advice*. The adolescent should be advised to stop using substances entirely, with added education linking substance use to negative health effects and risk of DWI (driving while intoxicated). For those who screen positive for problem use or abuse, the primary care APN should refer to a child and adolescent psychiatric APN for further *assessment*. Again, in order to determine whether the adolescent meets criteria for an SUD, the assessment includes pattern of use, negative consequences of use, and attempts to stop using. The APN also *assesses* the adolescent's readiness for change (Levy, Vaughn, et al., 2002; Miller & Rollnik, 2002). Adolescents who refuse to stop or reduce their substance use or are unable to reduce their use should be referred for more intensive treatment, perhaps to an inpatient treatment facility.

Table 20.4 contains levels of treatment intervention and provides the APN with guidelines to assist with decision making when determining the most appropriate level of care needed by the youth based on clinical presentation (AAP, 2008; AACAP, 2005; American Society of Addiction Medicine [ASAM], 2007; SAMSHA, 1999).

Evidence-Based Treatment

Psychosocial interventions for SUDs in adolescents include individual, group, and family interventions. Family-based interventions have been the most extensively studied and have the most empirical support (Deas, 2008; Hogue & Liddle, 2009; Perepletchikova, Krystal, & Kaufman, 2008). Reviews of studies comparing family-based treatment to at least one other modality (Becker & Curry, 2008; Hogue & Liddle; Vaughn & Howard, 2004; Waldron & Turner, 2008) have concluded that family-based treatments (FBT) are effective in treating adolescents with AOD conditions. Benefits of FBTs include positive treatment engagement, treatment impact across a range of outcome domains, and durability of treatment effects. In addition, a small number of FBT studies among minority populations support their use (Hogue & Liddle).

Family-based interventions take into account the adolescent's functioning within the family, patterns of communication, and relationships with extended family members and other social systems. Family-based approaches include multisystemic therapy (MST), integrated family therapy and cognitive-behavioral therapy (CBT), multidimensional family therapy (MDFT), and brief strategic family therapy. MDFT and MST have similar treatment foci and assume that the adolescent is involved in multiple domains that are associated with distinct risk factors relevant to substance use (Deas, 2008). Each uses a multisystemic

approach in which the intervention aims to change youth behavior but also to reduce risk factors for substance use in the adolescent's family, school, peers, or community. Chapters 16 and 17 in this text contain additional information about these treatment interventions.

Becker and Curry (2008) examined the strength of the evidence regarding outpatient interventions for adolescent substance abuse. They compared family-based interventions, motivational enhancement therapy (MET) or motivational interviewing (MI), behavioral therapy, and CBT. They found that the strongest evidence for FBTs was motivational interventions and CBT. Among the family-based interventions, the best outcomes were achieved using ecological models that expanded the boundaries of treatment beyond the family and that used individualized strategies to target adolescent substance use in the *context* of multiple interrelated systems (similar to Bronfenbrenner's Bioecological System as discussed in Chapter 1 of this text).

Individual therapies also are effective treatments and include behavioral treatments that teach adolescents to identify internal and external stimuli that trigger AOD use and then provide skill training in refusal skills, relaxation techniques, and behavioral management. In behavioral interventions, the treatment focus is on identifying triggers for substance use and developing alternate coping skills through reinforcement conditions. Behavioral interventions play a major role in relapse prevention. Cognitive therapies focus on distorted thoughts and maladaptive perceptions that lead to problem use behaviors. CBT explicitly aims to modify cognitive processes, beliefs, individual behaviors, and environmental reinforcers that are associated with adolescent substance use. In both MET and brief motivational interventions, the goal is to resolve ambivalence about whether the adolescent has a substance use condition and to improve his or her motivation to change (Deas, 2008). MET's emphasis on a collaborative or proactive communication style has theoretical appeal as an intervention for adolescents (O'Leary, Tevyaw, & Monti, 2004). MI helps build motivation toward behavior change. Brief motivational interventions consisting of one or two sessions targeted toward increasing the adolescent's motivation to decrease substance use also produced favorable outcomes in comparison studies. Numerous studies indicated the efficacy and effectiveness of brief MI interventions (Baer, Garrett, Beadnell, Wells, & Peterson, 2007; D'Amico, Miles, Stern, & Meredith, 2008; Gray, McCambridge, & Strang, 2005; McCambridge, Slym, & Strang, 2008; Thush et al., 2009; Walker et al., 2006).

In a meta-analysis of studies examining individual and family treatments for adolescent SUDs, all tested interventions were effective in reducing alcohol use (Tripodi, Bender, Litschge, & Vaughn, 2010). Large effect sizes were

Table 20.4 Levels of intervention

Level	Description	Reference
Outpatient Level 1	Not at risk for withdrawal except from nicotine. Is stable and not at risk of harm to self or others.	American Society of Addiction Medicine (ASAM), 2007
Intensive outpatient Level 2	At high risk for relapse without close monitoring and support.	
Partial hospitalization (PH) or day treatment (DT)	Most structured. PH may consist of several hours/day up to 5 days / week. PH can include a residential halfway program for nonacute substance users.	
Medically monitored intensive inpatient Level 3	For those at high risk for withdrawal, need 24-hour structure and monitoring, and are unable to control use; environments may be dangerous for continued use. Logistics problems for outpatient program.	
Medically managed intensive inpatient Level 4	For those needing 24-hour medical and nursing care perhaps due to severe risk of withdrawal or psychiatric care and addiction treatment.	
Residential	Long-term treatment including psychosocial rehab for those with multiple problems. Duration of 30 days to a year.	
Aftercare	Ongoing support for transition to home community and family; includes relapse prevention.	
Group homes	May follow treatment program or be part of it. Transitional living with staff and consumer participation in responsibilities, governance, school, or work.	
Psychosocial	Includes family treatments (multisystemic), integrated family therapy, and CBT. Individual psychoeducation for refusal skills, identification of triggers and learning alternative options. CBT may also be included. 12-Step programs include AA and NA.	AACAP, 2005; Becker & Curry, 2008; Deas 2008; Hogue & Liddle, 2009; Kaminer, 2001; Tripodi et al., 2010
Pharmacological	Withdrawal protocol from alcohol includes benzodiazepine taper, multivitamins, and seizure precautions Medically supervised withdrawal from opiates includes clonidine, methadone, and buprenophine (Naltrexone)	Fournier & Levy 2006; SAMHSA/CSAT, 2006; NIDA, 2009; Woody et al., 2008

found for CBT plus a 12-step approach, brief MI, CBT with active aftercare, MDFT, and brief interventions with the adolescent and parent. CBT was found to be superior to group interactional therapy and comparable to FBT and group psychoeducation. While the effects tended to fade over time, behavioral treatment had more enduring effects than supportive counseling, and effects of MDFT lasted longer than family education or group therapy. Behavioral treatment and MDFT had significant reductions in alcohol use at twelve months. Behavior-based treatments, whether individual or family based, were most beneficial in attaining long-term change (Tripodi et al.).

In the Cannabis Youth Treatment study, the largest treatment trial to date among adolescents with substance use conditions, CBT combined with either five or twelve sessions of MET; combined CBT, MET, and family support; and behavioral therapy were compared. Clinical outcomes were comparable across interventions while cost effectiveness favored CBT with MET (either five or twelve sessions) and behavioral therapy (Dennis et al., 2004). In other studies, CBT has produced rapid short-term effects, especially when combined with MET. Adding CBT to family-based interventions may lead to longer-term efficacy (Perepletchikova et al., 2008).

12-Step Programs

Many programs incorporate Alcoholics Anonymous (AA) or Narcotics Anonymous (NA) into their treatment program (SAMHSA/CSAT, 1999). No well-controlled studies to date have evaluated the effectiveness of attendance at 12-step programs for adolescents with SUDs; however, several studies have found benefits of AA and NA attendance. Generally, duration of treatment, including completing a treatment program and attending an aftercare program or AA meetings, is associated with more positive treatment outcomes (AACAP, 2005; Kaminer, 2001).

Pharmacological Interventions

Pharmacological interventions are *rarely used* in the treatment of adolescents with AOD use disorders (Deas & Clark, 2009). However, several medications are available for treating alcohol dependence, tobacco dependence, and opioid dependence. Medications may be used during detoxification to prevent serious sequelae of abrupt withdrawal or to prevent relapse by reducing cravings or by blocking the effects of illicit substances. Other medications are prescribed for comorbid psychiatric disorders (Simkin & Grenoble, 2010). The APN should be aware that most medications specific for treating substance dependence and used routinely in adults lack safety and efficacy data for use in children or adolescents.

Compared to psychosocial treatments, there is little evidence supporting the use of pharmacological agents for the treatment of substance use disorders in adolescents (Deas, 2008; Deas & Clark, 2009; Perepletchikova et al., 2008). Small controlled studies provided preliminary support for the use of disulfiram and acamprosate with alcohol-dependent adolescents in inpatient settings and suggested that the opioid antagonist naltrexone is an effective and well-tolerated adjunct to psychosocial interventions for alcohol-dependent adolescents (Perepletchikova et al.). The small number of studies, with small sample sizes, limits their usefulness in guiding practice.

Detoxification

Alcohol detoxification is rarely required for adolescents. Adolescents are more likely to require emergency treatment for alcohol poisoning after binge drinking. If an adolescent does require medically managed withdrawal from alcohol, the protocol typically includes a benzodiazepine taper, multivitamins, and seizure precautions. Opioid dependence is treated most effectively with a combination of behavioral and pharmacological treatments; however, the usual treatment offered to opioid-dependent youth is a short-term detoxification and individual or group therapy in residential or outpatient settings (Woody et al., 2008).

Medically Supervised Opiate Withdrawal (MSW)

MSW is a set of interventions to manage acute intoxication and withdrawal with the goals of relieving withdrawal symptoms and minimizing the physical harm caused by the abuse of substances. MSW consists of evaluation, stabilization, and fostering the patient's entry into treatment. Detoxification is not treatment; it is the first step toward treatment in either a drug-free program or one that uses pharmacotherapy (NIDA, 2009). Medications used during MSW of opiates include clonidine, methadone, and buprenorphine.

Methadone is the most frequently used agent approved for medically supervised withdrawal of heroin and all other opioids (SAMHSA/CSAT, 1999; 2006). Methadone is approved for children younger than eighteen only if they have relapsed twice following medication taper or short-term rehabilitation (Fiellin, 2008). Methadone is a long acting mu-opioid receptor agonist that displaces heroin or other opioids, suppresses withdrawal and drug craving for twenty-four to thirty-six hours (SAMHSA/CSAT, 2006), and prevents some of the euphoric effects of heroin. Methadone must be dispensed daily at a special SAMHSA-approved methadone clinic unless the patient is being hospitalized for a comorbid condition. Methadone is approved for both short-term detoxification and for use in longer-term substance abuse treatment. Continued methadone replacement is effective in reducing relapse rates in adults, and observational studies have found positive results with adolescents. Methadone stabilization is the treatment of choice for pregnant opioid-dependent patients. Methadone must be dispensed from licensed methadone clinics; however, many states restrict adolescents' access to methadone clinics (Fournier & Levy, 2006; Minozzi, Amato, & Davoli, 2009; SAMHSA/CSAT, 2006).

Clonidine is an alpha-2 agonist that has been used for opiate MSW since 1978. It relieves some of the symptoms of opiate withdrawal but is usually ineffective for common symptoms such as insomnia, body aches, and craving (SAMHSA/CSAT, 2006).

Buprenorphine is a schedule III mu-opioid partial agonist at the mu receptor and an antagonist at the kappa receptor. Buprenorphine has a greater margin of safety than methadone because it has a ceiling effect that prevents larger doses from producing larger agonist effects (SAMHSA/CSAT, 2006; Woody et al., 2008). It causes less physical dependence than methadone, so patients experience fewer withdrawal symptoms when discontinuing the drug. Buprenorphine precipitates withdrawal in patients who have recently used opioids, so it should not be initiated until a patient has begun to experience withdrawal symptoms. Buprenorphine/ naloxone combination is designed to minimize abuse by blocking the effects of crushing and injecting it. Buprenorphine/naloxone is taken sublingually once or twice a day and can be prescribed by specially trained physicians in an office setting (Fournier & Levy, 2006). It is approved for adolescents over sixteen years of age for detoxification and for opioid maintenance treatment.

Only two studies of buprenorphine use in opioid-dependent adolescents have been published. Woody et al. (2008) compared fourteen-day detoxification with buprenorphine/naloxone and twelve-week treatment. Continuing treatment patients reported less opioid use, less injecting, and a higher proportion remained in treatment at week twelve. However, high levels of opioid use occurred after discontinuation of the drug.

Naltrexone is an opioid antagonist that blocks the effects of other opioids, including heroin, morphine, and methadone. It should not be started until the patient is opioid free for seven to ten days, to prevent severe, sudden withdrawal. When used as directed, naltrexone effectively prevents relapse, but poor patient compliance has been reported (SAMHSA/CSAT, 2006).

Relapse Prevention

Even with the use of evidence-based interventions, the risk of relapse is significant. Half of adolescents treated for AOD conditions relapse within three months of completing treatment, and about two-thirds relapse within six months, with boys more likely to relapse than girls (Wagner, 2008). Developmental variables that may be associated with treatment outcomes include pubertal status, development of executive mental functions, social relationships, and developmental transitions (e.g., getting a driver's license, starting high school) (Wagner). Despite having better coping behaviors, African-American adolescents are more likely to relapse than white adolescents, illustrating the need

for programs addressing their different resource needs (Ciesla, Valle, & Spear, 2008).

Major predictors of relapse for adolescents include polydrug use and peer relationships following treatment. Adolescents whose friends use drugs were almost ten times as likely to return to regular drug use in one study (Ciesla, 2010), while having new friends post-treatment, attending support groups, and returning to school were protective factors following treatment (Ciesla et al., 2008). Persistent smokers are at higher risk for relapse with alcohol and marijuana than are those who quit smoking (deDios et al., 2009).

Relapse is viewed as a result of complex, dynamic interactions among multiple risk factors and situational determinants (Witkiewitz & Marlatt, 2004). Relapse prevention strategies includes CBT approaches focusing on skill-building in recognizing and avoiding high-risk situations when possible, and coping effectively with risky situations and emotional states (Carroll & Onken, 2007). CBT with internal cue exposure aims to bridge the gap between clinic and home behaviors by weakening the link between emotions and drug-craving and use and promoting nondrug responses to feelings of distress (Otto, O'Cleirigh, & Pollack, 2007). Incentive therapies also have been effective in maintaining abstinence from drugs following treatment (Caroll & Onken).

Collaborative Nursing Care

Much of the prevention and early intervention for adolescents at risk for tobacco, alcohol, and other drug use, abuse, and dependence can be completed in primary care settings through screening and brief interventions. For adolescents who require specialty treatment, primary care APNs can use their initial screening and assessment to refer adolescents to the appropriate specialists for further assessment and treatment. During outpatient treatment, primary care APNs should be involved in monitoring physical health status, especially assessing for potential consequences of AOD use. Following completion of specialty treatment, primary care APNs should be involved in follow-up care and continued screening for substance relapse.

A number of barriers prevent quality health care for many adults as well as adolescents with substance use conditions. Among the barriers are the separate systems of care for mental health, substance abuse, and general health conditions. Providing quality care for substance use conditions requires making collaboration and communication among primary care and specialty care providers the norm. Developing linkages among primary care and specialty providers is essential. Primary care and psychiatric mental health APNs are well-suited to develop such linkages. Practice models that foster such collaboration include practice agreements among primary care and specialty providers; collocation of mental health, substance use, and primary health care services; or clinically integrated practices of mental health/substance use and primary care.

Implications for Advanced Practice Nurses

Few education programs for APNs, physicians, or other health care providers include sufficient information about substance use conditions in their curricula. Nevertheless, primary care APNs can use the online education programs provided by the NIAAA, NIDA, and SAMHSA and websites for assistance with tobacco cessation, such as those of the CDC (2011), the National Cancer Institute (n.d.), and the American Lung Association (2011) to begin educating themselves about screening, brief intervention, treatment in primary care, and appropriate referral to specialty assessment and treatment. All adolescents should be screened for tobacco, alcohol, and prescription, OTC, and illicit drug use at least at annual physical examinations, and preferably at each appointment, using valid, age-appropriate screening instruments and procedures. Responses to brief interventions and referrals should be monitored consistently and documented. Family education and support are important components of treatment. Awareness that relapse occurs for most adolescents who attempt to quit smoking or who are treated for AOD abuse or dependence helps APNs remain nonjudgmental in the face of setbacks. Monitoring progress as well as potential risk factors such as stress is an important component of supportive follow-up care.

Case Exemplar

Paul is a sixteen-year-old high school sophomore who arrived at his primary care provider's office for an annual physical examination. As part of the history and examination, the primary care APN asked Paul the preliminary questions for the CRAFFT: Had he ever used tobacco, drank alcohol, used marijuana, or anything else to get high? Paul told her that he sometimes drank beer when he attended a party or if he went camping with his friends. He denied that he drank very much or often. When questioned further, he reported that he typically drank two or three times a week, and on most occasions he drank about five or six beers. The APN then asked specifically about use of tobacco, marijuana, inhalants, OTC drugs, or any illicit drugs. Paul denied using any illicit drugs, but said he did smoke cigarettes and occasionally drank high caffeine drinks when he was drinking beer "so he wouldn't fall asleep." He had "borrowed"

a classmate's Ritalin to study for a test a few times. In response to the CRAFFT questions, he reported that he had been in a car when the driver had been drinking or high and that he had once fallen into a window when he was drinking and cut his hand when the glass broke. Paul's CRAFFT score was positive on questions about car, friends, and trouble. The APN shared the results with Paul and initiated a brief intervention. Paul was advised to refrain from driving after drinking or from riding in a car with someone who had been drinking. She educated him about amounts of alcohol that were considered high risk and binge drinking; she asked him if he could abstain from drinking for a month. Paul seemed hesitant but agreed to abstain from alcohol and tobacco for two weeks. The APN arranged a follow-up visit in two weeks.

Paul rescheduled for two weeks later but did not keep the appointment. Three months later, Paul finally returned to the office complaining of a sore throat and fever, accompanied by his mother. Paul met with another APN, who again used the CRAFFT to screen for AOD use, but this time Paul denied ever riding in a car with a driver who had been high, drinking any alcohol, using tobacco, or misusing any OTC or prescription drugs. Paul was reminded about his reports at the previous office visit. Paul said that he had not made any changes and really thought that people were making a big deal out of nothing. He didn't think his drinking was a problem—all his friends drank as much or more than he did, and he didn't appreciate being told to stop. The APN asked if he had been able to stop or cut down on his drinking at all during the past three months. Paul said he had abstained for a week but then was invited to a party where everyone was drinking, so he did too. The APN expressed empathy about Paul's feelings about not drinking when with his friends but also expressed concern about Paul's difficulty abstaining from drinking. He reviewed Paul's previous screening results and the additional information gleaned from this interview and recommended referral for additional assessment. Paul refused to schedule an assessment appointment with a specialist. The APN continued to use motivational interviewing strategies to encourage Paul to consider changing his behavior. He also reminded Paul that his riding in cars when the driver has been drinking was a safety issue. He told Paul he wanted to discuss his concerns with Paul's mother. Paul argued that his mother did not need to be brought into their conversation. The APN told Paul that he was referring him for further assessment, not treatment; but because of the safety concern, Paul's parents should be aware of his riding in cars with others who were drinking. They discussed what information would be shared with Paul's parents.

They agreed that Paul's mother would be informed of the concerns about Paul's safety and the recommendation that Paul be assessed by a specialist. Paul agreed to stop riding in cars when the driver had been drinking or was high and agreed to the assessment. After discussing his concerns and recommendations with Paul's mother, the primary care APN scheduled Paul for an assessment appointment with an psychiatric APN and scheduled a follow-up visit in one month.

Paul completed the assessment. He was diagnosed with generalized anxiety disorder and alcohol abuse and was prescribed fluoxetine 20 mg by mouth every morning. The psychiatric APN planned to continue to see Paul for CBT and medication management, referred him to an alcohol education program with his parents, and referred them all for family therapy. Paul continued the outpatient therapy at the specialty clinic and was followed by his primary care APN for routine health status care and periodic blood and urine tests.

Summary

SUDs are complex chronic illnesses that are characterized by compulsive use that persists despite devastating consequences. Unlike other chronic illnesses, SUDs involve not only physical and psychological symptoms and distress, but also illegal behavior and consequences that can complicate treatment plans and add an additional financial burden for the adolescent's family. SUDs involve stigma that often causes both the adolescent and the family to experience embarrassment and shame. Many adolescents and their families view their drug- or alcohol-seeking behaviors as willful expressions of a moral failing, rather than as symptoms of a chronic illness. Adolescents are typically brought to treatment by their parents or other caregivers. By the time a family presents for treatment of their adolescent's SUD, multiple areas of their lives have been affected, and often their family relationships have been disrupted. Effective treatment approaches target not only the immediate issues of stopping AOD use and preventing severe withdrawal, but also teaching the adolescent how to prevent relapse and maintain a drug-free lifestyle while becoming productive at school or at work. In addition, treatment involves assisting the family in rebuilding their relationships.

Experimentation leading to hazardous and harmful use, abuse, and dependence on alcohol and other drugs is a developmental condition that typically arises during adolescence. Adolescents are at high risk of developing substance use conditions because of their propensity to take risks, the continuing development of brain areas important for decision making, their unique physiological responses to alcohol and other drugs, and their high-risk patterns of AOD use. Adolescents differ from adults in their physiological responses to AOD, in that they are more responsive to positive effects and are less sensitive to negative effects of alcohol intoxication.

Adolescents also have increased sensitivity to long-term behavioral and physiological consequences of AOD use, including greater vulnerability to alcohol-related neurodegeneration with accompanying disruptions in memory, learning, and executive functioning. Adolescents with AOD abuse and dependence can be treated as effectively as adults but have exceedingly high relapse rates within a short period of time. Integrating developmental considerations in the design and implementation of interventions for adolescent substance use conditions is essential for improving treatment effectiveness and reducing relapse rates. Among the most effective interventions for substance use conditions in primary care settings are screening and brief intervention, with referral to specialty treatment for adolescents exhibiting signs of AOD abuse or dependence.

Effective treatment requires attention to the multiple environmental risk and protective factors influencing adolescents' AOD use and the transition to abuse and dependence, including the adolescent's self-regulation abilities, current stressors, and family and peer influences, including parenting education. Important features of treatment are sufficient length of treatment, a focus on relapse prevention, including stress-management skills, and attendance at aftercare and/or a 12-step support program.

Resources

The federal government has published guidelines for screening for substance use on several websites. These include the Substance Abuse and Mental Health Services Administration (SAMHSA), National Institute on Alcohol Abuse and Alcoholism (NIAAA), and the National Institute on Drug Abuse (NIDA) at http://www.niaaa.nih.gov/Publications/EducationTrainingMaterials/Pages/guide.aspx#clinician.

The NIDA program, NIDAMED (http://www.drugabuse.gov/nidamed/) provides resources to assist primary care clinicians in screening patients for substance use using online and print versions of *NM ASSIST*, the NIDA modified version of the *Alcohol, Smoking, and Substance Involvement Screening Test* (ASSIST) (WHO ASSIST Working Group, 2002). Other resources can be found at the CDC (2011) site, the National Cancer Institute (n.d.), and the American Lung Association (2011).

References

American Academy of Child & Adolescent Psychiatry (AACAP). (2005). Practice parameter for the assessment and treatment of children and adolescents with substance use disorders. *Journal of the American Academy of Child & Adolescent Psychiatry, 44,* 609–621.

American Academy of Pediatrics (AAP). (2000). Indications for management and referral of patients involved in substance abuse. *Pediatrics, 106,* 143–148. Retrieved from http://aappolicy.aappublications.org/cgi/reprint/pediatrics;106/1/143.pdf

American Academy of Pediatrics (AAP). (2008). Statement of Endorsement: Treating tobacco use and dependence. *Pediatrics, 122*, 471.

American Lung Association. (2011). *Freedom from smoking online.* Available at http://www.ffsonline.org/

American Society of Addiction Medicine (ASAM). (2007). *ASAM PPC–2R patient placement criteria for the treatment of substance-related disorders* (Mee-Lee, D. [Ed.]). Philadelphia, PA: Lippincott, Williams & Wilkins.

Babor, T.F., Higgins-Biddle, J.C., Saunders, J.B., & Monteiro, M.G. (2001). *AUDIT: The alcohol use disorders identification test: Guidelines for use in primary care* (2nd ed.). Geneva, Switzerland: World Health Organization.

Baer, J.S., Garrett, S.B., Beadnell, B., Wells, E.A., & Peterson, P.L. (2007). Brief motivational intervention with homeless adolescents: Evaluating effects on substance use and service utilization. *Psychology of Addictive Behaviors, 21*, 582–586.

Becker, S.J., & Curry, J.F. (2008). Outpatient interventions for adolescent substance abuse: A quality of evidence review. *Journal of Counseling & Clinical Psychology, 76*, 531–543.

Bohn, M.J., Babor, T.F., & Kranzler, H.R. (1995). The alcohol use disorders identification test (AUDIT): Validation of a screening instrument for use in medical settings. *J Stud Alcohol, 56*, 423–432.

Budney, A.J., Hughes, J.R., Moore, B.A., & Vandrey, R.G. (2004). Review of the validity and significance of cannabis withdrawal syndrome. *American Journal of Psychiatry, 161*, 1967–1977. Retrieved from http://ajp.psychiatryonline.org/cgi/reprint/161/11/1967

Budney, A.J., Roffman, R., Stephens, R.S., & Walker, D.W. (2007). Marijuana dependence and its treatment. *Addiction Science & Clinical Practice, 4(1)*, 4–16. Retrieved from http://www.ncbi.nlm.nih.gov/pmc/articles/PMC2797098/

Carroll, K.M., & Onken, L.S. (2007). Behavioral therapies for drug abuse. *American Journal of Psychiatry, 162*, 1452–1460.

Centers for Disease Control and Prevention (CDC). (2011). *Quit smoking.* Available at http://www.cdc.gov/tobacco/quit_smoking/index.htm

Centers for Disease Control and Prevention (CDC). (2010). *Unintentional drug poisoning in the United States.* Atlanta, GA: Author. Retrieved from http://www.cdc.gov/HomeandRecreationalSafety/pdf/poison-issue-brief.pdf

Chan, Y.F., Dennis, M., & Funk, R.R. (2008). Prevalence and comorbidity of major internalizing and externalizing problems among adolescents and adults presenting to substance use treatment. *Journal of Substance Abuse Treatment, 34*, 14–24.

Ciesla, J.R. (2010). Evaluating the risk of relapse for adolescents treated for substance abuse. *Addictive Disorders & Their Treatment, 9*, 87.

Ciesla, J.R., Valle, M., & Spear, S.F. (2008). Measuring relapse after adolescent substance abuse treatment: A proportional hazard approach. *Addictive Disorders & Their Treatment, 7*, 87–97.

Clark, D.B., Cornelius, J.R., Kirisci, L., & Tarter, R.E. (2005). Childhood risk categories for adolescent substance involvement: A general liability typology. *Drug & Alcohol Dependence, 77*, 13–21.

Clark, D.B., Thatcher, D.L., & Tapert, S.F. (2008). Alcohol, psychological dysregulation, and adolescent brain development. *Alcoholism: Clinical & Experimental Research, 32*, 375–385.

D'Amico, E., Miles, J.N.V., Stern, S.A., & Meredith, L.S. (2008). Brief motivational interviewing for teens at risk of substance use consequences: A randomized pilot study in a primary care clinic. *Journal of Substance Abuse Treatment, 35*, 53–61.

Deas, D. (2008). Evidence-based treatments for alcohol use disorders in adolescents. *Pediatrics, 121*(Suppl 4), S348–354.

Deas, D., & Clark, A. (2009). Current state of treatment for alcohol and other drug use disorders in adolescents. *Alcohol Research & Health, 32*, 76–82. Retrieved from http://pubs.niaaa.nih.gov/publications/arh321/76-82.pdf

deDios, M.A., Vaughn, E.L., Stanton, C.A., & Niaura, R. (2009). Adolescent tobacco use and substance abuse treatment outcomes. *Journal of Substance Abuse Treatment, 37*, 17–34.

Dennis, M.L., Godley, S.H., Diamond, G., Tims, F.M., Babor, T., Donaldson, J., Funk, R. (2004). The Cannabis Youth Treatment (CYT): Main findings of two randomized trials. *Journal of Substance Abuse Treatment, 27*, 197–213. doi: 10.1016/j.jsat.2003.09.005

Dick, D.M., & Agrawal, A. (2008). The genetics of alcohol and other drug dependence. *Alcohol Research & Health, 31*, 111–118. Retrieved from http://pubs.niaaa.nih.gov/publications/arh312/111-118.htm

DiFranza, J.R., Savageau, J.A., Fletcher, K., Pbert, L., O'Loughlin, J., McNeill, A.D., et al. (2007). Susceptibility to nicotine dependence: The development and assessment of nicotine dependence in youth 2 study. *Pediatrics, 120*, e974–983. DOI: 10.1542/peds.2007–0027

Feldstein, S.W., & Miller, W.R. (2006). Substance use and risk-taking among adolescents. *Journal of Mental Health, 15*, 633–643.

Felgus, M.A., Caldwell, S.B., & Hesselbrock, V. (2009). Assessing alcohol-involved adolescents: Toward a developmentally-relevant diagnostic taxonomy. *Journal of Substance Use, 14*, 49–60.

Fiellin, D.A. (2008). Treatment of adolescent opioid dependence: No quick fix. [Editorial]. *JAMA, 300*, 2057–2059.

Fournier, M.E., & Levy, S. (2006). Recent trends in adolescent substance use, primary care screening, and updates in treatment options. *Current Opinion in Pediatrics, 18*, 352–358.

Gelhorn, H., Hartman, C., Sakai, J., Stallings, M., Young, S., Rhee, Crowley, T. (2008). Toward DSM-V: An item response theory analysis of the diagnostic process for DSM-IV alcohol abuse and dependence in adolescents. *Journal of the American Academy of Child & Adolescent Psychiatry, 47*, 1329–1339.

Gilpin, N.W., & Koob, G.F. (2008). Neurobiology of alcohol dependence: Focus on motivational mechanisms. *Alcohol Research & Health, 31*, 185–195. Retrieved from http://pubs.niaaa.nih.gov/publications/arh313/185-195.pdf

Gray, E., McCambridge, J., & Strang, J. (2005). The effectiveness of motivational interviewing delivered by youth workers in reducing drinking, cigarette and cannabis smoking among young people: Quasi-experimental pilot study. *Alcohol and Alcoholism, 40*, 535–539.

Hingson, R.W., Heeren, T., & Edwards, E.M. (2008). Age of drinking onset, alcohol dependence, and their relation to drug use and dependence, driving under the influence of drugs, and motor-vehicle crash involvement because of drugs. *J Stud Alcohol Drugs, 69*, 192–201.

Hingson, R.W., Heeren, T., & Winter, M.R. (2006). Age at drinking onset and alcohol dependence: Age at onset, duration, and severity. *Archives of Pediatrics & Adolescent Medicine, 160*, 739–746.

Hogue, A., & Liddle, H.A. (2009). Family-based treatment for adolescent substance abuse: Controlled trials and new horizons in services research. *Journal of Family Therapy, 31*, 126–154.

Jaycox, L.H., Morral, A.R., & Juvonen, J. (2003). Mental health and medical problems and service use among adolescent substance users. *Journal of the American Academy of Child & Adolescent Psychiatry, 42*, 701–709.

Johnston, L.D., O'Malley, P.M., Bachman, J.G., & Schulenberg, J.E. (2009). *Monitoring the future national results on adolescent drug use: Overview of key findings, 2008.* (NIH Publication No. 09-7401). Bethesda, MD: National Institute on Drug Abuse. Retrieved from http://monitoringthefuture.org/pubs/monographs/overview2008.pdf

Johnston, L.D., O'Malley, P.M., Bachman, J.G., & Schulenberg, J.E. (2010). *Monitoring the future national results on adolescent drug use: Overview of key findings, 2009*. (NIH Publication No. 10-7583). Bethesda, MD: National Institute on Drug Abuse. Retrieved from http://monitoring-thefuture.org/pubs/monographs/overview2009.pdf

Kaminer, Y. (2001). Alcohol & drug abuse: Adolescent substance abuse treatment: Where do we go from here? *Psychiatric Services, 52*, 147.

Kandel, D.B., Hu, M.C., Griesler, P.C., & Schaffran, C. (2007). On the development of nicotine dependence in adolescence. *Drug and Alcohol Dependence, 91*, 26–39.

Knight, J.R., Sherritt, L., Harris, S.K., Gates, E.C., & Chang, G. (2003). Validity of brief alcohol screening tests among adolescents: A comparison of the AUDIT, POSIT, CAGE, and CRAFFT. *Alcoholism: Clinical and Experimental Research, 27*, 67–73. DOI: 10.1111/j.1530-0277.2003.tb02723.x

Knight J.R., Sherritt, L., Shrier, L.A., Harris, S.K., & Chang, G. (2002). Validity of the CRAFFT substance abuse screening test among adolescent clinic patients. *Archives of Pediatrics & Adolescent Medicine, 156*, 607–614.

Knight, J.R., Shrier, L.A., Bravender, T.D., Farrell, M., Vander Bilt, J., & Shaffer, H.J. (1999). A new brief screen for adolescent substance abuse. *Archives of Pediatric & Adolescent Medicine, 153*, 591–596.

Kulig, J.W., & Committee on Substance Abuse. (2005). Tobacco, alcohol, and other drugs: The role of the pediatrician in prevention, identification, and management of substance abuse. *Pediatrics, 115*, 816–821. doi: 10.1542/peds.2004-2841

Leslie, F.M., Loughlin, S.E., Wang, R., Perez, L., Lotfipour, S., & Belluzzi, J.D. (2004). Adolescent development of forebrain stimulant responsiveness: Insights from animal studies. *Annals of the New York Academy of Sciences, 1021*, 148–159.

Levy, S., & Knight, J.R. (2008). Screening, brief intervention, and referral to treatment for adolescents. *Journal of Addiction Medicine, 2*, 215–221.

Levy, S., Vaughan, B.L., & Knight, J.R. (2002). Office-based intervention for adolescent substance abuse. *Pediatric Clinics of North America, 49*, 329–343.

Maggs, J.S., Patrick, M.E., & Feinstein, L. (2008). Childhood and adolescent predictors of alcohol use and problems in adolescence and adulthood in the National Child Development Study. *Addiction, 103*(Suppl 1), 7–22.

Martino, S., Grilo, C.M., & Fehon, D.C. (2000). Development of the drug abuse screening test for adolescents (Dast-a). *Addictive Behaviors, 25*, 57–70.

Masten, A.S., Faden, V.B., Zucker, R.A., & Spear, L.P. (2008). Underage drinking: A developmental framework. *Pediatrics, 121*(S4), S235–S251.

McCabe, S.E., Boyd, C.J., & Young, A. (2007). Medical and nonmedical use of prescription drugs among secondary school students. *Journal of Adolescent Health, 40*, 76–83.

McCambridge, J., Slym, R.L., & Strang, J. (2008). Randomized controlled trial of motivational interviewing compared with drug information and advice for early intervention among young cannabis users. *Addiction, 103*, 1809.

Miller, W. R., & Rollnick, S. (2002). *Motivational interviewing: Preparing people for changes* (2nd ed.). New York, NY: Guilford.

Minozzi, S., Amato, L., & Davoli, M. (2009). Detoxification treatments for opiate dependent adolescents. *Cochrane Database of Systematic Reviews 2009*(2). Art. No.: CD006749. DOI: 10.1002/14651858.CD006749.pub2

Mokdad, A.H., Marks, J.S., Stroup, D.F., & Gerberding, J.L. (2004). Actual causes of death in the United States, 2000. *JAMA, 291*, 1238–1245.

Moritsugu, K.P., & Li, T.K. (2008). Underage drinking: Understanding and reducing risk in the context of human development. [Foreword]. *Pediatrics, 121* (Suppl 4), S231–232.

National Association of Pediatric Nurse Practitioners (NAPNAP). (2009). NAPNAP position statement on prevention of tobacco use and effects in the pediatric population. *Journal of Pediatric Health Care, 24*(2), 13A–14A. doi:10.1016/j.pedhc.2009.10.004

National Cancer Institute. (n.d.). *Quit smoking today*. Available at http://www.smokefree.gov

National Institute on Alcohol Abuse and alcoholism. (2005). *Helping patients who drink too much*. Retrieved from http://www.niaaa.nih.gov/Publications/EducationTrainingMaterials/Pages/guide.aspx#clinician

National Institute on Drug Abuse (NIDA). (2005). *Heroin: National Institute on Drug Abuse research reports*. (NIH Publication No. 05-4165). Bethesda, MD: Author. Retrieved from http://www.drugabuse.gov/ResearchReports/Heroin/Heroin.html

National Institute on Drug Abuse (NIDA). (2008). *NIDA InfoFacts: Understanding drug abuse and addiction*. Retrieved from http://www.drugabuse.gov/Infofacts/understand.html

National Institute on Drug Abuse (NIDA). (2009). *Principles of drug addiction treatment: A research based guide* (2nd ed.) (NIH Pub No. 09–4180). Bethesda, MD: Author. Retrieved from http://www.drugabuse.gov/PODAT/PODATindex.html

National Institute on Drug Abuse (NIDA). (2010c). *Drugs, brains, and behavior: The science of addiction*. (NIH Pub. No. 10–5605). Bethesda, MD: Author. Retrieved from www.drugabuse.gov/scienceofaddiction/sciofaddiction.pdf

National Institute on Drug Abuse (NIDA). (2010a). *NIDA infofacts: Nationwide trends*. Retrieved from http://www.drugabuse.gov/infofacts/nationtrends.html

National Institute on Drug Abuse (NIDA). (n.d.). *Addiction science: From molecules to managed care*. Retrieved from http://www.drugabuse.gov/pubs/teaching/Teaching6/Teaching.html

National Institute on Drug Abuse (NIDA). (n.d.). *NIDAMED*. Retrieved on 4/29/11 from http://www.drugabuse.gov/nidamed/

National Institute on Drug Abuse (NIDA). (2010b). *NIDA Infofacts: Heroin*. Retrieved from http://www.drugabuse.gov/Infofacts/heroin.html

Newbury-Birch, D., Walker, J., Avery, L., Beyer, F., Brown, N., Jackson, K., Gilvarry, E. (2009). *Impact of alcohol consumption on young people: A systematic review of published reviews*. Nottingham, UK: Newcastle University, Department for Children, Schools and Families. Retrieved from http://www.education.gov.uk/publications/eOrderingDownload/DCSF-RR067.pdf

Nixon, K., & McClain, J.A. (2010). Adolescence as a critical window for developing an alcohol use disorder: Current findings in neuroscience. *Current Opinion in Psychiatry, 23*, 227–232.

Nonnemaker, J.M., Mowery, P.D., Hersey, J.C., Nimsch, C.T., Farrelly, M.C., Messeri, P., & Haviland, M.L. (2004). Measurement properties of a nicotine dependence scale for adolescents. *Nicotine & Tob Research, 6*, 295–301. doi: 10.1080/14622200410001676413

O'Connell, M.E., Boat, T., & Warner, K.E. (Eds.). (2009). (2009). *Preventing mental, emotional, and behavioral disorders among young people: Progress and possibilities*. Washington, DC: The National Academies Press.

O'Leary Tevyaw, T., & Monti, P.M. (2004). Motivational enhancement and other brief interventions for adolescent substance abuse: Foundations, applications and evaluations. *Addiction, 99*(Suppl 2), 63–76.

Otto, M.W., O'Cleirigh, C.M., & Pollack, M.H. (2007). *Science & Practice Perspectives, 3*(2), 48–56. Retrieved from http://archives.drugabuse.gov/PDF/Perspectives/vol3no2/Attending.pdf

Palmer, R.H.C., Young, S.E., Hopfer, C.J., Corley, R.P., Stallings, M.C., Crowley, T.J., & Hewitt, J.K. (2009). Developmental epidemiology of drug use and abuse in adolescence and young adulthood: Evidence of generalized risk. *Drug and Alcohol Dependence, 102*, 78–87. doi:10.1016/j.drugalcdep.2009.01.012

Patton, G.C., Coffey, C., Lynskey, M.T., Reid, S., Hemphill, S., Carlin, J.B., & Hall, W. (2007). Trajectories of adolescent alcohol and cannabis use into young adulthood. *Addiction, 102*, 607.

Perepletchikova, F., Krystal, J.H., & Kaufman, J. (2008). Practitioner review – Adolescent alcohol use disorders: Assessment and treatment issues. *Journal of Child Psychology & Psychiatry, 49*, 1131–1154.

Peterson, K. (2004/2005). Biomarkers for alcoholic use and abuse – A summary. *Alcohol, Research & Health, 28*, 30–37. Retrieved from http://pubs.niaaa.nih.gov/publications/arh28-1/30-37.htm

Prokhorov, A.V., Koehly, L.M., Pallonen, U.E., & Hudmon, K.S. (1998). Adolescent nicotine dependence measured by the modified Fagerström tolerance questionnaire at two time points. *Journal of Child and Adolescent Substance Abuse, 7*, 35–47.

Rehm, J., Taylor, B., & Room, R. (2006). Global burden of disease from alcohol, illicit drugs and tobacco. *Drug Alcohol Review, 25*, 503–513.

Rose, R.J., & Dick, D.M. (2004/2005). Gene-Environment interplay in adolescent drinking behavior. *Alcohol, Research & Health, 28*, 222–229. Retrieved from http://pubs.niaaa.nih.gov/publications/arh284/222-229.htm

Shields, A.L., Campfield, D.C., Howell, R.T., Wallace, K., & Weiss, R.D. (2008). Score reliability of adolescent alcohol screening measures: A meta-analytic inquiry. *Journal of Child & Adolescent Substance Abuse, 17*(4), 75–97.

Shiffman, S., Waters, A.J., & Hickcox, M. (2004). The Nicotine Dependence Syndrome Scale: A multidimensional measure of nicotine dependence. *Nicotine & Tobacco Research, 6*, 327–348.

Simkin, D.R., & Grenoble, S. (2010). Pharmacotherapies for adolescent substance use disorders. *Child & Adolescent Psychiatric Clinics of North America, 19*, 591–608.

Stahl, S. (2008). Disorders of reward, drug abuse, and their treatment. In *Stahl's essential psychopharmacology: Neuroscientific basis and practical applications.* New York, NY: Cambridge University Press.

Substance Abuse & Mental Health Services Administration Office of Applied Studies (SAMHSA/OAS). (2009b). *Results from the 2008 national survey on drug use and health: National findings.* (NSDUH Series H-36, HHS Publication No. SMA 09-4434). Rockville, MD: Author. Retrieved from http://oas.samhsa.gov/nsduh/2k8nsduh/2k8Results.cfm#TOC

Substance Abuse & Mental Health Services Administration (SAMHSA). (2010). *Results from the 2009 National Survey on Drug Use and Health: Volume 1. Summary of national findings.* (Office of Applied Studies, NSDUH Series H-38A, HHS Publication No. SMA 10-4586Findings). Rockville, MD: Author. Retrieved from http://oas.samhsa.gov/NSDUH/2k9NSDUH/2k9ResultsP.pdf

Substance Abuse and Mental Health Services Administration Center for Substance Abuse Treatment (SAMHSA/CSAT). (1999). *Treatment of adolescents with substance use disorders.* Treatment Improvement Protocol (TIP) Series 32. Rockville, MD: Author. Retrieved from http://www.ncbi.nlm.nih.gov/books/NBK14221/

Substance Abuse & Mental Health Services Administration Center for Substance Abuse Treatment (SAMHSA/CSAT). (2006). *Detoxification and substance use treatment.* Treatment Improvement Protocol (TIP) Series 45. (DHHS Pub. No. (SMA) 06-4131). Rockville, MD: Author. Retrieved from http://www.ncbi.nlm.nih.gov/books/NBK14497/

Substance Abuse & Mental Health Services Administration Office of Applied Studies. (SAMHSA/OAS) (2009a). *The NSDUH Report: Marijuana use and perceived risk of use among adolescents 2002 to 2007.* Rockville, MD: Author. Retrieved from http://www.oas.samhsa.gov/2k9/MJrisks/MJrisks.htm

Tapert, S.F., Aarons, G.A., Sedlar, G.R., & Brown, S.A. (2001). Adolescent substance use and sexual risk-taking behavior. *Journal of Adolescent Health, 28*, 181–189.

Tapert, D.F, Caldwell, L., & Burke, C. (2004/2005). Alcohol and the adolescent brain – Human studies. *Alcohol, Research & Health, 28*, 205–212. Retrieved from http://pubs.niaaa.nih.gov/publications/arh284/205-212.htm

Thatcher, D.L., & Clark, D.B. (2008). Adolescents at risk for substance use disorders: Role of psychological dysregulation, endophenotypes, and environmental influences. *Alcohol Research & Health, 31*, 168–176. Retrieved from http://pubs.niaaa.nih.gov/publications/arh312/168-176.htm

Thush, C., Wiers, R.W., Moerbeek, M., Ames, S.L., Grenard, J.L., Sussman, S., Stacy, A.W. (2009). Influence of motivational interviewing on explicit and implicit alcohol-related cognition and alcohol use in at-risk adolescents. *Psychology of Addictive Behaviors, 23*, 146–151.

Tingen, M.S., Andrews, J.O., & Stevenson, A.W. (2009). Primary and secondary tobacco prevention in youth. *Annual Review of Nursing Research, 27*, 171–193.

Tripodi, S.J., Bender, K., Litschge, C., & Vaughn, M.G. (2010). Interventions for reducing adolescent alcohol abuse: A meta-analytic review. *Archives of Pediatrics and Adolescent Medicine, 164*, 85.

Toumbourou, J.W., Stockwell, T., Neighbors, C., Marlatt, G.A., Sturge, J., & Rehm, J. (2007). Interventions to reduce harm associated with adolescent substance use. *Lancet, 369*, 1391–1401. DOI:10.1016/S0140-6736(07)60369-9.

Vaughn, M.G., & Howard, M.O. (2004). Adolescent substance abuse treatment: A synthesis of controlled evaluations. *Research on Social Work Practice, 14*, 325.

Wagner, E.F. (2008). Developmentally informed research on the effectiveness of clinical trials: A primer for assessing how developmental issues may influence treatment responses among adolescents with alcohol use problems. *Pediatrics, 121*(Suppl 4), S337–S347.

Waldron, H.B., & Turner, C.W. (2008). Evidence-based psychosocial treatments for adolescent substance abuse. *Journal of Clinical Child & Adolescent Psychology, 37*, 238–261.

Walker, D.D., Roffman, R.A., Stephens, R.S., Wakana, K., Berghuis, J., & Kim, W. (2006). Motivational enhancement therapy for adolescent marijuana users: A preliminary randomized controlled trial. *Journal of Consulting & Clinical Psychology, 74*, 628–632.

Wand, G. (2008). The influence of stress on the transition from drug use to addiction. *Alcohol Research & Health, 31*, 119–136. Retrieved from http://pubs.niaaa.nih.gov/publications/arh312/119-136.pdf

WHO ASSIST Working Group. (2002). Alcohol, Smoking and Substance Involvement Screening Test (ASSIST): Development, reliability, & feasibility. *Addiction, 97*, 1183–1194. DOI. 10.1046/j.1360-0443.2002.00185.x

Wheeler, K.C., Fletcher, K.E., Wellman, R.J., & DiFranza, J.R. (2004). Screening adolescents for nicotine dependence: The hooked on nicotine checklist. *Journal of Adolescent Health, 35*, 225–230. doi:10.1016/j.jadohealth.2003.10.004

Witkiewitz, K., & Marlatt, G.A. (2004). Relapse prevention for alcohol and drug problems: That was Zen this is Tao. *American Psychologist, 59*, 224–235. DOI: 10.1037/0003-066X.59.4.224

Winters, K.C., & Lee, C.Y. (2008). Likelihood of developing an alcohol and cannabis use disorder during youth: Association with recent use and age. *Drug and Alcohol Dependence, 92,* 239–247.

Woody, G.E., Poole, S.A., Subramaniam, G.A., Dugosh, K., Bogenschutz, M., Abbott, P., Fudala, P. (2008). Extended vs short-term buprenorphine-naloxone for treatment of opioid-addicted youth: A randomized trial. *JAMA, 300,* 2003-2011.

World Health Organization (WHO). (2011). Lexicon of alcohol and drug terms published by the World Health Organization. Retrieved from http://www.who.int/substance_abuse/terminology/who_lexicon/en/index.html

World Health Organization (WHO). (1992). *The ICD-10 classification of mental and behavioural disorders: Clinical descriptions and diagnostic guidelines.* Retrieved from http://www.who.int/classifications/icd/en/bluebook.pdf

World Health Organization (WHO). (1994/2006). Mental and behavioural disorders due to psychoactive substance use. *The international statistical classification of diseases and related health problems tenth revision: Version for 2007.* Retrieved from http://apps.who.int/classifications/apps/icd/icd10online/

Zucker, R.A., Donovan, J.E., Masten, A.S., Mattson, M.E., & Moss, H.B. (2008). Early developmental processes and the continuity of risk for underage drinking and problem drinking. *Pediatrics, 121*(Suppl_4), S252–S272.

21

Child and Adolescent Victims of Trauma

Angela Amar, Natalie McClain, and Carol Anne Marchetti

Objectives

After reading this chapter, APNs will be able to

1. Provide an overview of childhood and adolescent trauma and the resulting health effects.
2. Outline current and emerging developments in clinical and research findings among children and adolescents who have experienced trauma.

3. Discuss clinical parameters for the identification, assessment, and psychotherapeutic intervention with children and adolescents who have experienced trauma.
4. Describe practice, research, and education implications related to an advanced practice nursing approach to the treatment of traumatized children and adolescents.

Introduction

Childhood and adolescence are times of continuous emotional, psychological, cognitive, and physical development. In this chapter, the word "child" refers to both children and adolescents unless otherwise stated. Ideally, when children face stressors or events that challenge their feelings of safety, they will have the necessary skills and support to get through these difficult times and have a positive outcome. Yet, many children face stressful or traumatic situations every day that test the limits of their resilience and coping skills. Overwhelming or chronic traumatic experiences during childhood can disrupt the normal progress of development and may result in ongoing psychological and physical illness. Traumatic events can be acute, short-lived in nature, or chronic, occurring multiple times over a period of time. Examples of traumatic events or situations include violence (community, school, family/domestic, war, rape), natural/manmade disasters (earthquakes, floods, hurricanes, fire), accidents (motor vehicle, plane crashes), death of a loved one (murder, suicide, illness), child maltreatment (neglect, sexual, physical or emotional abuse), and medical trauma (illness/medical procedures). Traumatic experiences have pervasive effects on the lives of children and adolescents and profoundly affect physical, psychological, emotional, and cognitive domains.

Description of the Issue

The Diagnostic and Statistical Manual of Mental Disorders (DSM-IV-TR) defines a traumatic event as

> One that involves actual or threatened death or serious injury, or a threat to one's physical integrity, or witnessing an event that involves death, injury, or a threat of the

Child and Adolescent Behavioral Health: A Resource for Advanced Practice Psychiatric and Primary Care Practitioners in Nursing,
First Edition. Edited by Edilma L. Yearwood, Geraldine S. Pearson, and Jamesetta A. Newland.
© 2012 John Wiley & Sons, Inc. Published 2012 by John Wiley & Sons, Inc.

physical integrity of another person; or learning about unexpected or violent death, serious harm, or threat of death or injury experienced by a family member or close associate and the person's response to the event must involve intense fear, helplessness, or horror (American Psychiatric Association, 2000, p. 463).

By far, the most common traumatic experience for children involves violence. Children can experience violence within their homes and families, such as child abuse, neglect, and sibling violence. They may also witness intimate partner violence. Outside the home, in school and community life, experience with violence is through bullying, dating violence, gang membership or exposure, and as a victim and/or witness to crime. Children in many parts of the world endure oppression and traumatic experiences including being enslaved, sex trafficking, or war crimes. Many individuals immigrate to the United States following trauma in another country. Despite the variance of traumatic experiences, there is often consistency in the response to trauma. While myriad events comprise this topic, this chapter will use as an exemplar interpersonal violence, such as child maltreatment, dating violence, and exposure to family violence, with the understanding that the basic effects of, responses to, and interventions can apply to multiple types and forms of traumatic experiences.

The Centers for Disease Control and Prevention define *child maltreatment* as "any act or series of acts of commission or omission by a parent or other caregiver that results in harm, potential harm or threat of harm of a child" (Leeb, Paulozzi, Melanson, Simon, & Arias, 2008, p. 19). This includes physical abuse, neglect (emotional, physical, medical, educational), sexual abuse, emotional abuse, abandonment, and substance abuse. Not surprisingly, a large number of children who experience trauma do so at the hands of family members including parents or caretakers (Gilbert, 2009a). While maltreatment of children by parents and caregivers is an age-old problem, it was not brought to light until 1962. That year the landmark publication by Dr. C. Henry Kempe and colleagues titled "The Battered Child Syndrome" made child abuse a health concern. The Child Abuse Prevention and Treatment Act (CAPTA), first introduced into law in 1974 and later amended and reauthorized, provided federal funding to states for prevention, identification, investigation, prosecution, and treatment. Furthermore, every state in the United States has child abuse laws that mandate that all nurses and those in advanced practice specialty areas report instances of suspected child abuse.

In recent decades, researchers have expanded their attention to focus on dating violence. Dating is often viewed as a carefree time of exploration and experimentation, but the experience can also be traumatic for many adolescents. Dating violence (DV) is defined as physical, sexual, or psychological violence within a dating relationship (Black, Noonan, Legg, & Eaton, 2006). DV may occur as a single episode, such as date rape, or as a pattern of behavior, such as physical violence or stalking (Groves, Ausustyn, Lee, & Sawirds, 2002). Researchers propose that 30% of teens and college students report experiencing violence by a previous or current partner (Halpern, Oslak, Martin, & Kupper, 2001).

In the DV literature, adolescent violence is accepted as bidirectional (Harned, 2002). Research on physical violence in adolescent intimate relationships has consistently found that the majority of female victims also report the perpetration of physical aggression against male partners (Halpern et al., 2001). Despite this reciprocal nature, dating violence consequences are not necessarily symmetrical or mutual in that girls are more likely to be physically injured than boys (Amar, 2007; Cleveland, Herrera, & Stuewig, 2003). Younger women, ages sixteen to twenty-four, are more at risk for nonfatal injury from an intimate partner than are women in any other age group and their risk for murder by an intimate partner increases as these women age (Rennison, 2001).

Bullying is a form of aggression characterized by an imbalance of power that tends to peak in middle childhood. Prevalence estimates suggests that as many as half of students from grades six to ten experience some form of bullying with verbal and social bullying being most common (Wang, Iannotti, & Nansel, 2009). Although all children may experience bullying, children who appear weak, insecure, sensitive, isolated, or "different" are at an increased risk of victimization from bullying. Other forms of school violence include verbal and physical assault, threats with or without a weapon, and sexual victimization (including harassment). Instances of bullying increase in frequency with age peaking in preteens to adolescents. Cyberbullying is the latest expression of bullying and uses technology such as cell phones and the Internet to repeatedly contact and harass another person (Smith et al., 2008).

Sexual minority youth are at an increased risk for bullying and sexual harassment contributing to the negative mental health consequences experienced by these youth (Berlan, Corliss, Field, Goodman, & Austin, 2010; Gruber & Fineran, 2008). Practitioners should inquire about sexual orientation and experiences of bullying, harassment, or violence directed to sexual minority youth. If possible, provide resources and referrals that meet the unique needs of the traumatized sexual minority youth.

Numerous studies have established a link between traumatic experiences in childhood and negative psychological outcomes (Chan & Yeung, 2009; Schilling,

Aseltine, & Gore, 2007). The earliest linkages were identified by the landmark work of Felitti and Anda in the Adverse Childhood Experiences study. This joint CDC–Kaiser Permanente study is considered the largest investigation to determine associations between child maltreatment and later life health and well-being (CDC, 2006). Begun in 1995, the study continues prospectively to track outcomes and has determined associations between adverse childhood experiences and alcoholism, depression, health-related quality of life, suicide attempts, risk for intimate partner violence, and illicit drug use (Felitti et al., 1998).

Not all children display physical or psychological symptoms following a traumatic event. Following most trauma, the majority of children demonstrate resilience and have no resulting symptomatology. About half of child abuse survivors demonstrate resilience in childhood, which for nearly one-third of them persists into young adulthood (DuMont, Widom, & Czaja, 2007). In contrast to risk factors, protective factors buffer the negative consequences from violence. Protective factors include parental recognition of the problem, parental support, supportive grandparents, and accessible mental health care (Dubowitz & Bennett, 2007).

Literature examining the physical and psychological aftermath of trauma in children reports wide variation in prevalence of psychological and physical symptoms. The differences in outcomes can be attributed to several factors such as the type of trauma, frequency of the trauma, personality/temperament of child, coping abilities, the relationship of the child and perpetrator, and social support. Differences can exist regarding the severity of the stressor, chronicity of exposure, relationship to the offender, if appropriate, and occurrence of previous and subsequent distressful events. Multiple victimizations, five or more types in a one-year period, can predict higher rates of trauma-related symptoms (Finkelhor, Ormrod, & Turner, 2007; Finkelhor, Ormrod, Turner, & Holt, 2009a). Certain events, such as interpersonal violence in the form of physical and sexual abuse, are associated with more adverse effects than other events, such as natural disasters (Pine & Cohen, 2002; Wethington et al., 2008). Further, evidence of psychopathology before traumatic exposure and disruptions in social networks consistently emerge as strong predictors of psychopathology after exposure to trauma (Pine & Cohen).

Epidemiology

Exposure to traumatic events during childhood is far too common. Violence is prevalent in the everyday lives of children living in the United States; children are more likely than adults to be exposed to violence

(Finkelhor, Turner, Ormrod, & Hamby, 2009b). Several large national surveys of children and adolescents report rates of direct and indirect exposure to violence as high as three of five children exposed in a year and seven out of eight children exposed in their lifetimes (Finkelhor et al.). Not surprisingly, exposure to one form of violence increases the likelihood of future victimization (Rich, Gidycz, Warkentin, Loh, & Weiland, 2005).

In 2007, 3.2 million referrals were made to child protection agencies with 794,000 children who had been determined to be victims of child maltreatment (U.S. Department of Health and Human Services [USDHHS], 2009). Referrals to child protection agencies does not represent the total picture of child maltreatment, only that which is recognized, reported, responded to, and substantiated. The estimated cost for services and care to children and families of maltreatment in 2007 was $104 billion (USDHHS). Rates of victimization decrease with age with the youngest children accounting for the largest percentage of substantiated cases (birth to three years: 31.9%, four to seven years: 23.8%, eight to eleven years: 19%, twelve to fifteen years: 18.4%, sixteen to seventeen years: 6.7%) (USDHHS). Children under age four are at greatest risk of death and serious injury resulting from child maltreatment (Gilbert et al., 2009b). Females are more likely to be victims in substantiated cases (51.5%) with 46.1% of victims who are white, 21.7% African-American, and 20.8% Hispanic (USDHHS).

According to the 2007 data, the majority of child maltreatment cases are neglect (59%) followed by physical abuse (10.8%), sexual abuse (7.6%), and psychological maltreatment (<5%). In 2007, the rates of child fatalities were 2.35 deaths per 100,000 children (USDHHS, 2009). Neglect is the failure of the offender to care for the child and to meet the basic needs of the child. Physical abuse is the use of physical force with the intention and result of hurting the child. Sexual abuse includes any attempted or completed sexual act, contact, or sexual interaction between a child and adult. Psychological abuse is any behavior that intentionally undermines the child's sense of self and self-worth. Examples include belittling, degrading, terrorizing, isolating, and rejecting.

Most often, perpetrators of child maltreatment are the people who are closest to the child, including parents and caretakers (79.9%), with 56.6% of offenders being women and 42.2% men (USDHHS, 2009). Parents constitute the largest group of offenders (80%) with biological parents comprising nearly 90% of the parent offender group. The race and ethnicity of the perpetrators tend to mimic that of the victim.

Research has begun to explore the pervasiveness of childhood exposure to violence within the communities. A nationally representative sample of children revealed that more than 60% were exposed to violence either directly or indirectly (Finkelhor et al., 2009b). Indirect exposure occurs through witnessing or learning about a violent act. Research suggests that increased aggression is associated with witnessing community violence in young children (Guerra, Huesmann, & Spindler, 2003). Emerging literature has documented the mental health consequences of exposure to intimate partner violence via one's parents. Children as young as infants can experience traumatic symptoms in response to incidents of partner abuse between parents (Bogat, DeJohnghe, Levendosky, Davidson, & von Eye, 2006). A review of published literature from 1995 to 2006 found that children and adolescents living with domestic violence had an increased risk of experiencing emotional, physical, and sexual abuse, of developing emotional and behavioral problems, and of increased exposure to other adversities in their lives (Holt, Buckley, & Whelan, 2008).

Etiology

There are many possible causes of child trauma. Children across all racial, ethnic, cultural, religious, and socioeconomic groups experience interpersonal violence. As discussed, children and adolescents may be exposed to a variety of potentially traumatic situations. The risk of potential repercussions will vary greatly depending on the type of trauma. It is helpful to explore features that contribute or cause trauma from multiple perspectives on multiple levels. At the individual level, research documents risk factors that can predispose children to be victimized and parents to abuse their children. In addition, individual level factors include risk factors predictive of victimization and perpetration of dating violence, bullying, and other forms of interpersonal violence. Factors that occur at a family level can predict exposure to violence. Finally, at a societal and community level, risk factors for violence include cultural and societal norms as well as theoretical perspectives that explain the experience of violence.

At the individual level, characteristics that make a child more likely to experience child abuse include age (younger children at greater risk of severe injury and adolescents at greater risk of sexual abuse), disabilities, chronic illness, difficult temperament, and prior maltreatment exposure (Gilbert et al., 2009a; Stith et al., 2009). Risk factors for teen dating violence include alcohol or drug use, association with violent friends, witnessing violence at home, inability to manage anger, and poor social skills (Cornelius & Ressiguie, 2007).

At a family level, risk factors that identify parents at risk for violence include personality characteristics such as low self-esteem, external locus of control, and poor impulse control (Stith et al., 2009). Parental predictors of being a perpetrator include history of child abuse, limited information about growth and development of children, lack of education, single parents, mental illness, and history of drug or alcohol use (Fluke, Shusterman, Hollinshead, & Yuan, 2008). Other family attributes that increase the likelihood of child abuse are households with marital conflict, domestic violence, and lower income (Stith et al., 2009). Several programs are available for parents and families deemed at risk of child abuse. In particular, early childhood home visitation programs and parent education programs demonstrate some success at preventing child abuse (MacMillan et al., 2009).

At a community level, factors such as stress and poverty are associated with increased risk of child abuse (Stith, et al., 2009). Poverty, unemployment, and violent communities are all conditions that increase stress levels and decrease the resources and options available to families (Margolin & Gordis, 2000). Living in communities with increased violence may create a social norm that suggests acceptance of violence (Guerra et al., 2003). Increased stress can lead to feelings of powerlessness and set a cycle of the strong preying on the weak in an effort to feel powerful. Power and control are issues at the core of violence. Children living in communities with high rates of criminal activity are at higher risk of exposure to direct or indirect forms of violence including child maltreatment (Finkelhor et al., 2009b).

The U.S. demographics continue to change with the percentage of non-white individuals increasing. The change or "browning of America" also changes perceptions, attitudes, and beliefs regarding child maltreatment, child rearing, and discipline from the current Eurocentric perspective. As culture creates the lens through which an individual's experiences are interpreted, it is important to attempt to understand the unique perspectives of children, parents, caregivers, and families whose cultural and ethnic background is different from one's own. It is through the family that the individual learns about culture, and both cultural and familial features influence our definitions and perceptions of trauma, violence, and abuse. Ethnicity is a significant predictor of attitudes regarding parenting and definitions of child abuse (Ferrari, 2002). Cultural practices may be considered in the differential diagnosis of child maltreatment (Dubowitz & Bennett, 2007).

Theoretical perspectives commonly attributed to interpersonal violence include social cognitive theory, intergenerational transmission, feminist theory, and ecological approach. Social cognitive theory suggests that violence arises from social and contextual factors within one's world and is a learned behavior. It is a popular explanatory theory that suggests that individuals learn how to behave from exposure to and experience of violence. This leads to the intergenerational transmission of violence perspective that suggests that violence continues through generations in families as a learned behavior (Roberts, Gilman, Fitzmaurice, Decker, & Koenen, 2010). Feminist theory places an emphasis on power dynamics and the use of power to oppress the weak (Straka & Montminy, 2008). An ecological approach offers a broad contextual framework that considers individual, interpersonal, familial, community, and sociocultural factors and suggests that different levels of factors interact to cause violence (Gilbert et al., 2009a).

Research has explored psychobiology related to child maltreatment (Gilbert et al., 2009a). In particular, researchers have explored the effects of trauma on the development and regulation of the neurobiological stress system and alterations in brain maturation. As childhood and adolescence are periods of neurological growth and development, any stress in this period has the potential to disrupt typical neurodevelopmental processes and contribute to long-term negative consequences. A review of existing research suggests that "the overwhelming stress of child maltreatment is associated with alterations of the biological stress systems, which, in turn, leads to adverse effects on brain development and delays in cognitive, language, and academic skills" (Watts-English, Fortson, Gibler, Hooper, & DeBelis, 2006, p. 728).

Research has explored neurobiological influences of aggression and violent behavior, specifically, failures in the brain systems that modulate aggressive acts. Specific areas of promise include imbalances between the prefrontal regulatory influences and hyperresponsivity of the amygdala, excessive catecholaminergic stimulation, subcortical imbalances of glutamatergic/GABAminergic systems, and pathology in neuropeptide systems that regulate affiliative behavior (Siever, 2008). Dysregulation in brain function manifests itself in anxiety, impulsivity, poor affect regulation, and motor hyperactivity (DeBellis, 2001).

Identifying the causes and risk factors associated with interpersonal violence and trauma proves to be very challenging. No specific or singular cause has been identified. Rather, the interaction of factors on multiple levels creates conditions that may be favorable for child trauma to occur. Identification is facilitated by an exploration of associated risk factors that make children and families more vulnerable to abuse and neglect.

Profile of the Traumatized Child and Adolescent

Although not all children who experience trauma will appear to develop clinical symptoms following the event, research suggests that a significant number of children will develop immediate and long-term clinical symptoms of a stress reaction following a traumatic experience (Bogat et al., 2006; Kenardy, Spence, & Macleod, 2006; Mongillo, Briggs-Gowan, Ford, & Carter, 2009). Much research has documented children's behavioral, emotional, and psychological responses to trauma. Common mental health disorders include depression, post-traumatic stress disorder, anxiety, somatization, and adjustment disorders. As children often lack the cognitive ability to discuss trauma, consequences of stress are most often seen in their behavior. Adolescents also often demonstrate behavioral manifestations of trauma responses. Findings from studies suggest that even children who indirectly witness violence or traumatic events may develop symptoms of PTSD upon evaluation (Otto et al., 2007). Children as young as six months who are exposed to violence or traumatic life events display clinical symptoms consistent with post-traumatic stress response and one year olds have had documented trauma symptoms following hearing or witnessing intimate partner violence (Bogat et al., 2006; Mongillo et al., 2009).

Responses to trauma during childhood can vary depending on a number of factors including if the events were acute or chronic, developmental maturity of the child, presence or absence of family/social support, the perceived threat, loss from the trauma, and prior experience with trauma. Immediately following a traumatic event, children may appear stunned, numb, or unaware of the event. As they attempt to process the trauma event and associated emotions, they may demonstrate a number of symptoms (Table 21.1). Research suggests that the greater the number of traumatic experiences or adverse childhood events, the greater the risk of developing mental health disorders (Finkelhor et al., 2007). In other words, the toll of traumatic experiences has a cumulative effect on mental health.

The cardinal sign that signals psychopathology and that trauma could have occurred is a change from usual behavior (Hess & Orthmann, 2009). This can be seen in a change in school performance and in behavior at home or school. Common signs that could signal that a child has experienced abuse include withdrawn behavior, aggressive or angry behavior, and fearful behavior particularly if it is attached to a person or place (Cohen & Mannarino, 2008). Children may also demonstrate regressive behavior such as bedwetting or thumb sucking in response to trauma (Gilbert et al., 2009b).

Health consequences to trauma can occur in multiple domains that all can potentially influence the mental health of the child. Physical injury related to abuse can be quite severe, disfiguring, and enduring. The process of obtaining the required medical treatments can be

Table 21.1 Symptoms seen with child abuse

Symptoms	
Emotional	Anxiety, depression, despair, hopelessness, low self-esteem, fearfulness, withdrawn, attachment difficulties, impulsivity, eating disorders
Behavioral	Aggression, anger, delinquent behaviors, self-destructive behavior, defiance, noncompliance, personality disturbances, peer conflict, sexual acting out, substance use, truancy, compulsive or obsessive behavior, suicide thoughts/attempts
Cognitive	Attention/concentration problems, ADHD symptoms, difficulty making decisions, memory lapses, academic difficulties
Physical	Sleep disturbances, low energy, somatic symptoms (gastrointestinal disturbances, pain, headache, etc.)

isolating, traumatic, and frightening. The psychological impact of treatment can complicate recovery from the initial traumatic event.

Recognition of the Behavioral Patterns of Abused Children

Children and adolescents who have experienced physical abuse may demonstrate behavioral signs such as extreme rage, passivity, running away from home, cheating, lying or low achievement in school, regression, and inability to form satisfactory peer relationships (Margolin & Gordis, 2000). Children who have been sexually abused frequently present in a distinctive way, often with no external signs of child sexual abuse but with behavioral manifestations. These include unusual interest in or avoidance of all things of a sexual nature; seductiveness; statements that their bodies are dirty or damaged, and fear that there is something wrong with them in the genital area. Other signs include refusal to go to school; delinquency/conduct problems; secretiveness; aspects of sexual molestation present in drawings, games, fantasies; and unusual aggressiveness; or suicidal behavior (Margolin & Gordis, 2000).

Exposure to intimate partner violence (IPV) can cause specific mental health symptoms in children and adolescents. Preschool children may manifest yelling, irritability, stuttering, somatic complaints, attachment behavior, sleep disturbance, and signs of terror. School-age children may respond to exposure to IPV by demonstrating a greater willingness to use violence, distractibility, feeling responsible for violence, and lability. Adolescents often act out feelings of rage, shame and betrayal, and show decreased attention span (Berman, Hardesty, Lewis-O'Connor, & Humphreys, 2011).

Implications for Clinical Practice

Assessment

A thorough assessment for past and current victimization, which includes the child, family members, and others close to the child, is essential. Gathering information from at least two sources, the child and a parent or caregiver, is necessary to obtain a complete picture (Hess & Orthmann, 2009). Often, parents and children process the event and the aftermath differently and may report on different consequences. Children tend to report more internal manifestations and developmentally appropriate responses; parents tend to report the external and observable manifestations. Gathering information from multiple sources will enhance the diagnostic ability of the provider (AACAP, 2010). While information is often gathered from parents, care must be taken when the parent is the suspected abuser to ensure that the child has a free and open place to discuss the abuse in a confidential manner.

The use of a standardized interview and diagnostic tool may aid in gathering information about the violence and the resulting symptoms (Pine & Cohen, 2002). It is important to inquire about experiences using questions containing specific behaviors as opposed to using labeling words. Words such as child abuse and victim can trigger societal reactions and stigma. Research suggests that individuals may not think of themselves as "abused" even if they have experienced abusive behaviors (Amar & Gennaro, 2005). The use of behavioral questions such as, Have you been hit or punched?, is preferred (Groves et al., 2002). Posing questions in a direct manner can serve to normalize the experience and lead to an assault disclosure that would not have occurred otherwise, to attenuate the patient's concern about shocking the clinician. Conversely, many children assume that their experiences must represent the norm and, therefore, will not be forthcoming about details of an assault because of a perception that the information is not relevant or important. Often, children who display behavioral or externalizing manifestations commonly associated with traumatic events are referred for treatment. Thus, the use of screening questions with all children is necessary. Screening tools are useful in assessing a history of exposure to trauma and the impact of the event on the child or adolescent. The Traumatic Events Screening Instrument (TESI) is an easy to use screening tool for children ages 4–18 and is found in Figure 21.1.

Figure 21.1.   Traumatic Events Screening Instrument (TESI)

Recommended use: Screening for trauma history in children or youth in clinical, educational, juvenile justice, or research settings.

Special features: Administered as a semi-structured interview to children (TESI-C) or parents (TESI-PRR), or as a staff-assisted self-report questionnaire to adolescents (ages 11–18; TESI-C-SR).

General Description Information:

Measure format: Comes in both semi-structured interview and questionnaire formats.

Targeted age group: Children ages 4–18.

Events assessed: Wide range of potentially traumatic events including accidents, severe illness and hospitalization, physical or sexual abuse, separation from caregivers, neglect and emotional abuse, natural disaster, community violence, witnessing domestic violence, and traumatic losses.

Number of items; Time to administer: 15 items on TESI-C, 19 items on TESI-PRR, 26 items on TESI-C-SR; 10–30 minutes, depending on number of traumatic experiences endorsed.

Response format: Initial response choices are "yes", "no", and "pass" (with additional choices on the Interview versions, "not sure", "refused", and "questionable validity"). "Yes" and "not sure" responses are followed up with open-ended questions about what happened and closed-ended questions to establish Criterion A from the DSM-IV (See Aspects of Trauma Assessed below).

Training required to administer: All versions are designed to be administered only by qualified mental health or juvenile services professionals or advanced trainees supervised by a qualified professional. The critical qualifications are licensure for independent practice or job classification with responsibilities for behavioral health screening and counseling with children or youth, **and** *supervised experience in assessment or counseling with child or youth trauma survivors.*

Sample items:

> **TESI-C-SR:** Have you ever had a time in your life when *you did not have the right care* – like not having enough to eat or drink, being homeless, being left alone when you were too young to care for yourself, or being left with someone using drugs? Or have you ever been left in charge of your younger brothers or sisters for long periods of time, sometimes for several days? ❑Yes ❑No ❑Pass
>
> IF YES→   How old were you? The first time:_____ The last time:_____ The worst time:_____
>
> Self-appraisal of fear/helplessness/horror [DSM-IV Criterion A2]:
>
> Did you feel really bad, upset, scared, sad, or mixed up the worst time this happened? ❑Yes ❑No ❑Pass

TESI-C: Have you ever been in a really bad accident, like a car accident, a fall, or a fire? How old were you when this happened? Were you hurt? [What was the hurt?] Did you go to the doctor or hospital? Was someone else really hurt in the accident? [Who? What was the hurt?] Did they go to the doctor or the hospital?

Clinician appraisal of objective physical threat [DSM-IV Criterion A1]: Interviewer: In your clinical judgment, was each incident life-threatening? Was or could the child or another person have been killed/ severely injured?

Child's appraisal of fear/helplessness/horror [DSM-IV Criterion A2]: When [event] was happening, did you feel as scared as you'd ever been, like this was one of the scariest things that EVER happened to you? [If no, ask:] When [event] happened, did you feel really confused or mixed up? [If no, ask:] Did [event] make you feel sick or disgusted?

TESI-PRR: Has your child ever been in a serious accident like a car accident, a fall, or a fire? What happened? How old was your child when this happened? Was your child hurt? If so, what were the injuries? Was an ambulance/paramedic called? Did your child go to the doctor or hospital? Was someone else in the accident? If so, were they seriously injured or killed?

Parent's appraisal of the event [DSM-IV Criterion A1]: Was or could someone have been killed or seriously physically injured in the accident?

Parent's appraisal of child's fear, helplessness, or horror [DSM-IV Criterion A2]: Did your child feel extremely scared or afraid? Did your child feel sick/disgusted? Did your child appear to be really confused or mixed up?

Parent's appraisal of own fear, helplessness, or horror: Did YOU feel extremely scared or afraid? Did YOU feel helpless? Did YOU feel sick/disgusted or horrified?

Scoring: Each Item can be scored as a single *traumatic event* (or recurrent events, if multiple events occurred), based on the DSM-IV PTSD Criterion A for exposure to a traumatic stressor:

A1: Traumatic events must involve one of the following forms of **objective danger/harm:**

  a. **actual death** that is premature given the age of the person (*not* including death due to natural causes or expectable illness of an older adult) *or*
  b. imminent **threat of death** due to illness, accidental injury, or intentional violence *or*
  c. prolonged **separation from or loss of or failure to provide adequate basic safety and care by a primary caregiver** (including parents, other adults to whom a child's care is entrusted, or older youths including siblings) *or*
  d. **sexual acts** (witnessed or directly experienced) initiated by or involving person(s) five or more years older than the child.

and

A2: Traumatic events must include or be followed soon after by a **subjective state** *or* automatic bodily reaction of severe fear, helplessness, or horror.

Note: children exposed to recurrent traumatic events or events that began in infancy or toddlerhood (e.g., prolonged abuse or domestic or community violence) may become sufficiently emotionally numbed or dissociated or hopeless that they do not recall ever having felt distressed and will deny these reactions or simply not be able to remember having experienced them. While it cannot be assumed that such "resilient copers" have experienced a traumatic stressor and cannot or will not acknowledge having felt emotional or bodily distress reactions when events occurred, for clinical and rehabilitative purposes these youth may be classified as having a "probable" trauma history if they (or their parents) describe:

  A. An A1 event before age 6 for which they cannot recall their emotional or bodily reaction, or

  B. A recurrent or series of A1 events that began before age 2.

Composite Trauma History Classifications:

  A. **Physical Abuse:** Item 1.8 if the perpetrator(s) were family members or caregivers

  B. **Sexual Abuse:** Items 5.1 *or* 5.2

C. **Physical Assault:** Items 1.8 (if by a non-family member or non-caregiver), 2.2 (if occurred to the child/youth), *or* 2.3

D. **Domestic Violence:** Items 3.1 *or* 3.2

E. **Community Violence:** Items 2.2 (if witnessed a family member or close friend) *or* 4.1 *or* 4.2

F. **Emotional Abuse:** If by a primary caregiver or close emotional relationship, Items 2.1 or 6.1

G. **Neglect:** Items 6.2 *or* 6.3 (the latter only if by a primary caregiver)

H. **Interpersonal Victimization Trauma:** Any of A–G

I. **Traumatic Loss:** If a primary caregiver or primary emotional relationship, Items 1.4, *or* 1.6, *or* 1.7, *or* 3.3

J. **Traumatic Accident:** Items 1.1 *or* 1.2

K. **Traumatic Disaster:** Item 1.3

L. **Traumatic Illness/Medical Care:** Item 1.5

M. **Non-Interpersonal Trauma:** J, K, L, or Item 2.4

N. **Witnessed Trauma:** If witnessed but not directly harmed/threatened, Items 1.4 *or* 1.7. *or* 2.2 *or* 3 *or* 4 *or* 5.2 *or* 6.3

M. **Early Childhood Trauma:** If age of onset was 5 years old or younger

N. **Childhood Trauma:** If age(s) of occurrence was 12 years old or younger

O. **Adolescent Trauma:** If age(s) of occurrence was 13–17 years old

P. **Intra-Familial Victimization:** Any traumatic event(s) from category D (domestic violence) or (if family members were involved) A, B, C, F, or G (physical or sexual abuse or assault, emotional abuse or neglect)

Time frame assessed: Lifetime.

Correspondence with DSM: Assesses DSM-IV PTSD Criterion A-1 (experiencing or witnessing actual injury or threat of death/injury) and Criterion A-2 (subjective fear, helplessness, or horror).

Psychometric Information:

Validation populations: Child psychiatry and pediatric trauma patients, juvenile justice youth.

Reliability: TESI-C inter-rater agreement reported by Daviss et al. (2000) and Ford et al. (2000).

Validity: Convergent/Criterion validity reported by Daviss et al. (2000), Ford et al. (2000, 2008).

Daviss, W.B., Mooney, D., Racusin, R., Ford, J. D., Fleischer, A., & McHugo, G. (2000). Predicting post-traumatic stress after hospitalization for pediatric injury. *Journal of the American Academy of Child and Adolescent Psychiatry, 39*, 576–583.

Daviss, W.B., Racusin, R., Fleischer, A., Mooney, D., Ford, J. D., & McHugo, G. (2000). Acute stress disorder symptomatology during hospitalization for pediatric injury. *Journal of the American Academy of Child and Adolescent Psychiatry, 39*, 569–575.

Ford, J.D., Racusin, R., Ellis, C., Daviss, W.B., Reiser, J., Fleischer, A., & Thomas, J. (2000). Child maltreatment, other trauma exposure, and posttraumatic symptomatology among children with oppositional defiant and attention deficit hyperactivity disorders. *Child Maltreatment, 5*, 205–217.

Ford, J. D., Hartman, J. K., Hawke, J., & Chapman, J. (2008). Traumatic victimization, posttraumatic stress disorder, suicidal ideation, and substance abuse risk among juvenile justice-involved youths. *Journal of Child and Adolescent Trauma, 1*, 75–92.
Reprinted with permission from J. D. Ford.

Screening tools exist to measure the traumatic events. These tools have been carefully developed and tested to account for the developmental and intellectual capacity of children. They may be useful in supplementing the clinical interview. The Childhood PTSD Interview (Fletcher, 1996), Childhood PTSD Inventory (Saigh et al., 2000), and University of California Los Angeles (UCLA) PTSD Reaction Index (Pynoos, Rodriguez, Steinberg, & Frederick, 1998) measure both exposure to trauma and resulting PTSD symptoms. The first three are for children and adolescents while the latter has three versions, for children, adolescents, and parents. The When Bad Things Happen Scale (WBTHS) (Fletcher, 1996) and the UCLA PTSD Reaction Index are both self-reported, while the others are clinician administered. All tools have been widely used with a variety of populations and are well tested. Other measures for exposure to sexual abuse include the Anatomical Doll Questionnaire (Levy, Markovic, Kallinowski, Ahart, & Torres, 1995). Finally, other measures screen for history of trauma. The Child Trauma Questionnaire (Bernstein & Fink, 1998) can be used with adolescents twelve and older and assesses for emotional, physical, and sexual abuse and emotional and physical neglect. The Trauma Events Screening Inventory (Ribbe, 1996) measures child maltreatment, domestic violence, community violence, disasters, and previous injuries and hospitalization in children and adolescents. For a complete discussion of trauma measures for children and adolescents, refer to Strand, Sarmiento, and Pasquale (2005).

Commonly used psychometric instruments, with favorable psychometric properties for the evaluation of trauma in children, can be helpful. These include the Trauma Symptom Checklist for Children (Briere, 1996), Los Angeles Symptom Checklist-Adolescent (King, King, Leskin, & Foy, 1995), the Child Report of Post-Traumatic Symptoms, and the Parent Report of Post-Traumatic Symptoms (Greenwald & Rubin, 1999). The Child PTSD Symptom Scale (Foa, Johnson, Feeny, & Treadwell, 2001) is a widely used measure of DSM-IV symptoms in children. Most of the above-mentioned measures are derived from the DSM-IV-TR criteria for psychiatric symptoms and disorders commonly associated with trauma. The measures are age appropriate and have been widely used so that reliability and validity have been determined.

While empirical assessment methods are ideal, sometimes the assessment cannot proceed in this manner due to a variety of etiologies that can stem from developmental, psychological, or emotional issues. In addition, there may be other inhibiting factors such as denial or parental interference. Denial on the parent's part can occur because the parent is unaware of the trauma, because the parent is the offender, or for other reasons (AACAP, 2010). Children are often unable to verbalize their symptoms in a meaningful way. Often, children have an easier time discussing somatic symptoms resulting from trauma. Assessment of the child away from the parent using age-appropriate questions is warranted. In such cases, a clinician should rely on clinical judgment and use other, less formal strategies such as the use of art and play. In analyzing the content and process of the play patterns, elements of repetition, reenactment, and developmental inappropriateness should be of concern. For example, a traumatized preschool child might display regressive behaviors such as thumb sucking and bed-wetting; older children might present with somatic complaints and cognitive difficulties.

Interviews for the purposes of forensic evaluation and/or legal documentation should only be conducted by specially trained personnel; however, screening for trauma or exposure to violence should be part of a routine primary care and mental health evaluation. Practitioners need to provide children, regardless of their age, with an opportunity to talk about their trauma experiences without others, including family members, present. It is not uncommon for children to withhold details of trauma or abuse if they feel it will upset the family or parent (Hershkowitz, Lanes, & Lamb, 2007). Providing a private place where the practitioner and child can talk not only gives the child a chance to discuss traumatic events without a potential perpetrator present but also allows the child the opportunity to freely discuss their experiences without the child's concern for upsetting the parent.

When talking to children about their trauma experiences practitioners must be sensitive to the allegations, the child's developmental level, and the child's current mental state. The advanced practice psychiatric nurse (APN) can begin screening for less-threatening or traumatic experiences or begin with general statements that are not specific to the child. By also asking open-ended questions, the child is allowed to direct the conversation. It is helpful to use terms the child uses to refer to body parts or acts of violence or abuse. For example, it is helpful to begin a conversation with an adolescent patient about violence by stating, "I don't know if this is a concern for you, but many teens I see are dealing with violence or bullying issues, so I've started asking questions about violence routinely" (Groves et al., 2002). The provider can then follow with additional direct questions, such as, "Does anyone make you afraid? Is anyone hurting you?"

The notion of fear and being hurt can elicit responses from young children about normal daily activities. For example, a child may affirmatively respond to questions about being hit and then, through more questioning, the culprit is revealed to be a classmate or sibling. While sibling abuse should be evaluated, the nurse will also have to inquire further to determine if other incidences of violence occurred. Older children are capable of understanding the distinction between abusive touch as opposed to routine activities requiring touch. For example, parents routinely touch the private areas of children during bathing and toileting. The nurse may have to ask more probing questions to uncover abuse and determine inappropriate touch.

Once a child has disclosed a traumatic event, the clinician can then ask for more information such as details about onset, frequency, and duration. In screening for PTSD symptoms, it is important to use clear language about reexperiencing and avoidance items. For example, the clinician can ask the child if he or she becomes upset when in the specific place where the event occurred (AACAP, 2010).

Children may display psychiatric symptoms that could indicate trauma. APNs are encouraged to explore other psychiatric and physical conditions that may mimic PTSD, such as attention deficit hyperactivity disorder, endocrine disturbances, or seizure disorder (AACAP, 2010). Children who present with symptoms suggestive of trauma but with no confirmed reports of trauma should be referred for a forensic evaluation (AACAP, 2010).

Prevention

Primary prevention that can include education about the prevalence and impact of childhood trauma is imperative among all individuals in our society, particularly those who are trusted with the care of children and young people. Public awareness campaigns have continued to increase the public's awareness of traumatic stress in childhood and adolescence. Yet societal misperceptions about violence and stigma about seeking mental health treatment continue to exist. Advanced practice psychiatric nurses are in a position to educate the public and the health care system about new developments in the treatment of traumatic stress. In this time of advancing technology and knowledge explosion, education and training of APNs to remain current are critical.

Programs designed to reduce and prevent child maltreatment have received mixed reviews over the past twenty years. However, there is growing literature to support comprehensive, evidence-based home visitation programs led by professionals, such as nurses, delivering frequent and intense interventions as cost-effective measures in preventing child maltreatment

(Donelan-McCall, Eckenrode, & Olds, 2009; Reynolds, Mathieson, & Topitzes, 2009). In addition, programs exist to prevent dating violence in middle and high school students. While many programs report success at changing attitudes, few programs report sustained behavior change (Cornelius & Resseguie, 2007). For a review of available programs, the reader is referred to Cornelius and Resseguie (2007). An understanding of the risk factors associated with children, families, and parents enables the nurse to implement prevention programs targeted to high-risk individuals.

Intervention

Early intervention in responding to child and adolescent trauma is essential (Gilbert et al., 2009a). Families that provide support and a safe, nurturing environment as soon as possible following a traumatic event effectively limit the influence of the trauma on the child or adolescent. Common mental health disorders resulting from interpersonal violence include post-traumatic stress disorder, depression, somatization, general anxiety, and dissociative disorder. Outpatient management is appropriate for all of these symptoms; however, children and adolescents who demonstrate behavior that is harmful to self or others need inpatient hospitalization. Early treatment can alleviate symptoms of mental illness and mitigate long-term consequences. As previously stated, it is important to remember that not all who experience trauma develop mental health symptoms. The APN who works with a child immediately after trauma can work to foster the child's resilience and help the family provide optimal support to mitigate potential health consequences.

Psychotherapy is a vital treatment modality for children's emotional, behavioral, and social problems and within the scope of the psychiatric APN. Generally, the goal of psychotherapy following trauma is to allow the child or adolescent to talk about and integrate the event so that he or she is better able to cope with the pain or loss. Additionally, a goal of talk therapy (particularly among older patients) is to help the patient describe his or her feelings in order to recognize his or her own behaviors, symptoms, and characteristic responses to trauma. Moreover, talk therapy can help the patient gain perspective and understand the trauma within a given context.

Experiencing violence can disrupt the normal growth and development trajectory of children (Margolin & Gordis, 2000). In therapy, the clinician can effectively use this knowledge to help children meet their developmental tasks. For example, preschool-age children are beginning to learn right from wrong, which makes them focused on punishment and rewards. When abuse occurs for children this age, it can be very confusing, causing them to feel that it is their fault. Therapists can work to restore their normal curiosity and openness while helping to repair a healthy sense of self.

Techniques used in individual psychotherapy include psychoeducational strategies, cognitive-behavioral therapy (CBT), insight-oriented therapy, and trauma-focused techniques. Recent reviews of randomized control trials found strong evidence for the efficacy of CBT in treating PTSD and other psychiatric symptoms occurring after multiple traumatic experiences (Pine & Cohen, 2002; Wethington et al., 2008). Another review of all psychosocial treatments for children exposed to traumatic events found effectiveness in trauma-focused CBT and school-based group CBT. Evidence suggests that trauma-focused therapies are more effective in treating PTSD symptoms (Wethington et al., 2008). Further, treatment is essential when considering PTSD, depressive symptoms, anxiety symptoms, and externalizing behavior programs that result from traumatic experiences (Silverman et al., 2008).

Fundamental components of CBT include cognitive processing, exposure, and stress inoculation procedures. Cognitive processing provides opportunities to explore the child's cognitions about the event with the goal of correcting cognitive distortions. Exposure techniques help the child to disconnect thoughts and reminders of the traumatic events from overwhelming emotions using techniques such as gradual encouragement to share details of the trauma and the memories evoked (Pine & Cohen, 2002). Stress inoculation techniques can include relaxation, visualization and imagery, diaphragmatic breathing, and self-talk. The effectiveness of CBT has been documented in children as young as two years of age and was most commonly used in children aged 4.7 to 22 years (Wethington et al., 2008).

Trauma-focused CBT (TF-CBT) is a highly structured program that uses an individual format that includes education on cognitive and behavioral procedures, exposure through the use of narratives, drawings, or other imaginative methods, and cognitive reprocessing of the trauma and resultant symptoms (Silverman et al., 2008). The core elements of TF-CBT provide opportunities for the child to construct a detailed trauma narrative, engage in significant cognitive processing of the event, address behavioral manifestations of PTSD, and provide a parental treatment component (Cohen, 2003; Cohen, Mannarino, & Deblinger, 2006). "The trauma narrative, usually a book, song, poem, or other written narrative, helps the child to overcome avoidance of the traumatic memories, identify cognitive distortions, and contextualize the experience within the larger framework of the

child's life (Cohen & Mannarino, 2008, p. 160). TF-CBT was demonstrated to be effective for use with multiple traumatic experiences and has been adapted for use with children and adolescents across the age ranges. Parental involvement in TF-CBT often consists of education on the use of effective parenting skills and about incidence of trauma, common reactions to trauma, and the treatment approaches (AACAP, 2010). Please see Chapter 17 for a complete review of CBT.

Research suggests that school-based group CBT may be an effective treatment strategy for anxiety and depression in children exposed to trauma. Within this technique, emphasis centers on psychoeducation, graded exposures using writing and/or drawing, cognitive, and coping skills training, and social skills training (Silverman et al., 2008). Another CBT technique that holds promise for resolving symptoms associated with disturbing and painful events is eye movement desensitization and reprocessing. This treatment combines exposure and cognitive psychodynamic, and somatic therapies using an eight-phase approach (Shapiro & Maxfield, 2002). Effective use is reported with children as young as six years of age (Wethington et al., 2008).

Play therapy is another type of psychotherapy that can be beneficial for the assessment of young children who may lack the verbal or emotional skill to access and articulate their emotions, thoughts, and fantasies regarding the traumatic event. In addition, play therapy provides a vehicle for the child to connect his or her concrete experience with abstract thought (Wethington et al., 2008). For example, the child might reenact the event using dolls or via artistic expression, such as through drawing or painting. Although play therapy has been found to be beneficial to participants, insufficient evidence exists to conclude effectiveness (Wethington et al.). Please see Chapter 15 for further discussion of play therapy.

Children who have experienced the same trauma (e.g., surviving the same fire) can benefit from group therapy. In addition, group therapy can be efficacious among children who have experienced similar traumas (e.g., victims of sexual abuse or domestic violence). Group therapy is particularly useful for adolescents as it complements the developmental emphasis on peers. A review of outcome studies for adolescent girls who had been sexually abused revealed that psychodrama models decreased depressive symptoms and CBT and group therapies using exposure were associated with PTSD reduction (Avinger & Jones, 2007). Again, the focus of the group approach can include a combination of the following treatment modalities: psychoeducation, CBT, family therapy, and problem-focused therapy. However, the most effective group treatment modality appears to be CBT (Wethington et al., 2008). Please see Chapter 15 for a complete review of group therapy.

In some instances, children benefit from the use of psychotherapy in conjunction with medication to treat symptoms of PTSD, anxiety, and depression, which are diagnoses that are associated with trauma. It is not surprising that many of these diagnoses occur in clusters since, from a neurobiological perspective, it has yet to be determined if and how the body and brain distinguish among distinct trauma responses. In particular, children with persistent symptoms that do not respond to other forms of therapy may need pharmacological treatment. Examples of commonly prescribed medications include antidepressant medications, such as fluoxetine (Prozac), sertraline (Zoloft), and citalopram (Celexa) and antianxiety medications such as benzodiazepines, clonazepam (Klonopin), and other antianxiety agents such as clonidine (Catapres) and guanfacine (Tenex) (Preston, O'Neal, & Talaga, 2008). It is important to note that children are prescribed medications based on evidence and dosage recommendations that were researched with adult populations and often target adults. Selective serotonin reuptake inhibitors (SSRIs) are approved for adult use in PTSD to decrease all symptom clusters. Preliminary evidence suggests that SSRIs may be beneficial in treating children with PTSD but insufficient evidence exists to draw conclusions (Wethington et al., 2008). Existing evidence has demonstrated effectiveness of SSRIs in treating childhood depression and anxiety disorders (AACAP, 2010). It is important for the prescribing clinician to keep abreast of research evidence and new findings regarding psychotropic medication use with children and adolescents. Additionally, the child and adolescent brain is undergoing rather rapid development. Thus, vigilant surveillance is recommended to monitor for medication side effects and treatment response, preferably by a psychiatric APN with expertise in pediatric psychopharmacology. Please refer to Chapter 6 for a more detailed discussion of psychopharmacological management for the treatment of these symptoms and diagnoses.

As children and adolescents often live with parents or caregivers, interventions are necessary at the family level. A safe and stable environment is essential for the child and adolescent to manage the trauma and resulting symptoms. Anxious parents may need assistance to be able to provide for their child's emotional and security needs. Lower levels of parental distress are associated with a more positive response to treatment by the child (AACAP, 2010). When possible, emphasis should be placed on having the parents or caregivers maintain a close adherence to the usual structures and schedules of the home life so that the child can feel a sense of safety in his or her environment. Caregivers must also be taught to recognize the symptoms of escalating mental illness so they know when to bring in their child for treatment. The therapist can also ensure that the family has support systems in place to help them manage the stress associated with their child's adjustment. TF-CBT can include a parental treatment component. Inclusion of parents was found to be effective in improving the child's self-reported depressive symptoms (Cohen, 2003). Parents can be taught strategies for coping with their own emotional difficulties resulting from their child's trauma and can learn to model coping skills. Attachment-based interventions may improve insensitive parenting and infant attachment insecurity (MacMillan et al., 2009). Child- and parent-focused psychotherapy is indicated in families who also had exposure to domestic violence and for young children under age seven (AACAP, 2010). Please see Chapter 16 for a complete discussion of family therapy.

Providing Specialized Care

Intervention with clients who have experienced traumatic events will be most effective when the health care team works together. While many health providers, including those in primary care, may recognize trauma symptoms, providing mental health treatment for children and adolescents who have experienced trauma requires a trained psychiatric practitioner. This is especially true when children require medications to manage symptoms such as depression and anxiety, as many of these medications require close follow-up and management. In routine assessments, appointments, and physical exams, pediatric and family nurse practitioners may uncover signs of abuse and trauma. These primary care providers have the necessary skill set to document the physical findings and to testify in court if needed. However, only mental health providers have the necessary skill set for assessment and treatment of psychiatric symptoms. Further, clinicians unfamiliar with or lack the necessary skills to assess, treat, or manage these children should refer patients and families to experts in the area of child trauma.

Forensic Implications

Psychiatric clinicians are involved in court proceedings usually by requests to confirm a diagnosis of child abuse or to assess for damages to the child. Though definitions of what constitutes child abuse and neglect can vary by state, they include the minimum standards established by the federal government. The Federal Child Abuse Prevention and Treatment Act (CAPTA) (42 U.S.C.A. §5106g), as amended by the Keeping

Children and Families Safe Act of 2003, provides a seminal definition of child abuse and neglect. At minimum, a definition should include the following: Any recent act or failure to act on the part of a parent or caretaker which results in death, serious physical or emotional harm, sexual abuse or exploitation; or an act or failure to act which presents an imminent risk of serious harm (Gilbert, 2009b). While definitions may vary from state to state, every state has laws that designate nurses and advanced practice nurses as mandatory reporters.

An increasing numbers of cases of child maltreatment and abuse are under investigation and in the courts. Accordingly, advanced practice psychiatric nurses, child psychiatrists, and other qualified professionals make evaluations during legal proceedings. This can include evaluation of the competency of the child to testify, the credibility of the child's allegation, whether it is in the child's best interest to have contact with the alleged perpetrator and under what circumstances, if any, prior to court proceedings, particularly if the perpetrator is a relative. Clinicians may also evaluate whether the child is emotionally disturbed and in need of treatment, what emotional preparation is required for court testimony, whether the child will be able to cope with the stress of giving testimony, and whether the child would be further damaged psychologically by giving testimony.

Implications for Research and Education

Myriad studies document the extensive and detrimental influence of childhood trauma within social, psychological, and physical domains throughout the life span. Research is required on both diagnosis and treatment of children and adolescents who are at risk for abuse. Most of the findings on the impact of childhood trauma come from cross-sectional research. Hence, there is a need to examine and to measure the effects of the abuse over an extended period of time and within the context of a developmental framework (Gordis, 2000). As many cases of child maltreatment are undetected, it is essential that research examine the benefits of screening and interventions.

Additionally, research within the area of neurobiology offers hope for a better understanding of childhood abuse and more effective treatment strategies that utilize advances in technology. For example, transcranial magnetic stimulation (TMS) (Cohen et al., 2004) and immersive virtual reality (VR) therapy for the treatment of PTSD have shown promise among various populations, including combat victims and 911 victims (Difede & Hoffman 2002). TMS is a noninvasive technique that directly stimulates cortical neurons to create a therapeutic effect that, through testing with children under age

eighteen, was found to be effective (Quintana, 2005). VR uses virtual reality technology to treat patients with PTSD; research suggests that it is effective in treating adults, although randomized controlled trials are not available. Well-designed studies can determine if these progressive treatments hold promise for children and adolescents.

The rapid expansion of knowledge in the basic sciences impacts research needs for practice. The increased understanding of genetics and genomics expands the need for research on familial and biological causes of mental illness and responses to trauma. The pathways between trauma and consequences such as neurostructural alterations and abnormal neuropsychological responses are important areas of study. The field could benefit from studies that examine the relationships among trauma and disruptions in cognitive and affective processes and their associated neural circuits (Pine & Cohen, 2002). In addition, there is optimism that growing research in this field will lead to a better understanding of neurobiological development of children, adolescents, and young adults. The use of more extensive neuropsychological testing will help in this area.

Research on children and adolescents and especially research on victimized children and adolescents is not without ethical and practical obstacles (see Chapter 25). It would be useful to understand the effects of participating in research with children and adolescents and if it is harmful, helpful, or neutral to the recovery process. Despite the difficulties in this research, it is important to design prospective studies that describe long- and short-term outcomes and benefits to treatment. Randomized controlled trials are needed to determine the efficacy of treatment approaches including medication use and the effectiveness of prevention programs.

Key emerging trends include culture, treatment, and research. Cultural issues include increased use of ethnopsychology, ethnopsychiatry, ethnobiology, and ethnopharmacology, all of which entail an understanding of ethnic differences and approaches to therapy. Educational efforts must focus on readying the workforce to deal with clients of increasing diversity. Clinicians will need an understanding of the ways in which one's ethnic and racial background can affect perceptions and treatment of mental illness. These efforts include recruitment of a more diverse workforce and cultural sensitivity training for all APNs. Further, emphasis on culture-bound syndromes and on culturally relevant and sensitive assessment, diagnosis, and treatment is important. The changing demographics of the United States necessitate that clinicians understand cultural and ethnic expression of mental health symptoms, strategies for effective relationship building, and the influence of family and community structures in diverse groups. Research that includes diverse individuals can assist in the development and testing of interventions that are tailored for minority populations. Research involving child trauma must also pay attention to the sociocultural impact of religion, spirituality, health disparities, socioeconomic status, and sexual orientation on child treatment.

Technological advances bring new areas of intervention, such as the use of telehealth to expand child protection services. Trends within interpersonal violence include the influence of emerging technologies used in perpetration. Internet-based crimes include child predators targeting children and adolescents through the use of chat rooms and social networking sites. Pornography of children broadcast over the Internet provides a challenge to criminal justice investigations and includes the problem of the long-term nature of pictures and videos on the web. Bullying, stalking, and harassment can also include technology, in the form of text messaging, instant messaging, and social networking sites. A major problem is the intrusive, pervasive, and persistent effects of technology-assisted IPV. More research can aid in understanding prevention and intervention strategies related to technology-assisted violence.

A plethora of public policy issues exists. Due to the possibility of long-term neurological consequences, it is essential that child trauma and resulting psychiatric symptoms are identified early and intervention and treatment occur. School health nurses and school counselors can be instrumental in identifying children at risk and those who demonstrate behavioral profiles consistent with trauma. These children and their families need referrals and linkages with mental health providers, services, and resources. Programs that identify high-risk individuals and provide home visitation, education, and other social services can be helpful in preventing child abuse (Bilukha et al., 2005; Gilbert et al., 2009a; MacMillan et al., 2009). School-based programs can also be helpful in providing prevention and intervention with bullying and resources and referrals for offenders and victims.

Case Exemplar

Eric was a twelve-year-old Vietnamese American boy whose parents (Tan and Vivian) immigrated to the United States fifteen years ago. Tan worked in, owned, and operated a small construction company and Vivian worked full-time as an LPN in a nursing home. Eric had a nine-year-old sister (Julie) who was described by Vivian as "the perfect child—no trouble at all." The family lived in an urban community known for its high crime rate and poor community resources.

Tan and Vivian requested an evaluation for Eric because "the school said they don't know what to do because he can't be kept back again and we're worried about him crying all the time." During the initial telephone intake with Greta, the APRN, Vivian, an earnest and articulate young woman, expressed profound concern and frustration that "Eric will not do his school work and is so lazy and disrespectful." She explained that she and Tan believe that Eric is very smart and can do the work if he tries. Vivian reported that Eric has always been very "hyper" but that when he was younger "people always liked him."

Vivian shared that she "noticed a big change in Eric during the last year." She said, "Now, he seems angry all the time and he always annoys the other kids and grownups—even when they're being really nice to him. We don't know what to do. We tried everything and nothing works. We're afraid he will end up in prison because he has no respect for anything, not even himself. He eats all the time and he doesn't care that he's too fat. I know the kids at school make fun of him. The rest of us are so skinny." Vivian also expressed concern because Eric had been isolating himself in his room and crying a lot. "I know teenagers are moody and cry, but this seems to be way too much. He seems so different lately. I'm afraid something happened that he's not telling us."

Past Medical/Developmental History

Eric was born prematurely at thirty-three weeks' gestation and 4.5 lb. with Apgar scores of 6, 8, and 10. After about a three-week hospitalization in the NICU, he experienced no known complications related to his prematurity and low birth weight. He reached early motor and language milestones at developmentally appropriate times.

Initial Evaluation

During the initial evaluation, Greta, the APRN, reviewed the limits of confidentiality with Eric and his parents. Greta informed Eric that she had spoken at length with his mother via telephone and requested that the parents leave the office while she talked with Eric. Initially, Eric was withdrawn, made poor eye contact, and appeared anxious as evidenced by nail biting and foot tapping. About ten minutes into the session, Eric appeared to relax and requested that Greta, once again, review the limits of confidentiality. Eventually, Eric disclosed that Scott, the "guy" at the drop-in center had been sexually molesting him during the past year. Further, he stated that the molestation began as fondling, progressed to forced oral sex, and while he looked troubled, refused to say anymore.

Interventions for Acute Sexual Assault

Eric, aware that Greta was required to inform his parents and report to authorities, expressed relief "to have it off my chest." Eric stated that he did not fear retaliation from Scott and explained, "This is what makes it so bad. I'm bigger than he is, so it's not as if I couldn't resist. I just really wanted to impress him—it's so sick. I never thought it would go this far, though." Greta assured Eric that none of this was his fault and that Scott had victimized him. Additionally, she explained that people have a variety of different responses to sexual assault and that there is not a "normal" reaction to this type of trauma. Greta commended Eric for disclosing this information and suggested that they will be able to work through his feelings about this trauma together in therapy, but that her immediate suggestion was to speak with Eric's parents and inform them of the assault.

Next, Greta suggested that she arrange for Eric to be seen in an emergency department by a pediatric sexual assault nurse examiner. Once there, he would possibly have forensic evidence collected and receive appropriate preventative medication. Eric agreed to the plan and stated that he wanted to report the assault to the police "so that he doesn't do this to other kids." The APRN provided positive reinforcement to Eric and explained the role of the local child advocacy center.

Eric agreed to continue to see Greta for individual therapy. His parents were also involved in TF-CBT. He later disclosed anal perpetration by Scott and was again referred to a pediatric sexual assault nurse examiner at the local child advocacy center. In therapy, Eric was able to describe the event and his distressed feelings. He was able to discuss his eating and use of food as a protective measure. Most important, in therapy he was able to address his feelings of guilt and blame, correct distorted beliefs, and see that it was not his fault.

Summary

While many regard childhood and adolescence as carefree periods, this is not true for all youths. For some individuals like Eric, traumatic experiences mark childhood and adolescence. Far too many children and adolescents deal with traumatic experiences and the resulting psychiatric symptoms and distress. Greta was aided with an understanding of the risk factors and causes that allowed her to identify that Eric had experienced trauma. Early identification and treatment can mitigate the health consequences of trauma. A variety of therapy options exist that can aid the APN in helping children, adolescents, and their families to manage and recover from trauma. By remaining current with research and practice trends, the APN can provide individualized and targeted therapy to children, adolescents, and families and develop and implement prevention and intervention strategies.

Recommended Resources

Child Trauma Academy is a not-for-profit organization, based in Houston, Texas, that works to improve the lives of high-risk children through direct service, research and education. http://www.childtrauma.org/index.php/home

Prevent Child Abuse (PCA), America: Prevent Child Abuse (formerly the National Committee to Prevent Child Abuse) is nationally recognized as one of the most innovative leaders in child abuse prevention. It has a nationwide network of chapters and their local affiliates in hundreds of communities. www.preventchildabuse.org

Child Welfare League of America (CWLA): CWLA is an association of more than 1,000 public and private nonprofit agencies that assist over 2.5 million abused and neglected children and their families each year with a wide range of services. http://www.cwla.org/

American Professional Society on the Abuse of Children (APSAC) works to ensure that everyone affected by child maltreatment receives the best possible professional response. http://www.apsac.org/

National Clearinghouse for Child Abuse and Neglect (NCCAN) is a national resource for professionals seeking information on the prevention, identification, and treatment of child abuse and neglect, and related child welfare issues. http://www.calib.com/nccanch Email: nccanch@calib.com

The National Child Traumatic Stress Network works to raise the standard of care and improve access to services for traumatized children, their families, and communities throughout the United States. http://www.nctsn.org/nccts/nav.do?pid=ctr_main

The Red Cross has a long history of helping children, families, and communities recover from disasters. http://www.redcross.org/

Cohen, J. A., Mannarino, A. P., & Deblinger, E. (2006). Treating trauma and traumatic grief in children and adolescents. New York: Guilford Press.

References

Amar, A.F. (2007). Dating violence: comparing victims who are also perpetrators with victims who are not. *Journal of Forensic Nursing*, 3(1), 35–41.

Amar, A.F., & Gennaro, S. (2005) Dating violence in college women: associated physical injury, healthcare usage, and mental health symptoms. *Nursing Research*, 54(4) 235–242.

American Academy of Child and Adolescent Psychiatry (AACAP). (2010). Practice parameter for the assessment and treatment of children and adolescents with posttraumatic stress disorder. *Journal of the Academy of Child and Adolescent Psychiatry*, 49(4) 414–430.

American Psychiatric Association. (2000). *Diagnostic and statistical manual of mental disorders*, fourth edition, text revision. Washington, DC: Author

Avinger, K.A., & Jones, R.A. (2007). Group treatment of sexually abused adolescent girls: a review of outcome studies. *The American Journal of Family Therapy*, 35, 315–326.

Berlan, E.D., Corliss, H.L., Field, A.E., Goodman, E., & Austin, S.B. (2010). Sexual orientation and bullying among adolescents in the growing up today study. *Journal of Adolescent Health*, 46, 366–371.

Berman, H., Hardesty, J.L., Lewis-O'Connor, A., & Humphreys, J. (2011). Childhood exposure to intimate partner violence. In

J. Humphreys & J.C. Campbell. *Family violence and nursing practice* (second edition) (pp. 279–318).

Bernstein, D., & Fink, L. (1998). *Childhood trauma questionnaire: a retrospective self-report.* San Antonio: The Psychological Corporation.

Bilukha, O., Hahn, R.A., Crosby, A., Fullilove, M.T., Liberman, A., Moscicki, E., Task Force on Community Preventive Services. (2005). The effectiveness of early childhood home visitation in preventing violence: a systematic review. *American Journal of Preventive Medicine, 28*(2S1), 11–39.

Black, M.C., Noonan, R., Legg, M., & Eaton, D. (2006). Physical dating violence among high school students: United States, 2003. *MMWR, 55*(19), 532–535.

Bogat, G.A., DeJohghe, E., Levendosky, A.A., Davidson, W.S., & von Eye, A. (2006). Trauma symptoms among infants exposed to intimate partner violence. *Child Abuse & Neglect, 20,* 109–124.

Briere, J. (1996). *Trauma Symptom Checklist for Children (TSCC) professional manual.* Odessa, FL: Psychological Assessment Resources.

Centers for Disease Control and Prevention. Atlanta: CDC; 2006. *Adverse Childhood Experiences Study.* Available from: http://www.cdc.gov/nccdphp/ace/index.htm

Chan, Y., & Yeung, J.W. (2009). Children living with violence within the family and its sequel: A meta-analysis from 1995–2006. *Aggression and Violent Behavior, 14,* 313–322.

Cleveland, H.H., Herrera, V.M., & Stuewig, J. (2003). Abusive males and abused females in adolescent relationships: risk factor similarity and dissimilarity and the role of relationship seriousness. *Journal of Family Violence, 18*(6), 325–339.

Cohen, H., Kaplan, Z., Kotler, M., Kouperman, I, Moisa, R., & Grisaru, N. (2004). Repetitive transcranial magnetic stimulation of the right dorsolateral prefrontal cortex in posttraumatic stress disorder: A double-blind, placebo-controlled study. *American Journal of Psychiatry, 161,* 515–524.

Cohen, J.A. (2003). Treating acute posttraumatic reactions in children and adolescents. *Society of Biological Psychiatry, 53,* 827–833.

Cohen, J.A., & Mannarino, A.P. (2008). Trauma-focused cognitive behavioural therapy for children and parents. *Child and Adolescent Mental Health, 13*(4), 158–162.

Cohen, J.A., Mannarino, A.P., & Deblinger, E. (2006). *Treating trauma and traumatic grief in children and adolescents.* New York: Guilford Press.

Cornelius, T. L., & Ressiguie, N. (2007). Primary and secondary prevention programs for dating violence: a review of the literature. *Aggression and Violent Behavior, 12,* 364–375.

Daviss, W.B., Mooney, D., Racusin, R., Ford, J.D., Fleischer, A., & McHugo, G. (2000). Predicting post-traumatic stress after hospitalization for pediatric injury. *Journal of the American Academy of Child and Adolescent Psychiatry, 39,* 576–583.

Daviss, W.B., Racusin, R., Fleischer, A., Mooney, D., Ford, J.D., & McHugo, G. (2000). Acute stress disorder symptomatology during hospitalization for pediatric injury. *Journal of the American Academy of Child and Adolescent Psychiatry, 39,* 569–575.

DeBellis, M.D. (2001). Developmental traumatology: the psychobiological development of maltreated children and its implications for research, treatment, and policy. *Development and Psychopathology, 13,* 539–564.

Difede, J., & Hoffman, H. G. (2002). Virtual reality exposure therapy for World Trade Center post-traumatic stress disorder: A case report. *CyberPsychology & Behavior, 5,* 529–535.

Donelan-McCall, N., Eckenrode, J., & Olds, D.L. (2009). Home visitation for the prevention of child maltreatment: lessons learned during the past 20 years. *Pediatric Clinics of North America, 56,* 398–403.

Dubowitz, H., & Bennett, S. (2007). Physical abuse and neglect of children. *Lancet, 369,* 1891–1899.

DuMont, K.A., Widom, C. S., & Czaja, C.J. (2007). Predictors of resilience in abused and neglected children growing up: the role of individual and neighborhood characteristics. *Child Abuse and Neglect, 31,* 255–274.

Felitti, V.J., et al. (1998). Relationship of childhood abuse and household dysfunction to many of the leading causes of death in adults: the adverse childhood experiences (ACE) study. *American Journal of Preventative Medicine, 14*(4), 245–258.

Ferrari, A.M. (2002). The impact of culture upon child rearing practices and definitions of maltreatment. *Child Abuse and Neglect, 26,* 793–813.

Finkelhor, D., Ormrod, R.K., & Turner, H.A. (2007). Polyvictimization: a neglected component in child victimization. *Child Abuse and Neglect, 31,* 7–26.

Finkelhor, D., Ormrod, R., Turner, H., & Holt, M. (2009a). Pathways to poly-victimization. *Child Maltreatment, 14*(4), 316–329.

Finkelhor, D., Turner, H., Ormrod, R., & Hamby, S. (2009b). Violence, abuse, and crime exposure in a national sample of children and youth. *Pediatrics, 124*(5), 1–13.

Fletcher, K. (1996). Psychometric review of the When Bad Things Happen Scale (WBTH). In B.H. Stamm (Ed.), *Measurement of stress, trauma, and adaptation* (pp. 435–437). Lutherville, MD: Sidran Press.

Fluke, J.D., Shusterman, G.R., Hollinshead, D., & Yuan, Y.T. (2005). *Rereporting and Recurrence of Child Maltreatment: Findings from NCANDS.* Washington, D.C.: U.S. Department of Health and Human Services, Office of the Assistant Secretary for Planning and Evaluation.

Foa, E., Johnson, K., Feeny, N., & Treadwell, K.R. (2001). The child PTSD in children and adolescents. *Journal of Clinical Child Psychology, 30*(3), 376–384.

Ford, J.D., Racusin, R., Ellis, C., Daviss, W.B., Reiser, J., Fleischer, A., & Thomas, J. (2000). Child maltreatment, other trauma exposure, and posttraumatic symptomatology among children with oppositional defiant and attention deficit hyperactivity disorders. *Child Maltreatment, 5,* 205–217.

Ford, J.D., Hartman, J. K., Hawke, J., & Chapman, J. (2008). Traumatic victimization, posttraumatic stress disorder, suicidal ideation, and substance abuse risk among juvenile justice-involved youths. *Journal of Child and Adolescent Trauma, 1,* 75–92.

Gilbert, R., Widom, C. S., Browne, K., Ferguson, D., Webb, E., & Janson, S. (2009a). Burden and consequences of child maltreatment in high-income countries. *Lancet, 373,* 68–81.

Gilbert, R., Kemp, A., Thoburn, J., Sidebotham, P., Radford, L., Glaser, D., & MacMillan, H. L. (2009b). Recognising and responding to child maltreatment. *Lancet, 373,* 167–180.

Gordis, E. (2000). The effects of family and community violence on children. *Annual Review of Psychology, 1(41),* 445–479.

Greenwald, R., & Rubin, A. (1999). Brief assessment of children's posttraumatic symptoms: Development and preliminary validation of parent and child scales. *Research on Social Work Practice, 9,* 61–75.

Groves, B.M., Ausustyn, M., Lee, D., & Sawirds, P. (2002). *Identifying and responding to domestic violence: consensus recommendations for child and adolescent health.* San Francisco: Family Violence Prevention Fund.

Gruber, J.E., & Fineran, S. (2008). Comparing the impact of bullying and sexual harassment victimization on the mental and physical health of adolescents. *Sex Roles, 59*(1), 1–13.

Guerra, N.G., Huesmann, R., & Spindler, A. (2003). Community violence exposure, social cognition, and aggression among urban elementary school children. *Child Development, 74*(5), 1561–1576.

Halpern et al. (2001). Partner violence among adolescents in opposite-sex romantic relationships: findings from the National Longitudinal Study of Adolescent Health. *American Journal of Public Health, 91*(10), 1679–1685.

Harned, M.S. (2002). A multivariate analysis of risk markers for dating violence victimization. *Journal of Interpersonal Violence, 17*(11), 1179–1187.

Hershkowitz, I., Omer, L., & Lamb, M.E. (2007). Exploring the disclosure of child sexual abuse with victims and their parents. *Child Abuse and Neglect, 31*, 111–123.

Hess, K.M., & Orthmann, C.H. (2009) *Criminal investigation.* New York: Delmar.

Holt, S., Buckley, H., & Whelan, S. (2008). The impact of exposure to domestic violence on children and young people: a review of the literature. *Child Abuse and Neglect, 32*, 797–810.

Kenardy, J.A., Spence, S.H., & Macleod, A.C. (2006). Screening for posttraumatic stress disorder in children after accidental injury. *Pediatrics, 118*(3), 1002–1009.

King, L.A., King, D.W., Leskin, G., & Foy, D.W. (1995). The Los Angeles Symptom Checklist: a self-report measure of posttraumatic stress. *Assessment, 2*, 1–17.

Leeb, R.T., Paulozzi, L., Melanson, C., Simon, T., & Arias, I. (2008). *Child maltreatment surveillance: uniform definitions for public health and recommended data elements, Version 1.0.* Atlanta, GA: Centers for Disease Control and Prevention, National Center for Injury Prevention and Control.

Levy, H., Markovic, J., Kallinowski, M., Ahart, S., & Torres, H. (1995). Child sexual abuse interviews: the use of anatomical dolls and reliability of information. *Journal of Interpersonal Violence, 10*(3), 334–353.

MacMillan, H.L., Wathen, C.N., Barlow, J., Fergusson, D.M., Leventhal, J.M., & Taussig, H.N. (2009). Interventions to prevent child maltreatment and associated impairment. *Lancet, 373*, 250–266.

Margolin, G., & Gordis, E.B. (2000). The effects of family and community violence on children. *Annual Review of Psychology, 51*, 445–479.

Mongillo, E.A., Briggs-Gowan, M., Ford, J.D., & Carter, A.S. (2009). Impact of traumatic life events in a community sample of toddlers. *Journal of Abnormal Child Psychology, 37*, 455–468.

Otto, M.W., Henin, A., Hirschfeld-Becker, D.R., Pollack, M.H., Biederman, J., & Rosenbaum, J.F. (2007). Posttraumatic stress disorder symptoms following media exposure to tragic events: Impact of 9/11 on children at risk for anxiety disorder. *Journal of Anxiety Disorders, 21*, 888–902.

Pine, D.S., & Cohen, J.A. (2002). Trauma in children and adolescents: Risk and treatment of psychiatric sequelae. *Society of Biological Psychiatry, 51*, 519–531.

Preston, J.D., O'Neal, J.H., & Talaga, M.C. (2008). *Handbook of clinical and psychopharmacology for therapists* (fifth edition). Oakland, CA: New Harbinger Publications, Inc.

Pynoos, R., Rodriguez, N., Steinberg, A., Stuber, M., & Frederick, C. (1998). *The UCLA PTSD reaction index for DSM IV (Revision 1).* Los Angeles: UCLA Trauma program.

Quintana, H. (2005). Transcranial magnetic stimulation in persons younger than the age of 18. *The Journal of ECT, 21*(2), 88–95.

Rennison, C. (2001). *Intimate partner violence and age of the victim: 1993–1999* (No. NCJ 187635). Washington, D.C.: U.S. Department of Justice.

Reynolds, A J., Mathieson, L.C., & Topitzes, J.W. (2009). Do early childhood interventions prevent child maltreatment? A review of research. *Child Maltreatment, 14*(2), 182–206.

Ribbe, D. (1996). Psychometric review of Traumatic Events Screening Inventory for Children (TESI-C). In B. H. Stamm (Ed.), *Measurement of stress, trauma, and adaptation* (pp. 386–387). Lutherville, MD: Sidran.

Rich, C.L., Gidycz, C.A., Warkentin, J.B., Loh, C., & Weiland, P. (2005). Child and adolescent abuse and subsequent victimization: a prospective study. *Child Abuse and Neglect, 29*, 1373–1394.

Roberts, A.L., Gilman, S.E., Fitzmaurice, G., Decker, M.R., & Koenen, K.C. (2010). Witness of intimate partner violence in childhood and perpetration of intimate partner violence in adulthood. *Epidemiology, 21*(6).

Saigh, P.A., Yasik, A., Oberfield, R., Green, B., Halamandaris, P., Rubenstein, H., et al. (2000). The children's PTSD inventory: development and reliability. *Journal of Traumatic Stress, 13*(3), 369–380.

Schilling, E.A., Aseltine, R.H., & Gore, S. (2007).Adverse childhood experiences and mental health in young adults: A longitudinal survey. *BMC Public Health*, 7, 30.

Shapiro, F., & Maxfield (2002). Eye movement desensitization and reprocessing (EMDR): information processing in the treatment of trauma. *JCLP/In Session: Psychotherapy in Practice, 58*(8), 933–946.

Siever, L. (2008). Neurobiology of aggression and violence. *American Journal of Psychiatry, 165*, 429–442

Silverman, W.K., Ortiz, C.D., Viswesvaran, C., Burns, B.J., Kolko, D.J., Putham, F.W., et al., (2008). Evidence-based psychosocial treatments for children and adolescents exposed to traumatic events. *Journal of Clinical Child and Adolescent Psychology, 37*(1), 156–183.

Smith, P.K., Mahdavi, J., Carvalho, M., Fisher, S., Russell, S., & Tippett, N. (2008). Cyberbullying: its nature and impact in secondary school pupils. *Journal of Child Psychology, 49*(4), 376–385.

Straka, S.M., & Montiminy, L. (2008). Family violence: through the lens of power and control. *Journal of Emotional Abuse, 8*(3), 255–279.

Strand, V.C., Sarmiento, T.L., & Pasquale, L.E. (2005). Assessment and screening tools for trauma in children and adolescents. *Trauma, Violence, and Abuse, 6*(1), 55–78.

Stith, S. M., et al., (2009). Risk factors in child maltreatment: a meta-analytic review of the literature. *Aggression and Violent Behavior, 14*, 13–29.

U.S. Department of Health and Human Services, Administration on Children, Youth and Families. (2009). *Child Maltreatment 2007.* Washington, D.C.: U.S. Government Printing Office.

Wang, J., Iannotti, R.J., & Nansel, T.R. (2009). School bullying among adolescents in the United States: physical, verbal, relational, and cyber. *Journal of Adolescent Health, 45*, 368–375.

Watts-English, T., Fortson, B.L., Gibler, N., Hooper, S.R., & DeBellis, M.D. (2006). The psychobiology of maltreatment in childhood. *Journal of Social Issues, 62*(4), 717–736.

Wethington, H.R., et al. (2008). The effectiveness of interventions to reduce psychological harm from traumatic events among children and adolescents. *American Journal of Preventative Medicine, 35*(3), 287–313.

22

Children in Out-of-Home Placement

Diane M. Caruso, Charlotte A. Herrick, Robin Bartlett, and Carolyn Schmidt

Objectives

After reading this chapter, APNs will be able to

1. Describe types of formalized placements for children living out of their homes.
2. Explain the potential complex physical, developmental, and mental health care needs of the children living in an out-of-home placement.
3. Examine alternatives to out-of-home placement for children living in distressed families.
4. Describe the multifaceted role of the advanced practice nurse in caring for children at risk for or in an out-of-home placement.

Introduction

A child's healthy growth and development occur best in a safe, stable, and nurturing environment. Yet every year millions of children are abused so reprehensibly that they are removed from their homes by the state's welfare system or Department of Children and Family Services (DCFS) and placed in foster care (Bass, Shields, & Behrman, 2004). They are among the most vulnerable populations in the United States, often overlooked by policy makers (Marx, Benoit, & Kamradt, 2003). Children in foster care have considerably more medical, developmental, social, behavioral, and emotional problems when compared to their peers who are not in foster care (Vig, Chinitz, & Shulman 2005). In order to coordinate the health care resources necessary to meet these complex needs, children in foster care require supervision by a primary care provider (PCP) experienced in working collaboratively with other health care professionals and knowledgeable about the complexities of the foster care system.

The Current State of the U.S. Child Welfare System

The foster care system is a combination of many overlapping and interacting agencies, which include federal and state-supported agencies responsible for the protection of the foster child's welfare (Schneiderman, 2005). Because of this, health care for foster children is fragmented, insufficient, and poorly coordinated. An inherent problem is the lack of medical records that follow a child from one health care setting to another, whether within a locale, within a state, or when a child moves from state to state (Schneiderman, 2008). The inability to obtain comprehensive records compromises continuity and quality of health care.

Child and Adolescent Behavioral Health: A Resource for Advanced Practice Psychiatric and Primary Care Practitioners in Nursing,
First Edition. Edited by Edilma L. Yearwood, Geraldine S. Pearson, and Jamesetta A. Newland.
© 2012 John Wiley & Sons, Inc. Published 2012 by John Wiley & Sons, Inc.

Child welfare services are chronically underfunded across the country. Social workers have more children than they can adequately handle and caseloads have doubled during the past several years (Sadock & Sadock, 2009). Many caseworkers lack training about complex health and mental health issues; they do not understand medical jargon or the intricacies of the health care delivery system. Therefore, the health care needs of these children and adolescents are frequently overlooked.

Children in Foster Care

Data on children in foster care vary depending on the source; however, it is clear that over the last decade there has been growing concern about the increase in the number of children admitted to foster care with complex medical and emotional problems (Bruskas, 2008; Hansen, Mawjee, Barton, Metcalf, & Joye, 2004). The system is burgeoning; as many as 500,000 to 700,000 children are in foster care in the United States. This number has more than doubled in the past two decades (Sadock & Sadock, 2009). The majority of referrals are children under four years of age; 53% are male and 47% are female. Forty percent of children in foster care are Caucasian, 30% are African American, 20% are Hispanic, 2% are Alaska Native/American Indian, 1% are Asian American, and the remaining are multiracial or of "unknown" race/ethnicity (U.S. Department of Health and Human Services [USDHHS], 2010). The statistics are alarming; and if the present trends continue, by the year 2020 nearly 14 million reported cases of child abuse and neglect will be confirmed, and 22,500 children will die from abuse or neglect prior to their fifth birthday (USDHHS, 2007). With the anticipated increased numbers of children in foster care, caseloads will rise to untenable levels, and caseworkers may not be able to provide the attention and support that children need, diminishing quality of care. A shortage of licensed family foster homes would further exacerbate this situation. Caseworkers will have to scramble to find appropriate placements, posing much higher costs to states and the federal government (The Pew Commission on Children in Foster Care, 2004).

Legislation

President William Clinton signed the Adoption and Safe Families Act (ASFA) of 1997, which created the most sweeping changes since the establishment of the child welfare program. The act was designed to emphasize children's health and safety by limiting the time that biological parents had to participate in rehabilitation to twelve months and requiring that child welfare departments develop timely permanency placement plans to decrease the length of stay in foster care without long-term planning. Almost a decade later, the U.S. Congress passed the Safe and Timely Interstate Placement of Foster Children's Act of 2006. States were provided incentives for efforts to place children across state lines. The act provided for an increase in the number of caseworkers to complete home studies and required that the child's health and school records be supplied to new foster parents in a safe and timely fashion. The act also provided for the right of the parent, foster parent, preadoptive parent, and any relative to speak in court hearings on behalf of the foster child (USDHHS, 2007).

In 2008, Congress passed the Fostering Connections to Success and Increasing Adoptions Act. The new law provided major reforms, including the following:

1. Supports for relatives to care for foster children in their own families and homes
2. Educational opportunities for children transitioning from adolescence into adulthood
3. Increased funding to foster care families living on reservations to care for Native American children within their own communities
4. Reauthorizing the Adoption Incentives Program so that adoptive parents can receive assistance when adopting older or special needs children
5. Requirements for states to make a concerted effort to place siblings in the same setting

The most recent legislation proposed to the Senate Finance Committee is the Foster Care Mentoring Act of 2009 (U.S. Department of Justice, 2009). This legislation supports the authorization of funding to establish a network of both public and community agencies that will provide staff and volunteers acting as role models to mentor youth aging out of foster care. The emphasis will be on improving foster children's academic achievements through tutoring and providing assistance with access to public and private community resources to reduce drug and alcohol abuse, teenage pregnancy, delinquency, and homelessness (U.S. Department of Justice).

Annie E. Casey Foundation

Socially innovative programs directed at offering services that advocate for vulnerable children are equally as important as legislation mandating services. The Annie E. Casey Foundation is an advocacy organization for disadvantaged children. The primary mission of the Casey Foundation is to improve the lives of the most vulnerable children by recommending public policies, advocating human service reforms, providing community support, and identifying the barriers to adequate health care services. The foundation funds grants to help states, cities, and neighborhoods develop innovative cost-effective programs to promote the delivery of the best quality of care for the most disadvantaged families and children by emphasizing interdisciplinary education and practice between social workers, policy makers, providers, foster care families, and fragile parents. In light of the current numbers of children placed in foster care, the Casey challenge is to reduce the number of children in foster care by 50% by the year 2020 (Annie E. Casey Foundation, 2009).

Types of Out-of-Home Placements

Although family preservation is always the goal, efforts to preserve the family will frequently fail and children will require temporary out-of-home placement (Sadock & Sadock, 2009) in traditional foster care, therapeutic foster care, kinship care, group homes, or permanent placement through adoption. Placements are based on the needs of the child and the resources of the state.

Traditional Foster Care

Placement in a traditional foster home is necessary when parents are unwilling or unable to provide adequate care for their child or children. In the case of either abuse or neglect, removal of the child from the biological family is a court-ordered intervention, which is meant to be a temporary rather than a long-term solution (Greater Hope Foundation for Children, Inc., 2007). Adults over the age of twenty-one years can apply to be foster parents. They are carefully screened for drug and alcohol use and a past history of child abuse and criminal behavior. Caregivers must then be licensed or certified as a foster family upon completion of a foster parent training program, a home study conducted by the state's DCFS, and other licensing requirements.

Foster parents are regularly supervised and evaluated every few months according to local and state laws and may be dismissed upon a court order. If the birth parents' rights are not terminated, visitation rights are in place for the parents to see the child. Foster parents may act on behalf of the child for anything concerning the child's welfare such as meeting with specialists in health or mental health services, attending individual educational planning (IEP) meetings at school, or meetings at the welfare department.

Therapeutic Foster Care

Therapeutic foster care (TFC) was developed to provide specialized treatment within the context of a nurturing family environment. The foster parents are members of an interdisciplinary health care team and must commit to working collaboratively to develop all therapeutic treatment plans (Child & Family Focus, Inc., 2003). The TFC parent must meet all of the requirements of traditional foster parents but must have more extensive training in the treatment of children with special needs. The TFC parent must be twenty-five years old, and if there are two parents in the home, both must be involved in the training. Two siblings may be placed in the same home, but two children are the maximum allowed for each family.

TFC parents are expected to keep a systematic and descriptive daily record of the child's behavior and progress, medication administration, and all other services that the child receives in the plan of care. The foster parents also attend the permanency placement planning meetings, where they are able to contribute their observations and predictions of how well the child may adjust to a transition to a permanent home. The foster parents also assist the child in maintaining an ongoing relationship with biological family members and friends.

Kinship Care

Approximately 2.4 million grandparents are the primary caregivers of their co-resident grandchildren under eighteen years of age (USDHHS, 2000; U.S. Census Bureau, 2003). Kinship families tend to be more effective foster families because they are more committed to the child and can provide the child with a culturally sensitive and more familiar environment. When children remain with their own families, the stigma is less than when a child is placed in a foster home (Bailey & Letiecq, 2008). The kinship family often continues to have relationships with the child's parents, providing a sense of continuity for the child, which supports a sense of identity. In addition, children living with extended families showed improved outcomes in their overall emotional, physical, spiritual, and cognitive development (Crumbly & Little 1997).

Frequently, the DCFS is not involved with kinship placement of a child in the grandparents' home because the parents still have legal custody of the child. Therefore, they do not undergo the same scrutiny that is demanded of foster parents, unless they have been selected by the court to care for the child. One disadvantage of not meeting foster care requirements is that the grandparents or relatives are not eligible for the financial support that would be provided if they were officially designated as foster parents (Allen, DeVooght, & Geen, 2008). Children in kinship care experience fewer moves but are more likely to remain in out-of-home placement (USDHHS, 2000). Consequently, the number of grandparent-headed households has increased tremendously. However, kinship care is not a panacea. Many grandparents struggle both emotionally and financially with care-giving responsibilities and experience higher rates of anxiety and depression, neglect their own health, and experience an increase in financial problems (Bailey & Letiecq, 2008; Crumbly & Little, 1997).

Group Homes

The purpose of a group home is to simulate a family environment; therefore, they are frequently found in residential neighborhoods. House parents have received training in child development and behavior modification and are responsible for the residents twenty-four hours per day. The goals of a group home are to provide a nurturing family-type environment, integrate the residents into the school and local community, provide daily structure, coordinate all necessary community services, and prepare each resident for independence through reinforcement of daily living and self-care skills. Any facility that houses six or more children is considered a group home (California Alliance of Child and Family Services, 2004). Medicaid and other state and local funds support group homes; therefore, they are subject to federal regulations and assigned a case manager from the public health department or a mental health center.

Therapeutic Group Home

A therapeutic group home (TGH) houses children who are difficult to place because of complex physical and mental health problems, such as a diabetic child with mental illness. The TGH is similar to TFC because of the additional training house parents receive in behavior management and child development. Training is also provided to parents related to the specific physical needs of each child. Consequently, TFC and the TGH have demonstrated improved outcomes by a reduction in delinquent and risky behaviors exhibited by the foster child and by an increased number of children who are able to return to their relatives or to traditional foster care (Ashe, n.d.; Adopting.org, n.d.).

Residential Treatment

Residential treatment settings are rarely located where the child's family resides so the child is often isolated from family and friends. Residential treatment programs are staffed by social workers, psychologists, psychiatrists, and nurses. They are the most costly, provide the most structure, and are the most restrictive of all child protective service out-of-home placements. The residents are usually older children who are medically ill, severely mentally ill, or who may have been involved with the juvenile justice system (Cadena, 2008).

Residential programs are comprehensive, providing educational and recreational activities and clinical treatment programs. Treatment may include individual and group therapies, stress management, recreational therapy, and physical and occupational therapies to meet the complex needs of each child (Cadena, 2008). Prior to discharge, social workers in the treatment centers work across the continuum of care to coordinate probation, court recommended mental health care, medical care, and the juvenile justice system (Pearson, 2006).

Adoption

Approximately 2% of children grow up in adoptive families who are not biological relatives; foster parent adoptions account for over half of the adoptions of children from foster care. These children are more likely to be older children from minority groups or a sibling group; they are also more likely to have a history of abuse or neglect (Rushton & Dance, 2006). Early childhood adoption increases the probability of positive parent and child bonding and normal child development compared with adoption in middle or late childhood (Sadock & Sadock, 2009). Prolonged efforts to return children to their biological parents should be carefully examined, especially when there may be little chance of success. The longer the child remains in out-of-home placement, the more difficult is the adjustment to adoption (Rushton & Dance, 2006). All out-of-home placements are provided by the state's DCFS. States have their own laws governing out-of-home placements, but several federal laws (Child Welfare Information Gateway [USDHHS, n.d.]) supersede individual state laws. Ultimately, it is the responsibility of each state to provide a safe and healthy environment for the child in foster care.

The Complex Needs of Children in Out-of-Home Placements

Foster children suffer from physical assaults, emotional abuse, and sexual abuse. However, neglect is the most frequent type of maltreatment in childhood (Sadock & Sadock, 2009). Unfortunately, the complex health care needs associated with abuse and neglect are frequently overlooked, unidentified, or untreated (Justin, 2003; Kools & Kennedy, 2003; Marx et al., 2003). In addition, numerous placements from one home to another interfere with continuity of care, contributing to poor outcomes in the foster child's physical and mental health.

Physical and Developmental Health Care Needs

The maltreatment of children results in cognitive and developmental delays and a complexity of health problems. This begins in utero, if the child's developing brain is exposed to toxins such as drugs or alcohol. Alcohol causes the greatest assault on the fetal brain (Vig et al., 2005), especially when alcohol use by the mother results in fetal alcohol spectrum disorder (FASD). FASD describes a continuum of permanent birth defects that occur during pregnancy, including alcohol-related neurodevelopmental disorder and fetal alcohol syndrome. FASD is often underdiagnosed; alcohol exposure in utero can result in a myriad of abnormal physical findings including prenatal and postnatal growth deficiency, microcephaly, facial and hand anomalies, heart defects, and a wide range of cognitive deficits from mild developmental delay to extreme problems with language, memory, judgment, impulse control, and aggression (Vig et al.). Maternal drug and alcohol use also increases a child's risk for congenital infections such as HIV, syphilis, hepatitis, and herpes (Schneiderman, 2003; Vig et al.) because pregnant women using drugs and alcohol may be less likely to seek adequate prenatal care where treatments could be provided to significantly diminish fetal transmission of disease.

Children may suffer from multiple injuries secondary to physical abuse. The most profound is shaken baby syndrome. This form of abuse is a result of excessive shaking of a crying infant leading to a shearing injury to the brain causing subdural hemorrhages. The mortality rate can be as high as 40%, but over half of surviving infants have significant neurologic abnormalities and visual impairment (Vig et al., 2005).

If emotionally abused or neglected, children in foster care may regress to an earlier stage of growth and development following abuse. They may become delayed in speech and language acquisition skills and develop adaptive behavior deficits that result in bullying, lying, and disruptive behavior in social situations (Craven & Lee, 2006). By the time these children attend grade school, they may be unable to meet academic requirements, resulting in school failure and paving the way for teen truancy.

Other medical problems found in children in foster care are failure to thrive, malnutrition, lead toxicity, asthma, anemia, dermatological problems, vision and hearing deficits, underimmunization, and growth delay (Schneiderman, 2003; Vig et al., 2005). Despite placement in foster care with documented health care need, 32% of children have at least one unmet health care need after placement in foster care (Vig et al.). Given this, it is important that all children in foster care receive early childhood intervention services such as those provided by the Early and Periodic Screening, Diagnosis, and Treatment Program (EPSDT) designed to detect and treat health problems through regular medical, dental, vision, and developmental screenings (Child Welfare Information Gateway, 2006). School-aged children in foster care frequently require individual tutoring and special education testing and services.

Mental Health Needs

Many foster children suffer from emotional and behavioral problems requiring mental health services. Emotional problems found in many of the children at a young age are attachment disorders and anxiety disorders, including separation anxiety. Some foster children experience school phobias; many fear they will be abandoned. Foster children frequently suffer from low self-esteem and feelings of personal rejection (Bruskas, 2008; Kools & Kennedy, 2003).

Abused and neglected children may suffer from symptoms of posttraumatic stress disorder, including hypervigilance, startle responses to noise, nightmares, and depression. Depressed children may have thoughts of suicide or exhibit self-destructive behaviors. Continuing losses from many different out-of-home placements traumatize children, which interferes with their ability to establish positive interpersonal relationships. This is particularly difficult for children entering the teenage years because of the importance of the development of peer relationships (Kools & Kennedy, 2003). Adolescents in foster care often exhibit disruptive or antisocial acts that are oppositional and aggressive. Many engage in risky behaviors, including drugs, alcohol, tobacco use, and promiscuity, resulting in an increased incidence of teen pregnancy and sexually transmitted infections (Gramkowski et al., 2009; Kools & Kennedy, 2003; Sadock & Sadock, 2009).

Educational Needs

Because of the poor educational achievement outcomes of children in foster care, early intervention services in childhood, special education services in the school-age years, and aftercare services are critical for youth and those aging out of foster care. In order to reduce barriers to educating children in foster care, such as lack of collaboration between child protective services and local education agencies, formal procedures need to be in place to access specialized educational programs (Weinberg, Zetlin, & Shea, 2009). Agencies should begin life skills classes as soon as the child is developmentally capable, usually the early teen years. These classes should include education on finding employment, budgeting and managing money, going grocery shopping, finding a place to live, accessing medical and mental health services, and preventing sexually transmitted infections and pregnancy (Racusin, Maerlender, Sengupta, Isquith, & Straus, 2005). Teen parents require parenting classes.

Transition From Out-of-Home Placement to Adulthood

As adolescents transition from adolescence to young adulthood, they experience numerous challenges, such as completing their education, contemplating future careers, beginning full-time employment, living independently, and choosing a partner. Few foster children have family or peer support systems for these developmental transitions and are at risk for becoming homeless, unemployed, destitute, and incarcerated (Foster & Gifford 2004). Some programs phase out young people gradually while others end services abruptly; however, transitioning to adulthood means leaving the programs they have been dependent on for many years without actually demonstrating readiness for independent living. Completion of high school or the graduation equivalency diploma (GED), availability of financial resources for further education, absence of learning problems and substance abuse, and low rates of long-standing serious emotional problems are associated with positive transitions from the foster care system to adulthood (Racusin et al., 2005).

Intensive Family Preservation

Intensive family preservation services (IFPS) is known by many names including family-based services and family preservation, but IFPS is the most current nomenclature used in the literature. IFPS focuses on preventing unnecessary foster care placement of minor children by providing comprehensive, short-term, in-home treatment using a family-centered approach (Berry, Cash, & Brook, 2000). The primary goal of IFPS is to prevent out-of-home placement by adhering to key design elements and values (Table 22.1).

Families served by IFPS are those with children from birth through seventeen years who are considered at imminent risk of being removed from the home (Berry et al., 2000; National Family Preservation Network [NFPN], 2003, 2009). Situations that constitute imminent risk may be lack of effective parenting and family instability, abuse, neglect, law enforcement involvement, academic truancy, developmental disabilities, mental health issues, family violence, and health problems, especially those related to medical neglect and complications of teen pregnancy. The case is then accepted based on several inclusion criteria. Family members must be willing and able participants in the IFPS process. At least one child must be at imminent risk of removal from the home, and IFPS services will be implemented to protect the child or children from abuse or neglect in the short-term future. The child or children cannot concurrently be in the custody of any public agency.

Exclusionary criteria for IFPS may include parental substance abuse, mental illness, cognitive delay, or a history of sadistic or sexual abuse where the abuser still lives in the home (Berry et al., 2000). IFPS is not appropriate for children not at high risk for removal from the home because there are less intensive service models available for family support (NFPN, 2009). Ultimately, the family preservation caseworker and supervisor make the final decision whether IFPS intervention can safely meet the needs of the child and family.

The essential core program components of IFPS are based primarily on the HOMEBUILDERS model, the most widely used model of family preservation in the United States (NFPN, 2009). There are specific service components characteristic of innovative family preservation services in the child welfare system; these are listed in Table 22.2.

IFPS programs are required to provide certain interventions in order to increase the probability that a family will remain unified successfully. The interventions may vary but should include the basic fundamental elements listed in Table 22.3.

Table 22.1 Key design elements and values in intensive family preservation services

1. Maintain safety of clients, providers rendering services, and the community
2. Raise children within their own families when possible and when not possible, seek permanent placement
3. Work in partnership with clients, treating them as colleagues with unique cultural characteristics, strengths, and challenges
4. Recognize that all people are influenced by many factors such as environment, skills they possess, and social support
5. Recognize that all people can change as a result of planned learning
6. Use crisis to evoke change and teach clients new coping skills
7. Be accountable to clients for quality of care
8. Reduce barriers to care in order to assist clients in obtaining all necessary services and bring services into the home if possible
9. Provide services that are both concrete, such as food and housing, and therapeutic such as counseling

Sources: Arbuckle & Herrick, 2006; National Family Preservation Network [NFPN]-*IFPS Toolkit*, 2009; and Stroul, 1996

Table 22.2 Program components of intensive family preservation services

1. Availability of an IFPS caseworker or therapist to make a face to face family visit within 24 hours, obtain the family's willingness to participate, and ensure safety of all family members

2. Staff availability 24 hours a day, seven days a week for crisis intervention and support

3. Services delivered in the child's home to increase adherence

4. Services provided 5 to 20 hours per week to promote safety

5. Evening and weekend contact by the caseworker via phone or pager allowing for diffusion of potentially unsafe situations

6. Services that are time limited to 4 to 8 weeks, although this is a guideline determined by the family's needs

7. Small client to staff ratios, generally two to four families at a time because of the intensity of the services required

8. Use of a single caseworker and a back-up supervisor creating a stronger relationship with the family and enhancing accountability to the family

9. Utilization of ongoing training and quality assurance processes by caseworkers and supervisors

Sources: Fraser, Nelson, & Rivard, 1997; NFPN, 2003; NFPN-*IFPS Toolkit*, 2009

Table 22.3 Program interventions in intensive family preservation services

1. An initial family safety and crisis planning assessment giving the client as much time for the first visit as needed, when needed

2. Completion of a comprehensive family assessment tool such as the North Carolina Family Assessment Scale (NCFAS) upon initial contact or within one to two weeks of family contact, in order to determine imminent risk of out-of-home placement

3. Concrete interventions including assistance in meeting basic needs of food, clothing, shelter, and finances

4. Therapeutic interventions such as parenting and anger management classes to assist clients with developing life skills

5. Educating clients on interacting with other support systems in the community such as schools, medical providers, juvenile justice, and other social service programs

6. Referring clients to ongoing community resources or government agencies for support

Sources: Kirk, Kim, & Griffith, 2005; NFPN-*IFPS Toolkit 2009*; North Carolina Family Assessment Scale, n.d

High-fidelity models such as the HOMEBUILDERS program have consistently demonstrated the success of IFPS and that it works equally well in a variety of circumstances including families of color and those involved with abuse and neglect (Blythe & Jayaratne, 2002; Kirk & Griffith, 2004, 2008). Although IFPS may vary considerably with respect to program characteristics; all programs seek to stabilize families, improve family functioning, use community resources for family support, and assist caregivers with developing the skills needed to nurture and protect their children.

Intensive Case Management by an Interdisciplinary Health Care Team

In response to the daunting challenges the child welfare system faces in the twenty-first century, professionals are being asked to engage in interdisciplinary health care leadership teams to improve accessibility and quality of care to children in foster care (Bass et al., 2004; Magyary & Brandt, 2005). Competencies required to accomplish this goal include the development of collaborative relationships between multiple health care team providers, the recognition of the significant contributions made by each member of the interdisciplinary team, and incorporation of evidence-based practice in the development of a comprehensive and culturally sensitive intensive case management program by all interdisciplinary team members.

System of Care

Implementing models of care that represent a philosophy about the way services should be delivered to children and families can provide a framework for case management services essential to ensure the best medical and mental health outcomes for the foster care child. One model that provides this framework is the System of Care (Arbuckle & Herrick, 2006). Although the organizational configuration of the System of Care may vary between communities, the system is guided by core values essential to the operations of a System of Care (Stroul, 1996). The system must be child centered and family focused, community based in the most normative environment possible, and culturally competent. Clients must be provided with comprehensive care coordination of multiple services delivered in a therapeutic manner.

The Interdisciplinary Health Care Team

Even though the terms "multidisciplinary team" and "interdisciplinary team" are often used interchangeably, there is a distinct difference between the two concepts. Multidisciplinary teams work with clients independently of one another and share information about clients with each other. Interdisciplinary teams collaborate and are interdependent and complex, including professionals from many backgrounds who provide a variety of services (Table 22.4). Each member of the team addresses a particular need of the child and family, and every person's role in the process is clearly identified and mutually respected (Arbuckle & Herrick, 2006).

Intensive Case Management

The purpose of all case management services provided to a child and family is to deliver a coordinated System of Care (Arbuckle & Herrick, 2006). However, the process of case management differs significantly from that of intensive case management. Case management focuses on provision of medical care and utilization management of services. Intensive case management provides attention to patients' medical and social conditions; therefore, it is more comprehensive in its scope of services (Issel, 1997).

Effective intensive case management interventions must be flexible and tailored to meet the specific needs of each family. The process is based on a core set of functions that allow for a collaborative model, one of the most effective in delivering health care (Arbuckle & Herrick, 2006). These functions should be seen as a sequential process with overlapping tasks that are highly personalized and family focused (Stroul, 1996).

First, all agencies involved in addressing the child's and family's current health care needs must be identified and coordinated. Second, a plan of care must be developed in partnership with the family within the context of a multiagency team of professionals. Third, implementation of service delivery must be done in a timely and appropriate manner. Fourth, services must be coordinated by linking the various agencies, systems, and individuals involved with the care of the family. Finally, services must be monitored and evaluated for adequacy and appropriateness over time. Advocacy for the individual child and family is incorporated throughout the entire case management process (California Alliance of Child and Family Services, 2004; Stroul, 1996).

Several case management models have developed around the country with wide variations. However, the wrap-around method of delivering coordinated and collaborative care to children requiring services of an interdisciplinary team (Arbuckle & Herrick, 2006) uses the most family-centered approach to the case management process through the development of a child and family team (CFT). The CFT is led by a parent or caregiver and guided by specially trained individuals such as public health nurse case managers (referred to as case coordinators among System of Care experts) who assist caregivers in partnering with professionals (Pumariega, Winters, & Huffine, 2003). Wrap-around emphasizes extensive outreach and unconditional family-centered services, especially for those imminently at risk or already in out-of-home child placements (Pumariega et al.). The wrap-around process makes it possible to combine services that can provide for the intensity of inpatient or residential settings without actually removing a child from a foster home or an at-risk environment.

Table 22.4 Dimensions of services provided by an interdisciplinary team

1. Primary health care services ensuring a medical home model of care that is "accessible, continuous, comprehensive, family centered, coordinated, compassionate, and culturally effective" (American Academy of Pediatric [AAP], 2002, p. 184)

2. Mental health services such as counseling and treatment of diagnosed mental health disorders

3. Case management services using public health nurses as care coordinators in liaison roles to pediatric health systems, family support services, and early intervention programs

4. Social services using social workers coordinating child protective service issues

5. Substance abuse services incorporating professionals providing care to substance abusing clients

6. Vocational rehabilitation services for career education and job finding especially for transitional youth

7. Educational services incorporating school officials involved in student educational interventions

8. Recreational services such as after school programs and summer camps

Sources: AAP, 2002; Arbuckle & Herrick, 2006; Stroul, 1996

Outcome Measures

Once the interdisciplinary care team is established and intensive case management services are coordinated, planned, and implemented, outcomes must be measured. It has been a challenge to develop a practical, ongoing tracking mechanism for intensive case management of children in foster care and their families. However, four general domains of outcome measures include clinical outcomes, functional outcomes, system outcomes, and family satisfaction (Stroul, 1996). The interdisciplinary team should, through consensus, determine which outcomes to evaluate in the quality assurance process based on what the system is trying to accomplish. It is important to evaluate the individual service components within the context of the overall system because it is the synergy between the components and the coordination among the components that leads to enhanced outcomes (Stroul). The results of outcome evaluations remain an ongoing challenge for all professionals involved in the intensive case management process because children and their families traditionally need long-term services and support. However, following children in foster care and their families throughout the foster care experience and into the child's adulthood will provide important information about the long-term implications of foster care and the benefits of strategies to promote successful development for these vulnerable persons.

The concept of intensive case management by an interdisciplinary team is fraught with many challenges. These include replication and sustainability of the model, the potential breakdown of agencies, financial barriers that prevent a true System of Care approach, the integration of evidence-based interventions into practice, and accountability mechanisms for the system. These challenges need to be met through a combination of education, research, policy formation, and advocacy efforts. The core values of a family-centered, community-based System of Care need to guide professionals caring for foster children and their families in these efforts.

The Role of Advanced Practice Nurses (APNs)

Care of the foster child by a nurse practitioner (NP) should be guided by the American Academy of Pediatrics (AAP) statement on the delivery of health care services to children in the foster care system. These services are divided into four components: (1) an initial health screening, (2) a comprehensive medical and dental screening, (3) a developmental and mental health evaluation, and (4) provision for ongoing primary care in a medical home model (AAP, 2002).

Initial Health Screening

If a child is placed in the foster care system, an initial health screening must be conducted immediately before the child is placed or within two weeks of the most recent placement. Identification of any urgent medical needs of the child and including the foster parent and caseworker in planning treatment is essential (AAP, 2002). It is imperative that the review of the history includes details that led to the placement and, if possible, the past medical history. Careful measurements of height, weight, and head circumference are important to assess general nutritional status and growth. All body surfaces require an exam while unclothed to note for trauma, bruises, scars, deformities, or limitations in body function. Genital and anal exams should be conducted and, when necessary, photography documentation should be obtained. Screening lab work should be obtained if clinically indicated, such as for HIV infection or other sexually transmitted diseases. Infections and communicable diseases should be noted and treated promptly (AAP, 2002). The NP should discuss all findings and care instructions with the foster parent and caseworker directly and clarify the role that the foster parent has in meeting the health care needs of the foster child.

Comprehensive Health Assessment

Within one month of placement, a comprehensive health assessment should be conducted by a PCP with whom consistent care will be established. When possible, the biological parent should provide information about the past health status of the child and be kept informed of the child's present health status (AAP, 2002). Particular attention should be paid to assessing the child's adjustment to the foster home and any new health problems that have developed since the initial visit. In addition, periodic visits should be scheduled according to the AAP Recommendations for Preventive Pediatric Health Care (AAP, 2008).

Immunization records should be reviewed. These records may have to be pieced together from several sources including prior providers, schools, or vaccine registries. Many foster care children are unimmunized or incompletely immunized; therefore, they should be considered susceptible and immunized (AAP, 2002) according to the AAP Immunization Guidelines (AAP, 2009).

As part of the comprehensive health assessment, the PCP must also ensure that the foster child is provided with dental services. Foster children may require an array of dental services from routine care to intensive treatment. Periodic dental screenings should be included as part of the ongoing process of care.

Developmental and Mental Health Evaluation

A child's growth and development should be assessed by the PCP at every well-child encounter or more frequently if indicated. This assessment may be based on a structured interview that is age adjusted and developmentally specific, through the use of a standardized screening tool or review of school records (AAP, 2002). All children with identified developmental delays or problems should be referred to early intervention services, local consultants, or school resources. Some communities have established multidisciplinary programs that include professionals knowledgeable in evaluating children in foster care and should be used in diagnosing and treating children with developmental, mental health, and educational problems.

The prescribing provider must closely monitor any child prescribed psychotropic medication for potential adverse effects. The social worker should receive periodic updates on the child's progress, and the PCP should remain in close contact with the family to coordinate this effort.

Provision for Ongoing Care in a Medical Home Model

All children in foster care should have a medical home in which they receive ongoing primary care and assessments of their growth and development to determine if any changes in their health status requires additional services or interventions. The AAP recommends that reassessments should occur "monthly for the first 6 months of age, every 2 months for ages 6 to 12 months, every 3 months for ages 1 to 2 years, every 6 months for ages 2 years through adolescence" (AAP, 2002, p. 539), and at times of change in foster care placements or as indicated.

In order to enhance continuity of care in the primary care setting, several states have developed an abbreviated health record called a medical passport. The passport provides a brief description of the child's health, social, and family history and is designed to enhance the transfer of essential information among health professionals. Foster parents keep the document and bring it to all health care visits in order for the record to be updated. If the child changes foster homes, the record stays with the child to be used in a new medical home (AAP, 2002).

Case Exemplar

Cary is a six year old of mixed race who was placed in an emergency foster placement after her mother was unable to care for her due to incarceration for drug trafficking.

Cary's grandmother is unable to provide a placement for her and there are no other relatives. Her child welfare social worker took her to the emergency home, where there were several other young children. The foster mother was made aware of her daytime and nocturnal enuresis and her extreme thinness. It was unclear if she had ever had well child care. She had not gone to school and no immunization records were available. Cary is mute and sucks her thumb clutching a blanket. She quickly warmed to the nurturance of the foster mother, and the social worker left her sitting beside the mother, reading a book.

Within 48 hours Cary's social worker arranged a physical exam screen at a local federally qualified health center (FQHC). The Pediatric NP who did her physical noted that she had numerous round burns on her back, was underweight (in 6th percentile for weight and 45th for height), and had severe dental caries in her baby teeth. The PNP arranged for further evaluation by a pediatrician experienced in assessing physical and sexual abuse. They worked together on this part of the evaluation. The police were notified about the burns. Appointments with a psychiatric APN trained in play therapy and the dental clinic associated with the FQHC were arranged. The social worker also arranged for Cary to begin attending a diagnostic, therapeutic kindergarten aimed at identifying developmentally delayed children's specific problems. A nutritionist met with the foster mom to discuss eating and increasing calories.

This case exemplifies the interdisciplinary approach to a young child in placement.

Conclusion

Advanced practice nurses including certified family, pediatric, or psychiatric/mental health NPs, certified nurse midwives, and clinical nurse specialists face significant barriers when providing services to children in the foster care system. Barriers include lack of past medical history, social workers unable to provide details about the child's placement, foster care parents with limited training in health care issues, children with complicated physical and mental health conditions, lack of funding for needed services, and prior fragmentation of the child's care. To avoid some of these barriers, the APN should provide health care coordination, communicate effectively with all professionals, and provide compassionate support and education to foster and birth parents. APNs should be involved in the planning and development of a System of Care for children in foster care (AAP, 2002) and recognize the important role they play in all aspects of the foster care system.

References

Adopting.org. (n.d.). *Therapeutic foster care and group homes.* Retrieved from http://www.adopting.org/adoptions/therapeutic-foster-care-therapeutic-group-homes.html

Adoption and Safe Families Act of 1997. P. L. 105-89, 111 Stat 2115 (1997).

Allen, T., DeVooght, K., & Geen, R. (2008). Findings from the 2007 Casey Kinship Foster Care Policy Report. *Child Trends,* Retrieved from http://www.childtrends.org/Files/Child_Trend2009_02_24_FR_KinshipCare.pdf

American Academy of Pediatrics. (2002). Health care of young children in foster care. *Pediatrics, 109,* 536–541.

American Academy of Pediatrics. (2008). *Recommendations for preventive pediatric health care.* Retrieved from http://pediatrics.aappublications.org/cgi/data/120/6/1376/DC1/1

American Academy of Pediatrics. (2009). Recommended childhood and adolescent immunization schedule–U.S. Retrieved on from http://pediatrics.aappublications.org/cgi/content/full/123/1/189

Annie E. Casey Foundation. (2009). *Rebuild the National Child Welfare System.* Retrieved from http://www.aef.org

Arbuckle, M., & Herrick, C. (2006). *Child and adolescent mental health: Interdisciplinary systems of care.* Boston, MA: Jones and Bartlett Publishers.

Ashe, N.S. (n.d.). *Therapeutic foster care and group: Overview.* Retrieved from http://www.adopting.org/adoptions/therapeutic-foster-care-therap.

Bailey, S.J., & Letiecq, B.L. (2008). The mental health of rural grandparents rearing their grandchildren. *Focal Point, 22*(2), 22–25.

Bass, S., Shields, M., & Behrman, R. (2004). Children, families, and foster care: Analysis and recommendations. *The Future of Children, 14*(1), 5–29.

Berry, M., Cash, S., & Brook, J. (2000). Intensive family preservation services: An examination of critical service components. *Child and Family Social Work, 5,* 191–203.

Bruskas, D. (2008). Children in foster care: A vulnerable population at risk. *Journal of Child and Adolescent Psychiatric Nursing, 24,* 70–77.

Blythe, B., & Jayaratne, S. (2002). *Michigan Families First effectiveness study.* Retrieved from http://www.michigan.gov/fia/o,1607,7-124-55458-7695-8366- 21887-,oo.html

Cadena, C. (2008). *Foster parenting the child in residential care housing.* Retrieved from http://www.associate content.com/article/794305/foster_parenting_the_child_in_residential.html?cat=17

California Alliance of Child and Family Services. (2004). *Group homes for foster children.* Retrieved from http://www.cacfs.org/Advocacy/PublicPolicy.html S:\WORD\DOUG\GHRATEST\Group Home Fact Sheet 1-16-04CSedits.doc

Child Welfare Information Gateway. (2006). *Enhancing permanency for older youth in out-of-home care.* Washington, DC: U.S. Department of Health and Human Services. Retrieved from www.childwelfare.gov

Child & Family Focus, Inc. (2003). *Building communities and strengthening families.* Retrieved from http://www.childandfamilyfocus.org/index.shtm

Craven, P.A., & Lee, R E. (2006). Therapeutic interventions for foster children: A systematic research synthesis. *Research on Social Work Practice, 16,* 287-304.

Crumbly, J., & Little, R.L. 1997. Relatives raising children: An overview of kinship care. Washington, DC: The Child Welfare League.

Fraser, N.M., Nelson, K.E., & Rivard, J.C. (1997). Effectiveness of family preservation services. *Social Work Research, 21,* 138–152.

Foster, E.M., & Gifford, E.J. (2004, October). *Challenges in the transition to adulthood for youth in foster care, juvenile justice and special education* (Policy Brief, Issue 15). Philadelphia, PA: University of Pennsylvania, Department of Sociology, MacArthur Foundation Research Network.

Foster Care Mentoring Act of 2009, S. 986, 111th Cong. (2009).

Fostering Connections to Success and Increasing Adoptions Act of 2008. P. L. 110–351 (2008).

Gramkowski, B., Kools, S., Paul, S., Boyer, C.G., Monasterio, E., & Robbins, N. (2009). High risk behavior of youth in foster care. *The Journal of Child and Adolescent Psychiatric Nursing, 22,* 77–85.

Greater Hope Foundation for Children Inc. (2007). Retrieved on September 4, 2010, from http://www.greaterhopefoundation.com/home.html

Hansen, R.L., Mawjee, F.L., Barton, K., Metcalf, M.B., & Joye, N.R. (2004). Comparing the health status of low-income children in and out of foster care. *Child Welfare, 83,* 367–380.

Issel, L. (1997). Measuring comprehensive case management Interventions: Development of a tool. *Nursing Case Management, 2,* 132–140.

Justin, R.G. (2003). Medical needs of foster children. *American Family Physician, 67,* 474.

Kirk, R.S., & Griffith, D.P. (2004). Intensive family preservation services: Demonstrating placement prevention using event history analysis. *National Association of Social Workers Inc., 28*(1), 5–16.

Kirk, R.S., & Griffith, D.P. (2008). Impact of intensive family preservation services on disproportionality of out-of-home placement of children of color in one state's child welfare system. *Child Welfare League of America, 87*(5), 87–105.

Kirk, R.S., Kim, M.M., & Griffith, D.P. (2005). Advances in the reliability and validity of the North Carolina Family Assessment Scale. *Journal of Human Behavior in the Social Environment, 11,* 157–176.

Kools, S., & Kennedy, C. (2003). Foster child health and development. Implications for primary care. *Pediatric Nursing, 289,* 39–46.

Magyary, D., & Brandt, P. (2005). A leadership training model to enhance private and public service partnerships for children with special healthcare needs. *Infants and Young Children, 18*(1), 60–71.

Marx, L., Benoit, M., & Kamradt, B. (2003). Foster children in the child welfare system. In A. J. Pumariega and N. C. Winters (Eds.), *The handbook of child and adolescent system of care: The new psychiatry* (pp. 332–350). San Francisco, CA: Jossey-Bass.

National Family Preservation Network. (2003). *Intensive family preservation services protocol.* Retrieved from http://www.nfpn.org/images/stories/files/ifps_protocol.pdf

National Family Preservation Network. *2009 IFPS ToolKit.* Retrieved from http://nfpn.org/images/stories/files/ifps_toolkit.pdf

National Family Preservation Network. (n.d.) *North Carolina Family Assessment Scale: Sample scale and definitions* (v. 2.0). Retrieved from http://nfpn.org/images/stories/files/ncfas_scale_defs.pdf

Pearson, G. (2006). System of care with the juvenile justice population: The interface between justice and behavioral health. In M. Arbuckle & C. Herrick (Eds.), *Child and adolescent mental health: Interdisciplinary systems of care* (pp. 221–245). Sudbury MA: Jones & Bartlett.

Pumariega, A., Winters, N.C., & Huffine, C. (2003). The evolution of systems of care for children's mental health: Forty years of community child and adolescent psychiatry. *Health Community Mental Journal, 39,* 399–425.

Racusin, R., Maerlender, A. C., Sengupta, A., Isquith, P.K., & Straus, M.B. (2005). Psychosocial treatment of children in foster care: A review. *Community Mental Health Journal, 41,* 199–221.

Rushton, A.,& Dance, C. (2006). The adoption of children from public care: A prospective study of outcomes in adolescence. *Journal of the American Academy of Child and Adolescent Psychiatry, 45*, 877–883.

Sadock, B.J., & Sadock, V.A. (2009). Adoption and foster care: Child maltreatment and abuse. In B.J. Sadock & V.A. Sadock (Eds.), *Kaplan and Sadock's concise book of child and adolescent psychiatry* (pp. 214–225). Philadelphia, PA: Wolters Kluwer/Lippincott Williams & Wilkins.

Safe and Timely Interstate Placement of Foster Children Act of 2006. P. L. 109–239, §2, 120 Stat 508 (2006).

Schneiderman, J.U. (2003). Health issues of children in foster care. *Contemporary Nurse, 14*, 123–128.

Schneiderman, J.U. (2005). The child welfare system: Through the eyes of public health nurses. *Public Health Nursing, 22*, 354–359.

Schneiderman, J.U. (2008). Qualitative study on the role of nurses as health case managers of children in foster care in California. *Journal of Pediatric Nursing, 23*, 241–249.

Stroul, B. (1996). *Children's mental health: Creating systems of care in a changing society.* Maryland: Paul H. Brooks Publishing Co.

The Pew Commission on Children in Foster Care. (2004). *Fostering the future: Safety, permanence and well-being for children in foster care.* Retrieved from http://pewfostercare.org/research/docs/FinalReport.pdf

U.S. Census Bureau. (2003). *Grandparents living with grandchildren: Census 2000 Brief.* U. S. Department of Commerce Economics and Statistics Administration. Retrieved from www.census.gov/population/www/socdemo/grandparents.html

U.S. Department of Health and Human Services [Administration for Children and Families]. (n.d.).*Child welfare information gateway* [Library search]. Washington, DC: Government Printing Office. Retrieved from http://library.childwelfare.gov/cwig/ws/library/docs/gateway/ResultSet?upp=0&rpp=10&w=+NATIVE%28%27sti+%3D%22Index+of+Federal+Child+Welfare+Laws%22%27%29&r=1&%20order=+NATIVE%28%27year+%2F+descend%27%29

U.S. Department of Health and Human Services [Administration for Children and Families]. (2000). *Report to the Congress on kinship foster care.* Washington, DC: Government Printing Office. Retrieved from http://aspe.hhs.gov/HSP/kinr2c00/

U.S. Department of Health and Human Services [Administration for Children and Families]. (2007). *National child abuse and data on children and youth: Child maltreatment.* Washington, DC: Government Printing Office. Retrieved from http://www.americanhumane.org/about-us/newsroom/fact-sheets/child-abuse-neglect-data.html

U.S. Department of Health and Human Services [Administration for Children and Families]. (2010). *Foster care statistics.* Washington, DC: Government Printing Office. Retrieved from http://www.childwelfare.gov/pubs/factsheets/foster.cfm

U.S. Department of Justice [Office of Justice Programs-Office of Juvenile Justice and Delinquency Prevention (OJJDP)]. (2009). *OJJDP FY 2009 mentoring initiative for foster care youth.* Washington, DC: Government Printing Office. Retrieved from http://ojjdp.ncjrs.gov/grants/ solicitations/FY2009/MIFCY.pdf

Vig, S., Chinitz, S., & Shulman, L. (2005). Young children in foster care: Multiple vulnerabilities and complex service needs. *Infants and Children, 18*, 147–160.

Weinberg, L.A., Zetlin, A., & Shea, N.M. (2009). Removing barriers to educating children in foster care through interagency collaboration: A seven county multiple-case study. *Child Welfare, 88*(4), 77–111.

23

Chronic and Palliative Care Pediatric Populations

Penelope R. Buschman-Gemma, Jean Nelson Farley, and Cynda H. Rushton

"There are lots of living things in our world. Each one has a special lifetime. All around us, everywhere, beginnings and endings are going on around us all the time. So, no matter how long they are, or how short, lifetimes are really all the same. They have beginnings and endings, and there is living in between."

Lifetimes—A Beautiful Way to Explain Death to Children, by Bryan Mellonie and Robert Ingpen

"Palliate," from the Latin *pallio, palliare* (v.) meaning "to disguise, cloak, or mask"

Objectives

After reading this chapter, APNs will be able to

1. Define pediatric palliative care and discuss its development.
2. Explore concepts relevant to pediatric palliative care.
3. Identify and understand barriers to the provision of pediatric palliative care.
4. Describe end-of-life and bereavement care for children, adolescents, and families.
5. Understand the risk factors for families of children receiving palliative and end-of-life care.
6. Explore cultural, spiritual, ethical and legal issues unique to pediatric palliative care.
7. Discuss collaborative possibilities for primary care practitioners and advanced practice psychiatric nurses in the palliative care of children and families with chronic and life-shortening diseases.
8. Elucidate areas of research that will inform practice and education in pediatric palliative care.

Introduction

Seldom does a topic evoke more intense emotions and feelings than the discovery that a child has a serious illness that will shorten the full, long life that he or she was expected to live. It is very likely that at some point in their practice, advanced practice nurses (APNs) will encounter a child who is diagnosed with a life-limiting or life-threatening illness. While caring for these children, they will experience a roller coaster of emotions ranging from pure joy to profound sorrow. The goal of this chapter is to familiarize APNs with the state of the art and science of pediatric palliative care, so that equipped with this knowledge they can meaningfully contribute to the care of a child and family facing a life-limiting or life-threatening diagnosis. Thus, this chapter will focus on the most crucial skills needed by the APN caring for a seriously ill child: competencies in discussing the range

---

Child and Adolescent Behavioral Health: A Resource for Advanced Practice Psychiatric and Primary Care Practitioners in Nursing,
First Edition. Edited by Edilma L. Yearwood, Geraldine S. Pearson, and Jamesetta A. Newland.

of therapeutic and palliative options available to families, formulating realistic goals as a child's prognosis changes, and facilitating connection to the resources available to achieve the goals of care.

History and Evolution of Pediatric Palliative Care in the United States

In the past, offering palliative care for children (and adults) was often delayed until patients were very close to death, and cure-focused treatment to extend length of life was deemed futile and stopped. However, as the number of children who are surviving serious illness for longer periods of time has continued to increase, numerous advocacy organizations and professional groups have recognized the need to define pediatric palliative care more broadly—as both a philosophy of care and an organized and structured system for delivering services. Current opinion in the field, which began to evolve in the past decade, ideally views palliative care as a continuum, whose trajectory extends from the *time of diagnosis* of a life-limiting or life-threatening condition to the time of death, including the phase of family bereavement. Under this contemporary philosophy, the mandate for palliative care now focuses on preventing and relieving distressing symptoms experienced by the child with a life-limiting condition, *regardless* of his place on the illness trajectory. Consequently, although palliative care originated from the hospice model, it is not simply a synonym for hospice (Morgan, 2009). Thus, the new paradigm of palliative care focuses on improving the *quality of life* of the seriously ill child and "adding life to their years, rather than years to their life" (American Academy of Pediatrics, 2008, p. 353).

Although deaths in childhood are fortunately rare, the significant emotional discomfort accompanying childhood illness and death experienced by families and health professionals alike has often resulted in these children becoming "medical orphans in a health system geared to cure, and a culture where only the elderly die" (Trafford, 2002, p. A7). Recommending palliative care is one of the most difficult topics for pediatric health care providers to broach with families of seriously ill children. This is most likely due to a variety of reasons. In addition to equating palliative care with hospice, our Western cultural heritage generally rejects the notion that children suffer and die. It is simply too difficult to conceive that a child would die before a parent and it is uncomfortable to imagine a life of such unrealized potential coming to an early end. Society and health care professionals have slowly begun to recognize that such denial of suffering and death in childhood abandons the family to negotiate the perilous waters of serious childhood illness and eventual death alone.

Attention to the support needed by seriously ill children and their families gained further national attention with publication of the Institute of Medicine's 2003 report "When Children Die: Improving Palliative and End-of-Life Care for Children and Their Families." This report, researched and written by a panel of experts in the fields of pediatrics and palliative care, stressed five crucial themes:

- The death of a child has a devastating and enduring impact.
- Too often, children with fatal or potentially fatal conditions and their families fail to receive competent, compassionate, and consistent care.
- Better palliative care is possible now, but current methods of organizing and financing palliative, end-of-life, and bereavement care complicate the provision and coordination of services to help children and families and sometimes require families to choose between curative or life-prolonging care and palliative services, in particular, hospice care.
- Inadequate data and scientific knowledge impede efforts to deliver effective care, educate professionals to provide such care, and design supportive public policies.
- Integrating effective palliative care from the time of a child's life-threatening or life-limiting medical problem is diagnosed will improve care for children who survive, as well as children who die—and will help the families of all these children (IOM, 2003, p. 3).

Childhood death is a rare occurrence compared to death in adults. Approximately 50,000 to 55,000 infants, children, and adolescents die yearly in the United States from congenital defects, complications of prematurity, accidental injury, cancers, and a wide variety of other life-limiting and life-threatening illnesses (Himelstein, Hilden, Boldt & Weissmann, 2004). More significant is the number of children who suffer from chronic, complex health conditions that limit their life span. It is estimated that there are approximately 2 million children living in the United States with these life-limiting illnesses, who, together with their families, face a gamut of distressing symptoms and emotional upheaval (Torkildson, 2008). The gradual increase in this population of seriously ill children is primarily attributed to technological and medical advances that have produced new curative and palliative therapies previously unavailable (Friebert, 2009). These advances have prompted the need for a paradigm shift in care for this population, as more children who were unlikely to live past infancy now survive for months, years, or decades. It is this growing group of children who has primarily prompted the need to expand the definition of palliative care in the pediatric population just described.

The need for holistic, reimbursable care throughout the life span of seriously ill children has not kept pace with this expanded view of pediatric palliative care, and the number of pediatric palliative care programs that do exist are often neophytes and still small in number. Fiscal constraints make it difficult to create and continue palliative care programs that encompass true life span care. Many insurers reimburse for palliative care only when curative therapies have been stopped (Torkildson, 2010). However, the need to allow for a *dual focus* of care for seriously ill children was recently recognized by the Centers for Medicaid and Medicare Services (CMS) as legitimate for reimbursement under the Patient Protection and Affordable Care Act of 2010. In September 2010, CMS issued a state medical director letter instructing that children receiving Medicaid or Children's Health Insurance Program (CHIP) health insurance coverage who have elected a hospice benefit can continue to receive all other services, *including curative therapies for which the child is eligible* (CMS, 2010). This change will hopefully prompt more private insurers to follow suit and will make sustainability for pediatric palliative care programs a more attainable goal.

How Does Need for Palliative Care Place Children and Families at Risk?

There are risk factors for children and families in need of palliative and end-of-life care. While fewer psychiatric risk factors have been identified for children with chronic life-threatening illness, many more have been noted for parents and well siblings. It is recognized that most children with chronic physical illness do not have comorbid psychiatric diagnoses. However, the overall risk of emotional disorders in the chronically ill is considered to be somewhat greater than in the general pediatric population (Wallender, 2003). Of interest is that severity of physical illness is less of a factor in the child's adjustment and sense of vulnerability than is the nature of the disease itself. Children with diseases affecting the central nervous system are viewed at greatest risk for psychiatric disorders (DeMaso et al., 2009).

Families of these children bear the burdens and stressors associated with palliative and end-of-life care sometimes over an extended period of time. While there is a dearth of research measuring specific changes in families providing palliative care, several studies look at the impact of child death on family members (Arnold, Gemma, & Cushman, 2005; Li, Precht, Mortensen & Olsen, 2003; Sanders, 1980). In her landmark study comparing adult bereavement after the death of a parent, spouse, and child, Sanders (1980) identified significantly higher intensities of grief among those adults surviving the death of a child. Arnold, Gemma, and Cushman (2005) explored an understanding of parental grief on the death of a child, not as episodic but as complex and ongoing. Li, Precht, Mortensen, and Olsen (2003) reported an association between the death of a child and an overall increase in the mortality of mothers as well as a slightly increased early mortality in fathers. The authors posit that stress over the long term may result in pathophysiological changes, which increase susceptibility to infectious and cardiovascular disease. In addition, prolonged exposure to stress may affect changes in lifestyle contributing to mortality (2003).

When a child dies, the impact is most profound for parents and surviving siblings (Arnold & Gemma, 1994). While the authors describe the short-term effects on these siblings as those of horror, sadness, distress, relief, and guilt (1994), there are no longitudinal studies of surviving siblings to measure effects over their lifetimes. Arnold and Gemma (1994) note that surviving siblings, of all ages, may feel emotionally abandoned as parents struggle with their own grief. Indeed, the pain of losing a brother or sister is felt deeply, and parental presence and comfort may not be sustaining. There is much work to be done to better understand risk factors for families providing palliative and end-of-life care for their children and to provide interventions to mitigate the risks to all surviving family members.

Ethical Foundations and Legal Issues

Questions and discussion about what constitutes appropriate medical and surgical treatment for children of all ages whose conditions are severe, chronic, and life threatening have become topics in the pediatric bioethics literature as well as subjects for serious consideration by bioethics committees. Not what can be done but what ought to be done is central to any ethical consideration of treatment options as rapidly exploding knowledge and advances in technology expand possibilities for intervention in the care of children with chronic illness. Juxtaposed against those expanding possibilities is the issue of quality of life, defined by the wishes, hopes, and goals for treatment established by the child, family, and caregivers. Here the developmental needs and capabilities of children, adolescents, and families converge with wishes, belief systems, and cultural values, adding richness and complexity to the decision-making process. A goal of palliative care is to mitigate conflicts that may arise as a result of failures in communication, inadequate goal setting and care planning, and inappropriate care giving (IOM, 2003). Institutional efforts to identify situations posing a high risk of conflict; to develop protocols for ethics consults for patients, families, and all staff; and to draft evidence-based practice guidelines that will help clarify risks and benefits of new or experimental medical interventions are necessary to ensure a strong ethical foundation for palliative care decisions.

These are only some of the questions to be considered in the decision-making process in pediatric palliative care:

1. What constitutes informed consent and/or assent by the child, adolescent, and family?
2. When and how can a child or adolescent participate in decision making?
3. Who determines what is in the best interest of a child?
4. If parent- or child-voiced wishes for care are at odds with medical recommendations, how is the conflict resolved?
5. How are risks and benefits of medical treatment determined at end of life?
6. What factors affect accessibility of palliative care?
7. What effect does the reality of limited resources have on palliative and end-of-life care?

While adults are encouraged to create advanced directives in the form of living wills and health care proxies, no state recognizes a formal advanced directive signed by a person under the age of eighteen years (IOM, 2003). In most situations, parents have the legal right to make medical treatment decisions for their children.

The complex and difficult decisions to be made in pediatric palliative care can have repercussions for caregivers. Shepherd (2010) notes that conflict between external forces (including families, institutions, and religious belief systems) and ethical principles can result in "moral distress" for the caregiver, defined as knowing the right course of action and being prevented from pursuing it. Specific bioethical principles such as beneficence, autonomy, and nonmalfeasance may be in conflict with aggressive care and may be overlooked in the effort to provide intervention. Referring conflicts to a pediatric bioethics committee or consultant may provide a context in which discrepant views can be discussed, ethical principles reviewed, "moral distress" addressed, and wishes, including the child's, heard.

Basic Concepts and Quality Indicators

When investigating a referral source for pediatric palliative care, the APN should seek a provider who embraces certain philosophical principles within an organized framework for care delivery. Friebert (2009) and Huff (2010) propose that a viable and appropriate model of pediatric palliative care should encompass the following principles:

- The services are provided across a care trajectory that ideally starts at the *time of diagnosis* and extends to the period of bereavement, not only close to end of life.
- The services should incorporate a *holistic philosophy* and method of care delivery.
- The plan of care should be *individualized* and *family centered.*
- The goals of care are aimed at enhancing *quality of life* and day-to-day function of the child, *minimizing suffering,* and promoting opportunities for personal and spiritual growth.

Additionally, a pediatric palliative care program that supports these principles ideally implements services that are:

- Sensitive to personal, cultural, and religious practices
- Helpful to families as they make decisions and choices based on best practices and ethical principles
- Delivered by an interdisciplinary team
- Inclusive of the child's and family's community and environment
- Able to offer grief counseling for bereaved families
- Willing to support curative therapies concurrent with palliative treatment, if that is the family's wish
- Committed to providing children and families with options and choices regarding treatment and involvement in decision making
- Willing to offer effective pain and symptom management as paramount to optimizing quality of life (Friebert, 2009; Huff, 2010).

Settings for Provision of Pediatric Palliative Care

Palliative care for children can be provided in a variety of models and settings and is often determined by several factors, including age at diagnosis, complexity of symptom burden, family resiliency, access to resources, location of legal residence, and, finally, insurance coverage. Corr, Torkildson, and Horgan (2010), editors of the Children's Project on Palliative and Hospice Services (ChiPPS) Newsletter, have developed an overview of the range of programs, services, and pioneering collaborations that have evolved in the United States to expand and meet the unique needs of children and families requiring palliative care services (p. 6):

- **Pediatric Palliative Care Waivers**: These are created to address a gap in state plan services, usually through Medicaid, aimed at specific populations prevalent in a certain geographic locations.
- **Coalitions**: Statewide groups that typically focus on advocacy, education, and access to services.

- **Hospital-Based Services**: This is the most frequent setting for provision of palliative, hospice, and end-of-life care for children. Typically, the child remains under the care of the clinical service team that has been managing his illness, while specific palliative care recommendations and connection to resources are offered through consultation to that team and family.

- **Home-Based Care**: Once a child is stabilized and symptoms are under control, transition to home-based palliative care is an option that is often preferred by the child and family. Having the security and proximity of familiar surroundings and ready access to family and friends provides comfort and security to a sick child. It also offers convenience to families who must continue to meet a host of other responsibilities related to siblings, household management, work, and community. Unfortunately, the majority of palliative and hospice home care agencies provide services only for adults or have only a limited number of staff who are competent and comfortable giving care to seriously ill children. Also, home care agencies that want to offer care to children and families who wish to receive hospice and end-of-life benefits must apply for a special license allowing them to provide these types of home-based services.

- **School as Partner**: The inclusion or return of a seriously ill child to the school setting is a key factor in maintaining the quality of life of a child receiving palliative care. School can be an appropriate activity for children who have a serious, chronic, or terminal illness because "it provides a sense of normalcy, opportunities for socialization and personal achievement" (Selekman & Vessey, 2010, p. 57). It can be particularly stressful when a previously healthy child returns to school after diagnosis and treatment for a life-limiting or life-threatening illness. Anxiety and fear may be greater when the child's appearance has been altered because of his condition, such as weight change, hair loss, disfigurement, or the need for special devices or equipment (Hutton, Levetown, & Frager, 2008). The child may also require special adjustments to his school routine to accommodate a diminished energy level, medication administration, or skilled nursing procedures. All of these factors may contribute to the perception of the child as "different" and increase his risk of becoming physically and socially isolated or even bullied in the school setting (Van Cleave & Davis, 2006). Promoting a smooth transition to school is an appropriate and integral role for the APN to assume as the time approaches for the child to initially enter or return to the educational setting. The child with special needs is entitled to have an Individualized Education Plan (IEP), mandated under the Individuals with Disabilities Education Act (IDEA) and/or a 504 plan authorized under the Rehabilitation Act (American Academy of Pediatrics, 2010). Although IDEA exempts schools from providing "medical services," it still stipulates that the "provision of intermittent care necessary for the student's participation cannot be used as grounds for exclusion from school" (AAP, 2010, p. 1074).

Selekman and Vessey (2010) recommend that the following preparation for a seriously ill child's school entrance and transition be considered:

- A plan is developed regarding how and when information about the child's condition will be disclosed to school staff, classmates, and other parents.
- When developmentally appropriate, the child's wishes regarding this should be respected.
- When developmentally appropriate, the child should be involved in developing achievable academic and extracurricular goals while in the school setting, thus allowing him more choices and control over his life.
- Educational programming is adapted to the child's needs so that school remains relevant, especially if his condition is deteriorating. For example, a child who has deteriorating mobility and is an athletic team member could be offered an opportunity to serve other important functions, such as team manager, maintaining team statistics and records, managing equipment and transportation, scheduling practices, etc.
- Efforts are made to help the child maintain positive self-esteem, especially if he is experiencing changes in appearance and function, due to weight fluctuations, hair loss, disfigurement, cognitive decline, or diminished stamina and energy level (p. 38).

A common source of anxiety for school staff when a seriously ill child returns to school is fear that he will experience a medical crisis while in the classroom. It will be crucial to include information about what problems could occur, and a plan for dealing with such situations should be clearly delineated, put in writing, and made accessible to all who will interact with the child during the school day. When designing an IEP and IHCP (Individualized Health Care Plan), it is also essential to determine what the parents' wishes are regarding resuscitation of their child, should cardiac or respiratory arrest occur in the school setting. If a "Do Not Resuscitate (DNR)" order is in place, it must be determined if the local school board will honor such a directive. [Note: In some health facilities and agencies, the acronym DNR has been replaced by AND, or "Allow Natural Death" (AAP, 2010).] If this is not the case, the APN should consider acting as an advocate with the school jurisdiction to modify policies and regulations to allow the parents' and child's wishes regarding resuscitation to be honored. Advocacy efforts to achieve such a policy change should begin with systematic identification of the infrastructure needed to ensure that school personnel, the child, and the parents are supported if a DNR/AND order is in place. The National Education Association (NEA) has also published guidelines that ensure that the needs of all stakeholders will be respected when such a decision is made (NEA, 2000). It is important to bear in mind, however, that "Do Not Resuscitate" does not equate to "Do Not Care." When a DNR or AND order is in place, a clear strategy must be devised that specifies the plan for communication and comfort care for the child, should cardiopulmonary arrest occur. Preparations should also be developed to support the child's classmates and teachers, should a medical crisis or death occur in the school setting.

- **Free-Standing Hospice**: At present, "Dr. Bob's House" in Baltimore, Maryland, and the George Mark House in San Leandro, California, are the only free-standing centers that exclusively provide palliative and hospice care for children in the United States. Exceptional Care for Children, in Newark, Delaware, initially opened in 2004 with the intent of exclusively providing end-of-life care to children. However, this agency was unable to maintain fiscal stability with this single service focus and has now expanded its role to provide care to children requiring skilled respite, transitional, and palliative nursing care.

Assessment of Child and Family

The provision of pediatric palliative and end-of-life care is based on a complete and in-depth assessment of the family, who with the ill child is the focus of care. To develop an active partnership with the family, palliative team members gain an understanding of the family system, the factors and forces that form and impact it, and the multiple systems with which it interacts. Families are composed of the clusters of persons with whom the child lives and by whom care is given including parents, grandparents, siblings, extended family members, godparents, and friends. Who has legal responsibility for decisions made for and about the child? Who is the custodial parent or legal guardian? Constructing a genogram with the help of the child and family members helps to organize information gained and to clarify relationships among members. Physical and mental illness patterns can be traced, as can patterns of addicted or aberrant behavior. Exploring with family members their ethnicity, culture, and language as well as their religious beliefs, practices, and important family rituals provides information and lends rich texture to an understanding of the family fabric.

In addition, information about living environment is essential in planning a context for ongoing care. Families may live in their own homes or apartments, in rooms with extended family members, or in shelters. Some families are nondomiciled. Does the child attend school? Is that school a source of normalcy, enjoyment, and socialization with peers? Are teachers aware of the child's diagnosis and plan for care so that they can support and accommodate changing needs? In addition, the team should be aware of resources in the community providing social support, including churches, community agencies, and good neighbors. Immigrant families, particularly those who are undocumented, are at risk. While they desire the utmost care for their sick children, the exposure in the hospital and community adds the risk of detention and deportation to their lives. Undocumented families may be reticent to share with the pediatric palliative care team details of their precarious lives. This reticence and fear may limit the sick child's ability to communicate his needs and wishes.

Integral to an assessment of child and family is a careful exploration of symptoms and manifestations of disease that contribute to suffering and decreased quality of life. Hillstein and Kane (2006) suggest that such an assessment should include parental observations, the child's own physical, emotional, and social complaints in combination with the health care providers' knowledge of the pathophysiology of the underlying disease. Commonly reported symptoms include fatigue, anorexia, sleeplessness, anxiety, depression, social isolation, agitation, dyspnea, pain, and gastrointestinal complaints.

Exploration of the history of the illness, the family's understanding of causative factors and specific pathophysiology, as well as the child's theories and notions about his disease will help the pediatric palliative care team appreciate the meaning of the child's illness to the family. Including the child in this exploration and eliciting his lived experience of illness and how it affects his life, his wishes, hopes, and dreams will open a pathway for discussion of symptoms and management including traditional medical treatment, remedies tried by the patient and family, and alternative methods of care.

Barriers to Pediatric Palliative Care

Despite the growing acceptance of palliative care for children whose conditions are chronic and life threatening, there are significant barriers both systemic and deeply personal that limit access. Rushton (2010) writes that such barriers exist in clinical, educational, financial, regulatory, and attitudinal forms. In addition, Rushton (2010) notes that in this country, the denial of child death serves as a powerful barrier. Indeed, children are not supposed to die. In the early years of this nation, the death of children was so commonplace that families had many offspring in the hope that some would survive to contribute to the work and care of the family (Gemma & Arnold, 2002). With advances in public health and modern medicine, child death has become less frequent and an atmosphere of denial has developed, a wish to cover and hide the horror that children and adolescents can and do die. Himelstein et al. (2004) describe the challenges of prognosticating for children whose rare disorders and complex medical conditions would have resulted in early death without advanced care. The authors posit that medical caregivers view the death of these children as a "therapeutic misadventure" (p. 1758) rather than a natural outcome of disease, thus delaying or preventing consideration of palliative and end-of-life care.

The overall lack of pediatric palliative care educational programs also serves as a major barrier. While nursing has taken the lead in developing teaching and training models in palliative care, there are few such models that are interdisciplinary in nature. Without a designated and well-prepared pediatric palliative care team to provide guidance, consultation, and education, care providers are ill equipped to offer children and families the benefits of true palliative and end-of-life care.

Funding for pediatric palliative care programs in major children's hospitals has been in short supply as the marketing of advanced lifesaving technology and care has greater public appeal than support for children with chronic illness for which there is no cure. A major impediment to the provision of pediatric palliative care rests in the federal Medicare model, which was used as the basis for state Medicaid hospice benefits (AAP, 2000). Based on an adult patient with cancer model, hospice admission was restricted to patients with a life expectancy of six months or less. This stipulation has severely restricted hospice services for children because of the difficulty in predicting survival (AAP, 2000). These regulations have financial implications for families who would benefit from palliative and end-of-life care services for which there is no reimbursement (Rushton, 2010). Davies, Contro, Larson, and Widger (2010) note that cultural and linguistic differences may impede communication between families and health care providers, preventing family members from participating fully in decision making for their children. Without clear understanding of the nature of their child's chronic disease or condition and the options for treatment, including a full explanation of the nature of palliative care, families may misunderstand and feel demeaned, believing that such care is less valuable and less effective for their child.

When moderate to severe pain or dyspnea necessitates the use of opioids, considering their use can elicit a variety of fears and myths for both families and professionals. Apprehension regarding respiratory depression and hastening the time of death may lead health care providers to delay opioid initiation or dosage increases for appropriate pain relief (Brenneis & Brown, 2006). Parents may interpret that a plan to use opioids signals worsening of their child's condition or imminent approach of death. Families may also worry that their child could become addicted to this type of medication, especially when opioids are referred to as "narcotics." Another common fear is that too early introduction of opioids for pain relief may lead to tolerance and ineffectiveness when the child approaches the end of life.

Facilitators of Pediatric Palliative Care

Integral to pediatric palliative care is the notion of partnership between child, parents and family members, school teachers, clergy, and health care providers (AAP, 2000). Pediatric palliative care with its focus on family and child is most effective when offered by a well-educated and -prepared multidisciplinary team engaged in open and clear communication. Pediatric palliative care is proactive, engaged care that can be introduced at the time of diagnosis of a chronic and life-threatening disease. Pediatric palliative care may supplement active, curative care with an ongoing focus on comfort and quality of life, or it may stand alone as aggressive care is ended. Himelstein et al. (2004) describe palliative care planning as a four-step process that includes the identification of decision makers, careful determination of the child's and family's understanding of disease and prognosis, the establishment of goals of care, and, finally, discussion of the use or not of aggressive medical interventions. Advance directives are discussed with family and, if appropriate, with children and adolescents.

Communication

Approaching children and families with a diagnosis of a chronic and life-shortening illness is a Herculean task. Finding language that conveys medical information accurately and, understandably, assessing the parents' level of comprehension, and determining how much and in what way to communicate with the child and adolescent are among the greatest challenges for all pediatric caregivers. Families come with their own histories and experiences of illness and death and with their own ways of relating and communicating. Just as one considers the family system when giving difficult diagnoses, one must assess carefully the child or adolescent, considering chronological age, developmental level, and special factors contributing to cognitive and emotional status. Some of these same factors contribute to the child's and adolescent's understanding of death. Himelstein et al. (2004) present a helpful table depicting concepts of death based on normal cognition in designated age groupings (Table 23.1).

Much attention in the pediatric literature has been devoted to the impact of telling versus not telling the child about diagnosis and prognosis. In the past, caregivers have colluded with parents to protect the child from knowing, believing that disclosure would cause great distress. Within the past two decades, there has been a shift toward more open communication with children in an effort to reduce isolation and open conduits for communication of wishes and fears. Sourkes (1995) writes, "While the diagnosis is an event in time, 'telling' is a process over time" (p. 33), one in which the APN can be involved. The child's development and age, as well as relationship with parents, are factors to consider in explaining the diagnosis. Sourkes (1995) notes that the diagnosis of a serious, life-threatening illness catapults the child into an "irreversibly altered reality" (p. 32). The diagnosis itself marks the line dividing before from after.

Children respond to hearing a diagnosis with a wide range of emotions, including anger, shame, sadness, and sometimes a measure of relief. Sourkes (1995) notes

that "where ramifications of illness emanate from the physical to the psychological, the body is its focal site" (p. 50). Not surprisingly, the chronically ill child develops a heightened awareness of his body that both strengthens a sense of control and maintains vigilance over his changing symptoms.

It is this heightened awareness even in very young children with chronic life-threatening disease that with cognitive and emotional developmental factors contributes to the child's understanding of illness and, in time, of impending death. Communication with children of all ages requires an understanding of normal cognitive and emotional development as well as an appreciation for the lived experience of illness. Such communication requires the use of age-appropriate language, an appreciation of bodily gestures and manner, expressive play, and drawings or writings. Frequently, children and adolescents speak in metaphors that require acceptance without explanation. Siblings should be included in the process of telling. There may be an enormous burden of guilt carried by a child whose actions or inability to protect contributed to a sibling's injury or illness. For children whose guilt is great by virtue of their real actions or fantasies, there is a need for a careful listening and discussion. This work may include parents and can be facilitated by a child therapist (Arnold & Gemma, 1994).

Table 23.1 Development of death concepts and spirituality in children

Age Range	Characteristics	Predominant Concepts of Death
0–2 yr	Has sensory and motor relationship with environment Has limited language skills Achieves object permanence May sense that something is wrong	None
>2–6 yr	Uses magical and animistic thinking Is egocentric Thinking is irreversible Engages in symbolic play Developing language skills	Believes death is temporary and reversible, like sleep Does not personalize death Believes death can be caused by thoughts
>6–12 yr	Has concrete thoughts	Development of adult concepts of death Understands that death can be personal Interested in physiology and details of death
>12–18 yr	Generality of thinking Reality becomes objective Capable of self-reflection Body image and self-esteem paramount	Explores nonphysical explanations of death

Modified from Himelstein et al., 2004, with permission from the *New England Journal of Medicine*

Goals of Care

In partnership with child and family, the difficult news of diagnosis is given, and discussion shifts to formulation of goals of care. Bluebond-Langner and colleagues (2010) suggest an approach for involving children in decision making and goal setting. This approach focuses on understanding the abilities and vulnerabilities of children and respecting their relationship with parents. Indeed, the child, parents, and caregivers are involved in a communication process described by the authors as "shuttle diplomacy" (p. 336). Communication among the three major parties allows for the actual involvement of children in the decision-making process without the burden falling on one party's shoulders. In the "shuttle diplomacy" model, there is room for negotiation, dissent, and renegotiation. While the authors do not establish age as a criterion for involvement in this process, certainly some ability to understand and communicate is required for participation.

Throughout the course of the child's illness, palliative care providers continue their responsibility of "telling," explaining changes in condition, offering new treatment options, discussing comfort measures, eliciting wishes and hopes, and renegotiating goals. Recognizing the partnership with child and family, the palliative care provider acts as advocate, strengthening the family's stance and helping their wishes and goals to remain upper most in the medical setting and in the plan of action. In the recent past, disclosure of information to children was believed to increase fear and anxiety. However, there has been a welcome shift toward more open communication.

Education and Advocacy

While pediatric palliative care programs are developing in major hospitals, there are few educational programs preparing health care providers for this work. Incorporating pediatric palliative content and experience into curricula in graduate nursing and medical programs and creating opportunities for shared learning will enhance an appreciation for team work in this area. Pediatric palliative care does not belong to one specialty! To counter the impression that pediatric palliative care is offered when nothing more can be done, both education and information on advocacy are needed for health care providers and for the public.

Case Management

As the interdisciplinary approach has become increasingly recognized as a key standard of pediatric palliative care, it has also generated a need for a delivery model that can facilitate care coordination for the seriously ill child and his family. One role that is gaining increasing recognition as an effective facilitator of these services is that of *patient navigator* (PN). The PN concept was originally introduced by Freeman and colleagues in the early 1990s to improve access to health care for vulnerable populations whose cancer screening results indicated the need for follow-up diagnostic services (Freeman, Muth, & Kerner, 1995). As this service delivery model has grown over the years, the primary goal of the PN role evolved to simplify access to care. Thus, responsibilities typically consisted of identifying gaps in needed services and locating appropriate information, resources, and education to fill these gaps, especially with groups of patients with complex, chronic health conditions. Other crucial responsibilities frequently assumed by the PN include conducting patient needs assessments, providing education and treatment support, serving as liaison with other care providers throughout the illness trajectory, and assisting patients in navigating the health care system to access needed care and resources (Pedersen & Hack, 2010; Seek & Hogle, 2007). Effective PNs must have a range of core competencies and skills, including that of an expert communicator and educator who is extremely knowledgeable about the system in which the patient is seeking care. As this care delivery role has continued to expand over the years, the literature reveals a diverse range of individuals fulfilling this function, including nurses, social workers, peer supporters, and specially trained community members (Pedersen & Hack, 2010).

End-of-life Care

Close to the end of life, advanced care planning of the family may guide overarching decisions. However, immediate, day-to-day decisions will have to be made, which may involve withdrawal of hydration and nutrition and the stoppage of procedures causing pain and discomfort. Within the context of the palliative care partnership with child and family, decisions are made about pain and symptom relief, presence of family members and staff, and the granting of special wishes.

Case Exemplar

Ten-year-old James asked his parents and nurse to fulfill three wishes before his impending death. He begged to have his adoption finalized, his puppy brought from home, and a guarantee that his organs would go to a living child. At the request of parents, a family court judge in full regalia came to his bedside and with great ceremony, finalized James's adoption. Under cover of darkness, James's puppy arrived and settled in his hospital bed. Finally, James's attending physician gained formal permission from James and his parents for organ donation after his death. James died soon after his work was finished and his wishes granted.

Issues to be discussed with family members at the end of life include permission for autopsy and organ donation. Families may determine that they want nothing more to be done to their child's body and thus refuse to consider autopsy or discussion of organ donation. However, some families hope for information that will serve as rationale for physical changes in their child and for further understanding of a disease process. They may welcome the opportunity to give permission for autopsy, sometimes stipulating the extent of the procedure. Some families may wish to donate their child's healthy organs to needy recipients, believing that their child's life in this way continues. Occasionally, remarkable children, such as James, will initiate the request for organ donation, ensuring their own legacy.

While families may be reticent to initiate discussion about funeral planning, they may welcome the opportunity to gain information and do preliminary work while they are able to think clearly. Pediatric palliative care team members can offer information about community resources including affordable funeral homes to assist with cremation or burial and available clergy. In addition, families may welcome guidance for inclusion of surviving siblings in the funeral and burial rituals being planned. Arnold and Gemma (1994) note that participation of siblings in the family's rituals of mourning their dead child serves to strengthen relationships for survivors who must continue as a family together. The authors posit that these early decisions and the degree to which a family's grief is shared set the stage for the way in which the family members will deal with their loss in the years ahead. Surviving children who are excluded from planning and participation in rituals can think of their presence as unimportant, providing no comfort. Their grief goes unrecognized.

Grief and Bereavement

Arnold and Gemma (1994) note that the death of a child affects all members of a family and the system itself, causing significant alterations in structures and roles. Death of a child member becomes an essential identifying piece of information about a family. It is woven into its history while affecting day-to-day functioning of the family. Parents are forever parents of their dead child. Grief for their child who has died becomes an abiding connection between parents and child (Arnold, Gemma, & Cushman, 2005). While parental grief is experienced universally, the manifestations in ritual and behavior are family and culture bound (Gemma & Arnold 2002).

When a child dies, parents lose a part of themselves, leaving an empty space that can never be filled. In addition, parents lose the separate person their child was to become, their connection to the future, the embodiment of their hopes and dreams. Parental grief is profound and lifelong regardless of the age of the child, the cause of death, and the years since death (Arnold et al., 2005). Grieving is a process through which parents learn to live without their child, and with that specific emptiness in their lives.

While the family's grief is lifelong, their acute pain lessens. Birthdays, special holidays, and anniversaries will reactivate sharp feelings of grief. For some families whose children have suffered greatly, there may be a sense of relief that the child's pain is no more. Families whose children have been cared for in hospitals and residential hospice programs may experience as well the sadness of losing a network of caregivers. Bereavement follow-up for families becomes an essential component of pediatric palliative and end-of-life care. Good bereavement care for families requires a multidisciplinary approach that guides the grieving family from hospital/hospice to home/community providing support, linkages, and referrals as necessary. A small model program developed by one of the authors in conjunction with the nursing and social work leadership staff of a large urban hospital with maternal child, neonatal, and pediatric services is described:

1. Bereavement care begins in hospital with nursing, social work, and pastoral care providing comfort, requested rituals at end of life, and information about funeral services and cremation. A designated social worker refers the bereaved family to the advanced practice psychiatric nurse (APPN) bereavement consultant.

2. The APPN contacts family by phone at home, assessing each member of the family, providing comfort and information, and presenting resources for support and ongoing care. Phone calls are repeated at the family's request. The APPN invites parents (and grandparents) to a monthly parent support group that she leads. If the family requests additional counseling or psychiatric treatment, referral is made to a psychiatric nurse practitioner or a licensed family therapist, both of whom are experienced caring for grieving families.

3. A parent support group is held monthly in a community space in close proximity to the hospital.

4. Bereaved families are invited to attend an annual memorial service where they may share memories of their children and affix leaves with their children's names to a tree of life.

5. The bereavement committee composed of nursing and social work leadership meets quarterly to evaluate the program and plan the memorial service.

For families, there is no such thing as a good child death. However, there is compassionate and informed pediatric palliative care that guides the bereft family through their intense grief to a place where they can live with their loss and continue to grow. Arnold and Gemma (2008) note that bereft parents live without their dead child in a new and transformed reality.

Compassion Fatigue

As Figley (1995) aptly states, "There is a cost to caring" (p. 1), and caring for children who are seriously ill is particularly demanding for all stakeholders involved. Practicing in the field of pediatric palliative care requires complex knowledge, competencies, and the ability to engage in courageous advocacy (Rushton, 2004). These professionals must also be skilled in sustaining relationships, as the needs of children with life-limiting and life-threatening illness and their families often extend over protracted periods of time, for as the number of children who are surviving with chronic, complex health conditions grows, providers are now "more immersed and linked to their patient's experience than ever before" (Meadors & Lamson, 2007, p. 24). As the longevity of these children has increased, so has the probability for health professionals experiencing protracted exposure to the distressing symptoms and suffering which threaten the identity of these children and families. These factors can generate a high level of stress and dysfunctional behavior in the professional who is not vigilant about meeting her needs for self-care. "Compassion fatigue" is a term first coined by Figley in 1995 to describe the inability of an individual to maintain physical and/or emotional homeostasis because of the stress resulting from helping a suffering person. During his work with trauma victims, Figley observed that health professionals who witnessed and absorbed the distressing symptoms and suffering of trauma patients sometimes experienced a type of secondary traumatic stress themselves, "resulting from helping or wanting to help a traumatized or suffering person" (p. 7.) Previously, this emotional cost of caring had been described by a variety of terms, such as "burnout" and "caregiver stress." Figley (1995) also noticed that the amount of stress experienced by helping professionals was relative to the level of proximity, intensity, and duration of their exposure to the patient's distress. Health professionals who regularly witness the suffering experienced by ill children and their families are clearly at risk for experiencing compassion fatigue (Meadors & Lamson, 2007).

The most effective tool for preventing compassion fatigue in pediatric health professionals is the ability to regularly engage in self-assessment and self-recognition of increased risk factors. It is crucial to educate providers to identify signs and symptoms of physical or emotional distress in themselves before it begins to interfere with their ability to give care. Symptoms associated with compassion fatigue include a range of physical, emotional, and spiritual warning signs, such as anxiety, sleep disturbances, irritability, anger, depression, hopelessness, anorexia, headaches, substance abuse, and feelings of general emotional and physical exhaustion (Keene et al., 2010; Meadors & Lamson, 2007; Pfifferling & Gilley, 2000). Another hallmark of compassion fatigue is its propensity to spill over to the health professional's personal relationships, social networks, and other aspects of their professional lives (Meadors & Lamson, 2007, p. 25). Wright (2004) also observed that for professionals experiencing compassion fatigue, there "comes a point when we are so well defended against further pain, we become defended against the care and insights we might receive from one another and ourselves" (p. 3).

Pfifferling and Gilley (2000) developed a short instrument that health professionals can administer as a self-assessment for their personal risk of compassion fatigue. Although the tool has not been validated, it can be used as a quick screen of the caregiver's state of mind (Table 23.2).

Self-awareness and early recognition of the signs and symptoms of compassion fatigue are the keys to prevention or early detection of its occurrence, so that the health professional can continue to assist patients in relieving their symptom burden. Some interventions that can foster self-awareness include journaling or organizing and participating in a well-facilitated peer group where sharing personal experiences and stories is encouraged in a safe and supportive atmosphere. Identifying a mentor who is a good listener and with whom there exists an inner "connection" provides an objective observer who can serve as an early warning system when she perceives behaviors or symptoms that may indicate compassion fatigue. Other aspects of a "self-care plan" that are recognized to prevent or alleviate compassion fatigue include arranging for regular, personal time to enjoy "guilty pleasures," such as listening to preferred music, reading a favorite author, and engaging in recreational and leisure activities. Consistently meeting the body's physiologic requirements for balance in nutrition, exercise, and rest promotes both physical health and emotional well-being, both of which are crucial for maintaining a level of health that allows provision of compassionate, effective care to others.

Pfifferling and Gilley (2000) also strongly recommend health care providers enhance their professional

Table 23.2 Self-assessment for compassion fatigue

Screening Statement	Yes	No
Personal concerns commonly intrude on my professional life		
My colleagues seem to lack understanding		
I find even small changes enormously draining		
I can't seem to recover quickly after association with trauma		
Association with trauma affects me very deeply		
My patients' stress affects me every day		
I have lost my sense of hopefulness		
I feel vulnerable all the time		
I feel overwhelmed by unfinished personal business		

Answering "yes" to four or more questions may indicate that you're suffering from compassion fatigue.
Reprinted with permission from "Overcoming Compassion Fatigue," April 2000, Family Practice Management. Copyright © 2000 American Academy of Family Physicians. All Rights Reserved

resilience by developing a personal mission statement and "principles of practice" that articulate the boundaries within which they are comfortable providing care (p. 4). It may be helpful to post these personal values where they can be easily reexamined and provide a visible "moral compass" toward what is congruent with the professional's mission and values. Having these clear principles articulated also allows the APN the freedom to say "no" without guilt when demands on time and energy are not aligned with personal philosophy of care and priorities for practice (Pfifferling & Gilley, 2000).

Finally, the APN should also be alert to signs that professional colleagues also may be experiencing compassion fatigue and be prepared to offer support and referral for assistance. The Resource section at the end of this chapter provides information on organizations where health professionals can find support to prevent or treat compassion fatigue.

Case Exemplar

Carolyn, a seventeen-year-old with complicated and lifelong chronic illness, had been referred to the pediatric palliative care consultation team by her pulmonologist who requested help with end-of-life care. Carolyn was an only child of parents who separated ten years ago. Since that time, she had limited contact with mother, and father was her primary custodial caregiver. She attended high school and was home on hospital instruction.

Diagnosed with cystic fibrosis at age three years, Carolyn received her first lung transplant at age thirteen, and when that failed, a second at age sixteen. At the time of her referral for palliative care, Carolyn's condition had worsened. She was ventilator-dependent and had severe pancreatitis and liver disease. She was aware of her impending death and in discussion with her physician asked to remain in the tertiary care hospital where she felt most at home. Carolyn and her father had agreed to a DNR order. Carolyn became increasingly dyspneic and anxious. She stated that she was afraid of falling to sleep, believing she would not wake up.

Members of the pediatric palliative care team met with the physicians, nurses, and child life personnel caring for Carolyn. (One member noted the number of very young, newly graduated nurses assigned to Carolyn's care.) The team was asked for help with symptom relief for Carolyn's increasing dyspnea and anxiety and for information to prepare them for Carolyn's ultimate death. Several of the staff addressed their own emotional involvement with this adolescent patient that now compromised their ability to care for her. The pediatric palliative care team responded by:

1. Providing the pediatric team information requested about Carolyn's end-of-life course.
2. Offering suggestions for relief of increasing symptoms of dyspnea and anxiety.
3. Suggesting that newer and inexperienced nurses caring for Carolyn work in teams for support and respite.
4. Following Carolyn's death, which was imminent, meeting with staff to discuss and process the experience of caring for Carolyn and to support the staff in their grief.
5. Planning bereavement follow-up for the parents.

Illustrated by this clinical example is the opportunity for a palliative care team to assist pediatric colleagues with information, symptom management, intervention, and psychiatric support. In so doing, the palliative care team contributed to Carolyn's well-being at end of life and care of the family after death.

A question to consider is, What difference would it have made for Carolyn, her parents, and the pediatric staff to have had palliative care consultation at the time of diagnosis or earlier in the course of her illness?

Future Directions

Clinicians who care for children with life-threatening conditions and those who are dying need systematic processes and structures to provide quality pediatric palliative care. Integration of palliative care into pediatric practice requires specific strategies focusing on clinical practice and care delivery models, professional education, research, and policy reform.

The provision of pediatric palliative care has been integrated into many tertiary pediatric centers across the United States but is still insufficient to meet the needs of children and families. Similarly, there are more hospices providing care to pediatric patients and their families (NHPCO, 2009). Through a collaborative effort among leaders in pediatric palliative care, a National Network for Pediatric Palliative Care was established as an interactive, grassroots community for those providing pediatric palliative care in the United States. This network is designed to link services and expertise of clinicians across the care continuum, with state-of-the-art knowledge, current events in the field, resources, education, and research (www. network4pedspallcare.org).

Similarly, Standards for Pediatric Palliative and Hospice Care have been developed to provide guidance to those who will contribute to improving the lives of children living with life-threatening conditions (NHPCO, 2009, http://www.nhpco.org/i4a/ pages/index. cfm?pageid=5874). These standards provide the basis for designing pediatric palliative care programs and care provision nationwide.

Health care professionals face unique challenges when caring for dying children and their families. In particular, health care professionals may not have the requisite knowledge and skills to provide care in an ethically grounded and clinically competent manner (IOM, 2003; Solomon et al., 2005). Although education in this area is improving, studies documenting the effectiveness of specific models and content are sparse. Innovative curricula have been developed for pediatric palliative care. Two focus on essential content, while providing structure and process: (1) the Pediatric End of Life Nursing Education Consortium (ELNEC) provides extensive outlines and slide content that reflect key elements of pediatric palliative care nursing and (2) the Children's Project on Palliative/Hospice Services (ChiPPS) offers essential resources and references for pediatric palliative care. The Initiative for Pediatric Palliative Care (IPPC) is an interdisciplinary model; it provides a holistic framework for family-centered pediatric care that engages parents as co-facilitators of the process. The IPPC curriculum includes facilitation guides, videos, and educational models, designed to facilitate individual and interdisciplinary learning and to serve as a vehicle for cultural transformation.

Innovative models of teaching and learning must be evaluated and disseminated. To capture the depth of impact of these methods, novel models for evaluating the impact on health care professionals and their patients and families will need to be devised. Interdisciplinary research teams including parents can be instrumental in utilizing, evaluating and disseminating family-centered, experiential palliative care curricula such as IPPC (Solomon et al., 2009). Educational programs that offer interdisciplinary teams the opportunity to reflect on their experiences in caring for dying children and their families and to assess the effect of providing this care on their own emotional and spiritual well-being and quality of care are particularly promising. Collaborative research models are necessary to assess adequately the impact of these interventions on important individual and patient/family outcomes.

Similar to other areas of pediatric palliative care research, interventions should be developed with preliminary data supporting their efficacy before being subjected to randomized trials. A particular challenge is to identify outcome measures that authentically reflect the lived experience of both patients and families and health care professionals and are able to capture the complex interplay of intellectual, emotional, and spiritual dynamics.

Anticipating the possibility of dying for children living with life-threatening conditions continues to be challenging. Researchers need to develop methods for earlier integration of palliative care processes and interventions and to evaluate the impact of these interventions on key areas such as earlier pain and symptom management, ongoing communication about goals of care, advance care planning, quality of life, and holistic emotional, psychosocial, and spiritual support (Mack & Wolfe, 2006).

Summary

This chapter presented pediatric palliative care both as a philosophy of care and as a structured system for delivering services that have as a focus on children and families whose conditions and diseases cannot be cured and who face shortened lives. There is no greater opportunity for APNs in primary care pediatrics and child psychiatry to collaborate than in the care of the chronically ill and dying child or adolescent. The APNs' shared valuing of the unit of care being the child and family and their commitment to continuing care from time of diagnosis to end of life and beyond for the family forges potential for rich and satisfying collaboration. Recognizing that each brings unique perspective to the table, APNs are challenged to find ways to contribute to the wholeness of pediatric palliative care by promoting innovative clinical practice, and by participating in educational and research initiatives.

Resources

Family Resources

- **Family Voices:** A national grassroots network of families and friends speaking on behalf of children with special care needs.

  Contact Information:
  Internet: www.familyvoices.org
  E-mail: kidshealth@familyvoices.org
  Phone: 888-835-5669

- **Compassionate Friends:** This is an international support organization for families who have experienced death of a child.

  Contact Information:
  Internet: www.compassionatefriends.org
  Phone: 877-969-0010

- **Candlelighters' American Childhood Cancer Foundation (ACCF):** This organization was formed in 1970 to provide support and information to families experiencing childhood cancer. It also advocates for children facing this disease and supports research related to childhood cancer.

  Contact Information:
  Internet: www.candlelighters.org
  E-mail: staff@accf.org
  Phone: 800-366-2223

- **Americans for Better Care of the Dying (ABCD):** This organization is dedicated to ensuring that all Americans can count on good, end-of-life care. The mission of ABCD is to build momentum for reform, explore new methods and systems for delivering care, and shape public policy through evidence-based understanding.

  Contact Information:
  Internet: www.abcd-caring.org
  E-mail: info@abcd-caring.org

- **Bandaides and Blackboards:** This site was developed by a nurse to help sensitize children to what it is like to grow up with a medical problem. There are also topics that would be of interest for adults who parent a child with a chronic health condition.

  Contact Information:
  Internet: www.lehman.cuny.edu/faculty/jfleitas/bandaides/cont-kids.html

- **Kidsaid: 2 Kids, 4 Kids, By Kids:** This is a site for children and teen grief support, including "kid-to-kid" grief support that is administered by a clinical psychologist who is a certified traumatologist.

  Contact Information:
  Internet: www.kidsaid.com
  E-mail: cendra@griefnet.org

- **Now I Lay Me Down to Sleep:** This organization provides remembrance photography to parents suffering the loss of a child, with the free gift of professional portraiture. The volunteer professional photographers who participate in this program believe that these images serve as an important step in a family's healing process by honoring their child's legacy.

  Contact Information:
  Internet: www.nowilaymedowntosleep.org
  E-mail: headquarters@nilmdts.org
  Phone: 877-834-5667

- **Partnership for Parents:** This site serves as an internet source of support for parents with children experiencing serious illness, to assist them in finding the information they need to cope with this journey.

  Contact Information:
  Internet: www.partnershipforparents.org
  Phone: 831-763-3070

- **Make a Wish Foundation of America:** The mission of this organization is to grant wishes of children with life-threatening medical conditions, to enrich the human experience with hope, strength, and joy.

  Contact Information:
  Internet: www.wish.org
  Phone: 800-722-9474

- **Inspire:** Builds and manages online communities where patients, family members, and caregivers support and communicate with one another in a safe, secure, privacy-protected environment.

  Contact Information:
  Internet: www.inspire.com
  Phone: 703-243-0303

- **Center for Professional Well Being, Durham, NC**

  Contact Information:
  Internet: www.cpwb.org
  Phone: 919-489-9167

- **Professional Renewal Center, Lawrence, KS**

  Contact Information:
  Internet: www.prckansas.org
  Phone: 877-978-4772

Professional Resources

- **The Initiative for Pediatric Palliative Care (IPPC):** The goal of the organization is to enhance family-centered care for children living with life-threatening conditions through education, research, and quality improvement.

  Contact Information:
  Internet: www.ippcweb.org
  E-mail: ippc@edc.org
  Phone: 617-618-2388

- **End of Life Nursing Education Consortium (ELNEC):** A national initiative to provide nurse educators with training in end-of-life care so that they can teach this essential information to nursing students and professional nurses practicing across the country.

  Contact Information:
  Internet: www.aacn.nche.edu/elnec
  Phone: 202-463-6930

- **Children's Hospice International (CHI):** Mission is to so ingrain the hospice concept of care into health care for children, that it is considered an integral part of pediatric health care, rather than a separate specialty.

  Contact Information:
  Internet: www.chionline.org
  E-mail: info@chionline.org
  Phone: 800-242-4453

- **Children's Project on Palliative and Hospice Services (ChiPPS):** This organization is a division of the National Hospice and Palliative Care Organization and works to enhance the science and practice of pediatric hospice and palliative care and to increase the availability of state-of-the-art services for families.

Contact Information:
Internet: www.nhpco.org
E-mail: nhpco_info@nhpco.org
Phone: 703-837-1500

- **National Hospice and Palliative Care Organization (NHPC):** This is the largest nonprofit membership organization representing hospice and palliative care programs and professionals in the United States. The organization is committed to improving end-of-life care and expanding access to hospice care with the goal of profoundly enhancing quality of life for people dying in America and their loved ones.

Contact Information:
Internet: www.nhpco.org
E-mail: nhpco_info@nhco.org
Phone: 800-658-8898/Multilingual Helpline: 877-658-8896

- **Hospice and Palliative Nurses Association (HPNA):** HPNA is a collaborative, professional hospice and palliative specialty nursing organization that utilizes evidence-based educational tools to assist members to deliver evidence-based care to palliative and hospice care patients.

Contact Information:
Internet: www.hpna.org
Phone: 412-787-9301

- **American Society for Pain Management Nursing (ASPMN):** The American Society for Pain Management Nursing's mission is to advance and promote optimal nursing care for people affected by pain by promoting best nursing practice, through education, standards, advocacy, and research.

Contact Information:
Internet: www.aspmn.org
E-mail: aspmn@goamp.ocm
Phone: 888-342-7766

- **Association of Pediatric Hematology/Oncology Nurses (APHON):** APHON provides and promotes expert practice in pediatric hematology/oncology nursing to its members and the public at large.

Contact Information:
Internet: www.aphon.org
E-mail: info@aphong.org
Phone: 847-375-4724

- **Center to Advance Palliative Care (CAPC):** The Center to Advance Palliative Care (CAPC) provides health care professionals with the tools, training, and technical assistance necessary to start and sustain successful palliative care programs in hospitals and other health care settings. CAPC is a national organization dedicated to increasing the availability of quality palliative care services for people facing serious illness.

Contact Information:
Internet: wwww.capc.org
E-mail: capc@mssm.edu
Phone: 212-201-2670

- **Children's Organ Transplant Association (COTA):** This organization helps children and young adults who need a life-saving transplant by providing fundraising assistance and family support.

Contact Information:
Internet: www.cota.org
E-mail: cota@cota.org
Phone: 800-366-2682

- **Children's Hospice and Palliative Care Coalition:** This advocacy organization works with hospitals and community organizations to improve pediatric palliative care by promoting compassionate, all-inclusive medical treatment.

Contact Information:
Internet: www.childrenshospice.org
Phone: 831-763-3070

- **International Children's Palliative Care Network:** An international resource providing information about pediatric palliative care services for fundraisers, professionals, caregivers, and families, to raise the profile of children's palliative care while fostering an awareness of the worldwide need for children's palliative care services.

Contact Information:
Internet: www.icpcn.org
E-mail: hpca@iafrica.com
Phone: +27(0)21 5310277

References

American Academy of Pediatrics. (2000). www.aap.org.

American Academy of Pediatrics. (2008). www.aap.org.

American Academy of Pediatrics Council on School Health & Committee on Bioethics (2010). Honoring do-not-attempt resuscitation requests in schools. *Pediatrics, 125*(5), 1073-1077. doi:10.1542/peds.2010-0452

Arnold, J.H., & Gemma, P.B. (1994). *A child dies: a portrait of family grief.* Philadelphia: Charles Press.

Arnold, J.H., Gemma, P.B., & Cushman, L.F. (2005). Exploring parental grief: combining quantitative and qualitative measures. *Archives of Psychiatric Nursing, 19*(6), 245–255.

Arnold, J.H., & Gemma, P.B. (2008). The continuing process of parental grief. *Death Studies, 32,* 658–673.

Bluebond-Langner, M.B., Belasco, J.B., & Wander, M.D. (2010). "I want to live, until I don't want to live anymore": involving children with life-threatening and life-shortening illnesses in decision making about care and treatment. *Nursing Clinics of North America, 45*(3), 329–343.

Brenneis, C., & Brown, P. (2007). International models of excellence. In B.T. Ferrell & N. Coyle (Eds.), *Textbook of palliative nursing* (second edition). Oxford: Oxford University Press.

Centers for Medicare & Medicaid Services. *Concurrent care for children.* Retrieved from www.cms.gov/smdl/downloads/SMD10018.pdf.

Corr, C., Torkildson, C., & Horgan, M. (2010, May). Pediatric hospice and palliative care in the United States: The current state of the art. *ChiPPS E-News.* Retrieved from http://www.nhpco.org/files/public/ChiPPS/ChiPPS_enews-19_May_2010.pdf

Davies, B., Contro, N., Larson, J., & Widger, K. (2010). Culturally-sensitive information-sharing in pediatric palliative care. *Pediatrics, 125*(4), e859–e865.

DeMaso, D.R., Martini, D.R., Cahen, L.A., Bukstein, O., Walter, H.J., Benson, S., Medicus, J. (2009). Practice parameters for the psychiatric assessment and management of physically ill children and adolescents. *J. Am. Acad. Child Adolesc. Psychiatry, 48*(2), 213–233.

Figley, G. (Ed.). (1995). *Compassion fatigue: coping with secondary traumatic stress disorder in those who treat the traumatized.* New York: Taylor & Francis Group.

Freeman, H., Muth, B., & Kerner, J. (1995). Expanding access to cancer screening and clinical follow-up among the medically underserved. *Cancer Practice, 3*(1), 19–30.

Friebert, S. (2009). *NHPCO Facts and figures: pediatric palliative and hospice care in America.* Alexandria, VA: National Hospice and Palliative Care Association.

Gemma, P.B., & Arnold, J.H. (2002). Loss and grieving in pregnancy and the first year of life: A caring resource for nurses. New York, NY: March of Dimes.

Hillstein, M.B., & Kane, J. (2006). Symptom management in pediatric palliative care. In B.R. Farrell & N. Coyle (Eds.), *Textbook of palliative nursing* (second edition). New York: Oxford University Press.

Himelstein, B.P., Hilden, J.M., Boldt, A.M., & Weissman, D. (2004). Pediatric palliative care. *New England Journal of Medicine, 350*(17), 1752–1762.

Himelstein, B. (2006). Palliative care for infants, children, adolescents and their families. *Journal of Palliative Medicine, 9*(1), 163–181. doi:10.1089/jpm.2006.9.163

Huff, S. (2010, September). *Standards of care for pediatric palliative and hospice care.* Paper presented at the District of Columbia Pediatric Palliative Care Collaboration, Washington, D.C.

Hutton, N., Levetown, M., & Frager, G. (2008). School and community issues. In C.P. Storey (Ed.), *The hospice and palliative medicine approach to caring for pediatric patients* (pp. 27–28). Glenview, IL: American Academy of Hospice and Palliative Medicine.

Institute of Medicine (2003). *When children die: improving palliative and end-of-life care for children and their families.* Washington, D.C.: The National Academies Press.

Keene, E., Hutton, N., Hall, B., & Rushton, C. (2010). Bereavement debriefing sessions: An intervention to support health care professionals in managing their grief after the death of a patient. *Pediatric Nursing, 36*(4), 185–189.

Klick, J., & Hauer, J. (2010). Pediatric palliative care. *Current Problems in Pediatric and Adolescent Health Care, 40*, 120–151. doi:10.1016/j.cppeds.2010.05.001

Li, J., Precht, D.H., Mortensen, P.B., & Olsen, J. (2003). Mortality in parents after death of a child in Denmark: A nationwide follow-up study. *Lancet, 361*(9355), 363–367.

Mack J.W., & Wolf, J. (2006). Early integration of pediatric palliative care: for some children, palliative care starts at diagnosis. *Current Opinions in Pediatrics, 18*, 10–14.

Meadors, P., & Lamson, A. (2007). Compassion fatigue and secondary traumatization: Provider self care on intensive care units for children. *Journal of Pediatric Health Care, 22*(1), 24–34.

Mellonie, B., & Ingpen, R. (1983). *Lifetimes: A beautiful way to explain death to children.* St. Louis, MO: Turtleback Books.

Morgan, D. (2009). Caring for dying children: Assessing the needs of the pediatric palliative care nurse. *Pediatric Nursing, 35*(2), 86–91.

National Education Association. (2000). *Providing safe health care: The role of educational support personnel.* Retrieved from www.nea.org/home/20779.htm

National Hospice and Palliative Care Organization (NHPCO). (2009). *Standards for pediatric palliative and hospice care: Advancing care for America's children.* Author.

Pedersen, A., & Hack, T. (2010). Pilots of oncology health care: A concept analysis of the patient navigator role. *Oncology Nursing Forum, 37*(1), 55–60. doi:0.1188/10.ONF.55-60

Pfifferling, J., & Gilley, K. (2000). Overcoming compassion fatigue. *Family Practice Management 7*(4). Retrieved from www.mdconsult.com/das/article/body/219754151-4/jorg

Rushton, C.H. (2010). Pediatric palliative care: coming of age. *Innovations in End-of-Life Care, 2*(2). http://www.edc.org/lastacts

Rushton, C. (2004). The other side of caregiving: Caregiver suffering. In B. Carter & M. Levetown (Eds.), *Palliative care for infants, children and adolescents.* Baltimore: Johns Hopkins Press.

Sanders, C. (1980). A comparison of adult bereavement in the death of a spouse, child, and parent. *Omega, 10*, 303–322.

Seek, A., & Hogle, W. (2007). Modeling a better way: Navigating the healthcare system for patients with lung cancer. *Clinical Journal of Oncology Nursing, 11*(1), 81–85. doi:10.1188/07.CJON.81–85

Selekman, J., & Vessey, J. (2010). School and the child with a chronic condition. In P. Allen, J. Vessey, & N. Shapiro (Eds.), *Primary care of the child with a chronic condition* (fifth edition) (pp. 42–59). St. Louis: Mosby-Elsevier.

Shepard, A. (2010). Moral distress: a consequence of caring. *Clinical J of Oncology Nursing, 14*(1), 25–27.

Solomon, M.Z., Sellers, D.E., Heller, K.S., Dokken, D.L., Levetown, M., Rushton, C., Fleischman, A.R. (2005). New and lingering controversies in pediatric end-of-life care. *Pediatrics,* (116), 872–883.

Sourkes, B.M. (1995). *Armfuls of time.* Pittsburgh: University of Pittsburgh Press.

Torkildson, C. (2010, May). Models of pediatric hospice and palliative care in the United States. *ChiPPS E-News, 19*, 4–8. Retrieved from http://www.nhpco.org/files/public/ChiPPS/ChiPPS_enews-19_May_2010.pdf

Trafford, A. (2002, August 6). Second opinion: Medical orphans. *The Washington Post, pp.* F1, F7.

Van Cleave, J., & Davis, J. (2006). Bullying and peer victimization among children with special needs. *Pediatrics, 118*(4), e1212–1219. doi:10.1542/peds.2005–3034.

Wallender, J.L., Thompson, R.J., & Alriksson-Schmidt, A. (Eds.), (2003). Psychological adjustment of children with chronic physical conditions. *Handbook of pediatric psychology.* New York, Guilford Press.

Wright, R. (2004). Compassion fatigue: How to avoid it. *Palliative Medicine, 18*, 3–4.

SECTION 4

Special Issues

24

Collaborative Treatment with Primary Care

Jamesetta A. Newland and Kathryn K. Ellis

Objectives

After reading this chapter, APNs will be able to

1. Define the concept of collaborative treatment within the context of meeting the behavioral and primary care health needs of children and adolescents.
2. Describe roles of team members and different models of an interprofessional approach to provide services to these children.

3. Recognize facilitators and barriers to implementing collaborative treatment models.
4. Examine issues related to patient privacy, provider responsibility, and disclosures.

Introduction

Children and adolescents traditionally access medical health care services through a primary care provider (PCP), who is a pediatric or family nurse practitioner (PNP/FNP), a family physician, or a pediatrician. Services for behavioral health care needs, alternatively, can be provided by the PCP but might more appropriately be delivered by a psychiatric mental health (PMH) specialist, such as a psychiatric mental health advanced practice nurse (APN), psychologist, social worker, psychiatrist, or other person trained to manage behavioral and mental health needs of children and adolescents. The separation of care for medical and behavioral and mental health needs often creates a situation where children and adolescents receive disconnected care from different health care professionals in various settings. They are repeatedly shuttled between providers who face difficulty in trying to communicate

with each other because of obstacles such as physical location, reimbursement issues, and legal restrictions. Or these children receive minimal or no services for behavioral and mental health needs. Few providers are equipped to individually address the multiple needs of this population. Major organizations and individuals have called for the integration of behavioral health services in primary care (American Academy of Child and Adolescent Psychiatry [AACAP] and American Academy of Pediatrics [AAP], 2009; Collins, Hewson, Munger, & Wade, 2010; Institute of Medicine [IOM], 2006; World Health Organization, 2008).

In *Crossing the Quality Chasm: A New Health System for the 21st Century*, the IOM (2001) made recommendations for clinicians and institutions to "actively collaborate and communicate to ensure an appropriate exchange of information and coordination of care" (p. 9). In the report, the committee encouraged clinicians and organizations in the U.S. health care system to develop

---

Child and Adolescent Behavioral Health: A Resource for Advanced Practice Psychiatric and Primary Care Practitioners in Nursing,
First Edition. Edited by Edilma L. Yearwood, Geraldine S. Pearson, and Jamesetta A. Newland.
© 2012 John Wiley & Sons, Inc. Published 2012 by John Wiley & Sons, Inc.

creative strategies to link services and communications for physical, mental, and substance use diagnoses; medications and treatments; and all aspects of clinical care for patients to decrease the increasing fragmentation of care. The IOM (2006) further stated in *Improving the Quality of Health Care for Mental and Substance Use Conditions*, "collaboration is multidimensional and requires the aggregation of several behaviors" (p. 212)—a shared understanding of goals and roles, effective communication, and shared decision making. Teams were to be composed of professionals with distinctive roles and skills who agreed to work together in a mutually respectful environment toward common goals. Communication involved the sharing of information relevant to meeting the patient's needs. Information could be shared through traditional means, verbally or in writing, or through new avenues using information technology, such as electronic health records. These actions were proposed to ultimately improve the quality of care for patients, the common goal. The most vulnerable groups who received fragmented care were identified as older adults, *children and adolescents*, ethnic minorities, uninsured or low income persons, and individuals with mental health problems who presented with primarily physical symptoms (Bartlett, Herrick, & Greninger, 2006; Unutzer, Schoenbaum, Druss, & Katon, 2006).

This chapter will present background information and discussion of issues in providing integrated behavioral health and primary care services through collaborative treatment models. The most common collaborative and integrated practice models are presented. Barriers and facilitators to successful integration of behavioral health and primary care are reviewed. The chapter ends with a case exemplar.

Traditional Health Care

Parents readily take children to a PCP for physical complaints of illness. Because recommendations and regulations for immunizations and well physical examinations are part of routine health care and school attendance requirements, children and adolescents have multiple visits over the course of their natural growth and development. Parents are comfortable with the PCP and feel the provider knows them; the physical and emotional environment is viewed as safe (AACAP & AAP, 2009). Parents in this familiar setting are more likely to introduce concerns about a child's behavioral and mental health to a trusted PCP. In one study, physicians likewise were more comfortable initiating a conversation about their observations of a child's behavioral, emotional, or developmental issues with a parent they had known for a period of time (Cooper, Valleley, Polaha,

Begeny, & Evans, 2006). In busy pediatric practices, the time assigned to each patient might be too brief to assess any behavioral or mental health disorder that is not overtly recognized. Time for comprehensive mental health assessments is limited (Guevara, Greenbaum, Shera, Bauer, & Schwarz, 2009). Thus, a parent's comment about a behavior or mental health concern might be the first indication to a PCP that a problem must be addressed.

Signs and symptoms of mental disorders, substance abuse conditions, and psychosocial problems fall along a continuum that complicates distinguishing acceptable from unacceptable behaviors. Cultural beliefs and norms influence parents' perceptions of normal versus not normal. Factors identified that have been presumed to be influential in preventing parents from seeking care for behavioral and mental health concerns about their child include stigma, family conflict or dysfunction, cultural differences, being uninsured or underinsured, or not knowing where to go for specialty mental health services (Foy & AAP Task Force on Mental Health, 2010). Parents might assume that a PCP does not address these types of "mental" issues and are thus reluctant to mention their concerns. They are confused about where to go in a complex health care system that does not clearly explain how or where to access certain services, whether insured or uninsured. A parent may also be reluctant to label the child for fear their "untrained" diagnosis and inability to deal with the problem will make them appear weak to the world around them (Pincus, 2003). Society also attaches biases to conditions or behaviors that have been judged unacceptable (Pincus). Integration of behavioral health and primary care might serve to remove the stigma associated with seeking care for mental health needs and reduce health disparities (Earls, 2010; Rainwater, 2009).

Whether a primary care practitioner refers a child or adolescent to a psychiatric professional depends on several factors. The AACAP (2010) offers the following reasons, which might include one or more: (a) clinical presentation of the patient, (b) training, skill, and experience of the practitioner, (c) family and environmental situation, (d) availability of support services and personnel, and (e) availability of a child and adolescent psychiatrist (or other qualified professional) with relevant experience.

Defining Integrated Health Care

Various authors and groups have defined integrated health care (behavioral health and primary care) and components of the concept. The descriptions are similar although the terminology varies slightly. Understanding the concept of integrated care is important in designing and implementing programs. Health care delivery falls along a continuum from complete separation on one end to total integration on the other end.

Collaboration

In 1996, Doherty, McDaniel, and Baird (as cited by Integrated Behavioral Health Project [IBHP], 2007) described collaboration between primary and behavioral health care professionals along a continuum with five levels. In Level One, there is *minimal collaboration*. Mental health and other health care professionals operate in silos, with neither communicating with the other, and services are rendered in separate locations. This is the traditional method that results in fragmented care. In Level Two, the providers practice *basic collaboration at a distance*. They operate in separate locations and in separate systems; communication is through telephone calls or letters when there is a particular patient issue. This works well for straightforward problems such as a patient with asthma and anxiety being treated independently by each without any shared decision making. In Level Three, *basic collaboration on-site*, different providers still maintain separate systems but share the same facility. Communication might be face-to-face because of co-location of services; coordination of treatment might occur but shared decision making is not part of the interactions.

In Level Four, there is *close collaboration in a partly integrated system*. Mental health and other providers share the same space and some parts of their systems, such as computer scheduling. There are more face-to-face meetings with the team and members acknowledge the roles and skills of other providers. The degree of shared decision making is influenced by logistics such as the power hierarchy of the organization, differences between the organizations in areas of insurance reimbursements, or allocated visit time. Level Five is the desired model, *close collaboration in a fully integrated system*. In this situation, mental health and other professionals share the same sites, the same vision, and the systems of care are seamless for the provider and the patient. Each provider is valued for what their role and expertise bring to the team (IBHP, 2007). These five levels are represented across the various settings in which health care services are delivered, and others have categorized service delivery similarly.

Blount (2003) also discussed the relationship between medical and behavioral health services in primary care in three levels: *coordinated, co-located, and integrated*. These levels were not mutually exclusive but fell along a continuum of care (collaboration). Coordinated services existed in different locations, completely separated;

co-located services were provided in the same physical location but by different providers in behavioral health and primary care who operated more or less independently of each other. Integrated services could be provided in different locations or at the same location; the distinguishing feature of integrated services versus the other models was that medical and behavioral health professionals mutually developed a treatment plan for a specific patient or population of patients.

Blount (2003) further distinguished the difference in providing care by designating whether services were offered as targeted or nontargeted problems. Behavioral health services to a targeted problem, for instance substance abuse, might be more resource-full and accepted by patients identified for these services compared to services that were not targeted to any particular patient populations and were available to the general population. Blount made a final distinction between specified and unspecified treatment modalities, such as a prescribed medication protocol for all patients diagnosed with depression versus a treatment plan that was dependent upon the individual provider's knowledge and skill. Comparisons were more difficult when the treatment a patient received was not known; specified treatments were more standard and consistently administered to patients. These categorizations were intended to facilitate efforts to collect meaningful information that reflected, on comparable terms, the impact of one particular model over another in meeting patients' needs so that systems of care could be modified accordingly (Blount).

Integrated Health Care

A widely accepted definition of "integrated health care" is attributed to Alexander Blount, therapist and educator:

> It's a coordinated system that combines medical and behavioral services to address the whole person, not just one aspect of his or her condition. Medical and mental health providers partner to coordinate the detection, treatment, and follow-up of both mental and physical conditions. Combining this care allows consumers to feel that, for almost any problem, they've come to the right place (Integrated Behavioral Health Project [IBHP], 2009, p. 6).

The *IBHP Toolkit* contains a list of forty-two reasons why primary care and mental health professionals should collaborate. Four examples include (a) more cohesive service delivery system and better continuity of care, (b) better mental health outcomes when a physical condition is managed, (c) a "full picture" about patients being treated by both medical and behavioral professionals, and (d) easier access for patients to mental health facilities through primary care clinics.

Other conceptualizations of integrated health care use strategies and algorithms for applying the chronic care principles to the care of children with mental health and substance abuse problems as the PCP would apply these interventions to a child with a chronic medical condition (Foy & AAP Task Force on Mental Health, 2010; Foy, Kelleher, Laraque, & AAP Task Force on Mental Health, 2010). One modified chronic care model, the Four Quadrant Clinical Integration Model, is an approach that uses stepped care to integrate primary and behavioral health care (National Council for Community Behavioral Healthcare [NCCBH], 2009). Behavioral health services are rendered within the primary care setting depending on the [patient] population, the variant of the model, and the providers. The model has four quadrants, each representing along a continuum the behavioral health/risk complexity (BH) and the physical health/risk complexity (PH) of the patient. In Quadrant I (QI) are low BH and low PH individuals; Quadrant II (QII) includes high BH and low PH individuals; Quadrant III (QIII) represents low BH and high PH individuals; and Quadrant IV (QIV) contains high BH and high PH individuals.

Primary responsibility for managing health conditions depends on severity and whether the knowledge and skills of behavioral or primary health care is the more urgent need. Low BH and low PH (QI) individuals can be managed by the PCP through use of routine screening tools and consultation with a PCP-based behavioral health professional. Low BH and high PH (QIII) individuals should be managed by the PCP in collaboration with specialty medical/surgical experts and PCP-based behavioral health professionals. For both QI and QIII categories, psychiatric consultation is indicated when the patient is not showing improvement. High BH and low PH (QII) individuals should be managed by a behavioral health professional in collaboration with a medical provider such as an NP or physician who is located at the behavioral health site. High BH and high PH (QIV) individuals should be managed collaboratively by a medical professional at the behavioral health site with the assistance of a nurse care manager and behavioral health clinician/case manager. Medical and behavioral specialists would also participate in the care of these QIV complex patients (NCCBH, 2009). The model proposes that service delivery should depend on the needs of the individual, personal choice, and available community and collaboration resources. As stated before, consultation among behavioral and primary care professionals is appropriate when indicated no matter who has primary responsibility for coordinating the patient's care. Table 24.1

Table 24.1 Examples of patients in categories of the Four Quadrant Clinical Integration Model

Q	Patient	BH Risk	PH Risk	Management
I	4 years	ADHD [L]	Eczema [L]	PCP
II	12 years	Bipolar disorder [H]	Acne [L]	BH/MP
III	9 years	School anxiety[L]	Sickle cell disease [H]	PCP/CM
IV	17 years	Self-harm [H]	Cystic fibrosis[H]	PCP/BH

Q = Quadrant; BH = Behavioral Health; PH = Physical Health; H = High; L = Low; PCP = Primary Care Provider; MP = Medical Provider at BH site; CM = Case Manager for PH and BH

includes an example of a child or adolescent in each of the four categories and the primary team member.

The IMPACT model (Improving Mood–Providing Access to Collaborative Treatment) is an example of a team approach that integrates evidence-based depression treatment into primary care and other medical settings (University of Washington, n.d.). Implementation of the model occurred in a randomized clinical trial in eighteen primary care clinics at seven study sites. The model has been shown to be effective with depressed patients of diverse demographic characteristics, including adolescents. The program demonstrated greater effectiveness than traditional means of treating depression, has improved quality of life for patients, and has resulted in a reduction in overall health care costs (Saur et al., 2002). The IMPACT program has five key components: (a) collaborative care between the PCP and care managers; (b) use of a depression care manager who can be a nurse, social worker, or psychologist, supported by a medical assistant or other paraprofessional; (c) a designated psychiatrist; (d) an outcome measurement for depression; and (e) stepped care or treatment adjustments based on clinical outcomes and evidence-based algorithms (University of Washington). Sites are also implementing the program for treatment of other common mental disorders, such as anxiety disorder. Information and materials for clinicians and organizations in implementing IMPACT in a variety of settings are available on the web site (http://impact-uw.org).

Although the population was the elderly, Saur et al. (2002) demonstrated the effectiveness of nurses working collaboratively as depression clinical specialists in primary care settings. The master's-prepared PMH clinical nurse specialist, as a nurse psychotherapist, was able to implement the IMPACT model without additional specialized training, while the baccalaureate-prepared

PMH nurse generalist needed only minimal additional training. Both were valued members of the health care team in the primary care setting, which included the PCP and a psychiatrist, because of the knowledge and skills they lent to the care of elderly patients with depression from the framework of therapeutic nurse-patient relationships.

Patient-Centered Health Home

The AAP (2002) issued a policy statement describing the pediatric medical home; the statement was based on previous policy statements issued by AAP. A medical home for infants, children, and adolescents was to be accessible, family-centered, continuous, comprehensive, coordinated, compassionate, and culturally effective. It was a "home base" where patients could feel comfortable in the health care process. PCPs and specialists, when consultation or referral was indicated, were expected to collaborate and share management in partnership with the child and the family. Primary care was defined as per the IOM and entailed integrated, accessible health care services, partnership with patients, and practice within the context of the family and community. Comprehensive care did include assessment and intervention for behavioral and mental health care needs. This policy statement was reaffirmed in 2008 (http://aappolicy.aappublications.org/cgi/content/full/pediatrics;110/1/184).

Although pediatric medical homes were implemented for both well and special needs children, Cooley (2004) conducted a review of studies on special needs children to determine whether medical homes actually existed and whether the care provided was more efficient, effective, and satisfying to patients. Cooley reviewed a report of data from the 2001 National Survey of Children with Special Health Care Needs, which revealed that 52.6% of them did indeed receive care in a pediatric medical home, having met five criteria: "having a usual source of care; having a specific, primary care provider; having timely access to needed specialty care; having effective care coordination when needed; and receiving care that is family-centered" (p. 890). Yet significant racial/cultural and economic disparities were discovered. Non-Hispanic white children were more likely to have a medical home than poor children. Cooley reviewed a report that determined that care coordination and continuity of care improved the quality of primary care and was dependent on five factors: adequate medical records, continuity of personnel, practitioner-patient communication, clinical quality of care, and advocacy for patients.

Davis, Schoenbaum, and Audet (2005) proposed seven characteristics of patient-centered primary care practices. *Patient-centered* connoted that the health system would be more responsive to patients' preferences, needs, and values and not operate on the principle of business as usual. The seven points were:

- Superb access to care
- Patient engagement in care
- Clinical information systems that support high-quality care, practice-based learning, and quality improvement
- Care coordination
- Integrated, comprehensive care and smooth information transfer across a fixed or virtual team of providers
- Ongoing, routine patient feedback to a practice
- Publicly available information on practices (p. 954)

To meet these criteria would require a major shift in how health care is delivered in the United States. Putting everything in perspective, practice for infants, children, and adolescents has been a task undertaken by AAP in collaboration with other agencies and organization, including the federal government. Malouin and Merten (2010) examined various tools available and in use to identify, recognize, and evaluate a practice as a pediatric medical home. Difficulties encountered in collecting information were the absence of a standard definition for a pediatric medical home, tools that did not necessarily measure the stated concept or construct, and lack of parallel formats of a tool that could be used with different stakeholders including patients, providers, families, and others. Valid and reliable measures that can generate data about health care delivery can only facilitate continued support for the concept of patient-centered medical homes.

The Centers for Medicare and Medicaid Services (CMS) (2011) currently has demonstration projects in eight states under the Advanced Primary Care Practice Demonstration for Multipayers and the Federally Qualified Health Centers Advanced Primary Care Practice Demonstration for Medicare. Plans are under way to test the patient-centered medical home model under the new Innovation Center created through the Patient Protection and Affordable Care Act. The AAP statements and other papers, however, refer to physicians only as PCPs and coordinators of care through medical homes. The Preserving Patient Access to Primary Care Act of 2009 introduced a model that would allow clinicians other than physicians to qualify as coordinators of medical homes. This bill would amend the definition of PCP to include an NP and a physician assistant on a physician-directed or NP-directed team, who provided first contact, continuous, and comprehensive care to patients. The shortage of primary care clinicians of all types helped to move this bill forward. The bill was still in process in early 2011 and had support from several main nursing organizations and physician groups. Debate continues over what to call this "home"—medical home, health home, patient-centered home, or other. Likewise, providers struggle with how best to provide health care services to their pediatric patient populations.

Examples of Different Models of Care

Examples of collaborative teams can be found in the literature (Campo et al., 2005; Connor et al., 2006; Valleley et al., 2007). Campo et al. (2005) described a primary care–based program that employed a stepped-care approach in a collaborative model between a mental health (MH) psychiatric clinic and primary care clinicians (PCCs) in a rural pediatric practice in Pennsylvania. The approach to each child depended on the child's type of disorder and severity, complexity, and response to treatment. The goal of this program was to integrate MH professionals into a primary care practice. The on-site team included a PCC, an APN (FNP with training in psychiatry), a psychiatric social worker, and a part-time pediatric psychiatrist. The PCC identified children with emotional and behavioral problems, made a diagnosis, and managed the less complex mental conditions (e.g., attention deficit hyperactivity disorder [ADHD], depression, and anxiety) and functional somatic symptoms. The APN coordinated management of care by the PCC and acted as liaison between the PCC and other members of the MH team. The APN triaged patients to the MH team where indicated (e.g., parenting skills, learning problems, tics, and eating problems), providing patient and family education and treatment support. The social worker delivered focused therapeutic interventions, while the psychiatrist handled psychopharmacological management. Patients received on-site routine care (PCC only) or collaborative care (PCC and MH team), or specialty mental health care (off-site).

Connor et al. (2006) described a model of primary clinician-child psychiatry collaborative care instituted in one state to assist PCPs without access to child psychiatry consultation in managing children with complex ADHD, depression, anxiety disorders, and pediatric psychopharmacology. Targeted Child Psychiatric Services offered real-time telephone consultation to 139 primary care physicians and nurse practitioners in 22 primary care practices that provided pediatric care to over 100,000 children and adolescents in central Massachusetts. Child psychiatrists or "pediatric mental health nurse clinicians" completed initial psychiatric evaluations on children who were referred for in-person evaluation. Of the direct patient referrals, 63% were for diagnosis. The authors concluded that in their limited population, PCPs were able to identify children and adolescents with moderate to severe psychiatric symptoms, serious psychopathology, and significant functional impairment but wanted help from a child psychiatrist in managing these children. Other collaborative consultation programs have targeted the common diagnosis of ADHD (Epstein et al., 2007; Leslie, Weckerly, Plemmons, Landsverk, & Eastman, 2004).

Valleley et al. (2007) described an integrated primary care–behavioral health program in rural communities where limited mental health resources were available. Authors found three benefits to the integration: affiliation with trusted physicians, ease of referral, and increased confidentiality. An established physician-patient relationship contributed to the likelihood of patients, adults and children attending appointments when referred for behavioral health services. Second, the co-location of services made it easier for patients to attend appointments. And finally, the stigma of seeking mental health services was removed because services were not accessed in a distinctly identifiable location but in the same (accepted) location where regular medical services were rendered. Patients were again more likely to attend appointments. Referrals were made by PCPs to behavioral health specialists on-site. The team used progress notes, informal hallway consultation, and in-session meeting to share information and decision making about treatment. Children with higher functional impairment were more likely to attend their appointments. Of all children referred over a two-year period ($N = 807$), 87% scheduled an appointment and 81% attended the initial behavioral health visit. Authors recommended scheduling appointments as soon after a referral as possible and to institute some type of reminder system for patients, such as a phone call several days before the appointment.

A well-established community-based integrated health system has been in place for approximately thirty years in Tennessee. In the Cherokee Health Systems, a behavioral health consultant is available at the primary care visit for assessment, triage, and intervention. Patients are comfortable in the familiar surroundings of the primary care practice and more open to referrals for mental health services when referred by a trusted PCP to a behavioral health consultant at the same location. PCPs appreciate the presence of a mental health specialist with a different set of skills to help in patients. Patient and provider satisfaction was increased (Freeman, 2007).

Working collaboratively improved access to mental health specialists for the children in these communities. One advantage of having different models is the flexibility to modify the model used to meet the needs of the providers and the patients. APNs in integrated health settings bring the perspective of a holistic approach to providing care and with specialized training in psychiatric nursing become invaluable members of interprofessional teams, and often the leaders. Inherent in innovation, however, are challenges and barriers.

Challenges and Barriers

Challenges to integrating behavioral health and primary care are similar no matter what the model: a fragmented health delivery system, cultural differences between disciplines, restrictive confidentiality laws about sharing information related to substance abuse and mental health issues, and separate payment structures (Campo et al., 2005; Collins et al., 2010; Pincus, 2003). Collins et al. highlight three major challenges concerning information sharing, confidentiality laws, and reimbursement. Other authors present similar challenges.

Health professionals in the past were trained in silos (Blount & Miller, 2009; Gunn & Blount, 2009; Pincus, 2003). Members in different disciplines were introduced to practice and matured in isolated silos, each discipline developing separate cultures and norms for practice. Education has been so focused on competencies related to one specialty that providers have limited knowledge and skills outside of their domain, even for basic needs. Part of the culture has been the secrecy surrounding behavioral health records and reluctance and legal restrictions for sharing the information with a primary care or other professional. Sharing of information rarely occurs even in practices where primary care and behavioral health are co-located. After a referral, the records are more often maintained separately. Correspondence might range from a verbal exchange to a formal consultation letter but not full access to the written notations of providers in the other discipline, whether on paper or in an electronic record. Only in a truly integrated system is documentation accessible to both types of providers.

The Health Insurance Portability and Accountability Act of 1996 (HIPAA) (U.S. Department of Health and Human Services [DHHS], Office for Civil Rights [OCR], 2003) was enacted to protect an individual's privacy rights by establishing rules that safeguard one's protected health information (PHI) when accessing health care services. Covered entities must comply with the rules; these include health plans, health care clearinghouses, and any health care provider who transmits health information in electronic form in connection with standard transactions such as filing claims and obtaining authorization for referrals. The HIPAA rules are intended to ensure that an individual's PHI is protected while still giving providers the capability to share health information needed to deliver high-quality health

care to persons seeking care. Protecting public safety is also part of the process.

But federal and state (varying) confidentiality laws related to substance abuse and mental health are usually more restrictive than those pertaining to physical health. Although primary care and mental health practitioners have used these more restrictive rules as a reason for not sharing information, HIPAA permits the exchange of information for treatment, payment, or health care operations for a covered entity. Generally, written permission from the individual authorizing disclosure of psychotherapy notes is necessary before these notes can be shared. In two circumstances psychotherapy notes may be disclosed by a covered entity without the individual's authorization—(a) use for treatment and (b) use for training by the covered entity, for defense in legal proceedings, and several other broader circumstances (DHHS, OCR, 2003, p. 9). Therefore, primary care and mental health providers are able to share information for the purposes of care coordination. A comprehensive discussion of issues related to confidentiality and sharing of information can be found in Chapter 25 of this book on legal and ethical issues in providing care to children and adolescents.

A significant barrier to integrated health systems is current reimbursement practices for services rendered. Pincus (2003) noted that mental health services in the past were largely funded in the public sector and were always underresourced, and insurance reimbursement was limited at best. The advent of community mental health centers, private psychiatric hospitals, psychoanalysis, and behavioral health special programs created further separation from primary care in practice and payment systems. Alternately, patient visits for medical care were covered by insurance plans and mental health services were compromised, thus resulting in disparate systems. Differences encompass separate deductibles, high co-pays, and annual spending limits lower than those for medical services (AAP & AACAP, 2009). Some states and insurers separated billing codes for primary care and behavioral health by specialty, preventing a specialist in one discipline from accessing and using codes from a different specialty. For pediatrics, available diagnostic codes do not adequately describe the developmental and behavioral problems of children; thus, primary care clinicians are not reimbursed for the time spent identifying, treating, and managing these problems in children (AAP & AACAP). Regular consultation between specialties and care management might not be funded (Unutzer et al., 2006). Also excluded from reimbursement were the administration and interpretation of health risk assessments as well as other evidence-based treatment plans, interventions that had demonstrated utility in dealing with mental health. Time-restricted primary care clinicians cannot spend the time needed for behavioral assessments even if they have the skill set to address both physical and mental health issues, especially if they are not going to be reimbursed. Discussing solutions to the current payment system is beyond the scope of this chapter.

Implications for Practice, Research, and Education

Providers can no longer be educated, trained, or work in silos. Future PCPs and PMH professionals, which include APNs, must be acculturated to collaborative interprofessional models of care. The implications for practice, research, and education to create change are compelling. Efforts to introduce health care reform to improve the U.S. health system have been met with resistance from stakeholders in every sector, including providers, patients, legislators, and insurers. But as always noted, the ultimate goal of change is to improve the quality of care and patient health outcomes.

Collins et al. (2010) make recommendations for health care system and policy changes. The authors suggest that the broad spectrum of stakeholders come together to plan, design, and implement new systems. An often overlooked or underused partnership is between public and private entities (philanthropies); they caution not to exclude the consumer. Professional organizations might also work together to promote the adoption of evidence-based standards in primary care for [adults and] children in the areas of mental health and substance abuse. A key element in moving forward is the ability to demonstrate to stakeholders, based on data and particularly providers and payers, that integrated care is "clinically beneficial and financially viable." Usual parameters reported in the past have been "improved *access* to services, *clinical outcome, maintained improvement,* improved *adherence to treatment regimens, patient satisfaction, provider satisfaction, cost effectiveness* or *medical cost offset*" (Blount, 2003, p. 121). The burden lies in documenting the impact [improvement] related to delivering care in an integrated system.

Much too often nursing has not been at the table with decision-makers (Newland, 2010). The Patient Protection and Affordable Care Act of 2010 has given APNs an opportunity to take a seat at the table and be key stakeholders in shaping health care reform. The concept of the medical home, health home, or patient-centered home is an ideal setting for APNs to step into clinical leadership roles and develop intraprofessional models to improve care delivery to the many U.S. citizens with limited or no access to health care. *The Future of*

Nursing (IOM, 2010) has called into action nurses and other health professionals to center the focus of health care once again on the patient, to educate and train students from different disciplines to work together, to remove barriers to practice to allow nurses to practice to the full scope of their education and training, and to elevate the level of education for all nurses.

In 2001, Bower, Garralda, Kramer, Harrington, and Sibbald conducted a systematic review of 25 studies from the United States and the United Kingdom that included randomized clinical trials and before/after studies with and without controls. The researchers questioned the effectiveness of interventions for child and adolescent mental health problems in primary care and [educational] interventions designed to improve the skills of primary care staff. Methodological flaws in study designs limited interpretation; further research to develop evidence-based policy and service delivery models was recommended.

Weiss, Haber, Horowitz, Stuart, and Wolfe (2009) advocated for integrated care for physical and psychiatric health needs, stating that "mental-physical" were intricately connected; individuals with mental illness seemed to have a high prevalence of physical illness, leading to increased morbidity and mortality. A fragmented health care system and separate payment mechanisms for physical and mental health were also contributing factors for these outcomes. The authors proposed four creative strategies to deal with the situation: (a) "restore adequate behavioral health content to basic nursing licensure exam," (b) "promote the role of the advanced practice psychiatric nurse in all primary care settings," (c) "establish competency-based coursework across graduate specialties that incorporates the knowledge and skills necessary for integrative care," and (d) "develop and evaluate integrated systems of care" (pp. 376–377).

Just as important as equipping new nursing graduates with basic knowledge and skills needed to be able to recognize and appropriately address mental health issues is the need to incorporate mental health content into curricula of nonpsychiatric graduate specialties. Giving APNs certified in PMH the opportunity and responsibility to manage mental health needs of patients, as NPs do in primary care, would increase the numbers of accessible mental health professionals to render services to a growing population that needs such services. Other experts advocate for formal mental health competencies in practical curricula—knowledge, skills, and attitudes—training for pediatric PCCs (pediatricians) during medical school and residency programs (AAP, 2009) and for physicians, nurses, social workers, and psychologists (Blount, DeGirolamo, & Mariani, 2006; Unutzer et al., 2006).

Conclusion

New models of health care delivery are emerging, and existing models are being adapted to accommodate behavioral and medical [primary] health within a primary care setting. The particular model implemented by providers from both primary care and behavioral health will depend on many factors, including access to either professional in the community, retooling for current providers and training for new practitioners, opportunities for and willingness to collaborate, financial and reimbursement structures, and patient acceptance. With each new IOM report, the mandate is given to change how we deliver today's health care services, to coordinate, collaborate, and integrate these services. With a currently limited workforce, all types of providers must work better. Guidance is available through many resources offered by governmental agencies, special foundations, and professional and specialty organizations. Goals are multifaceted: (a) increased access to behavioral health care for those in need; (b) earlier identification and treatment of behavioral health problems; (c) creation of a less complex point of access to behavioral health services for patients when they seek primary care services, and vice versa; (d) increased training among disciplines to improve interprofessional collaboration and co-management of appropriate patients; and (e) improved patient outcomes. Health care reform and revamping the financial/insurance health system must be priorities. These goals might be achieved by establishing integrated health care systems where providers from primary care, behavioral health, and other disciplines share information and decision making, including documentation, in delivering care to patients.

Case Exemplar

Molly was an eleven-year-old fifth grader who lived at home with her mother and two older brothers. She was delivered at thirty-eight weeks via repeat cesarean section and weighed 8 lb 4 oz. Her mother's gestational diabetes was treated with diet modification and did not require insulin. Pediatric records indicated that Molly was consistently in the ninetieth percentile for height and weight during her early childhood. However, at her nine-year-old checkup, her weight jumped to greater than the ninety-fifth percentile and has continued in this range over the past two years. Molly consumed large amounts of carbohydrates and fats on a daily basis, including cookies, chips, regular soda, and fruit juices. Several nights a week the family ate fast food—burgers, fries, and pizza. She was sedentary and spent at least three hours per day watching television or playing games on the computer. Although she enjoyed a good relationship with her mother, her brothers teased her incessantly about "being fat and ugly." Molly's father lived out of state and had little contact with her.

Over a three-week period, her mother reported that Molly had been waking up on school days with stomach aches, headaches, and other minor complaints. She was refusing to go to school and complained that the kids made fun of her and excluded her from activities. Molly's teachers noted a change in her school performance manifested by missed assignments, poor test grades, and lack of concentration. Her mother reported that Molly had become withdraw and isolated, spending most of her time in her bedroom by herself.

Molly's mother made an appointment with the family nurse practitioner (FNP) at the school-based clinic for a physical examination and evaluation. On physical exam, the FNP noted that Molly had skin changes consistent with acanthosis nigricans at the base of her neck. Her height was 4 ft 9 in and weight was 155 lb (BMI 33.5). Her affect was flat and she did not seem engaged in the conversation. In addition to the physical examination, the FNP conducted a comprehensive history and screening for depression and lab work. Lab results revealed an elevated fasting glucose level of 106 mg/dl and elevated total cholesterol of 245 mg/dl. The FNP initiated several referrals based on these findings. The first referral was to a pediatric psychiatric mental health nurse practitioner (PMHNP) for evaluation of depression. Additionally, a consultation with a nutritionist who specializes in children with obesity was scheduled. Both providers, also located on the campus, worked with the school-based clinic. The school counselor was also contacted, made aware of the situation, and agreed to meet with Molly on a regular basis.

The PMHNP diagnosed Molly with major depressive disorder (mild) and initiated therapy on a weekly basis. Molly and her mother also saw the nutritionist and attended "Healthy Eating" classes together for several months. The FNP communicated with the interdisciplinary team to assure that Molly's care was coordinated and that resources were available for the family. At her three-month follow-up exam, Molly's mood had improved and she was attending school regularly. She had also changed her diet significantly and had lost 4 lb. Her mother and brothers joined Molly in family group therapy sessions.

This exemplar demonstrates several themes related to children and health care delivery:

- Childhood obesity
- Impaired fasting glucose (prediabetes)
- Social isolation
- Depression

- Coordination by PCP for patient-centered care
- Co-location of health services
- Interdisciplinary team
- Shared information and decision making

The collaborative efforts of the entire team resulted in improved mental and physical health for Molly. Her medical, behavioral, and mental health needs were addressed by team members.

Resources

Agency for Healthcare Research and Quality. (2008). *Integration of Mental Health/Substance Abuse and Primary Care*: http://www.ahrq.gov/clinic/tp/mhsapctp.htm

Cherokee Health Systems: http://www.cherokeehealth.com

Collaborative Family Healthcare Association: http://www.cfha.net

Hogg Foundation for Mental Health: http://www.hogg.utexas.edu/

ICARE Partnership: http://www.icarenc.org

IMPACT (Improving Mood – Providing Access to Collaborative Treatment): http://impact-uw.org

Integrated Behavioral Health Project (IBHP): http://www.ibhp.org

Integrated Primary Care, Inc.: http://www.integratedprimarycare.com

Intermountain Behavioral Health Program: http://www.intermountainhealthcare.org

National Council for Community Behavioral Healthcare: http://www.nccbh.org

[The] Patient Centered Primary Care Collaborative: http://www.pcpcc.net

Technical Assistance Partnership for Child and Family Mental Health—Sustaining Systems of Care: http://tapartnership.org/SOC/SOCsustaining.php

World Health Organization. (2008). *Integrating Mental Health Into Primary Care: A Global Perspective*: http://www.who.int/mental_health/resources/mentalhealth_PHC_2008.pdf

References

American Academy of Child & Adolescent Psychiatry [AACAP}. (2010). *When to seek referral or consultation with a child adolescent psychiatrist*. Retrieved from http://www.aacap.org/cs/root/member_information/practice_information/when_to_seek_referral_or_consultation_with_a_child_adolescent_psychiatrist

American Academy of Child & Adolescent Psychiatry and American Academy of Pediatrics. (2009). *Improving mental health services in primary care: Reducing administrative and financial barriers to access and collaboration—Background*. Retrieved from http://www.aacap.org/galleries/LegislativeAction/Final%20Background%20paper%203-09.pdf

American Academy of Pediatrics, Medical Home for Children With Special Needs Project Advisory Committee. (2002). The medical home. *Pediatrics, 110*, 184–186. Retrieved from http://www.pediatrics.org/cgi/content/full/110/1/184

American Academy of Pediatrics [AAP], Committee on Psychosocial Aspects of Child and Family Health and Task Force on Mental Health. (2009). The future of pediatrics: Mental health competencies for pediatric primary care. *Pediatrics, 124*, 410–421. doi:10.1542/peds.2009-1061

Bartlett, R., Herrick, C.A., & Greninger, L. (2006). Using a system of care framework for the mental health treatment of children and adolescents. *The Journal for Nurse Practitioners, 2*, 593–598.

Blount, A. (2003). Integrated primary care: Organizing the evidence. *Families, Systems & Health, 21*, 121–134. Retrieved from http://test.pcpcc.net/files/organizing_the_evidence.pdf

Blount, A., DeGirolamo, S., & Mariani, K. (2006). Training the collaborative care practitioners of the future. *Families, Systems, & Health, 24*, 111–119.

Blount, F.A., & Miller, B.F. (2009). Addressing the workforce crisis in integrated primary care. *Journal of Clinical Psychology in Medical Settings, 16*, 113–119.

Bower, P., Garralda, E., Kramer, T., Harringtton, R., & Sibbald, B. (2001). The treatment of child and adolescent mental health problems in primary care: A systematic review. *Family Practice, 18*, 373–382. Retrieved from http://fampra.oxfordjournals.org/content/18/4/373.full.pdf+html

Campo, J.V., Shafer, S., Strohm, J., Lucas, A., Gelacek Cassese, C., Shaeffer, D., & Altman, H. (2005). Pediatric behavioral health in primary care: A collaborative approach. *Journal of the American Psychiatric Nurses Association, 11*, 276–282. Doi: 10.1177/1078390305282404

Centers for Medicare and Medicaid Services [CMS]. (2011). *Medicare demonstrations*. Retrieved from http://www.cms.gov/DemoProjectsEvalRpts/MD/itemdetail.asp?filterType=none&filterByDID=99&sortByDID=3&sortOrder=descending&itemID=CMS1199247&intNumPerPage=10

Collins, C., Hewson, D.L., Munger, R., & Wade, T. (2010). *Evolving models of behavioral health integration in primary care*. New York, NY: Milbank Memorial Fund. Retrieved from http://www.milbank.org/reports/10430EvolvingCare/EvolvingCare.pdf

Connor, D.F., McLaughlin, T.J., Jeffers-Terry, M., O'Brien, W.H., Stille, C.J., Young, L.M., & Antonelli, R.C. (2006). Targeted child psychiatric services: A new model of pediatric primary clinician – child psychiatry collaborative care. *Clinical Pediatrics, 45*, 423–434. doi:10.1177/0009922806289617

Cooley, W.C. (2004). Redefining primary pediatric care for children with special health care needs: The primary care medical home. *Current Opinions in Pediatrics, 16*, 689–692.

Cooper, S., Valleley, R.J., Polaha, J., Begeny, J., & Evans, J.H. (2006). Running out of time: Physician management of behavioral health concerns in rural pediatric primary care. *Pediatrics, 118*, e132-e138. doi:10.1542/peds.2005-2612

Davis, K., Schoenbaum, S.C., & Audet, A. (2005). A 2020 vision of patient-centered primary care. *Journal of General Internal Medicine, 20*, 953–957.

Earls, M. (2010, January). *Mental health integration in primary care: Opportunities for LAUNCH projects*. Paper presented at Project LAUNCH Grantee Meeting, New Orleans, LA. Retrieved from http://projectlauch.promoteprevent.org/webfm_send/1446

Epstein, J.N., Rabiner, D., Johnson, D.E., Fitzgerald, D.P., Chrisman, A., Erkanli, A., Conners, K. (2007). Improving attention-deficit/hyperactivity disorder treatment outcomes through use of a collaborative consultation treatment service by community-based pediatricians: A cluster randomized trial. *Arch Pediatr Adolesc Med, 161*, 835–840. Retrieved from http://archpedi.ama-assn.org/cgi/reprint/161/9/835

Foy, J.M., Kelleher, K.J., Laraque, D.; for the American Academy of Pediatrics Task Force on Mental Health. (2010). Enhancing pediatric mental health care: Strategies for preparing a primary care practice. *Pediatrics, 125*, S87–S108. doi:10.1542/peds.2010-0788E

Foy, J.M., & the American Academy of Pediatrics Task Force on Mental Health. (2010). *Pediatrics, 125*, S109–125. doi:10.1542/peds.2010-0788F

Freeman, D.S. (2007, Fall). Blending behavioral health into primary care at Cherokee Health Systems. *The Register Report*, 32–35.

Gabel, S. (2010). Child and adolescent psychiatrists addressing the needs of underserved youth through technology and a new program model [Letters]. *Academic Psychiatry, 34,* 240–241. Retrieved from http://ap.psychiatryonline.org/cgi/reprint/34/3/240

Guevara, J.P., Greenbaum, P.E., Shera, D., Bauer, L., & Schwartz, D.F. (2009). Survey of mental health consultation and referral among primary care pediatricians. *Academic Pediatrics, 9*(2), 123–127.

Gunn, W.B., & Blount, A. (2009). Primary care mental health: A new frontier for psychology. *Journal of Clinical Psychology, 65,* 235–252.

Institute of Medicine (IOM). (2001). *Crossing the quality chasm: A new health system for the 21st century* [Electronic Version]. Washington, DC: National Academies Press. Retrieved from http://books.nap.edu/openbook.php?record_id=10027

Institute of Medicine (IOM). (2006). *Improving the quality of health care for mental and substance use conditions.* Washington, DC: National Academies Press. Retrieved from http://books.nap.edu/openbook/0309100445/gifmid/212.gif

Institute of Medicine (IOM). (2010). *The future of nursing: Leading change, advancing health.* Washington, DC: The National Academies Press.

Integrated Behavioral Health Project (IBHP). (2007). *Levels of integrated behavioral health care.* from http://www.ibhp.org/index.php?section=pages&cid=85

Integrated Behavioral Health Project (IBHP). (2009). *Partners in health: Primary care/County mental health collaboration tool kit* (1st ed.). San Francisco, CA: The California Endowment and the Tides Center. Retrieved from http://www.ibhp.org/uploads/file/IBHP%20Collaborative%20Tool%20Kit%20final.pdf

Leslie, L.K., Weckerly, J., Plemmons, D., Landsverk, J., & Eastman, S. (2004). Implementing the American Academy of Pediatrics attention-deficit/hyperactivity disorder diagnostic guidelines in primary care settings. *Pediatrics, 114,* 129–140. doi:10.1542/peds.114.1.129

Malouin, R.A., & Merten, S.L. (2010). *Measuring medical homes: Tools to evaluate the pediatric patient- and family-centered medical home* [Monograph]. Elk Grove Village, IL: American Academy of Pediatrics/National Center for Medical Home Implementation.

National Council for Community Behavioral Healthcare [NCCBH]. (2009). *Behavioral health/Primary care integration and the person-centered healthcare home.* Washington, D.C.: Author. Retrieved from http://www.thenationalcouncil.org/galleries/resources-services%20files/Integration%20and%20Healthcare%20Home.pdf

Newland, J.A. (2010). [Editor's Memo]. Our sphere of influence: Are we doing all we can? *The Nurse Practitioner, 35*(5), 6.

Patient Protection and Affordable Care Act of 2010, Pub. L. No. 111–148, 124 Stat. 119 (2010). Available at http://www.gpo.gov/fdsys/pkg/PLAW-111publ148/pdf/PLAW-111publ148.pdf

Pincus, H.A. (2003). The future of behavioral health and primary care: Drowning in the mainstream or left on the bank? *Psychosomatics, 44,* 1–11. Retrieved from http://psy.psychiatryonline.org/cgi/reprint/44/1/1

Preserving Patient Access to Primary Care Act of 2009, H.R. 2350, 111th Cong. (2009).

Rainwater, M. (2009, June). *Integrated primary care & behavioral health programs.* Paper presented at the meeting of California Mental Health Planning Council, San Jose, CA. Retrieved from http://www.ibhp.org/uploads/file/IBHPCAMHPlanningCouncilPresentation.pdf

Saur, C.D., Harpole, L.H., Steffens, D.C., Fulcher, C.D., Porterfield, Y., Haverkamp, R., Unutzer, J. (2002). Treating depression in primary care: An innovative role for mental health nurses. *Journal of the American Psychiatric Nurses Association, 8,* 159–167. doi:10.1067/mpn.2002.128680

University of Washington, Department of Psychiatry & Behavioral Sciences. (n.d.). *IMPACT key components.* Retrieved from http://impact-uw.org/about/key.html

Unutzer, J., Schoenbaum, M., Druss, B.G., & Katon, W.J. (2006). Transforming mental health care at the interface with general medicine: Report for the president's commission. *Psychiatric Services, 57,* 37–47. Retrieved from http://www.ps.psychiatryonline.org/cgi/reprint/57/1/37

U.S. Department of Health and Human Services, Office for Civil Rights. (2003). *Summary of the HIPAA privacy rule.* Washington, D.C.: Author. Retrieved from http://www.hhs.gov/ocr/privacy/hipaa/understanding/summary/index.html

Valleley, R.J., Kosse, S., Schemm, A., Foster, N., Polaha, J., Evans, J.H. (2007). Integrated primary care for children in rural communities: An examination of patient attendance at collaborative behavioral health services. *Families, Systems, & Health, 25,* 323–332.

Weiss, S.J., Haber, J., Andrews Horowitz, J., Stuart, G.W., & Wolfe, B. (2009). The inextricable nature of mental and physical health: Implications for integrative care. *Journal of the American Psychiatric Nurses Association, 15,* 371–382. doi:10.1177/1078390309352513

World Health Organization (WHO). (2008). *Integrating mental health into primary care: A global perspective.* Retrieved November 22, 2010, from http://www.who.int/mental_health/resources/mentalhealth_PCH_2008.pdf

25

Legal and Ethical Issues

Margaret Hardy and Sarah B. Vittone

Objectives

After reading this chapter, APNs will be able to

1. Identify specific ethical and legal foundations in clinical practice with children and adolescents in primary care.
2. Describe basic legal obligations of advanced practice nurses in primary care and associated ethical practice implications.

3. Apply legal and ethical principles in managing child and adolescent issues in primary care.

Introduction

The delivery of health care to children is heavily dependent on the relationships between the providers, the children, and their parents, guardians, and caretakers. Like all relationships, each participant brings his or her own personal values, moral agency, and expectations to the interactions. An understanding of the many factors that may impact the formation and maintenance of those relationships is an important first step in caring for children, in both the pediatric and the mental health setting. In addition, advanced practice nurses (APNs), as primary care providers of children, have a prevailing sensibility toward a "best interests" definition in planning care. In the ideal "shared decision-making model of care," the best interest plan for any child is the collaborative effort of the child, family, and the provider. It is with this consideration that this chapter speaks to specific issues frequently encountered in practice. Further, APNs provide primary care adhering to professional

obligations set by society to protect individual patients and families. These obligations are at the intersection of three points of view: first, as defined by certification and licensure (*legal*); second, through professional standards of practice (SOP) and boundaries as defined by nationally recognized authorities in evidence-based clinical practice (*clinical*); and third, as defined in professional ethics obligations (*ethical*). This chapter will introduce the legal and ethical considerations for the APN providing care to children in primary care settings and suggest methods for resolving practical concerns that confront the APN.

Description of the Issue

Historically speaking, society defines the scope and boundary of safe and acceptable practice in health care. Society changes current expectations of care and practice through legal case precedent as well as through professional deliberation and consensus building. Professional

---

Child and Adolescent Behavioral Health: A Resource for Advanced Practice Psychiatric and Primary Care Practitioners in Nursing,
First Edition. Edited by Edilma L. Yearwood, Geraldine S. Pearson, and Jamesetta A. Newland.
© 2012 John Wiley & Sons, Inc. Published 2012 by John Wiley & Sons, Inc.

nursing, through the American Nurses Association (ANA) *Code of Ethics* (2001), describes its mission as the prevention of illness, alleviation of suffering, and the promotion, protection, and restoration of health. This mission is accomplished through individuals and organizations attentive to social, ethical, and legal boundaries.

The legal status of children in the United States has undergone a major change in the last century but, in many ways, is still poorly defined in state and federal legislation. Laws such as those restricting the use of child labor and instituting compulsory education moved society away from a mindset that children were the property of their parents, to be treated as the parents saw fit. However, the extent to which children have autonomy in making life decisions, including those related to their health care, is not always clear and, in many cases, varies from state to state.

Historically, mental health services for children began as institutions, then transitioned over time to community programs and integrated systems. The institutionalization of children in the United States with mental "defect", disorder, or disability has been documented since the early 1780s. Court-ordered involuntary treatment was available only in inpatient settings until the mid-1960s when the expectation of "least restrictive environment" began to prevail. In the actionable case of Willowbrook State School in Staten Island, New York, children were institutionalized for mental "defect" from 1930 to 1987 without regard to their safety or therapeutic needs (Rothman & Rothman, 2005). Their deplorable care and use as research subjects stand out as an example to practitioners and consumers alike of the specific need for legislative protection of children. Through the study of the deinstitutionalization of these residents and children, we began to see the mainstreaming of children with disabilities, including those with behavioral health diagnoses, into schools as a continuing work in progress regardless of legislative requirements.

Community programs and school-based services have become a recommended standard of practice since the 1970s. Pediatric health and mental health needs are often overlapping but not addressed or met in any one program. Currently, children seen in primary care settings may be identified with acute or chronic behavioral health issues through general screening. However, poor funding, lack of adequately prepared health care providers, and poor or irregular utilization of services have impacted the overall health of these children. What is known is that intervention during childhood is key to limiting the growing population of emotionally, psychiatrically, and behaviorally disabled adults.

Finally, behavioral health, mental health, and mental illness are all used to identify the services described here.

It is in these names that stigma may arise for the child and the family. The APN must be aware and intervene to provide secure and private opportunities to reach children in need as well as to enhance their adherence to recommended treatment regardless of stigma.

Legal and Ethical Issues: Risks to Children

Our society views all children as a vulnerable population, to be afforded the highest protection and value. Individually, children may also fall within other at-risk populations, including the poor and impoverished, the disabled, those with learning difficulties, those in foster care or in dysfunctional families, the abused, and those with chronic or serious illness.

According to Hudspeth (2009), complaints received and investigated by boards of nursing generally fall into one of four categories: exceeding or some breach in scope of practice, drug diversion or problematic alcohol/substance use, ethical and moral issues or boundary violations, and other criminal activity outside of nurse practitioner (NP) clinical practice, such as assault (p. 366). The most common causes for NP disciplinary action were related to patient abuse, abandonment, and boundary violations (Hudspeth).

Health care professionals are obligated to comply with the laws and regulations that govern the scope of practice as defined by their state of practice. According to the National Council of State Boards of Nursing (ncsbn.org, 2010), the state board of nursing is the regulatory body for NPs in forty-seven jurisdictions. In 2008, five states including Alabama, Maryland, North Carolina, South Dakota, and Virginia reported sharing duties with their board of medicine, and two states, Nebraska and Rhode Island, have separate APN practitioner boards.

Ethical issues for children in the primary care setting cover issues related to their dependence as minors including adherence to appointments and treatment regimens, insurance constraints and access to health care, and quality of care; identification of safety issues related to physical, emotional, cognitive, and social abuse and neglect; as well as identification of developmental delays and other behavioral concerns, and guardians being misinformed about treatment options. All these issues may be influenced by the professional practice and ethical response of the health care providers and guardians.

Who Is the Client?

When the client is a child, the APN must consider the provider relationship within the legal relationship of the guardian. Fisher (2009) suggests that in addition to clarifying this question, another question should be posed. Due to at least two persons being in this relationship with the APN, the APN should consider what ethical obligations are owed to each person, a step beyond a single relational professional obligation. In behavioral health settings, where family involvement and participation may be a vital component of a child's treatment, it is important to clarify expectations and to be forthcoming regarding disclosure obligations and the confidentiality (or lack thereof) of information shared by the minor to the APN. When providing care to a minor (in most states, an individual under the age of eighteen years), the APN must keep in mind that most states permit minors to consent to the diagnosis and treatment of specific conditions, including mental health and substance abuse treatment, but state laws vary as to the minimum age requirement and the nature and extent of treatment to which they may consent (Vukadinovich, 2004). The cognitive developmental maturity of minors with regard to capacity in decision making is discussed later in the chapter.

Who Is the Guardian?

Essential to providing care to children is the identification of the person or persons with the legal right to have access to the child's health information and to make decisions on behalf of the child. In most instances, it is the parent(s) who has this right and responsibility. A provider cannot assume that that is the case, however. Client intake forms should ask for the identity of the child's guardian(s). In the event that someone other than a parent is identified, the provider should request a copy of the documentation appointing the guardian and defining the parameters of the guardianship. In some instances, parental rights may have been terminated at the time a legal guardian was appointed, for example, in cases of severe abuse or neglect. Such information must be clearly documented in the treatment record and communicated to members of the treatment team. Providers should obtain clarification from the child's legal guardian regarding the person or persons authorized to act on the child's behalf. APNs should be mindful of the fact that the person who accompanies the child to medical appointments, while perhaps not the legal guardian but a grandparent or babysitter, provides significant daily care and can be a valuable source of information for the provider.

Obligations of Children and Their Guardians

In the health care relationship, the client is obligated to provide accurate and truthful history and pertinent information to help inform the treatment. The child and guardian are obligated to participate in clinical planning of care and to make responsible decisions. They must be honest in reporting relevant clinical symptoms and adherence to treatment. The client must meet also financial obligations as discussed with the provider. These obligations and other expectations must be shared with the client at the beginning of the relationship and reviewed as necessary thereafter. Guardians must always act in the best interests of their children. As such, a child's guardian/decision maker/surrogate must be available at all times and is required to provide consent for treatment unless an emergency exists requiring immediate treatment. Guardians as surrogates for their children are obligated to provide care that relieves suffering, preserves and restores function, as well as improves the quality and extent of the child's life. The APN must be cognizant of the fact that guardians sometimes fail in their duties as guardians either intentionally, through neglect, as a result of poor communication, or through confusion. When the provider becomes aware of such a situation there are ethical and legal duties required of the provider in order to protect the child, including a possible report to Child Protective Services in accordance with state law and regulations.

Foundations for Practice: Legal

Duties to Patients

Each state defines the scope of practice for nurses within their state. Sometimes but not always referred to as Nurse Practice Acts, these rules are most often set in both laws and regulations adopted by the state. The specificity of the rules varies between states but generally describes the licensure requirements, practice parameters, and means and methods of disciplinary actions within the state. Because the scopes of practice for APNs vary widely between states, every APN must be familiar with his or her state's rules, copies of which are available from the licensing authority of each state.

In addition to state law, some APN activities are governed by federal law, to the extent that federal law has authority or jurisdiction over the specific activity. For example, federal law requires that APNs register with the Drug Enforcement Administration (DEA) prior to prescribing controlled substances. Health care reform, changing reimbursement schedules, consumer expectations, and simple supply and demand create constant flux in the laws and regulations that apply to APNs. Typically, APNs and the groups that advocate for them support the expansion of the APN role to permit more autonomy or a broader scope of practice, while other groups with conflicting interests oppose that expansion.

Duties to Others

When considering the duties of an APN, one generally thinks of the duties owed to patients for whom the nurse is providing care. The duties of an APN may reach beyond his or her patients, however, to third parties or to the general public. All fifty states have a law mandating the reporting of child abuse and neglect. These laws are in place to protect children but they are also required in order to qualify for funding under the Child Abuse Prevention and Treatment Act (CAPTA). Originally passed in 1974, CAPTA has been amended several times since then. CAPTA establishes threshold definitions for child abuse and sexual abuse, but individual states may choose to adopt more expansive definitions. While every state requires that certain professionals, including health care providers, report suspected child abuse, the extent of the knowledge that triggers the duty to report varies between states. For example, in some states, providers must report whenever they have a "reasonable cause to believe" that abuse has occurred, while other states require that providers report "known or suspected" abuse. CAPTA also requires that each state enact legislation that provides immunity from prosecution for reporting abuse. All states provide some form of immunity from criminal and civil liability for those persons who, acting in good faith, report suspected child abuse (U.S. Department of Health and Human Services [DHHS], Child Welfare Information Gateway, 2008). In a majority of states, reporters of child abuse are presumed to be acting in good faith.

In some circumstances, a provider may have a reporting duty to individuals other than his or her patients. In 1976, the Supreme Court of California recognized a health provider's duty to respond to potential danger that a patient might present to a third party. In *Tarasoff v. Regents of the University of California, et al.* (1976), the parents of Tatiana Tarasoff sued, among others, a therapist named Dr. Lawrence Moore for the murder of their daughter by Prosenjit Poddar. Two months prior to the murder, Mr. Poddar had confided to Dr. Moore that he intended to kill Ms. Tarasoff, who had refused Mr. Poddar's romantic advances. Dr. Moore contacted the police and reported the threat. The police detained Mr. Poddar and questioned him but released him when he appeared to be rational and promised to stay away from Ms. Tarasoff. Neither Dr. Moore nor the police, who were also sued, notified Ms. Tarasoff or her parents of the threats made by Mr. Poddar. Despite the fact that Dr. Moore had no patient-physician relationship with Ms. Tarasoff, had never met her, and had a duty to confidentiality to Mr. Poddar, the Supreme Court of California held that Dr. Moore had a legal obligation to take steps to protect Ms. Tarasoff from being harmed by Mr. Poddar.

Since the court's ruling in Tarasoff, a majority of states have enacted laws that impose a duty on health care providers, including APNs, in most cases, to take steps to protect third parties who may be in danger as evidenced by threats from patients. The laws define when the duty arises; for example, some states require only that the health care provider know that a potential danger exists, while others impose a duty to act only on threats that are directly communicated to the provider. In most cases, a provider can comply with the duty in several ways, including notifying the object of the threat, contacting the police, and hospitalizing the patient. Most states provide protection from malpractice or disciplinary actions for the provider resulting from a breach of the patient's confidentiality when taking action in good faith as required by the law; failure to comply with the law can result in either or both actions being taken against the provider (Geske, 1989).

In addition to the duties imposed by the Tarasoff-based statutes, some states also impose statutory duties on nurses to report other health care providers who may have violated the rules or regulations governing their practice. Depending on the state, the duty may include reporting health care providers who have been hospitalized for substance abuse or psychiatric conditions or have practiced in such a way to pose a danger to patients (Gafney, 2001).

Potential Liabilities for the Nurse

Like other health care providers, APNs can be and are sued for malpractice. While malpractice law varies to some degree by state, all malpractice cases have four basic elements (Physicians, Surgeons, and Other Healers, *American Jurisprudence*, 2002). The first of these elements is the presence of a duty that was owed by the provider to the plaintiff. This duty may arise from common law or from statutes like those based upon the Tarasoff case. For APNs, the duty may arise from direct care provided or from the supervision of others who provided care.

The second element in a malpractice action is negligence, defined as a breach of the standard of care by the health care provider. Such a breach goes beyond merely what may, in hindsight, have been an error but had been justified at the time. In order to rise to the level of a breach of the standard of care, a nurse's actions or inactions must have failed to comply with what a reasonable nurse would have done under the same or similar circumstances. Generally, expert testimony from a nurse is required in a malpractice action to establish the standard of care and to testify to the defendant nurse's compliance with the statute. It is important to note that the standard is based upon what a *reasonable* APN would have learned, known, and done, not on the particular APN being sued.

The third element in a malpractice action is harm to the patient/plaintiff that was proximately caused by the alleged negligence. Without that connection, a malpractice action cannot be established. Such a connection cannot be assumed based merely on the alleged negligence of the defendant nurse, but must be proved, usually through the use of expert testimony. For example, it may be negligent for an APN to fail to follow up on an abnormal laboratory result, but that negligent act may bear no causal relationship to the patient's adverse outcome.

The fourth and final element of a malpractice action is damages that resulted from the harm. Such damages can include pain and suffering, medical bills, and, in some cases, emotional or mental anguish. Although this element may appear to be very straightforward, disputes often arise as to whether specific damages were caused by the harm alleged, preexisted the alleged negligence of the provider, or were caused by contributory negligence of the patient or their guardian. Psychiatric mental health practitioners may be able to defend against malpractice claims or at least apportion the damages if it is shown that the client and/or their family caused some of the harm. An example of contributory negligence occurred when a patient's family violated the contraband policy, hid cigarettes and a lighter, and gave them to a patient who suffered cognitive impairments. The patient accidentally set their clothes on fire while smoking in a wheelchair and suffered third-degree burns. Self-harm such as cutting or suicide attempts are not generally considered to be contributory negligence if the potential for self-harm is one of the reasons for treatment. The courts are reluctant to impose liability for outpatient suicide attempts unless the patient was recently discharged without appropriate documentation of risk (Yorker, 1995). Psychiatric nurses who work with children and adolescents in group settings should also be aware that they may be liable for negligence if one patient harms another, e.g., sexual molestation or physical assault (Yorker, 1997).

Generally speaking, an employer is responsible for the negligent acts of employees. Therefore, hospitals, medical practices, and other employers are generally liable for acts of negligence by the APNs they employ, provided the APN was acting within the scope of his or her employment at the time of the alleged negligence. The APN may or may not be actually named as a defendant in the lawsuit. APNs, NPs, and registered nurse anesthetists are more frequently named individually as defendants in malpractice actions than registered nurses although their employers are also generally liable for their negligent acts (Negligence, *American Jurisprudence*, 2002).

APNs may be required by their employers to maintain malpractice insurance or the employers may provide such insurance. Insurance companies offer malpractice coverage to all levels of nurses, which includes coverage for both the cost of defending a malpractice action, as well as indemnity for any judgment that may be entered against the nurse. Adverse or unexpected outcomes are inevitable in health care. Fearing a malpractice suit or licensing complaint, the health care provider's first response to such an outcome is often avoidance—avoiding the patient and family and everyone else involved. In some situations, talking with the patient and family about the adverse outcome may diffuse the anger or mistrust that could otherwise result in a lawsuit or disciplinary action. The health care provider should carefully consider the information to be communicated, the method of the communication, and the individuals who should be included in the communication. Depending upon the nature and severity of the adverse event, or the patient's and family's reaction to it, it may be wise to seek the advice of a health care attorney.

Historically, expressions of sorrow or regret by a health care provider following an unanticipated outcome could be used against the provider in a subsequent malpractice action as an admission of negligence. However, a majority of states have now enacted legislation that protects health care providers who express sympathy to a patient or family after such an outcome (Ebert, 2008). Often referred to as "I'm sorry laws," the actual protections provided by such laws vary from state to state. For example, some states protect only verbal, not written, expressions by the health care provider. Other states protect only statements made within a certain period of time after the unanticipated outcome. Still other states protect expressions of sympathy, but not apologies. Every health care provider should be aware of whether his or her own state has such a law and, if so, what protections the law offers.

Disciplinary Actions

Each state nursing board has its own rules and regulations regarding the processing of complaints and the investigatory and disciplinary process. Complaints can be filed by patients or their family members, employers, colleagues and others, and in most cases can be made anonymously. Some disciplinary actions are initiated upon receipt by the state licensing board of a report that a malpractice claim against a nurse has been settled or resulted in a judgment entered against the nurse. The laws and/or regulations of each state specify those actions that may result in discipline being imposed against a nurse. Often, insurance policies that provide coverage for nursing malpractice actions also provide coverage for license protection, which may cover all the legal costs and fees associated with defending oneself in a disciplinary proceeding.

Facing a disciplinary action before the state licensing board is always difficult. The possibility of having disciplinary action taken against one's license is stressful enough, but nurses who find themselves in that situation should realize that the consequences of an adverse decision by a licensing board may have far-reaching consequences. Nurses who have disciplinary actions taken against their licenses may face discipline from other states in which they are licensed, which can be imposed administratively without the opportunity to defend themselves (Aspinwall, 2007). Depending upon the nature of the allegations, other consequences may include criminal prosecution, revocation of the provider's DEA registration number, and exclusion from participation in federal health care programs such as Medicare and Medicaid (Collins & Mikos, 2008). Because of the potential impact that a disciplinary action may have, it is important that nurses seek the advice of an experienced attorney when faced with a licensing complaint, even though the complaint appears to be without merit.

Importance of Documentation

Nursing schools stress the importance of documentation in practice, and for good reason. The medical record is one of the most important means of communication between health care providers. The documentation in an inpatient chart provides vital information regarding the plan of care, the implementation of that care, and the patient's response, as well as important historical information regarding the patient. In the primary care setting where multiple providers may be seeing the patient, the record is equally important. The record contains not only the documentation of the care provided in the office but also the record of communication with other providers who are involved in the patient's care.

Documentation takes on additional importance when a malpractice or disciplinary action arises. Nurses often hear the adage, "If it's not written, you didn't do it." Although in most cases a nurse would be permitted to testify during a malpractice action regarding care she provided but did not contemporaneously document, a document written at the time the care was provided, prior to any action being filed, obviously may be more persuasive and allow the nurse to avoid having to answer the question as to why if it was important enough to remember, but it was not important enough to document. While the time during which a patient has to file a medical malpractice action varies by state, years may elapse from the time a nurse provided care to a patient until the time she learns she has been named as a defendant in a malpractice action. By then, the nurse may have no independent recollection of the patient or the care provided. In those situations, a well-documented record may be crucial to defending the care.

Documentation can be equally important in disciplinary actions. Typically, a copy of the medical record is obtained during the investigation of any disciplinary action involving allegations related to patient care. Documentation that is clear, understandable, and consistent with the nurse's testimony will greatly assist the nurse in a subsequent disciplinary action. On the other hand, documentation that is missing or inaccurate may lead to additional allegations to which the nurse must respond.

It is often challenging to keep up with the documentation demands in a busy primary care setting. Providers who are overly concerned about the legal and disciplinary consequences of poor documentation may be tempted to focus more on that documentation than providing quality care. On the other hand, those who discount the importance of documentation may focus instead on providing care to the detriment of documenting that care. Neither of those extremes is appropriate. Providers must find the balance along that spectrum that fits their clinical setting, the care being provided, and the types of records being maintained.

Some general rules apply to nursing documentation, regardless of the clinical setting. Ideally, documentation should be contemporaneous with the provision of care. While that may not be realistic in every setting, it is important that care be documented as soon as possible after the care is provided. When circumstances require that late entries be added to the medical record, those entries should be clearly identified as having been added at a later time and dated and timed when actually made, while referencing the date and time of the care being documented. Entries should be patient-specific and nonjudgmental. Avoid entries in the record that reference family members or others, unless those entries are relevant to the care of the patient. To the extent possible, use direct quotes from the patient or guardian, rather than characterizing the patient using judgmental terms, such as describing the patient or family using terms such as "demanding" or "difficult." As more and more medical records are maintained electronically, the use of templates is increasingly common. Often, providers are given the option of choosing to import and repeat information recorded previously by other providers. APNs must be very careful not to import information that may not be accurate for their entry.

Foundations for Practice: Ethical

Health care ethics is the application of ethical philosophy and/or moral guidelines within health care situations. Philosophical motivation for ethical practice may include tenets of deontology, virtue ethics, utilitarianism, or an ethics of care. These theories may guide motivation in ethical clinical practice. Ultimately, it is the applied principles, as defined here, in ethical and moral values and guidelines that produce the most successful outcomes. Ethical and moral guidance define the motivation that produces "right or wrong" behavior. Moral guidance is generally formed by society through influence of values, culture, religion, and the law. Our society has accepted a moral code of conduct for individuals to exist peacefully. The values of honesty, dignity, integrity, compassion, fairness, self-control, and duty are generally appreciated in our society (Killinger, 2007).

Health care ethics adheres to applied principles for professional guidance specifically including autonomy, beneficence, nonmaleficience, and justice (Fletcher, Lombardo, & Spencer, 2005). More specifically, professional ethics are defined through codes of conduct within health care organizations and professional societies. Professional ethics for the APN is most broadly defined by the ANA *Code of Ethics (Code)* (2001) available at www.nursingworld.org. The ANA *Code* includes obligations to the patient's dignity through accountability, advocacy, respect, and a commitment of the nurse to the patient. Provisions in the ANA *Code* also articulate obligations to continue professional education, maintain professional integrity, and improve health care environments. In addition, APNs practice globally and in this respect should also embrace the four-part *The ICN Code of Ethics for Nurses* by the International Council of Nurses available at www.icn.ch/. The ICN publication identifies elements related to human rights, values, and customs and specifically identifies responsibility for supporting the health and social needs of vulnerable populations (ICN, 2006).

In the United States, professional nursing specialties speak to standards of practice and clinical concerns for children with behavioral health issues. These pertinent professional organizations include the American Psychiatric Nurses Association (APNA), the International Society of Psychiatric-Mental Health Nurses (ISPN), as well as the National Association of Pediatric Nurse Practitioners (NAPNAP). Yet these organizations *do not* propose separate codes of ethics for APNs, apart from the ANA *Code* (2001). Further, the most obvious ethical issues for APNs that are not addressed by the ANA *Code* include issues related to collaboration and consultation, clearly a role for the APN.

Yet, there has been discussion of this need. In 2004, Peterson and Potter considered that the mixed role of the NP with influences from both nursing and medicine required an APN code of ethics with mixed obligations. But, they further suggested that a standardized scope of practice must be defined prior to creating an advanced practice ethical code for nurses. As of yet, the scope of practice for the APN is still left to various state interpretations. There has been no movement for national standards for scope of practice at this time.

While ethical principles and professional codes are foundations for resolving ethical dilemmas, ethical dilemmas within health care are best resolved with thoughtful and careful reflection and may be best resolved through dialogue with colleagues. It is valuable to create professional relationships for reflection and discussion of common ethical concerns in practice. Ethics committees and consultants are available for conference on an individual case basis.

Moral Distress

Moral agency is generally defined as having the personal values for knowing the difference between right and wrong. The moral agent in a health care relationship will use personal values and the professional ethics as described previously to engage with clients. Nurses and APNs most commonly value the use of guiding principles of respect for persons (which include autonomy, individual rights and human dignity, confidentiality, privacy, veracity, and informed consent), freedom, equality, and justice. Decision making is a frequent action for an APN and yet this can be a difficult task depending on the nature of the client and the decision involved. Laabs (2007) considered issues of moral distress in nursing, contending that at some point in a morally distressing action (even in the face of patient autonomy and strong beneficence), the moral integrity of the nurse comes at odds with the personal self. Nurses' use of reflection and discernment may assist them in defining the limits of which their moral agency may be stretched. Laabs suggested that in the event that no successful resolution can occur, then the practitioner should be prepared to address what degree of personal moral distress would be acceptable. APNs must be prepared to draw the line between acceptable and unacceptable actions when asked to participate in morally distressing actions. Clearly there is a risk to the relationship with the client and in such, the APN must be clear about the role and in what situations the relationship is at risk. The American Association of Critical Care Nurses has developed a product, *The 4A's to Rise Above Moral Distress* Toolkit (2006), which APNs may find helpful.

Ethical issues common to APNs in primary care include insurance constraints, managed care policies, access to health care, quality of care, guardians being misinformed about treatment options, and APNs feeling caught between managed care rules and advocacy for the patient's care. When asked in a study by Ulrich et al. (2006), 47% of APNs and physician assistants admitted that patients had asked them to mislead insurers in receiving care. In an additional question, the respondents replied that insurance companies interfered with their ability to provide quality patient care.

Basic Professional Ethics Obligations

As derived from the above basic tenets of bioethical guidance, the basic professional ethics obligations for health care providers including APNs are derived from a principle of respect for persons and include:

- Informed consent
- Privacy and confidentiality
- Communication, truth telling, and disclosure
- Capacity of the client (in this case the minor and of the guardian)

These four areas have developed over time, historically defined by society through interpretation of the law, and creation of protections through new law (Rothstein, 2009). Ethical tenets through the ANA *Code* (2001) partner with the law to ensure that these basic obligations are upheld.

Complex Ethical Risks in Health Care

In health care, there are many areas in which society, health professions, and the law have been well defined, as in confidentiality and privacy. There are other areas that are less well defined, leaving room for interpretation by stakeholders. These complex areas include:

- Beginning of life concerns—reproduction, sterilization, genetic therapy, artificial reproductive technology, maternal-fetal conflicts
- End of life concerns—withholding and withdrawing life-sustaining therapy, refusal of indicated therapy, palliative sedation, euthanasia, and assisted suicide
- Relational issues such as patient sovereignty and paternalism
- Professional relationships related to managed care and fees
- Allocation of resources

The areas with specific implications when working with children and particularly with children in the behavioral health setting will be discussed later in the chapter.

Patient's Rights and Basic Obligations of Providers

With respect to ethical and legal foundations, all patients expect a certain degree of respect in the health care environment including their right to:

- Privacy
- Health information (medical records)
- Make their own health care decisions
- Informed consent
- Refuse treatment

These rights and obligations are founded in the ethical and legal frameworks as defined in society (Rothstein, 2009). They are generally accepted and may be without written standards. In addition, the APN as a primary health care provider should disclose the nature and length of the health care relationship and the expected outcome of the relationship. The APN is obligated to provide honest disclosure of information received from third parties (referrals). Documentation must be timely and available as the information within is owned by the patient. The APN who collaborates with other medical services and makes and/or receives referrals relating to this patient must be open and disclose such to the patient. Fair billing practices and information related to billing and payment should be confidential and timely. The patient seeks your care as safe, expert, and qualified in this specialty. Information about your practice should be readily available to your patient population.

Sovereignty vs. Abandonment

Patient sovereignty is a model of a health care relationship in which the patient directs the clinical care and may request or demand therapy, medication, and treatment (Cohen & Cesta, 2005). The APN may consider withdrawal from the case for conscientious objection or refuse such demands by patients based on scientific SOP. An APN is not to be forced, coerced, or compelled in any way by the patient, family, colleague, or the court to provide interventions or treatment to patients that the provider considers unsafe or inappropriate. The provider should make every effort to educate the patient/family as to the standard of care. Yet, in the event of an impasse, the patient's care should be transferred to another qualified provider. The APN must, however, take the steps necessary to transfer the care to another provider, including the transfer of treatment records.

Implications for Practice

While the following concepts are based in legal and ethical foundations, the application of such in the clinical setting will be considered, including

- Confidentiality/right to information/disclosure
- Decision making
  - Capacity/competence
  - Informed consent
  - Right to refuse treatment
- Involuntary treatment
- Restraint
- Reproductive treatment

Confidentiality and the Right to Information

Like other health care providers, nurses who fall within the definition of covered entities under the Health Insurance Portability and Accountability Act (HIPAA) of 1996 (DHHS, n.d.) must comply with the HIPAA Privacy Rule of 2002. The basic premise behind the HIPAA Privacy Rule—that patients have a right to privacy in their personal health information—is nothing new. The right to patient confidentiality has long been recognized in statutory and common law and is an emphasized part of nursing education at all levels. While HIPAA does not provide for private causes of action by patients for violations, meaning that a patient cannot sue a provider for a HIPAA violation, providers can face significant civil and criminal penalties for violations of the Privacy Rule. In addition, the circumstances of a violation may also be sufficient to establish a basis for civil liability under state law.

Between the Privacy Rule's compliance date in April 2003 and the end of 2009, over 48,000 complaints of HIPAA violations were received by the DHHS Office of Civil Rights, the agency responsible for investigating such complaints. Over 80% of those complaints have been resolved. Of those, more than half were determined to be ineligible for enforcement, either because (1) the activity complained of did not violate the rule, (2) the complaint was untimely, withdrawn, or not pursued by the complainant, or (3) the Office of Civil Rights lacked jurisdiction under HIPAA, such as complaints regarding an activity that preceded the compliance date for the Privacy Rule or complaints made against an entity not covered by the Privacy Rule. Approximately 5,000 of the complaints received were investigated and resulted in a finding that no violation had occurred. The remainder or approximately 20% of the complaints that have been resolved resulted in some enforcement activity, which can include substantial civil and criminal penalties for more egregious violations. The most commonly investigated issue is the impermissible use and disclosure of protected health information; the most common type of covered entity that has been required to take corrective action is private practice.

In addition to the federal Privacy Rule, most states have their own laws protecting the confidentiality of patient information. Since 2003, many of those laws have been amended to be consistent with the requirements of the HIPAA Privacy Rule. When considering confidentiality issues, it is helpful to keep in mind that a patient's health information belongs to the patient. As such, patients are entitled to access to their own information, unless there is reason to believe they could be harmed by it. The release of confidential information to anyone other than the patient or, in the case of a minor, a legal guardian must fall within the definition of a permitted or authorized disclosure. Generally speaking, health care providers are permitted to use and disclose information to the extent necessary for purposes of (1) treatment, including the release of information necessary for consultations and follow-up with other providers, (2) payment, including the submission of bills to insurers, and (3) health care operations, such as quality review, without the express consent of patients or their representatives. In some instances, state and federal law not only permit but require that information be disclosed when necessary for public health or safety reasons, such as the reporting of child abuse or certain communicable diseases. Other exceptions exist for complying with court orders, such as a subpoena for medical records, protecting third parties from patients who may present a danger, and certain law enforcement purposes. In situations where the disclosure of information is not permitted or required under state or federal law, a patient or someone permitted to act on his or her behalf must authorize the release of medical information.

Generally speaking, privacy laws recognize the right of a parent to access the health information of his or her child. As described above, however, in some instances a biological parent may not be the legal guardian of the child and may no longer have the right to obtain or authorize the disclosure of the child's health information. Whenever custody and/or guardianship of a child has been transferred to someone other than the parent, health care providers must make sure that the treatment team is aware of the person or persons who are entitled to access the child's information and that the medical record clearly reflects that right to access.

It is important to remember that access to medical information includes more than just a copy of the medical record; it includes verbal communications from health care providers, as well. Health care providers must also be mindful of the risk of unintended disclosure of information, such as the potential compromise to an adolescent's confidentiality by billing a parent's health insurance for treatment sought by the adolescent without the parent's knowledge.

When working with children in the behavioral health setting, it is important to establish clear policies and procedures for maintaining the confidentiality of patient information that are both consistent with state and federal law and understood by the patient, to the extent possible. While certain protections must be in place for all private health information, health care providers must recognize and be able to respond to unique situations. For example, the HIPAA Privacy Rule permits a parent to agree that a minor child may obtain confidential treatment. The HIPAA Privacy Rule also permits a covered health care provider to choose not to provide parental access to a child's health care information if the provider is concerned about abuse or harm to the child. The HIPAA Privacy Rule imposes very specific requirements for written authorizations for the release of medical information. Those requirements include a description of the relationship of the person authorizing the release to the patient, when signed by someone other than the patient.

Problem Solving and Decision Making

Problems within the context of health care require sensitivity and care. Each problem may have ethical as well as legal components in which resources may be sought to provide support and direction. The provider must weigh the outcomes from each element of an individual decision. The final decision making comes down to the provider and the guardian in a shared decision-making model seeking the best interest of the child as the outcome. The provider must collaborate with the guardian to seek the most successful outcome for the child with respect to the family as well. There must be consideration of evaluating the benefits and burdens of treating and not treating the child. The provider and guardian must consider the physical and emotional effects of treatment on the child, any pain or suffering that might be involved, any effect of the treatment on the child's life expectancy, and the potential for recovery and restorations, with and without the treatment. The indications, risks, side effects, and benefits of the treatment are included in the consent process. Finally, the decision overall should be based on family goals and values as reflected in previous health care decisions.

Independent providers, such as APNs, must consider routine methods for solving problems including using peers and mentors to voice concerns and to seek guidance. The APN may have access to organizational ethics committees or consultants who may provide assistance in difficult matters. When in a leadership position with staff, the APN should seek the input of all clinical parties with concerns so as to gain any pertinent or additional information necessary to formulate a solution.

General models for solving ethical problems are similar to clinical problem solving methods such as collecting data, considering possible outcomes, and deriving a best outcome through engaging the appropriate persons for decision making. When ethical principles are at risk or have been violated outright, some of the various elements may be considered using the following method. The following model was developed and used in practice by one of the authors:

1. Identify the clinical and personal data—engage the client and family in their perspective related to the clinical data. Clarify the client and the guardian.
2. Consider the needs of the client and others with ethical standing including the health care team and the family.
3. Identify the ethical principles with potential or actual violations—a moral diagnosis. Consider basic obligations as well as more complex issues. Use principles and an ethical code to evaluate and support successful options. Articulate your concerns in the medical record and in person to the client and guardian.
4. For each problem, identify a goal or outcome and set of implementation strategies.
5. If there is no desirable outcome possible or there is an impasse, consider the least burdensome outcomes and strategies. If necessary, consider legal options and consult with legal counsel.
6. Evaluate the context and situational data that led to the problem. Identify any preventative strategies that could have been used and report such to those in authority.

Capacity and Competence

There is a presumption of competence in the law (Physicians, Surgeons and Other Healers, *American Jurisprudence*, 2002). Adult guardians and those over the age of majority are presumed competent and capable of making health care decisions for their children when engaged in the elements of consent and the decision-making process. The determination that an individual guardian is incompetent, and therefore incapable of giving informed consent, is a judicial one. Concurrent with a determination of incompetence is the appointment of a guardian to serve as the individual's legal representative. When the practitioner is concerned about the soundness of a guardian's decision making or whether the guardian is acting in the best interest of the child, it may be necessary to seek the input from another guardian, if one exists, or obtain guidance from a child protective agency or a court, if the situation warrants such intervention.

When creating a sensitive professional relationship with a young child or adolescent, the provider may be motivated to allow this child some latitude in participation in decision making, based on the child's developmental age. It is at this time when the APN and guardian support the young person in their growth, playing a more active role in their care. Specifically, the adolescent has the right to a protected period in which to develop his or her decision-making skills (Mercurio, 2007). The basic four elements of capacity include the ability to understand the information being presented, the ability to communicate and appreciate the decisions and reason between options, using personal values (Fletcher, 2005). Young children are capable of participating in decisions at a basic threshold showing some evidence of choice. As the child matures, the child is more able to identify a reasonable outcome in order to base a choice. As the child matures, the child will base a choice on rational reasons and then will begin to show evidence of understanding. Finally, as an adult, the child is able to exhibit actual understanding.

When assessing the child for developmental capacity in decision making, consider a developmental assessment of cognitive and social elements. Assess the child for cognitive development, their use of preoperational versus concrete versus formal operations (Piaget & Inhelder, 1969). The child must be able to form an understanding of hypothetical reasoning as in the formal operations in order to participate fully in weighing options in decisions. Further, the APN should consider elements of information processing including attention span and memory in the child. Capacity assessment of a child should also consider a social assessment looking for examples of conformity versus nonconformity behavior, examples of identity development, identification of personal values and resiliency, and previous experience with decisions (McCabe, 1996). Children over fourteen years of age but under the age of majority who are developmentally capable should be engaged in all disclosure elements. The guardian and APN should consider an individualized threshold for participation in decision making. Children of the ages seven to fourteen years should be engaged in disclosure to their level of capacity for participation but should use strictly an assent/dissent model with regard to plan of care. If the plan is not to be disclosed to the child, the provider should document the nature of the decision. Finally, children as they approach the age of majority may be engaged by the practitioner and guardian to enact a psychiatric advanced directive (PAD) to specify their wishes for therapy should their ability to participate in the decision making be impaired related to their mental health or other reasons.

Informed Consent

One of the first and most fundamental steps in providing care to any patient is obtaining informed consent of the patient, or someone authorized to act on behalf of the patient. In the case of a minor child, we usually assume it is the parent who must provide that consent, and in most instances, that is true. In fact, the Fourteenth Amendment of the U.S. Constitution protects the fundamental right of parents to make decisions concerning the care, custody, and control of their children. That right is not absolute, however, and it may be waived or supplanted by circumstance or government action.

As a general rule, parents must provide consent for the treatment of a child until the child reaches the age of majority. One exception to that rule is created by a change in the legal status of the child. Most, but not all, states have laws in place that permit a minor to become emancipated, thereby separating the minor from the control of his or her parents and relieving the parents from responsibility for the minor. An emancipated minor has the legal right to consent to treatment, regardless of the parents' wishes (Parent and Child, *American Jurisprudence*, 2002). The procedure and requirements for becoming emancipated vary between the states that permit it but can result in documentary evidence of emancipation. A health care provider should not act on the belief that a child is emancipated without a copy of that evidence. In addition to legal emancipation, some states recognize the rights of homeless minors and/or those fitting the statutory definition of mature to consent to medical treatment.

State and federal law creates other exceptions to the rule of parental consent. For example, a minor has the right to obtain HIV testing in every state without having parental consent. Depending upon the state, minors may also have the right to seek testing, counseling, and treatment for other conditions, such as pregnancy, sexually transmitted disease, sexual assault, substance abuse, and mental health issues. A health care provider offering any of these services to minors should know the laws of his or her state regarding parental consent and have clear policies and procedures in place for when these issues arise.

Another exception to the need for parental consent arises in the case of an emergency. If a minor presents to a health care provider in need of emergency treatment, the parents are deemed to have given "implied consent" for that treatment (Parent and Child, *American Jurisprudence*, 2002). It is the same concept that allows health care providers to render treatment to patients who are unconscious; there is an assumption that the patient or parent of the patient would consent to the treatment if he or she were able to do so. Obviously, there can be disagreements over what constitutes an emergency. Generally speaking, if the patient is at risk for serious harm or death without immediate treatment, the implied consent rule applies. If, however, treatment can be delayed until someone with the authority to provide consent can be contacted, without harm to the patient, efforts should be made to obtain consent.

Even in the absence of any of the exceptions described above, the issue of parental consent is not always simple. In the case of divorced or unmarried parents, the parent with legal custody is authorized to provide consent. Health care providers cannot assume that the parent with physical custody also has legal custody. Therefore, before consent to treatment is obtained, the parent with the legal right to provide that consent must be identified. For some children, there may be a guardian or governmental entity, such as a department of social services, that has the right to consent to treatment, not the biological parents. In those instances, the health care provider must obtain documentation describing the parameters of the parental rights that have been transferred to the guardian or entity and what, if any, rights the biological parents continue to have.

Once the person authorized to provide consent is identified, the next step is to provide the information necessary to allow an informed decision. Such information generally includes the indications for, the risks and benefits of, and the alternatives to the proposed therapy. The depth of the information to be provided is dependent, in large part, on the nature of the proposed therapy. Various standards for disclosure are described in practice, but the "reasonable person standard" is most widely accepted. Significant risks, likely side effects, and those therapies that require invasive procedures also require that more information be given to the guardian in advance. It is important that children and their guardians be given the opportunity to ask questions and obtain clarity regarding the proposed therapy. Consent for more complex or invasive procedures should be written, along with documentation of the information provided. Finally, the consent must be voluntary without undue influence based on the decision maker's value system.

Right to Refuse Treatment

Inherent in the concept of informed consent is the right to withhold consent. The right to refuse treatment is based upon more than just the doctrine of informed consent, however. The right of a patient, or in the case of a minor, a guardian, to refuse treatment is also rooted in the constitutionally protected right to privacy (*Cruzan v. Missouri Department of Health*, 1990). In most instances, declining to consent to treatment is, in essence, a refusal

of treatment and absent an emergency of some sort, the matter is closed. Situations do arise, however, where public policy or safety override one's right to refuse certain treatment. In the behavioral health setting, situations most often involve patients who are deemed to be a danger to themselves or others and in need of involuntary detention and treatment by means of a civil commitment. The standards for involuntary commitment are established by state law, but most require some degree of immediacy of the threat of self-harm or harm to others. The more difficult situations often involve the refusal of treatment that may be vital, even lifesaving, in the absence of immediate danger or any suicidal or homicidal threat. News stories have detailed the accounts of parents who have refused treatment for their children on religious or other grounds. In some instances, providers have petitioned the courts for the right to treat without the patient's or parents' consent; in other instances, the state has assumed legal custody of the child to ensure that treatment was given. Some courts have upheld the patients' and/or parents' rights to refuse treatment, regardless of the likely outcome of that refusal. Each of these situations is fact-specific and the options available to the health care providers dependent on state law. It is important in each of these situations, however, that the treatment team work together, with input from an ethics committee, if available, and legal counsel to determine the best course to take.

Involuntary Patients

In the case of court-mandated outpatient therapy (MOT) or inpatient treatment, the APN must provide the assessment and therapy as defined by the involuntary commitment and the provisions of the state Nurse Practice Act. Much of the recent trend in involuntary therapy is in the outpatient environment. Guardians and children must be informed with full disclosure of the nature of this order and the consequences. Nonadherence to therapy recommendations is common in clinical settings but in the case of children in involuntary therapy, nonadherence must be documented and reported to the legal authorities. Clearly, adherence to the appointment schedule and medication therapy are crucial, as would be attendance in a school setting and group sessions outside the provider's supervision.

Chemical or Physical Restraint

In the event that a child must be restrained or put into seclusion, there must be clear documentation of the danger to self, and the provider must assess and agree with the need. It is preferable that therapeutic holding be used should the situation require it. Yet, the provider must follow state law and organizational policies governing the restraint of minors, including any disclosure to the guardians and to the patient. Restraints should be limited and appropriate with respect to the escalation and danger and removed as soon as the child has regained control and the provider's assessment deems it so. Emergency restraint may be applied if necessary to protect the child while the appropriate medical care or provider is en route. This must be time-limited and the child must be informed of the safety and concerns requiring the restraint throughout (Baren et al., 2008). Documentation in the narrative is valuable to the review of the care during a restraint or seclusion episode.

Reproductive Issues

Providing reproductive care and advice to minors presents a special challenge for health care providers. Although the days of forced sterilization are long past, the pendulum has not swung so far as to permit minors full autonomy in making decisions regarding reproductive issues. Most states have laws concerning a minor's rights to birth control, but the specifics of those laws vary between states. Fewer than half of the states permit minors to obtain contraceptive services without restrictions, although some of those states permit the health care provider to notify the parents without the consent of the minor. A few states permit only married minors to obtain contraceptive services without parental consent, while others require only a determination that the minor is mature. As with many aspects of health care governed in whole or in part by state law, it is essential that providers who prescribe contraceptive services to minors familiarize themselves with the laws of their state.

Implications for Research

Historically research with children has had some unfortunate outcomes as exemplified by Willowbrook (Rothman & Rothman, 2005). While there are requirements based on individual institutional review boards (IRBs) as well as federal and other funding agencies, according to Emmanuel, Wendler, and Grady (2000), there are seven requirements that ethical research must satisfy, including:

1. Value—for the knowledge from the work itself
2. Scientific validity
3. Fair subject selection
4. Favorable risk-benefit ratio
5. Independent review
6. Informed consent
7. Respect for the enrolled subjects

Further, with the enrollment of children in studies, specifically within the behavioral health context and with respect to informed consent (proxy consent), researchers need to include the child in a process of "informed assent." Assent has been recognized historically within clinical and research areas for adults and children. The American Academy of Pediatrics (AAP) published their findings and recommendations for assent in 1995 (which were reaffirmed in 2006); these recommendations have been widely referred to since. Securing assent for the child's participation in a research study, especially when the study outcome has a low benefit impact for the child, is in the general sense securing an agreement by the child to participate. The information shared with the child should include age-specific language and a brief explanation of the child's role as a subject. The child must be informed that she/he can stop participation whenever she/he needs to and that any questions she/he has will be answered. The child should also understand that there is no penalty for not participating. Further, a lack of disagreement by the child does not indicate an agreement or assent to participate (AAP). The child's assent should be in conjunction with the guardians' consent. Guardians must be confident that participation is consistent with the child's interests and values. In relation to proxy consent, caution should be used when the actual individual benefit is low and the risks or uncertainty of risks/benefits are unknown. Guardian consent as proxy for the child should also be scrutinized for obvious power influences, that is, persuasion by the guardian (Coyne, 2010). APNs who serve as primary investigators should not enroll their own clients for obvious influential persuasion. The research team and process should include many checks and balances to ensure that respect for subjects includes options for subjects to opt out, for subjects to gain information as gleaned from the study, and for subjects to be given information about harms or benefits during the course of the study (which may influence their willingness to continue).

Implications for Education and Continuing Education

Continuing education of practitioners is a professional obligation as stated in the ANA *Code* (2001) as well as legally required by many state boards of nursing. It is recommended that an official review of licensure, scope of practice, and change in state statute occur annually as part of routine continuing education. Ethical issues that arise from legal precedent and various other avenues should be reviewed annually as well. One of the core competencies in *The Essentials of Master's Education for Advanced Practice Nurses*, originally stated by Shugars,

O'Neil, and Bader, is the ability for all health professions' graduates to "provide counseling for patients in situations where ethical issues arise, as well as participate in discussions of ethical issues in health care as they affect communities, society and the health professions" (as cited in American Association of Colleges of Nursing [AACN], 1996, p. 9). Ethical decision making may be enhanced through the networking with peers and colleagues and should be encouraged especially where APNs practice in solo and further in rural and remote areas.

Accreditation of Educational Programs

Several nursing organizations recommend content for undergraduate and graduate curricula related to ethical and legal knowledge and application. Content at the baccalaureate level should include professional values including altruism, autonomy, human dignity, and integrity, as well as social justice (AACN, 2008). Additional material should include ethical and legal frameworks, professional accountability, and the ANA *Code of Ethics for Nurses* (2001). Legal information at the undergraduate level should include Nurse Practice Acts and scope of practice. Ethical content for the undergraduate should also include moral agency, privacy, confidentiality, self-reflection, and professional accountability. Content for graduate programs specific to ethics should include identification and analysis of ethical dilemmas, decision-making process, personal and organizational perspectives, conflict of interest, dilemma resolution, and professional accountability (AACN, 1996, 2011). Surprisingly, there has been no mention of legal content or education recommendations. This seems to be an oversight on the part of the graduate recommendations where scope of practice and liability issues are accentuated due to the independent role of the APN.

Implications for Primary Care—Ethical Situations

Primary care has in its nature the true basic relationship of provider to client and client to provider in a total trusting relationship based on integrity, altruism, and loyalty by both parties. The provider is required both ethically and legally to document an accurate reflection of the assessment, diagnosis, plan, therapy intervention, and an evaluation of such. The relationship in most instances is ongoing and this continuity is a basic foundation for both. In part due to the private nature of this relationship, ethical concerns are generated. Jeremy Sugarman in 2000 published *Twenty Common Problems: Ethics in Primary Care,* which provides more detail referred to here. In this section we will consider additional primary care issues including:

- Requests for nonindicated therapy and tests
- Requests for medical exemptions and privileges
- Adherence to therapeutic regimen
- Managed care
- Conflicts of interest and obligations
- Consultation and referral
- Request for therapy outside of the client relationship

Requests for Nonindicated Therapy and Tests

The concept of patient sovereignty as expressed previously lends itself to the issues for providers in which the client and/or family requests therapy or tests that are not indicated. While the provider is obligated to engage the client and guardian in a collaborative plan of care, the APN should not shirk professional liability and acquiesce to the requests of clients that are not clinically indicated. Should the issues of power be so forceful, the provider with support of beneficence and nonmaleficence must insist on following clinically sound judgment, decline to prescribe the requested therapy, and, if necessary, assist the client in obtaining a second opinion and /or transfer the care to another provider.

Requests for Medical Exemptions and Privileges

Similarly, with regard to clients and guardians requesting medical exemptions and privileges, the APN is supported through sound clinical judgment and ethical tenets of beneficence and nonmaleficence in a decision to decline from providing exemptions or privileges to patients upon their request. This is common in caring for children who must frequently miss school or sports activities for health reasons, and yet in missing those activities, the APN is accountable for the health of the child. The APN should use sound judgment when considering such requests and work collaboratively with the family as a unit.

Adherence to Therapeutic Regimen

Adherence to medical recommendations can be complicated when working with clients who are children. Many times the lack of adherence to therapy may be a result of the child's inability to cooperate, the guardian's inability to follow therapy based on finances, or perhaps even a misunderstanding of instructions or the like. Nonadherence can have significant implications: (1) it can be dangerous for the client not to take prescribed medications; (2) it can cause the provider to misinterpret clinical assessment and (3) perhaps even make further unnecessary recommendations based on misinformation. Interventions for children who are not adhering to therapy includes an evaluation of the home setting and guardian's ability to provide the care required, including making appropriate follow-up appointments and being at the appointments on time.

Managed Care

Managed care and the role of primary providers have led to various issues for clinicians in maintaining access to patients balanced with sound clinical practice. Previously, it was a common practice to provide care as available without regard for cost. It is the accountable professional who will provide beneficent clinical sound care while taking into account the cost to the society as a whole. For example, diagnostic procedures that will provide information that will not be used in treatment planning need not be performed. Information for the sake of information is not necessary. Sabin in 1994 addressed four rules for primary providers that were particularly valuable and have been extrapolated now for use within the APN's practice. First, the APN should view her dual duty as advocating for both the individual patient and other patients in the group by resource decisions. Second, always use the least expensive treatment unless there is substantial evidence that a more expensive treatment will be more effective. Third, spend some time reviewing the rules and practices of the managed care plan to assure the practices are fair. Finally, if the plan does not provide reimbursement for a therapy the provider believes would be beneficial, the provider should discuss the therapy, including the clinical indications, benefits, and costs, with the guardian to allow the guardian to make an informed decision on how to proceed.

Conflicts of Interest and Obligation

Clinicians have primary duty to their clients; in the case where a provider's own interests conflict with such, an ethical conflict exists. Conflicts of interest as identified by Goold (2000) included investment in medical facilities, reimbursements for services, gifts from commercial or industry (pharmaceuticals), industry sponsorship of research, pursuit of nonmonetary goods (power, reputation), and peer pressure. Goold also identified conflicts of obligations as in clinical research, educating clinicians in training, needs of other patients for more time, and family needs. In considering the implications of these conflicts, the APN should consider the following questions: Is the conflict avoidable or unavoidable? Is the conflict reasonable or unreasonable? What is the strength or intrusiveness of the conflict on the relationship and client trust?

Consultation and Referral

APNs as primary providers may have opportunity to refer or consult with other APNs, physicians, or other specialists related to the care of their clients. This stems from an ethical responsiveness to nonmaleficence. If the APN deems that she or he is not the best suited to diagnose or treat the client, then the APN must in an intention of "do no harm" engage another, more-qualified clinician for the client. Employment concerns over self-referral or fee splitting are valid in these times where health care organizations are often large and can be an obvious referral empire. The client must be aware of financial relationships that the APN or the organization may have. Clients should be offered a choice where possible related to referrals.

Request for Therapy Outside of the Client Relationship

This is a common request known as the "curb side" consult or "neighbor" friendly advice. In this relationship, the APN is not engaged in a professional relationship and should therefore be cautious about providing treatment or opinion for persons and children for whom there is no assessment or history taken or implications for relational veracity between this person and the APN. Further, documentation of this type of interaction would be unlikely and may cause then further moral, ethical, or legal conflict for the APN. An obvious exception to this would be in the event of urgent or emergency care for a person's life and safety.

Case Exemplars

It is the hope of these authors that the material presented here is applicable to your practice and will be beneficial to your client base in a successful practice. The following two cases are presented along with the various actual and potential risks and violations or legal and ethical foundations. The resolution to each case is obviously dependent on many variables. Outcomes should be based on best interest standards with the balance of burdensome outcomes in the negative. Further, it should be noted that legal and/or ethical consultation may be warranted. Table 25.1 contains definitions of terms used in chapter.

Concept Illustration 1

This example involves disclosure of information to a minor. In this type of challenge, the guardian requests the clinical diagnosis or perhaps the rationale for medication being withheld from the child/adolescent. The primary legal concerns are related to a potential breach of duty to the patient. If the patient is a minor, the patient relationship is to both the guardian and the minor. As the primary provider, it is your obligation to be clear about the impact of nondisclosure of vital information and the liability that may be incurred for doing so. Further, the ethical concerns for this type of nondisclosure includes a risk to dignity of the child, risk

Table 25.1 Glossary of ethical and legal terms

Term	Definition
Assent	In the case of categorical or functional incapacity, this is the general agreement to understanding and agreement to cooperation with treatment by the minor child. Informed consent is required from the guardian.
Autonomy	An ethical principle that is derived from a principle of respect for persons. Persons have the right to self-determination and choice about actions that impact their life and livelihood.
Benefits/ Burdens Balance	Desired outcome in ethically challenging decisions, with benefits outweighing burdens for the identified client as well as others with ethical standing.
Beneficence	An ethical principle that intends that actions will promote good.
Best Interest	An ethical standard for decision making used with clients who have not reached mature adult capacity or competence. Best interest is generally thought to be best defined by the family and gradually by the child as he/she matures. In health care, the primary provider has considerable influence in defining this through the collaborative nature of the relationship with the child and family.
Capacity	A clinical assessment for capability to make independent decisions. Adults achieve a categorical definition of capacity by age of majority. Childhood as a category is defined as incapacitated. Elements of capacity include an ability to understand, communicate, reason, and appreciate the information/decision being considered with a set of personal values. Threshold for capacity required for certain decisions may be flexible depending on the significance of the decision.
Confidentiality/Privacy	Derived from a principle of respect for persons in which personal information shared in any form with any person representing the health care relationship may not be repeated or disclosed except by the client who owns all personal health information in any form.
Conflict of Interest	A situation in which a provider's interests, whether professional, personal, economic, or otherwise, conflict with that of the patient.
Deontology	A moral philosophy credited to Immanuel Kant in which the moral actions are based on specific moral duties or obligations. More recent use of this philosophy incorporates use of a variety of duties and with these an evaluative nature of consequences in order to achieve a balance or right over wrong.
Disclosure	An element of informed consent in which information pertinent to the decision is shared with those involved with the decision. The content of the disclosure may be based on various standards including the professional standard and the reasonable person standard. Disclosure should include nature of the therapy, purpose, risks, benefits, and alternatives.
Dissent	In the case of categorical or functional incapacity, this is the general agreement to understanding and disagreement to cooperation with treatment. Informed consent is required from the guardian.
Ethic of Care	While similar in foundations to feminist ethic, this ethical theory is based on relationships and engages communication and cooperation as strategies for problem solving. This theory does emphasize sensitivity and emotion, and while this is a valid motivator for clinical practice, its use in challenging decision making is limited.
Ethical Dilemma	A potential or actual violation of an ethical principle with regard to an individual client in a health care relationship, whether intentional or unintentional; with actual or potential for burdensome outcome.
Ethical Standing	Also referred to as moral standing or ethical right, it is the claim by someone other than the legal guardian that their perspective or information is valuable to the care of the patient. This may be a consistent caregiver in the case of a child.
Feminist Ethic	A contextual theory that highlights the relationship of the provider and the client with regard to actions from a sense of justice and care. Decision making itself in the health care arena is embedded in this relationship, and for this reason this theory does not provide specific guidance in decision making—more in the context of the relationship usually specific to power and vulnerable groups.
Fidelity	An ethical value in a trusting relationship from which loyalty and accountability is derived.

(continued)

Table 25.1 (cont'd)

Term	Definition
Informed Consent	Derived from the principle of respect for persons; an ethical ideal with intended outcome to engage the person to make efficient and effective decisions with regard to beneficial outcomes as defined by the person. Elements generally include a voluntary and capable decision maker (capacity), as well as the adequate disclosure and comprehension of information.
Integrity	A self-actualized set of values including accuracy, honesty, and truthfulness as a professional in clinical practice and professional relationships.
Justice	A general ethical principle that intends that actions are fair with equal impact and outcome. In health care, specifically, distributive justice as a principle considers the allocation of scarce resources such as access to providers and outpatient therapy.
Least Restrictive Environment	One of six principles included in the protection of students with disabilities as defined by the Individuals with Disabilities Education Act (2004), which is interpreted that children with disabilities should be included in classrooms with nondisabled students to the extent possible.
Malpractice	Professional misconduct; the failure to exercise the degree of skill and education that would be expected of a reasonable professional in the same situation.
Moral Distress	With respect to health care professionals, this anguish may not only be professional but also personal and may violate one or more various personal values of self-defined moral agency. This distress may not be an ethical dilemma for the client but rests solely as dilemma for the professional.
Negligence	The failure to act as a reasonable person would act under given circumstances, or the taking of action that a reasonable and prudent person would not.
Nonmaleficence	An ethical principle that intends that actions will not cause harm.
Paternalism	An ethical principle for which the practitioner makes independent clinical treatment decisions without the input of the client or with disregard of the client's input.
Patient Sovereignty	Power demanded by the patient to make clinical requests for care regardless of the practitioner's judgment in the health care context.
Professional Ethics	In health care professions certain societal obligations of a caregiver are paramount including a duty to help; that actions will promote health and palliate illness and distress.
Power	A dynamic force at work in relationships, as a result of individual perception and conflict of authority. This force may be overt or discrete. In the case of an imbalance, the individuals may choose to address this and resolve it or not. The choice to address the imbalance is dependent on the obligation of the individual to advocate for an outcome.
Respect for Persons	A principle highly valued in Western society in which human beings are highly valued as individuals and in that various principles and values are derived including self determination, autonomy, privacy, and veracity.
Shared Decision-Making Model of Care	This blends respect for autonomy and clinical expertise as defined by both clinicians and other persons. The success of treatment plans depends on the adherence and motivation of the client as well as the expertise and flexibility of the provider.
Truth Telling/ Veracity	Derived from a principle of respect for persons. Disclosure with fundamental intent on sharing information as well as meaning and recommendation; this differs from "telling the truth" which may be described as sharing only the most comfortable knowledge with a trend toward paternalism. This may be to individual clients or in professional relationships.
Utilitarianism	A moral theory credited to Jeremy Bentham and John Stuart Mill in which the morality of an action is based on its consequences moreover that the balance of good outweighs any costs.
Virtue Ethics	An ethical theory that is based in the character of the person and their actions based in this character. Virtuous behavior is motivated by such values as honesty, kindness, fairness, and loyalty. Decision making is not from principles or obligations but from the person's sense of value in personal virtues. This theory, while providing motivation in clinical practice, is difficult to apply to an ethical dilemma.

to the assent rights of the child, risk or violation of your obligations to provide disclosure and for the client to receive disclosure, risk to a beneficent outcome though collaboration between provider/guardian and child and the potentials for an autonomy breach, veracity breach, and for abuse of confidentiality. Each of the risks and potential risks to the ethical relationship are real and for your consideration in each individual case. Specifically, withholding the information from the child may impact his or her ability for self-care as well as readiness to participate in the plan of care.

Concept Illustration 2

This example involves the guardian identified as at-risk for noncompliance/nonadherence with the minor's care. In this challenge, the provider is concerned about noncompliance or nonadherence with the child's therapeutic regimen and, with this, creating a nonconducive relationship with the clinician. The legal concerns here relate mostly to a potential for bad outcome giving rise to a malpractice claim or disciplinary complaint. It is the obligation of the clinician to consider possible implications for noncompliance including lack of resources, knowledge limitations, and poor continuity/follow-up. Further, the ethical concerns in the case relate to a risk to professional integrity, potential risk to abandonment of client, potential risk to beneficence in therapy outcomes, risk to collaboration in therapeutic relations, and potential risk for maleficent outcomes. It is the obligation of the clinician to maintain the relationship with the client to the end that a therapeutic outcome can be achieved successfully. If this is not the case, the provider should consider alternative options for referral to a skilled provider to ensure that the child receives successful therapy in collaboration with the guardian. If the guardian appears to be disinterested in participating in a way that serves the child's best interest, the provider may have a legal and ethical obligation to engage others who share guardianship responsibility or report the situation to the local child protective services agency.

Summary

The APN providing care to children in the pediatric or mental health setting has a unique relationship to his or her patients, one that presents both great opportunity and great responsibility. While it is essential for the APN to always consider the best interests of the child, he or she is often confronted with diverse, and sometimes competing, interests. The APN must have an understanding of the potential legal and ethical challenges that may arise, and be cognizant of the way in which his or her own personal values and ethical code of practice may impact decision making and interactions with patients, families, and colleagues. Establishing procedures and protocols that are based on sound clinical practice and compliant with state and federal law and regulations are a critical first step. Knowledge of what, when, and where to document information not only is important clinically but also necessary for sound risk management. While unexpected outcomes are inevitable in health care, a practice that incorporates sound clinical decisions, respect for patients and their families and guardians, and an awareness of one's ethical and legal obligations provides a solid foundation to enable one to respond appropriately when dealing with those outcomes. When a provider is confronted with a situation that presents ethical or legal challenges that are unusual or beyond the experience of the provider, it is important that the provider reach out for guidance. Depending upon the situation, colleagues, ethical advisors, and/or a health care attorney may be able to provide valuable support to assist in protecting both the interests of the patient and the provider.

References

American Academy of Pediatrics [AAP], Committee on Bioethics. (1995). Informed consent, parental permission, and assent in pediatric practice. *Pediatrics, 95,* 314–317.

American Association of Colleges of Nursing [AACN]. (2008). *The essentials of baccalaureate education for professional nursing practice.* Washington, DC: Author. Retrieved from http://www.aacn.nche.edu/Education/pdf/BaccEssentials08.pdf

American Association of Colleges of Nursing. (1996). *The essentials of master's education for advanced practice nurses.* Washington, DC: Author. Retrieved from http://www.aacn.nche.edu/Education/pdf/MasEssentials96.pdf

American Association of Colleges of Nursing. (2011). *The essentials of master's education in nursing.* Washington, DC: Author. Retrieved from http://www.aacn.nche.edu/education-resources/MastersEssentials11.pdf

American Association of Critical Care Nurses, Ethics Work Group. (2006). *The 4A's to rise above moral distress toolkit.* Aliso Viejo, CA: Author.

American Nurses Association. (2001). *Code of ethics for nurses with interpretive statements.* Silverspring, MD: Author. Available at http://www.nursingworld.org

Aspinwall, T. (2007). Preventing the cascade: Dealing successfully with the collateral consequences of professional discipline. *Journal of Nursing Law, 11,* 75–79.

Baren, J., Mace, S., Hendry, P., Dietrich, A., Goldman R., & Warden, C. (2008). Children's mental health emergencies: Part 2. *Emergency Department Evaluation and Treatment of Children with Mental Health Disorders, 24,* 485–498.

Child Abuse Prevention and Treatment Act of 1974 (CAPTA), 42 U.S.C. §5101 et seq. (1974).

Cohen, E. & Cesta, T. (2005). *Nursing case management: From essentials to advanced practice applications* (4th ed.). St. Louis, MO: Mosby.

Collins, S. & Mikos, C. (2008). Evolving taxonomy of nurse practice act violators. *Journal of Nursing Law, 12,* 85–91.

Coyne, I. (2010). Research with children and young people: The issue of parental (proxy) consent. *Children & Society, 24,* 227–237.

Cruzan v. Missouri Department of Health. 492 U.S. 261, 271 (1990).

Ebert, Robin E. (2008). Attorneys, tell your clients to say they're sorry: Apologies in the health care industry. *Indiana Health Law Reiew, 5,* 337.

Emmanuel, E., Wendler, D., & Grady, C. (2000). What makes clinical research ethical? *Journal of the American Medical Association, 283,* 2701–2711.

Fisher, M. (2009). Replacing "who is the client" with a different ethical question. *Professional Psychology: Research and Practice, 40,* 1–7.

Fletcher, J., Lombardo, P. A., & Spencer, E. M. (2005). *Fletcher's introduction to clinical ethics* (3rd ed.). Hagerstown, MD: University Publishing Group.

Gafney, T. (2001). *Regulation of Nursing Practice* [The Nursing Risk Management Series]. Silverpring, MD: American Nurses Association Continuing Education. Online at http://nursingworld.org

Geske, M. R. (1989). Statutes limiting mental health professionals' liability for the violent acts of their patients. *Indiana Law Journal, 64,* 391–399.

Goold, S. (2000). Conflicts of interest and obligation. In J. Sugarman, *Twenty common problems: Ethics in primary care* (pp. 93–102). New York, NY: McGraw-Hill.

Hudspeth, R. (2009). Understanding discipline of nurse practitioners by boards of nursing. *Journal for Nurse Practitioners, 5,* 365–371.

International Council for Nurses. (2006). *The ICN code of ethics for nurses.* Geneva, Switzerland: Author.

Laabs, C. A. (2007). Primary care nurse practitioners' integrity when faced with moral conflict. *Nursing Ethics, 14,* 795–809. doi. 10.1177/0969733007082120

Killinger, B. (2007). *Integrity: Doing the right thing for the right reason.* Montreal, Quebec: University Press.

Mercurio, M. R. (2007). An adolescent's refusal of medical treatment: Implications of the Abraham Cheerix case. *Pediatrics, 120,* 1357–1358.

McCabe, M. (1996). Involving children and adolescents in medical decision making: Developmental and clinical considerations. *Journal of Pediatric Psychology, 21,* 505–516.

Negligence. In *American Jurisprudence* (2nd ed., 57B, §1106). (2002).

Parent and Child. In *American Jurisprudence* (2nd ed., 59, §792). (2002).

Peterson, M., & Potter, R. (2004). A proposal for a code of ethics for nurse practitioners. *Journal of the American Academy of Nurse Practitioners, 16,* 116–124.

Physicians, Surgeons, and Other Healers. In *American Jurisprudence* (2nd ed., 61, §§158, 167, 287). (2002).

Piaget, J., & Inhelder, B. (1969). *The psychology of the child* (2nd ed.). New York, NY: Basic Books.

Rothman, D., & Rothman, S. (2005). *The Willowbrook wars: Bringing the disabled into the community.* New Brunswick, NJ: Transaction Publishers.

Rothstein, M. (2009). The role of law in the development of American bioethics. *International Journal of Bioethics, 20,* 73–84, 110–1.

Sabin, J. (1994). A credo for ethical managed care in mental health practice. *Hospital Community Psychiatry, 45,* 859–860.

Sugarman, J. (2000). *Twenty common problems: Ethics in primary care.* New York, NY: McGraw-Hill.

Tarasoff v. Pregents of the University of California, et al., 551 P, 2d 334 (1976).

U.S. Department of Health and Human Services. (n.d.). *Summary of the HIPAA Privacy Rule.* Retrieved from http://www.hhs.gov/ocr/privacy/hipaa/understanding/summary/index.html

U.S. Department of Health and Human Services, Child Welfare Information Gateway. (2008). *Immunity for reporters of child abuse and neglect: Summary of state laws.* Retrieved from http://www.childwelfare.gov/systemwide/laws_policies/statutes/immunity.cfm

U.S. Department of Health and Human Services, Office for Civil Rights. (n.d.). *Health information privacy: Enforcement data.* Retrieved from http://www.hhs.gov/ocr/privacy/hipaa/enforcement/data/index.html

Ulrich, C., Danis, M., Ratcliffe, S. J., Garrett-Mayer, E., Koaiol, D., Soeken, K. L., & Grady, C. (2006). Ethical conflicts in nurse practitioners and physician assistants in managed care. *Nursing Research, 55,* 391–401.

Vukadinovich, D. M. (2004). Minors' rights to consent to treatment: Navigating the complexity of state laws. *Journal of Health Law, 37,* 667.

Yorker, B. (1995). Liability issues for nurses who work with psychiatric mental health patients. *Journal of Nursing Law, 2,* 7–20.

Yorker, B. (1997). Institutional liability for children who molest other children. *American Professional Society on the Abuse of Children-Advisor, 10,* 9–15.

26

Evidence-Based Nursing Practice

Donna Hallas and Elizabeth Bonham

Objectives

After reading this chapter, APNs will be able to

1. Describe current issues related to the implementation of evidence-based practice in pediatric and adolescent primary care and mental health practice settings.
2. Describe the significance of using evidence-based practice in clinical settings.
3. Describe the evidence-based process for use in clinical practice settings:

   a. Formulate clinically relevant PICO questions.
   b. Describe strategies to search for the best available evidence.
   c. Discuss the use of critical appraisal tools in the evidence-based process.
4. Identify national and international resources in order to provide care to clients and their families using best available evidence.

Introduction

Evidence-based medicine (EBM) was first described by Sackett, Rosenberg, Muir Gray, Haynes, and Richardson in 1996: "Evidence-based medicine is the conscientious, explicit, and judicious use of current best evidence in making decisions about the care of individual patients. The practice of evidence-based medicine means integrating individual clinical expertise with the best available external clinical evidence from systematic research" (p. 71). The underpinnings of this work have been the analysis of the results of research studies conducted to examine the efficacy of interventions and treatments using an experimental treatment and control group design. Included in the description of evidence-based practice (EBP) was the concept of considering patient preferences in the decision-making process (Sackett, Straus, Richardson, Rosenberg, & Haynes, 2000).

EBM has evolved into an EBP framework that has been embraced by nursing, the social sciences including psychology, and other allied health professions. Evidence-based nursing has adopted Sackett et al.'s definition of EBM. Thus, nurses make clinical decisions on the basis of the best available current research evidence, his or her own clinical expertise, and the needs and preferences of the patient (Melynk & Fineholt-Overholt, 2010).

Implementation of EBP requires a commitment from each health care provider to search for and use the best available evidence to establish the diagnosis and care management plans for each patient encountered in every practice setting. For each pediatric patient, implementation includes assessing the preferences of the child and

---

Child and Adolescent Behavioral Health: A Resource for Advanced Practice Psychiatric and Primary Care Practitioners in Nursing,
First Edition. Edited by Edilma L. Yearwood, Geraldine S. Pearson, and Jamesetta A. Newland.
© 2012 John Wiley & Sons, Inc. Published 2012 by John Wiley & Sons, Inc.

family members and incorporating these preferences into care management plans to achieve optimum health care for each individual and family.

Analysis of the interrelatedness of primary health care and the mental and emotional health care for each patient encountered in primary care and mental health settings is a new endeavor for pediatric nurse practitioners (PNPs), family nurse practitioners (FNPs), psychiatric nurse practitioners (PMHNPs), or psychiatric clinical nurse specialists (PMHCNSs). Collaborative practice between these providers has the potential to improve the care provided to each child, adolescent, and family with a focus on both the physical and emotional care. Pediatric, family, and psychiatric practitioners (referred to as advanced practice nurses [APNs] throughout this chapter) who understand the significance of these interrelationships are able to enhance their care management plans through critical analysis of the best available evidence for both primary care management and the mental health care management of patients.

This chapter describes current issues related to the implementation of EBP for APNs in their individual and collaborative practices. The steps for implementing EBP in practice settings are presented. National and international resources for using EBP in primary and mental health practice settings are also highlighted in Table 26.1.

Table 26.1 Evidence-based resources

Agency for Healthcare Research and Quality; http://www.ahrq.gov/

AGREE collaboration; http://agreecollaboration.org/

American Academy of Child and Adolescent Psychiatry (AACAP); http://www.aacap.org

American Academy of Pediatrics (AAP); http://www.aap.org

American Psychiatric Association (APA); http://ww2.psych.org/MainMenu/PsychiatricPractice/PracticeGuidelines_1.aspx

Clinical trials; http://clinicaltrials.gov/

Cochrane Collaboration; http://www.cochrane.org

DARE of Abstracts of Reviews of Effects (DARE); http://mrw.interscience.wiley.com/cochrane/cochrane_cldare_articles_fs.html

Joanna Briggs Institute; http://www.joannabriggs.edu.au

National Guideline Clearinghouse; http://www.guideline.gov

National Health Services Critical Appraisal Skills Program (CASP); http://www.casp-uk.net/

PubMed; http://www.ncbi.nlm.nih.gov/pubmed/

Significance of Implementing Evidence-Based Practice

APNs who continuously raise relevant evidence-based formatted questions (see information in this chapter under Evidence-Based Process), analyze each phase of the evidence-based care management process, and use the best available evidence for each clinical decision to provide care that is scientifically based. EBP is based on the use of interventions for which there is consistent scientific evidence showing that the interventions improve health care outcomes (Drake et al., 2001). When patient preferences are integrated within the clinical decision-making process, patients achieve improved health care outcomes (Ganz, 2002). Thus, APNs who incorporate EBP for each patient encounter have the potential to significantly improve patient outcomes, patient satisfaction with their care, and the overall physical and emotional health of their patients.

Comparison of Evidence-Based Practice to Traditional Clinical Practice

The fields of evidence-based mental health practice and evidence-based pediatric primary care practice are in the earliest stages of development and refinement. Most practicing practitioners were educated as passive learners in a traditional teacher-directed lecture format. Clinical experiences included observing an experienced clinician perform an assessment and design a treatment plan based on what was learned in an educational program. Students would then return demonstrations and reiterate treatment plans. The more complex, puzzling cases would be discussed, and students and practitioners would consult textbooks for answers to their questions and search for an exemplary case study to explain the clinical findings and determine a treatment plan.

Practicing in an evidence-based classroom and clinical environment is considerably different. Faculty, preceptor, and clinical mentors are facilitators of learning and are expected to embrace student and clinician inquiries, offering students and clinicians opportunities to explore all diagnostic and treatment possibilities for an individual patient presentation. Students and clinicians are expected to be active lifelong learners who critically question everything and search for the best available literary evidence to diagnose and treat the pediatric and adolescent patient and family. Textbooks are resources but database searches for the best available evidence are daily occurrences in an EBP environment. In clinical EBP environments, new and experienced clinicians who have embraced the EBP practice model explore established and intentional inquisitive processes to design treatment plans for patients that include individual patient preferences as well as expert opinion. In contrast, in a traditional practice environment, while patient preferences are considered, the patient is most often given a provider-designed treatment regimen and is expected to be "compliant" with the treatment plan. There is considerable evidence that traditional treatment plans are most often ineffective with less-than-ideal health care outcomes for children, while using an evidence-based approach in practice has improved health care outcomes (Jones, 2009).

The Evidence-Based Process

The evidence-based process for clinical practice includes using the following strategies: (1) develop the relevant clinical question in PICO format; (2) search the databases for systematic reviews of the literature, meta-analyses, practice guidelines, and randomized controlled studies or case studies that address the clinical question; (3) appraise the literature using CASP tools or the AGREE Tool (for practice guidelines); (4) combine the best available evidence, the APN's clinical expertise, and patient preferences to make and implement the practice decision; and (5) evaluate the clinical decision (Melynk & Fineout-Overholt, 2010).

Formulating Relevant Clinical (PICO) Questions

Successful implementation of the evidence-based process in clinical practice is dependent on formulating a relevant clinical question, using a format commonly referred to as a PICO question. The PICO mnemonic refers to the following: Population (P), Intervention (I), Comparison (C) intervention, and Outcome (O) (Melnyk & Fineout-Overholt, 2005). PICO questions emerge directly from clinical practice during daily encounters with patients and their presenting problems. Raising relevant PICO questions is an integral component of clinical practice in the EBP process and requires APNs to develop an "inquiring mind"—where everything is questioned, researched, and evaluated throughout the clinical decision-making process. The outcome is rendering care based on the best available clinically based research evidence.

Identifying the population of interest is a necessary first step in formulating a relevant clinical question. By defining the specific population, the database search will be narrowed and more precise. An example of a population is: "children with a diagnosis of attention deficit hyperactivity disorder (ADHD)." Once the population is identified, the APN questions which interventions (I) are based on the best available evidence for treatment, i.e., medications versus therapy for management of children with ADHD, thus comparing (C) the two interventions

to determine the best management (O) for the child with a particular presenting problem.

To summarize, the final PICO question is: "In children with a diagnosis of ADHD (P), is medication management (I) more effective than therapy (C) in improving the child's focus in school (O)?"

Searching for the Best Available Evidence

To find the best available evidence, practicing APNs must develop two essential new skills: (1) the ability to conduct database searches based on the PICO question and (2) the ability to understand and use techniques for critical appraisal of the research evidence identified in the database searches. Ideally, practicing APNs and all clinicians should have access to a health science librarian to help with the database searches. However, lack of access to librarians and or university libraries is not a barrier to implementing EBP. APNs can perform searches in some databases that are free to the public and readily available on the Internet.

The U.S. government offers EBP treatment guidelines at the National Guideline Clearinghouse (guideline.gov). The Clearinghouse is an initiative of the Agency for Healthcare Research and Quality (ahrq.gov) and provides outcomes research information. Outcomes research seeks to acquire an understanding of the end results or outcomes for specific health care practices and interventions. Outcomes research provides information about risks, benefits, and treatment results so that informed decisions are made by the clinician, the patient, and the family. Last, outcomes research is directly related to the quality of care provided to an individual and family. In addition to these web sites, the U.S. government offers the results of ongoing government clinical trials (clinicaltrials.gov).

The Cochrane Collaboration (cochrane.org) has established standards for reviews of medical, health, and mental health treatments. The Cochrane Collaboration also provides systematic reviews of the research literature.

Another excellent free Internet resource is PubMed (available at ncbi.nlm.nih.gov/pubmed). PubMed contains more than 19 million articles from MEDLINE and other science journals, making it an invaluable resource for all clinicians using an EBP model to deliver high-quality care to each client.

The American Psychiatric Association (APA) provides a number of practice guidelines for use by clinicians. Their web site can be found in Table 26.1 along with other evidence-based resources. Part A of each APA practice guideline is first published in a supplement to the *American Journal of Psychiatry*. The APA web site is an excellent resource to search for practice guidelines and current practice parameters including excerpts from the Diagnostic and Statistical Manual of Mental Disorders-IV-TR (DSM-IV-TR; APA, 2000) and the planned new edition of the DSM-V scheduled for 2013.

The American Academy of Pediatrics (AAP) web site (aap.org) provides an excellent resource for the assessment, treatment, and management of children's physical health issues. The American Academy of Child and Adolescent Psychiatry (AACAP) web site (aacap.org) also provides exemplary mental health resources for providers and families.

It is best to start a search with the databases that contain clinical practice guidelines since an answer for the clinical PICO question often can be found within five minutes of beginning the search, a significant advantage for an APN in a busy practice environment.

The best available evidence can be found in the literature as critically appraised synopses; systematic reviews and meta-analyses of randomized controlled trials (RCTs), and clinical practice guidelines (DiCenso, Guyatt, & Cilika 2005; Melynk & Fineout-Overholt, 2010). If none can be found for the PICO question under investigation, then the next best available evidence is from at least one RCT (randomized control trial). If an RCT is not available, then the best evidence may be case studies and/or reports based on expert clinical opinions, both of which are considered lower levels of evidence.

APNs with access to a health science university library can search multiple databases simultaneously. Efficient, refined searches can also yield results in these databases in less than five minutes. Two commonly used databases are CINAHL and MEDLINE. Searches on these databases can be refined using Boolean search strategies in which "AND" and "OR" are used between the keywords that are being searched. Mileham (2009) provides a helpful discussion on how to do a literature search as well as a list of commonly used databases.

Searching for an Answer to Our PICO Question

As you recall, our PICO question exemplar is: "In children with a diagnosis of ADHD, is medication management more effective than therapy in improving the child's focus in school?"

Searching the National Guidance Clearinghouse using the keywords "ADHD AND Medication Treatment" provided seven relevant articles in less than one minute. Searching PubMed using the same keywords provided fifty-four articles. Searching the Cochrane Library using the keywords "ADHD AND Medication Treatment" provided six relevant articles. Searching the AAP web site for our PICO question immediately retrieved a journal article that assessed the use of practice guidelines for these children (pediatrics.aappublications.org). Likewise, searching the APA web site (aap.org) for answers to our PICO question provided numerous up-to-date references for review by APNs and all health care providers.

Thus, several options are available to APNs to search for the best available evidence including free government-sponsored web sites that provide access to practice guidelines. However, once this evidence is identified, the APN must critically appraise the evidence to determine if the particular practice guideline or specific evidence "fits" the PICO question that is under investigation and the population in the APN's practice setting.

Understanding the Evidence

Systematic reviews of the literature were defined by Evans and Kowanko (2000) as "scientific tools which are used to summarize and communicate the results and implications of otherwise unmanageable quantities of research" (p. 35). Systematic reviews of the literature examine the best available evidence for a specific clinical question and the particular methods used. A systematic review of the literature provides a thorough search of the primary studies that pertain to the question. Furthermore, systematic reviews communicate and summarize study results and make recommendations based on the findings.

If a systematic review of the literature is not available, a search for a meta-analysis should be conducted.

Table 26.2 Rating system for hierarchy of evidence

Level of Evidence	Type of Evidence
Level 1	A systematic review or meta-analysis of all relevant randomized controlled trials (RCTs), or evidence-based clinical practice guidelines based on systematic reviews
Level II	At least one well designed RCT
Level III	Well designed controlled trials without randomization
Level IV	Well designed case control or cohort study
Level V	Systematic reviews of descriptive and qualitative studies
Level VI	A single descriptive or qualitative study
Level VII	Opinion of authorities and/or reports of expert committees

Reprinted from Melynk & Finehout-Overholt, 2010, with permission from Lippincott, Williams & Wilkins

Table 26.3 Summary of filtered and unfiltered evidence

Type of Evidence	Description	Filtered Information *	Unfiltered Information **	Evaluation
Systematic Review	Authors raise a specific question, perform a comprehensive search of all available literature, review the materials from the search, set particular criteria for acceptance or elimination of the studies from the systematic review, determine the levels of evidence in the study, and often make recommendations for practice based on the outcomes of the analysis	Yes	NO	CASP Tools
Critically Appraised Evidence (referred to as synthesized evidence)	Authors evaluate and synthesize multiple research studies based on a particular topic	Yes	No	CASP Tools
Critically Appraised Individual Articles	Authors evaluate and provide a synopsis of one article	Yes	No	CASP Tools
Randomized Controlled Trial (RCT)	An experimental test for a new treatment or intervention includes random assignment to treatment or control group, and a large and diverse sample	No	Yes	"The gold standard" Evaluates for rigor in research design CASP Tool
Cohort Study	A study that focuses on a particular subpopulation	No	Yes	Evaluates for rigor in design
Case Controlled Study	A study of one individual case	No	Yes	Evidence is not sufficient to make recommendations for practice
Expert Opinion	No formal studies are available. Recommendations are based on the opinions of experts. The opinion may be made by one individual or a group of experts	No	Yes	Evidence is not sufficient to make recommendations for practice

*Filtered information has been appraised formally
** Unfiltered information has not been formally appraised

A meta-analysis is a powerful research methodology that uses statistical techniques to combine results from different studies that have addressed the same clinical question. A meta-analysis provides a quantitative estimate of the overall effect of the intervention under study for the desired outcome (McGraw-Hill, 2002). A meta-analysis provides a more powerful estimate and conclusion of the effects of the proposed interventions since several studies are included in the meta-analysis rather than just one study (Cannon & Boswell, 2007; Mileham, 2009).

Melnyk and Fineout-Overholt (2010) rate evidence from systematic reviews and meta-analyses as Level I, or the most reliable evidence, on the hierarchy of evidence. This rating indicates that these reviews have examined relevant randomized clinical trials (RCTs), long considered the gold standard of empirical evidence. Table 26.2 contains the hierarchy of evidence for all seven levels of evidence. Table 26.3 provides a summary of filtered and unfiltered evidence. Filtered evidence is evidence that has been critically appraised by researchers and includes systematic reviews of the

Table 26.4 Levels of evidence for assessing practice guidelines

A	The recommendation is strongly recommended for a specific population or condition
B	The intervention is recommended for eligible populations
C	No recommendation can be made for the intervention
D	Not recommended for the population
I	Insufficient evidence to make any recommendations

Reprinted with permission from the National Guideline Clearinghouse, retrieved October 4, 2010, from http://www.guideline.gov

literature, authors who evaluate and synthesize multiple research studies, or authors who have evaluated an individual research study. Unfiltered evidence has not been critically appraised and includes randomized controlled trials, cohort studies, case reports, and expert opinions. Table 26.4 provides descriptors for assessing practice guideline evidence. Other reviews include integrative reviews and narrative reviews. Integrative reviews synthesize and generalize a set of studies, while narrative reviews are more subjective and describe study results written in trade or lay publications.

Evidence-based experts from Canada rate critically appraised evidence referred to as synthesized evidence or synopses rather systematic reviews. Synthesized evidence is a critical appraisal of multiple research studies based on a particular topic that has been evaluated and synthesized by a group of expert authors/researchers (DiCenso et al., 2007).

Finally, clinical practice guidelines are a mechanism to transform knowledge—that is, results from individual studies into a clinical protocol from the systematic research reviews (Brown, 2009). Practice guidelines may be institution specific, which by definition limits generalization to other populations and contexts but works well for the facility. Practice guidelines may be developed by expert clinicians who, after systematic reviews, develop guidelines for a professional organization (e.g., ACAPN Guidelines for Care and Practice). These are accessible to the public and other practitioners.

To summarize, using the PICO question: "In children with a diagnosis of ADHD (P), is medication management (I) more effective than therapy (C) in improving the child's focus in school (O)?" as an exemplar, the literature search revealed a practice guideline from the AAP that was developed from a systematic review of the literature (Level 1 evidence) (AAP, 2000, 2001). Thus, the systematic review, Level 1 evidence, specifically addresses the PICO question.

Evaluating the Evidence through Critical Appraisals

A critical appraisal of a research article (i.e., systematic review, RCT, or practice guideline) that the APN is considering implementing in practice assures that the evidence is not flawed and may be appropriate for implementation in her or his practice. Several questions are considered during the critical appraisal including: Is the research population consistent with the population of patients in my practice? Was the research methodologically sound and rigorous by design? What were the study results? Were the results valid? Will the results benefit my patients? (DiCenso, Guyatt, & Ciliska, 2005; Melynk & Fineout-Overholt, 2010).

The National Health Services Critical Appraisal Skills Program (CASP) provides tools that can be used for appraising the different types of studies (National Health Services, 2001). The CASP tools are available (see Table 26.1 for evidence-based resources). Using the CASP tools, the research evidence is judged for credibility, clinical significance, and applicability (Brown, 2009). Study results are reviewed for credibility. For example, are the results from one study similar to another? If not, a knowledge gap may be identified or flawed methodology may be determined.

Reviewing a study that uses a quantitative methodology requires a different appraisal than reviewing a study that uses a qualitative methodological approach. In addition, clinical practice guidelines and integrative research reviews result in evidence that impacts a clinical population with the appropriate intervention. When results demonstrate clinical significance, the results are sizable enough to make practical differences and demonstrate validity (Brown, 2009; Salmond, 2007).

Finally, applicability is determined by implementing the study findings in the practitioner's own setting. The study recommendation or intervention works well for the APN when the evidence from the study being implemented "fits" the APN's setting, the client population, and institution (Stetler, 1994). Other components that are in place for applicability include feasibility (the setting result is similar to the study result), safety (few risks are identified for the patient), and expected benefits for improved patient outcomes.

Practice Guidelines

Practice guidelines are developed as mechanisms to ensure that a certain intervention for a particular population will have the desired outcome, which, in turn, will result in better care as well as a best practice. While there is no standardized way of developing a practice guideline, there are similarities in their development. Brown (2009) describes a twenty-two–step method for producing evidence-based clinical practice guidelines. After a comprehensive search of the literature, the best available evidence for the research (PICO) question under investigation is systematically examined, categorized by the levels of evidence (see Table 26.2 for hierarchy of evidence), analyzed, and then recommendations for practice are presented in the guideline based on the review of the best available evidence and expert opinions.

For the PICO question, "In children with a diagnosis of ADHD (P), is medication management (I) more effective than therapy (C) in improving the child's focus in school (O)?", the AGREE Tool (agreecollaboration.org) should be used to critically appraise the AAP practice guideline for the diagnosis and treatment of school-aged children with ADHD. The analysis of the practice guideline with the critical appraisal tool revealed that the practice guideline met the criteria for an EBP guideline.

Implementation and Evaluation of Practice Guidelines

AGREE (Appraisal of Guidelines Research & Evaluation) is an international collaboration of researchers and policy makers whose goal was to improve the quality and effectiveness of clinical practice guidelines. Countries that participate in this collaboration include Denmark, Finland, Germany, Italy, the Netherlands, Spain, Switzerland, the United Kingdom, Canada, New Zealand, and the United States. The AGREE collaboration produced and validated an instrument that is used to evaluate the quality of clinical practice guidelines. Categories of the instrument include scope and purpose, stakeholder involvement, rigor of development, clarity, applicability, and editorial independence (Brown, 2009).

Systematic research reviews offered by the AHRQ also offer appraisal guides (AHRQ, 2009). The Cochrane Collaboration (cochrane.org) and the Joanna Briggs Institute (joannabriggs.edu.au/) are two organizations that offer standards and methods that can be developed into evaluation measures of practice guidelines.

Barriers to Implementing Evidence-Based Practice

While EBP was introduced into medical and nursing practice in 1996, many practicing practitioners were educated before EBP was introduced as a significant part of the curriculum in academic programs. Therefore, many currently practicing practitioners are unfamiliar with the evidence-based process and, thus, unable to implement EBP into their current practice. A practice guideline may be read but without the skills to critically appraise it and the evidence presented; the clinician may or may not use the guideline within his or her clinical practice. Therefore, one major barrier to nationwide implementation of EBP in all practice settings is unfamiliarity with the evidence-based process by a major portion of the health care workforce.

A second barrier to EBP is the time and commitment of all providers to implement and evaluate the process in various settings. Primary care settings, whether private or public care centers, with multiple health care providers offer a unique challenge. First, the providers need to make a commitment to change to EBP, and a time commitment to make the change, and then to evaluate the outcomes of the EBP.

A major barrier to implementation of EBP within both pediatric primary care and mental health settings is the general lack of experimentally designed studies with children as participants. Children are viewed as a vulnerable population; thus, inclusion of children in experimentally designed studies has been a challenge and a major barrier to finding the best available evidence to care for children. Many of the treatment interventions used in the pediatric and adolescent populations have primarily been studied in the adult population with only a limited number of case studies reporting on the efficacy of the treatment in one or two children. For example, a recent systematic review of the literature that focused on interventions for children with pervasive developmental disorders revealed that the majority of the studies had weak experimental designs and included only a small number of children in the treatment and control groups (Opsina et al., 2008). Thus, whether those interventions could be generalized to the general pediatric and adolescent autistic populations were rightly questioned.

Implications for Future Directions

The evidence clearly shows that health care outcomes improve when clinical decision making is guided by an EBP model (AHRQ, 2010). To use the best available evidence, future experimental studies need to be rigorously designed and implemented to include children and adolescents as participants to obtain the best evidence for clinical decision making for the pediatric and adolescent populations.

All clinical educational programs need to provide experiences for students to acquire EBP competencies and to implement care based on the best available clinical evidence. National and international professional organizations that provide continuing education for clinicians also need to provide educational programs that assist the membership to acquire EBP competencies.

Summary

EBP requires the use of a systematic way to raise relevant PICO (clinical) questions, search for the best available evidence relevant to the question, and identify the best available evidence and/or practice guidelines for treatment of the patient. Systematic reviews, RCTs, and practice guidelines are appraised by the APN using standardized critical appraisal tools (agreecollaboration.org) to determine the goodness of fit for implementation in the APN's practice. APNs who implement the tenets of EBP in their clinical practice settings are using the best available evidence for the assessment, diagnosis, and clinical decision making for the treatment of their patients. Research studies examining the implementation of EBP in practice settings have demonstrated an improvement in patient health care outcomes in practices that consistently use an evidence-based approach in their practice settings.

References

Agency for Healthcare Research and Quality (AHRQ). Retrieved from http://www.ahrq.gov/

AGREE Collaboration. *The AGREE Tool*. Retrieved from http://agreecollaboration.org/

American Academy of Child and Adolescent Psychiatry (AACAP). Retrieved from www.aacap.org

American Academy of Pediatrics (AAP). Retrieved from http://www.aap.org

American Academy of Pediatrics (AAP). 2001. Committee on Quality Improvement, Subcommittee on Attention Deficit/Hyperactivity Disorder. Clinical practice guideline: Treatment of the school-age child with attention-deficit/hyperactive disorder. *Pediatrics, 108*, 1033–1044.

American Psychiatric Association. (2000). *Diagnostic and Statistical Manual of Mental Disorders TR-IV* (revised fourth edition). Washington, D.C.: Author.

Association of Child and Adolescent Psychiatric Nursing (AACPN). *ACAPN Guidelines for Care and Practice*. Retrieved from http://www.ispn-psych.org/html/acapn.html

Brown, S.J. (2009). *Evidence-based nursing: The research-practice connection*. Sudbury, MA: Jones and Bartlett Publishers.

Cannon, S. & Boswell, C. (2007). Application of evidence-based nursing practice with research. In C. Boswell & S. Cannon (Eds.), *Introduction to nursing research: Incorporating evidence-based practice* (pp. 317–332). Sudbury, MA: Jones and Bartlett Publishers.

DiCenso, A., Guyatt, G., & Ciliska, D. 2005. *Evidence-based nursing: A guide to clinical practice*. St. Louis, MO: Elsevier.

Drake, R.E., Goldman, H.H., Leff, H.S., Lehman, A.F., Dixon, L., Muser, K.T., & Torrey, W.C. (2001). Implementing evidence-based practices in routine mental health service settings. *Psychiatric Services, 52*(2), 179–182. Retrieved from http://psychservices.psychiatryonline.org/cgi/content/full/52/2/179

Evans, D., & Kowanko, I. (2000). Literature reviews: Evolution of a research methodology. *The Australian Journal of Advanced Nursing, 18*(2), 33–38. Retrieved from http://www.ncbi.nlm.nih.gov/pubmed/11878498

Ganz, P.A. (2002). What outcomes matter to patients: A physician-researcher point of view. *Medical Care, 40*(6): Suppl: III-11-III-19. Retrieved from http://www.jstor.org/pss/3767708

Jones, S.K. (2009). Pediatric evidence-based practice: Using the best available evidence to improve patient outcomes. *AACN Advanced Critical Care, 20*, 19–25. DOI. 10.1097/NCI.0b073e37819436ba

McGraw-Hill. (2002). *McGraw-Hill concise dictionary of modern medicine*. New York, NY: The McGraw-Hill Companies. Retrieved from http://medical-dictionary.thefreedictionary.com/meta-analysis

Melynk, B.M., & Fineholt-Overholt E. (2010). Evidence-based practice in nursing and healthcare: A guide to best practice (second edition). Philadelphia, PA: Lippincott Williams & Wilkins.

Mileham, P. (2009).Finding sources of evidence. In N.A. Schmidt & J.M. Brown, (Eds.). *Evidence-based practice for nurses: Appraisal and application of research* (pp. 75–104). Sudbury, MA: Jones & Bartlett Publishers.

National Health Services Critical Appraisal Skills Program (CASP). Retrieved from www.phru.nhs.uk/casp/critical_appraisal_tools.htm

Ospina, M. B., Seida, J.K., Clark, B., Karhaneh, M., Hartling, L., Tjosvold, L., Vandermermeer, B., Smith, V. (2008). Behavioural and developmental interventions for autism spectrum disorder: A clinical systematic review. *PLoS One, 3*(11), e3755.

Sackett, D., Rosenberg, W., Muir Gray, J., Haynes, R., & Richardson, W. (1996). Evidence based medicine: What it is and what it isn't. *British Medical Journal, 312*, 71–72. Retrieved from http://cebm.jr2.ox.ac.uk/ebmisisnt.html

Sackett, D.L., Straus, S.E., Richardson, W.S., Rosenberg, W., & Haynes, R.B. (2000). *Evidence-based medicine: How to practice and teach EBM*. London, UK: Churchill Livingstone.

Salmond, S. (2007). Advancing evidence-based practice: A primer. *Orthopaedic Nursing, 26*(2), 114–123. Retrieved from http://www.ncbi.nlm.nih.gov/pubmed/17414381

Stetler, C.B. (1994). Refinement of the Stetler/Marram model for application of research findings to practice. *Nursing Outlook, 42*, 15–25. Retrieved from http://www2.kumc.edu/instruction/nursing/RTaunton/Article/Stetler.pdf

27

Influence of Culture/Needs of Immigrant Children

Edilma L. Yearwood and Ellen Carroll

Objectives

After reading this chapter, APNs will be able to

1. Define culture and understand the cultural context of mental health.
2. Explain unique psychosocial experiences and needs of immigrant youth.
3. Describe common behavioral and psychiatric disorders seen in immigrant youth and youth of immigrant parents.

4. Identify ways that primary care and psychiatric-mental health APNs can collaborate to deliver seamless quality care to immigrant youth.
5. Develop personal learning strategies aimed at developing and refining culturally informed nursing care and practice based on knowledge of the complexity of working with immigrant youth.

Introduction

Discussion of culture is complex and, within a mental health context, can be controversial. Some prefer not to engage in the conversation, professing that everyone is the same; others minimize the role and impact of culture on presenting behaviors, while others embrace and value their own culture but disrespect or marginalize the culture of others, and some are eager to learn more about culture and how it works within different contexts in order to maximize care rendered. This chapter will discuss the changing demographics of children, adolescents, and their families in the United States; define culture, acculturation, and marginalization; explore cultural factors of which advanced practice nurses (APNs) must be aware that impact the mental/behavioral health of immigrant children or children of immigrant parents;

and formulate culturally informed treatment strategies to enhance the mental health of immigrant youth. The chapter will also include practice, education, and research implications and recommendations for nurses working with immigrant populations and will conclude with a case exemplar of an adolescent immigrant.

Changing U.S. Demographics

Of the 75 million children in the United States, approximately 19 million are immigrants, with that number expected to rise to 33 million of the anticipated 100 million youth population by 2050 (Passel, 2011). First-generation U.S. immigrant children are children born in another country who then migrate to the United States; their parents are foreign born. Generation 1.5 immigrant children refers to youth with the following characteristics: (a) not

---

Child and Adolescent Behavioral Health: A Resource for Advanced Practice Psychiatric and Primary Care Practitioners in Nursing,
First Edition. Edited by Edilma L. Yearwood, Geraldine S. Pearson, and Jamesetta A. Newland.

born in the United States; (b) migrated to the United States at an early age; (c) have resided in the United States for a long period of time; (d) have foreign-born parents; and (e) are sociologically closer in behaviors to second-generation youth (Portes & Rivas, 2011). Second-generation immigrant children are children born in the United States who have at least one immigrant parent, and third-generation immigrant children are children born in the United States of U.S.-born parents (Perreira & Ornelas, 2011). Children who reside in mixed legal status households (with one or both parent (s) an undocumented immigrant) are more at risk for accessing health care later, not having a primary care health provider, experiencing stress, anxiety, and depression related to documentation status, and not having health insurance (Perreira & Ornelas).

In 2008, 16.5 million children aged seventeen years and younger had at least one immigrant parent; 56% of the children of immigrants were Hispanic; 29% were poor, and 49% resided in low-income households (Urban Institute, 2010). Forty-three percent of these children aged zero to eight years have parents from Mexico; 20% have parents from Central America, the Caribbean, and South America combined; 22% have parents from Asia and the Middle East; and 15% have parents from Africa, Europe, Canada, and Australia combined; with at least one-third of young children of immigrants living in linguistically isolated households (non–English speaking) (Fortuny, Hernandez, & Chaudry, 2010). Sixty-five percent of immigrants to the United States live in California, New York, Florida, Texas, New Jersey, or Illinois (Urban Institute, 2010).

The process and characteristic of *planned migration*, or the move from one country to another country with the intent of living in the new country, differ from the process involved in resettlement as a refugee. Refugees are defined as "people who have been persecuted or fear they will be persecuted due to race, religion, nationality, and/or membership in a particular social group or political opinion" (U.S. Citizenship and Immigration Services, n.d.). The United Nations High Commission for Refugees (as cited in Downes & Graham, 2011) adds that a refugee lives in a country other than the one of his/her nationality or last residence and is concerned about safety and protection from the country being fled. Having to emigrate quickly and inconspicuously from a country poses physical and psychological challenges for refugees who experience multiple losses during resettlement (i.e., place, family and friends, and culture); uncertainty (i.e., where to live, how to earn a living, and fear about the safety and status of those left behind), and change in personal status (i.e., socioeconomic, professional, and possible change from majority to minority status).

Specific to child and adolescent refugees, children are increasingly victims of torture or witnesses to mass tragedy associated with wars or persecution. They can become refugees by virtue of these experiences. As a result, they may have had to live in refugee camps, endure multiple moves, or be separated from parents or caretakers in order to remain safe. Food, warmth, clothing, stability, ability to attend school, and unconditional and predictable parental "presence" may have been lacking or compromised (Birman & Chan, 2008; Llabre & Hadi, 2009). Over time, posttraumatic stress, depression, anxiety, sleep disturbance, substance abuse, and suicidality are some of the mental health consequences of these traumatic experiences (Downes & Graham, 2011).

A cultural practice that has been condemned by many throughout the world is female genital mutilation (FGM), for which girls, adolescent females, and young women are at risk in many societies (Africa, Latin America, Asia, and the Middle East). The practice entails removal of healthy and normal female genital tissue, with four levels of removal possible. Needless to say, the practice is painful, unsterile, done with little or no preparation of the child, and without anesthesia. The International Society of Psychiatric Nurses (ISPN) developed a position statement against the practice of FGM and described the psychological trauma that girls and women carry with them for a lifetime as a result of the practice (2009). Nurses working with immigrants are likely to encounter young girls and women on whom FGM was done as part of cultural practices. Issues of betrayal, mistrust, anger, anxiety, and depression may be part of the client presentation and the focus of psychological work with a psychiatric APN. The primary care APN may identify that this practice was done during routine physical examination or post procedure when medical complications may arise.

Stages of Migration

There are three distinct stages involved with planned migration or the move from one country to another. *Premigration*, or the period before the move, involves making the decision to move, planning, discussion with family and friends, and leave taking. Premigration can be stressful because of uncertainty about the new place of residence, economic hardship, or if significant people, things, or status is being left behind (Perreira & Ornelas, 2011). *Intramigration*, or the period during travel to the new country, can evoke anxiety if the travel is difficult, long, circuitous, or uncertain or if family members are separated during the process. *Postmigration* involves settling in the new country; maneuvering a new environment without the usual source of social support; acculturation stress; adjusting to a different educational system, and possibly dealing with changes in language, roles, downward mobility, and/or undocumented status (Perreira & Ornelas; Suarez-Orozco & Todorova, 2003; Thompson & Gurney, 2003). Many refugees and immigrants spend time in other countries before immigrating to the United States, which prolongs the uncertainty and disruption they experience.

Why Knowledge of Culture Matters

There are many definitions of "culture." Definitions included here provide the reader with an understanding of how comprehensive and complex the concept is. Cross, Bazron, Dennis, and Isaacs defined culture as "the integrated pattern of human behavior that includes thoughts, communication styles, actions, customs, beliefs, values and institutions of racial, ethnic, religious or social group" (1989, p. iv.). Keesing and Strathern (1998) and Helman (2007; cited in Andrews et al., 2010) viewed culture as a contextual system of shared ideas and learned guidelines that affect how the individual or group views the world and thus behaves. Hall (1984; cited in Andrews et al., 2010) stated that there are three levels of culture: primary (made up of rules followed by group members but which are rarely stated), secondary (foundational rules known by members but rarely shared with nonmembers), and tertiary (explicit rules and behaviors of the group or individuals seen by others). Primary and secondary levels of culture are more intrinsic and difficult to change.

An understanding of culture matters because culture influences how individuals understand health and illness and the contextual practices they use to manage their illness (Anderson et al., 2010; Bronfenbrenner, 1994; 2005; Campinha-Bacote, 1998; Kleinman, 1988). Those in some cultures believe that physical or mental illness is caused by bad spirits visiting the individual or family, while others believe that illness occurs when the body is not in harmony or as a punishment for wrong doing (Andrews et al., 2010). It is the belief of the co-authors of this chapter that an understanding of the cultural context must be acknowledged and factored into health encounters and interventions as it serves as a foundation for positive health outcomes.

Acculturation

Nurses working with immigrant youth and their families must understand the concept of acculturation and be able to determine where the child and/or family is on the acculturation trajectory. This knowledge helps the nurse fully grasp the social, cultural, emotional, and interactional experiences and stressors that the child, adolescent, or family is dealing with in their status as immigrants. The place where the child, adolescent, and/or family is on the acculturation trajectory has been implicated in health, health practices, and health inequities (disparities) (Campinha-Bacote, 1998; Lopez-Class, Castro, & Ramirez, 2011).

Berry (1997) described the acculturation process as two cultures coming into contact resulting in conflict within the individual from the nondominant (nonhost) culture. As a result of this interaction over time, the individual adopts one of four behaviors: integration (embraces behaviors and values from both cultures), assimilation (embraces behaviors and values of the dominant culture and rejects own culture of origin), separation (immerses self in own culture of origin, rejecting behaviors and values of the dominant culture), or marginalization (rejects both cultures). McDermott-Levy's concept analysis of acculturation emphasized that the process is bidirectional but uneven, occurs over time (can occur over several generations), and is a phenomenon that is, "interactive, multifactorial, developmental and multidimensional" (2009, p. 283).

Choi (2001) developed a concept analysis of cultural marginality from a thorough literature review. Attributes of the concept (factors found repeatedly) included passive "betweeness," the correct term for forging new relationships in the midst of old relationships, emotional conflicts, and struggles, and anxious/hopeful promise. Passive betweeness was defined as straddling both cultures without feeling comfortable or empowered in either. An example illustrating this element would be a child or adolescent brought to the United States by parents with the child/adolescent having no say in the migration decision. The second element, forging new relationships in the midst of old relationships, can be illustrated by how adeptly children/adolescents learn the new language and make friends in the new country, while parents and older siblings tend to hold onto old friendships from the country of origin and have more difficulty fitting into the new culture. The third element, emotional conflicts and struggles, refers to feelings of helplessness, anxiety, depression, loss, and alienation experienced by many new immigrants. Last, the element of anxious/hopeful promise speaks to uncertainty and apprehension about the future mixed with hope about new possibilities. If immigrants are successful in navigating these elements, Choi further proposed that they develop a good sense of self and have positive psychological and cognitive growth. However, if they have difficulty navigating these elements, they experience psychological degradation, withdrawal from others, and identity confusion.

Kim (2004) conducted a grounded theory study on the experiences of young Korean immigrants to the United States looking at negotiation of social, cultural, and generational boundaries. Qualitative interview data were obtained from nineteen youths with a mean age of

21.5 years who had been in the United States between four and nineteen years. A major theme identified was negotiating boundaries. Participants spoke of conflicts they encountered that made them painfully aware of the cultural differences between their culture and the dominant culture; difficulty they had with parents and peers; difficulties at home and school; navigating both the Korean and English languages; and, because of the length of time in the United States, feeling that they were neither first-generation nor second-generation immigrants. Participants also reported feeling that they were a visible minority when not living in or going to school in Korean cultural enclaves. Participants who were less than ten years of age when they migrated to the United States reported having less difficulty with social, cultural, and generational boundaries than did participants who migrated when they were fifteen years or older.

As illustrated previously by McDermott-Levy (2009), Choi (2001), and Kim (2004), acculturation is an ecologically dynamic process that affects cultural identity and the psychological state of individuals and groups (Berry, 2005). Researchers and clinicians have moved away from a simplistic and unidimensional view of acculturation that included a focus on language or generational factors. Current acculturation research, which is a good fit with nursing research, focuses on attitudes, values, behaviors, stress, identity, discrimination, economics, family relationships, values, and security (Berry; Lopez-Class et al., 2011).

Marginalization

Marginalization is described by Phinney, Berry, Vedder, and Liebkind (2006) as having little interest in cultural maintenance and little interest in having relations with other groups as a result of being excluded or discriminated against. Individuals who are marginalized do not feel embraced by others and are not integrated into the fiber of the culture, the group, or the environment. They experience isolation when ignored and made to feel inconsequential. Ultimately, these individuals are at risk for poor self-esteem, depression, and self-harm (Barber & Vega, 2011).

Immigrant Paradox

The immigrant paradox (healthy immigrant phenomenon) refers to a frequently observed trend that, compared to children from native-born families, first-generation "immigrant children present with better physical health, less involvement in risky behaviors and similar or greater academic achievement and psychological well-being" (Fuligni, 1998, p. 100). Cultural foods, complementary and alternative health practices, being raised in more supportive community environments, and a more phys-

ically active lifestyle in the country of origin are reasons offered for these findings (Mendoza, 2009).

Unfortunately, the longer immigrants are in the United States (shift from first generation to second or third generation), the further they navigate away from high academic aspirations and good physical and emotional health (Suarez-Orozco, Rhodes, & Milburn, 2009) and experience lower self-esteem (Smokowski, Rose, & Bacallao, 2010). Findings from a Canadian study of 4,069 students in three generations of immigrant youths from grades seven through twelve revealed that drug use, harmful drinking, and delinquency increased with second- and third-generation immigrants; however, psychological distress was higher in the first-generation youth, possibly due to migration stress and uncertainty (Hamilton, Noh, & Adlaf, 2009). This shift toward poorer outcomes with longer residence is believed to occur as a result of acculturation and adoption of behaviors, values, and lifestyles of the host or dominant culture. APNs need to know the medical and psychosocial history of the child or adolescent but also understand the community climate where the child lives, specifically issues of tolerance or intolerance that the child and family experience.

Child Fostering

APNs working with immigrant populations may encounter a rare phenomenon known as "child fostering" that might impact the parent-child relationship. The child's sense of belonging within the family may be affected and can result in behavioral and psychological symptoms such as anger, isolation, anxiety, and depression. Child fostering, or what Leinaweaver refers to as "outsourcing care" (2010), refers to the "informal care and placement of children in a household where their biological parent does not reside" (Miller, 1998, p. 36). This practice appears to have originated during the time when African slaves were brought to the United States and their children were given to other adults to be cared for. It continues as a frequent practice in Latin America and the Caribbean when primarily single parents migrate to another country for employment and to establish a home prior to sending for the children. In the current child fostering process, parents working in the United States, Canada, or other resource-rich or high-income environments send money back to the country of origin to the adult raising their children for the care being rendered (Leinaweaver; Yearwood, 1998).

While there are clearly economic advantages to this practice, the length of separation from the child can extend from weeks to years, causing a disruption in the parent-child bond and establishing a level of uncertainty for the child as to when and whether they will see their parent again. Compounding this practice might be the undocumented status of the parent who cannot return to the country of origin to visit the child for fear of not being allowed back into the country where they are now working and living. In addition, the child left behind in the care of a friend or acquaintance might be at risk for sexual, physical, or emotional abuse and/or abandonment. When unification with the biological parent does occur, the child then experiences the loss of the person who was caring for them while their parent was away, anger toward the biological parent over the delay in reunification and new rules and behavioral expectations, and worry that she/he may be separated from the parent again. This adds increased risks to disturbances in mental wellness and adjustment to their new environment.

Transnationals

Transnationals are individuals who maintain contact and ties with their country of origin through frequent visits (cyclical migration), frequent communication via technology, and by sending goods and money to friends and relatives who remain in the country of origin. There may be confusion as to where these individuals "fit" and challenges to their experience of acculturation. Transnationals may be at risk for relational stress secondary to frequent separations and reunions, and to generational stress secondary to contact with several generations each having beliefs and values that may challenge those held by the transnational (Falicov, 2007).

Discrimination

Discrimination, racism, and various levels of aggression are other experiences immigrant youth report as newcomers to the United States. Rousseau, Hassan, Measham, and Lashley (2008) looked at prevalence and types of conduct disorders in 252 Caribbean Canadian and Filipino Canadian adolescents aged twelve to nineteen years. A notable characteristic of the participants was that these youth had experienced a long parent-child separation as a result of immigration. The researchers concluded that adolescents with high levels of perceived racism and low self-esteem displayed more behavioral problems.

In a study conducted in Switzerland with 568 boys and 522 girls, the researchers looked at peer acceptance, victimization, and language competences of immigrant and Swiss children in kindergarten. They found that lack of language competence in immigrant children is a risk factor for low peer acceptance and higher peer victimization. In addition, poor language skills were found to impede integration into the host country and were a barrier to development of social competence (Grunigen, Perren, Nagele, & Alsaker, 2010). They recommended assessment of the cause of the language difficulties, additional personnel in classrooms in earlier grades to support language acquisition in immigrants, and working with nonimmigrant children around issues of tolerance and understanding others.

Garcia and Lindgren conducted a descriptive study to obtain parent and adolescent perspectives on mental health stressors. Focus groups ($N = 8$) were used for data collection with fifty-three participants. There were three stressors identified: discrimination, immigration, and familial disconnection (2009).

In another study, Peguero looked at whether immigrant generational status is associated with in-school victimization of Latino and Asian immigrant children. Data were from the Educational Longitudinal Study of 2002 and the sample included 1,628 Latino, 1,129 Asian, and 5,626 white Americans. Victimization was defined as violence, property crime, and fear. Findings indicated that first-generation Latino children felt that their school was unsafe and that third-generation Latino children experienced more property crime and violence directed at them compared to their white peers. First- and second-generation Asian children felt their school was unsafe and were the victims of violence and property crime more frequently than their white peers (2009). The researcher stressed the importance of school policies that develop, implement, and enforce safe learning environments in schools.

Asian American immigrants have been referred to in the literature as the "model immigrant" group primarily because of their educational and economic success and well-behaved presentation (Qin, Way, & Mukherjee, 2008; Suarez-Orozco & Carhill, 2008). However, Qin et al. caution that Asian American youth reported poor social and psychological adjustment as immigrants in the United States. Their conclusion was based on data from two longitudinal studies of 120 first- and second-generation Chinese students they conducted in two large cities in the northeastern part of the United States. Data were collected between 1996 and 2001 using semistructured and structured interviews. Youth reported frustration with and alienation from their parents in the area of communication; long duration of parent work hours, which left little time for family activities; a language barrier with parents who spoke the native language and expected the adolescents to maintain skills and fluency in that language; anger over high academic expectations their parents held for them; harassment from peers over their inability to speak English properly; and their smaller stature (Qin et al.). The discrepancy between how this cultural group is viewed and the reality of the youths' experiences highlight the importance of a comprehensive assessment of *each* youngster and his or her family and that the APN cannot make any assumptions based on ethnic or cultural group membership.

Social Determinants of Health

Efforts to improve this population's health and mental health call for an awareness of the social determinants of health that serve as barriers or facilitators to health status. First-generation immigrant children and youth migrating to the United States are frequently leaving a low- or middle-income country to enter a high-income country (i.e., United States). Globally, social, political, and economic challenges are contributing to imbalances in human and other resources and play a significant role in health inequity and mental and behavioral disorders with which children and adolescents present. Global epidemiological data on prevalence rates for child and adolescent behavioral and psychiatric disorders are fair or inconsistent at best. Therefore, when APNs are assessing both first-generation and generation 1.5 children, gathering data about possible psychiatric assessment, diagnosis, and treatment while in the country of origin along with cultural views on mental health and stigma surrounding mental illness is essential. This information will inform the plan of care and assure the youth and family that both the primary care and psychiatric APNs are respectful of the culture of origin and open to a creative plan of care that safely incorporates cultural values.

The World Health Organization (WHO) endorsed the Social Determinants of Health, which says that psychological and physical health of populations is dependent on the following factors that must be addressed at the individual, family, community, policy, and national levels:

1. Healthy conditions of daily life (clean and safe environments; a ready supply of clean water and adequate food sources; opportunities for work; an end to violence, and availability of resources to support growth and development across all age groups)
2. Equitable distribution of power, money, and resources for both men and women
3. Educational opportunities for all, a trained workforce, and public knowledge and awareness of the importance of the social determinants of health (WHO, 2008; Yearwood & DeLeon Siantz, 2010)

Poverty

As stated previously, many immigrant children and families live in poverty. With poverty status comes the lack of health insurance, worse health outcomes, poorer living situations, risk for not completing school, future job insecurity, and lower wages (Tienda & Haskins, 2011). Poorer community environments have little or no resources to meet the complex needs of individuals and families residing in those environments. For example, schools may lack human and material resources to have smaller classroom sizes staffed with bilingual or English as a second language (ESOL)-proficient teachers. A five-year mixed method longitudinal study on 408 immigrant children from Central America, China, Haiti, the Dominican Republic, and Mexico was conducted to identify academic trajectories across the study population. Researchers found that high achieving and academically successful immigrant children were from families that had structure and family capital to support the child's school success, were in less segregated schools, and had stronger English skills (Suarez-Orozco, Bang, et al., 2010). However, at year four of the study, most of the participants displayed a significant decline in their academic grades with the exception of the children from China who consistently maintained good academic achievement (Suarez-Orozco, Rhodes, et al., 2009).

Children and adolescents raised in poverty are more at risk for anxiety and depression, violence, gang involvement, substance abuse, food insecurity, and sleep difficulties (Suarez-Orozco & Carhill, 2008; Suarez-Orozco, Rhodes, et al., 2009). Having knowledge of the socioeconomic status of the child will help the nurse understand potential risk for poor health and mental health outcomes. However, it should also prompt the nurse to assess further for presence of any protective factors or strengths (which are often overlooked) that can mitigate a negative outcome.

Potential Protective Factors

Suarez-Orozco, Rhodes, et al. (2009) identified several protective factors that promote success, social self-efficacy, and resilience in immigrant youth. These factors include academic self-sufficiency, English language proficiency, residing in a two-parent household, having a positive relationship with parent(s) with clear and respectful communication, being female, positive relationships with teachers at school, and social supports (peers, nonparental supportive adult, extended and supportive family members). Other researchers (Fung & Lau, 2010; Leidy, Guerra, & Toro, 2010; Smokowski et al., 2010) endorse one or more of the protective factors described by Suarez-Orozco et al.

In a study of 227 high-risk Hispanic adolescents in the eighth grade, Schwartz et al. (2009) examined whether family and school functioning and personal and ethnic identity were associated with conduct problems, drug use, and sexual risk taking. The researchers found that positive accomplishments in school were a protective factor in preventing conduct difficulties, drug use, and early and risky sexual activity. The researchers also found that adolescents who were experiencing difficulty with ethnic identity confusion displayed more problem behaviors, while positive ethnic and personal identity was protective against behavioral acting out.

In addition, Han and Huang (2010) looked at the relationship between language status and externalizing and internalizing behaviors of Asian school-age children when compared to a white non-Hispanic U.S.-born comparison group. The data were from a large longitudinal data set of 12,586 children. Findings indicated that bilingual language skills predicted (protective) a slower rate of internalizing and externalizing behavior problems in this sample.

Behavioral and Psychiatric Presentations of Immigrant Youth

Globally, what is known about behavioral and psychiatric disorders in children and adolescents is limited due to a lack of age and culturally appropriate screening tools; inconsistent epidemiological data-gathering methods across countries; lack of adequately trained mental health practitioners in low- and middle-income countries; and myopic priorities of medical and communicable diseases despite evidence that psychiatric disorders are a significant component of the noncommunicable disorders seen worldwide (Patel, Flisher, Hetrick, & McGorry, 2007; Yearwood & DeLeon Siantz, 2010). Research conducted with immigrant youth in the United States has focused on youth behaviors in the school; parent-child behaviors; the protective role of healthy parenting; behaviors associated with level of acculturation the youth is navigating; common behavioral or psychiatric presentations; and the youth's perception of host country discrimination/racism.

Mood disorders are expected to be the second largest contributor to global burden of disease by 2020 with a significant increase of mood symptoms and diagnoses expected in adolescence (Lewinsohn et al. and WHO as cited in Yearwood, Crawford, Kelly, & Moreno, 2007). Immigrant youth must be carefully assessed for pre-, intra-, and postmigration stressors, untreated premigration psychopathology; behavioral and psychological responses to perceived losses; cultural stigma surrounding mental illness; academic competence; self-concept; and parent-child relationship (Yearwood et al., 2007). All of these issues have the potential to affect emotional, social, relational, and psychological development of the child or adolescent. In clinical practice, presentations will include isolation, anger, irritability, self-harm, poor self-esteem, depression, and anxiety. Additional information about mood disorders and recommended management approaches are found in Chapter 9 of this text.

A frequently cited cultural behavioral presentation of distress described in the DSM-IV (American Psychiatric Association, 2000) is *ataques de nervios*. Nurses working with immigrant children should have an understanding of how this behavioral presentation is viewed as a "normal" response to stressful events within the Latino cultural context. Symptoms of this episodic behavior include trembling, crying, convulsions, screaming, and at times falling to the ground. It differs from panic attacks in that it occurs around other people, and after the episode the person verbalizes feeling better. Triggers appear related to loss, discord, or disruption (Lopez et al., 2009). Lopez and colleagues were interested in assessing the lifetime prevalence and psychiatric correlates of *ataques de nervios* of five- to thirteen-year-old youths living in the south Bronx section of New York and San Juan, Puerto Rico.

There were a total of 1,138 New York children and 1,353 Puerto Rican children in the sample. Data collection measures included the Diagnostic Interview Schedule for Children (DISC-IV), the Parent Interview Child Global Assessment Scale, the Stressful Life Events Scale, the Exposure to Community Violence Scale, and the Hispanic Stress Inventory, which measured parental cultural stress. Study findings included no difference by site (New York versus Puerto Rico) in the prevalence of the disorder, with approximately 5% of the sample at each site meeting the criteria for *ataques de nervios*, and no gender difference in occurrence. However, all children who experienced *ataques* symptoms had more psychological impairment than their peers, putting them at greater risk for meeting the criteria for a psychiatric disorder; had higher exposure rates to violence; and exhibited behaviors not associated with depressive symptoms (Lopez et al., 2009).

Assessment and Screening Tools

A useful cultural assessment tool that helps the practitioner understand the immigrant's (or any other individual or group) experience and beliefs about his/her illness is Kleinman's Explanatory Model. The questions posed try to elicit what the person believes causes the illness, how the illness is explained in the culture, how the illness affects the social world of the individual or group, and how the illness is usually managed. The illness can be either physical or psychological. Specific questions include (Anderson et al., 2010; Kleinman, 1988; Kleinman & Benson, 2006):

1. What do you call the problem?
2. What do you think is wrong?
3. What do you want the health care practitioner to do?
4. Why do you think you are experiencing these symptoms at this time?
5. How has the illness affected your life?
6. What about this illness worries you the most?
7. What do you think needs to be done to treat the illness?
8. How do people in your culture talk about and understand the illness?
9. How long do you think the illness will last?
10. Does the illness serve a purpose?

Table 27.1 Recommended screening tools

Name of Tool	Developed by	Targeted Age	Characteristics
Strengths and Difficulties Questionnaire SDQ	Goodman (1999)	3- to 16-year-olds	25-item brief behavioral screening tool for positive and negative behaviors. Screens for emotional, conduct, hyperactivity, peer relationship, and prosocial behaviors. Translated into 66 languages
Child Self-Rating Scale (CSRS)	Hightower et al., 1987	5- to 13-year-olds	40-item self-report measure. Screens for rule compliance and acting out, anxiety and withdrawal, friend and peer relationships, and school interest
Pediatric Symptom Checklist (PSC)	Jellinek et al., 1988	6- to 16-year-olds	35-item screening tool that parents respond to. Available in several languages and takes approximately 10 minutes to complete
Behavioral Assessment System for Children (BASC)	Reynolds & Kamphaus, 1992	2- to 21-year-olds	Screens for both adaptive and maladaptive thought and behaviors. Available for teachers, parents, and the child to complete. Version 2 of the scale is more comprehensive. Parent and teacher scales take 1 to 20 minutes to complete and child self-report takes 30 minutes to complete
Child Behavior Checklist (CBCL)	Achenbach, 1991	4- to 18-year-olds	Multiple versions of the scale in many languages. Can be used by parent, teacher, and child. Measures internalizing and externalizing behaviors
War Trauma Questionnaire	Macksoud, 1992	3- to 16-year-olds	45-item scale that is grouped into the following: exposure to shelling or combat, separation from parents, bereavement, witnessing violence, suffering injuries, victim of violence, emigration, displacement, involvement in violence and deprivation
PTSD-Reaction Index	Pynoos et al., 1998	7- to 18-year-olds	22-item self-report scale that takes approximately 30 minutes to complete. Translated into many languages. Assesses symptoms of PTSD within the last month
Depression Self-Rating Scale	Birleson, 1981	8- to 14-year-olds	18-item scale to measure childhood depression
*Child and Adolescent Functional Assessment Scale (CAFAS)	Hodges & Wong, 1996	7- to 17-year-olds	*This scale is used by a **trained clinician**. It assesses child functioning over the prior 3 months in school, home, community, behavior towards others, and behavior towards self, mood, substance abuse and thinking. Scale also assesses strengths. Caregiver strengths and problems can also be assessed

Reprinted from Birman & Chan, 2008, with permission from the Center for Health and Health Care in Schools at George Washington University.

The APN must be aware that in some cultures, direct conversation with the child or adolescent about the illness experience is not endorsed by adults because of the low status children may have within the culture.

The explanatory model questions can be modified by the health care practitioner to facilitate age-appropriate interaction, if there is a need to gather additional data or a need to better translate the questions to ensure understanding. The questions, however, are expected to facilitate communication between the care provider and the individual seeking care, broaden the provider's understanding of the cultural world of the patient/client, and deter the usual provider dominant or top-down conversation style. As can be seen by the questions, the model is quite conducive to understanding how older children and adolescents understand their behavioral and or psychological difficulties within their cultural context.

Table 27.1 provides a brief overview of recommended screening tools for use with immigrant children and adolescents.

Collaborative Care Delivery

As is clear from the information discussed in this chapter, work with immigrant children, adolescents, and families is complex and informed by multiple layers of cultural experiences. In 2005, the American Academy of Pediatrics revised their Position Statement on Providing Care for Immigrant, Homeless, and Migrant Children. The revised document advocates for a "community-based approach to health care delivery" (p. 1095). This approach endorsed knowledge of the special mental and physical health problems faced by immigrant children, cultural barriers that interfere with achieving optimal health, the need to support enrollment of immigrant children in available health insurance plans; and the importance of comprehensive, coordinated, and continuous health services.

Immigrant youth receiving health care may access those services in primary care and be treated by a primary care APN. Conducting routine medical care and obtaining a comprehensive medical, developmental, family, and psychosocial assessment are the purview of the pediatric or family APN. However, with the often complex presentations of these youngsters, additional in-depth psychosocial and psychiatric assessments may be warranted followed by brief or long-term psychiatric supportive interventions. Psychiatric-mental health APNs are trained to provide these services. Given the issues of loss and transitions that many immigrant children deal with, we support a health care model based on collaboration between practitioners and community care providers who work together over time to meet the changing medical and psychosocial needs of youths.

Specific strategies for both primary care and psychiatric-mental health APNs would include active listening to the child and parents, an open and respectful interaction style, an awareness of community resources to support changing needs, and valuing and providing continuity of care. In addition, this population may need assistance with transitions, which may need to begin at the point of assessment with clear planning and education. Last, APNs working with immigrant youth must recognize the critical role both parents (and significant adults) and school play in the development, socialization, and self-concept formation of these youths. The APN can foster communication between school and parents; support development of positive parenting skills and knowledge of normal child and adolescent development, and teach the importance of healthy parent-child communication and relationship development. These interventions would provide a better foundation for emotional, psychological, social, and behavioral competence in first-, second-, and third-generation immigrant youth.

The Robert Wood Johnson Foundation has been active in supporting programs across the United States that have developed strategies aimed at engaging families, schools, youth, community programs, and mental health agencies in supporting healthy development and success of immigrant and refugee children in response to changing demographics. Information on these programs can be found at www.rwjf.org and at www.healthinschools.org.

Research, Education, and Practice Implications

Mendoza (2009) described three priority areas for research with immigrant youth that nurses can and should pursue in order to develop the science on effective health care and outcomes for this population. These include developing and testing strategies to improve access to care, describing components of quality health care for individuals with complex needs, and understanding cultural factors that support positive development and health outcomes. Additional areas for research include comparison of behavioral and psychiatric presentations of stress associated with migration, acculturation, and trauma; immediate, short-term and long-term effects of social disruption; immigrant strengths across age groups; methods to improve early and accurate identification of immigrant mental health needs, and behavioral outcome comparison in youth across types and duration of parent involvement in schools. Nursing research should consist of qualitative, quantitative, and longitudinal studies.

Personal education efforts to develop skills working with immigrant populations should include immersion in the cultural activities of the immigrant group and curiosity and openness to learning about the other. Nursing education can make it a priority to include more opportunities for students to work with a variety of immigrant groups in public health, offering community-based learning experiences and supporting cultural immersions abroad.

APNs are in a unique position to develop culturally informed practice skills by virtue of their increased interaction with a variety of children, adolescents, and families from multiple countries who have emigrated to the United States. As stated earlier, there have been dramatic increases in the number of immigrants and this contact provides opportunities for nurses to learn about other cultures and cultural practices and to develop person-specific care interventions developed in collaboration with the youth and parent to ensure respect and acknowledgment of cultural values.

Conclusion

This chapter has described factors that APNs need to know about the unique and complex experiences of immigrant children and families before, during, and after migration to better understand their mental health and behavioral presentations and needs. The pervasive and far-reaching impact of culture and acculturation have been explored to provide a context for this understanding. In addition, the importance of providing care using a collaborative model that embraces continuity of care, youth and family inclusion in the development of care, and respect for the values of the immigrant unit has been provided. The chapter ended with a discussion of areas of research awaiting nurse scientists that would be an immense contribution to knowledge development and evidence-based practice with this population.

Case Exemplar

Jef, a seventeen-year-old boy, recently emigrated from Yemen. He is in the initial months of his second year attending a New York City public school when he presented at the school-based health center for an immunization update and a preparticipation sports physical examination. Initial assessment of the high school athlete included a review of history, review of systems, psychosocial assessment, and physical exam with attention to the neuromusculoskeletal exam. Jef was at ease from the onset of the interview; his answers to assessment questions were clear and forthcoming. When asked about where he lived, he assumed the APN wanted to know about where he came from and shared that his hometown was wrought with violence and warlord/gang style activities. Regarding his current home, he reported that he lived with his father, uncle, mother, and two siblings in an apartment in Brooklyn. He was the oldest son with a younger sister and brother. He reported he was Muslim and adhered to Muslim principles for prayer, diet, and socialization. He wanted to be a member of the school bowling club and, because of the rules for participation, he was having his physical today.

During the initial history while on the topic of hospitalization Jef reported he was hospitalized at age nine years for "bullettothehead." It was at first unclear to the practitioner what he was saying when he remarked "bullettothehead." When asked to repeat what he said for the third time he stated, "I was shot in the head by some gang involved people in the neighborhood where I lived."

When asked to describe the incident further, he told of how he was playing outside of his home, and then was struck in the head by something, and then saw the blood on his hand when he reached up to check the place that was struck. He related that he ran home and his mother quickly took him to the local hospital, where they were told, "yes," he was shot in the head, the bullet probably was still inside, and there was nothing they could do to help them. Jef's mother and some other family members took him further to the next town and received the same response. The mother continued to a still further third town, and at that hospital, there were surgeons visiting from India who were able to perform surgery and remove the bullet from his skull. Jef assured the nurse practitioner that nothing vital was injured and, except for the ridge on his skull, there were no further complications. He restated he was indebted to the doctors from India and agreed with the practitioner that he was very lucky to be alive without residual trouble.

Jef's review of systems was relatively benign and free from physical complaints to any body system. Under nutrition he revealed that he was keeping a strict fast and that he had to wake at 4 AM if he was going to have any nutrition in order that he didn't break the fast. He further related that this early morning ritual was very difficult because he worked until midnight at his family's business, and sometimes the sleep was more important than the food. His weight and height were at the fiftieth percentile. When asked if he had time for the after-school bowling team in addition to his required hours at the family business, he assured the nurse practitioner that work didn't start until 7 PM, and he knew from his peers that the team was a lot of fun and a good place to socialize. The way Jef related the story it became apparent that Jef was burning the candle at both ends, attending high school from 7:25 AM to 2:15 PM and working an evening shift of about five hours until midnight each night. During holy times of fasting he would go without eating or interrupt his sleep by rising at about 3 or 4 AM to take in some nutrition before another full day of school work and fasting. The picture was adding up to an overall imbalance and yet the young man was looking to "enrich" his already tight schedule with extracurricular activity.

The interview section of the encounter concluded with the psychosocial review, which is formulated as a HEADDSS assessment that inquires about Home, Education, Affiliations, Depression, Drugs, Sex, and Suicidal ideation. During this assessment Jef conveyed that he felt safe at home and could speak with his parents, he felt that he and his parents wished for the same things and that he would continue to "be a good Muslim." He shared that he felt he was provided for. School was a relatively benign topic for Jef who was working on the language issues but intended to do well because his parents wanted him to be successful and go to college and not have to only work in the family business. He reported that he paid attention and did his work and found school "good to be here." When considering affiliations, Jef shared that he had friends at school and spent leisure time with extended family and cousins both older and near to his age. He reported that he abstains from alcohol and drugs. Jef denied feeling depressed and reported no intent to hurt himself or others. He remarked, "There is no need to feel depressed," adding that "if you work at school and at work then you can be successful." He admitted he might feel tired and sorry to have to go to work but it was necessary for the family to stay in the United States and be together.

The topics of sex and sexuality caused Jef to be a bit more evasive as he considered his answers. He reported he has been sexually active and observes, "There are a lot of female classmates I like, and many of the girls here are very friendly and they are not so strict." He shared that he has a "girlfriend" from outside his culture and that they see each other mostly during school hours and at times later in the day. When asked if abstinence from fornication as part of his religion-culture was problematic to this relationship and his relationship with his parents, he avoided providing a direct answer.

Physical exam included hearing and vision assessment and were within normal limits. Immunizations were updated, which included the Tdap vaccine and the Mantoux test for tuberculosis screening. Physical assessment and lab findings were all within normal limits. When Jef returned and was provided his paperwork; he was pleased to be able to join the bowling club.

This case exemplar depicts the story of a young man who continues to try to operate within a traditional religious cultural tract although he is displaced in metropolitan New York and wants to be a part of majority culture normal adolescent behaviors. Having attended more than a year of high school he has initiated affiliations with those he might normally consider outsiders. His devoutness and religiosity are readily conveyed in his history, as are the considerations of living in a more secular, diverse, and permissive environment. He shrugs off the near death nature of his past injury and commits himself to the family plan of becoming successful in the majority culture through educational success.

Resources

Anderson, N., et al. (2010). Culturally based health and illness beliefs and practices across the life span. *Journal of Transcultural Nursing, 21*(Suppl. 1), 152S- 235S.
Andrews, M., et al. (2010). Theoretical basis for transcultural care. *Journal of Transcultural Nursing, 21*(Suppl. 1), 53S-136S.
Annie E. Casey Foundation: http://www.aecf.org
Center for Health and Health Care in Schools: www.healthcarein schools.org

Chaudry, A. et al. (2010). Facing the future: children in the aftermath of immigration enforcement. The Urban Institute.
Holtz, C. (2010). Global health issues. *Journal of Transcultural Nursing, 21*(Suppl. 1), 14S-38S.
Howard, P., & El-Mallakh, P. (Eds.). Mental health across the lifespan. *Nursing Clinics of North America, 45*(4).
National Institute on Minority Health and Health Disparities (NIMHD): htpp://www.nimhd.nih.gov/
PEW Hispanic Foundation: www.pewhispanic.org/
Robert Wood Johnson Foundation: www.rwjf.org
Immigrant Children. (2011). *The Future of Children, 21*(1).
Urban League: http://www.urban.org

References

Achenbach, T.M. (1991). *Manual for child behavioral checklist.* Burlington, VT: University of Vermont.
American Academy of Pediatrics. (2005). Providing care for immigrants, homeless, and migrant children. *Pediatrics, 115*, 1095–1100.
American Psychiatric Association. (2000). *Diagnostic and statistical manual of mental disorders* (fourth edition) (DSM-IV). Washington, DC: APA.
Anderson, N., Andrews, M., Bent, K., Douglas, M., Elhammoumi, C., Keenan, C., & Mattson, S. (2010). Culturally based health and illness beliefs and practices across the life span. *Journal of Transcultural Nursing, 21* (Suppl. 1), 152S-235S.
Andrews, M., Backstrand, J., Boyle, J., Campinha-Bacote, J., Davidhizar, R., Doutrich, D., & Zoucha, R. (2010). Theoretical basis for transcultural care. *Journal of Transcultural Nursing, 21*(Suppl. 1), 53S-136S.
Barber, C., & Vega, L. (2011). Conflict, cultural marginalization, and personal costs of filial care giving. *Journal of Cultural Diversity, 18*(1), 20–28.
Berry, J. (1997). Immigration, acculturation and adaptation. *Applied Psychology, 46*, 5–34.
Berry, J.W. (2005). Acculturation: Living successfully in two cultures. *International Journal of Intercultural Relations, 29*, 697–712.
Birleson, P., Hudson, I., Buchanan, D., & Wolff, S. (1987). Clinical evaluation of a self-rating scale for depressive disorder in childhood. *Journal of Child Psychology and Psychiatry, 28*, 43–60.
Birman, D., & Chan, W. (2008). Screening and assessing immigrant and refugee youth in school-based mental health programs. *Center for Health and Health Care in Schools* (Issue Brief #1). Retrieved from www.healthinschools.org
Bronfenbrenner, U. (2005). *Making humans beings human: Bioecological perspectives on human development.* Thousand Oaks, CA: Sage.
Bronfenbrenner, U. (1994). Ecological models of human development. *International Encyclopedia of Education, 3*, 1643–1647.
Campinha-Bacote, J. (1998). The process of cultural competence in the delivery of healthcare services (third edition). Cincinnati, OH: Transcultural C.A.R.E. Associates.
Choi, H. (2001). Cultural marginality: A concept analysis with implications for immigrant adolescents. *Issues in Comprehensive Pediatric Nursing, 24*, 193–206.
Cross, T., Bazron, B., Dennis, K., & Isaacs, M. (1989). *Towards a culturally competent system of care: A monograph on effective services for minority children who are severely emotionally disturbed.* Washington, DC: CAASP Technical Assistance Center, Georgetown University Child Development Center.
Downes, E.A., & Graham, A.R. (2011). Health care for refugees resettled in the US. *Clinician Reviews, 21*(3), 25–31.

Falicov, C. (2007). Working with transnational immigrants: Expanding meanings of family, community and culture. *Family Process, 46,* 157–171.

Fortuny, K., Hernandez, D., & Choudry, A. (2010). Young children of immigrants: The leading edge of America's future (Issue Brief #3). Retrieved from www.urban.org

Fuligni, A. (1998). The adjustment of children from immigrant families. *Current Directions in Psychological Science, 7,* 99–103.

Fung, J., & Lau, A. (2010). Factors associated with parent-child (dis) agreement on child behavior and parenting problems in Chinese immigrant families. *Journal of Clinical Child and Adolescent Psychology, 39,* 314–327.

Garcia, C., & Lindgren, S. (2009). "Life grows between the rocks": Latino adolescents' and parents' perspectives on mental health stressors. *Research in Nursing and Health, 32,* 148–162.

Goodman, R. (1999). The extended version of the Strengths and Difficulties Questionnaire as a guide to child psychiatric case-ness and consequent burden. *Journal of Child Psychology and Psychiatry, 40,* 791–799.

Grunigen, R., Perren, S., Nagele, C., & Alsaker, F. (2010). Immigrant children's peer acceptance and victimization in kindergarten: The role of local language competence. *British Journal of Developmental Psychology, 28,* 679–697.

Hamilton, H., Noh, S., & Adlaf, E. (2009). Adolescent risk behaviours and psychological distress across immigrant generations. *Canadian Journal of Public Health, 100,* 221–225.

Han, W., & Huang, C. (2010). The forgotten treasure: Bilingualism and Asian children's emotional and behavioral health. *American Journal of Public Health, 100,* 831–838.

Hightower, A., Cowen, E., Spinell, A., & Lotyczewski, B. (1987). The Child Rating Scale: The development of a socioemotional self-rating scale for elementary school children. *School Psychology Review, 16,* 239–255.

Hodges, K., & Wong, M. (1996). Psychometric characteristics of a multidimensional measure to assess impairment: The Child and Adolescent Functional Assessment Scale. *The Journal of Child & Family Studies, 5,* 445–467.

Holtz, C. (2010). Global health issues. *Journal of Transcultural Nursing, 21*(Suppl. 1), 14S-38S.

International Society of Psychiatric Nurses (ISPN). (2009). *Position statement on the practice of female genital mutilation (FGM): Implications for health and psychiatric mental health nursing.* Madison, WI: Author. Retrieved from http:www.ispn-psych.org.

Jellinek, M.S., Murphy, J.M., & Robinson, J. (1988). Pediatric symptom checklist: Screening school-age children for psychosocial dysfunction. *Journal of Pediatrics, 112,* 201–209.

Kim, S. (2004). The experiences of young Korean immigrants: A grounded theory of negotiating social, cultural, and generational boundaries. *Issues in Mental Health Nursing, 25,* 517–537.

Kleinman, A. (1988). *The illness narratives: Suffering, healing & the human condition.* New York, NY: Basic Books.

Kleinman, A., & Benson, P. (2006). Anthropology in the clinic: The problem of cultural competency and how to fix it. *PLoS Med, 3(e294)* 1673–1676.

Leidy, M., Guerra, N., & Toro, R. (2010). Positive parenting, family cohesion, and child social competence among immigrant Latino families. *Journal of Family Psychology, 24,* 252–260.

Leinaweaver, J. (2010). Outsourcing care: How Peruvian migrants meet transnational family obligations. *Latin American Perspectives, 37*(5), 67–87.

Llabre, M., & Hadi, F. (2009). War-related exposure and psychological distress as predictors of health and sleep: A longitudinal study of Kuwaiti children. *Psychosomatic Medicine, 71,* 776–783.

Lopez, I., Rivera, F., Ramirez, R., Guarnaccia, P., Canino, G., & Bird, H. (2009). Ataques de nervios and their psychiatric correlates in Puerto Rican children from two different contexts. *The Journal of Nervous and Mental Disease, 197,* 923–929.

Lopez-Class, M., Castro, F., & Ramirez, A. (2011). Conceptions of acculturation: A review and statement of critical issues. *Social Science & Medicine.* doi:10.1016/j.socscimed.2011.03.011

Macksoud, M. (1992). Assessing war trauma in children: A case study of Lebanese children. *Journal of Refugee Studies, 5,* 1–15.

McDermott-Levy, R. (2009). Acculturation: A concept analysis for immigrant health. *Holistic Nursing Practice, 23,* 282–288.

Mendoza, F. (2009). Health disparities and children in immigrant families: A research agenda. *Pediatrics, 124,* S187-S195.

Miller, A. (1998). Child fosterage in the United States: Signs of an African heritage. *The History of the Family an International Quarterly, 3*(1), 35–62.

Passel, J. (2011). Demography of immigrant youth: Past, present, and future. *The Future of Children: Immigrant Children, 21,* 19–41.

Patel, V. Flisher, A., Hetrick, S., & McGorry, P. (2007). Mental health of young people: A global public health challenge. *Lancet, 369,* 1302–1313.

Peguero, A. (2009). Victimizing the children of immigrants: Latino and Asian American student victimization. *Youth & Society, 41,* 186–208.

Perreira, K., & Ornelas, I. (2011). The physical and psychological well-being of immigrant children. *The Future of Children: Immigrant Children, 21,* 195–218.

Phinney, J.S., Berry, J.W., Vedder, P., & Liebkind, K. (2006). The acculturation experience: Attitudes, identities, and behaviors of immigrant youth. In J. W. Berry, J. S. Ohinner, D. L Sam, & P. Vedder (Eds.), *Immigrant youth in cultural transition* (pp. 71-116). Mahwah, NJ: Lawrence Erlbaum Associates.

Portes, A., & Rivas, A. (2011). The adaptation of migrant children. In The Future of Children. *Immigrant Children, 21,* 219–246.

Pynoos, R., Rodriguez, N., Steinberg, A., Stuber, M., & Frederick, C. (1999). *Reaction index-revised.* Unpublished psychological test, University of California Los Angeles.

Qin, D., Way, N., & Mukherjee, P. (2008). The other side of the model minority story: The familial and peer challenges faced by Chinese American adolescents. *Youth & Society, 39,* 480–506.

Reynolds, C., & Kamphaus, R. (1992). *Behavior assessment system for children.* Circle Pines, MN: American Guidance Service.

Rousseau, C., Hassan, G., Measham, T., & Lashley, M. (2008). Prevalence and correlates of conduct disorder and problem behavior in Caribbean and Filipino immigrant adolescents. *European Child and Adolescent Psychiatry, 17,* 264–273.

Schwartz, S., Mason, C., Pantin, H., Wang, W., Brown, C., & Szapocznik, J. (2009). Relationships of social context and identity to problem behavior among high-risk Hispanic adolescents. *Youth & Society, 40,* 541–570.

Smokowski, P., Rose, R., & Bacallao, M. (2010). Influence of risk factors and cultural assets on Latino adolescents' trajectories of self-esteem and internalizing symptoms. *Child Psychiatry and Human Development, 41,* 133–155.

Suarez-Orozco, C., Bang, H., O'Connor, E., Gaytan, F., Pakes, J., & Rhodes, J. (2010). Academic trajectories of newcomer immigrant youth. *Developmental Psychology, 46,* 602–618.

Suarez-Orozco, C., & Carhill, A. (2008). Afterword: New directions in research with immigrant families and their children. In H. Yoshikawa & N. Way (Eds.), *Beyond the family: Contexts of immigrant children's development :New directions for child and adolescent development* (pp. 87-104). Hoboken, NJ: Jossey-Bass.

Suarez-Orozco, C., Rhodes, J., & Milburn, M. (2009). Unraveling the immigrant paradox: Academic engagement and disengagement among recently arrived immigrant youth. *Youth & Society, 41,* 151–185.

Suarez-Orozco, C., & Todorova, I. (2003). The social worlds of immigrant youth. In C. Suarez-Orozco & I. Todorova (Eds.), *New directions for youth development: Understanding the social worlds of immigrant youth, 100* (Winter), 15–24.

Thompson, N., & Gurney, A. (2003). "He is everything": Religion's role in the lives of immigrant youth. In C. Suarez-Orozco & I. Todorova (Eds.), *New directions for youth development: Understanding the social worlds of immigrant youth, 100* (Winter),75–90.

Tienda, M., & Haskins, R. (2011). Immigrant children: Introducing the issue. *The Future of Children: Immigrant Children, 21,* 3–18.

Urban Institute. (2010). *Children of immigrants drive the increase in America's youth population, but almost half live in low-income families.* Retrieved from http://www.urban.org

U.S. Citizenship and Immigration Services. (n.d.). *Refugees and asylum.* Retrieved from www. Uscis.gov/portal/site/uscis

World Health Organization, Commission on Social Determinants of Health. (2008). *Closing the gap in a generation: Health equity through action on the social determinants of health.* Geneva, Switzerland: World Health Organization.

Yearwood, E.L., & Siantz, M.L.D. (2010). Global issues in mental health across the life span: Challenges and opportunities. In P. Howard & P. El-Mallakh (Eds.) [Special Issue], *Mental Health Across the Lifespan. Nursing Clinics of North America, 45,* 501–519.

Yearwood, E.L., Crawford, S., Kelly, M., & Moreno, N. (2007). Immigrant youth at risk for disorders of mood: Recognizing complex dynamics. *Archives of Psychiatric Nursing, 21,* 162–171.

Yearwood, E.L. (1998). *'Growing up' children: Current child rearing practice among immigrant Jamaican families* (Doctoral dissertation). Available from ProQuest Dissertations and Theses database. (UMI No. 9907831)

28

Conducting Research with At-Risk and High-Risk Children and Adolescents

M. Katherine Hutchinson and Elizabeth Burgess Dowdell

Objectives

After reading this chapter, APNs will be able to

1. Discuss the roles of advanced practice nurses as consumers, collaborators, and initiators of research.
2. Identify sources of funding for APNs who wish to conduct behavioral health research.
3. Describe the relationship between theory and intervention design for health behavior change.
4. Describe the ethical responsibilities of the APN, as an investigator or research team member, when conducting research with human subjects.

Introduction

Injury-related incidents such as motor vehicle accidents (occupants and pedestrians), homicides, suicides, malignant neoplasms, and heart disease are the leading causes of death in children and adolescents, ages five to nineteen years (Minino, 2010). Many risky health-related behaviors that contribute to morbidity and mortality begin in childhood and adolescence. The 2009 Youth Risk Behavior Surveillance System (YRBSS) reported the most common risky behaviors of teens and young adults—unintentional injuries and violence, tobacco use, alcohol and other drug use, sexual behaviors that contribute to unintentional pregnancy and sexually transmitted diseases, including human immunodeficiency virus (HIV) infection; unhealthy dietary intake, and physical inactivity (Centers for Disease Control and Prevention [CDC],

2010). Although these risk behaviors occur across all groups, some populations are disproportionately affected.

Health behavior research seeks to describe the prevalence of a health-related behavior in a specific population, compare patterns across groups, and examine factors that promote or inhibit the occurrence of risky or protective health behaviors. The ultimate goals are to understand why individuals engage in behaviors that place them at risk for adverse health consequences and identify the individual-, family-, and community-level factors that contribute to these risk behaviors in order to design interventions to prevent health risk behavior, change behavior, and reduce adverse health outcomes. This chapter will discuss the different roles of advanced practice nurses (APNs) in research and the process of conducting health behavior research with at-risk children and adolescents.

Child and Adolescent Behavioral Health: A Resource for Advanced Practice Psychiatric and Primary Care Practitioners in Nursing,
First Edition. Edited by Edilma L. Yearwood, Geraldine S. Pearson, and Jamesetta A. Newland.
© 2012 John Wiley & Sons, Inc. Published 2012 by John Wiley & Sons, Inc.

Advanced Practice Nurses as Research Consumers, Contributors, and Collaborators or Investigators

With a graduate-level education, training, and leadership roles as health care providers and coordinators of care, APNs are the frontline practitioners at the intersections of behavioral health practice and research with at-risk children, adolescents, and families. APNs frequently assume one or more of three primary roles in relation to research—as consumers of research, contributors to ongoing research endeavors, and/or as collaborators or generators of research studies.

Research Consumers

As consumers of research, APNs review and critically evaluate current research and findings in the nursing and behavioral health literature in order to guide evidence-based practice in their work settings (LoBiondo-Wood & Haber, 2009). Readers are referred to Chapter 26 in this text for a thorough discussion of evidence-based practice.

Research Contributors

In addition to being informed consumers of nursing and behavioral science research and promoting the dissemination and use of evidence-based practice, APNs often work in clinical sites and agencies where clinical trials and other research studies with children, adolescents, and families are being conducted. These nurses and APNs are able to contribute to the generation of new knowledge through their participation as research team members. However, nurses and APNs must be very clear about what their roles and responsibilities are, if any, on an ongoing research project and be knowledgeable about the rules and regulations that are associated with each research team role. For example, research team members who are involved in recruiting participants, completing informed consent procedures, and collecting data from research participants must complete training and certification in the ethical conduct of research and the protection of human subjects. Online training/certification programs are available through most universities and major medical centers as well as through the National Institutes of Health (www.nih.gov).

In addition to ensuring that they have completed any required individual training, nurses and APNs who are asked to participate as team members of ongoing research studies should first verify that the study has been reviewed and approved by the appropriate authorities. All research studies that involve human subjects require approval by the institutional review board (IRB) of the university, medical center, or other community institution where the study is being conducted. Depending on the level of risk to patients or subjects that is associated with participation in the study, the IRB may grant the study "exempt" status, conduct an expedited review, or conduct a full-board review. If information from a patient's medical record is being used in a study, then the rules governing the confidentiality of patient information must also be observed. Such studies must comply with the Health Insurance Portability and Accountability Act of 1996 (HIPAA) regulations (www.hhs.gov/ocr/privacy/).

Research Collaborators and Investigators

Beyond being research consumers and team members, there is a growing need for APNs themselves to collaborate and initiate research studies to investigate research questions that are of significance and relevance to nursing. These individuals provide the impetus for new research and the generation of new knowledge by taking on lead roles as principal and co-investigators and guiding the design and implementation of behavioral research with children, adolescents, and families. Many of the most important research questions are derived from experience, observations from practice, and knowledge of the population with whom one works. As research investigators, APNs can further the development of nursing science and promote nursing's voice in the development of interdisciplinary science in order to promote positive health behaviors among at-risk children, adolescents, and families. With its longstanding commitment to health promotion and prevention, nursing is uniquely qualified to assume a lead role in interdisciplinary behavioral health research as the national emphasis continues to shift in that direction.

How does one initiate a research study? It all begins with a question. As was previously mentioned, research questions often come from practice and clinical observations. From personal observations in practice, it may "seem" to the APN that certain youth are more likely to engage in a certain behavior, X, than other youth. Likewise, the APN may question the best way to intervene with a specific ethnic or cultural group. He/she should first search through the published literature and find what is already known. If there are gaps in the literature, if little is known about a question of interest that is significant to nursing and health (see NINR priorities and Healthy People 2010 priorities [Department of Health and Human Services, 1999]), then research on the question may be warranted.

This is not to say that the APN with no research experience (and a full-time job) should "go it alone." Research is time-consuming and demanding. It is easy for an inexperienced researcher to become mired down in the time and work required for even the simplest of studies. It is also easy to overlook potential problems and flaws in study design. In order to be worthwhile, research needs to be rigorous and methodically executed. An experienced researcher can anticipate study flaws and confounds and assist in the development of the best possible study to answer the research question. The practicing nurse with a researchable question should identify experienced researchers who could serve as potential collaborators and develop a research team. Collaboration is an excellent way to capitalize on many people's individual expertise and also distribute the workload. Thus, roles and responsibilities need to be made very clear from the start to avoid common problems later. Every research team should include at least one member who is an expert in research design (quantitative or qualitative) and an expert in data analysis. If you are planning a quantitative study in which data will be statistically analyzed, then a statistician should be consulted from the outset.

Building a Research Team

Important questions to answer when developing a research team include:

- Who will be the lead or principal investigator?
- Who will be the co-investigators or other research team members?
- What will be each person's contribution to the project?
- Who will receive credit and be included in publications or presentations of research results? (Who will be first author, second author, etc.?)
- What is the question to be answered?
- What type of data will be collected? How will the data be collected?
- How will the data be analyzed and by whom?

Potential research collaborators may already be present in the clinical practice site. Many large medical centers have research centers and research directors; many have directors of nursing research. These individuals may be able to provide direct assistance or refer the neophyte to other experienced researchers who may be of assistance. Other clinicians, practitioners, physicians, administrators, and leaders within the clinical site may be interested in participating on a research team. While these individuals may be valuable research team members who are able to provide both clinical expertise and access to patient populations, they may or may not be experts in research design and data analysis. In order to be successful, the research team needs to have members who are experienced researchers and methodological experts. If there are experienced researchers present in the clinical setting, they may be ideal choices as collaborators. These

persons bring an additional benefit as they are likely to be knowledgeable about the procedures and approvals needed to conduct a research study in that specific clinical practice site.

Research collaborators may also be identified at a local university; this is particularly true if it is a research-intensive university. Many universities have faculty web pages that provide an overview of the individual's research interests and experience. Another way to identify potential collaborators is through reviewing published research reports in nursing and interdisciplinary journals and by attending research conferences. It is important to bear in mind that research collaborators do not have to be located in the same city or state. Experienced researchers who have similar interests may be willing to serve as co-investigators or consultants for your project. Whether or not they are local, experienced researchers may be familiar with how to best ask the questions of interest. They may have or know of reliable and valid instruments or questionnaires that can be used to measure behaviors and attitudes of interest. Experienced researchers may have research staff with whom they work and may be able to identify statisticians or others who can help plan the data analysis for the project. Finally, if the focus of the research study is to develop and/or test an intervention to change behavior or support behavior change, then the team should seek out an experienced intervention researcher, someone who is knowledgeable and experienced in the design and evaluation of behavioral interventions.

In addition to building a research team, it is necessary to identify what other resources are needed to conduct a research study. For the APN in primary care or mental health, key questions include:

- What other resources (time, personnel, equipment, space) will be needed to conduct the study?
- Will research grant funding be needed? If so, how much money is needed? Where might the needed funding be obtained?
- How will a researcher gain access to the population of interest?

Sources of Research Funding for Nurses

For more than twenty years, the National Institute of Nursing Research (NINR) has been one of the primary funders of nursing research in the United States. NINR grew out of the findings from two federal studies and related public acts. "A 1983 report by the Institute of Medicine concluded that nursing research be included in the mainstream of biomedical and behavioral science, and a 1984 National Institutes of Health (NIH)

Task Force study found nursing research activities to be relevant to the NIH mission" (www.nih.gov/ninr). In response to these recommendations, the National Center for Nursing Research (NCNR) was established at NIH in 1986. In 1993, the name was changed to the National Institute of Nursing Research to reflect a change in its status to that of an institute.

NINR supports research training for nurse scientists and provides research grant funding to support basic and clinical research. The research priorities of NINR include health promotion, disease prevention, quality of life, health disparities, and end-of-life care (http://www.ninr.nih.gov/AboutNINR/NINRMissionandStrategicPlan). According to its Congressional Budget Justification (http://www.ninr.nih.gov/AboutNINR/BudgetandLegislation/), NINR awarded more than $99 million in research project grants in fiscal year 2009 to conduct research in a wide variety of areas of interest to nursing.

In addition to NINR, there are a number of other NIH institutes and centers whose missions overlap areas that may be of interest to APNs with a focus on child and adolescent behavioral health. Some of these include:

- National Cancer Institute (NCI)
- National Institute on Alcohol Abuse and Alcoholism (NIAA)
- National Institute of Allergy and Infectious Diseases (NIAID)
- Eunice Kennedy Shriver National Institute of Child Health and Human Development (NICHD)
- National Institute on Drug Abuse (NIDA)
- National Institute of Mental Health (NIMH)
- National Institute on Minority Health and Health Disparities (NIMHD)

Many other federal and nonfederal agencies, foundations, and private organizations also fund research in child and adolescent behavioral health that is consistent with their particular mission. The CDC awards millions of dollars in research grants every year to enhance understanding of the mechanisms of disease and health-risk behaviors. The CDC also funds the widespread distribution of effective behavior change interventions. For example, Dr. Loretta Sweet Jemmott, a nurse researcher from the University of Pennsylvania School of Nursing, developed an HIV prevention intervention for urban adolescents entitled, "Be Proud! Be Responsible!" This intervention was then disseminated nationally by the CDC as part of its "Programs that Work" initiative (Jemmott, Jemmott, & Fong, 1992).

Nongovernment organizations that frequently fund nursing research include the Robert Wood Johnson Foundation, the American Nurses Foundation (ANF), Sigma Theta Tau International (STTI), local chapters of STTI, and many state nurses' associations. National and local specialty nursing organizations also offer research grants that might be of interest to APNs with a focus on child and adolescent behavioral health, including the American Academy of Nurse Practitioners, American Association of Critical Care Nurses, National Association of Pediatric Nurse Associates and Practitioners, Academy of Neonatal Nursing, and the Association of Women's Health, Obstetric and Neonatal Nurses. These organizations tend to fund research in their particular areas of interest. Most have web sites or publications that provide specifics on their research grant programs, funding cycles, and eligibility requirements. While most NIH research grants require that the principal investigator holds a doctorate or other terminal degree, many foundations, specialty organizations, and regional research foundations accept research grant applications from nurses and nurse practitioners with master's degrees.

Conducting Health Behavior Research with At-Risk Children, Adolescents, and Families

Health behavior research seeks to describe patterns of health behavior and understand why individuals engage in behaviors that place them at risk for adverse health consequences. Ultimately, information gathered is used to design interventions to change behavior, support behavior change, and to reduce adverse health outcomes.

However, health behavior is complex. Knowledge alone does not determine behavior. For example, most adolescents and young adults "know" the facts about smoking; they are knowledgeable about the adverse effects of cigarette smoking on their health. So why do adolescents smoke cigarettes? Similarly, why do adolescents drink alcohol? Exhibit unhealthy eating behaviors (e.g., overeating, anorexia, bulimia)? Engage in unprotected sex? Because health behavior is complex and knowledge alone does not determine behavior, simplistic interventions that seek to change behavior by increasing knowledge are unlikely to succeed; they are equally unlikely to be funded.

In order to be effective, behavioral interventions must be theory based, culture specific, developmentally appropriate, and rigorously evaluated (Jemmott, Jemmott, & Hutchinson, 2001; Pequegnat & Scapoznik, 2000). Behavioral interventions that are theory based are more likely to be effective than those that are not theory based (Ammerman, Lindquist, Lohr, & Hersey, 2002; Fishbein, 2000).

Using Health Behavior Theories and Models to Guide Behavioral Health Research and Interventions

Theories and models of health behavior help the APN in both clinical practice and research by providing structure for understanding health-related behaviors and highlighting factors that are likely influences of the behavior. Although it is beyond the scope of this chapter to provide a comprehensive or in-depth discussion of health behavior models and theories, a brief summary of some of the leading health behavior theories is provided below. For more detailed coverage, readers are referred to *Health Behavior and Health Education: Theory, Research and Practice* (Glanz, Rimer, & Viswanath, 2008a, 2008b) and *Emerging Theories in Health Promotion Practice and Research* (DiClemente, Crosby, & Kegler, 2002).

Individual-Level Models

Many of the most widely used models for understanding health behavior focus on the individual and have their roots in disciplines such as psychology and social psychology. Three examples include the transtheoretical stages of change model (TTM) (Prochaska, Redding, & Evers, 2008), the theory of planned behavior (TPB), and its precursor, the theory of reasoned action (TRA) (Ajzen, 1985, 1991, 2005; Ajzen & Fishbein, 1980; Montano & Kasprzyk, 2008).

In brief, the TTM posits that behavior change is a process that evolves through a series of stages. The process itself involves an individual recognizing the need for change, developing intentions to change, and ultimately undertaking and maintaining the behavior change (Prochaska et al., 2008). Widely used for studies of addiction, smoking cessation, dietary change, and exercise behavior, the implication for behavioral intervention is that programs are more likely to be effective if they are designed to address the individual's needs at his or her current stage in the change process.

The five stages identified in the TTM include (a) precontemplation (a defensive and resistant phase in which the individual may not acknowledge the problem or the need to change; (b) contemplation (an ambivalent phase in which the individual may be thinking about taking action but the negatives associated with changing are seen as greater than the benefits of behavior change); (c) preparation (a planning phase in which the individual may want to change and develops a plan to take action); (d) action (the phase in which the individual makes specific changes in behavior); and (e) maintenance (the long-term postchange phase during which the individual works to prevent relapse to earlier behaviors (Prochaska et al., 2008). Behavior change interventions

for persons in the earlier stages might focus on assessing attitudes toward behavior change, developing awareness for risk reduction if not elimination, promoting the positive aspects of behavior change and helping individuals to work through their fears related to change (Prochaska et al.).

In contrast, the TPB (Ajzen, 1985, 1991, 2005) and its predecessor, the TRA (Ajzen & Fishbein, 1980), focus on how an individual's beliefs and attitudes influence his/her intentions and likelihood of performing a specific behavior (Ajzen, 1985, 1991, 2005; Ajzen & Fishbein; Hutchinson & Wood, 2007; Jemmott et al., 2001; Montano & Kasprzyk, 2008). The TRA and TPB have been widely used to model a variety of health-related behaviors including HIV-related sexual risk behavior and condom use (Hutchinson, Jemmott, Jemmott, Braverman, & Fong, 2003; Jemmott, Jemmott, & Villarruel, 2002; Villarruel, Jemmott, Jemmott, & Rodis, 2004), smoking (Godin, Valois, Lepage, & Desharnqais, 1992; Hanson, 1997), and adolescent eating practices (Fila & Smith, 2006).

The TPB asserts that intentions are the primary determinants of behavior and intentions are, in turn, influenced by the individual's attitudes/behavioral beliefs, normative beliefs, and perceived behavioral control/control beliefs regarding the behavior (Ajzen, 2005; Ajzen & Fishbein, 1980; Hutchinson & Wood, 2007; Montano & Kasprzyk, 2008). Attitudes refer to the tendency to favor or disfavor the behavior, whereas behavioral beliefs refer to perceptions about the likely consequences of performing the behavior (Ajzen, 1985, 2005). Normative beliefs are an individual's perceptions of whether people who are important to him/her would approve or disapprove of him/her performing the behavior (Ajzen, 1985, 2005). Control beliefs are the individual's perceptions as to whether he/she has the skills to perform the behavior and perceived behavioral control refers to perceptions of how easy or difficult it is to perform the behavior (Ajzen, 1985, 2005).

Multilevel Models

Other models focus more broadly on the individual's interactions with others or the environment and how these interactions influence his or her health-related behaviors. Examples of these types of theories and models include social cognitive theory (Bandura, 1997; McAllister, Perry, & Parcel, 2008), ecological models (Bronfenbrenner, 1989; Sallis, Owen, & Fisher, 2008), social networks and social support models (Heaney & Israel, 2008; Olds, Henderson, Chamberlin, & Tatelbaum, 1986; Olds, Robinson, et al., 2002), and more recently, the theory of gender and power (Wingood & DiClemente, 2000). These types of multilevel models have several added benefits: (a) they are particularly relevant for understanding the behavior of children and adolescents who live within family systems (Hutchinson & Wood, 2007); (b) they add to our understanding of health disparities among racial and ethnic minorities and marginalized populations by highlighting the community-level and society-level factors that contribute to adverse health outcomes (Hutchinson, Thompson, & Cederbaum, 2006; Wingood & DiClemente); and (c) they identify multiple potential targets with whom one can intervene to ameliorate health problems in addition to the individual. As a result, these multilevel models may be more likely to lead to effective interventions (DiClemente & Wingood, 2000; Hutchinson, Thompson, et al., 2006; Hutchinson & Wood, 2007; Pequegnat & Szapocznik, 2000) than individual-level only designs.

For example, ecological models acknowledge that individuals live within a series of nested systems and they are in constant interaction with these systems and other individuals (Bronfenbrenner, 1989; Sallis et al., 2008). For children and adolescents, these systems would include families, school systems, communities, and the larger society. Children and adolescents may also be influenced by systems that they themselves may not have direct contact with (e.g., the parent's work environment) (Bronfenbrenner; Sallis et al.). Because of the ongoing interactions between children and these systems, multilevel intervention programs may include components directed to the children themselves, their parents, peer networks, schools, etc. By moving beyond the individual (DiClemente & Wingood, 2000), interventions that employ these "multiprong" or multilevel approaches may generate greater and/or more sustained effects than individual-only interventions (Hutchinson & Wood, 2007; Pequegnat & Szapocnik, 2000).

Applying Behavioral Health Models in Nursing Research

Nurse researchers who are interested in behavioral health often *adopt* interdisciplinary models and apply them to research contexts and problems that are of significance to nursing. For example, Flynn (1999) developed a family support intervention to reduce the incidence of low birthweight, reduce the risk for child abuse and neglect, and increase immunization rates among infants born to adolescent mothers in Newark, New Jersey, through the use of community support persons. The intervention design was derived from David Olds's models of family support (Olds et al., 1986, 2002). Program participants had significantly lower rates of low birthweight infants, significantly higher rates of infant immunization, and

lower scores on a risk assessment battery for child abuse and neglect than control group members who did not receive the intervention (Flynn).

Nurse researchers also *adapt* existing theories and models from nursing and other disciplines in order to enhance the understanding of a phenomenon or provide additional guidance to research and intervention design. For example, in a 2001 NIH-funded study (R03 MH63659, M. K. Hutchinson, PI), Hutchinson expanded the TPB into a dyadic model to illustrate that the intentions of both the male and female sexual partners can influence whether condoms are used during sexual intercourse. This model posited that the gender-power dynamic within the couple would moderate which partner's condom use intentions were enacted.

Later, Hutchinson and Wood (2007) expanded the TPB into a family-level model to illustrate the influence of parents on the sexual risk–related attitudes and beliefs of their adolescent children and the potential to intervene with both parents and adolescents in order to change adolescents' risk behaviors. This model, shown in Figure 28.1, was used to guide a research study examining the influence of urban African American mothers on the tobacco, alcohol, and substance use behaviors of their adolescent sons (R03 DA029707, Cederbaum & Hutchinson, Co-PIs), and studies of parent influences of sexual risk-related attitudes and behaviors among urban African American adolescent girls (Hutchinson et al., 2003) and African American college students (Hutchinson & Montgomery, 2007). As is described below, it also served as the framework for the development and testing of a mother-daughter HIV risk reduction intervention in Kingston, Jamaica (R01 NR010478, M. K. Hutchinson, PI).

Case Exemplar

This example involves developing a theory-based intervention to change behavior. Regardless of whether the focus is on nursing practice in an acute care setting or the development of a behavior change program, intervention development should always be a systematic process that is informed by what is already known and guided by an appropriate theoretical model (Jemmott et al., 2001; Whittenmore & Grey, 2002). The following is an example of the systematic development of a theory-based behavior change intervention.

In 2007, researchers developed the *Jamaican Mother-Daughter HIV Risk Reduction Intervention* and tested the intervention's effectiveness through a randomized controlled trial. The research proposal itself was the result of several years of collaboration, team-building, interviews with key informants in Jamaica, and focus groups

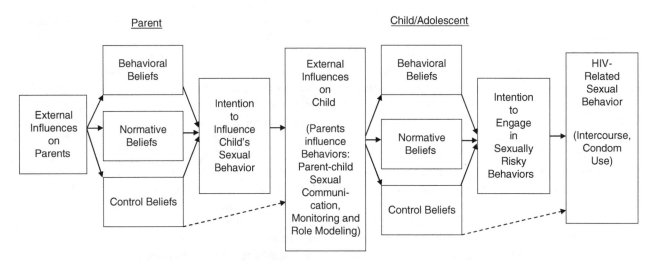

Figure 28.1 Parent-based expansion of the theory of planned behavior. Reprinted from Hutchinson & Wood, 2007, with permission from John Wiley & Sons, Inc.

with parents, teens, and teachers (Hutchinson et al., 2007). The goals of the intervention program were to (a) reduce the sexual risk behaviors and sexually transmitted infection (STI) rates among urban Jamaican girls, ages thirteen to seventeen years, and (b) increase their mothers' protective parenting behaviors, including sexual risk communication, supervision, and role modeling.

The four-year project was scheduled to occur in three distinct phases. Year 1 focused on strengthening existing collaborations between U.S. and Jamaican researchers, identifying community-based organizations and individuals who would serve on a community advisory board, and conducting additional focus groups with Jamaican mothers and adolescent girls to better understand what specific attitudes, beliefs, and behaviors should be addressed in the intervention and how the intervention should be structured and scheduled. Year 2 included adapting research instruments and questionnaires for use with urban Jamaican mothers and teens and pilot testing them. The other major focus for Year 2 was developing the actual intervention curricula for mothers and daughters. In Years 3 and 4, the interventions would be implemented with 360 pairs of urban adolescent girls, ages thirteen to seventeen, and their mothers or female guardians. The effectiveness of the intervention would be evaluated by comparing self-reported data on questionnaires that mothers and daughters would complete before the intervention, immediately after the intervention, and three and six months after the intervention. In addition to questionnaires, adolescent girls would provide urine specimens for STI testing before the intervention and again at the six-month follow-up session.

The Jamaican Mother-Daughter HIV Risk Reduction Intervention Curricula

Hutchinson and Wood's (2007) parent-based expansion of the TPB-guided development of the intervention. Separate curricula were developed specifically for Jamaican mothers and daughters based upon findings from the earlier elicitation and focus group research (Hutchinson et al., 2007). Each intervention curriculum included ten 50-minute sessions or modules that were scheduled over two consecutive Saturdays. All of the modules were scripted, led by trained facilitators, and included age- and culturally appropriate videos, music, games, activities, and discussions. Many of the activities and modules included in the intervention were adapted from HIV risk-reduction interventions developed by Loretta Sweet Jemmott, which had been effective in reducing HIV-related sexual risk with urban adolescents, women, and families in the United States. The initial intervention curricula were completed and pilot tested in August 2009. Final revisions were made based on the results of the pilot testing.

The intervention curricula corresponded closely to the parent-based expansion of the TPB (shown in Figure 28.1). The mothers' curriculum addressed behavioral beliefs, normative beliefs, and perceived behavioral control related to parenting behaviors such as mother-daughter sexual communication, supervision, and role modeling. The daughters' curriculum focused on girls' behavioral beliefs, normative beliefs, and perceived behavioral control related to abstinence and unprotected intercourse, partner negation, and refusal skills. Each 50-minute module addressed a specific component of the model. For example, one of the modules for mothers addressed sexual role modeling and mothers' beliefs and attitudes about how their own behavior might influence their daughters. Several modules addressed mother-daughter sexual risk communication, helped mothers identify their own beliefs and fears regarding sexual communication and led them through a series of activities and role-plays designed to increase their communication skills. Before initiating the study, researchers addressed several issues inherent in conducting research with children and adolescents.

Issues of Informed Consent with At-Risk Children and Adolescents Involved in Behavioral Health Research

APNs who participate as principal investigators (PIs), co-investigators (Co-Is), or as a research team member should understand that collecting data from human subjects can be a complicated process. All of data collection is governed by ethical principles on how human being should be and must be treated during the research process. In 1964, the Declaration of Helsinki was developed and adopted by the World Medical Association (WMA) as a statement to those conducting human research on the important use of ethical principles in their studies (O'Lonergan & Zodrow, 2006). Like the WMA, the American Nurses Association (ANA) also developed codes of scientific conduct by forming the Commission on Nursing Research which identified the rights of human subjects in three ways: (1) right to freedom from harm, (2) right to privacy and dignity, and (3) right to anonymity (Griffin & Titler, 2009). All nurses are charged with the responsibility of protecting the rights of all subjects in their care (Griffin & Titler).

The question of including children and adolescents, especially young children or at-risk children, as participants in research studies is one that has been debated for years and is coupled with the concern of whether a child can provide an informed consent for his /her own participation. Historically, children and adolescents were unable to receive health care or medical treatment, except in an emergency, without clear explicit consent from a parent or guardian. As evidenced by standing law, the consent of a parent is required to treat a child; providers who fail to obtain consent when it is required expose themselves to legal liability in terms of both malpractice (for failing to adhere to standards of care) and, in some cases, for medical battery (for touching and treatment of another person without consent) (Harty-Golder, 2008).

Although some types of research may differ from medical treatment, many clinical trials involve treatment as part of the research protocol. When recruiting subjects to participate in a clinical trial or in any research project, researchers must do a thorough assessment of the risk/benefit ratio. Risk may occur in any one of several domains, including physical, emotional, and privacy (Beigay, 2007). Institutional protocols and state and national laws require that all individuals be provided with detailed information prior to participating in any research project or study.

Consent

Research team members are responsible for making sure that each person understands the nature of the research project and the implications of participating. At the beginning of the 20th century Justice Benjamin Cardozo wrote, "Every human being of adult years, and sound mind, has the right to determine what shall be done with his body" (Naarden & Cissik, 2006, p. 194). With this statement, the foundation of informed consent for treatment or research participation was put into place.

In research, consenting to participate is based on two ethical principles, autonomy and beneficence. Autonomy refers to self-determination, an individual's right to assess the risks and benefits and then agree or disagree to participate in research (O'Lonergan & Zodrow, 2006; Simpson, 2009). Beneficence refers to protection of the research participant (Simpson). While these principles can be easily applied to adults who are considered competent and able to make decisions, extra steps are required when the potential research participant is a member of a vulnerable population (e.g., a child or an adolescent).

Informed Consent

Prior to beginning any research study or project, approval from the IRB that governs the research setting must be obtained. The IRB pays particular attention to the process of informed consent. Informed consent has evolved over time and is now universally accepted as a significant part of sample recruitment and data collection (O'Lonergan & Zodrow, 2006). Informed consent must include notifying participants:

- They may choose to participate or not participate in the study
- They may change their mind and withdraw from the study at any time without harm or consequences
- What the study is and what participation in the study entails
- What the potential benefits of participating in the study are
- What potential risks (physical, emotional, economic, social, or legal) may occur as a result of participating in the study

Informed consent must be written in simple language. If subjects cannot read, forms should be read to potential subjects by a member of the research team. Many studies may include individuals who identify English as a second language; consent form(s) for these individuals should be written in their native language or read and clearly explained by an interpreter. Finally, persons who are approached and invited to participate in a research study should have sufficient time to carefully think about whether to participate.

Children's Ability to Provide Informed Consent

The researcher must assess the developmental and cognitive capacity of the child or adolescent to ensure the individual has the ability to understand and appreciate the risk, benefits, and requirements of participation in the study before agreeing or declining to consent (Simpson, 2009). In 2005 the U.S. Department of Health and Human Services (USDHHS), in its Policy for the Protection of Human Subjects in subpart section 46.402, defined a child as "a person who has not attained the legal age for consent to treatments or procedures involved in the research, under the applicable law of the jurisdiction in which the research will be conducted" (p. 12). Usually there is an assumption that any person younger than eighteen years old is a child, since age eighteen years has generally been established as the legal age of consent. However, it is important to realize that the actual age limit can vary across states and across funding agencies (Beigay, 2007; Tillet, 2005).

In both law and ethics, children and adolescents have been presumed to lack the capacity to provide informed consent; a child is considered a "developing person" (Fisher, 2006). Depending upon where the child or adolescent is in his or her development, or chronological age, she or he may not be considered to be intellectually, emotionally, or cognitively capable of providing legal informed consent. It is the immaturity of his or her cognitive development that may be in question, or the lack of experiences in situations similar to what she or he is being asked to do in regards to participation in the research study.

The Common Rule (U.S. DHHS Title 45 CFR 46 Subparts A, B, C and D) is the baseline standard of ethics to which any government-funded research in the United States is held (Office for Human Research Protections [OHRP], 2010). The Common Rule requires parental permission and assent from children generally seven or older for federally regulated research (OHRP; O'Lonergan & Zodrow, 2006).

Child Assent

In addition to obtaining parental consent, most studies that involve children and adolescents must also obtain child assent. Child assent refers to a child's affirmative agreement to participate in a research study; assent is not the same as failure to object (O'Lonergan & Zodrow, 2006; ORHP, 2010). In order to obtain child assent, the child must be provided with the same basic information given during the process of informed consent. This information may need to be simplified or limited depending upon the child's comprehension level and ability to make decisions (Faux, Walsh, & Deatrick, 1988; O'Lonergan & Zodrow). IRB guidelines vary with regard to documentation of assent, and researchers should be certain they understand the requirements of their own IRBs. Some IRBs require children above age twelve or fourteen years to sign a separate youth consent/assent form (ORHP, 2010). For children and adolescents, the language used in an assent form must be at a developmentally appropriate level (O'Lonergan & Zodrow).

Emancipated Minors

Emancipation is a formal legal action in which an adolescent can petition to basically free him/herself (minor child) from the supervision of his or her adult parent(s). Emancipated minors can assume most of the legal rights of adulthood, including the right to enter into contracts and the ability to consent to medical care, if they are able to provide court documents to verify their status (Harty-Golder, 2008). The provisions that permit a minor to be considered emancipated vary from state to state and may depend upon the specific circumstances. For example, a minor can be considered emancipated for one specific purpose (e.g., for obtaining birth control) but not for others such as consenting to surgery or entering into a legal contract (Beigay, 2007). A suggested guideline for use with adolescents who state that they are emancipated is to request a copy of the emancipation order prior to enrollment into the research study and/or check with the IRB at your institution.

Summary

In summary, APNs who work in primary care or psychiatric and behavioral health settings must be knowledgeable about research. In their roles as direct care providers and leaders, APNs should, at the very least, be informed consumers of research who use research findings to guide evidence-based practice. In addition to being informed consumers, many APNs participate as research team members in studies that are being conducted in their clinical agencies. It is incumbent upon all nurses and APNs who interact with research participants to be aware of their responsibilities regarding the ethical conduct of research and treatment of human research subjects. Finally, because of their graduate education and front-line clinical practice, many APNs are in the unique position of being able to identify health behavior and intervention problems and questions that are in need of answers. As research co-investigators and collaborators, these APNs are able to initiate research projects that help to build nursing science and advance our knowledge of health behavior with at-risk children and adolescents.

References

Ajzen, I. (1985). From intentions to actions: A theory of planned behavior. In J. Kuhl & J. Beckmann (Eds.), *Action control: From cognition to behavior*, pp. 11–39. Berlin, Germany: Spring-Verlag.

Ajzen, I. (1991). The theory of planned behavior. *Organizational Behavior and Human Decision Processes, 50,* 179–211.

Ajzen, I. (2005). *Attitudes, personality and behavior* (2nd ed.). New York: Open University Press.

Ajzen, I., & Fishbein, M. (1980). *Understanding attitudes and predicting social behavior.* Englewood Cliffs, NJ: Prentice-Hall.

Ammerman, A., Lindquist, C., Lohr, K., & Hersey, J. (2002). The efficacy of behavioral interventions to modify dietary fat and fruit and vegetable intake: A review of the evidence. *Preventive Medicine, 35*(1), 25 – 41.

Bandura, A. (1997). *Self-efficacy: The exercise of control.* New York: W. H. Freeman.

Beigay, T. (2007). Children in research: Human subjects considerations for the inclusion of children as research participants. *Progress in Transplantation, 17,* 54–56.

Bronfenbrenner, U. (1989). Ecological systems theory. *Annals of Child Development, 6,* 556–581.

Centers for Disease Control and Prevention (CDC). (2010, June 4). 2009. Youth Risk Behavior Surveillance – United States, 2009. *MMWR, 59*(No. SS-5). Retrieved from http://www.cdc.gov/mmwr/pdf/ss/ss5905.pdf

DiClemente, R. J., Crosby, R. A., & Kegler, M. C. (Eds.). (2002). *Emerging theories in health promotion practice and research: Strategies for improving public health.* San Francisco, CA: Jossey-Bass.

Department of Health and Human Services (DHHS). (1999). *Healthy People 2010.* Washington, DC: U.S. Government Printing Office.

DiClemente, R., & Wingood, G. (2000). Expanding the scope of HIV prevention for adolescents: Beyond individual-level interventions. *Journal of Adolescent Health, 26,* 377–378.

Faux, S. A., Walsh, M., Deatrick, J. A. (1988). Intensive interviewing with children and adolescents. *Western Journal of Nursing Research, 10,* 180–194.

Fila, S., & Smith, C. (2006). *International Journal of Behavioral Nutrition and Physical Activity, 3,* 3–11.

Fishbein, M. (2000). The role of theory in HIV prevention. *AIDS CARE, 12*(3), 273–278.

Fisher, C. (2006). Privacy and ethics in pediatric environmental health research – Part 1: Genetic and prenatal testing. *Environmental Health Perspectives, 114,* 1617–1621.

Flynn, L. (1999). The adolescent parenting program: Improving outcomes through mentorship. *Public Health Nursing, 16*(3), 182–189.

Glanz, K., Rimer, B., & Viswanath, K. (Eds.). (2008a). *Health behavior and health education: Theory, research and practice* (4th ed.). San Francisco, CA: John Wiley & Sons.

Glanz, K., Rimer, B., & Viswanath, K. (2008b). The scope of health behavior and health education. In K. Glanz, K. Rimer, and K. Viswanath (Eds.), *Health behavior and health education: Theory, research and practice* (4th ed.)(pp. 3–22). San Francisco, CA: John Wiley & Sons.

Godin, G., Valois, P., Lepage, L., & Desharnais, R. (1992). Predictors of smoking behaviour: An application of Ajzen's theory of planned behaviour. *British Journal of Addiction, 87,* 1335–1343.

Griffin, E. & Titler. M. (2009). Using evidence through collaboration to promote excellence in nursing practice. In N.A. Schmidt and J.M. Brown (Eds.) *Evidence-based practice for nurses: Appraisal and application of research.* Sudbury, MA: Jones & Bartlett Publishers.

Hanson, M. (1997). The theory of planned behavior applied to cigarette smoking in African American, Puerto Rican and non-Hispanic white teenage females. *Nursing Research, 46*(3), 155–162.

Harty-Golder, B. (2008). Defining minors under the law. *Medical Laboratory Observer.* November. Available at http:www.mlo-online.com. Accessed on January 28, 2010.

Heaney, C., & Israel, B. (2008). Social networks and social support. In K. Glanz, K. Rimer, and K. Viswanath (Eds.), *Health behavior and health education: Theory, research and practice* (4th ed.) (pp. 189–210). San Francisco, CA: John Wiley & Sons.

Hutchinson, M. K., Jemmott, J. B., Jemmott, L. S., Braverman, P., & Fong, G. (2003). The role of mother-daughter sexual risk communication in reducing sexual risk behaviors among urban adolescent females: A prospective study. *Journal of Adolescent Health, 33*(2), 98–107.

Hutchinson, M. K., Jemmott, L. S., Wood, E., Hewitt, H., Kahwa, E., Waldron, N., & Bonaparte, B. (2007). Culture-specific factors contributing to HIV risk among Jamaican adolescents. *Journal of the Association of Nurses in AIDS Care, 18*(2), 35–47.

Hutchinson, M. K., & Montgomery, A. (2007). Parent communication and sexual risk among African Americans. *Western Journal of Nursing Research, 29,* 691–707.

Hutchinson, M. K., Thompson, A., & Cederbaum, J. A. (2006). Multisystem factors contributing to disparities in preventive health care among lesbian women. *JOGNN, 35,* 393–402.

Hutchinson, M. K. & Wood, E. (2007). Reconceptualizing adolescent sexual risk using a parent-based expansion of the Theory of Planned Behavior. *Journal of Nursing Scholarship, 39* (2), 141–146.

Jemmott, J. B. III, Jemmott, L. S., & Fong, G. T. (1992). Reductions in HIV risk-associated sexual behaviors among Black male adolescents: Effects of an AIDS prevention intervention. *American Journal of Public Health, 82,* 372–377.

Jemmott, L., Jemmott, J., & Hutchinson, M. (2001). HIV/AIDS: Prevention needs and strategies for a public health emergency. In R. Braithwaite (Ed.), *Health issues in the Black community* (2nd ed.) (pp. 309–346). San Francisco, CA: Jossey-Bass.

Jemmott, L., Jemmott, J., & Villarruel, A. (2002). Predicting intentions and condom use among Latino college students. *Journal of the Association of Nurses in AIDS Care, 13*(2), 59–69.

LoBiondo-Wood, G., & Haber, J. (2009). *Nursing research: Methods and critical appraisal for evidence-based practice.* Philadelphia, PA: Mosby.

Minino, A. M. (2010, May). Mortality among teenagers aged 12–19 years: United States, 1999–2006. *NCHS Data Brief, 37,* 1–8. Hyattsville, MD: National Center for Health Statistics. Retrieved from http://www.cdc.gov/nchs/data/databriefs/db37.pdf

McAllister, A., Perry, C., & Parcel, G. (2008). How individuals, environments and health behaviors interact: Social cognitive theory. In K. Glanz, K. Rimer, and K. Viswanath (Eds.), *Health behavior and health education: Theory, research and practice* (4th ed.) (pp. 169–188). San Francisco, CA: John Wiley & Sons.

Montano, D., & Kasprzyk, D. (2008). The theory of reasoned action, theory of planned behavior and the integrated behavioral model. In K. Glanz, K. Rimer, and K. Viswanath (Eds.), *Health behavior and health education: Theory, research and practice* (4th ed.)(pp. 67–96). San Francisco: John Wiley & Sons.

Naarden. A., & Cissik, J. (2006). Informed consent. *The American Journal of Medicine, 119*, 194–197.

Office for Human Research Protections (OHRP). (2010). Policy guidelines for the Common Rule: Title 45 CFR 46 (Public Welfare). The U.S. Department of Health and Human Services. Retrieved from http://www.hhs.gov/ohrp/researchfaq.pdf

Olds, D., Henderson, C., Chamberlin, R., & Tatelbaum, R. (1986). Preventing child abuse and neglect: A randomized trial of nurse home visitation. *Pediatrics, 78*(1), 65–78.

Olds, D., Robinson, J., O'Brien, R., Luckey, D., Pettitt, L., Henderson, C., Ng, R., Sheff, K., Korfmacher, J., Hiatt, S., & Talmi, A. (2002). Home visiting by paraprofessionals and by nurses: A randomized controlled trial. *Pediatrics, 110*, 486–496.

O'Lonergan, T., & Zodrow, J. J. (2006). Pediatric assent: Subject protection issues among adolescent females enrolled in research. *Journal of Law, Medicine & Ethics, 34*, 451–459.

Pequegnat, W., & Szapocznik, J. (2000). The role of families in preventing and adapting to HIV/AIDS: Issues and answers. In W. Pequegnat and J.Szapocznik (Eds.), *Working with families in the era of HIV/AIDS* (pp. 3–26). Thousand Oaks, CA: Sage.

Prochaska,J., Redding, C., & Evers, K. (2008). The transtheoretical model and stages of change. In K. Glanz, K. Rimer, and K. Viswanath (Eds.), *Health behavior and health education: Theory, research and practice* (4th ed.)(pp. 97–122). San Francisco: John Wiley & Sons.

Sallis, J., Owen, N., & Fisher, E. (2008). Ecological models of health behavior. In K. Glanz, K. Rimer, and K. Viswanath (Eds.), *Health behavior and health education: Theory, research and practice* (4th ed.) (pp. 465–486). San Francisco, CA: John Wiley & Sons.

Simpson. C. (2009). Decision-making capacity and informed consent to participate in research by cognitively impaired individuals. *Applied Nursing Research.* doi:10.1016/j.apnr.2008.09.002

Tillet, J. (2005). Adolescents and informed consent: Ethical and legal issues. *Journal of Perinatal & Neonatal Nursing, 19*(2), 112–121.

U.S. Department of Health and Human Services (DHHS). (2005). Public Welfare: Protection of Human Subjects. Retrieved from http://www.hhs.gov/ohrp/humansubjects/guidance/45cfr 46.htm

Villarruel, A., Jemmott, J., Jemmott, L., & Ronis, D. (2004). Predictors of sexual intercourse and condom use intentions among Spanish-dominant Latino youth: A test of the planned behavior theory. *Nursing Research, 53*, 172–181.

Whittemore, R., & Grey, M. (2002). The systematic development of nursing interventions. *Journal of Nursing Scholarship, 34*, 115–120.

Wingood, G., & DiClemente, R. (2000). Application of the theory of gender and power to examine HIV related exposures, risk factors and effective interventions for women. *Health Education Behaviors, 27*, 539–565.

29

Advanced Practice Nurses Interfacing with the School System

Ellen Carroll, Allison W. Kilcoyne, and Pamela Galehouse

Objectives

After reading this chapter, APNs will be able to

1. Discuss historical premise and rationale for behavioral health promotion within the school milieu for students with emotional or behavioral disorders.
2. Review federal legislation and special education mandates responsible for inclusion of in-school support services for students in need.
3. Present evidence-based collaborative practice models.
4. Describe the school-based health center model of care and how it improves access to behavioral health services, student success, and improved behavioral outcomes.
5. Identify APN roles and responsibilities for collaboration within the school community.

Introduction

School is central to the daily lives of children both in the United States and in other countries. Learning is the work of children, and because the majority of their time is spent in the care of schools, that environment can be considered a significant "home environment." Desmond O'Byrne of the World Health Organization made the declaration that education and health are inseparable due to their mutually supportive tendencies (WHO, 2004). This positive relationship between health and education and the logistics of schools being a center for access to school-aged and adolescent youth make it the ideal setting for integrating efforts directed at health promotion, prevention, and intervention.

This chapter will provide a historical context for the various federal laws affecting the education of children in school settings, present common behavioral presentations of youth seen in schools, describe roles for advanced practice nurses (APNs) in school-based practice models, highlight evidence on the effectiveness of collaborative models, and present a case exemplar illustrating how school-based programs can meet the mental health needs of youngsters.

Mental Health in the Education System

The U.S. education system is a federal, state, and local partnership mandated to serve the educational needs of all children. Schools play a major role in any comprehensive system of care for children with 125,000 schools educating 55 million school-aged youth across the United States (Coordinated School Health Programs [CSHP], 2008). There were 1909 identified school-based, school-linked, and mobile programs providing and coordinating comprehensive health care for

---

Child and Adolescent Behavioral Health: A Resource for Advanced Practice Psychiatric and Primary Care Practitioners in Nursing, First Edition. Edited by Edilma L. Yearwood, Geraldine S. Pearson, and Jamesetta A. Newland.

school-aged children in a 2007–2008 survey conducted by the National Assembly on School-Based Health Care (NASBHC, 2007–2008). The Office of Special Education and Rehabilitative Services (OSERS) of the U.S. Department of Education further estimates that there are approximately 6.5 million children who receive special education services for physical, emotional, behavioral, or psychological disabilities (n.d.). For an unknown number of persons with these disorders who may not have been identified, it is apparent that the effectiveness of comprehensive systems of care is dependent on the full and constructive participation of public schools (U.S. Department of Education, 1998). In fact, advocates for school-based mental health services argue that the school should be the core unit in which behavioral health care is implemented because school is the one constant environment that most youth attend (Allensworth, Lewallen, Stevenson, & Katz, 2011; Evans, 2009; Institute of Medicine [IOM], 2009; Lear, 2007). No longer is the task of education concerned only with the mastery of academics. Schools have more recently been recognized as the primary environment and home community for enrolled students, thereby making significant contributions to child socioemotional development, which, in turn, impacts academic success. Also, school is a focal point for addressing health inequities.

APNs concerned with the care of children whether in primary care or the subspecialty of mental health must consider this high level of integration between school and health in their assessment and planning of care for school-aged youths. The school environment is not only the context for a major portion of childhood experiences but it can also be a contributing factor, a measure of functioning, and mode of additional support for the successful implementation of behavioral health treatment plans. School, as part of its framework, is the predominant setting for the child's daily experiences—interactions with teachers, peers, classmates; enactment of roles and responsibilities, and of course engagement in academics. Cooperation, working within a structure, and learning are major expectations of the child attending school. Inability or decreased ability to function in school is often an early sign of an underlying health, emotional, behavioral, or psychological issue. In addition, each school has its own unique culture, its own unique rules, and therefore its own expectation for individual student functioning.

The school's infrastructure and specifically its specialized programming to meet the needs of all students as legislated by federal mandate provide additional resources that can be called on by health care providers in the implementation of their plan of care for the child experiencing a general health or mental health concern. Familiarity with the relevant education laws and school-based programs that support health and well-being and guide and delimit care is a necessary asset for the APN working in schools or interfacing with school-aged populations. Establishing relationships and working collaboratively with school personnel and external partners while having knowledge of resources enable the APN to offer comprehensive treatment to school-aged youth.

Attention to health, safety, and developmental needs of children in schools is historically linked to federal education legislation and, more directly, federal mandates for special education, which are included in Table 29.1.

Education, although federally legislated, is implemented on the state level. There are several levels between federal legislation and school implementation. State boards of education implement and enforce the mandates set forth by the federal government and state legislature, while their designees (local school districts) dispense regulations guiding practices in schools that will then be evaluated. Local school boards, or local educational agencies (LEAs), interpret state mandates and manage operating funds that are allocated by state-level entities and, in some cases, physical capital resources from federal, state, and local sources. School boards determine distribution of funds at the local level in many cases; however, there are districts whose budgets must be approved by a local populous vote. A superintendent, who serves as a chief executive officer, hired by local school boards, usually serves as the head of the school district. Schools with their administrators, faculty, and support staff are, in turn, charged with the implementation of directives from federal, state, and local authoritative bodies (U.S. Department of Education, n.d.). This review of educational legislation's "trickle down" is intended to provide a summary of the authorities involved with implementing the federal mandates. Because of differing state and municipal laws and policies, APNs are advised to become familiar with relevant governing principles of the school districts in the areas that they serve.

Newer federal initiatives following the No Child Left Behind Act of 2001 and recognition of the critical part schools must play in promoting mental health in children and adolescents by a presidentially convened commission (President's New Freedom Commission, 2003) have encouraged mental health professionals to approach schools from the perspective that mental health is intrinsic to academic success and academic success is a protective factor for high school graduation (Allensworth et al., 2011; Hoagwood et al., 2007; Trussell, 2008). In addition, health professionals should incorporate mental health services in schools using the

Table 29.1 History of special education

- **1965—Civil Rights Act Title VI of the Elementary and Secondary Education Act.** Created a Bureau of Education for the Handicapped.

- **1973—Section 504 of the Rehabilitation Act.** Protects qualified individuals from discrimination based on their disability.

- **1974—Family Educational Rights and Privacy Act (FERPA).** Allows parents to have access to all personally identifiable information collected, maintained, or used by a school district regarding their child.

- **1975—The Education for All Handicapped Children Act (EAHCA).**

  o 1975—Mandated all school districts to educate students with disabilities.

  o 1977—The final federal regulations are enacted at the start of the 1977–1978 school year; provides a set of rules to which school districts must adhere when providing an education to students with disabilities.

- **1986—The EAHCA is amended with the addition of the Handicapped Children's Protection Act.** Clarifies that students and parents have rights under EAHCA and Section 504.

- **1990—The Americans with Disabilities Act (ADA).** Adopts the Section 504 regulations as part of the statute; "504 Plans" for individual students have become more common in school districts.

- **1990—The EAHCA is amended and renamed the Individuals with Disabilities Education Act (IDEA).** School districts are now required to look at outcomes and assist students with disabilities in transitioning from high school to postsecondary life.

- **1997—IDEA.** Is reauthorized and requires students with disabilities to be included in state and district-wide assessments. Regular education teachers are required to be a member of the IEP (individualized education plan) team.

- **2001—No Child Left Behind Act.** Sets the goal that all students, including students with disabilities, are to be proficient in math and reading by the year 2014.

2004—IDEA. Requires more data on outcomes to assure greater accountability at the state and local levels; school districts must provide adequate instruction and intervention for students to help keep them out of special education.

Source: Peterson, J. (2007). A timeline of special education history. Available at http://admin.fortschools.org/PupilServices/ StaffInfo/A%20TIMELINE%20OF%20SPECIAL%20EDUCATION%20HISTORY.htm. U.S; Department of Justice. (2005). A guide to disability rights laws. Available at http://www.ada.gov/cguide.htm

framework provided by public health and endorsed by the IOM (1994, 2009) for preventing mental disorders. This framework considers three levels of prevention (universal, selected, and indicated) as well as treatment and seeks to expand the delivery of services beyond those mandated services for children with identified mental health needs discussed earlier in the chapter. The value of early identification and intervention of mental health problems has been endorsed by the 2007 No Child Left Behind Commission, which recommended that schools, when creating school improvement plans, be required to determine the availability of school and community supplemental education services to enhance academic achievement (Commission on No Child Left Behind, 2007). This recommendation was expanded by

legislators engaged in reviewing education initiatives to include mental health problems that interfere with academic achievement (Chu, 2010). In 2010, nearly $6 million was allocated to sixteen school districts in thirteen states to finance expansion of mental health services (U.S. Department of Education, 2010).

Findings indicated that while schools have demonstrated an ability to identify and respond to children who presented with externalizing problems, they were less capable of early identification of internalizing problems such as those associated with anxiety, depression, and trauma, which impact long-term functioning (Hoagwood et al., 2007). They were also less capable of consistently instituting evidence-based programs that might serve to promote healthy responses and reduce risk for low socioeconomic status children and youth (Kavanagh et al., 2009). Here, also, the "reciprocal relationship model" between emotional and academic competencies played a major role in achievement. The risk for poor academic outcomes for children residing in impoverished areas has been well documented as has the need to promote parent-school-community collaboration (Price & Lear, 2008). For these children, the protective factors provided by school organization, structure, and "climate" were anticipated to counter risks and expand personal socioemotional learning (SEL) factors important for academic advancement (Hunter et al., 2005; Zins, Bloodworth, Weissberg, & Walberg, 2004). However, Hoagwood et al. (2007) suggested that consensus on definitions of academic success and establishment of methods to measure context and climate variables were necessary to expand outcome studies in this area of mental health.

Description of the Issue

The centrality of school in the life of children and adolescents provides a natural opportunity for onsite delivery of services that support the biopsychosocial needs of children. Special education history seems to have evolved full circle from including and supporting children with disability or special needs in contained environments to requiring that all other options and supportive interventions and/or teaching methods be utilized to keep special needs students in mainstream environments. The requirement to add intervention and instruction to prevent students from needing segregated special education services must be inclusive of all students including those with emotional and behavioral disorders. This caveat opened the doors to expanding support services in the school environment and led to school systems collaborating with other domains to enrich the school community in order to facilitate functioning of children and adolescents who attend.

In addition to special education legislation, there have been other contributors to the movement for in-school support of children with special needs. The division of Adolescent and School Health at the Centers for Disease Control and Prevention (CDC) has been the leading advocate for health promotion and delivery of services in schools using the eight components of the Coordinated School Health Framework. The components include health education, physical education, healthy and safe school environment, health services, mental health and social services, health promotion for staff and faculty, family and community involvement, and nutrition services (CDC, n.d.).

The School Mental Health Project at the University of California at Los Angeles sought to understand a range of learners in schools and targeted barriers to healthy educational development (Adelman & Taylor, 2000). This approach worked by providing support, mental health, individualized instruction, and parental services in partnership with community-based health and human services organizations (Mulhall, 2007). Community-based collaborations for the provision of mental health services to students is one remedy that has been implemented in schools, as in the school-based health centers (SBHCs) and school-linked health centers. These formulations usually involved APN providers. On the occasion that a school health services team included both school nurses and APNs, school nurses were able to assist in the early identification of students with health problems, and primary care APNs and psychiatric-mental health APNs could treat health and mental health presentations (National Association of School Nurses [NASN], 2003, 2006). A Substance Abuse Mental Health Service Administration (SAMHSA) survey reported that school nurses are usually the first school staff member with knowledge of a child's mental health problems (Foster et al., 2005).

The landmark 2000 report from the U.S. Surgeon General stressed that mental health was critical to children's learning and general health, as important as immunizations, to ensuring that every child had the best chance for a healthy start in life. The report revealed additional notable statistics:

1. An estimated 21% of young people in the United States between ages nine and seventeen, about 15 million children, had diagnosable emotional or behavioral health disorders, but less than a third received help for these problems.
2. Only 16% of all children received any mental health services, and of these, 70% to 80% received that care in school settings by school counselors, nurses, and psychologists (U.S. Public Health Service, 2000).

School-Based Health Centers

Over the past thirty years, schools partnering with community-based health and mental health organizations and individuals have become the largest providers of mental health services to children. Among those children who receive mental health services, up to 80% access care at school. While many of these children and adolescents receive services by participating in special education programs, an increasing number are getting help through one of the SBHC models. Table 29.2 illustrates the services provided by three different SBHC models (NASBHC, 2007–2008).

SBHCs located within the school grounds are operated by or affiliated with an outside community health

Table 29.2 Models of school-based health centers

	Primary Care (1)	Primary Care and Mental Health (2)	Primary Care and Mental Health +
Services provided	Immunizations; asthma treatment; screening; sports physicals; risk and health assessments; acute and chronic illness management; med administration; nutrition counseling; referrals	Same as column 1 plus mental health assessment; crisis intervention; skill building; brief solution therapy; substance use counseling; psychoeducation; long-term therapy; psychiatric consultation; conflict resolution; case management	Same as column 2 but services are more comprehensive and presence of additional professional staff with adequate time on site
Usual staffing	APN or physician assistant with physician supervision; RN or LPN and health aide; some have social work and / or health education	Primary care APN; mental health provider; substance abuse counselor and staff as in column 1	Same as column 2; health educator; social services case manager; nutritionist

Source: NASBHC 2007–2008.

agency or hospital. The SBHC personnel consist of both medical and mental health providers. Of the 2.6 million employed nurses, 2.76 % are school nurses and of that number approximately 3% are APNs (NASN, 2007; U.S. Department of Health and Human Services [U.S.DHHS/HRSA], 2010).

Research and evaluations have demonstrated that SBHC greatly enhance children's access to health care. Kisker and Brown (1996) found that 71% of students in SBHCs reported having a health care visit compared to 59% of students who did not have access to an SBHC. Specifically related to behavioral health care needs, adolescents were 10 to 21 times more likely to use an SBHC for mental health services than a community health center network or HMO (Juszczak, Melinkovich, & Kaplan, 2003; Kaplan, Calonge, Guertnsey, & Hanrahan, 1998). National SBHC census data show that 30% of SBHCs partner with the school to support students with special health care needs (students with health issues that affect their ability to learn and/or attend school). SBHCs support the academic success of these students by monitoring medications, assisting in implementing the individualized health plan (IHP), and serving on individualized education plan (IEP) development committees (NSNA, 2008).

Etiology of Behavioral Health in Schools

The Individuals with Disabilities Education Act (IDEA, 2004), first enacted in 1990 and then amended in 1997 and 2004, is the current federal policy relevant to children with disabilities, including children with emotional and behavioral disorders (EBD), that assures "special education," via an IEP. For each child deemed eligible, schools must convene a multidisciplinary team of educators, specialty providers, family members, and when appropriate, the student, to develop an IEP that meets the student's learning and emotional needs in the least restrictive environment possible. The program should be designed to provide all additional health and related services necessary to allow that student to fully participate in his or her education.

The IEP describes the goals the team sets for a child during the school year, as well as any special support needed to help the child achieve the identified goals. Students struggling in school may qualify for support services, allowing them to be taught in a need-specific and individualized way, for reasons such as learning disabilities, attention deficit hyperactivity disorder (ADHD), emotional disorders, mental retardation, autism, hearing or visual impairment, speech or language impairment, and/or developmental delay. Children who are eligible for special education services under IDEA are also protected under Section 504. However, if the disability *does not adversely affect educational performance*, the child is *not* protected by IDEA and can be vulnerable to neglect of disability needs.

Section 504 of the Rehabilitation Act of 1973 enables qualified students with a disability (not otherwise qualified under the IDEA) to receive accommodations needed to enable them to participate in school programs to the extent of their nondisabled peers. To be eligible for protections under Section 504, the child must have a physical or mental impairment that *substantially limits* at least one major life activity (i.e., walking, seeing, hearing, speaking, breathing, learning, reading, writing, performing math equations, working, caring for oneself, and performing manual tasks). Under Section 504 and Title II of the Americans with Disabilities Act [ADA], school systems must accommodate the needs of students with disabilities. Modifications can include changing rules, policies or practices, removing architectural or communication barriers, and/or providing aids, services, or assistive technology (National Center for Learning Disabilities [NCLD], 2009).

The National Association of School Psychologists (NASP) endorsed the definition of EBD to identify students who were in need of specialized educational services (2005). The definition states that EBD is a condition in which behavioral or emotional responses of an individual in school are so different from his/her generally accepted, age-appropriate, ethnic or cultural norms that they adversely affect performance in such areas as self-care, social relationships, personal adjustment, academic progress, classroom behavior, or work adjustment; the response is more than a transient, expected response to stressors in the child's or youth's environment and would persist even with individualized interventions. This definition further requires that the identification of EBD be based on multiple sources of data about the individual's behavioral or emotional functioning with the behavior exhibited in at least two different settings, one of which is school related. EBD can coexist with other disabilities such as schizophrenia, affective disorders, and anxiety disorders, or other sustained disturbances of behavior, emotions, attention, or adjustment (NASP, 2005).

Historically, schools have educated children diagnosed with an EBD within special education environments and Section 504 designations, without significantly involving families and other organizations in the community. The special education and school support staff provided services to the special education population, and often the primary care provider in the community would be aware of the special education services, but further coordination or communication was rare and limited to prescriptive notations on school forms for specialized services. More recently, this isolationist view has dissipated, as evidence supports the interconnectedness of the child, family, and community environments (Cohen, Linker, & Stutts, 2006). Changes in service philosophy, including increased emphasis on providing care in the least restrictive setting, greater attention to involving families in service planning, and the emerging focus on building on existing strengths, as opposed to the traditional deficit-based approaches, have provided impetus for collaboration (Cohen et al.). Eighty-three percent of schools report providing case management for students with behavioral or social problems and nearly half of all schools contract with or make other arrangements with a community-based organization to provide mental health services to students (Center for Health and Health Care in Schools [CHHCS], 2011). The movement toward integrating mental health services in SBHC services has come to mean that comprehensive education services include the provision of case management and coordination of support services for students in need. Case management and care coordination are usually carried out by a designated school staff member who serves as the liaison between school, family, and community resources.

The School Team

School support personnel are a critical component of the school team, which includes school nurses or allied health professionals, guidance counselors, school social workers, school psychologists, and parent outreach/support workers. Other members of the community such as legal advocates, legal guardians, and representatives from the department of social services may also be involved in the support of an individual child. Engaged parents or caretakers who are advocates for their children should be kept informed at all times by the team and included in planning and decision-making meetings.

These professionals are the core to any school support collaboration and are likely already known to the student and family. This sense of affiliation and familiarity may augment the collaborative process and facilitate entry of the APN new to the school community, student, or family. The school nurse or allied health staff is generally engaged in routine health surveillance and in-school management of treatments for students in need. The nurse may be in daily contact with at-risk students and have experience in the school support team processes and thus can serve as a liaison for the APN collaborating on students' behalf. APNs who are not a part of a school or SBHC should obtain consent from parents and inform the child if they wish to communicate with school personnel.

Guidance counselors are often best known by students and are the first layer of support outside of the classroom; these persons are excellent resources for the APN interfacing with schools. The guidance counselor may have first-hand experience with the processes involved in responding to the special requirements of the student experiencing an emotional or behavioral disorder. Although the level of counseling associated with guidance counselors is usually more academically focused and less clinical, it is not uncommon for students to become accustomed to using the guidance office for counseling support. The school social worker is the next level of support with the social worker role varying from school to school but usually involving counseling, academic and developmental testing, and some level of case management for an identified caseload. The school psychologist may have a part-time presence and is often only involved in assessment with a very limited clinical or interventional role.

In many cases school support focuses on special education and Section 504 – related assessments and evaluation. When no school-based health or mental health care is available, the recommendations for nonacademic follow-up, assessment, counseling, and intervention are placed in the hands of parents and guardians. Acquisition of additional community-based medical, mental health, or developmental support services may be hindered by lack of availability within the region, parent or guardian inability to take time off from work to meet with outside providers, and/or lack of coverage for the cost of needed care.

When school-based treatment is not an option, the structure and process of case management become paramount. Although ongoing case management and coordination may be absent from the infrastructure of most schools, the school's willingness to partner with community providers and to establish processes has the potential to eliminate gaps between needs and service provision.

APN Collaboration

Although APNs represent a very small segment of nurses employed in schools or in SBHCs, their holistic approach to child and adolescent health is in concert with the philosophy of No Child Left Behind and the Affordable Health Care Act. Therefore, an increase in the number of APNs in SBHCs can be anticipated. The primary care (PC) and psychiatric mental health (PMH) APN collaboration has demonstrated effectiveness in meeting multiple needs in children with limited access to primary care as well as mental health interventions across prevention and treatment domains (Grossman et al., 2007; McClowry et al., 1996). As with the school nurse, the PC-APN serves as a referral source for mental health services and in many instances the PMH-APN is an appropriate consultant when children require additional screening, psychotropic medications, and treatment for serious mental health issues. In addition to providing services to individuals, PMH-APNs serve as school resources around such diverse issues as violence (Smith & Thomas, 2000), cultural dissonance (DeSocio, Elder, & Puckett, 2008), and inclusion of sexual minority status youth (Hirsch, Carlson, & Crowl, 2010).

Concerns have been voiced about the lack of evidence-based school mental health interventions. In response, nurses and others have started to develop and study programs that target those needs in underserved, minority populations in schools. Cummings, Ponce, and Mays (2010) compared racial and ethnic differences in mental health service use among adolescents. While no differences were found in school-based use of mental health service, significant differences were noted in clinical settings, indicating that schools may be critical avenues for reducing the unmet need for mental health services among racial/ethnic minorities.

One promising example of an indicated prevention model is a school and home visit program aimed at reducing depression and enhancing problem-solving abilities in Mexican American mothers and their children (Cowell, McNaughton, Ailey, Gross, & Fogg, 2009). A school-based selective prevention intervention program that targets children, parents, and teachers (McClowry, Snow, & Tamis-LaMonda, 2005) was discussed in Chapter 2.

Linkage With Behavioral/Psychiatric Profile of the Child and Adolescent

Examination of current general education and special education policies, as well as the theories behind these policies, clarifies why community collaboration (schools, human service agencies, families, and communities working together to more effectively and efficiently use resources to meet needs) is necessary to ensure that EBD students receive the quality of services that they deserve and are guaranteed to them by law (Cohen et al., 2006; White & Wehlage, 1995). The child with EBD may be of normal academic functioning but struggle in the school environment related to their emotional or behavioral disorder. The elements of support provided through IDEA and Article 504 legislation create the provision for all students to be supported through school case management and/or collaboration with the external therapeutic community.

APNs caring for children and adolescents with an EBD should be able to advise their client's families of special education resources and school supports that facilitate their child's functioning within their primary environment, the school. APNs involved in the care and treatment of youth with emotional health needs are often called upon by parents to participate in a dialogue with school staff and administrators, as part of the parental request for special education and in school supportive or adaptive services. In effect, the provider is asked to "prescribe" or "validate" considerations that are not academic in nature but are imperative for the optimal functioning of the individual child in the school setting. These range from validating indications for less restrictive settings, facilitating the administration of treatments necessary for safe and comfortable functioning in the school environment, and developing behavioral and logistic plans for adapting to stressors that may arise within the school environment. In most instances, the input of the APN will be provided through correspondence or by attendance and participation at the IEP or other student support team meetings. Parents concerned with their ability to be heard as advocates for their children may seek support from trusted members of the SBHC.

Many students experiencing emotional and behavioral health issues are not identified by the school system as special needs, although their diagnoses may clearly impact their ability to learn and, therefore, in most states, they are eligible for specialized accommodations and services. When these students are not serviced through special education and remain within the mainstream population, they struggle and often fail. These students may be the patients of APNs practicing in the community, in a school-based or school-linked health service, or recently discharged from an inpatient facility. The task of any APN is to consider the elements of school participation as part of the treatment planning for management of the individual child in order to promote both optimal health and academic success. There is a role for the APN to assist students and their families in obtaining the school-related supports entitled to them related to their functional disability or diagnosis.

The APN Role in School Collaboration

First and foremost, the APN must be knowledgeable of the medical and behavioral health resources already available within the school and the community. Assessment of school functioning is part of the comprehensive health assessment for school-aged and adolescent youth; therefore, when establishing a plan of care, school-related issues and supports should be a natural consideration for this age group. Not all cases call for in-school collaboration; however, for the child who is struggling socially or exhibiting behavioral or emotional issues, the incorporation of school support through direct consultation or through facilitation of the parent role as advocate through education, documentation, or consultation is an appropriate intervention. The APN or other providers collaborating with the school system whether from the outside community or from within a school-linked/school-based service arrangement must, together with school administration, work in the spirit of mutual respect and consideration in developing guidelines for the collaborative processes involved with the service.

The increase in school-based support programs and the expansion of school mental health services have created unique professional opportunities for APNs to be employed directly or through subcontracts within the school environment. This role may be endorsed through employment in the role of school nurse or mental health provider, as a primary care provider or mental health provider of an SBHC, or as a provider/employee of a primary care or mental health practice linked with a school through subcontract for the provision of support services to school students. Depending on the level of integration of the health services, the APN may be positioned to be a key player in the development of team processes and planning that promote stability and consistency of approach in facilitating the treatment and support of the student with an EBD.

In any of these circumstances, the role of the APN is directed by professional standards of care and scope of practice requirements of the regional board of nursing. School policies about information sharing in the academic milieu are often less rigid than the level of care required through an organization's patient confidentiality and Health Insurance Portability and Accountability Act (HIPAA) regulations. APNs should clearly explain their role and responsibility in the care of the students and highlight the boundaries of the communication process. These requirements should be explained initially and reinforced throughout the process of interfacing with the school staff and administration, so that professional requirements related to scope of care and communication are better understood and tolerated within the collaborative process. Empirical evidence has suggested that given the intense levels of service required, a team approach is not only more effective for children with EBD but also reduces the risk of burnout among educators and other service providers (Cohen & Cohen, 2000).

Participation as part of a team or network of school administrators, educators, and health service providers can be both challenging and rewarding. The collective impact of these endeavors is potentially much farther reaching than what is possible when providing services without collaboration. When school-based or school-linked arrangements exist, the APN working within the school system has a unique perspective from the shared experience of the school environment. Socialization with school staff and administrators as well as integration as a community member through roles in various schoolwide activities, planning meetings, or committee participation can be instrumental in promoting credibility as a collaborator. Additionally, the experience provides first-hand understanding of the systems at work in the coordination of student-focused services.

The school-based model of care has important advantages to treatment planning for students in need. Scheduled appointments at a school or school-based health center may increase treatment plan compliance; parents may be engaged via telephone contact, alleviating the stress of missed work or transportation issues. Referral and consultation with affiliates of the professional staff providing care in the school enhance access to specialty providers and other resources through that agent's network.

Parents and guardians are the gatekeepers in the process of interfacing with schools; their consent is critical to outsiders' entry and access to school records and strategy sessions. The APN's knowledge, experience, and ability to assist parents and family members in understanding the complex issues regarding etiology and course of treatment of their child's condition are great assets to the process of achieving comprehensive services through school and community services. The APN serves as advocate and mentor; parents and guardians, empowered by the information and resources from the APN, are better prepared to advocate for their children. The parents' improved understanding of the clinical issues, combined with their knowledge of what works for their child, assists them in informing others of their child's special needs and considerations. Once collaborating with "in-school" support persons, it is imperative that the APN not turn her back on the parental role and, in fact, should facilitate parental adaptation to the advocate role for the child.

Evidence-Based Implications for Practice, Research, and Education in Child and Adolescent Behavioral Health in Primary Care

One evidence-based program of note, which identifies the application of overall system guidance and directed intervention for behavioral concerns in the school setting, is the School Wide Positive Behavioral Supports (SW-PBS) program. SW-PBS is a multifaceted intervention that merges decades of research on effective instruction, behavior management, and systemic school change. Initially developed and disseminated at the University of Oregon by Drs. Horner and Sugai, SW-PBS encourages schools to take a proactive approach aimed at promoting socially appropriate behavior and preventing problem behavior (Borgmeier, 2007).

The goal of SW-PBS is to create systems in schools that infuse best practices in behavior management throughout the school. Using a three-tiered prevention model, primary prevention is available to 100% of the school and 80% of the school population is expected to be successful behaviorally. The remaining students in the top two tiers are those who do not successfully respond to the primary system and require additional interventions and supports to be successful. These two tiers of students are matched with interventions that will effectively meet their behavioral support needs. Secondary prevention includes specialized groups for student with at-risk behaviors, whereas tertiary prevention group interventions are more intensive and includes matching interventions to address unique individualized needs (Borgmeier).

The care and treatment of the two tiers of students identified as needing more supports form the priority group that schools usually focus on, either through structured programs for early identification and intervention or by natural course as the at-risk child self-identifies or is "picked up" through the intuition or experience of school support personnel. In both cases, once it is apparent that a higher level of care is required to support student academic function, collaboration with clinical service providers is needed.

The format of the PBS plan has a prescriptive value that affords easy delineation of roles for the APN operating within this system. Primary prevention, assessment, education, and promotion may be carried out by both the PC- and PMH-APN; assessment of behavioral and emotional health risk is part of each provider's routine assessment whether completed individually or through a schoolwide screening. Both types of APNs may run health education and social support type groups for a school's general population and for high-risk students. This service acts as a supportive measure for the child with EBD who is seen by an outside provider as a means to augment other behavioral or medication components of her or his plan of care. Tertiary prevention care whether individualized or delivered as a group intervention is within the domain of the PMH-APN alone as the specific knowledge and skills required for behavioral intervention, counseling, and psychopharmacology fall within the domain of that practice. The supportive functions in this domain include routine follow-up of medication management/compliance and periodic laboratory assessment for symptoms and side effects; education regarding medications may be carried out by either the PC- or PMH-APN, providing the information is communicated consistently.

Best practices associated with successful school collaborations concerning the provision of mental health include, but are not limited to:

1. Developing procedures for the identification, referral, and disposition of students needing assistance.
2. Communicating with students, teachers, and families to obtain views on problems and concerns and their suggestions for addressing them.
3. Coordinating as available the provision of prevention and intervention programs.
4. Participating in school support team meetings, discussing ongoing problems of students in treatment,

and sharing knowledge and recommendations to improve care and meet IEP goals.

5. Developing a "reentry" plan of care for students who are returning from treatment for an EBD in an inpatient or partial hospitalization setting.

6. Developing educational programs for teachers and school staff on EBD and how to manage these children in the school milieu (American Academy of Child and Adolescent Psychiatry [AACAP], 2005; Hurwitz & Weston, 2010; Lear, 2007; NASN, 2007, 2008, 2011).

When considering *identification and referral procedures* it is best to be clear about what level of support the APN is able to offer. If the APN is already the primary care provider or the mental health provider overseeing the behavioral health treatment plan for the child with an EBD, the identification is more of an introduction of self to school personnel as an established support with an interest in coordination of all aspects of the individual student's care. In this model the provider, with the parent's consent, attempts to collaborate with in-school supports in order to share information, consult on interventions, and coordinate services to ensure augmentation of all available resources on the patient's behalf. For instance, the APN in the community may contact school support via telephone, e-mail, or letter to request the further evaluation of a potential learning disability, share information regarding any organic entities that may be related to the child's school function, or request support in the day-to-day management of a student's established treatment plan. This approach may require only brief interface initially with a plan for periodic communication of progress and review or revision of planned strategies.

APNs working within the school or SBHC or contracted through schools may be instrumental in the schoolwide establishment of procedures for identification and referral of students that exhibit need of support, as well as planning for intervention. Clear referral and communication policies should be established at the onset of the collaborative relationship and carried out in a consistent manner.

Communicating with the school community and family usually means the APN would go to the family, visit the school, and hold forums or focus groups as part of a school community offering. Providers based in schools and providers from the surrounding community can gain introduction through parents' associations or, in the case where the group of interest is intrinsic to the school community, the principal or their designee may act as the central mediator of passage within the school walls and for access to staff. It is important to identify the key stakeholders within an individual school—those individuals who have the power to make decisions and promote change. There are a number of staff meetings and enrichment offerings over the course of a school year where an APN from in-house or the community may seek a forum to reach school staff, provide education, and request support or feedback. These opportunities can also be used as an arena to gain referral and promote the available services of the APNs and affiliated programs.

Coordination of services is at the heart of the nursing process. After carefully assessing the child or adolescent, a nursing diagnosis and treatment plan is formulated; this often includes other services and supports for the student who is central to the encounter. Understanding the individual needs for services and assuring that services are provided in a timely manner with a focus on quality care are core to that process. Often the APN is the most aptly informed about the progress and involvement of support services. The APN may ensure this role as coordinator, liaison, and organizer of services directed at the success of the centrally place student/patient. The school-based model may include the APN's assumption of additional roles that promote consultation and/or education regarding a schoolwide behavioral intervention.

Participation in school-based meetings concerning the student being served is a forum for collaboration considered to be the key to success. The APN's participation can range from correspondence to attendance at IEP meetings. In the case of the community-based APN provider, it is advised that a format for collaboration be decided after consultation with the school-based support liaison or the coordinator of special education services. In the case of providers who share space in the school or who are contracted for referral directly from the school, a more routine presence in this team process may be expected and planned for as the APN or other provider may be utilized in a consultative manner for the schoolwide management of this process.

Developing a reentry plan should be incorporated as part of discharge planning for the student returning to school from inpatient or partial hospitalization. Students should be aware of additional supports or plans to alleviate the stress of reentry to the school milieu. School staff can benefit from understanding that the absence was related to a health issue so that their plans and expectations regarding makeup assignments and remediation should be assistive to the student's reentry. Generally, this communication need not be too specific or revealing about the nature of the absence but should be clear to eliminate the possibility of overwhelming the student with academic expectations relative to making up the work. Hospitalizations and inpatient treatment stays may result in a revised treatment plan. Health and behavioral professions should also plan for the student's reentry that may include additional sessions, assessments, and advocacy for the newly returned student.

Developing educational programs for teachers and school staff on EBD may include providing staff development offerings of an educational nature to provide insight and overview of the issues involved in EBD in the school setting, or informally where the provider offers self as a resource to staff who may be struggling through classroom management issues generally, or related to EBD students. The time required to meet this goal may make this level of involvement unrealistic for the collaborating community-based provider but can be configured as part of the in-kind contribution of a school-based provider.

Developing and providing educational programs for students is a crucial health promotion and disease prevention role of the APN. The following are topics that are particularly applicable in the school environment:

- Bullying awareness and prevention
- Stigma
- Depression and anxiety
- Respectful communities
- Preventing violence
- Coping skills
- Identifying and communicating feelings
- Physical and emotional effects of substance use

It is relevant to note that evidenced-based treatment protocols for the care and management of a variety of EBDs in the child and adolescent population have been developed and tested. The problems and disorders for which evidence-based treatments now exist encompass the concerns that bring the great majority of children and adolescents into clinical care. Tested treatments have now been developed to address multiple internalizing conditions within the anxiety-depression spectrum, multiple externalizing conditions ranging from chronic disobedience and aggression to the disruptive behavior disorders, autism and related developmental disorders, habit problems such as enuresis and obesity, anorexia nervosa, and some forms of substance misuse (Kazdin & Weisz, 2003). Development and dissemination of evidence-based treatments, treatment that has been evaluated and shown to be effective, provide a resource that enhances clinicians' ability to provide best practice in the care of the school-age and adolescent youth and to inform nonclinical persons about treatment.

Case Exemplar

One of the initial referrals to the SBHC with expanded mental health services (SBHCMH) presented to the program after attending only one period of the third academic day of the new school year. The student was escorted to the area by a school security guard after he "explosively" disrupted the classroom using strong curse words and throwing items around the room; the tantrum culminated in his throwing his own body up against the wall and doorways before falling to a crouched position against the wall where he covered his head into his folded arms across his knees and tuned out. This sixth-grader, a new student at the school, will be referred to as Billy. Billy was escorted to the APN who also served as the program director by a school administrator with a hint of sarcasm about this student being "just what you were asking for". After assuring that the student had no injuries and was in a calmer frame of mind, the APN provided school staff with the formal referral request that was to be completed and sent to the SBHMH office so that the outreach worker could contact the parent and initiate enrollment. In the meantime, the student was to be treated by usual disciplinary processes associated with the schoolwide Positive Behavior System (PBS). Billy was enrolled in the SBHC and the program's outreach worker supported his mother in navigating the processes within the school milieu for the handling of this "disruptive-conduct disorder student" (the school's terms, not that of the program). This involved activation of the Student Support Team where Billy's mother, teachers, a school administrator, psychologist, school nurse, the APN, and school support staff reviewed his history and developed his IEP. HIPPA requirements and the limitations on sharing specific information about Billy's diagnosis and treatment without his and his parent's consent were reviewed with the family. Both Billy and his mother provided consent to have his case discussed. Over the course of the intake it became apparent that Billy, who had been in special education throughout his public school career, was scholastically able as evidenced by his test scores but emotionally and socially challenged. It was also discovered that his promotion to the middle school resulted in his reclassification with special education and the loss of his 1:1 paraprofessional staff support. The school planned a review of that reclassification and Billy's enrollment in the SBHCMC was expected to be assistive in his continued transition to middle school.

As mental health services were on site in the school and were an extension of the health center, Billy was able to have a comprehensive physical by the PC-APN and baseline laboratory assessment prior to his initial treatment meeting with the PMH-APN. Initially, Billy was diagnosed as depressed with r/o conduct disorder and the treatment plan included medication management, individual psychotherapy, and participation in a social skills group. Consent for psychotropic medications as well as briefing about the side effects and risks was initiated by the PMH-APN. The PC-APN as the sole professional nurse and program coordinator provided further education about medications in use at the clinic to mental health staff, parent, and participants. As treatment progressed, symptoms of a bipolar disorder became apparent, medication was changed to Abilify, and the PC-APN continued to monitor response to medication and for symptoms of medication side effects. Clonazepam was also prescribed for use in the case of muscle spasms associated with a dystonic reaction to the Abilify; this drug was kept in the care of the PC-APN. Education regarding the new medication was provided and a plan for accessing the medical suite in case of signs of medications neuromuscular side effects was established in conjunction with the PC-APN, Billy, and the adult responsible for him. One episode of dystonia did occur during Billy's enrollment in the program. The availability of a dose of Clonazepam was instrumental in providing quick relief of his symptoms, which started as ocular "cramping and twitching" and quickly progressed to neck cramping and posturing.

Throughout this time Billy continued to maintain his treatment program with his primary mental health care provider-social worker, his support group, and the psychiatrist. Monthly school support team meetings about Billy's progress were part of the routine and by the mid-year break, in-school support with a 1:1 paraprofessional was reinstated and Billy was progressing in school and tolerating his treatment plan. Improvement in classroom behavior and academic performance was noted.

Sometimes staff would question Billy in front of the class, "Are you taking your medication because it doesn't seem to be working?" Billy saw these types of inappropriate comments as an obstacle to his treatment in the school. Program staff met with school administration to address more appropriate ways that teachers could work with students with special needs and keep information about them confidential. Again, school staff and administration were reminded that program staff could not share specifics of Billy's care but that he was actively participating in his treatment and showing progress. A lot of time and follow-up discussion was necessary to reshape the processes and change the tone that was considered usual to the school environment. The PBS intervention that was being implemented during that same time was helpful in addressing the negative postures and biases that were part of the school's culture. Overall expectations and rules of the road that promoted respect, safety,

and responsibility were integrated school wide and applied to students and staff.

Eventually Billy stabilized. He was compliant with medication and therapies and, with the exception of a few dose changes and concerns about the neuromuscular side effects of the medication, he was complaint free about his treatment plan. He improved in his ability to make eye contact, demonstrated socially acceptable manners, and came to be known as a fairly jovial youngster. His mother was relieved by her son's progress at home and by the less frequent complaints from school administration. More and more of the school staff began to engage Billy in a more facilitative and appropriate way.

By the end of sixth grade Billy's school functioning had flourished to the point that reclassification to a contained classroom without the 1:1 support was planned for seventh grade. Continued treatment and participation in the SBHMHC supported further movement to partial mainstreaming for science and math, which was initiated in the second half of the seventh grade, and additional mainstream classes were added in eighth grade. Meetings concerning his IEP became more and more productive as his tenor at the middle school progressed. Billy's graduation to high school meant the end to his special education classroom placement, and he transitioned to full program regular education. His involvement with mental health services continued through his participation in a community-based adolescent mental health service that was affiliated with the SBHMHC.

Much of the success sustained by Billy in the exemplar can be credited to the ease of access to mental health services, timeliness of enrollment to mental health support services, appropriateness of diagnosis, and the subsequent treatment plan. The structure and function of the SBHMHC and the integration of providers in the school system were facilitative in the overall developmental and scholastic progress realized by Billy. The program's clarity of mission and focus coupled with the APN's ability to clarify roles and maintain boundaries gave credibility to the program and eased tensions of the family and school administrators who appreciated access to such intensive resources.

Summary

The APN engaged in the care of the child/adolescent with behavioral health needs is in a unique position to facilitate child/adolescent assessments, management, reentry, transition, and stabilization to the school environment. Nursing's core roles of advocate, educator, and liaison are instrumental in formulating a plan of care that is considerate of the child/adolescent's primary environment, the school.

Although the practitioner and the school administrators and counselors may agree to work in the best interest of the child and their mental health and educational needs, it must be recognized that these types of collaborations are a new concept and engender potential complications, many of which are at the communication level. Concerns tend to occur around levels of disclosure, specificity of roles, systems for access, consultation, and consistency in adhering to treatment plans.

Promoting an understanding of the role and intention of the APN in the care of students experiencing emotional behavioral disorder can be invaluable to the APN in the process of school collaboration; putting the student centrally in the process gives all participants a chance to contribute to the overall outcome of student success. APNs should take the time to explain their role and the nature of the advanced practice classification in order to clarify the professional conduct expectations and distinguish the client-centered focus of care that drives their participation with school and community in the care of the individual student. Keeping the focus on the common goal of the successful student allows all participating team members to envision their contribution to the process and can keep the tone of the collaboration positive and proactive.

Resources

Education of All Handicapped Children Act of 1975, Pub. L. No. 94–142 § 689 Stat. 773 (1975).

Educators for Social Responsibility: http://www.esrnational.org/

Individuals with Disabilities Education Improvement Act of 2004 (IDEA), Pub. L. No. 108-446, 118 Stat. 2647 (2004).[Amending 20 U.S.C. §§ 1400 et seq.].

Center for Health and Health Care in Schools: http://www.healthinschools.org

Council for Exceptional Children's "Understanding the Differences Between IDEA and Section 504"

For kids: http://www.DoSomething.org

For kids: http://kidpower.org/SERVICES/Children.html

Massachusetts General Hospital School Psychiatry Program: www.schoolpsychiatry.org: The site will help clinicians, educators and parents meet the needs of young people with depression, bipolar disorder, attention deficit / hyperactivity disorder, autism spectrum disorders, and anxiety disorders, including panic disorder and obsessive-compulsive disorder. Mental health care for youth. Who gets it? How much does it cost? Who pays? Where does the money go? RAND Health. Santa Monica, CA. 2002: http://www.rand.org/publications/RB/RB4541/National Assembly of School-Based Health Care: http://www.nasbhc.org

National Association of State Boards of Education: http://www.nasbe.org. National Institute of Mental Health (NIMH): http:/ /www.nimh.nih.gov/topics/topic-page-children-and-adolescents.shtml

National Association of School Nurses: http://www.nasn.org

No Child Left Behind Act of 2001, Pub. L. No. 107–110, 115 Stat. 145 (2002).

SAMHSA's National Mental Health Information Center: http://mentalhealth.samhsa.gov/child/childhealth.asp

School Mental Health Project provides a introduction to mental health services and programs located in schools: http://smhp.psych.ucla.edu

Teaching Tolerance (Southern Poverty Law Program): http://www.tolerance.org/index.jsp

National Dissemination Center for Children with Disabilities: http://www.nichcy.org/

University of Maryland's Center for School Mental Health offers prepared Power Point presentations, classroom education material and other clinical references for clinicians: http://www.schoolmentalhealth.org

U.S. Department of Health and Human Services, The Center for Mental Health Services and the National Institute of Mental Health sponsor a web site contains mental health information related to HHS research programs, policies, and media campaigns and highlights the latest research findings and policy efforts. See Mental Health: The Cornerstone of Heath: http://www.mentalhealth.org/cornerstone

Bright Futures/ Mental Health: information on early recognition and intervention for specific mental health problems and mental disorders; provides a tool kit for use in screening, care management, and health education: http://brightfutures.org/mentalhealth/pdf/tools.html

References

Adelman, H.S., & Taylor, L. (2000). Promoting mental health in schools in the midst of school reform. *The Journal of School Health, 70*, 171–178.

Allensworth, D., Lewallen, T., Stevenson, B., & Katz, S. (2011). Addressing the needs of the whole child: What public health can do to answer the education sector's call for a stronger partnership. *Preventing Chronic Disease, 8*(2), 1–6.

American Academy of Child and Adolescent Psychiatry (AACAP). (2005). Practice parameters for psychiatric consultation to schools. *Journal of the American Academy of Child and Adolescent Psychiatry, 44*, 1068–1083.

Borgmeier, C. (2007). A school-wide approach to promoting young adolescent social and behavioral success in middle school. In S. Mertens, V. Anfara, & M. Caskey (Eds.). *The young adolescent and the middle school* (pp. 343–365). Charlotte, NC: IAP- Information Age Publishing Inc.

Center for Health and Health Care in Schools (CHHCS). (2011). *Children's mental health needs, disparities, and school-based services: A fact sheet.* Retrieved from http://www.healthinschools.org/NewsRoom/Fact-Sheets/MentalHealth.aspx

Centers for Disease Control and Prevention (CDC). (n.d.). *Coordinated school health.* Retrieved from http://www.cdc.gov/HealthYouth/CSHP/# 5

Chu, J. (2010). *Strengthening our schools: A new framework and principles for revising school improvement grants.* Retrieved from http://chu.house.gov/SOS%20Report%20FINAL.pdf

Cohen, R., & Cohen, J. (2000). *Chiseled in sand: Perspectives on change in human services organization.* Belmont, CA: Wadsworth.

Cohen, R., Linker, J., & Stutts, L. (2006). Working together: Lessons learned from school, family, and community collaborations. *Psychology in the Schools, 43*, 419–428.

Commission on No Child Left Behind. (2007). *Beyond NCLB: Fulfilling the promise to our nation's children.* Queenstown, MD: Aspen Institute. Retrieved from http://www.aspeninstitute.org/policy-work/no-child-left-behind/beyond-nclb

Coordinated School Health Programs (CSHP). (2008). *Healthy youth 2008.* Retrieved from http://www.cdc.gov/healthy/youth/about/healthyyouth.htm

Cowell, J.M., McNaughton, D., Ailey, S., Gross, D., & Fogg, L. (2009). Clinical trial outcomes of the Mexican American problem solving program (MAPS). *Hispanic Health Care International, 7*, 179–189. doi:10.1891/1540–4153.7.4.178

Cummings, J.R., Ponce, N.A., Mays, V.M. (2010). Comparing racial/ethnic differences in mental health service use among high-need subpopulations across clinical and school-based settings. *Journal of Adolescent Health, 46*, 603–606.

DeSocio, J., Elder, L., & Puckett, S. (2008). Bridging cultures for Latino children: School nurse and advanced practice nurse partnerships. *Journal of Child and Adolescent Psychiatric Nursing, 21*(3), 146–153.

Evans, M.E. (2009). Prevention of mental, emotional, and behavioral disorders in youth: The Institute of Medicine report and implications for nursing. *Journal of Child and Adolescent Psychiatric Nursing, 22*, 154–159.

Foster, S., Rollefson, M., Doksum, T., Noonan, D., Robinson, & G. Teich, J. (2005). *School mental health services in the United States, 2002–2003.* (DHHS Pub. No. [SMA] 05–4068). Rockville, MD: Center for Mental Health Services, Substance Abuse and Mental Health Services Administration.

Grossman, J., Laken, M., Stevens, J., Hughes-Joyner, F., Sholar, M., & Gormley, C. J. (2007). Use of psychiatric nurse practitioner students to provide services in rural school-based health clinics. *Journal of Child and Adolescent Psychiatric Nursing, 20*, 234–242.

Hirsch, J.A., Carlson, J.S., & Crowl, A.L. (2010). Promoting positive developmental outcomes in sexual minority youth through best practices in clinic–school consultation. *Journal of Child and Adolescent Psychiatric Nursing, 23*, 17–22. doi:10.1111/j.1744–6171.2009.00212.x

Hoagwood, K.E., Olin, S.S., Kerker, B.D., Kratochwill, T.R., Crowe, M. & Saka, N. (2007). Empirically based school interventions targeted at academic and mental health functioning. *Journal of Emotional and Behavioral Disorders, 15*(2), 66–92.

Hunter, L., Hoagwood, K., Evans, S., Weist, M., Smith, C., Paternite, C., the School Mental Health Alliance. (2005). *Working together to promote academic performance, social and emotional learning, and mental health for all children.* New York, NY: Center for the Advancement of Children's Mental Health at Columbia University.

Hurwitz, L., & Weston, K. (2010). *Using coordinated school health to promote mental health for all students.* Retrieved from http://www.nasbhc.org

Individuals with Disabilities Education Act of 2004 (HR 1350). (2004). Retrieved from http://thomas.loc.gov/cgi-bin/query/z?c108h.1350.enr

Institute of Medicine (IOM). (2009). *Preventing mental, emotional, and behavioral disorders among young people: Progress and possibilities.* Washington, D.C.: National Academies Press.

Institute of Medicine (IOM). (1994). *Reducing risks for mental disorders.* Washington, D.C.: National Academies Press.

Juszczak, L., Melinkovich, P., & Kaplan, D. (2003). Use of health and mental health services by adolescents across multiple delivery sites. *Journal of Adolescent Health, (32S)*, 108–118.

Kaplan, D., Calonge, B., Guernsey, B., & Hanrahan, M. (1998). Managed care and SBHCs: Use of health services. *Archives of Pediatric and Adolescent Medicine, 152*, 25–33.

Kavanagh, J., Oliver, S., Lorenc, T., Caird, J., Tucker, H., Harden, A., Oakley, A. (2009). School-based cognitive-behavioural interventions: A systematic review of effects and inequalities. *Health Sociology Review, 18*, 61–78.

Kazdin, A.E., & Weisz, J.R. (Eds.). (2003). *Evidence-based psychotherapies for children and adolescents.* New York, NY: Guilford Press.

Kisher, E.E., & Brown, R.S. (1996). Do school-based health centers improve adolescents' access to health care, health status, and risk-taking behavior? *Journal of Adolescent Health, 18*, 335–343.

Lear, J.G. (2007). Health at school: A hidden health care system emerges from the shadows. *Health Affairs, 26*, 409–419.

McClowry, S.G., Snow, D.L., & Tamis-LeMonda, C.S. (2005). An evaluation of the effects of INSIGHTS on the behavior of inner-city primary school children. *Journal of Primary Prevention, 26*, 567–584.

McClowry, S.G., Galehouse, P., Hartnagle, W., Kaufman, H., Just, B., Moed, R., & Patterson-Dehn, C. (1996). A comprehensive school-based clinic: University and community partnership. *Journal of Society of Pediatric Nurses, 1*, 19–26.

Mulhall, P. (2007). Health promoting high performing middle level schools: The interrelationships and integration of health education for young adolescent success and well-being. In S. Mertens, V. Anfara, & M. Caskey (Eds.), *The young adolescent and the middle school* (pp. 1–26). Charlotte, NC: IAP- Information Age Publishing Inc.

National Assembly on School-Based Health Care (NASBHC). (2007–2008). *School-based health centers: National census school year 2007-2008.* Retrieved from http://www.nasbhc.org/site

National Association of School Nurses (NASN). (2011). *The role of the school nurse and school-based health centers* (Position Statement). Silver Spring, MD: Author. Retrieved from http://www.nasn.org

National Association of School Nurses (NASN). (2008). *Mental health of students* (Position Statement). Silver Spring, MD: Author. Retrieved from http://www.nasn.org

National Association of School Nurses (NASN). (2007). *Coordinated school health programs* (Position Statement). Silver Spring, MD: Author. Retrieved from http://www.nasn.org

National Association of School Nurses (NASN). (2006). *School nursing management of students with chronic health conditions* (Position Statement). Silver Spring, MD: Author. Retrieved from http://www.nasn.org

National Association of School Nurses (NASN). (2003) *The role of the advanced practice registered nurse in the school setting* (Position Statement). Silver Spring, MD: Author. Retrieved from http://www.nasn.org/Default.aspx?tabid=197

National Association of School Psychologists (NASP). (2005). *Position statement on students with emotional and behavioral disorders.* Bethesda, MD: Author. Retrieved from http://www.nasponline.org/about_nasp/pospaper_sebd.aspx

National Center for Learning Disabilities (NCLD). (2009). *Section 504 and IDEA comparison chart.* Retrieved from http://www.ncld.org/at-school/your-childs-rights/iep-aamp-504-plan/section-504-and-idea-

Peterson, J. (2007). *A timeline of special education history.* Retrieved from http://admin.fortschools.org/PupilServices/StaffInfo/A%20TIMELINE%20OF%20SPECIAL%20EDUCATION%20HISTORY.htm

President's New Freedom Commission on Mental Health (2003). *Achieving the promise: Transforming mental health care in America.* Rockville, MD: Department of Health and Human Services.

Price, O.C., & Lear, J.G. (2008). *School mental health services for the 21st century: Lessons from the District of Columbia school mental health program.* Washington, D.C.: Center for Health and Health Care in Schools at George Washington University.

Smith, H., & Thomas, S.T. (2000). Violent and nonviolent girls: Contrasting perceptions of anger experiences, school, and relationships. *Issues in Mental Health Nursing, 21*, 547–575.

Trussell, R.P. (2008). Promoting school-wide mental health. *International Journal of Special Education, 23*, 149–155.

U.S. Department of Education. (2010). *Grants for the inclusion of mental health services: 2010 Awards.* Retrieved from http://www2.ed.gov/programs/mentalhealth/awards.html

U.S. Department of Education. (n.d.). *Mission and federal role in education.* Retrieved from http://www.2.ed.gov/about/overview/fed/role.html?src=ln

U.S. Department of Education. (1998). *Twentieth annual report to Congress on implementation on the individuals with disabilities education act.* Washington, D.C.: Author.

U.S. Department of Health and Human Services, Health Resources and Services Administration (USDHHS/HRSA). (2010). *The registered nurse population: Findings from the 2008 national sample survey of registered nurses.* Retrieved from http://bhpr.hrsa.gov/healthworkforce/rnsurvey/2008/

U.S. Department of Justice. (2005). *A guide to disability rights laws.* Retrieved from http://www.ada.gov/cguide.htm.

U.S. Public Health Service. (2000). *Report of the surgeon general's conference on children's mental health: A national action agenda.* Washington, D.C.: Department of Health and Human Services.

Weist, M., Ambrose, M., & Lewis, C. (2006). Expanded school mental health: A collaborative community-school example. *Children & School, 28*(1), 45–50.

White, J.A., & Wehlage, G. (1995). Community collaboration: If it is such a good idea, why is it so hard to do? *Educational Evaluation and Policy Analysis, 17*(1), 23–38.

World Health Organization (WHO). (2004). *The World Health Organization's information series on school health.* Retrieved from www.who.int'school_youth_health/media/en/sch_local_action_en.pdf

Zins, J.E., Bloodworth, M.R., Weissberg, R.P., & Walberg, H.J. (2004). The scientific base linking social and emotional learning to school success. In J.E. Zins, R.P. Weissberg, M C. Wang, & H.J. Walberg (Eds.), *Building academic success on social and emotional learning: What does the research say?* (pp. 3–22). New York, NY: Teachers College Press.

30

Child and Adolescent Mental Health Policy

Sally Raphel and Kathy Ann Sheehy

The mentally sound child works well, plays well, feels well, loves well, copes well and hopes well.

Anthony and Cohler, 1987

Objectives

After reading this chapter, APNs will be able to

1. Describe the history of children's rights.
2. Identify major policy areas related to child and adolescent mental health.
3. Explore partnerships within nursing to expand focus on child and adolescent mental health promotion.
4. Propose collaborative advocacy for child and adolescent mental health policy implementation in primary care settings.

Introduction

Fostering social and emotional health in children as a part of healthy child development has become a national priority (U.S. Public Health Service Office of the Surgeon General, 2000). Fifteen million children need mental health services of some kind; however, it is estimated that only 20% (3 million) receive any type of help. Of that number, only 20% are treated by clinicians actually trained in child mental health (Stroul, 2007). Policy development is key to meeting these mental health needs. While mental health policy formation had a very slow start in the United States (National Commission on Children, 1993), it stands at the forefront of change around children's mental health. Yet, policies should not be considered as eternal truths but as hypotheses subject to modification and replacement by better ones (Wildavsky, 1979). Block tells us that the public policymaking process and results are influenced by many

factors. It is critical to first identify the problem(s) (2004, p. 13). For example, the current heightened awareness of health, limited access to care, run-away costs, and quality factors have added an impetus to policy development at a national level. Mental health is now recognized as a critical component of children's well-being and overall general health.

Insurance coverage/payment for mental health services is often a barrier to access. It is obvious to many experts that children with mental health issues, especially from low-income families, are not able to access needed care due to gaps and flaws in state Medicaid and State Children's Health Insurance Programs (SCHIP). According to Kronebusch (2004), policymakers and administrators face many difficulties guaranteeing that children below the poverty line who need Medicaid assistance are enrolled for benefits. His study looked at whether Medicaid coverage for low-income children was preserved as intended with welfare reform laws of

---

Child and Adolescent Behavioral Health: A Resource for Advanced Practice Psychiatric and Primary Care Practitioners in Nursing,
First Edition. Edited by Edilma L. Yearwood, Geraldine S. Pearson, and Jamesetta A. Newland.
© 2012 John Wiley & Sons, Inc. Published 2012 by John Wiley & Sons, Inc.

1996; only a few states accomplished holding the line for coverage. He stated "it is probable that both policy choices, such as the overall eligibility limits and administrative activities, such as the very difficult nature of the application process will affect the use" (p. 291). The evidence points out that states have failed in the task of protecting Medicaid coverage for low-income children. Recent research has uncovered serious problems in private insurance coverage (Busch & Barry, 2009). All of this contributes to lack of availability of mental health services. This chapter will review historical and current child and adolescent mental health policy issues influencing nursing care provided in primary care and psychiatric settings.

Children's Rights

For centuries, children were seen as property rather than as individuals. Some societies viewed them as resources of the state, or disposed of them due to infirmity or gender. Children were not identified by society as vulnerable and in need of protection until the beginning of the 20th century with the enactment of the first children's laws in Western countries (Benporath, 2003; Takanishia, 1978). Child protection laws identified the child as vulnerable and in need of societal protection. In time, child protection shifted to a focus on the children's rights movement. The child was no longer seen as powerless and without responsibility, but as an autonomous being with the right to participate in society (King, 2007; Matthews & Limb, 1998; Miljeteig-Olssen, 1990; Such & Walker, 2005; Wilcox & Naimark, 1991). The importance of the child rights movement has been keenly felt in the area of child and adolescent mental health. Advanced practice nurses (APNs) need to be prepared to consider including children's rights, an undertheorized domain of social science and research efforts, particularly as they relate to mental health treatment (Raynaert, Bouvenve-deBie, & Vandevelde, 2009).

The changing status of children in society has led to a change in family dynamics. Support of children's rights can be conflictual with the rights of the parents (Cohen & Naimark, 1991; Howe, 2001; Huntington, 2006; Melton, 1996, 2005; Roose & Bouverne-de Bie, 2008; Thomas & O'Kane, 1998; Tomanovic-Miljajlovic, 2000). The APN's keen assessment of family dynamics can provide a family-centered approach leading to early assessment and treatment. Parent and family bias specific to mental health stigma needs to be explored while respecting the rights of both child and parent.

In 1989, the United Nations General Assembly adopted a much expanded version to its own 1959 Declaration of the Rights of the Child, expanding the original protocols for food, shelter, lodging, health, and education to include:

1. The child must be given the means requisite for its normal development, both materially and spiritually.
2. The child that is hungry must be fed, the child that is sick must be nursed, the child that is backward must be helped, the delinquent child must be reclaimed, and the orphan and the waif must be sheltered and succored.
3. The child must be the first to receive relief in times of distress.
4. The child must be put in a position to earn a livelihood, and must be protected against every form of exploitation.
5. The child must be brought up in the consciousness that its talents must be devoted to the service of its fellow men (UNICEF, 1998; retrieved from http://www.unicef.org/crc/?q=printme).

Recognizing the special vulnerability of children, the United Nations issued a *Convention on the Rights of the child* (CRC). All of the CRC goals were expressed with respect to a child's age and evolving capacities, with the child's best interests always the paramount concern. The convention repeatedly emphasized the primacy and importance of the role, authority, and responsibility of parents and family. In general, the convention called for:

- Freedom from violence, abuse, hazardous employment, exploitation, abduction, or sale
- Adequate nutrition
- Free compulsory primary education
- Adequate health care
- Equal treatment regardless of gender, race, or cultural background
- The right to express opinions and freedom of thought in matters affecting them
- Safe exposure/access to leisure, play, culture, and art (UNICEF, 2008; retrieved from: www.Amnestyusa.org/children/crn_faq.html)

The CRC was the first legally binding international treaty to give universally recognized norms and standards for the protection and promotion of children's rights (http://www.un.org/cyberschoolbus/treaties/child.asp). As of December 2008, 193 nations of the world had adopted it. Only the United States and Somalia have not (http://en.wikipedia.org/wiki/Convention_on_the_Rights_of_the_Child, p. 3).

Certainly the tenants of the Children's Rights Convention promoted mental health of growing children with each having a right to—Be wanted; Be born healthy; Live in a healthy environment; Have basic needs met; Experience continuous loving care; and, Acquire the cognitive skills needed for life. While treatment of illness and behavioral problems is an urgent need, it is now known that prevention is equally important. A 2004 World Health Organization (WHO) report found that since early days of mental hygiene (early 20th century) many ideas have been offered to prevent behavioral problems and mental disorders in children. The document states, "Some experimental programs were instituted in primary health care and schools; however, systematic development of science-based prevention programs and controlled studies to test their effectiveness did not emerge until 1980" (p. 7). The evidence points out that for people in positions of authority to significantly influence a change in primary prevention and early intervention ... "it is only possible through successful collaboration between multiple partners involved in research, policy and practice, including community leaders and consumers" (p. 7).

Stroul (2007) observed, "Based on current clinical evidence, the time has come and passed to integrate the training and practice of pediatricians and other clinicians with mental health professionals" (p. 2). Improved communication between mental health and primary care practitioners will improve ongoing communication between providers, families, and financing entities, resulting in improved quality of care.

Policy Formation

Policy and mental health policy in particular set out the vision, values, and principles of the issue. Policy craftsmanship is very important, and the need is initiated by several means: public stimulus, research substantiation, or governmental/organizational request. The process requires backing up the information gathered and forecasting. A cost-benefit analysis must be incorporated for the results the policy envisions, as well as the attempt to answer what action is morally right. It is crucial to consider affected societal groups (e.g., children, parents, their support systems, providers) or constituent wishes (Stanley, 1994). Policy vision sets what is desirable for the mental health of a country's citizens and what is possible according to available resources and technology. Values and principles are the basis of governmental objectives and goals, and from these flow strategies and courses of action.

The WHO has defined the key points of mental health policy as (1) improving the health of the population, in this case children and adolescents, by responding to people's expectations with respect for confidentiality and autonomy; (2) having a client-centered focus; and (3) providing financial protection from mental and behavioral problems through equity in distribution of resources and allocation of an appropriate percentage of the health budget to mental health (WHO, 2004). Examples of values and principles in mental health policies include: psychological well-being, mental health as indivisible from general health, community care and participation, cultural relativism, protection of vulnerable people, accessibility, and equity. A few accompanying principles are that mental health promotion should be integrated (1) into social and educational services; (2) into the general health system; (3) with a least restrictive form of care; and (4) with intersectoral collaboration and linkages with community development (WHO, 2004).

The main areas for action in all mental health policy are: human rights, organization of services, financing, collaboration (of providers/agencies), human resources and training for caregivers/clinicians, promotion, prevention, treatment and rehabilitation, essential drug (medication) procurement and distribution, advocacy, quality improvement, information systems, research, and evaluation of policies and services. Adequate financing is one of the most critical global factors in the implementation of mental health policy (WHO, 2003). Integral to the field of mental health policy is a strong support for human rights legislation.

Legislation is essential to guarantee that the dignity of people with mental disorders is preserved and protected (WHO, 2003). In the U.S., childhood mental illness and behavioral problems, including substance abuse, must be approached on parity with medical health problems (Bee & Gibson, 1998; Mental Health America, 2008) and expanded to non traditional settings (home, school, community clinics). With the passage of the landmark *Mental Health Parity and Addiction Equity Act of 2008* introduced by Senators Paul Wellstone and Pete Domenici, mental health coverage was mandated. As Public Law 110–343 enacted October 2008 is intended to end health insurance benefits inequity in the U.S., group plans of 51 or more employees can be no more restrictive than the predominant requirements and limitations placed on substantially all medical/surgical benefits (Mental Health America). Authorized services should include a continuum of health promotion and illness prevention services; least restrictive interventions should be employed; and concepts of **quality, cultural sensitivity, access, cost-effectiveness, provider choice, and continuity of care must drive the systems**.

Another national advocacy organization, the National Community Mental Healthcare Council (NCMHC), recommends that child/adolescent mental health policy can be structured into three sections: (1) organizational issues, (2) service provision, and (3) operations. In the first section of the NCMHC policy document, one finds vision and values, governance and management, personnel policies and practice, public involvement and advocacy, and accountability of public agencies. The second section has statements of consumer-centered care, supporting families and caregivers, needs assessment and service utilization, care coordination and linkage, and integration of care. The operations area covers payment mechanisms and financial operations, quality assurance and improvement, accountability, recording, maintaining and exchanging information and provider partnerships, networks and alliances (NCMHC, http://www.thenationalcouncil.org/cs/groups_networks).

Why Is Policy Important?

The statistics concerning psychiatric problems among children and adolescents are alarming. The Global Burden of Disease Study indicates that by 2020, childhood neuropsychiatric disorders will increase by more than 50% internationally to become one of the five most common causes of morbidity, mortality, and disability among children in the world (Murray & Lopez, 1996). Although the number of children receiving care has doubled in the last decade, the extent of unmet needs is still great (Pottick, 2002). It is well established that without treatment, psychological problems disrupt the child's social, academic, and emotional development and results in family turmoil. Also 7.5 million parents are affected by depression every year. This puts at least 15 million children at risk for a wide range of problems (IOM, 2009). Additional policy reports from the Office on Youth Violence (USDHHS, 2001b), Suicide Prevention (USDHHS, 2001a), and Risk of Drinking (USDHHS, 2007) each spotlight grave concerns and offer action plans.

A seven-year longitudinal study (1998–2001) of 1,088 youth in residential, outpatient, and inpatient treatment for drug use showed that 43% reported receiving no mental health services in the three months after admission despite severe mental health problems. In each of three sites surveyed where mental health services would be provided at no additional costs, the percentage of youth who received services was 6%, 28%, and 79%, respectively. The same period found rates of general health care services at 64% to 71% (Jaycox, Moralar, & Juvonen, 2003). Failure to provide effective and timely care has serious personal and societal consequences as the evidence supports.

Focusing on importance, a study funded by the U.S. Department of Health and Human Services (2009) published in *Children and Youth Services Review* found that 45% of youth with prior involvement with the child welfare system had at least one mental health problem as they transitioned to adulthood. The study sampled over 5,000 children from 92 child welfare agencies across the country. More than a quarter of the youth were in the clinical range for depression. The study also examined the youths' surrounding life circumstances, finding that at least 60% lived in households at or below the national poverty line, and only about a quarter lived with one or more parent. The study's authors called for policymakers, researchers, clinicians, and service system administrators to acknowledge these extreme needs and work better with this vulnerable population (USDHHS).

Finally, at least 2.4 million young adults aged eighteen to twenty-six years experienced a serious mental illness. To help this population access needed services and make a successful transition to adulthood, proposed legislation would provide planning and implementation grants to the states to develop statewide coordination plans to help adolescents and young adults with serious mental illness. States would be urged to target specific populations, including but not limited to those involved with the child protection and juvenile justice systems. The legislation would establish a federal committee to coordinate service programs helping young adults with mental illness and provide technical assistance to states. A Senate companion bill has not yet been reintroduced. Child Welfare League of America (CWLA) strongly supports this legislation, along with the Bazelon Center for Mental Health Law, the American Psychological Association, First Focus, and Mental Health America (CWLA, 2005).

Timeline of Existing Policy Development

Nursing has been at the forefront of policy development for mental health in a formal way since the 1990s. The strong impetus for policy in this area came from *Nursing's Agenda for Health Care Reform* (American Nurses Association [ANA], 1991), in the policy document *Health Care Reform: Essential Mental Health Services* (Krauss, 1993), and in the strong voices of nurse leaders (Stanley, 1994). Nursing's plan addressed the need for reform in areas such as primary-mental health service delivery, universal access to a basic mental health benefits package, and structure and financing of the public mental-health system for continuous care (Krauss). Children and adolescents were one of the life span target groups. The belief was stated that primary care clinics, school health clinics, community health centers, and pediatric offices were the most likely places where children and adolescents would receive care. This included services for those with behavioral, emotional, and mental health concerns. Nursing's policy statement proposed the integration of mental health promotion and mental illness prevention into existing primary care settings using nurses already in the system to conduct routine mental health assessments and refer to child mental health APNs for treatment. The vision in this policy was that funding would be directed to the local central authority, making the authority responsible for delivery of services, thus creating an organized system for continuous community-based care. Krauss (1993) presented childhood risk factors and extrinsic and intrinsic protective factors pivotal to developmental mental health to make the case for comprehensive care.

Government policy bodies have taken steps to provide for children's mental health, as one can see in Box 30.1. In 1999, the Surgeon General of the United States released the landmark first national U.S. mental health policy document *Mental Health: A Report of the Surgeon General* with a major section dedicated to children and adolescents. The overarching themes in the policy report were to take a life span approach; to use a public health perspective; to stress that mental disorders were disabling; to promote mind and body as inseparable; to acknowledge that effective treatments existed; and, consumer and family movements were critical to advocacy. In Chapter 3, *Children and Mental Health*, specific concerns and issues were laid out. The first

major point of the conclusions was that there was a wide range of normal for children. Efficacious psychosocial and pharmacologic treatments existed and primary care and schools were major settings for recognition and treatment of mental disorders. The document pointed out that the number of trained clinicians was limited and contributed to access barriers to effective treatment options. It went further to state that multiple problems associated with serious emotional disturbance required a systems approach, cultural differences exacerbated problems of access, and families were essential partners in the treatment process (USDHHS, 1999).

In 2000, an important policy delineation of children and mental health came from Surgeon General David Satcher, in the form of a Report of the Surgeon General's Conference on *Children's Mental Health: A National Action Agenda* (Raphel, 2001; USDHHS, 2000). The overarching vision was that mental health was a critical component of children's learning and general health. Fostering social and emotional health in children as a part of healthy child development must be a national priority. Both the promotion of mental health in children and the treatment of mental disorders were identified as major public health goals (USDHHS, Surgeon General). To achieve these goals, the National Action Agenda had as guiding principles a commitment to:

1. Promoting the recognition of mental health as an essential part of child health
2. Integrating family-, child-, and youth-centered mental health services into all systems that serve children and youth
3. Engaging families and incorporating the perspectives of children and youth in the development of all mental health care planning
4. Developing and enhancing a public-private health infrastructure to support these efforts to the fullest extent possible (pp. 5–6)

Goals for policy implementation by government and agencies followed. These were to:

1. Promote public awareness of children's mental health issues and reduce stigma associated with mental illness
2. Continue to develop, disseminate, and implement scientifically proven prevention and treatment services in the field of children's mental health
3. Improve the assessment of and recognition of mental health needs in children
4. Eliminate racial/ethnic and socioeconomic disparities in access to mental health care services
5. Improve the infrastructure for children's mental health services, including support for scientifically proven interventions across professions

---

Box 30.1 Decades of mental health policy statements

1993 *Health Care Reform: Essentials of Mental Health Services.* Nursing's Mental Health Policy Statement

1999 *Mental Health: A Report of the Surgeon General* published with a major section dedicated to children and adolescents

2000 *Children's Mental Health: a National Action Plan* released by Dr. David Satcher

2001 *Youth Violence: A Report of the Surgeon General* was released

2001 *A National Strategy for Suicide Prevention: Goals and Objectives for Action*

2001 *Crossing the Quality Chasm: A New Health System for the 21st Century.* Institute of Medicine Committee on Quality of Health Care in America

2003 *Achieving the Promise: Transforming Mental Health Care in America.* Report of the President's New Freedom Commission on Mental Health

2004 *Prevention of Mental Disorders: Effective Interventions and Policy Options.* Report of WHO Department of Mental Health and Substance Abuse

2006 *Improving the Quality of Health Care for Mental and Substance-use Conditions* from the Institute of Medicine Quality Chasm Series

2007 *The Surgeon General's Call to Action to Prevent and Reduce Underage Drinking* was released

6. Increase access to and coordination of quality mental health care services

7. Train frontline providers to recognize and manage mental health issues, and educate mental health care providers about scientifically proven prevention and treatment services

8. Monitor the access to and coordination of quality mental health care services (p. 6)

This was a clear message to the nation that children and adolescents were important. The national focus on vulnerable children and adolescents was maintained by a number of subsequent government policy statements including: *A National Strategy for Suicide Prevention: Goals and Objectives for Action* (USDHHS, 2001a) and *Youth Violence: A Report of the Surgeon General* (USDHHS, 2001b). Although a national dialogue about evidence-based practice and empirically validated treatments for children had been ongoing for a decade, youth and families continued to suffer because of missed opportunities for prevention of psychiatric disorders and early interventions in behavioral problems. Mental health professionals identified culturally relevant clinical standards and implementation guidelines as needing to be included in the dialogue on child and adolescent mental health (USDHHS, 2000).

In 2002, the President's New Freedom Commission on Mental Health identified policies that could be implemented by federal, state, and local governments to maximize the use of existing resources, improve coordination of treatments and services, and promote successful community integration for children with serious emotional disturbance. They reported the current system "a patchwork relic—the result of disjointed reforms and policies … with barriers that often add to the burden of mental illness for individuals, their families and our communities" (New Freedom Commission, 2003, p. 4). They identified that services remained fragmented, disconnected, and inadequate. To address some of these issues, a special coalition was formed entitled the Annapolis Coalition on Behavioral Health Workforce Education to address training issues. This was a collaborative effort to identify a set of core or common competencies as a key strategy for advancing behavioral health education, training, and workforce development initiatives. The Annapolis Coalition received grant funding from the Substance Abuse and Mental Health Services Administration (SAMHSA) to commission a series of position papers and to convene a body of experts in a summit to develop competencies (http://www.annapoliscoalition.org/pages/images/Conference_Recommendations.pdf).

Building on *Crossing the Quality Chasm: A New Health System for the 21st Century* (IOM, 2001), additional gaps in treatment knowledge were defined by the IOM. Evidence-based clinical practice guidelines were unavailable for many mental/substance use problems and illnesses, especially for individuals at both ends of the age continuum, children and older adults (IOM, 2006). This policy document put forward an agenda for change with strategies for filling knowledge gaps and actions needed for quality improvement at all levels of the health care system. The failures to treat persist (IOM, 2006); this is especially true from data reported for gaps in effective treatment for children and adolescents. The IOM policy work group labeled the critical features of an ideal system of care for depressed parents and their children as: (a) multigenerational, (b) comprehensive, (c) available across settings, (d) accessible, (e) integrative, (f) developmentally appropriate, and (g) culturally sensitive. The goals from mental health policy for treating depression would be to provide hope, foster resilience, and promote health, general/mental, and recovery (Evans, 2009; IOM, 2009).

In 2006, after more than a decade, the key concepts for policy change were again reported to include comprehensive identification of needs and strengths; family driven, individualized care in the least restrictive setting; family voice, choice, and engagement; local systems' partnerships, accountability, and overall health status monitoring in the context of mental health treatment. Identification of a level of care for each child in need, outreach through ongoing case managers and health care managers, and interventions with an integrated plan and quality measures were recommendations from the Georgetown Institute Forum (Stroul, 2007).

Child and Adolescent Mental Health Promotion

Policy statements are useless without action plans and implementation. Because policy formation includes input from vested groups, key stakeholders, and child advocates, the opportunities for partnerships between public (government)-private partnerships should follow. For example, public policy integrating mental health into primary care settings is getting considerable and deserved attention. It is agreed that children and adolescents are the populations with unique service needs, requiring specialized planning and coordinated service delivery approaches. As far back as 1995, the American Psychiatric Association (APA) published the *Diagnostic and Statistical Manuel of Mental Disorders- Primary Care Version (DSM-IV-PC)* in collaboration with 10 national organizations for primary care providers. Chapter seven of that manual addresses Disorders Usually First Diagnosed in Infancy, Childhood or Adolescence, noting that the primary care presentation can be extremely diverse. Consideration of developmental variation is key to accurate identification. One should refer to the appropriate section based on presenting symptoms for the suggested algorithm (p. 176). This work led to collaboration between the American Academy of Pediatrics (AAP) and APA for a *DSM-PC Child and Adolescent Version* (AAP, 1996). In October 1996, the Academy introduced the *Diagnostic and Statistical Manual for Primary Care: Child and Adolescent Version (DSM-PC)*. The manual is a compendium that blends developmental, behavioral, and primary care pediatrics for diagnosing and assessing mental health issues in primary care.

In 2006, the Georgetown University Training Institute developed recommendations for policy and technical assistance to support communities implementing effective mental health service delivery in primary care settings. Experts facilitated discussion focusing on strategies for policy, services, financing, advocacy, information development/dissemination and training, and technical assistance. They called for policy implementation through specific actions, such as (1) providing consultation to primary care clinicians on behavioral health issues, (2) increasing the role of primary care clinicians in identifying and addressing behavioral health needs, (3) co-locating mental health specialists in primary care settings for increased access and consultation to primary care clinicians, (4) implementing a medical home approach to ensure mental health, physical care, dental, eye care, etc. are accessible, and (5) providing health and mental health services through school-based clinics (Stroul, 2007, p. 6).

In this decade, we have moved from policy to action plans and implementation, as various collaborative primary care-mental health promotion constituent models have been put forward. Nurses through the National Association for Pediatric Nurse Practitioners (NAPNAP) stepped up with the Keep Your Children Safe and Secure (KySS). This prevention program was based on the philosophy that comprehensive health care that includes prevention efforts and early recognition and treatment of mental health problems in children will result in an optimal level of functioning and development as a foundation for productive adult years (NAPNAP, 2001). KySS partners included: Society of Pediatric Nurses (SPN), the Honor Society of Nursing - Sigma Theta Tau International, the National Assembly of School Based Health Care (NASBHC), and the National Youth Anti-Drug Media Campaign. A key issue explored was primary care and specialty referrals for mental and physical health. Through efforts to raise awareness, disseminate information, educate health professionals, teachers, and the public; and continued development of effective partnerships, the hard work of this core group continues. One

southwestern university was awarded a grant for a national KySS Fellowship for NPs in Underserved U.S.: Improving Child & Teen Mental Health (NAPNAP, 2008). This was a collaborative endeavor between Arizona State University College, Healthcare Innovation, and NAPNAP's KySS Program. Another example of enactment of policy related to training and education programs for primary care NPs and other nurses was the publishing of mental health curriculum for pediatric nurses in the primary care setting (Melnyk et al., 2009; NAPNAP, 2008).

As we expand from nursing actions, there are other community strategies, such as the Massachusetts Mental Health Services Program for Youth (MHSPY) started in 1998. This is a program of wraparound care and a variety of non traditional interventions to create a complete, expanded benefit package. It recognizes that youth are connected to a family or caregivers and require services and support from a variety of sectors. The various agencies and clinicians need visibility with each other. The system of care partners includes agencies such as Parent Advocacy League, Department of Mental Health, Department of Education, Juvenile Justice, Child Protection (Department of Social Services), Medicaid, Department of Public Health, and local school districts (Stroul, 2006, p. 3). According to Katherine Grimes of the Harvard Department of Psychiatry, overall health status has to be monitored in the context of mental health treatment given that medications have adverse general health effects, and medical conditions influence mental health conditions (Stroul, 2006).

Another example of a comprehensive approach to child mental health treatment is the partnership between the Bureau of Milwaukee Child Welfare, the County Delinquency and Court Services, Behavioral Health Division, and the State Division of Heath Care Financing, which operates Medicaid (Wells, Miranda, Bruce, Algeria & Wallerstein, 2004). Funds from the four agencies are pooled to create maximum flexibility and a sufficient funding source to meet the comprehensive needs of the families served. A planned program for Milwaukee County was built with partners from health care industry and both private and public sectors. Work with one health maintenance organization developed business processes for serving Medicaid populations, in particular children in out-of-home placements. The system relies on Wraparound Milwaukee, an existing program for behavioral health that establishes mental health assessment teams and expanded provider network. The initial challenges the program faced were lack of technology at the provider level, establishing trust between medical and mental health providers, privacy concerns, and access including waiting lists and unavailability of services (Stroul, 2006).

Collaborative Advocacy

Nursing has a professional, ethical, and social directive to advocate as part of the nursing process (Schlairet, 2010). Typically, nurses see this as part of their job and one of the primary reasons they entered the profession. Although advocacy is considered a part of daily clinical nursing practice, the concept is not well defined in measurable terms and often vague. The *Oxford Dictionary of Nursing* (McFerran, 2003) defines advocacy as an integral part of the professional health care practitioner's role. The ANA includes advocacy within Nursing's Social Policy Statement, stating that nurses provide "advocacy in the care of individuals, families, communities, and populations" (2003, p. 6).

Advocacy is also included in the ANA Code of Ethics for Nursing. The ANA Code of Ethics Provision 3 and 8 state, "The nurse promotes, advocates for, and strives to protect the health, safety and rights of the patient, and the nurse collaborates with other health professionals and the public in promoting community, national, and international efforts to meet health needs" (ANA, 2001). Advocacy is also recognized in almost all major nursing professional organizations, with a separate committee or division for advocacy, heath care policy, or government affairs.

Although nursing advocacy behaviors, such as analyzing, counseling, and responding, have been identified in the literature, until recently there has not been an instrument that measures the nursing advocacy process especially as it impacts the role of the advocate, advocate activities and outcomes, and the perspective of the nurse and patient (Vaartio, Leino-Kilpi, Suominen & Puukka, 2009). The literature supports that when nurses advocate, they can experience loss of control and self-determination, as well as conflict (O'Connor & Kelly, 2005; Wheeler, 2000). Based on the number of titles and keywords extracted from database searches, there is limited research on the behaviors and the time nurses advocate during their daily practice (Vaartio et al., 2009).

APNs need to understand and practice advocacy behaviors that result in positive professional and clinical outcomes, as well as the policy that shapes them. Further research into the understanding of nursing advocacy education and implementation will provide APNs with empiric data supporting the influence of nursing as a change agent in health care. The concept of "Leading the Way" (Cohen et al., 1996) applies to political involvement but also applies to all areas of professional and clinical practice where nursing initiates change. The APN can use these behaviors and strategies in many different roles within health care delivery and conduct research regarding the resulting outcomes.

Advocacy has a wide range of definitions and use in nursing. Advocacy can occur at the bedside as the APN empowers the child or family to gain information or influence. Advocacy can relate to professional goals and advancement. Advocacy also can occur within a social or political context. The following five types of nurse advocacy (Kubsch, Sternard, Hovarter & Matzke, 2004) can be used to develop a foundation for incorporating short and long term goals into a professional and clinical advocacy strategy.

1. Legal advocate
2. Moral-ethical advocate
3. Spiritual advocate
4. Substitutive advocate
5. Political advocate

Advocacy knowledge and behaviors are necessary both clinically and politically to effect change. APNs can no longer be passive and attempt to effect change at the distal end of the health policy system, where frustrations can lead to negative consequences such as conflict with colleagues, poor communication, reprimand, loss of professional control, and for some nurses, pressure to resign, or a decision to leave the profession (Chaowalit, Hatthakit, Nasae, Suttharansee & Parker, 2002; McDonald & Ahern, 2000; O'Connor & Kelly, 2005; Sundin-Huard, 2001; Wheeler, 2000).

Advocating beyond the bedside and into the public and political environment will lead to improved patient outcomes, enhanced professional empowerment and professionalism. In the United States, health care has become a political issue. Politics and policy drive health care coverage, health care organization regulation, and clinical practice policies. Mason, Leavitt, and Chaffee, in their chapter, *Policy and Politics: A Framework for Action,* (2007), state, "Nursing is concerned with health; therefore every action and decision that influences health and the health system should be important to nurses" (p. 3). In order for APNs to be seen as health care leaders, they must politically advocate for the APN role regarding nursing image, clinical privileges, and reimbursement. Once the APN achieves heightened visibility and clinical practice, impact on child and adolescent mental health services will be easier to achieve.

Professional nursing organizations are also active in policy advocacy with a separate branch usually devoted to professional and public health care goals. The ANA House of Delegates and Board of Directors are charged with "setting policy in healthcare, the workplace, patient care, and other areas where nurses are engaged" (http://nursingworld.org/MainMenuCategories/Health careandPolicyIssues/ANAPositionStatements.aspx).

APNs should be members of the ANA and members of specialty organizations that support child and adolescent health issues and mental health agendas. Professional nursing organizations participate in policy development through collective membership, and both psychiatric and primary care APNs need to be actively engaged in current advocacy and policy discussions.

NAPNAP was established in 1973 and presently has 7,500 members. NAPNAP's mission is to promote optimal health for children through leadership, practice, advocacy, education, and research. The organization has championed many child health causes, including gun safety, access for contraception to avoid pregnancy, and access for children with special needs (http://www.napnap.org/aboutUs.aspx). Although the organization does not specifically address mental health issues, it has addressed youth suicide (Duderstadt, 2004) and has recently included mental health presentations at the annual conferences. NAPNAP utilizes its membership to speak to global issues related to child health care needs and is an excellent example of a specialty nursing organization where united primary care APNs and psychiatric APNs can achieve collaborative goals.

On October 5, 2010, the IOM released a ground breaking report: *The Future of Nursing: Leading Change, Advancing Health.* The report recommended overcoming practice barriers that prevent nurses from responding to a rapidly changing health care system.

More specifically, it states the following:

- Nurses should practice to the full extent of their education and training.
- Nurses should achieve higher levels of education and training through an improved education system that promotes seamless academic progression.
- Nurses should be full partners, with physicians and other health care professionals, in redesigning health care in the United States.
- Effective workforce planning and policy making require better data collection and information infrastructure (p. 4).

This report, equally applicable to child and adolescent primary care and psychiatric practitioners, has the potential to be a springboard for policy changes as health care transforms and changes. The report points out that responsibility for these changes rests on government, business, health care and insurance agencies, as well as the profession of nursing. Nursing is poised to initiate and participate in policy changes that will advance nursing practice (IOM, 2010, http://www.iom.edu/reports.aspx).

Summary

Fifteen million children need mental health services of some kind; only 20% (3 million) receive any type of help. Of that group, only 20% are treated by clinicians actually trained in child mental health (Stroul, 2007). Health policy statements for child and adolescent mental health exist and must be applied. Parity legislation has established equity between health and mental health care in the United States. The most urgent and difficult part of child mental health policy action and implementation still faces global health care systems. In this country, there are pockets of excellent mental health care. Many more are needed to meet the critical access problems that exist. It is decreed in multiple policy documents that primary care is the site for child and adolescent mental health care. Collaborations of all kinds are needed to effect changes in the current resource poor environment. Models have appeared at the state and county levels using co-ordination of dozens of agencies but funding methods are often uncertain or insufficient. Who can make it happen? Stakeholder nursing groups such as primary care and psychiatry APNs are well poised to lead the way.

References

American Academy of Pediatrics [AAP]. (1996). *Diagnostic and statistical manual for primary care: Child and adolescent version (DSM-PC)*. Washington D.C.: Author.

American Academy of Pediatrics [AAP]. (2001). The new morbidity revisited: A renewed commitment to the psychosocial aspects of pediatric care [Committee on Psychosocial Aspects of Child and Family Health]. *Pediatrics, 108*(5), 1227–1230.

American Nurses Association [ANA]. (1991). *Nursing's agenda for health care reform.* Washington DC: ANA Publishing.

American Nurses Association [ANA]. (2001). *Code of ethics for nurses with interpretive statements.* Retrieved from http://www.nursingworld.org/MainMenuCategories/EthicsStandards/CodeofEthicsforNurses/2110Provisions.aspx

American Nurses Association [ANA]. (2011). *ANA position statements.* Retrieved from http://nursingworld.org/ainMenuCategories/HealthcareandPolicyIssues/ANAPosition Statements.aspx

American Nurses Association. (2003). *Nursing social policy statement.* (2nd ed.). Washington, DC: Author.

American Psychiatric Association. (1995). *Diagnostic and statistical manual of mental disorders: Primary care version.* Washington, DC: APA Publishing.

Anthony, E. J., & Cohler, B. J. (1987). *The invulnerable child.* New York, NY: Guilford Press.

Bee, S., & Gibson, M. J. (1998). *Mental health parity: An overview of recent legislation.* Retrieved from http://aarp.org/research/health/carequality/aresearch-import-676-FS69.html

Benporath, S. R. (2003). Autonomy and vulnerability: On just relations between adults and children. *Journal of Philosophy of Education, 37*(1), 127–145.

Block, L. E. (2004). *Health policy: What is it and how it work.* In C. Harrington and C. L. Estes (Eds.), *Health policy: Crisis and reform in the U.S. health care delivery system* (4th ed.) (pp. 4–14). Boston, MA: Jones & Bartlett Pub.

Busch, S. H. & Barry, C. L. (2009). Does private insurance adequately protect families of children with mental health disorders? *Pediatrics, 124,* S399–S406. Retrieved from http://www.pediatrics.org/cgi/content/full/124/Supplement_4/S399

Chaowalit, A., Hatthakit, U., Nasae, T., Suttharansee, W., & Parker, M. (2002). Exploring ethical dilemmas and resolutions in nursing practice: A qualitative study in Southern Thailand. *The Journal of Nursing Research, 6,* 216–230.

Child Welfare League of America [CWLA]. (2005). *Standards for transition, independent living and self-sufficiency services.* Retrieved from http://www.cwla.org /programs/standards/cwstandardsindependentliving.htm

Cohen, C. P., & Naimark, H. (1991). United Nations Convention on the Rights of the Child: Individual rights concepts and their significance for social-scientists. *American Psychologists, 46*(1), 60–65.

Cohen, S., Mason, D., Kovner, C., Leavitt, J., Pulcini, J., & Sochalski, J. (1996). Stages of nursing's political development: Where we've been and where we ought to be. *Nursing Outlook, 44*(1), 20–23.

Duderstadt, K. G. (2004). Advocacy for children through activism. *Journal of Pediatric Health Care, 18*(5), 217–218.

Evans, M. E. (2009). Prevention of mental, emotional, and behavioral disorders in youth: The Institute of Medicine report and implications for nursing. *Journal of Child and Adolescent Psychiatric Nursing, 22,* 154–159.

Howe, R. B. (2001). Do parents have fundamental rights? *Journal of Canadian Studies/Revue d'etudes Canadiennes, 30*(3), 61–78.

Huntington, C. (2006). Rights myopia in child welfare. *UCLA Law Review, 53*(3), 637–699.

Institute of Medicine [IOM]. (2009). *Depression in parents, parenting and children: Opportunities to improve identification, treatment and prevention* [Report Brief]. Washington, DC: National Academies Press. Retrieved from http://iom.edu/cms/12552/45551/69567.aspx?printfriendly=true

Institute of Medicine [IOM]. (2010). *The future of nursing: Leading change, advancing health.* Washington, DC: National Academies Press. Retrieved from http://books.nap.edu/openbook.php?record_id=12956&page=4

Institute of Medicine Committee on Crossing the Quality Chasm [IOM]. (2006). *Improving the quality of health care for mental and substance-use conditions.* Washington, DC: National Academies Press.

Institute of Medicine Committee on Quality of Health Care in America [IOM]. (2001). *Crossing the quality chasm: A new health system for the 21st century.* Washington, DC: National Academies Press.

Jaycox, L. H., Moralar, A. R., & Juvonen, J. (2003). Mental health and medical problems and service use among adolescent substance users. *Journal of the American Academy of Child & Adolescent Psychiatry, 42*(6),701–709.

King, M. (2007). The sociology of childhood as communication: Observations from a social systems perspective. *Childhood, 14*(2), 193–213.

Krauss, J. B. (1993). *Health care reform: Essentials of mental health services.* Washington, DC: American Nurses Publishing.

Kronebusch, K. (2004). Medicaid for children: Federal mandates, welfare reform, and policy backsliding. In C. Harrington and C. L. Estes (Eds.), *Health policy: Crisis and reform in the U.S health care delivery system* (pp. 287–292). Boston, MA: Jones and Barlett, Pubs.

Kubsch, S. M., Sternard, M. J., Hovarter, R., & Matzke, V. (2004). A holistic model of advocacy: Factors that influence its use. *Complementary Therapies in Nursing Midwifery, 10*(1), 37–45.

Mason, D. J., Leavitt, J. K., & Chaffee, M. W. (2007). Policy and politics: A framework for action. In D. J. Mason, J. K. Leavitt, & M. W. Chaffee (Eds.), *Policy and politics in nursing and health care* (5th ed.) (pp. 1–18). St. Louis, MI: Saunders Elsevier.

Matthews, H., & Limb, M. (1998). The right to say: The development of youth councils/forums within the UK. *Area, 30*(1), 66–78.

McDonald, S., & Ahern, K. (2000). The professional consequences of whistleblowing by nurses. *J Professional Nursing, 16,* 313–321.

McFerran, T. A. (2003). *Oxford Dictionary of Nursing* (4th ed.). Oxford, UK: Oxford University Press.

Melnyk, B., Hawkins-Walsh, E., Beauchesne, M., Brandt, P., Crowley, A., Choi, M., & Greenburg, E. (2009). Strengthening PNP curricula in mental/behavioral health and evidence-based practice. *Pediatric Health Care,* published on line May 22, 2009. Retrieved from http://www. Jpedhc.org/article/S0891-5245(09)00028-5

Melton, G. B. (1996). The child's right to a family environment: Why children's rights and family values are incompatable. *American Psychologist, 51,* 1234–1238.

Melton, G. B. (2005). Building humane communities respectful of children: The significance of the convention on the rights of the child. *American Psychologist, 60,* 918–926.

Mental Health America. (2008). *Fact sheet: Paul Wellstone and Pete Domenici mental health parity and addiction equity act of 2008.* Retrieved from http://takeaction.mentalhealth america.net/site/PageServer?pagename=Equity_Campaign_d…

Miljeteig-Olssen, P. (1990). Advocacy of children's rights: The convention as more than a legal document. *Human Rights Quarterly, 12*(1), 148–155.

Murray, C., & Lopez, A. (1996). *The global burden of disease: A comprehensive assessment of mortality and disability from disease, injuries, and risk factors in 1990 and projected to 2020.* Cambridge, MA: Harvard University Press.

NAPNAP's KySS Program. (2008). *Fellowship for NPs in underserved in U.S.: Improving child and teen mental health.* Retrieved from http://napnap.dev.vtcus.com/aboutUs/AboutPNP/ProgramsAndInitiatives/KySSHome/KySSNews.aspx

National Association for Pediatric Nurse Practitioners (NAPNAP). (2001). *Keep your children/yourself safe and secure [KySS] program: A national effort to reduce psychosocial morbidities in children and adolescents.* Retrieved from www.Napnap.org/ProgramsAnd Initiatives/KySS/About KySS.aspx

National Commission on Children. (1993). *Just the facts: A summary of recent information on America's children and their families.* Washington, DC: National Commission on Children.

New Freedom Commission on Mental Health. (2003). *Achieving the promise: Transforming mental health care in America.* DHHS Pub No. SMA-03-3831. Rockville, MD: USDHHS.

O'Connor, T., & Kelly, B. (2005). Bridging the gap: A study of general nurses' perceptions of patient advocacy in Ireland. *Nursing Ethics, 12*(5), 453–467.

Pottick, K. J.(2002, Summer). Children's use of mental health services doubles, new research—policy partnership reports. In *Update: Latest findings in children's mental health, 1*(1), 1–3 [Brief]. Brunswick, NJ: Institute for Health, Health Care Policy and Aging Research.

Raphel, S. (2001). A national action agenda for children's mental health. *Journal of Child and Adolescent Psychiatric Nursing, 14,* 193.

Raynaert, D., Bouverne-de-bie, m., & Vandevelde, S. (2009). A review of children's rights literature since the adoption of the United Nations convention. *Childhood, 16,* 518. Retrieved from http://chd.sagepub.com/content/16/4/518

Roose, R., & Bouverne-de Bie, M. (2008). Children's rights: A challenge for social work. *International Social Work, 51*(1), 37–46.

Schlairet, M. (2009). Bioethics mediation: The role and importance of nursing advocacy. *Nursing Outlook, 57*(4), 185–193.

Stanley, S. R. (1994). Crafting mental health policy. *Nursing Clinics of North America, 29*(1) 19–27.

Stroul, B. A. (2007). *Integrating mental health services into primary care settings.* Summary of the Special Forum, National Tech Assistance Center for Children's Mental Health. Washington, DC: Georgetown University Center for Child & Human Development.

Stroul, BA. (July, 2006). Integrating mental health services into primary care settings. Retrieved from http://www.mockingbirdsociety.org/files/reference/Mental_Health_and_Foster_Care/integrating_mental_health_and_primary_care.pdf

Such, E., & Walker, R. (2005). Young citizens or policy objects? Children in the "rights and responsibiliies" debate. *Journal of Social Policy, 34*, 39–57.

Sundin-Huard, D. (2001). Subject positions theory: Its application to understanding collaboration (and confrontation) in critical care. *Journal of Advanced Nursing, 34(3),* 376–382.

Takanishi, R. (1978). Childhood as a social issue: Historical roots of contemporary child advocacy movements. *Journal of Social Issues, 34*(2), 8–28.

Thomas, N., & O'Kane, C. (1998). When children's wishes and feelings clash with their "best interest". *International Journal of Children's Rights, 6*(2), 137–154.

Tomanovic-Miljajlovic, S. (2000). Young people's participation within the family: Parent's accounts. *International Journal of Children's Rights, 8*(2), 151–167.

UNICEF. (2008). *Convention on rights of the child.* Retrieved on July 30, 2009, from http://www.unicef.org/crc/?q=printme

United States Department of Health and Human Services. (2001a). *A national strategy for suicide prevention: Goals and objectives for action.* Rockville, MD: USDHHS, Centers for Disease Control and Prevention, National Center for Injury Prevention and Control; Substance Abuse and Mental Health Services Administration, Center for Mental Health Service; National Institutes of Health, National Institute of Mental Health.

United States Department of Health and Human Services. (2001b). *Youth violence: A report of the surgeon general.* Rockville, MD: USDHHS, Centers for Disease Control and Prevention, National Center for Injury Prevention and Control; Substance Abuse and Mental Health Services Administration, Center for Mental Health Service; National Institutes of Health, National Institute of Mental Health.

United States Department of Health and Human Services [USDHHS]. United States Public Health Service Office of the Surgeon General. (2007). *The surgeon general's call to action to prevent and reduce underage drinking.* Rockville, MD: USDHHS, U.S. Public Health Service.

United States Department of Health and Human Services. (2009). *National Survey of Child and Adolescent Well-Being (NSCAW), 1997–2010.* Rockville, MD: USDHHS, Administration for Children & Families. Retrieved from http://www.acf.hhs.gov/programs/opre/abuse_neglect/nscaw/index.html

United States Public Health Service Office of the Surgeon General. (1999). *Mental health: A report of the surgeon general.* Rockville, MD: USDHHS, U.S. Public Health Service.

United States Public Health Service Office of the Surgeon General. (2000). *Children's mental health: A national action plan.* Rockville, MD: UDDHHS, U.S. Public Health Service.

Vaartio, H., Leino-Kilpi, H., Suominen, T., & Puukka, P. (2009). Nursing advocacy in procedural pain care. *Nursing Ethics, 16*(3), 340–362.

Wells K., Miranda, J., Bruce, M. L., Algeria, M., & Wallerstein, N. (2004). Bridging community intervention and mental health services research. *American Journal of Psychiatry, 161,* 955–963.

Wheeler, P. (2000). Is advocacy at the heart of professional practice? *Nursing Standard, 14*(24), 39–41.

Wilcox, B. L., & Naimark, H. (1991). The rights of the child: Progress towards human dignity. *American Psychologist, 46*(1), 49.

Wildavsky, A. (1979). *Speaking truth to power: The art and craft of policy analysis.* Boston, MA: Little Brown.

World Health Organization. (2004). *Mental health policy, plans and programmes: Mental health policy and service guidance package updated version.* Geneva, Switzerland: Author.

World Health Organization. (2003). *Mental health financing.* Geneva, Switzerland: Author.

Mental Health is a critical component of children's learning and general health
David Satcher, Surgeon General, 1999

Index

Note: Tables are noted with *t*.

---

self-esteem in children with, 8
self-regulation difficulties and, 26
stimulants and nonstimulants for,
   120–122
   contraindications, 121
   dosing, 121
   drug-drug interactions, 121
   indications for use, 121
   long-term use, 122
   monitoring, 121
   pharmacology, 120–121
   side effects of, 121
symptoms across the life span, 142t
treatment for, 30
   algorithm, 149
   comparison of nonstimulating
      drugs, 147t
   medications for, 145t–146t
   self-regulation with, 32
   in young children, 336, 340
Attention efficacy, successful self-
   regulation and, 24
Attention span, assessment of, 65
Atypical antipsychotics, 132
   for autism spectrum disorder, 252–253
   for bipolar disorder, 180
   complications from use of, 210
   FDA approved age, form, dosing range,
      side effects, duration, pros, and
      precautions, 136t
   monitoring, protocols for, 117t
   side effects of, 252, 253
Atypical autism, 246
AUDIT. See Alcohol Use Disorders
   Identification Test
Auditory hallucinations, 206
   children and adolescents with
      schizophrenia and, 206, 213–215
   very early onset schizophrenia and, 209
Auditory screening, intellectual
   disabilities assessment and, 267
Australian Scale for Asperger Syndrome,
   243t
Autism, 42
   atypical, 246
   diagnosis of, average age for, 241
   temperament profiles of children
      with, 30
Autism Co-morbidity Interview, 246
Autism Co-Morbidity Interview-Present
   and Lifetime Version, 247
Autism spectrum, ADHD diagnosis
   and, 140
Autism spectrum disorder, 3, 238–257,
   286
   associated conditions with, 246
   atypical antipsychotic agents for,
      252–253
   behavior approaches for, 324–325
   case exemplar, 256–257

clinical picture: screening and
   assessment, 241–242
   clinical features, 241
   delays in language and social skills,
      242
   red flags, 241–242, 242t
complementary and alternative
   medicine interventions for, 253,
   255, 255t
costs across the lifespan related to, 239
current diagnostic criteria for,
   245–246, 246t
direct instruction, 250
etiology, 239–241
   disruption in brain structure and
      function, 239
   genetic predisposition, 240–241
   parental age, 239–240
health care encounter and, 244
implications for practice, research, and
   education, 256
integration with primary care, 255
interventions
   for challenging behaviors, 251
   communication, 252t
   peer-mediated, 251
   psychopharmacology specific to
      ASD population, 252
   for sleep problems, 251–252
interventions and plan, 249–250
   for speech and language
      development, 249–250
laboratory and diagnostic
   investigations, 244–245
medical comorbidities, 248–249
overview, 238–239
physical and assessment, 243–244
   health care encounter, 244
psychiatric comorbidities, 246–248
psychopharmacology and, 254t
referrals, 244
repetitive and stereotyped patterns of
   behavior and restricted interests,
   242
screening tools for autism in older
   child, 243t
selective serotonin reuptake inhibitors
   and, 52, 253
for social skill development, 250
Social Story use and, 251
stimulants, 253
symptoms of ADHD and, 142
video modeling, 250–251
Autism Spectrum Screening
   Questionnaire, 243t
Autistic disorder, 238
   current diagnostic criteria, 245
   in infancy and early childhood, 338t
Autistic youth, naltrexone and self-
   injurious behaviors by, 199

Autonomy, 462, 471t
Autonomy vs. Shame and Doubt,
   toddlerhood and, 5
Autopsy, 435
Autoreceptors, 49
Axline, V., 280t
Axons, 46, 48
Azaspirones
   drug-drug interactions, 132
   FDA approved age, form, dosing range,
      side effects, duration, pros, and
      precautions, 134t
   indications for use, 131
   monitoring, 132
   pharmacology, 130
   side effects of, 131

Bacterial infections, autism spectrum
   disorder and, 241
BADDS. See Brown Attention Deficit
   Disorder Scale for Children and
   Adolescents
Bandaides and Blackboards, 439
Bandura, Albert, 314
Barbiturates, street names, DEA
   schedule/ingestion method(s),
   intoxication/withdrawal signs,
   health consequences, 381t
Basal ganglia, location, primary function,
   and primary connections, 45t
Basal nucleus, acetylcholine firing and, 3
BASC. See Behavioral Assessment System
   for Children
Basic collaboration at a distance, 447
Basic collaboration on-site, 447
Battelle Developmental Inventory
   Screening Tool, 266t, 341
"Battered Child Syndrome, The"
   (Kempe), 397
Bayley Infant Neurodevelopmental
   Screen, 266t
Bayley Scales of Infant Development, 341
Bayley III, 265
Bazelon Center for Mental Health
   Law, 525
BBB. See Blood-brain barrier
BDD. See Body dysmorphic disorder
BDI. See Beck Depression Inventory
BDI-ST. See Battelle Developmental
   Inventory Screening Tool
BDNF. See Brain-derived neurotrophic
   factor; Brain-derived
   neutrotrophic factor
Beck, Aaron, 279, 314
Beck Depression Inventory, 122, 178, 198
Beck Depression Inventory II, 178
Beck Hopelessness scale, 199
Behavioral approaches
   for anxious behaviors, 323
   for attention deficit disorder, 324

CPSIA information can be obtained
at www.ICGtesting.com
Printed in the USA
BVHW01s1238040918
526211BV00009B/8/P